European Manual of Medicine

Series Editors

W. Arnold, Munic, Germany
U. Ganzer, Düsseldorf, Germany

Presenting state-of-the-art procedures in all clinical medicine disciplines, the European Manual of Medicine book series aims to educate postgraduate students and residents in accordance with the U.E.M.S. charter on training medical specialists in the European Union. Each volume is a comprehensive reference devoted to a specific discipline, and the editors are internationally renowned specialists from different European Countries. The contents cover both diagnostic and therapeutic methods which are subdivided into essential procedures (those that are commonly employed in all European countries) and helpful procedures (which might be of further interest as well). The reader-friendly layout allows quick retrieval of information, and concise checklists and algorithms throughout each volume clearly present the pathway from patient complaint to diagnosis. This text book series is ideal for any practitioner in the European Union looking to gain a thorough understanding of the latest procedures in their field of interest. The European Union of Medical Specialists (U.E.M.S.) represents national associations of medical specialists in the European Union and its associated countries. Active at the European level since 1958, the UEMS promotes the free movement of European medical specialists while ensuring the highest quality of medical care for European citizens. More information can be found online at: www.uems.net

Antoinette am Zehnhoff-Dinnesen
Joseph Sopko
Marie-Claude Monfrais-Pfauwadel
Katrin Neumann
Editors

Phoniatrics II

Speech and Speech Fluency Disorders – Literacy Development Disorders

Springer

Editors
Antoinette am Zehnhoff-Dinnesen
Department of Phoniatrics and Pedaudiology
University Hospital Münster
Münster, Germany

Marie-Claude Monfrais-Pfauwadel
Hopital Europeen Georges Pompidou
Paris, France

Joseph Sopko
Basel, Switzerland

Katrin Neumann
Department of Phoniatrics and Pedaudiology
University Hospital Münster
Münster, Germany

ISSN 2626-7845 ISSN 2626-7853 (electronic)
European Manual of Medicine
ISBN 978-3-031-25174-0 ISBN 978-3-031-25175-7 (eBook)
https://doi.org/10.1007/978-3-031-25175-7

This Springer imprint is published by the registered company Springer Nature Switzerland AG
The registered company address is: Gewerbestrasse 11, 6330 Cham, Switzerland

Foreword of the Series Editors

The European Manual of Medicine (EMM) book series offers medical graduates and clinicians current state-of-the-art knowledge, in accordance with the charter of the European Union of Medical Specialists (UEMS) in Brussels, on training medical specialists in the European Union.

Like Volume *Phoniatrics I* (2020; ISBN 978-3-662-46,780-0), which presents the topics Fundamentals, Voice Disorders, Disorders of Language and Hearing Development, this volume *Phoniatrics II* offers phoniatric and ENT trainees as well as members of related disciplines a textbook/e-book of unique high quality.

Phoniatrics II includes the parts Dysglossia, Resonance Disorders, Velopharyngeal Insufficiency; Speech Fluency Disorders; and Literacy Development Disorders.

According to the principles of EMM, a standardised structure is used in addressing basics, special kinds of disorders, diagnosis/differential diagnosis, prevention, and rehabilitation/prognosis. Case studies, colour photos, tables, and supplementary audio and video samples, along with detailed reference lists, provide a substantial amount of up-to-date information to the reader.

Antoinette am Zehnhoff-Dinnesen, as editor-in-chief (Münster, Germany), and the associated editors Katrin Neumann (Münster, Germany), Joseph Sopko (Basel, Switzerland), and Marie-Claude Monfrais-Pfauwadel (Paris, France) have invited well-known, interdisciplinary experts from various countries to ensure the excellent quality of the book series.

Special thanks go to Springer Nature, especially to Wilma McHugh, Daniela Heller, Timo Lange, Aruna Sharma and Shanjini Rajasekaran for their precious help and assistance.

The signing series editors are extremely grateful for the work of all editors and especially for the immense, untiring effort our friend, editor-in-chief, Antoinette am Zehnhoff-Dinnesen, has shown in creating this unique textbook.

Munich, Germany — Wolfgang Arnold
Düsseldorf, Germany — Uwe Ganzer
Summer 2024

Preface

Volume II of the textbook *Phoniatrics* from the book series 'European Manual of Medicine' provides, after Volume I with its 181 contributions, another substantial basis for setting high standards and good quality in patient care and for improving training and education in phoniatrics. It is aimed at phoniatric trainees, ENT trainees, and specialised clinicians but—because of the interdisciplinary nature of phoniatrics—may also be of interest to medical students, physicians in other specialties with a special interest in phoniatrics and members of related disciplines. This book provides guidance and internationally recognised standards in the current situation, where the extent and intensity of phoniatric training vary across different countries.

In addition to the complete textbook, the reader is also offered individual e-chapters and e-books. To enhance understanding of the speciality, *Phoniatrics II* features a large number of colour photos, figures, tables, and case studies in 93 contributions, supplemented by audio and video samples. To achieve the aim of the book series, the majority of articles are written by more than one author, most of whom are from different countries. A total of 77 authors and co-authors contributed to this volume, representing 18 countries from four continents and 27 disciplines.

Volume I focused on the Fundamentals of Phoniatrics, Voice Disorders, and Disorders of Language and Hearing Development. Volume II highlights Dysglossia/Resonance Disorders/Velopharyngeal Insufficiency, Speech Fluency Disorders, and Literacy Development Disorders. All these topics have been prepared by following the training programme and logbook *Medical Speech, Voice and Language Pathology, and Hearing and Swallowing Disorders* within the Section Oto-Rhino-Laryngology of the European Union of Medical Specialists (UEMS) in Brussels.

We thank all authors and co-authors who invested time and effort in this project, for their valuable contributions and crucial support.

Thanks go especially to the external lectors who, in addition to the editors, provided in-depth research and analysis that significantly helped to achieve a high standard of knowledge transfer by their particular competence, proficiency, and expertise:

Joseph Agius (Malta), Per Alm (Sweden), Michael M. Bornstein (Hong Kong), Monika Brunner (Germany), Susanne Cook (USA), Philippe Dejonckere (Belgium), Mirela Duranovic (Bosnia and Herzegovina), Kurt Eggers (Belgium), Pascale Fichaux-Bourin (France), Anja Fiori (Germany), Dobrinka Georgieva (Bulgaria), Lynn Grames (USA), Alexander Hemprich

(Germany), Jenö Hirschberg* (Hungary), Thomas Lambrecht (Germany), Ben Maassen (The Netherlands), Rudolf Reiter (Germany), Saskia Rohrbach-Volland (Germany), Kenneth O. St. Louis (USA), Sabine Van Eerdenbrugh (Belgium), and J. Scott Yaruss (USA).

The editors are much obliged and deeply grateful to the editors of the manual series, Wolfgang Arnold (Munich, Germany) and Uwe Ganzer (Düsseldorf, Germany), who initiated and decisively supported this important project.

Our special thanks go to Springer Nature, especially to Wilma McHugh, Daniela Heller, Timo Lange, Aruna Sharma and Shanjini Rajasekaran, for their substantial assistance and valuable advice.

The editors are deeply indebted to Dr. Trevor G. Cooper, lector for English language, for his excellent work and continued invaluable support as experienced scientist. His input decisively helped to complete this book.

We also thank Nicole Neptun for her work on some book parts, especially concerning the layout and the reference lists; Ross Parfitt for his diligent help in clarifying copyright questions; and Peter Matulat for his valuable support and advice in technical and IT matters.

To have a comprehensive textbook and e-book on phoniatrics in the English language is one keystone to providing an international basis for standards, thereby improving training and education in this medical speciality. This activity supports the aim of the Union of the European Phoniatricians and the European Academy of Phoniatrics to establish a European Board Exam in Phoniatrics; we hope that *Phoniatrics II* will provide a comprehensive training tool for everyone interested in the field of communication disorders.

Münster, Germany	Antoinette am Zehnhoff-Dinnesen
Basel, Switzerland	Joseph Sopko
Paris, France	Marie-Claude Monfrais-Pfauwadel
Münster, Germany	Katrin Neumann
Summer 2024	

*Jenö Hirschberg was deceased at the time of publication.

Contents

About the Editors

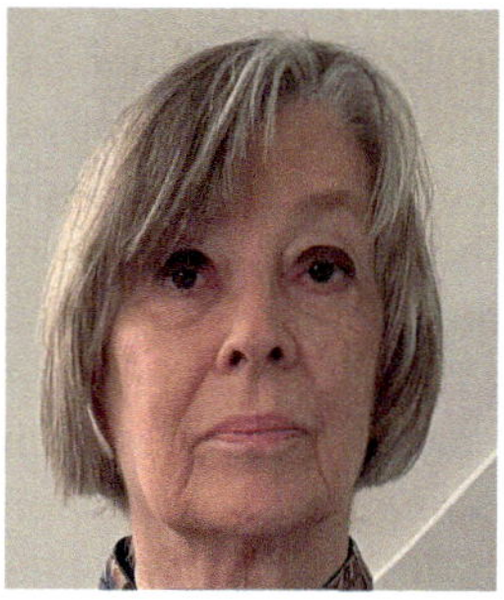

Antoinette am Zehnhoff-Dinnesen studied medical sciences in Düsseldorf and Bonn. In 1983, she became a medical specialist in ENT diseases, and in 1986, a medical specialist in phoniatrics and paedaudiology. In 1988, she gained her Habilitation from Düsseldorf University for her work on regulation of vocal amplitude and frequency during voice onset. In 1990, Dr. am Zehnhoff-Dinnesen was appointed Professor of Phoniatrics and Paedaudiology at the Medical Faculty of Philipps University in Marburg. The following year she became Professor at the Medical Faculty of the Westphalian Wilhelms University of Münster, where she was Head of the Clinic of Phoniatrics and Paedaudiology until her retirement in 2020. She is author or co-author of more than 160 original papers in German and English on various aspects of phoniatrics and paedaudiology and co-author of several books. She has been both Secretary and President of the German Society of Phoniatrics and Paedaudiology, President of the Union of the European Phoniatricians (UEP), and has initiated and promoted the foundation of the European Academy of Phoniatrics as the founding director. She and her team have received several awards. Antoinette am Zehnhoff-Dinnesen is the honorary chairwoman of the Union of European Phoniatricians and an honorary member of the Polish Society of Otorhinolaryngologists and Head and Neck Surgeons, the Czech Society of Otorhinolaryngology and Head and Neck Surgery, the German Society of Phoniatrics and Paedaudiology, the European Academy of Phoniatrics, and the Confederation of German Hearing Screening Centres. In 2025 she was appointed Vice-President of the German Section of the German-Indonesian Society of Medicine.

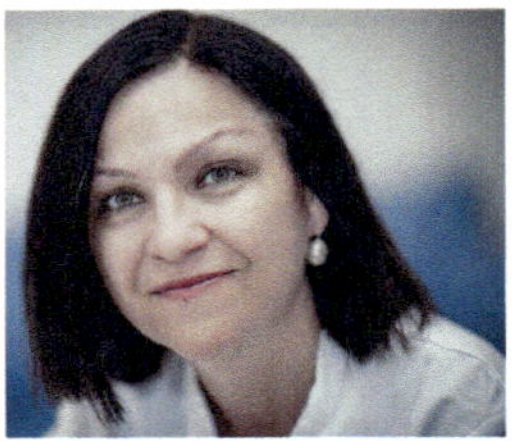

Katrin Neumann studied medicine at the University of Leipzig. She is Professor of Population Medicine of Communication Disorders at the University of Münster and Director of the Department of Phoniatrics and Paedaudiology at the University Hospital Münster, Germany. She is editor-in-chief of the *Journal of Fluency Disorders* (Elsevier) and co-editor of the journals *Communication Disorder Quarterly* and *LOGOS*. As a WHO expert advisor, she contributes to the work of the WHO Programme of Prevention of Deafness and Hearing Loss and of the WHO Rehabilitation Programme. She is WHO representative of the Union of European Phoniatricians (UEP), the German Society of Phoniatrics and Paedaudiology (DGPP), and the German Society of Audiology (DGA). She has published more than 270 original articles, monographs, guidelines, and book chapters and has received a number of national and international awards. Her research interests include neuroimaging and population medicine of hearing, speech fluency, developmental language, and voice physiology and pathology.

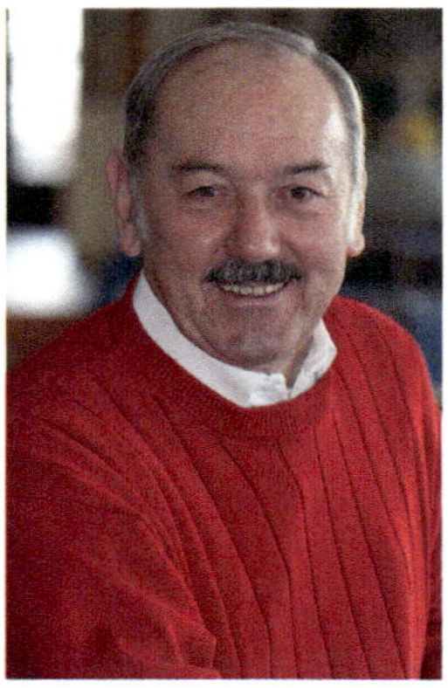

Joseph Sopko Prof. Dr. med. Dr. h.c., began his study of medicine in his native town of Košice, Slovakia. Later, he continued his studies at the University of Basel, Switzerland, where he habilitated with a speciality in phoniatrics, and in 1991, he was elected full professor (extraordinarius) for otorhinolaryngology and phoniatrics. In 1975, Professor Sopko founded the Phoniatrics and Paediatric Audiology Department in the ORL University Clinic, Basel, and worked there as head until 2003. He led the speech therapy school at the University Basel from 1975 to 2002. In 1995, he also founded the Phoniatric Department in the ORL-Clinic, Kantonsspital Aarau, and worked there for more than 20 years. He is the phoniatrician to the Basel Opera and Stadttheater and also has a private practice in Basel. In 2002, he received an Honorary Doctorate from the University of Košice. His scientific-publishing activity includes more than 80 articles and book contributions.

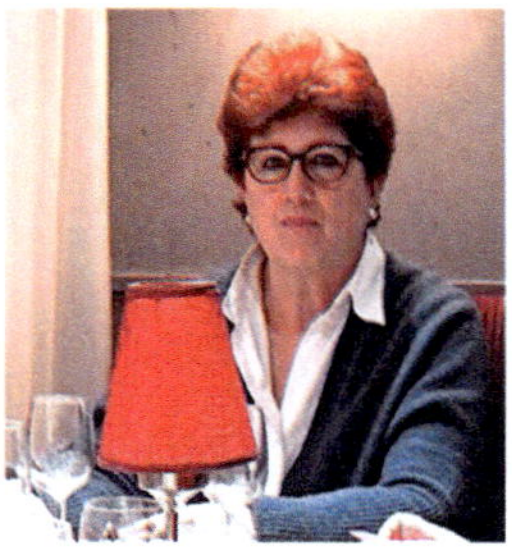

Marie-Claude Monfrais-Pfauwadel studied medicine at the René-Descartes University in Paris, then trained in ENT and phoniatrics, and graduated in 1978. She completed her education with degrees in Psychology and Psychoanalysis at Paris-6 University (MBS) and Linguistics and Phonetics at Paris-3 and Paris-6 Universities (MBS). She gained her degree in Phonetics by working on the nosology of disfluencies and their physiopathology. Later, she added a speciality degree in Muscle Physiology and Myopathies at the Pitié-Salpetrière Hospital in Paris. She worked for more than 10 years in the Voice/Speech/Language Clinic at the Pitié-Salpetrière Hospital in Paris, then created the Voice and Speech Laboratory in the new Georges Pompidou Hospital in 2000, alongside a 'Stuttering Clinic'. Meanwhile she obtained in 1985 the first scholarship from the Stuttering Foundation of America at Northwestern University to become acquainted with the latest techniques and research discoveries about speech motor control and stuttering. Back in France, she started teaching the clinical, physiological, linguistic, and phonetic aspects of stuttering and created a two-year MS degree devoted to Stuttering for Phoniatricians and Speech Therapists in 2005, which is still running. She has authored and co-authored several books on voice disorders, stuttering clinics, stuttering therapy, and neurolinguistics and many journal articles. She was twice elected President of the French Medical Phoniatric Society. She was one of the founding members of the International Fluency Association (IFA) in 1993 and was a member of the IALP Fluency Committee for 20 years since its founding. She retired from practice in 2012 but kept teaching clinics and phonetics for phoniatricians and speech pathologists. Recently, she was asked to join the ANR Programme at Montpellier-3 University, focussing on the role of the 'Frontal Aslant tract' in the genesis of stuttering. She is actually co-responsible for this programme, which will run for the next 3 years.

Abbreviations

%SS	Percent stuttered syllables
3D	Three-dimensional
4S	Self-stigma of stuttering scale
A/CMs	Active/compensatory misarticulations
AAA	American Academy of Audiology
AAC	Augmentative and alternative communication
AAF	Altered auditory feedback
ABA-2	Apraxia battery for adults (second edition)
ABR	Auditory brainstem response
AC	Auditory cortex
ACT	Acceptance and commitment therapy
ADD	Attention deficit disorder
ADHD	Attention deficit (and) hyperactivity disorder
ALR	Auditory late response
AMLR	Auditory middle latency response
AMPS	Assessment of motor and process skills
ANSD	Auditory neuropathy spectrum disorder
AOS/AoS	Apraxia of speech
AOS MFCC	AOS Mel-frequency cepstral coefficients
APA	American Psychiatric Association
APD	Auditory processing disorder
APM	Ambulatory phonation monitor
AQT	A quick test of cognitive speed
AS	Acquired stuttering
ASA	Acetylsalicylic acid
ASD	Autism spectrum disorders
ASDS	Asperger Syndrome Diagnostic Scale
ASHA	American Speech-Language-(and)-Hearing Association
aSTG	Anterior superior temporal (supratemporal) gyrus
ATLFF	Assessment tool for lingual frenulum function
AVLT	Auditory verbal learning test
AWNS	Adults who do not stutter
AWS	Adults who stutter
AWS	Adults whose stuttering improved without therapy
AWS+	Adults whose stuttering improved with therapy
AWSrs	Adults whose stuttering recovered unassisted
AWSt	Adults whose stuttering improved by treatment

BA	Brodmann area
BAB	Behaviour assessment battery
BAI	Beck anxiety inventory
BASC-3	Behaviour assessment scale for children (third edition)
BASS	Bochum-Aachener Stotterscreening
BCL	Behaviour checklist
BCLP	Bilateral CLP
BDAE	Boston Diagnostic Aphasia Examination
BDAE-3	Boston Diagnostic Aphasia Examination (third edition)
BDI-II	Beck Depression Inventory (second edition)
BG	Basal ganglia
BMPs/Bmps	Bone morphogenetic proteins
BRIED	Behavior Rating Inventory of Executive Function
BSA	British Society of Audiology
BTAT	Bristol Tongue Assessment Tool
CABC-WM	Comprehensive assessment battery for children—working memory
CAEs	Compensatory articulation errors
CAFET	Computer-aided fluency establishment trainer
CAPD	Central auditory processing disorders
CAS	Childhood apraxia of speech
CAT	Communication attitude test
CATA	Continuous Auditory Test of Attention
CBD	Corticobasal degeneration
CBGTC	Cortico-basal ganglia-thalamocortical
CBT	Cognitive behaviour (behavioural) therapy
CC	Corpus callosum
CCD	Charge-coupled device
CCT	Children's category test
CD	Conduct disorder
CDE	California Dyslexia Guidelines
CE	Conical elevations
CELF-5	Clinical Evaluation of Language Fundamentals
CGI	Clinical Global Impression
CHARGE	Coloboma, heart defect, atresia choanae, restricted growth and development, genital abnormality, and ear abnormality
CL	Cleft lip
CLA	Cleft lip alveolus
CL/P	Cleft lip or cleft palate
CLP	Cleft lip and palate
CMA	Chromosomal microarray analysis
CMOS	Complementary metal oxide semiconductor
CMS	Children's Memory Scale
CNS	Central nervous system
CNs	Cranial nerves
CNVs	Copy number variants
CO-OP	Cognitive orientation to daily occupational performance

COPM	Canadian Occupational Performance Measure
CP	Cleft palate
CPAP	Continuous positive airway pressure
CPT-3	Continuous performance test (third edition)
CR	Computerised rehabilitation
CRISPR	Clustered regularly interspersed short palindromic repeats
CRM	Continuous recognition memory test
CRT	Choice response time
CSL	Computerised Speech Lab
CT	Computed tomography
CTAP	Computerised index finger tapping
CTOPP-2	Comprehensive test of phonological processing (second edition)
CTRS	Conners' Teacher Rating Scale
CV	Consonant-vowel
CVs	Consonant-vocal clusters
CWS	Children with stuttering
DAF	Delayed auditory (aural) feedback
DAS-II	Differential Abilities Scale (second edition)
DBS	Deep brain stimulation
DCD	Developmental coordination disorder
DCM	Demands–capacities model
DD	Developmental dyslexia
DDG	Developmental dysgraphia
DDL	Developmental dyslexia
D-KEFS	Delis–Kaplan Executive Function System
DLB	Dementia with Lewy bodies
DM1	Myotonic dystrophy type 1
DME	Direct magnitude estimation
DNC	Delayed neural commitment
DO-80	Dénomination Orale d'images
DPW	Dorsal pharyngeal wall
DS	Developmental stuttering
DSM5/DSM-5	Diagnostic and Statistical Manual of Mental Disorders (fifth edition)
DTI	Diffusion tensor imaging
DTLA-4	Detroit Test of Learning Aptitude (fourth edition)
DTLA-5	Detroit Test of Learning Aptitude (fifth edition)
DVT	DoctorVox Voice Therapy Technique
DZ	Dizygotic
EAI	Equal-appearing interval
ECC3	Ectrodactyly, ectodermal dysplasia, and cleft lip/palate syndrome
ECD	Eruption control devices
ECE	Early childhood education
ECO	European Cleft Organisation
ED	Elimination disorder
EGG	Electroglottograph

EHFHL	Extended high-frequency hearing loss
EID	Elimination disorder
ELAN	Early left anterior negativities
EMA	European Medicines Agency
EMG	Electromyography
ENT	Ears, nose, and throat
ERPs	Event-related potentials
ES	Equivalent score
ESPEN	European Society for Clinical Nutrition and Metabolism
EYFP	Early years foundation profile
FA	Functional anisotropy
FAF	Frequency-altered feedback
FAR	Feifer Assessment of Reading
FDA	Frenchay Dysarthria Assessment
FGFR2	Fibroblast growth factor receptor 2 gene
FGFs/Fgfs	Fibroblast growth factors
FISH	Fluorescence in situ hybridisation
FM	Frequency modulated
FMPS	Frost Multidimensional Perfectionism Scale
fMRI	Functional magnetic resonance imaging
FOA	Fronto-orbital approach
FraDySc	Frankfurt Dysphagia Screening Score
FVNP	Flexible video-nasopharyngoscopy
G	Gingiva
GARS-3	Gilliam Autism Rating Scale (third edition)
GILCU	General increase in length of utterances
GM	Grey matter
GMV	Grey matter volume
GORT-5	Gray Oral Reading Test-5
GP	Globus pallidus
GPi/Gpi	Globus pallidus internus
GRB	Gamma band response
GRST	Gary's silent reading test
GWAS	Genome-wide association studies
HD	Huntington disease
HESA	Higher education statistical agency
HG	Heschl's gyrus
HH	Hedgehog family
HHIW	Here's How I Write
HHL	Hidden hearing loss
HMs	Hidden Markov models
HRNB	Halstead–Reitan neuropsychological battery
HVLT	Hopkins verbal learning test
ICD	International Classification of Diseases
ICF	International Classification of Function (Functioning, Disability and Health)
ICP	Intracranial pressure
IFG	Inferior frontal gyrus (gyri)

indels	Insertions and deletions
IPD	Idiopathic Parkinson's disease
IQ	Intelligence quotient
IQS	IQ screen
IRF6	Interferon inhibiting factor 6
ISCED	International Standard Classification of Education
ITPA-3	Illinois Test of Psycholinguistic Ability (third edition)
IVA + Plus	Integrated Visual and Auditory Continuous Performance Test
Jordan-3	Jordan left-right reversal test (third edition)
KABC-II NU	Kaufman Assessment Battery for Children (second edition)
KAIT	Kaufman Adolescent and Adult Intelligence Test
KCPT	Conners performance test
KES	Kinder Erleben ihr Stottern (kids experience their stuttering)
KeyMath-3 DA	KeyMath-3 Diagnostic Assessment
KiddyCAT	Communication Attitude Test for Preschool and Kindergarten Children
L_{AFmax}	Maximum sound pressure level
LAN	Left anterior negativities
LCD	Lowest common denominator
LCRs	Low-copy repeats
LD NOS	LD Not otherwise specified
LD	Learning disability
LD	Learning disorder
LL	Lower lip
LPC	Linear prediction coding
LPW	Lateral pharyngeal wall
Lv	Logopenic/phonological variant
lv-PPA	Logopenic variant primary progressive aphasia
MACI	Millon Adolescent Clinical Inventory
MAF	Masked auditory feedback
MAOIs	Monoamine oxidase inhibitors
MBS	Modified barium swallow
MCMI-IV	Millon Clinical Multiaxial Inventory (fourth edition)
MD	Multiple demand
MDVP	Multi-dimensional voice programme
MEG	Magneto-encephalography
MEPs	Motor-evoked potentials
MET	Multiple Errands Test
MFT	Myofunctional therapy
MGB	Medial geniculate body
MMN	Mismatch negativity
MMP2	Matrix metalloproteinase 2
MMPI	Minnesota Multiphasic Personality Inventory
MMPI-II-RF	Minnesota Multiphasic Personality Inventory-2-Restructured Form

MMS	Mini Mental State Examination
MMSE	Mini Mental State Examination
M-PACI	Millon pre-adolescent clinical inventory
mPT	Motion-sensitive planum temporale
MRA	Magnetic resonance angiography
MRI	Magnetic resonance imaging
MRS	Magnetic resonance spectroscopy
MS RES	MS rapidly evolving severe
MS	Mean score
MSA	Multiple system atrophy
MSC	Mesenchymal stem cells
MSI	Magnetic source imaging
MT-86	Montreal-Toulouse aphasia battery
mtDNA	Mitochondrial DNA
MVF	Multi-view videofluoroscopy
MVP	Mundvorhofplatte (oral vestibular plate)
MZ	Monozygotic
NAF	Non-altered auditory feedback
NAM	Nasal-alveolar moulding
NCCs	Neural crest cells
NDRT	Nelson Denny Reading Test, Forms I and J
NDT	Neurodevelopmental therapy
NE	Nasal emission
NEO-FFI	NEO-Five factor inventory
NEPSY-II	Neuropsychological assessment (second edition)
NG	Nasal grimace
NGS	Next-generation sequencing (high-throughput sequencing)
NLD	Non-verbal learning disabilities
NOT-S	Nordic orofacial test-screening
NS	Neurogenic stuttering
NSOMT	Non-speech oral motor treatment
NSRT	Non-verbal selective reminding test
NT	Narrative therapy
OAEs	Oto-acoustic emissions
OASES	Overall Assessment of the Speaker's Experience of Stuttering
OASES-A	Overall Assessment of the Speaker's Experience of Stuttering for Adults
OASES-S	Overall Assessment of the Speaker's Experience of Stuttering for School Age
OASES-T	Overall Assessment of the Speaker's Experience of Stuttering for Teens
OAVS	Oculo auriculo vertebral spectrum
OD	Other disfluencies
ODD	Oppositional defiant disorder
OECD	Organisation for Economic Co-operation and Development
OFD1	Oro-facial-digital syndrome 1
OMD	Oral motor devices

OMD	Orofacial myofunctional disorders
OMI	Oral motor intervention
OMIM	Online Mendelian Inheritance in Man
OMT	Orofacial myofunctional treatment
OOM	Orbicularis oris muscle
ORL	Otorhinolaryngology
OSA	Obstructive sleep apnoea
OSAS	Obstructive sleep apnoea syndrome
OT	Occupational therapy
OWLS II RC	Oral and Written Language Scales II Reading Comprehension
OWLS II WE	Oral and Written Language Scales II Written Expression
OWLS II	Oral and Written Language Scales II
PA	Phonological awareness
PAL	Paired associate learning
PAL-II M	Process Assessment of the Learner (second edition) Diagnostic for Math
PAL-II RW	Process Assessment of the Learner (2nd edn) Diagnostic for Reading and Writing
PANDAS	Paediatric Autoimmune Neuropsychiatric Disorders Associated with Streptococcal Infections
PASAT	Paced auditory serial addition test
PCA	Phonological components analysis
PCI	Parent–child interaction
PCT	Personal construct therapy
PD	Parkinson (Parkinson's) disease
PDS	Persistent developmental stuttering
PECS	Picture exchange communication system
PEP	Post-encephalitic Parkinsonism
PET	Positron emission tomography
PFS	Posterior fossa syndrome
PM	Pars marginalis
PN	Parenteral nutrition
PNAM	Pre-surgical naso-alveolar moulding
POSHA-CL	Public opinion survey of human attributes–cluttering
POSHA-S	Public opinion survey of human attributes–stuttering
PP	Pars peripheralis/Peripheral part
PPN	Partial parenteral nutrition
pre-SMA	Pre-supplementary motor area
PROMPT	Prompt of reconstructing oral muscular phonetic targets
PS	Pars superficialis
PSI	Perception of stuttering inventory
PSIO	Pre-surgical infant orthopaedics
PSNE	Phoneme-specific nasal emission
PSP	Progressive supranuclear palsy
PSW	Processing strengths and weaknesses
PT	Planum temporale
PWS	Person who stutters

RA	Retinoic acid
RAN	Rapid automatized naming
RC	Reading comprehension
RCOT	Royal College of Occupational Therapists
RD	Radial diffusivity
RD	Reading disabilities
RD	Reading disorder
RIAS	Reynolds Intellectual Assessment Scales
RNA	Ribonucleic acid
ROCF	Rey–Osterrieth complex figure
ROM	Range of motion
RSES	Rosenberg Self-Esteem Scale
rs-fMRI	Resting-state functional magnetic resonance imaging
RSs	Raw scores
RTI	Response-to-intervention
rTMS	Repetitive transcranial magnetic stimulation
RTP	Real-time pitch
SAAND	Stuttering associated with acquired neurological disorders
SAS	Supervisory attentional system
SCAN	Screening test for auditory processing disorders
SCAS	Spence child anxiety scales
SCESS	Satisfaction with communication in everyday speaking situations
SCL	Subepithelial cleft lip
SCWT	Stroop colour and word test
SD	Standard deviation
SDMT	Symbol digit modalities test
SES	Socio-economic status
Shh	Sonic hedgehog
SIRFES	Simultaneous radiological and fibre (flexible)-endoscopic evaluation of swallowing
SLD	Specific learning disorder(s)
SLD	Stuttering-like disfluencies
SLDM	SLD in mathematics
SLDT-A NU	Social language development test—adolescent
SLDT-E NU	Social language development test—elementary
SLI	Specific language impairment
SLP	Speech (and) language pathologist(s)/pathology
SMA	Spinal muscular atrophy
SMA	Supplementary motor area
SMART	Specific, measurable, achievable, relevant, and timed
SNP(s)	Single-nucleotide polymorphism(s)
SNr	Substantia nigra
SNVs	Single-nucleotide variants
SP	Substance P
SPECT	Single-photon emission computed tomography
SpLDs	Specific learning disabilities
SRS-2	Social responsiveness scale II

SRT	Simple response time
SSC	Speech situation checklist
SSC-ER	Speech situation checklist—emotional reaction
SSC-SD	Speech situation checklist—speech disruption
SSI	Stuttering severity instrument/index
SSI-4	Stuttering severity index-4
SSRI(s)	Selective serotonin re-uptake inhibitor(s)
SSS	Subjective screening of stuttering
ST	Speech therapy
STN	Subthalamic nucleus
Sv	Semantic variant
SVR	Simple view of reading
SWLP	Stabilised weighted linear prediction
TALENS	Transcription activator-like effector nucleases
TAPS-4	Language processing skills assessment-4
TAT	Thematic apperception test
TCAs	Tricyclic antidepressants
TCS	Treacher Collins syndrome
TD	Tourette disorders
TD	Typically developing
tDCS	Transcranial direct current stimulation
TEA-Ch	Test of everyday attention for children
TEWL-4	Test of early written language (fourth edition)
TMJ	Temporomandibular joint
TMS	Transcranial magnetic stimulation
TMT	Trail making tests
TNA	Total nutrient admixture
TOC	Test of orthographic processing
TOCS	Test of childhood stuttering
TOPS	Test of problem solving
TORC-4	Test of Reading Comprehension (fourth edition)
TOVA	Test of variables of attention
TOVA-9	Test of Variables of Attention (ninth edition)
TOWL-4	Test of Written Language (fourth edition)
TOWRE-2	Test of word reading efficiency (second edition)
TP	Test person
UCLP	Unilateral cleft palate
UIS	UNESCO Institute for Statistics
UL	Upper lip
UNESCO	United Nations Educational, Scientific and Cultural Organization
UNESCO-UIS	UNESCO Institute for Statistics; Eurostat
UTBAS	Unhelpful thoughts and beliefs about stuttering
V	Velum
VBM	Voxel-based morphometry
VC	Vowel-consonant
VCFS	Velo-cardio-facial syndrome (DiGeorge syndrome/ Sedlàçkovà syndrome)

VDW	von Willebrand disease
VET	Vocational education and training
VIM	Ventral (ventro) intermediate nucleus
VOT	Visual organisation test
VP	Velopharyngeal
VPC	Velopharyngeal closure
VPD	Velopharyngeal dysfunction
VPI	Velopharyngeal insufficiency (incompetence)
VPP	Velopharyngeal port
VRP	Voice range profile
VSRT	Verbal selective reminding test
VWS	Van der Woude syndrome
WAB	Western aphasia battery
WAIS-III	Wechsler adult intelligence scale (third edition)
WAIS-IV	Wechsler adult intelligence scale (fourth edition)
WAIS-R	Wechsler adult intelligence scale–revised
WASSP	Wright and Ayre stuttering self-rating profile
WCST	Wisconsin card sorting test
WE	Written expression
WES	Whole exome sequencing
WGS	Whole-genome sequencing
WHO	World Health Organization
WIAT-III	Wechsler Individual Achievement Test (third edition)
WISC-IV	Wechsler Intelligence Scale for Children (fourth edition)
WISC-V	Wechsler Intelligence Scale for Children (fifth edition)
WJ-IV	Woodcock-Johnson Tests of Achievement (fourth edition)
WJ-IV ACH	Woodcock-Johnson Tests of Achievement (fourth edition)
WJ-IV OL	Woodcock-Johnson Tests of Oral Language (fourth edition)
WJ-IV-COG	Woodcock-Johnson Tests of Cognitive Abilities (fourth edition)
WM	White matter
WM	Working memory
WMS-IV	Wechsler Memory Scale (fourth edition)
WRAMAL II	Wide Range Assessment of Memory and Learning (second edition)
XLP	Extended linear prediction
ZFN	Zinc finger nucleases

Part I

Dysglossia, Resonance Disorders and Velopharyngeal Insufficiency

Editors
Antoinette am Zehnhoff-Dinnesen and Joseph Sopko

Lectors
Michael M. Bornstein, Monika Brunner,
Philippe Dejonckere, Pascale Fichaux-Bourin,
Lynn Grames, Alexander Hemprich, Jenö Hirschberg,
Thomas Lambrecht, and Saskia Rohrbach-Volland

1 Basics of Dysglossia, Resonance Disorders and Velopharyngeal Insufficiency

Karen J. Golding-Kushner, Ute Pröschel, Saskia Rohrbach-Volland, Alan L. Shanske, and Robert J. Shprintzen

1.1 Definition, Epidemiology, Symptomatic Profile, Aetiology and Pathogenesis of Dysglossia

Saskia Rohrbach-Volland and Ute Pröschel

1.1.1 Definition

Dysglossia focuses on articulation disorders that are caused by *peripheral* organic abnormalities of the motor, peripheral-nerve or structural system (including the skeletal system) of the head and neck region. In contrast to dysglossia, dysarthria is caused by *central* sensorimotor deviances.

1.1.2 Epidemiology

Owing to its multiple causes, exact epidemiological data for dysglossia are not available. The incoherent nature of pre-and post-operative testing of the quality of speech and swallowing functions even limits the value of studies and reduces their comparability.

In children, the most common malformation causing dysglossia is cleft PALATE, with or without cleft LIP, in its various expressions. Its frequency varies depending on different regions of the world. The incidence of cleft lip with or without cleft palate is 1:1000 (Mitchell and Risch 1992), and the incidence of isolated cleft palate varies substantially by geography from 1.3 to 25.3 per 10,000 live births (Burg et al. 2016). Boys are more frequently affected with cleft lip or palate than girls. Malformations such as lymphangioma or haemangioma causing dysglossia are rare. Since the number of head and neck cancers is increasing, dysglossia caused by tumours or postoperative defects is also increasing steadily.

Supplementary Information The online version contains supplementary material available at https://doi.org/10.1007/978-3-031-25175-7_1.

K. J. Golding-Kushner (✉)
Golding-Kushner Consulting, LLC,
East Brunswick, NJ, USA

U. Pröschel
Vestische Kinder- und Jugendklinik Datteln,
Datteln, Germany
e-mail: u.proeschel@kinderklinik-datteln.de

S. Rohrbach-Volland
HNO Praxis, Berlin, Germany
e-mail: saskia@everskin.ch

A. L. Shanske · R. J. Shprintzen
The Virtual Center for Velo-Cardio-Facial Syndrome,
Manlius, NY, USA
e-mail: ashanske@aol.com;
robert.schprintzen@vcfscenter.org

A. am Zehnhoff-Dinnesen et al. (eds.), *Phoniatrics II*, European Manual of Medicine,
https://doi.org/10.1007/978-3-031-25175-7_1

1.1.3 Symptomatic Profile

Phonetic disorders can have a negative impact on social, academic and vocational development (Leme et al. 2014). The symptoms in dysglossia range from imprecise articulation, the inability to pronounce certain phonemes, with profoundly reduced speech intelligibility, to the inability to speak at all.

Depending on the localisation of the damage, dysglossia can be classified as labial, lingual, palatal, velopharyngeal or nasal dysglossia (Schröter-Morasch and Ziegler 2005). In contrast to dysarthria, distinct parts of articulation are mostly deteriorated. Whereas labial dysglossia causes phonetic problems of the first articulatory zone, dental dysglossia influences phonology of the second and lingual dysglossia of the second and the third articulatory zones. The velopharyngeal localisation of dysglossia affects the latter two articulatory zones, main symptom of velopharyngeal insufficiency (VPI) is hypernasality, while nasal dysglossia causes hyponasality (Friedrich 2013).

The degree of phonetic constraint reflects the magnitude of the defect: the size of a tumour, the extent of tissue resection and the healing of defects all influence the grade of dysglossia. Local defect healing provides better results concerning articulation than myo-or fasciocutaneous flaps (Schönweiler et al. 1996). Thus, injuries of the anterior tongue influence the correct generation of consonants, whereas resections of posterior lingual tissue reduce quality of vowel production (Leonard et al. 1992). Studies from Müller and Gebelein (2001) summarised the frequency of articulatory problems depending on the affected area: base of the tongue 100%, lower jaw 87.5%, base of the mouth 81%, tongue 72.7%, lips 28.6% and tonsils 27.3%. Nevertheless, even in hemi-glossectomy or glossectomy (aglossia), articulation can be realised by compensation of other tissues, e.g. parts of the oropharynx. The outcome depends on the motility of the rest of the tongue, on the mobility of the lips and on the activity of the oropharyngeal muscles.

In patients with tumours and surgery of the tongue and the base of the mouth, besides articulation, chewing and swallowing, oral sensitivity and sensation of taste are also deteriorated. These functions become even worse with radiochemotherapy (Koppetsch and Dahlmeier 2004). It can secondarily impair function by damaging peripheral cranial nerves, even years after therapy (Lin et al. 2002). In cases of defects of the palate and the upper jaw, with a connection between the nasal and oral cavities, a pronounced open rhinophonia and dysphagia results (Schröter-Morasch and Ziegler 2005).

1.1.4 Aetiology and Pathogenesis

Because of its multiple causes, the aetiology of dysglossia is variable. Three general groups of dysglossia can be differentiated by their causes:

1. Congenital disorders that cause craniofacial malformation (i.e. cleft lip or palate, lymphangioma, haemangioma) or syndromes (Böhme 2003).
2. Pre-or post-operative alterations in the head and neck (e.g. tumours, radio-chemotherapy, scars, other alteration of tissue).
3. Peripheral palsy of craniofacial nerves (especially facial and hypoglossal nerves) caused by inflammation (e.g. otitis media, zoster oticus), trauma (e.g. temporal bone fracture), carcinoma (e.g. parotis carcinoma) and surgery (e.g. after operation of the parotid gland or Bell's palsy).

In (1), mostly cleft lip or palate causes dysglossia, but all changes of the tongue (e.g. in macroglossia, trisomy 21, Beckwith–Wiedemann syndrome, Cornelia de Lange syndrome, muscular dystrophia Duchenne, endocrine diseases (hypothyrosis, acromegaly), storage diseases (e.g. mucopolysaccharidosis, amyloidosis)) can cause severe dysglossia. Concerning dysglossia, tongue-tie/anterior and posterior ankyloglossia (4–10% of all newborns: Ballard et al. 2002) with inhibited motility are discussed controversially

(Walsh and McKenna 2019), but all affect breastfeeding (O'Shea et al. 2017; Hong 2013). In such syndromes such as velocardiofacial syndrome (Shprintzen syndrome, 22q11 microdeletion) and Pierre–Robin sequence, cleft palate and VPI cause dysglossia and reduced speech intelligibility, associated problems like prominent upper jaw, underdeveloped lower jaw, thin upper lip and hearing loss may intensify the extent of phonetic constraint.

In (2), pre-or post-operative alterations in the head and neck, whether benign (e.g. haemangioma, lymphangioma) or malign (e.g. squamous cell carcinoma of the tongue, base of the mouth and oropharynx, others), cause dysglossia. Scars, flaps and skeletal defects after resections of parts of the mandible or the upper jaw can also cause dysglossia. Prosthetic application to defects of the upper jaw can effectively improve symptoms (Brown and Shaw 2010). Outcomes become worse if the velum is integrated in the resection area.

In (3), uni-and bi-lateral peripheral nerve defects and palsies of the buccal branch of the facial nerve, the hypoglossal nerve, but also the glossopharyngeal nerve, cause dysglossia by affecting the motility of the lips, the tongue and the velum. While unilateral paralysis of the buccal branch induces a mild constraint of labial phonemes, bilateral paralysis deteriorates all labial phonemes and changes /b/ to /w/, /p/ to /f/ and /m/ to /n/. Uni-and bi-lateral palsy of the tongue, owing to its variable motor and sensitive functions, induces effects on articulation by impeding contact with the teeth, the alveolar crest and the hard and soft palate. In unilateral peripheral hypoglossal palsy, the protruded tongue deviates to the side of the palsy and the labial phonemes /b/ and /p/, and the alveolar phonemes /d/, /t/, /n/ and /s/ are mildly influenced. In bilateral peripheral hypoglossal palsy, the tongue does not show any motility, the musculature is atrophic and it can show some fasciculations. Dysglossia in this case brings a pronounced articulation disorder with doughy, slurred speech, combined with dysphagia of the oral phase. Articulation of the phonemes /d/, /t/, /l/, /n/, /r/, /g/, /k/, /e/ and /i/ is especially affected, and /s/ and /sch/ are articulated imprecisely. Compensation can be achieved by lifting the mandible and guiding the tongue to its original articulatory destination.

1.2 Definition, Nomenclature and Symptomatic Profile of Velopharyngeal Insufficiency (VPI)

Karen J. Golding-Kushner

1.2.1 Introduction

When discussing velopharyngeal insufficiency, the automatic inclination is to think of individuals with clefts of the palate. This is probably related to the large amount of medical literature devoted to cleft palate surgery, cleft palate speech disorders (primarily hypernasality) and numerous descriptions of clinical care for people with cleft disorders. But clinicians should also be aware that VPI and dysfunction of the velopharyngeal mechanism occur in many other disorders, including neurological disorders, trauma, hearing impairment, congenital anomalies other than palatal clefts and disordered learning of speech mechanics. In this section, we will consider all of these problems and show that each may have its own clinical presentation, status over time, treatment options and treatment outcomes.

1.2.2 Nomenclature and Definition of Velopharyngeal Insufficiency

Some years ago, clinicians began a process of renaming a variety of forms of velopharyngeal dysfunction in an attempt to differentiate the root cause of excessive nasal resonance (hypernasality), and adopted the term 'velopharyngeal dysfunction', or VPD, differentiating it from velopharyngeal insufficiency (VPI). To us, this was a mental exercise that had no significance for the understanding or treatment of hypernasal resonance. VPI or VPD, or any other term applied to the absence of velopharyngeal closure during speech when it should be present, is simply a clinical observation. It is not a disease, not a symptom (hypernasality is a symptom) but is an observation or clinical finding that leads to the symptom.

We dislike the term VPD because the term 'dysfunction' is a judgement that implies there is a specific function, when we know that there are many possible ways for the velopharyngeal orifice to close during speech. There is not a single functional mechanism of how the palate and pharyngeal walls close that space. The point, however, is unimportant and as a good friend once said, scientists are often more likely to share their toothbrush than their terminology. In this section, we will refer to abnormalities of closure of the velopharynx during speech as VPI.

A term we use to designate the purpose of the structures in the velopharyngeal region is 'velopharyngeal valve'. A valve is a mechanism that controls the flow or rate of flow of a fluid (gas or liquid) through a passage or opening. This is precisely what the velopharyngeal valve does and the moving structures that constitute this valve include the velum (soft palate) and the pharyngeal walls (lateral and sometimes posterior). Whether we call the failure of this valve to cut off the airflow completely when it is supposed to do so, an inadequacy, an insufficiency or an incompetence is inconsequential. Regardless of the term attached, a good clinician will investigate thoroughly to find out exactly what the problem is, what causes it and how to treat it. Some brief definitions follow:

Velopharyngeal, Velopharynx: the terms used to describe the area of the upper airway in the region of the junction between the nasopharynx and oropharynx.

Velopharyngeal Orifice: a term often used to describe the opening between the nasopharynx and oropharynx, although it is not a structure per se but rather the components of the combined movement of the soft palate (velum), the lateral pharyngeal walls and posterior pharyngeal wall. The adenoid is a component of the posterior pharyngeal wall that is almost always a part of the velopharynx, or velopharyngeal orifice, in young children until the age when the adenoids involute, beginning as prepubertal changes begin. The term 'orifice', while descriptive and commonly used, is not really accurate in the sense that it implies a specific place when it is, in fact, variable both within a single person and highly variable between people.

Velopharyngeal Valve: this term accurately describes the function of the velopharynx for speech, swallowing and other airflow-related functions of the human upper airway. The movements of the velum and pharyngeal walls open and close the upper airway, thereby separating the nasal and nasopharyngeal airway from the oral, oropharyngeal and hypopharyngeal airways. Complete separation of the nasal airway from the lower portions of the airway (velopharyngeal closure) is the norm during the production of normally non-nasal speech sounds, during swallowing (both reflexive and purposeful), during blowing from the mouth, and during gagging, but the method of closing the velopharyngeal valve is not the same for each of those acts (Shprintzen et al. 1974).

Velopharyngeal Insufficiency (VPI): a failure of the velum, lateral pharyngeal walls and posterior pharyngeal wall to move and close sufficiently to separate the nasopharynx from the oropharynx. VPI is the most common cause of hypernasality but it does not always result in perceivable hypernasal resonance disorder. Some people use different terms for the causes of VPI, but we think the differentiation is inconsequential in terms of effect and treatment and, for that reason, do not distinguish them. They are described here only for reference, as the reader may encounter these terms. They are all abbreviated VPI, and the authors use the term velopharyngeal insufficiency and the abbreviation VPI regardless of aetiology:

Velopharyngeal insufficiency—VPI caused by abnormal structure, such as a cleft palate or removal of the adenoid; the authors usually use this as the generic term for all types of velopharyngeal dysfunction

Velopharyngeal incompetence—VPI due to abnormal movement, such as in cerebral palsy or other dysarthria.

Velopharyngeal inadequacy—a generic term that includes VPI resulting from any aetiology; also referred to as *velopharyngeal dysfunction* (VPD).

We do not believe that the addition of these subcategories is very helpful in terms of clinical care or the ability to describe these disorders to patients who are affected by the problem. They certainly do not help in devising treatment strategies. We prefer the use of a single term signifying that the velopharyngeal mechanism is not functioning normally, and that term would be *velopharyngeal insufficiency*, or VPI.

1.2.3 Symptomatic Profile of Velopharyngeal Insufficiency

VPI is associated with certain *obligatory speech characteristics* including hypernasality, nasal emission or turbulence, and reduced intra-oral air pressure. It is also associated with a class of learned articulation errors, sometimes called 'cleft palate speech' or maladaptive *compensatory articulation errors (CAEs)*. The CAEs can only be corrected with speech therapy; surgery does not resolve them. The obligatory errors typically require physical management, surgery or prosthetics (Golding-Kushner 2001a; Golding-Kushner and Shprintzen 2011).

1.2.3.1 Obligatory Speech Errors

These are a class of error directly caused by an anatomical or physiological condition. They are not amenable to correction by therapy but usually disappear when the condition is eliminated. If they do not self-correct when the condition is eliminated, they are generally amenable to therapy at that time. Examples are:

- (Passive) nasal emission and nasal turbulence
- Reduced intra-oral air pressure.
- Hypernasality due to VPI.

Nasal Emission (NE): a passive escape of air through the nasal cavity. Nasal emission should be present during production of nasal phonemes (/m, n, ng/ in English) but absent from other sounds. Nasal emission may be audible or silent. Silent nasal emission may be detected with a stethoscope or straw with one end placed in the nose and the other in the ear, or by looking for fogging on a mirror held beneath the nose. NE is usually an obligatory error. Oral sounds produced with accompanying NE usually sound better with the nares occluded.

Nasal Turbulence (NT) or Nasal Rustle: a nasal emission that passes through a narrow constriction causing a rustling noise. Like nasal emission, it is usually passive and is usually an obligatory error. Sounds produced with accompanying NT usually sound better with the nares occluded. NT is a consonant event because it is due to attempts at creating oral air pressure. In contrast, hypernasality is a vowel phenomenon-it is characterized by excessive nasal resonance during production of vowels.

Nasal Grimace (NG): a scrunching of the nose that often occurs with NE, NT or NS. It is probably an attempt to use the nasal muscles in order to prevent nasal escape of air. It usually stops without treatment when NE, NT or NS are eliminated. It is a consonant event, associated with production of sounds requiring oral air pressure.

Facial Grimace: the same as nasal grimace but involving accessory muscle movement noted in other facial features such as the eyes, eyebrows and forehead. It is probably an attempt to use the nasal muscles in order to prevent nasal escape of air. It usually stops without treatment when NE, NT or NS are eliminated.

1.2.3.2 Compensatory Articulation Errors (CAEs)

These are a class of error associated with cleft palate, VPI or both. These errors are rare in speakers without a history of cleft palate or VPI and are errors in learning. They include the following:

- Glottal stop.
- Pharyngeal stop.
- Pharyngeal fricative.
- Glottal fricative.
- Nasal snort (velar fricative).
- Mid-dorsal palatal stop.
- Mid-dorsal palatal fricative.

Glottal stop: a sound produced by abrupt closing of the vocal folds that momentarily stops the flow of air through the glottis (the space between the vocal folds) followed by the release of the air pressure built up during the temporary closure; because the acoustic event of the stop plosive has occurred, the oral gesture of the intended sound (lip closure for /p, b/, lingua-alveolar contact for /t, d/, lingua-velar contact for /k, g/) is frequently not produced, resulting in misperception that this is a sound omission, or that the speaker is 'apraxic' and unable to produce the oral gesture. This probably develops as a speaker's attempt to produce the acoustic event of a stop consonant in a part of the vocal tract where building up air pressure can be done, before the air flow leaks through the velopharyngeal valve resulting in reduced oral air pressure. The sound also occurs naturally as the onset of a word with a vowel as the first sound and is phonemic in some languages as the first sound and is phonemic in some languages. It may be produced as a substitution for a sound or coproduced with a sound.

Pharyngeal stop: a stop consonant produced by contraction of the pharyngeal walls or contact of the posterior part of the tongue to the pharynx; like the glottal stop, it is a speaker's attempt to produce the target sound below the velopharyngeal orifice and before the air leaks through the nose.

Pharyngeal fricative: the same as the pharyngeal stop but with constriction, rather than complete contact of the structures, often a substitute for fricative and sibilant sounds.

Glottal fricative: the same as the glottal stop but with the vocal folds approximating but not closing fully to replicate a fricative sound.

Nasal fricative or nasal snort (NS): air that is forcibly directed through the nasal cavity, usually during production of fricative or sibilant sounds. NS is a maladaptive compensatory error and is a learned articulation error. It is not obligatory and can only be corrected with speech therapy. Sounds produced as an NS usually sound worse (or cannot be produced at all) with the nares occluded. NS may be produced as an anterior nasal fricative, usually accompanied by nasal grimace and voiceless, or as a posterior nasal fricative, which is usually noisy and may or may not be accompanied by nasal grimace. NS is a consonant event. It is also referred to as velopharyngeal mis-learning, and sometimes when it occurs as an articulation error affecting one sound or one class of sounds, as phone-specific VPI. Of all the maladaptive compensatory errors, this is the one most likely to be produced in the absence of history of cleft palate or VPI.

Mid-dorsal palatal stop: a sound produced by contact of the tongue dorsum with an area of the palate between the alveolar ridge and the velum; it is often associated with an anterior fistula or malocclusion; it results in a sound that is not quite a /k, g/ and not quite a /t, d/ but something in between.

Mid-dorsal palatal fricative: the same as the mid-dorsal palatal stop but with constriction rather than contact of the structures, resulting in a fricative rather than a stop sound.

1.2.3.3 Resonance

Hypernasality: an excessive nasal resonance caused by failure of full separation of the nasal cavity from the oral cavity, and the nasopharynx from the oropharynx during normally non-nasal speech. It is usually caused by velopharyngeal insufficiency but may also result from a palatal fistula. Hypernasality is a vowel phenomenon and does not occur on consonants. Hypernasality may co-occur with hyponasality; they are not on a single continuum, and should be rated separately. Hypernasality alone does not generally cause speech to be unintelligible, and when it is the only speech symptom, a speech that excludes the nasal phonemes /n, m, ŋ/ will sound normal with the nares occluded. Hypernasality has many different causes including structural anomalies such as cleft palate and other congenital anomalies, trauma, neurological disorders, deafness, learning errors, hypertrophic tonsils, growths (benign or cancerous), and as a complication from palatal, maxillary or adenotonsillar surgery.

Hyponasality: insufficient or absent nasal resonance, on normally nasal sounds. Although most sounds in all languages are typically produced without nasal resonance, a small number of sounds must be produced with the velopharyngeal valve opened. These sounds include /m/, /n/,

/ñ/ and /ń/, /ŋ/, /ṇ/ (voice velar nasal), /ɲ/ (voice palatal nasal) and /ɴ/ (voice uvular nasal). Hyponasality is usually caused by nasal or nasopharyngeal obstruction, such as adenoid hypertrophy or deviated septum, or the presence of a neoplasia, or a complete blockage of the nasal cavity by chronic or temporary nasal congestion, enlarged turbinates, severe sinusitis, neoplasias or foreign objects. It may also be caused by insufficient duration of nasal consonants or omission of the nasal element of nasal-oral clusters, such as when saying 'mukkey' instead of 'monkey' or 'lap' for 'lamp'. Hyponasality may co-occur with hypernasality, they are not on a single continuum, and should be rated separately.

Cul-de-Sac Resonance: an atypical nasal resonance caused by a combination of VPI that results in pairing of oropharynx and nasopharynx but with a nasal obstruction, such as a severely deviated nasal septum, which separates the extended resonance cavities of the pharynx from the nasal cavity or at least the full nasal cavity.

Muffled or 'Potato-in-the-Mouth' Resonance: an atypical oral resonance also referred to as 'marshmallow in the mouth'. It may be caused by tonsil hypertrophy, excessive posterior tongue bunching, or other atypical tongue postures, and may co-occur with abnormal nasal resonance, either hypernasality or hyponasality. The pattern is most often prompted by partial obstruction of the oropharynx that dampens the vocal signal from the larynx, thereby reducing the resonance of the sound in the oropharynx and above. Palatine tonsil hypertrophy is the most common cause of this resonance pattern and is most often independent of other anomalies. Posterior tongue carriage or tongue "humping" is another cause. Some craniofacial disorders have reduced pharyngeal volume (Shprintzen et al. 1974) so that even mildly enlarged tonsils can result in the pattern. In some cases, congenital malformation syndromes, including Treacher Collins syndrome, Nager syndrome and craniosynostosis syndromes (Crouzon, Apert, Pfeiffer, Shprintzen–Goldberg syndrome as examples), which are known to have structurally small upper airways related to cranial base anomalies, can cause it (Sher et al. 1986). In these syndromes, even normal amounts of lymphoid tissue can cause obstructions in an airway that is structurally small.

1.2.3.4 Developmental Articulation Errors

This class of error includes sound production typical of an earlier stage of development, retained at a later stage. Examples are anterior lisp, which is developmentally appropriate for a 2-year-old but not an 8-year-old, and substitution of w/r. These errors are unrelated to cleft palate or VPI and should be treated if they persist beyond the typical age by which they are resolved. The nature of the error is critical to distinguishing between a compensatory error (that will not be 'outgrown' and must be treated with speech therapy at the earliest possible time) and developmental errors. Standard tests of articulation do not make this distinction, which is why a decision about the need for speech therapy cannot be based on a test score only.

For example, if the only error in the speech sample of a 3-year-old is on /s/, the test score would be in the average range for age. If the error was substitution of /th/ for /s/, one would monitor the child's development but would not recommend speech therapy. In contrast, if the error was production of a nasal snort for /s/, the test score would still be in the average range (because the score is quantitative, not qualitative), but one would need to intervene with speech therapy in order to eliminate the maladaptive compensatory error. The goal of speech therapy would be correct production of /s/ with elimination of the nasal snort. When the nasal snort was eliminated, the child might have an accurate /s/ or might then develop an interdental /s/ (lisp), which would be developmentally appropriate and acceptable. (It would not have been the goal, but could be the outcome.)

1.2.3.5 Other Speech Disorders

Dysarthria: a speech disorder caused by paralysis, weakness or incoordination of the entire speech mechanism related to central or peripheral nervous system disorders or damage. Dysarthria is often accompanied by VPI and hypernasality, articulation impairment and reduced intelligibility. Velopharyngeal insufficiency differs considerably from that seen in cleft disorders. While VPI in cleft cases is typically consistent with velopharyngeal closure never occurring during the production of normally non-nasal speech, in dysarthria there is often good closure of the velopharyngeal valve during production of pressure consonants; but in the vowels that separate pressure consonant sounds, the valve opens creating hypernasal resonance that is typically perceived as consistent VPI. Imaging of the velopharyngeal valve during speech (nasopharyngoscopy and videofluoroscopy) should include speech samples that include normal conversational speech when this pattern can be seen. This type of hypernasal speech does not respond well to typical surgical treatment because of the inconsistency of movements in the velopharyngeal valve and the slurring of speech production. Even if surgical correction totally obstructs the velopharyngeal orifice, intelligibility is not often improved. Eliciting a speech sample with the nares open and with the nares occluded can provide a sense of the degree to which speech intelligiblity will be improved with treatment of VPI.

Nasal Emission vs. Nasal Snorting: VPI is almost always accompanied by detectable emission of air from the nose unless the nose itself is blocked or congested, either permanently or temporarily. The presence of nasal emission is not always accompanied by significant hypernasality. Asymptomatic detectable airflow from the nose (i.e. during perceptually normal speech) is not unusual and should not require treatment. Nasal snorting is a form of nasal emission but is a compensatory articulation pattern when the air is pushed out of the nose forcefully in order to make a sound that is typically substituted for sibilant or fricative sounds (Golding-Kushner 2001a). This type of substitution, while seen in people with cleft palate and VPI, is also found in people with no structural anomalies, or in people with hypertrophic palatine tonsils. This type of nasal emission has also been labelled as phoneme-specific nasal emission. When the snort is associated only with fricative and sibilant sounds, the error is known as either a posterior or anterior nasal fricative. This type of substitution is actually an articulation error and is often easily resolved with specific type of speech therapy (Golding-Kushner 2001a; Golding-Kushner and Shprintzen 2011). A posterior nasal fricative is a sound made when air is forced out of the nose while the velum is in close approximation to the pharyngeal walls, but not closed tight. This sound is occasionally accompanied by a constriction of the nares which is usually called a grimace. An anterior nasal fricative is when air is forced through the nose on fricative/sibilant sounds, but the constriction creating the frication is at the nares, which is always seen as a grimace.

1.3 Epidemiology, Aetiology and Pathogenesis of Velopharyngeal Insufficiency

Robert J. Shprintzen

1.3.1 Introduction

Separation of the nasal airway from the oral and hypopharyngeal airways for speech is unique to the human species (Shprintzen 2003). Humans are the only species to have speech as we know it, meaning that we can make a large variety of consonant sounds that require the ability to impound oral pressure along with such continuant and nasal sounds such as /l/, /w/, /r/, /m/, /n/, /ñ/, /ń/, /ŋ/ and /ṇ/. Animal species' sound communications consist of a variety of vowels often described as hoots, howls, screams or purrs, and occasional use of nasal sounds, most often sustained /m/ sounds. Humans alone use velopharyngeal closure during speech, resulting in the ability to make pressure sounds, both as stops (such as /p/, /b/, /t/, /d/, /k/, /g/) and continuants (including fricative /s/, /z/, /f/, /v/; glides /j/, /w/, /r/, /l/, /h/ and others) allowing the production of transitions from fricatives to glides to stops, etc. (Shprintzen

2003). The large number of consonants and vowels that can be produced by humans allows the formation of innumerable words, and this sound production drives the unique ability in humans to have spoken language and have an average vocabulary of more than 30,000 words for the average person (López-Barroso et al. 2013; Shprintzen 2003).

Why is the structural development of the velopharyngeal mechanism unique to humans? As described by Davidson (2003) and Davidson et al. (2005), evolutionary changes in *Homo sapiens* that led us to walk upright were accompanied by the increased vertical inclination of the upper airway (Fig. 1.1).

The upper airway in humans becomes more vertical with age. More horizontal at birth, before the onset of speech, the airway is structured to allow an infant to breathe through the nose while simultaneously nursing (Sidoti and Shprintzen 1995). With growth and age, the head grows vertically, and the upper airway becomes more upright. At birth, there is little separation between the tongue and hard palate and the upper airway is relatively horizontal, but after 1 year of age there is significant increase in the vertical height of the airway so that the resonating chamber of the pharynx increases in vertical height (Fig. 1.2).

This increases the amount of space for the tongue to move and sound resonance to increase in tenor and variation. The first utterances of infants, including crying, are sounds with nasal resonance, mostly vowels and occasionally a sound that approximates the continuant /m/, but these sounds are all randomly produced and are not speech. The first appearance of sounds requiring velopharyngeal closure occurs when babbling begins. The sounds are usually voiced, such as /b/ and /d/ and /g/. As these sounds are recognised and reinforced by parents and siblings, those that are parts of the language are learned and remain in the child's speech repertoire, while those that are not included disappear over time because of non-reinforcement. For example, /r/ is

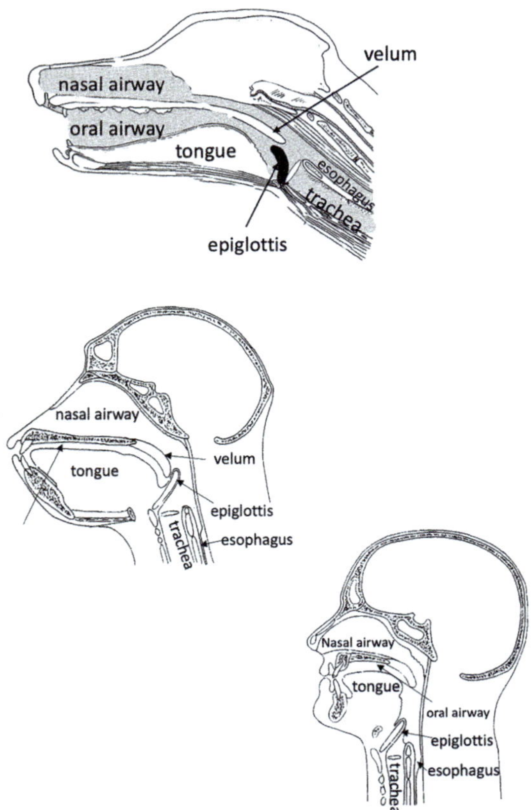

Fig. 1.1 A comparison of the adult human airway and that of the upper airway of a chimpanzee and a domestic dog. Note the difference in the angulation of the airway (Shprintzen©2021)

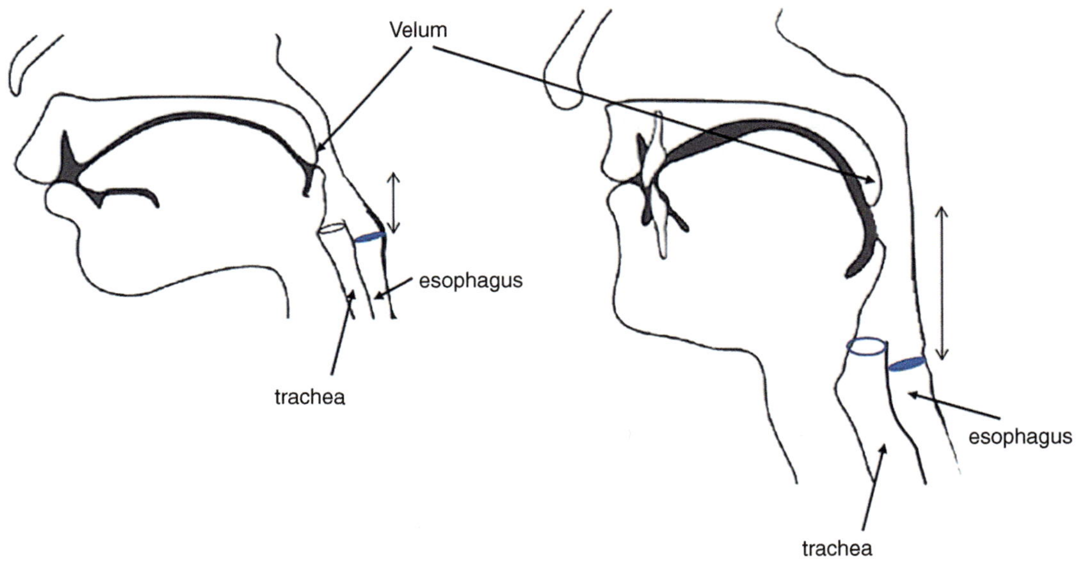

Fig. 1.2 The vertical compression of the upper airway in infants allows a newborn to eat and breathe simultaneously. With age, the airway lengthens with the increase in face height, removing the velum from the region just above the glottis (Shprintzen©2021)

in the sound repertoire of Japanese, but /l/ is not. Conversely, in both Mandarin and Cantonese Chinese, there is no /r/ but there is an /l/.

Velopharyngeal closure is essential to all languages in order to produce pressure consonants such as /p/, /b/, /t/, /d/, /k/, /g/, /ʃ/, /ʃ/, /θ/, /tʃ/, /ð/, /s/, /z/, /ʒ/, /dʒ/, /f/ and guttural sounds such as /x/. Vowels do not require velopharyngeal closure and when produced in isolation are often nasalised. Some vowels, such as high front vowels (e.g. /i/) have less nasal resonance than high back vowels (e.g. /u/). However, in connected speech, when vowels follow, precede or are surrounded by non-nasal consonants, the velopharyngeal closure achieved for the consonants carries over to the vowels. When surrounded by nasal consonants (e.g. /m/, /n/, /ŋ/), the vowels are nasalised and velopharyngeal closure does not occur.

The structure of the upper airway changes substantially with age until adult life, primarily related to vertical growth of the face and changes in angulation of the skull base (Shprintzen 2003). The vertical relationship of the palate to the cervical spine, the adenoid mass, the larynx and surrounding structures changes considerably (Shprintzen 1995, p.64). In the newborn and infant period, the velum hangs vertically into the oropharynx and is in close proximity to the epiglottis in the hypopharynx. This arrangement is necessary for nursing and allowing the infant to breathe and suck at the same time. With age, the vertical growth of the maxilla, cervical spine and pharyngeal soft tissues separates the velum from the hypopharyngeal airway, allowing a bolus of food to be accommodated in the oral cavity and oropharynx as diet progresses from a liquid to a solid diet (Fig. 1.2).

The first reported description of velopharyngeal closure was a direct observation of the velopharyngeal mechanism from above through a facial defect created by an encapsulated tumour that was spontaneously evulsed in an adult patient (Hilton 1836). This single case report was an accurate assessment of the movement of the velum and lateral pharyngeal walls, creating a sphincter like valve separating the nasopharynx from the oropharynx. It was not until the twentieth century (Scheier 1909) that observations of velopharyngeal closure were reported by radiography in the lateral view with still films. Lateral (mid-sagittal) view radiographs became the standard assessment procedure for the next six decades, moving from still radiographs, cephalographs (Subtelny 1957) and, eventually, cineradiography (Moll 1965). Although these procedures are still in use in some locations, they have been recognised as being inadequate. Still radiographs do not provide motion, which is critical to speech, and even cineradiography and videofluoroscopy in lateral view are merely two-dimensional representations of a three-dimensional region. Lateral radiographs cannot provide any evidence of the movement of the lateral pharyngeal walls that are critical to a full assessment of velopharyngeal closure (Golding-Kushner et al. 1990; Shprintzen and Golding Kushner 1989; Shprintzen et al. 1979b; Skolnick et al. 1973).

Two major advances were introduced in 1969, one radiographic and the other endoscopic. In two articles (Skolnick 1969; Skolnick and McCall 1972) Skolnick described fluoroscopic assessment of the velopharyngeal valve in three different views (Fig. 1.3): lateral (mid-sagittal), frontal (posterior-anterior or P-A) and base (submentovertical).

The three views were implemented serially during the procedure, using the same speech sample during all three, provided a three-dimensional assessment of all of the components of velopharyngeal valving. Since the description of multi-view videofluoroscopy by Skolnick, other views have been added to assist in the complete understanding of the movements of all components of velopharyngeal closure. These include left and right oblique views when asymmetry is noted in the frontal view, and Townes view when lateral view shows that the primary contact of the velum to the posterior pharyngeal wall is on a prominent adenoid mass (Golding-Kushner et al. 1990; Shprintzen 1995; Ysunza et al. 2016).

At the same time that multi-view videofluoroscopy was reported, so too was nasopharyngoscopy being developed with both flexible and rigid endoscopes (Pigott 1969; Pigott et al. 1969; Miyazaki et al. 1975). The use of rigid instruments was originally touted as providing a better image and in its infancy the external diameter of flexible instruments was no better than the external diameter of down-looking rigid endoscopes. However, after several years, the external diameter of forward-looking fibre-optic endoscopes was reduced to 3 mm (Shprintzen et al. 1979a) and eventually approximately 2 mm. The light-carrying capabilities of endoscopes and brightness of light sources made the examination of velopharyngeal insufficiency with very thin fibre-optic endoscopes commonplace, and flexible fibre-optic nasopharyngoscopy became the instrumentation of choice in most places.

The initial descriptions of nasopharyngoscopy all included methods for recording the studies on video media. Systems for video-nasopharyngoscopy have been developed, but it is also quite simple to set up a video system with any flexible fibre-optic endoscope, a light source, an endoscopic video camera and a notebook or desktop computer (Skolnick 1970). The total cost for the system (not including the endoscope and light source) can be well under U.S. $3000 for high-quality digital audio recording with sound (Shprintzen and Ysunza 2020). However, as reported by these authors, it is likely that half the examinations or more do not record the video of examinations, and of the examinations recorded on video, less than a third have sound recorded. They concluded that any endoscopic study of speech production without both video and sound is

> archaic, inadequate and not to be trusted—Shprintzen and Ysunza (2020), p. 201

It is well known that studies viewed by a single examiner cannot be presumed to be valid, and having a panel of diagnosticians reviewing such studies together is recommended (D'Antonio et al. 1989).

In reviewing methods of diagnosis of velopharyngeal insufficiency (VPI), it is clear that nasopharyngoscopy is the favoured imaging procedure. This author has visited more than 100 cleft palate/craniofacial centres in North America, South America, Asia, Europe, Africa and Australia. Only a small handful of those centres utilised multi-view videofluoroscopy to assess VPI, but all of them used nasopharyngoscopy, although techniques and the extent of the examination were highly variable. For example, in some locations, the endoscope was never passed

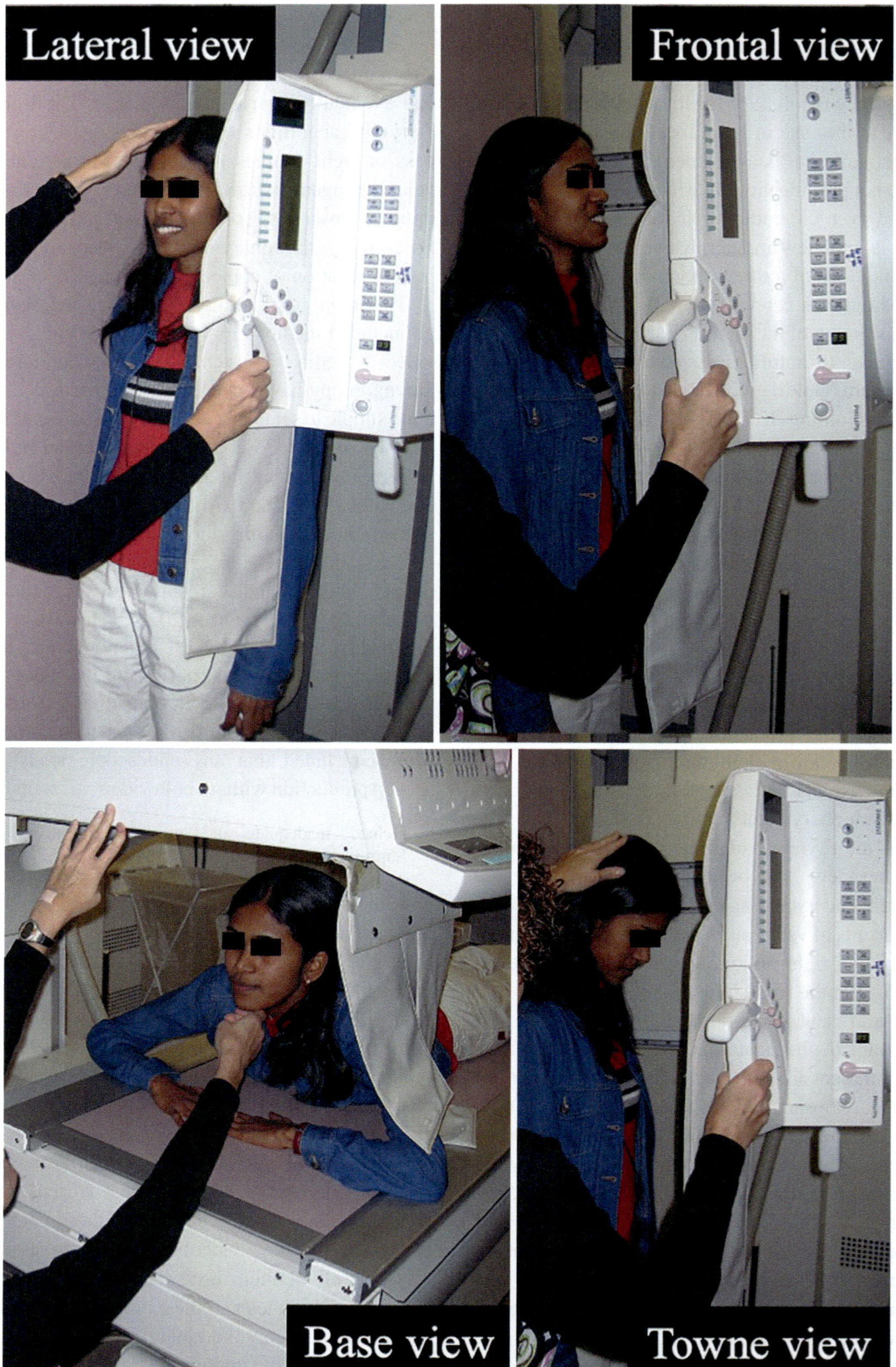

Fig. 1.3 Positioning for multi-view videofluoroscopy and resulting views (Shprintzen©2021)

beyond the nasopharynx so that the only portion of the upper airway seen was the nasopharynx. This prevents observations of the larynx and the full extent of lymphoid tissue in the oropharynx and hypopharynx. There was also variability in the use of speech samples. In some programmes, only isolated phonemes and syllables were used and connected conversational speech was not used. Because the outcome of treatments for VPI are judged on conversational speech, the use of isolated vowels, consonants and nonsense syllables makes little sense.

In 1988, an International Working Group was formed and spent 2 days together in order to develop a standardised protocol for assessing and reporting the results of visual VPI assessments. Held in New York, representatives from the United States, Mexico, Canada, the United Kingdom and Sweden, a total of 27 clinicians with extensive clinical, research and publication experience accepted the invitation to join the working group, and they included the pioneers in the development of both endoscopy and multi-view videofluoroscopy (Drs. Pigott, Skolnick and McCall). The task was to arrive at universal agreement over best practice standards as well as a way to standardise reporting of the results of the examination. A ratio system was devised for rating all components of movement in the velopharyngeal valve or each radiographic projection. For complete evaluation of VPI, it was recommended that both naso-pharyngoscopy and multi-view videofluoroscopy be used. Speech samples were also recommended to include syllable repetitions, production of sustained fricatives and sibilants and the use of conversational speech samples and repeated phrases that include all phonemes to the person's native language.

The results of the International Working Group meeting were written by Dr. Karen Golding-Kushner and circulated to the participants for approval, and then submitted to the Cleft Palate Journal where it was published in 1990 (Golding-Kushner et al. 1990). Subsequent studies showed validation of the work of the group's system for assessing and reporting assessments of VPI. However, because multi-view videofluoroscopy is used infrequently at most centres, the evaluation of velopharyngeal function remains limited in most locales. In part, this is because many if not most surgeons do not employ the notion that reconstructive procedures should be specific to the patient's type of VPI, including tailoring the operation for the size and location of the velopharyngeal gap (Shprintzen et al. 1979a; Ysunza et al. 2019). Another reason is that surgeons prefer to see living tissue rather than radiographic images. Nasopharyngoscopy provides an excellent view of the tissues of the pharynx. However, the entire upper airway and not all of the movements can be observed at one time, especially if the velum is elevating towards the posterior pharyngeal wall and blocking the view of the endoscope, limiting the observation to the nasopharynx. Seeing something through the endoscope does not mean one is seeing everything.

Note that the movement of the lateral pharyngeal walls cannot be determined from the endoscopic examination, but on frontal view videofluoroscopy excellent lateral pharyngeal wall motion can be seen.

Shprintzen (1995) reported that in his experience applying both procedures for all patients was mandatory for avoiding false negative errors in assessing the movements of the lateral and posterior pharyngeal walls. As with nasopharyngoscopy, all fluoroscopic examinations must be recorded with both video and synchronous sound. Because it is possible that velopharyngeal movements will be variable across phonemes, these variations can only be observed and noted if sound is recorded for the examination.

The examinations of the velopharyngeal mechanism by fluoroscopy and endoscopy should be reviewed by both the diagnosticians and the surgeons who will be treating patients with VPI. Multiple observers of the videos will ensure a more valid review of the examinations and will also allow the choice of treatment to be discussed by all involved in the process. Surgical management should be variable according to the size and location of the VPI (Shprintzen et al. 1979b; Ysunza et al. 2019). Moreover, the consistency of the movements may contribute to avoidance of surgery if complete closure is observed on some of the speech sounds being produced (Golding-Kushner 2001b). Because the implication of inconsistency and its importance would be most likely to have importance to speech-language pathologists or other specialists focused on speech productions, but may not be within the scope of study for surgeons, a panel of experts reviewing the recorded studies should be implemented for all cases.

1.3.2 Structure of the Velopharyngeal Valve

Rather than being a structure that is the same in all people, the velopharyngeal mechanism is highly variable from person to person. It should also be understood that the velopharyngeal valve is not a specific structure, but rather an area of the pharynx constituted of multiple structures. Specifically, the velopharyngeal valve is a combination of both ultrastructural components and multiple muscle groups. In addition, the structural components change very substantially over time (Siegel-Sadewitz and Shprintzen 1986). The structural components in early childhood include the velum, the adenoid and the lateral pharyngeal walls. In lateral view, the contact during velopharyngeal closure for young children is the velum against the adenoid pad (Fig. 1.4).

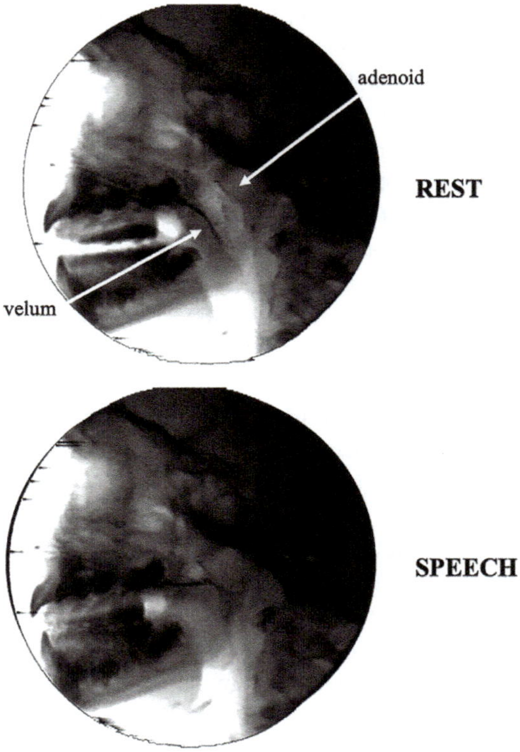

Fig. 1.4 Lateral view fluoroscopic view of velopharyngeal mechanism in a 4-year-old child showing velar contact with the adenoid (Shprintzen©2021)

In older children, the adenoid begins to involute, typically between 8 and 12 years of age, and the adenoid is no longer a component of velopharyngeal closure for almost all people. In many people, the adenoid is no longer present in adult life. The velopharyngeal valve also changes in its orientation, from relatively horizontal, to completely vertical. This is a gradual process over the first few years of life (Shprintzen 1995; Siegel-Sadewitz and Shprintzen 1986), and the involution of the adenoid becomes imperative because of the change of the pharynx from the relatively horizontal to vertical. As humans get older, the cranial base increases its flexion to a more acute angle related to growth of the posterior cranium and the expanding brain within the calvarium. As a result, the posterior pharyngeal wall, which is suspended from the cranial base, becomes more vertical relative to the palate, as well as being in closer approximation to the velum. The nasopharynx expands vertically, related to the height increase in the maxillofacial complex after puberty. The course of the uppermost fibres of the superior pharyngeal constrictor changes with age. In childhood, that muscle tends to follow a course parallel to the hard palate, while in adolescence, the fibres course forward and upward with the plane of the hard palate being higher than the uppermost fibres of the superior constrictor. This is important in applying muscular contractions to the movements of the various components of the velopharyngeal mechanism.

It is important to realise that when clinicians and scientists speak about the 'plane' of velopharyngeal closure, it is a concept that is completely false. Velopharyngeal closure is a three-dimensional activity. There is not only the mid-sagittal component (as seen in lateral view) and

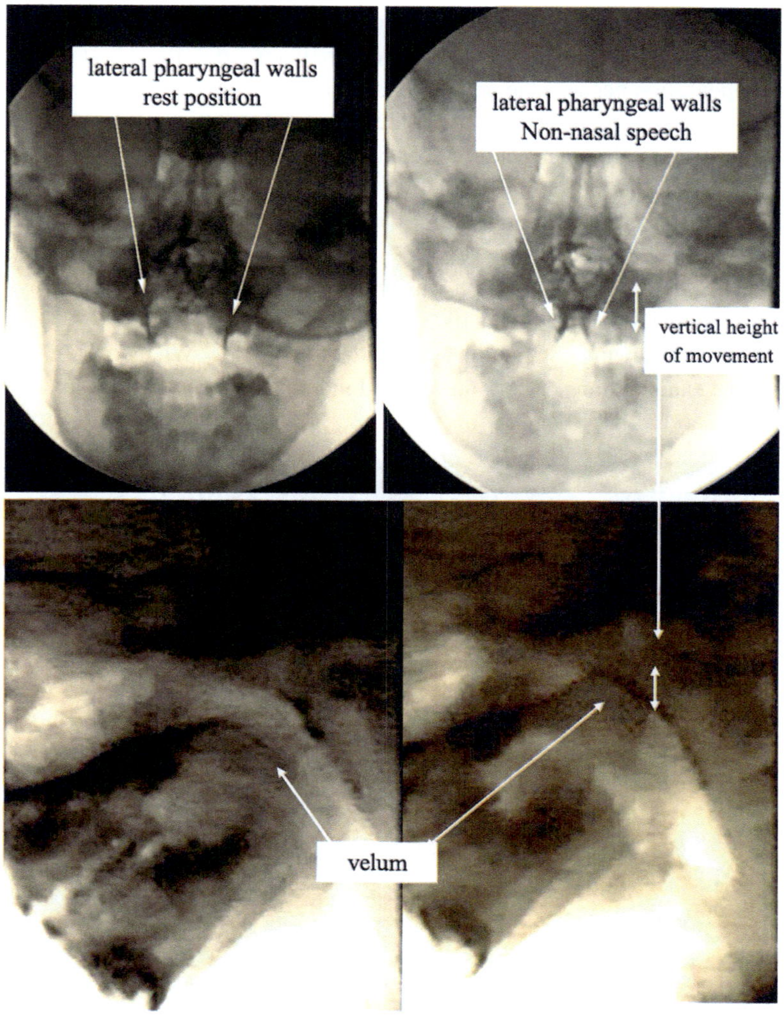

Fig. 1.5 Lateral and frontal view of velopharyngeal closure showing the vertical extent of velopharyngeal closure (Shprintzen©2021)

the transverse component (as seen in the P-A view), but also a vertical component (Fig. 1.5).

The velum can make a broad vertical contact with the posterior pharynx, and the lateral pharyngeal walls show medial motion over several centimetres of vertical height. The contact between the components of movement from the velum and the pharyngeal walls may require a vertically broad area of tissue in the vertical dimension in order to withstand the oral pressures during speech. Therefore, calculations of area for velopharyngeal gaps are not valid; measuring an area in mm^2 is therefore inappropriate: measurements should be in mm^3.

1.3.3 Is Velopharyngeal Closure Achieved the Same Way for Everyone?

During the era when the velopharyngeal mechanism was visualised only with lateral view radiography, the common perception of velopharyngeal closure was that the velum elevated and moved posteriorly to make contact with the posterior pharyngeal wall. In some cases, anterior movement of the posterior pharyngeal wall was seen, referred to as Passavant's ridge. This was usually thought of as a compensatory mechanism, although it was often unsuccessful in providing closure of the velopharyngeal valve, and hypernasal speech was occurring. This would contradict a compensation because the only purpose of a compensation is to yield success, or at the very least, improvement. In many cases, Passavant's ridge continues to be present in people who have large velopharyngeal gaps and severe hypernasality. What accounts for this?

The answer to that question was made evident by a landmark publication in 1973 (Skolnick et al. 1973). Reviewing 85 multi-view videofluoroscopic examinations of both normal and individuals with clefts of the palate and VPI, the authors described four different general categories of velopharyngeal closure: coronal closure, sagittal closure, circular closure and a true sphincteric closure, or circular closure with movement (Fig. 1.6).

The observations reported by Skolnick et al. (1973) were subsequently confirmed with data from both multi-view videofluoroscopy and nasopharyngoscopy examinations (Croft et al. 1981a).

What do these variations of velopharyngeal patterns of movement imply? Two concepts are in

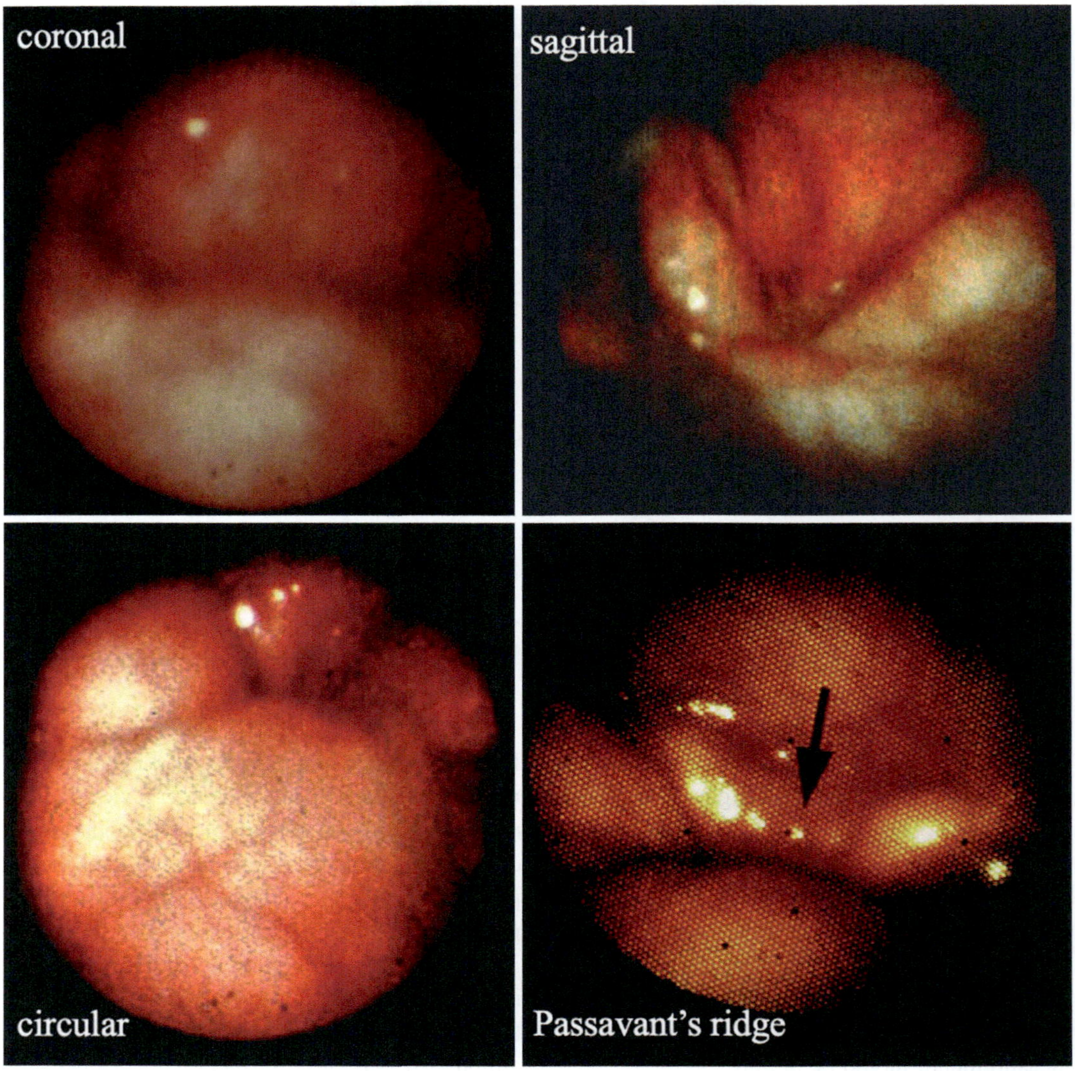

Fig. 1.6 Variable patterns of velopharyngeal closure showing coronal, sagittal, circular and Passavant ridge (sphincteric) closure (Shprintzen©2021)

effect for all people: variations in anatomical structure and the learning of velopharyngeal closure.

1.3.4 Anatomical Structure

As is true for all anatomical structures, no two people are identical in structure with the possible exception of monozygotic multiple births. The height of the pharynx and width of the pharynx is highly variable from person to person. It has been observed that the width of the nasopharynx is variable, especially in congenital anomalies that are expressed in the craniofacial complex (Shprintzen et al. 1985b). With increased or decreased width of the pharynx, the attachments, orientations and trajectory of contractions of the muscles involved in velopharyngeal closure will vary considerably among persons. Therefore, the degree of elevation of the velum, the vertical level of movement of the lateral pharyngeal walls and the presence or absence of posterior pharyngeal wall motion will not be the same for everyone. In patients with VPI, this variation implies that the location and size of velopharyngeal gaps are likely to be highly variable in part related to structural variation.

1.3.5 Learning

Although rarely considered, it is clear that velopharyngeal closure is learned (Siegel-Sadewitz and Shprintzen 1982). The process is as follows: babies are born with the velum in close approximation to the epiglottis and larynx. In other words, the vertical height of the pharynx is very small, so the palate can interlock with the epiglottis, allowing the infant to breathe through the nose while they are sucking and swallowing (Shprintzen 1995). This relationship between the pharyngeal and laryngeal structures is eventually lost as the pharynx grows vertically along with the face growing vertically (Fig. 1.2). As the infant matures and the pharynx brings the velum in closer approximation to the roof of the nasal cavity and the adenoid, the closure of the velopharyngeal valve becomes possible. As babies start babbling, making random noises as they vocalise, the movements of the velum and pharyngeal walls are random and not purposeful. Most early vocalisations are vowel sounds and eventually nasal sounds, most often /m/. During babbling, the use of voicing in the presence of the lips being closed is perceived by the parents as being an attempt to say 'ma-ma' or 'mom'. Eventually, as vocalisations are occurring, by chance, the palate will approximate to the pharyngeal structure by random movement while the baby is babbling. It will be heard as a non-nasal sound, usually a /b/, /p/ or /d/. When heard by parents, the production of a consonant sound is reinforced with smiles, hugs and happy repetitions of the sound. This reinforces the use of the sound in babbling, and eventually has meaning to it attached, such as saying dada or papa or baba, all words that in a variety of languages mean 'father'. Because the velopharyngeal closure was made by random movement that were reinforced, the baby will be likely to use the same pattern of movement after it has been reinforced to produce the same sound again, which will once again be reinforced by the parents. This classical operant learning and is how children learn speech sounds. Because this occurs in infancy, palate repair is recommended to occur before the first birthday of the child with a cleft palate. If the palate remains open, or if surgical repair is not successful in permitting velopharyngeal closure, children do not learn a specific pattern of closure of the velopharyngeal valve and correct production of non-nasal speech sounds will not be achieved, often requiring speech therapy and secondary surgery to correct aberrant patterns of speech.

Further evidence of learning in velopharyngeal valving comes from a number of studies that utilise nasopharyngoscopic visual biofeedback, which have demonstrated the ability to alter velopharyngeal closure patterns (Siegel-Sadewitz and Shprintzen 1982; Ysunza et al. 1997). This would only be possible if the movements made during velopharyngeal closure were learned as motor tasks, much like walking, writing, smiling, etc.

1.3.6 Physiological Components of Velopharyngeal Closure

The muscular contributions to the velopharyngeal valve during speech include the levator veli palatini, the uppermost fibres of the superior pharyngeal constrictor and the musculus uvulae. Although other muscles insert into the palate either as a small number of skeletal muscle fibres or ligamentous tissue, they do not contribute to closure of the velopharyngeal mechanism. The palatoglossus, salpingo-pharyngeus and palatopharyngeus play other roles in terms of modulating the height shape of the resonating cavity of the pharynx; they are active during swallowing but they do not contribute to speech-related movements within the velopharyngeal mechanism. The salpingo-pharyngeus muscle is not always present within the salpingo-pharyngeal fold which, when present, is comprised primarily of some glandular and connective tissue. The tensor veli palatini, which has often been thought to be the dilator of the Eustachian tube orifice, is not really in a position to do so because its location in relation to the Eustachian tube is in the bony portion of the skull base (Shprintzen and Croft 1981).

1.3.7 Levator Veli Palatini

The levator veli palatini is a paired muscle that runs from the lateral pharyngeal wall on each side of the pharynx. The muscle arises from the cranial base where it is attached to the temporal bone by a tendon. The muscle courses medially and anteriorly running along the cartilaginous portion of the Eustachian tube and then enters the superior aspect of the velum from beneath the torus tubarius. The fibres then attach to the palatal aponeurosis. During normal speech production, the two sides act in unison, like a sling, to lift or pull the velum postero-superiorly until the velum contacts the adenoid or posterior pharyngeal wall. In addition, because the levator normally enters the velum under the tail of the torus tubarius when it contracts, it impels the posterior aspect of the torus upwards and in so doing dilates the orifice of the Eustachian tube. Dilation of the Eustachian tube has often been attributed to the tensor veli palatini, but it seems more likely that the dilation of the tube is related to the movements of the levator during swallowing, which are more vigorous than those seen during speech. The levator is also active in swallowing to prevent solids and liquids from penetrating the nasal airway.

Is the contraction of the levator veli palatini sufficient to close the **velopharyngeal** port? Not by itself. As demonstrated in previous publications (Shprintzen 1995; Skolnick 1970), it is necessary for most people to have sufficient movement of the lateral pharyngeal walls to close off the spaces on either side of the velum to prevent air and sound leakage around either side of the pharynx. This is why, as stated earlier in this section, it is essential that the movement of the lateral walls can be defined by imaging before determining what treatment is necessary to resolve VPI.

1.3.8 Superior Pharyngeal Constrictor

The superior pharyngeal constrictor is highly variable in its location and course, dictated by the height and width of the upper airway and the overall length of the neck. The superior constrictor consists of two portions. The uppermost fibres originate on both sides of the pterygoid plates, coursing postero-laterally through the lateral pharyngeal walls submucosally, and attaching to the posterior pharyngeal wall in the midline (Fig. 1.7).

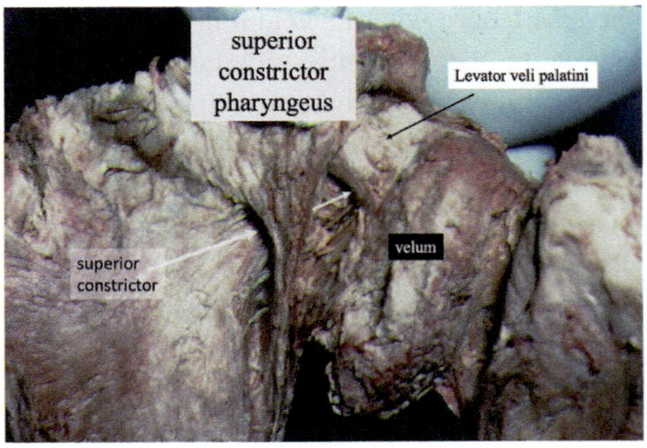

Fig. 1.7 The superior constrictor muscle showing the uppermost fibres that enter the velum and cause lateral pharyngeal wall motion (Shprintzen©2021)

The lower portion of the superior constrictor does not play a role in velopharyngeal closure because it is well below the palatal plane. It is the uppermost fibres that arise from the palatal plane that are responsible for the movements of the lateral pharyngeal walls and, if present, Passavant's ridge.

1.3.9 Musculi Uvulae

The role of the musculi uvulae in speech and how they function to contribute to velopharyngeal closure was first reported in 1979 (Croft et al. 1978) and in subsequent publications (Shprintzen 1979; Lewin et al. 1980). As nasopharyngoscopy progressed to become a common diagnostic procedure for VPI, large numbers of cases were examined and variations of anatomy and physiology became appreciated. In 1975, Kaplan reported a condition he labelled as the occult submucous cleft palate. He described four cases taken to surgery to resolve VPI and hypernasality. None of the cases had overt cleft palate or obvious submucous cleft palate (such as a bifid uvula or zona pellucida). He also carefully dissected the velum during his surgical reconstruction and found that the muscles were in abnormal position and course as seen in over and submucous clefts. Therefore, Kaplan (1975) hypothesised that the disorder was essentially a submucous cleft palate with none of the anatomical signs of the anomaly on oral examination, hence the term 'occult' (meaning mysterious or hidden). Of note, three of the cases shown in Kaplan's article are now known to have velo-cardio-facial syndrome (VCFS). Occult submucous cleft palate is a common finding in VCFS (Shprintzen 1982). Although overt clefts and obvious submucous clefts occur in VCFS, the majority of the palatal anomalies in VCFS are occult submucous clefts. Occult submucous clefts are expressed as a velum with reduced muscle mass, abnormal attachments of the levator veli palatini and either absence or severe hypoplasia of the musculi uvulae. The normal structure of the musculi uvulae is that of a paired muscle with each half in approximation arising from its attachment to the aponeurosis, just behind the posterior border of the hard palate and running longitudinally to terminate at the base of the uvula attaching to some fibrous tissue (Fig. 1.8).

The musculi uvulae, the only intrinsic muscle in the velum, had been regarded in the past as being vestigial tissue with no known purpose, but more recently, it has been found that this paired muscle is much larger in humans than any other species, leading to the hypothesis that the musculi uvulae is an important anatomical structure for the development of normal speech (Croft et al. 1978; Shprintzen 1979, 1982, 1995). The musculi uvulae are known to have their thickest portion overlying the levator veli palatini. When the levator contracts and is pulled towards the posterior pharynx, the musculi uvulae contract. Because the musculi uvulae do not have an attachment to a hard fixture at their distal end, they thicken at their bellies, thereby thickening the soft palate at the point where it would contact the posterior pharynx or adenoid pad. This thickening of the musculi uvulae increases the mass of the velum at the point where closure occurs, thereby making it a bigger target for the movement of the pharyngeal walls (Fig. 1.8). This only happens in humans, and

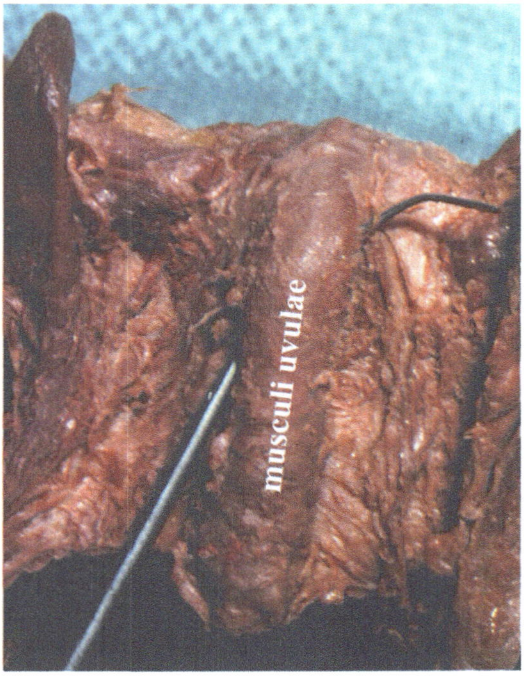

Fig. 1.8 The musculi uvulae (Shprintzen©2021)

humans are the only species that have the ability to create non-nasal consonants during vocalisation.

1.3.10 Tensor Veli Palatini

The tensor veli palatini have, for many years, been considered paired muscles that dilate the Eustachian tube. This supposition is related to an article published in 1920 (Rich 1920). However, this often-cited paper was based on a study of dogs, and the craniofacial and oropharyngeal anatomy and physiology of canines are very different from humans, and the function of the structures of the palate cannot be compared. It has been suggested that in humans, the tensor veli palatini has more to do with acoustic reflexes at the continuation of the muscle to the middle ear and tympanic membrane. It is now known that the tensor does not enter the velum as a muscle, but rather the muscle's tendon that hooks around the pterygoid hamulus and fans out into the soft palate as a sheet of connective tissue. As pointed our earlier, the levator is more likely to assist in the process of Eustachian tube function.

1.3.11 Cleft Palate

Palatal clefts are not all the same. Many are clinical findings in multiple anomaly syndromes. Several genetic and morphological studies of large populations of individuals with clefts found that approximately half of all clefts in children are found in the presence of other anomalies and are probably a part of a multiple anomaly syndrome (Skolnick et al. 1973; Shprintzen et al. 1985b). Many of these syndromes involve developmental delay, some so severe that speech is never developed. Other such syndromes have shortened life spans. But it is also true that the majority of children who have surgical repair of the palate develop normal speech after initial repair. Reported statistics indicate that 70–90% of children with cleft palate have normal speech after palatoplasty. A recent report indicated that approximately 80% of primary palatal repairs are likely to have positive outcomes without need for secondary surgery (Stein et al. 2019). It is also true that many, if not most, cases of submucous cleft palate do not have VPI and hypernasality (Shprintzen et al. 1985a). Therefore, although cleft palate is a relatively frequent major anomaly, only a relatively small percentage of cases have VPI, so that the prevalence of VPI is most likely to be approximately 1:5000 overt cleft cases present with hypernasal speech. A far more common cause of hypernasality may be the presence of a neurological abnormality ranging from cerebrovascular problems, such as strokes, other cerebrovascular accidents, brain malformations, nervous system disorders, including neurofibromatosis, velo-cardio-facial syndrome, hypoxic episodes and many more. Because VPI is often suspected in children with clefts, this population has much higher scrutiny by the medical community and detection will be more frequent as a result.

1.3.12 Submucous Cleft Palate and Occult Submucous Cleft Palate

Submucous cleft palate is not recognised in many instances, especially if speech is normal from its onset. Shprintzen et al. (1985) reviewed all cases in a large general paediatric practice and noted all cases with bifid uvula. All of these cases had a speech evaluation and were examined with nasopharyngoscopy to determine if they all had submucous clefts. It has been found that not all people with submucous cleft have the classic triad of findings of bifid uvula, zona pellucida and notching of the posterior border of the hard palate (Shprintzen 1982). It is now known that there is variability in the expression of submucous clefts ranging from all of the clinical signs to none of them. The one definitive sign is the absence or hypoplasia of the musculi uvulae, which is best determined by nasopharyngoscopy. Endoscopically, the normal palate has a prominent convexity on the nasal surface when the musculi uvulae are present (Fig. 1.9).

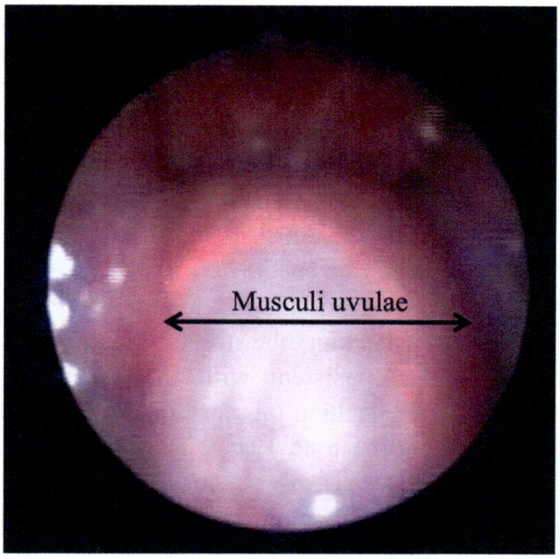

Fig. 1.9 Convex shape of the nasal surface of the velum demonstrating a prominent midline mass representing the musculi uvulae (Shprintzen©2021)

When absent, the nasal surface of the velum is either flat, or shows evidence of concavity, either U-shaped or V-shaped (Fig. 1.10).

Occult submucous cleft is characterised by the same endoscopic features as submucous cleft. Occult submucous cleft is a very common finding in velo-cardio-facial syndrome, and if a patient presents with hypernasal speech and no evidence of a palatal anomaly on nasopharyngoscopy, VCFS (also known as DiGeorge syndrome and in Eastern Europe as Sedlàçkovà syndrome) should be suspected. At this time, no one knows the population frequency of occult submucous cleft palate, nor do we know what percentage of people who have normal speech have the physical features of occult submucous cleft palate. However, the author has seen people who have normal speech without evidence of hypernasal resonance and normal oral examination results, and yet who do have occult submucous clefts. These cases were detected when having nasopharyngoscopy for disorders unrelated to speech, such as FEES, FEESST, complaints of globus or questions of upper airway obstruction. Is it important to know if someone has an asymptomatic occult submucous cleft palate? Absolutely.

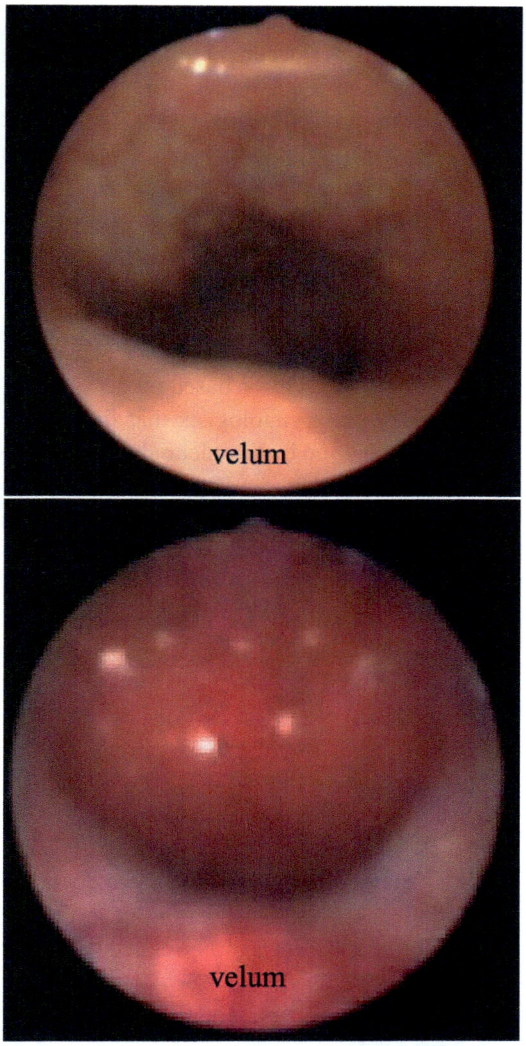

Fig. 1.10 Flat and concave nasal surfaces of the velum demonstrating an absent musculi uvulae and submucous cleft (Shprintzen©2021)

1.3.13 Lymphoid Tissue and Resonance Disorder

A relatively common occurrence is the onset of VPI and hypernasality following adenoidectomy or adenotonsillectomy (Croft et al. 1981b). Although there are multiple reasons that hypernasal speech may follow the removal of the adenoids or tonsils, the most common is the unmasking of an anatomical or functional disorder of the velopharyngeal sphincter. The most common anatomical problem is either submucous cleft palate or occult submucous cleft palate. Of course, if a person had a repaired overt cleft palate, removal of the adenoids would most likely result in VPI. Most otolaryngologists know that the presence of an obvious submucous cleft palate is something that should not be considered unless there is very strong evidence that VPI would not be the outcome of the surgery. One of the indications for adenoidectomy in opinion of many otolaryngologists is chronic middle ear disease. This is based on the supposition of many otolaryngologists that the middle ear disease is caused by the adenoid either blocking the Eustachian tube orifice in the nasopharynx, or somehow contaminating the Eustachian tube with pathogens. Of course, it would be possible to test this hypothesis by doing a nasopharyngoscopy so that the Eustachian tube orifice and adenoid can be visualised. That procedure would also potentially reveal the presence of a submucous cleft palate (occult or obvious). The presence of a cleft of any type can also be the cause of chronic middle ear disease, so assuming that the adenoid is the culprit is nothing more than a guess if imaging procedures are not utilised. It should also be noted that the association of middle ear disease and clefting of the palate should not be presumed to be related to abnormal muscle function. The Eustachian tube has been shown to be abnormal in individuals with cleft palate. Its cartilage and orifice has been found to be of abnormal structure (Fig. 1.11), with patency of the orifice being impaired as a result (Dickson and Dickson 1972; Dickson 1976; Maue-Dickson et al. 1976; Shprintzen and Croft 1981; Shprintzen 1982).

These observations of hypoplastic and abnormal Eustachian tube structure in the nasopharynx are consistent with the finding of obstructed Eustachian tube orifices in children with clefts (Bluestone 1971). The presence of chronic middle ear disease in young children should prompt exploration of a differential diagnosis that considers submucous or occult submucous cleft palate.

1.3.14 Resonance Disorders and Lymphoid Tissue

As discussed in the preceding paragraph, hypernasality can be caused by adenoid removal in individuals with cleft palate, submucous cleft palate or occult submucous cleft palate. The author has also seen several cases of individuals who had the faucial pillars macerated that resulted in hypernasality because of scar tissue

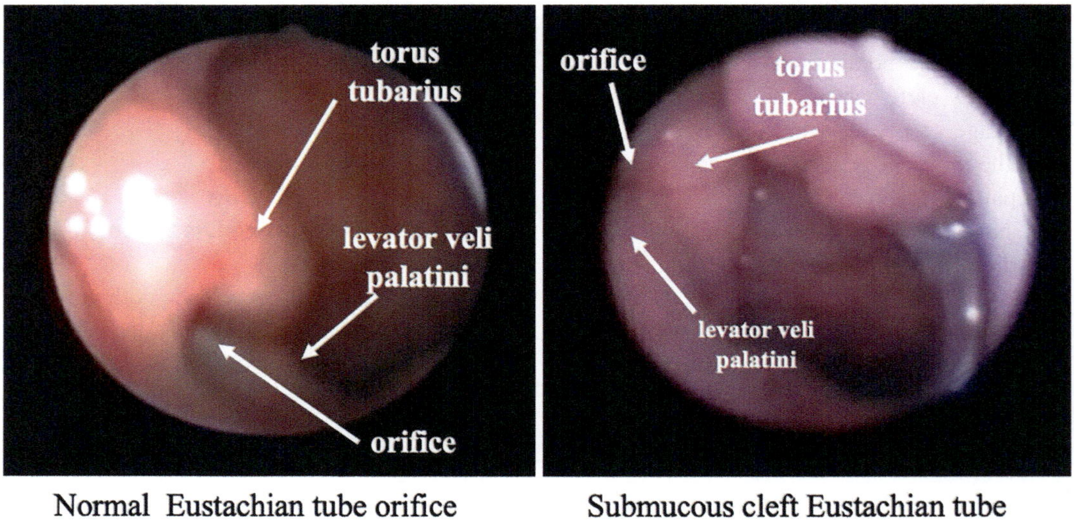

Fig. 1.11 Abnormal appearance of the Eustachian tube orifice in a case of submucous cleft palate. (Shprintzen©2021)

preventing the velum from elevating sufficiently. A more common cause of resonance disorders related to lymphoid tissue is hypertrophic or malpositioned tonsils (Shprintzen et al. 1987; MacKenzie-Stepner et al. 1987). Tonsils are often assessed for size by oral examination. The standard rating system is a 0 to 4+ rating scale with 0 defined as the absence or non-visibility of the tonsils on per-oral examination, 1+ meaning that the tonsils are confined to the space between the anterior and posterior faucial pillars, 2+ the tonsils extend medially less than half the distance to the midline, 3+ the tonsils extend more than halfway to the midline and 4+ referring to what is often called 'kissing tonsils' meaning that the tonsils are actually touching in the midline. The primary problem with this system is the assumption that when the tonsils grow larger, the only way they can go is medially. This is absolutely not true. The tonsils can grow downwards behind the tongue and into the hypopharynx, thereby blocking the passage of food and fluids into the pyriform sinus either unilaterally or bilaterally. We have often seen tonsils on endoscopic examination that touch the epiglottis either near the midline or laterally (Fig. 1.12), resulting in coughing during eating and drinking and chronic obstructive breathing issues during sleep and wakefulness, prompting constant mouth-breathing, a mouth-open posture resulting in vertical mandibular growth and vertical maxillary excess, fatigue and speech having a muffled oral resonance, often called 'potato-in-the-mouth' resonance pattern.

In cases that have muffled resonance or hypernasality caused by the tonsils' interfering with the movements of the velum or pharyngeal walls, tonsillectomy will resolve the problem. Another possible, but less frequent problem is when the tonsil grows upwards behind the velum reaching into the nasopharynx (Fig. 1.13) and the region where movements of the velopharyngeal valve are occurring (Shprintzen et al. 1987).

In most of these cases, hypernasal speech resulting from tonsillar obstruction is resolved with tonsillectomy. Tonsillectomy in these cases must be complete surgical removal. The above mentioned disorders caused by hypertrophic tonsils are not rare, but are easily diagnosed by nasopharyngoscopy and multi-view videofluoroscopy (Figs. 1.12 and 1.13). Besides the resonance disorder, tonsillar hypertrophy is almost always accompanied by problems with eating, including coughing, throat clearing and diet modification

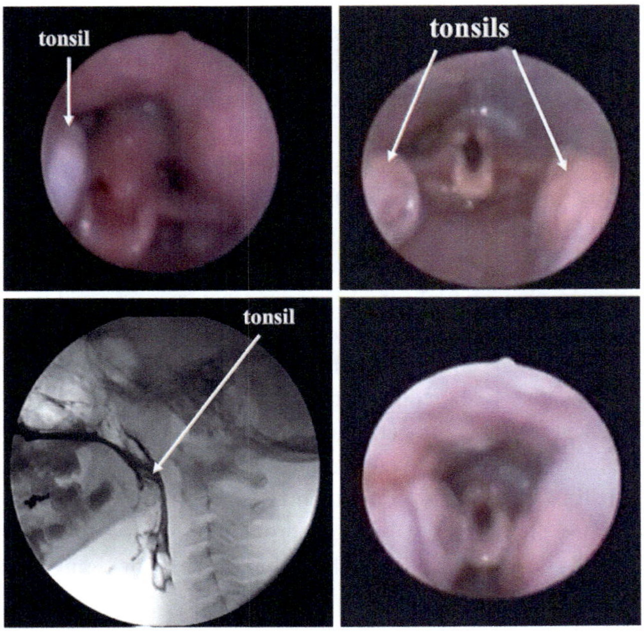

Fig. 1.12 Hypertrophic tonsils extending deep into the hypopharynx and coming into contact with the epiglottis (Shprintzen©2021)

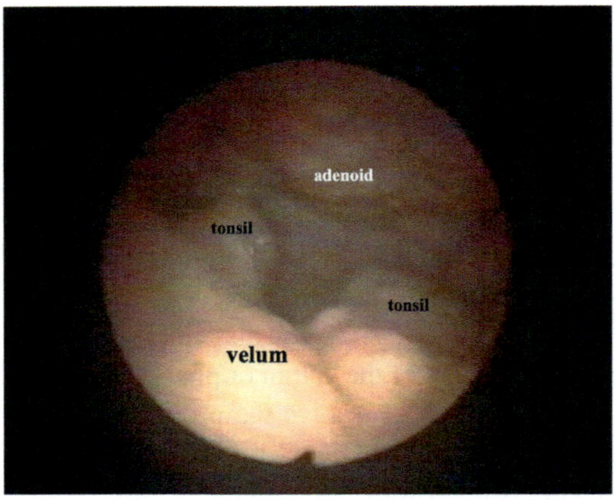

Fig. 1.13 Tonsils extending high into the nasopharynx interfering with velopharyngeal closure (Shprintzen©2021)

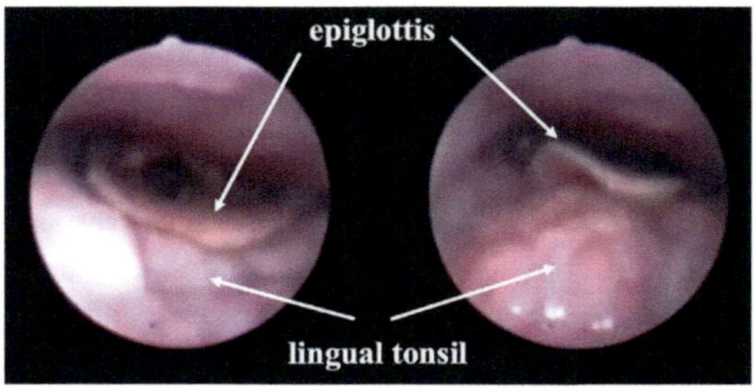

Fig. 1.14 Hypertrophic tonsil seen endoscopically (Shprintzen©2021)

with preference for soft, easy-to-swallow foods such as pasta, soups and purees.

Another problem related to lymphoid tissue is a hypertrophic lingual tonsil (Fig. 1.14).

Hypertrophic lingual tonsils can be related to reflux, infection, chronic irritation from smoking, medications or alcohol, or to chronic lymphatic system disorder or inflammation. In cases of hypertrophic lingual tonsil, speech resonance is muffled, deglutition is often a problem because the vallecula is obstructed and the pyriform sinuses may be blocked. Eating in these cases is often accompanied by chronic cough, gagging or diet modification with tendency towards eating soft foods and avoiding foods that are more difficult to chew and swallow. A chronic feeling of globus is also common when the problem is severe.

1.3.15 Hyponasality

Hyponasality is a result of the absence or restriction of nasal resonance on sounds that require nasal resonance. In English and many other languages, those sounds include /m/, /n/, /ñ/, /ŋ/, as well as isolated vowel production. The most common cause of hyponasality is nasal obstruction. If nasal obstruction is in the anterior nasal cavity, what is heard is cul-de-sac resonance, because sound will resonate in the nasal cavity during nasal sound production. However, if the obstruction is posterior and related to structural abnormalities of the posterior nasal cavity or enlarged adenoids, and sometimes a combination of hypertrophic tonsils and adenoids, speech lacks nasal resonance where it should appear. In some cases, the obstruction can be related to septal anomalies (such as an S-shaped septum) or a choanal atresia. Diagnosis can be accomplished with nasopharyngoscopy in almost all cases. Treatment is obviously removal of the obstruction, making sure that there is no velopharyngeal insufficiency. If velopharyngeal insufficiency is present, removal of the obstruction could unmask the insufficiency thereby causing hypernasal resonance.

1.3.16 Is Velopharyngeal Closure the Same for all Functions that Require It?

No. Velopharyngeal closure is achieved during speech, but also during swallowing, gagging, blowing air out of the mouth and other reflexes, such as the diving reflex. The physiology of velopharyngeal function can be divided into two basic classes: stopping fluids (liquids and air) from escaping out of the nose and stopping fluids from entering the lungs. It has been observed that the muscular movements are different for the protective mechanism of gagging and the act of swallowing than they are for speech and blowing (Shprintzen et al. 1974). For the mechanisms that are protective of the airway such as gagging and the diving reflex, the entire upper airway closes by the movements of the velum and all of the pharyngeal constrictors (superior, middle and inferior). At the same time, the larynx responds in unison by the glottis closing at both the vocal folds and the ventricular (false vocal) folds. The purpose of this response is to prevent fluids from penetrating into the lungs, and in the case of gagging, fluids and solids. These movements are reflexive, rapid and essentially immediate to the perception of exposure to a noxious or dangerous stimulus. For example, the diving reflex can be prompted by immersing the face in water or jumping into a swimming pool. The velopharyngeal valve's response to volitional or reflexive swallowing is the same. The contraction of the entire muscular system of the pharynx and larynx functions to prevent the airway from being penetrated with food or liquids, thereby preventing the aspiration of substances that would contaminate the lower airway. The movements of the velum and pharynx for speech are specific only to the velopharyngeal valve. This also true for blowing, because the hypopharyngeal and oropharyngeal airways must be patent for an airstream to be directed out of the mouth. However, blowing is not speech, and the use of blowing or swallowing exercises in speech therapy is a complete waste of time. The physiology of these is different and because speech is not involved in either blowing or swallowing, the useless approach of 'oral-motor exercises' to strengthen the palate or tongue or lips has been strongly criticised because of the ineffective outcomes and complete lack of reports of positive outcomes (Golding-Kushner 1995, 2001b).

1.3.17 What Problems Can Cause Velopharyngeal Insufficiency? Is Cleft Palate the Most Common?

Cleft palate is probably not the most common cause of VPI and hypernasal speech. Overt clefts of the palate with or without cleft lip probably occur in the range of 1:2000 to 1:1500 people, but that number does not include submucous cleft palate. Submucous cleft palate is frequently undetected in otherwise normal people, and occult submucous cleft palate is still rarely detected because it can only be adequately diagnosed by nasopharyngoscopy or other imaging procedures. Neurological disorders, whether congenital or acquired, are more common than cleft-related hypernasality, and congenital deafness also results in hypernasality. Neurological disorders can include cerebral palsy, dis-coordination caused by central nervous system anomalies, progressive neurological illnesses and multiple anomaly disorders that involve brain abnormalities, congenital craniofacial anomalies and birth injury.

Cerebral palsy, often caused by bleeding in the brain or hypoxic brain damage, results in major dis-coordination problems. Speech production is laborious and often slow, with prolonged production of vowels. Because vowels do not require velopharyngeal closure, the prolonged production of the sound causes the velopharyngeal valve to open during prolonged utterances, which is perceived as consistent hypernasal resonance. The author has seen such cases go to surgical correction of VPI that had little benefit in terms of the resonance characteristics.

Central nervous system anomalies such as pachygyria, polymicrogyria, microencephaly, milder forms of holoprosencephaly, arachnoid cysts, colloid cysts and other CNS abnormalities can also result in impaired development and impaired functioning of the brain, resulting in speech disorders. These anomalies can and often do result in impaired function of the velopharyngeal mechanism. Many multiple-anomaly congenital malformation syndromes will have these abnormalities of the brain as clinical features, and many of them have VPI as a clinical finding. In some cases, such as velo-cardio-facial syndrome, Down syndrome, CHARGE syndrome (**c**oloboma, **h**eart defect, **a**tresia **c**hoanae, **r**estricted growth and development, **g**enital abnormality, and **e**ar abnormality) and foetal alcohol syndrome, to name only a few, have both structural anomalies of the palate and a variety of brain anomalies. Therefore, differential diagnosis must consider that the source of hypernasal speech may have multiple aetiologies in a single case.

Hypernasality in severe or total deafness is very common, but it is not at all similar in either cause or management. Ysunza and Vazquez (1993) reported that approximately 92% of 53 people with prelingual deafness had some hypernasal resonance during speech. Of that number, 82% had severe hypernasality. They concluded that people who have profound or total deafness have a functional disorder of velopharyngeal function during speech caused by an absence of the ability to regulate resonance patterns or to compare their speech to normal speakers. People with 'deaf speech' are clearly not candidates for surgical treatment of VPI. Ysunza et al. (1997) noted that muscular movement of the velopharyngeal valve was present but dis-coordinated in relation to the timing and extent of the movements. With increasing use of cochlear implants, it is likely that speech is normalising with increased frequency in the population of individuals with profound hearing loss.

1.3.18 Summary

Although study of the velopharyngeal mechanism dates back more than a century, opinions about the anatomy and physiology underlying it have undergone a significant evolution. In the earliest days of study, the major emphasis was on the velum and its postero-superior movements, and little attention was paid to the possibility of variability from person to person. It took nearly 80 years and the development of new imaging procedures for researchers and clinicians to realise that there was significant variation of movements of the velopharyngeal mechanism, in terms of the production of both normal and disordered speech. This led to an expansion of a variety of treatment procedures and the development of new instrumentation that could be used in many clinical settings. Let us hope that progress continues so that outcomes are excellent in everyone's hands with minimal effort and cost.

1.4 Genetics of Craniofacial Disorders Including Counselling and Future Directions

Alan Shanske

1.4.1 Genetics in Medicine

A casual perusal of any speciality medical journal demonstrates the impact of genetics on every medical discipline. The elaboration of the genetic bases of rare genetic disorders and syndromes has grown exponentially in recent years. Of equal importance, our understanding of the heritability factors of common disorders of adult life has also grown exponentially with the emergence of genome-wide association studies (GWAS) and the isolation of the contributions of rare DNA mutations to diseases of ageing, such as cardiovascular disease, cancer and neurodegenerative diseases. The observation of possible hereditary traits has fascinated mankind since ancient times. The earliest written observation of the transmission of a human trait was recorded in the Babylonian Talmud in the second century CE. The Talmud instructs that a boy must not be circumcised on the eighth day if he had two brothers who died from excessive bleeding following their circumcisions. The twelfth century rabbi, philosopher and physician Maimonides instructed further that this excluded paternal half-brothers. Both strictures may have been due to a concern about haemophilia. The scientific basis of haemophilia was not described until the twentieth century.

1.4.2 Mendelian Genetics

The basis for our understanding of modern clinical genetics was established by Gregor Mendel, an Augustine friar and abbot, in the middle of the nineteenth century. Our current understanding of human genetics is largely based on the revolutionary breeding experiments on garden peas presented to the Natural History Society of Brunn in Bohemia (now Brno in the Czech Republic). These ground-breaking observations were published shortly after (in Mendel 1866) and remained unappreciated until 16 years after Mendel's death in 1884. The rediscovery of Mendel's Laws in 1900 led eventually to the identification and deciphering of the genetic code at the molecular level. This totally unanticipated trajectory of discovery began with the discovery of Mendel's work by three botanists, Hugo de Vries, Erich von Tschermak and Carl Correns, who independently confirmed Mendel's findings. Mendel's work represents nothing less than the discovery of the gene, the term first used by the botanist Johannsen in 1909, which was a derivative of the word pangenesis coined by Darwin in 1868. The genes responsible for contrasting traits came to be known as alleles, which can occur in the homozygous or heterozygous state. Mendel's publications and work were eventually recognised as the basis of a renewed interest in genetics by scientists across Europe, including William Bateson, Archibald Garrod and Erwin Baur. It is one of the ironies of scientific discovery that Darwin's Origin of Species, published in 1859 could not take into account Mendel's Laws. Had Darwin been aware of them, he would have been able to explain how organisms slowly acquire or evolve beneficial traits that bestow a survival or reproductive advantage.

1.4.3 Gregor Mendel's Laws of Inheritance: Law of Segregation, Dominance, Independent Assortment

Mendel performed his studies with the pea plant (*Pisum sativum*), which he chose for a number of reasons. Pea plants can finish one life cycle pretty quickly, so it was the perfect plant to use in order to observe a number of generations. Mendel selected seven distinct traits in the plants, purple flowers versus white ones, round seeds versus wrinkled, etc. He used crossbreeding of plants that differed in only a single trait, e.g. flower colour. One plant had purple flowers and the other had white flowers. When he bred these two together, all the plants of the first generation (called F1) had purple flowers. Fortunately for him, all the traits he selected bred true, and there was no blending of their effects. He then bred two plants from this F1 generation. Of the four plants that he got, three had purple flowers and one had white flowers. This is called the F2 generation. This type of cross or breeding is called a monohybrid cross. This simply displays the inheritance pattern of one character. He realised that purple flowers were dominant over white flowers, meaning that even if one gene for purple flowers was present in the plant, as is the case in the first generation, the flowers were purple. It essentially masked the effect of the gene for white flowers. These genes are known as alleles. They both decide the flower colour, but will give different colours to the plant. 'P' represents the dominant allele, and 'p' represents the recessive allele.

On the basis of this cross, Mendel came to certain conclusions; Gregor Mendel's Laws of Inheritance: Law of Segregation, Dominance, Independent Assortment:

- **Segregation** This law states that during the formation of the gamete or reproductive cell, the genes will segregate, without any mixing or blending of their effects.
- **Dominance** The second law states that when there are two different alleles in a cell, one will mask the effect of the other. This is the dominant gene, while the gene whose effect is masked is known as the recessive gene.
- **Independent segregation** The law of independent assortment states that during the formation of the gamete, the alleles of one character will segregate independently of the other character. Therefore, the colour and shape of the seeds are not dependent on each other.

These are the three basic laws of inheritance. They can be applied not only to plants, but to all living organisms that reproduce sexually. These laws allow us to make predictions on the transfer and inheritance of various traits, diseases etc. There are certain traits, such as blood group, which do not comply with these laws. We will discuss these exceptions a bit later. Although there are exceptions, these laws still form the basis of clinical genetics.

1.4.4 Online Mendelian Inheritance in Man®—OMIM®

OMIM (2021) is a comprehensive, authoritative compendium of human genes and genetic phenotypes, which is freely available. The full-text, referenced overviews in OMIM contain information on all known Mendelian disorders and over 15,000 genes. OMIM focuses on the relationship between phenotype and genotype. It is updated daily, and the entries contain copious links to other genetics resources. One's genotype, meaning the characterisation of all of our genes, is referred to as that person's genome. The expression of those genes, meaning anything that can be used to describe a person such as height, hair colour, IQ score or myopia, is the phenome.

1.4.5 Genetic Counselling

The discipline of genetic counselling began about 50 years ago. There are three critical steps in the process of providing information about a genetic disorder that includes details about the diagnosis, cause, recurrence risk and options available for prevention and treatment. Coming to a genetic diagnosis involves the three fundamental steps required in any medical evaluation: creating a medical history, making a complete and special physical examination, and finally making appropriate laboratory investigations. Genetic counselling services depend on the availability of many extensive services such as speciality referrals and the latest diagnostic and laboratory facilities. Today, laboratory investigations for genetic diseases require a knowledge of the latest molecular and biochemical technologies, advanced computational skills and familiarity with bioinformatics. However, given the use of all of the above, diagnostic confusion can often arise as a result of aetiological heterogeneity. This is most often seen in cases of non-specific neuro-developmental delay and neurosensory hearing loss. Genetic counsellors should be familiar with all patterns of Mendelian inheritance discussed above that predict the transmission of single gene disorders, and must have a thorough understanding of the origin and transmission of chromosomal abnormalities. They must also be aware of all of the more recently described patterns of non-Mendelian inheritance, which will be described below. Risk assessment and empirical risk calculation must be in a counsellor's toolbox. There have been dramatic technological advances in prenatal diagnosis, including pre-implantation genetic diagnosis and cell-free DNA analysis. Counsellors must be current in their understanding of these modalities. There are also a few conditions for which foetal therapy is available. Counsellors can now offer their patients new tools made available as a result of next-generation or multiplex sequencing. The multiplex or multigene technology was introduced in the United States in 2013 and enables simultaneous examination of dozens of genes at a cost that is comparable to that of tests for individual genes. Testing panels now include those for hereditary neuropathy, hereditary cancer, Ashkenazi Jewish Genetic Disease, epilepsy and hereditary deafness.

Counsellors are also responsible for understanding and resolving ethical dilemmas associated with the inheritance of complex disorders, as well as issues dealing with prenatal diagnosis and assisted reproductive technologies. A balance must be struck between a patient's autonomy to make a decision, and ethical and societal norms, especially in cases involving the termination of a foetus. Common issues include prenatal diagnosis for sex or non-disease traits, testing asymptomatic adults for late-onset diseases such as Huntington disease, or whether prenatal diagnosis and termination are justified in the case of deafness or mental retardation. Finally, ethical genetic counselling stands on the two pillars of privacy and non-coercion.

1.4.6 Non-Mendelian Inheritance

1.4.6.1 Codominance

Dominant disorders occur whether or not there is a normal gene product made by the normal allele. Codominance occurs when there is phenotypic expression of two different alleles at a locus. Each allele is said to be codominant. The ABO blood group is the best-known example of codominance, in which case each of the ABO alleles is expressed equally. The first example of human protein variation was detected in the blood group antigens. There are four major phenotypes in the ABO system determined by the presence of either, both or neither of the two antigens.

1.4.6.2 Epistasis

The interaction between a genetic disease at a specific locus and a modifier gene at a different locus is known as epistasis. Modifier genes interact with the disease locus and modify the phenotype. Modifier genes and environmental factors (diet, radiation, atmospheric pollution, microbes, teratogens, age, gender and the uterine environment) result in poor genotype-phenotype correlations. A well-known example of gene modification in humans is the hereditary persistence of foetal haemoglobin in patients with the beta thalassemia phenotype. Genetic variants that control the production of foetal haemoglobin can modify the beta thalassemia phenotype. An elevated level of foetal haemoglobin is thought to be protective and can delay the onset of symptoms of beta thalassemia.

1.4.6.3 Pleiotropy

A single gene may give rise to two or more phenotypic effects. A single biochemical defect, resulting from a deficiency of the enzyme phenylalanine hydroxylase that converts phenylalanine to tyrosine, is the cause of phenylketonuria (PKU). The impaired biochemical pathway can cause symptoms such as cognitive impairment, seizures, abnormal gait and posture, and delayed growth. Because tyrosine is used by the body to make melanin (a component of the pigment found in the hair and skin), failure to convert normal levels of phenylalanine to tyrosine can lead to fair hair and skin. These seemingly different traits in different tissues are an example of the pleiotropic effect of a single gene mutation.

1.4.6.4 Mitochondrial Inheritance

Human mitochondrial DNA (mtDNA) is a small, circular, double-stranded molecule 16.5 kb in length. It contains 37 genes, which specify two ribosomal RNAs (rRNAs), 22 transfer RNAs (tRNAs) and 13 polypeptides. All 13 polypeptides encoded by mtDNA are components of the respiratory chain or oxidative phosphorylation. These complexes also contain approximately 75 subunits encoded by nuclear DNA that are imported from the cytoplasm into the mitochondria. There are several distinctive features of mtDNA relevant to the understanding of mtDNA-related diseases. At fertilisation, all mitochondria are contributed by the oocyte; thus, mtDNA is inherited only from the mother. Most mtDNA point mutations are maternally inherited: a woman carrying an mtDNA point mutation will transmit it to all of her children, males as well as females, but only the daughters will transmit it to their progeny. In contrast to nuclear genes, each consisting of one maternal and one paternal allele, there are hundreds or thousands of copies of mtDNA in every cell. A deleterious mutation coexists with normal mtDNAs within a patient's tissues, a condition known as heteroplasmy. Homoplasmy is the situation when all mtDNAs are identical. Non-deleterious mutations of mtDNA (neutral polymorphisms) are homoplasmic, whereas pathogenic mutations are usually, but not always, heteroplasmic. A critical number of mutated mtDNAs must be present before tissue dysfunction and clinical signs become apparent (the so-called threshold effect). Tissues with high requirements for oxidative energy metabolism, such as muscle, heart, eye and brain, have relatively low thresholds and are particularly vulnerable to mtDNA mutations. Relatively low levels of mutated mtDNAs can affect the respiratory capacity of these tissues. It is therefore not surprising that most mtDNA disorders are encephalomyopathies, affecting primarily brain and muscle. At cell division, the proportion of mutant mtDNAs in daughter cells can shift—a phenomenon termed mitotic segregation. If and when the pathogenic threshold for a particular tissue is exceeded, the phenotype can change. Thus, in a patient who is heteroplasmic for a pathogenic mutation, the clinical phenotype can change during the course of time.

1.4.6.5 Epigenetics

One of the more interesting exceptions to Mendel's Laws is epigenetics. Organisms with identical genotypes, even identical twins, can have very different phenotypes. These changes involve non-Mendelian heritable changes in gene expression that are not mediated by alterations in the DNA sequence. Epigenetic regulation mediates adaptation to the environment by the genome resulting in plasticity in response to environmental conditions. This regulation is produced by chemical modification of the DNA sequence or nuclear histone proteins. The best understood examples of epigenetic changes are parent-of-origin specific gene expression and X-chromosome inactivation. The Prader–Willi and Angelman syndromes are very different in terms of phenotype, but are caused by the same microdeletion from the long arm of chromosome 15. The difference is that Prader–Willi syndrome, which has speech, language and developmental phenotypes associated with metabolic and eating disorders, occurs as a result the loss of DNA from the copy of chromosome 15 inherited from the father, while Angelman syndrome is caused by the same loss of DNA but from the maternal copy of chromosome 15.

1.4.6.6 Polygenic or Complex Inheritance and Multi-Factorial Inheritance

Mendelian traits involve only two alleles, one mutant and the other normal. Some traits and diseases are polygenic and result from changes in alleles in more than one gene. Technical advances in the use of multiple DNA probes have identified changes in many genes that can interact in a quantitative manner and produce so-called complex (polygenic, multi-factorial) inheritance. These traits are much more common than Mendelian disorders that conform to Mendel's laws of transmission. They include congenital anomalies such as cleft lip and palate, and late onset disorders (diabetes, hypertension, cancer, cardiovascular disease, neurodegenerative disorders and psychiatric illness) that account for the majority of the morbidity and mortality in developed countries. One model for multi-factorial inheritance for common malformations such as clefting, neural tube defects, clubfoot and pyloric stenosis, is based upon genetic susceptibility of a given defect secondary to many different genes, and a threshold determined by both genetic and environmental factors. Those individuals with a critical numbers of factors beyond a theoretical threshold will exhibit the abnormal phenotype. A second model of quantitative inheritance has been developed to explain the interaction of multiple genes such as those that are responsible for quantitative traits such as height and weight and skin colour. In this each gene exerts a small additive effect and the effects of the genes are cumulative, no one gene being dominant or recessive to another.

While genetic diseases are generally classified as being either simple (monogenic) or complex (polygenic), the distinction between Mendelian and complex disorders is becoming increasingly blurred. Mendelian disorders may demonstrate qualities more typical of multi-factorial diseases through shared clinical presentations such as in the case of isolated clefting deformities and the van der Woude syndrome, a dominant clefting syndrome (see below). Heterozygosity for a simple Mendelian disorder can be a risk factor for a seemingly unrelated complex disease. A recent example is the observation that mutations in glucocerebrosidase, the enzyme deficient in Gaucher disease, may be a risk factor for the development of Parkinson disease and other synucleinopathies. Other examples that result in an increased susceptibility to non-syndromic clefting include mutations in MSX1, which cause Witkop syndrome, and in TBX22, which is responsible for X-linked cleft palate with ankyloglossia. Insights gleaned from the study of Mendelian disorders may ultimately lead to a better understanding of factors influencing complex diseases.

1.4.7 Molecular Biology of Genetic Diseases

As interest in Mendelian inheritance grew, so did speculation on the physical basis and transmission of the heritable material. It has been known since the second half of the nineteenth century that the nucleus of the cell contained thread-like structures known as chromosomes. Around 1900, Sutton (1902) and Boveri (1904) proposed independently that chromosomes could be the physical bearers of the hereditary material. A few years later, Thomas Hunt Morgan (1911) transformed Sutton's and Boveri's chromosome theories into the theory of the gene. But, the precise chemical identity of the gene was still unknown. Morgan's thousands of experiments on the fruit fly led him to the idea of genetic linkage of genes and to hypothesise the phenomenon of crossing over. He theorised that the amount of crossing over between linked genes differs, and that crossover frequency might indicate the distance separating genes on a chromosome. In tribute, years later the English geneticist J.B.S. Haldane proposed that the unit of measurement of linkage be called the Morgan. But even with the acceptance of Morgan's theory of the gene, its biochemical structure still remained a mystery. DNA was discovered in 1868 by a medical student, Johann Friedrich Miescher (Dahm 2008), but its significance as the genetic material was not understood until nearly a century later. Its key role as the genetic material was established in the 1940s and attracted the efforts of Watson and Crick, who deciphered the structure in 1953. Until then, many believed that hereditary information was transmitted by proteins, especially because nucleic acids were known to contain only four base pairs, which were thought to be far too few to account for the observed degree of genetic variation. The helical double-stranded structure of DNA resembles a right-handed spiral staircase. The genetic information encoded in the human genome resides in the specific sequence of nucleotides. The genetic code consists of three nucleotide letters, each corresponding to one of the 20 amino acids, and allows the faithful transmission of the genetic code from cell generation to generation. The separation of the polynucleotide strands enables transcription of the code to messenger RNA and replication of the strands during mitosis and meiosis. The polynucleotide chains in the form of a double helix range in size from about 50 million base pairs for the smallest chromosome, chromosome 21, to 250 million base pairs for the largest, chromosome 1.

1.4.8 The Human Genome Project

The rapid advances in DNA technology inspired a group of investigators to persuade the United States Congress in 1988 to fund an international collaborative programme to sequence the entire human genome. It ran from 1990 to 2005 at a cost of at least US$3 billion. The draft sequence of DNA containing 3 billion base pairs was completed in 2000 and the complete sequence was published in 2004 under budget and almost 2 years earlier than expected.

1.4.9 Bioinformatics of Genetic Diseases

The success of the Human Genome Project was facilitated by the new discipline of bioinformatics, the establishment of resources for collecting, storing, organising, interpreting, annotating, analysing and sharing data. The project could not have succeeded without the freely disseminated access to the information. This was accomplished by establishing a large number of databases available on the World Wide Web. These resources include DNA and protein sequence databases, such as Gen Bank and EMBL; resources for human genetic mapping, such as GDB, CEPH and CHLC; and annotated genome data, such as Ensembl and UCSC Genome Bioinformatics; as well as the OMIM. Bioinformatics involves a combination of genetics, mathematics, statistics and computer science.

1.4.10 The Origin of Mutations and Copy Number Variations

Alterations in the genetic material may result in benign variation or to a pathological mutation. Genetic change can occur at the chromosome level, so-called genomic changes, which include errors in chromosome structure or their migration to resulting reproductive cells during meiosis. Genome mutations are by far the most common type of mutation. Mutations of the chromosomes that result from their rearrangement are the second-most common, followed by gene mutations that result from DNA base pair alterations. Most inherited genetic changes are benign variants. The vast amount of DNA sequence variation accumulated as a result of the Human Genome Project has resulted in catalogues of human DNA diversity.

The simplest and most common of all polymorphisms are *single nucleotide polymorphisms* (*SNPs*). These are common and occur on average once every 1000 base pairs, which means that there is an average of 3,000,000 differences between any two human genomes' DNA sequence variations. More than 100 million SNPs have been found in populations around the world. Most commonly, these variations are found in the DNA in between genes. They can be used as biological markers, helping scientists locate genes that are associated with disease. When SNPs occur within a gene or in a regulatory region near a gene, they may play a more direct role in disease by affecting the gene's function. Most SNPs have no effect on health or development. Some of these genetic differences, however, have proven to be very important in the study of human health, and may help predict an individual's response to certain drugs, susceptibility to environmental factors such as toxins, and risk of developing particular diseases. SNPs can also be used to track the inheritance of disease genes within families. More recently, *genome-wide association studies* (*GWAS*) on SNP markers have localised and often identified susceptibility genes for a range of complex common disorders, especially those associated with ageing. Future studies will be to identify SNPs associated with complex diseases such as heart disease, diabetes and cancer, and neurodegenerative diseases such as Alzheimer's and Parkinson's diseases.

The next most common DNA polymorphism results from the insertion or deletion of between two and 100 nucleotides (*indels*). A nucleotide is a base pair with the DNA backbone that supports the organic bases (Fig. 1.15).

Indels number in the hundreds of thousands in the genome. *Microsatellites* are a special class of indel polymorphism that constitute units of two to four nucleotides repeated between one and a few dozen times. The different alleles in a microsatellite are referred to as short tandem repeat polymorphisms. The final class of indel polymorphism results from the insertion of hundreds or

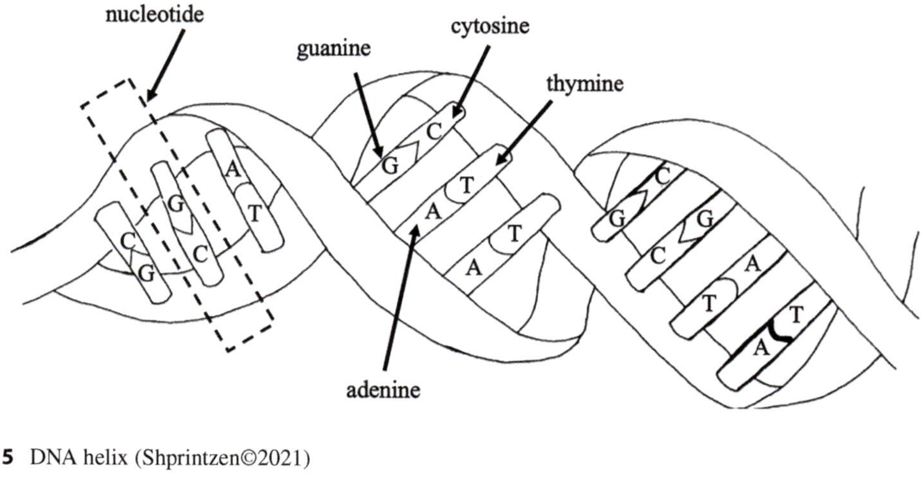

Fig. 1.15 DNA helix (Shprintzen©2021)

thousands of copies of a DNA sequence of 10–100 base pairs are known as *minisatellites*. However, these newly described susceptibility genes account for only a small fraction of trait heritability or risk in common diseases. The most recently described form of human polymorphism are *copy number variants* (*CNVs*) and are thought to account for almost 20% of human genetic variation (Stranger et al. 2007). These consist of variations in the number of copies of larger segments of the genome ranging from 200 to nearly two million base pairs. They are too small to be detected by cytogenetic examination and too large to be detected by DNA sequencing but can be discovered by comparative genomic hybridisation. Although first described in the 1980s, in the last few years, variation in gene copy number has been recognised as a common source of inter-individual variation that provides a background of common genetic variation.

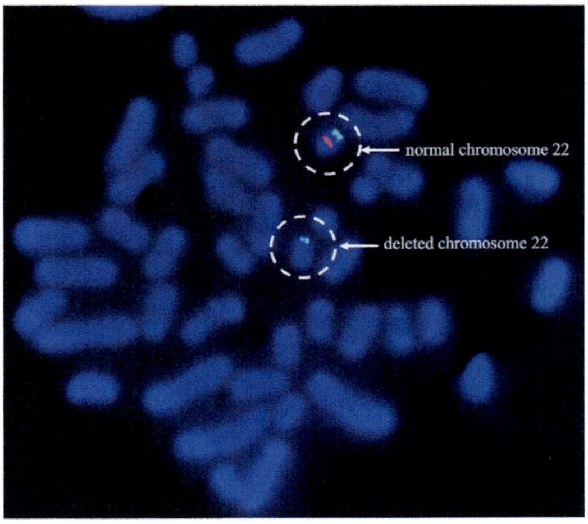

Fig. 1.16 Normal and deleted chromosome 22 verified by fluorescence in situ hybridisation FISH (Shprintzen©2021)

1.4.11 Detection of Chromosomal Aberrations and Decoding DNA

Since the inception of clinical cytogenetics in the 1950s, new methodologies have enabled us to detect smaller and smaller chromosome aberrations. The haploid complement of human chromosomes contains 3×10^9 base pairs (megabase pairs). The resolution of a Giemsa-stained banded chromosome preparation done at the 550 band level is 5–10 megabases (Mb). The average band contains about 6 Mb. *FISH* (*fluorescence* in situ *hybridisation*) has been used since the 1980s to increase the sensitivity of karyotype analysis (Fig. 1.16).

The size limit for FISH detection can be as low as 10 kilobases (kb). The ability to detect sub-microscopic imbalances results from the use of microarrays containing genomic clones and comparative genomic hybridisation. *Chromosomal microarray analysis* (*CMA*) was introduced in 2004. In essence these were artificial chromosome regions arranged on a slide, rather than the classical cytogenetic situation where whole chromosomes were spread on a glass slide and visualised by a banding technique. Genome-wide chromosomal microarray analysis enables detection of very small cytogenetic imbalances, such as CNVs. Cytogenetic imbalances detected by CMA are now described on the basis of the chromosomal location of the probes used to delineate the imbalance. An example is a deletion of ~1 Mb in band 16p11.2 is designated as 'arr 16p11.2 (29,500,000–30,500,000 × 1 (GRCh37/hg19)'. GRCh37/hg19 refers to the deletion's size and location in the genome, measured in nucleotides from the end of the short arm of chromosome 16. This information is compiled in a large constantly updated data base curated by the Genome Reference Consortium maintained by the NCBI and human genome (hg) from the UCSC Genome Bioinformatics Group. Online tools are available with assistance in interpreting the significance of these very small changes (ClinGen Dosage Sensitivity Map; and Database of Chromosomal Imbalance and Phenotype in Humans using Ensembl Resources [DECIPHER]). DNA sequences analysed by the Sanger di-deoxy nucleotide method can be used to sequence a relatively short fragment of DNA containing an area of interest.

So-called *next-generation sequencing* (*NGS*) generates masses of DNA sequencing data and is both less expensive and less time-consuming than traditional Sanger sequencing. Sequencing systems can deliver data output ranging from 300 kilobases up to multiple terabases (10^{12} bases) in a single run, depending on instrument type and configuration. NGS, also known as *high-throughput sequencing*, is the catch-all term used to describe a number of different modern sequencing technologies. They all use the concept of massive parallel sequencing to generate massive amounts of DNA sequencing data quickly. Whole exomes, as in *whole-exome sequencing* (*WES*), or entire genomes, as in *whole-sequencing*, can now be inexpensively sequenced in a very short time. The *exome* is the sum total of all exons in a person's genetic make-up, or the sum total of all exons in humans when dealing with large populations. Exons are a segment of a gene that encodes the RNA that will leave the cell and move to the ribosomes where a protein is created to perform a function in the person. Genes will have multiple exons within their DNA. These exons are separated by introns, segments of DNA that do not encode RNA. Introns are spliced out of DNA during RNA formation.

1.4.12 Craniofacial Biology

Approximately three quarters of children with birth defects have anomalies that affect the craniofacial structures. Many of these children have velopharyngeal insufficiency as a result of defective valving of the velopharyngeal apparatus. Defects in this area of the body result in lifelong disability, major challenges to families and society, and often a serious effect on life expectancy. Surgery has been the primary intervention for these disorders, with frequently less than optimal outcomes and risk for additional morbidity and mortality. The challenge for clinicians caring for these children is to develop new methods for the treatment and prevention of these disorders. An understanding of the evolution of the head and the finely tuned temporospatial signalling pathways involved is critical to understanding the origins of the vertebrates as well as of human craniofacial malformations. In the future, these new approaches will be based upon our enhanced understanding of the developmental tool kit and signalling networks fashioned by evolution, and the application of this knowledge towards the development of new diagnostic, pharmacological and genetic interventions for these disorders.

1.4.13 Introduction to the Evolution and Development of the Head and Face

> If it could be demonstrated that any complex organ existed, which could not possibly have been formed by numerous, successive, slight modifications, my theory would absolutely break down. But I can find out no such case.—Charles Darwin (1859)

More than one hundred and 50 years have passed since this salient observation on the importance of the uniqueness of the human face. The face is the most distinguishing feature of the vertebrate body as can be seen in the seven billion unique faces of the world's human population. Advances in craniofacial biology demonstrate that 'successive, slight modifications' in signalling pathways have resulted in the kind of diversity seen in the animal kingdom noted by Darwin, and at the same time, the extreme variations that result in craniofacial pathology. It has been some 350 million years since the first animal crawled out of the sea and onto the land. Ahlberg et al. (2005) recently demonstrated that this animal, Ichthyostega, might not have actually crawled but rather inched its way over the land, probably dragging its hind legs and long tail behind. This creature, with very short legs and long tail, may have propelled itself by arching its spine and propelling itself forward like an inchworm. Nonetheless, Ichthyostega possessed the already ancient tetrapod body form of paired fins/limbs and vertebrate head.

An understanding of the evolution of the head and the finely tuned temporospatial signalling pathways involved is critical to understanding the origins of the vertebrates as well as of human craniofacial malformations. Congenital anomalies are a major cause of infant mortality and childhood morbidity, affecting 2–3% of all babies.

Approximately 1% of these newborns have syndromes or multiple anomalies; craniofacial anomalies are often a component part. In fact, three-quarters of human birth defects have malformations involving the craniofacial region (see Centers for Disease Control 2010). Craniofacial anomalies other than cleft lip and palate occur in 1 in every 1600 newborns in the United States of America and include jaw deformities, malformed or missing teeth, defects in the ossification of facial or cranial bones, and facial asymmetries.

Clefting deformities, cleft lip or palate (CL/P) or isolated cleft palate (CP) is the aetiology in the majority of children with hypernasality. There are more than 400 syndromes associated with clefting deformities. The recurrence risk for non-syndromic clefting deformities is in the range of 3–5%. Syndromic clefting results from a wide range of mutations in genes that are part of the developmental pathways necessary for the growth of the derivatives of the pharyngeal arches and their transformation into the definitive structures of the oropharyngeal structures. Several examples of syndromic clefting are described below. A quick review of the embryology of the craniofacial region allows us to appreciate more fully the unfolding events and the contribution of unique genetic mutations.

The bony skull is formed from two components, the neurocranium and the viscerocranium, and comprises 22 separate bones, 20 deciduous and 32 permanent teeth. The whole viscerocranium and part of the neurocranium are formed from the neural crest. The elaboration of the neural crest probably represents the most important step in the evolution of the vertebrate head. Cranial neural crest precursors were present in the common ancestors of all extant chordates including vertebrates. The most primitive vertebrates did not have jaws. Though the paired fin/limb evolved shortly before jaws, there is remarkable overlap of the signalling pathways co-opted in head and limb development; so much so that genes involved in limb development are good candidates for genes that might be involved in errors of craniofacial morphogenesis. Sonic hedgehog (Shh) thus functions as a morphogen in both limb and craniofacial development. It is part of the Sonic Hedgehog-Patched Gli signalling pathway. Molecular defects anywhere along this pathway can result in a malformation syndrome. These diverse conditions include severe craniofacial defects such as holoprosencephaly, cancer syndromes and limb defects including split hand foot malformation. The embryo's multifarious utilisation of Shh and other signalling molecules such as the Nodal family, fibroblast growth factors (FGFs) and receptors, the wingless Wnt family, the bone morphogenic proteins (BMPs) and the hedgehog family (HH) reflect the limited tool kit of signal molecules available to extant organisms.

Most of the tissues and organs of the craniofacial region are derivatives of neural crest cells (NCCs). NCCs populate the frontonasal process, the first, second, third and fourth pharyngeal arches, and contribute to neural, skeletal, dermal and mesenchymal structures. Because of this pluripotency, the neural crest has been referred to as the fourth germ layer. A tightly regulated spatial and temporal signalling network is required for the induction, migration, proliferation and differentiation of NCCs that are the primordia of craniofacial structures. Aberrations in the complex multi-step processes result in craniofacial malformations. Individual populations of NCCs that populate the seven prominences comprising the vertebrate face react with adjacent cells required for normal craniofacial morphogenesis. NCC patterning within the pharyngeal arches is dependent upon a number of signalling pathways, including bone morphogenetic proteins (Bmps), fibroblast growth factors (Fgfs), endothelins and retinoic acid (RA). Recent advances in our understanding of primary cilia have shed light on the pathogenesis of additional craniofacial disorders such as the oro-facial-digital (OFD1). The primary cilium is a ubiquitous organelle which facilitates interactions between the cell and its environment much like signal transduction pathways.

The development of the craniofacial complex, just like that of any part of a multicellular organism, depends upon the communication between cells, mediated primarily by extracellular signal molecules. The delay of about 2.5 billion years between the appearance of prokaryotes and multicellular organisms probably reflects the difficulty of evolving a language of cellular communication and their evolutionary centrality. At the same time, it is now clear that an understanding of the general principles of cell communication can be translated into the elucidation of the pathogenesis of craniofacial disorders and, it is to be hoped, into therapeutic modalities. The emerging field of craniofacial biology is attracting scientists from a wide range of disciplines including clinical geneticists, developmental and evolutionary biologists, dentists, pharmacologists and surgeons. The future collaboration of members of these disciplines will add to our knowledge of how the highly conserved molecular pathways and their functions in craniofacial development create a face and not a limb bud, and enable new non-surgical options for the treatment and prevention of these complex disorders.

The treatment of the more than 700 recognised disorders with significant craniofacial malformations requires the integrated intervention of, among others, surgeons, dentists, audiologists, geneticists and psychologists, all treating patients sometimes over many years, and yet the outcomes are often variable and unsatisfactory.

1.4.14 Craniofacial Disorders Associated with Hypernasality

Many disorders associated with hypernasality. See Table 1.1 for a comprehensive list of these disorders.

Table 1.1 Syndromes with hypernasal speech as a possible feature (Shanske and Shprintzen©2021)

Phenotype	Location	Phenotype MIM number	Inheritance	Gene/Locus (if known)	Gene/Locus MIM number
Aarskog	Xp11.22	305400	XLR, AD, AR	FGD1	300546
Aase–Smith		147800	AD		
Abruzzo–Erikson	Xq21.1	302905	XL	TBX22	300307
Acrocallasol	15q26.1	200990	AR	KIF7	611254
Adams–Oliver syndrome 1	3q13.32–q33	100300	AD	ARHGAP31	610911
AEC	3q28	106260	AD	TP63	603273
Aicardi	3p21.31	235750	AD,AR	TREX1	606609
Ataxia-telangiectasia	11q22.3	208900	AR	ATM	607585
Baller–Gerold	8q24.3	218600	AR	RECQL4	603780
Bannayan–Zonana (Cowden Syndrome 1)	10q23.31	158350	AD	PTEN	601728
Basal cell nevus	9q22.32	109400	AD	PTCH1	601309
Beckwith–Wiedemann	11p15.5	130650	AD	ICR1,KCNQ10T1, CDKN1C	616816, 6014115, 600856
Bencze		141350	AD		
Berardinelli-Seip	9q34.3	608594	AR	AGPPAT2	603100
Brachial plexus neuropathy	17q25.3	162100	AD	SEPT9	604061
Carpenter	6p12.1-p11.2	201000	AR	RAB23	606144
Cat eye	22q11	115470	AD		
Catel–Manzke	13q32.1	616145	AR	TGDS	616146
Cerebro-costo-mandibular	20p13	117650	AD	SNRPB	182282
Cleidocranial dysplasia	6p21.1	119600	AD	RUNX2	600211
Cockayne syndrome A	5q12.1	216400	AR	ERCC8	609412
Craniofrontonasal	Xq13.1	304110	XLD	EFNB1	300035
Crouzon	10q26.13	123500	AD	FGFR2	176943

(continued)

Table 1.1 (continued)

Phenotype	Location	Phenotype MIM number	Inheritance	Gene/Locus (if known)	Gene/Locus MIM number
Cornelia de Lange syndrome 1	5p13.2	122470	AD	NIPBL	608667
Diastrophic dysplasia	5q32	222600	AR	SLC26A2	606718
Down	21q22.3	190685	Isolated cases	Trisomy of DCR (Down syndrome critical region)	
Dubowitz		223370	AR		
EEC3	3q28	604292	AD	TP63	603273
Escobar	2q37.1	265000	AR	CHRNG	100730
Facial-cardio-renal		227280			
Facio-scapulo-humeral	4q35	158900	AD	Contraction of D4Z4 repeat	
Familial dysautonomia	9q31.3	223900	AR	ELP1	603722
Femoral hypoplasia-unusual facies (BFD-UF)		134780			
Foetal alcohol	4q23	103700	Increased risk with metabolic defect	ADH1A	
Foetal hydantoin		617955	Increased risk with metabolic defect		
FG	Xq13.1	304450	XLR	MED12	300188
Filiform adhesion-cleft palate (AEC)	3q28	106260	AD	TP63	603273
Freeman–Sheldon		277720	AR		
Golabi–Rosen	Xq26.2	312870	XLR	GPC3	300037
Goldenhar (Oculo-auriculo-vertebral)	14q32	164210	AD		
Goldberg–Shprintzen	10q22.2	609460	AR	KIAA1279	609367
Hajdu–Cheney	1p12	102500	AD	NOTCH2	600275
HMC		239800			
Holoprosencephaly-1	21q22	236100	AD, IC	At least 12 loci	
Homocystinuria	21q22.3	236200	AR	CBS	613381
Johnson–McMillan		147770	AD		
Kallman syndrome 1	Xp22	308700	XLR	ANOS1	300836
Kearnes–Sayre		530000	mtDNA deletion		
Kniest	12q13.11	156550	AD	COL2A1	120140
Landau–Kleffner	16p13.2	245570	AD	GRIN2A	138253
Larsen	3p14.3	150250	AD	FLNB	603381
Lenz	8q22.1	151050	AD	PTDSS1	612792
Marden–Walker	18p11.22–p11.21	248700	AD	PIEZO2	613629
Marshall	1p21.1	154780	AD	COL11A1	120280
Mohr (OFD4)	10q24.1	258860	AR	TCTN3	613847
Nager	1q21.2	154400	AD	SF3B4	605593
NF1	17q11.2	162200	AD	NF1	613113
Niikawa–Kuroki (Kabuki)	12q13.12	147920	AD	KMT2D	602113
Noonan	12q24.13	163950	AD	PTPN11	176876
Oculo-dento-digital	6q22.31	164200	AD	GJA1	121014

(continued)

Table 1.1 (continued)

Phenotype	Location	Phenotype MIM number	Inheritance	Gene/Locus (if known)	Gene/Locus MIM number
Oculopharyngeal MD	14q11.2	164300	AD	PABPN1	602279
Opitz GBBB1	Xp22.2	300000	XLR	MID1	300552
Oral-facial-digital, type I	Xp22.2	311200	XLD	OFD1	300170
Oto-palatal-digital, types I and II	Xq28 Xq28	311300 304120	XLD XLD	FLNA FLNA	300017 300017
Pierre–Robin	17q24.3–25.1	261800	AR		
Pontobulbar palsy with SN hearing loss	20p13	211530	AR	SLC52A3	613350
Popliteal pterygium	1q32.2	119500	AD	IRF6	607199
Prader–Willi	15q11.2 15q11.2	176270 176270	AD AD	NDN SNRPN	602117 182279
Rapp–Hodgkin	3q28	129400	AD	TP63	603272
Robinow	9q22.31	268310	AR	ROR2	602337
Rubinstein–Taybi	16p13.3	180849	AD	CREBBP	600140
Saethre–Chotzen	7p21.1	101400	AD	TWIST1	601622
Seitelberger	22q13.1	256600	AR	PLA2G6	603604
Smith–Lemli–Opitz	11q13.4	270400	AR	DHCR7	602858
Spondyloepiphyseal dysplasia	12q13.11	183900	AD	COL2A1	120140
Steinert (myotonic dystrophy)	19q13.32	160900	AD	DMPK	605377
Stickler	12q13.11	108300	AD	COL2A1	120140
Treacher Collins	5q32–33	154500	AD	TCOF1	606847
Turner			Monosomy X chromosome		
Van der Woude	1q32.2	119300	AD	IRF6	
VCFS	22q11.2	192430	AD	TBX1	602054
Velofacioskeletal		600736	AD		
Velopharyngeal insufficiency		167500	multifactorial		
Weaver	7q36.1	277590	AD	EZH2	601573
Wolf–Hirschhorn	4p16.3	194190	IC		
X-linked M.R.			many loci		

MIM Mendelian inheritance in man, *p* and *q* are the short and long arm of chromosomes, *AD* autosomal dominant, *AR* autosomal recessive, *XLR* X-linked recessive, *IC* isolated cases

1.4.14.1 Velo-Cardio-Facial Syndrome, (VCFS)

The field of human genetics has been expanded to include genome mutations that result from mal-segregation of a chromosome pair that result in a microdeletion. VCFS (Shprintzen syndrome, DiGeorge syndrome, 22q11.2 deletion syndrome, Sedláčková syndrome) is the most common human microdeletion syndrome, and as a result it has been intensely studied at the molecular level. The molecular defect is usually a deletion of approximately 3 Mb at the 22q11.21 locus. The deletion occurs because this region of chromosome 22 is flanked by two identical sequences of DNA known as *low-copy repeats* (*LCRs*). LCRs occur frequently throughout the genome. During meiosis when the chromosomes align during the first stage and crossing over occurs resulting in recombination of the long arms of the two copies of chromosome 22. Because the flanking LCRs are identical, the chromosomes are prone to misaligning, resulting in the loss of a segment of DNA from one copy chromosome 22. This deleted region contains approximately 40 genes with many of them critical to normal human development and function. Two of the genes in the critical deleted region, Tbx1 and Crkl, are directly involved in causing anomalies as a result of their absence (Guris et al. 2001; Funato 2020), such as cleft palate (including submucous and occult submucous clefts), conotruncal heart anomalies, cranial structure variations and minor ear and nose findings. VCFS has an estimated population prevalence of approximately 1:2000 and the deletion occurs in 1:960 established pregnancies (Grati et al. 2015). People with milder phenotypic features, or who do not have congenital heart disease, may not present VCFS until later in life when speech disorders, specifically severe hypernasality and articulation disorders, become evident. The vast majority of cases arise as a de novo event (more than 90%) but there is a 50% recurrence risk in familial cases. Associated abnormalities include speech-language disorders, especially velopharyngeal insufficiency; developmental delay; hearing impairment; palatal abnormality; congenital heart defects, especially conotruncal defect; feeding problems; immune disorders or deficiencies; hypocalcaemia; learning disabilities or cognitive impairment; and a wide range of behavioural disorders, including psychosis. VCFS has been identified as the most common genetic cause of psychosis. It is interesting to note that there is a duplication 22q11.2 syndrome that results in the duplication of the same 3 Mb DNA segment. Theoretically it is the result of the same misaligned recombination of the LCRs that flank the critical region on 22q11.2 during meiosis. The disorder has a very variable phenotype but is not detected as frequently as VCFS.

1.4.14.2 CNVs (Copy Number Variants)

Over 90% of cases with velo-cardio-facial syndrome (also known as DiGeorge syndrome, Shprintzen syndrome and 22q11.2 deletion syndrome) have a deletion of approximately three million base pairs (3 megabases, 3 Mb) encompassing more than 40 genes. Smaller nested deletions have also been described. All patients with VCFS have detectable deletions of the proximal 1.5 Mb, often referred to as the DiGeorge Critical Region. There are some cases with clinical features of a 22q11 deletion including major anomalies such as conotruncal heart defects but with normal FISH results. Busse et al. (2011) analysed DNA from eight patients with normal 22q11 FISH results and identified copy number variants (CNVs) at different loci in four of eight patients. Two patients showed large CNVs in regions of known genomic disorders. A 3 Mb deletion of chr19p13.3, which includes a gene associated with conotruncal heart defects, was found in a third patient. Two potentially pathogenic CNVs were found in a fourth patient. Although there may be overlap of certain clinical features, this does not mean that the diagnosis of VCFS can be applied to such cases. For example conotruncal heart anomalies occur in CHARGE syndrome, Down syndrome and foetal alcohol syndrome, but the overall presentation of these syndromes is very different than VCFS.

1.4.14.3 IRF6 and Van der Woude Syndrome (VWS)

Originally reported by Van der Woude in 1954, this disorder is a dominantly inherited craniofacial developmental disorder characterised by pits or sinuses of the lower lip, with cleft lip or cleft palate (CL/P, CP) and hypodontia. Although velo-cardio-facial syndrome is the most common syndrome of cleft palate, Van der Woude is the most common syndrome that has cleft lip as a feature. The lower lip pits represent small openings to accessory salivary glands (Fig. 1.17).

The vast majority of cases have a mutation in the interferon inhibiting factor 6 (IRF6). In

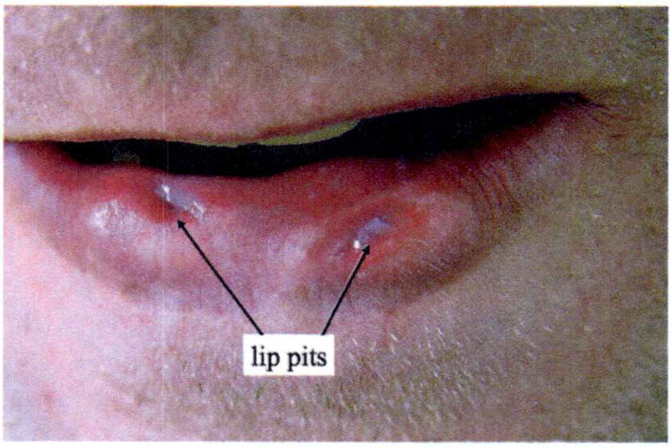

Fig. 1.17 Lip pits (Shprintzen©2021)

some affected families, because of the variable expressivity of the gene, the syndrome is expressed only as pits, while in others cleft lip or cleft palate without pits. VWS is one of the few malformation syndromes that has a mixing of cleft type in first degree relatives. It is not uncommon in VDW to see siblings where one has a cleft palate only, and another has clefting of both the lip and palate. Only few other malformation syndromes manifest this phenomenon, including Robinow syndrome, which is also an autosomal dominant disorder, EEC syndrome, popliteal pterygium syndrome (which also has lip pits as a feature and caused by a mutation in IRF6 gene as is VDW), Hay-Wells syndrome (or AEC syndrome) among a small number of others. Lip pits, the most common manifestation in VDW, are present in 88% of the affected individuals and were the only manifestation in 64%. Clefts of the lip and palate occur in 21% of cases. Conical elevations (CE) on the lower lip at the site of sinuses and lacking bicuspid teeth in some cases are minor anomalies associated with VDW, and may be the only signs of the syndrome in some cases. Birnbaum et al. (2008) analysed the IRF6 gene in 63 families with what was believed to be isolated CL/P or CP, and identified a deletion/insertion and duplication in two families. Screening for mutations in isolated CL/P is essential for genetic counselling because of the similarity in phenotypes between VWS and isolated CL/P, and the recurrence risk of VWS is higher than that for non-syndromic clefts. Mutations in IRF6 are also examples of phenotypic heterogeneity in that IRF6 mutations also result in the popliteal pterygium syndrome, sometimes in the same family. Traditionally, genetic disorders have been classified as either Mendelian diseases or complex diseases. This classification greatly simplified genetic counselling in the past. At the present time, the significant over-representation of variants, including copy number variations (CNVs) in complex disorders, suggests the important roles of CNVs in complex diseases and the vital role of accurate genetic counselling (Jin et al. 2012).

1.4.14.4 Crouzon Syndrome

Originally described in 1912 by Crouzon, this disorder of craniofacial development is characterised by shallow orbits, craniosynostosis, especially of the coronal, lambdoidal and sagittal sutures, and maxillary hypoplasia. The nose may be curved and parrot-like, and the palate has an inverted V shape. Patients occasionally have a cleft lip with or without cleft palate. Increased intracranial pressure may inhibit normal brain development. Crouzon is inherited as an autosomal dominant disorder with about one quarter of cases representing new mutations in the fibroblast growth factor receptor 2 gene (FGFR2). It is interesting to note that a variety of mutations of FGFR2 result in Pfeiffer syndrome, Apert syndrome and Beare–Stevenson cutis gyrate syndrome, a dramatic illustration of phenotypic heterogeneity (different mutations in the same gene resulting in different phenotypes).

1.4.14.5 Goldenhar Syndrome

Goldenhar syndrome (oculo-auriculovertebral, hemifacial microsomia) is a common birth defect involving the first and second branchial arch derivatives. It typically affects the external ear, middle ear, mandible and temporo-mandibular joint, muscles of mastication and facial muscles, and other facial soft tissues on the affected side. In some cases, other facial structures, such as the orbit, eye, nose, cranium or neck, may be involved. Velar asymmetry in both structure and function is common (Shprintzen et al. 1980) and CL/P occurs in some cases. Involvement is usually limited to one side, but bilateral involvement is not uncommon. In addition to craniofacial anomalies, there may be cardiac, vertebral and central nervous system defects. The phenotype is highly variable. Most cases are sporadic and occur as a result of multi-factorial inheritance, but there are rare familial cases that exhibit autosomal dominant inheritance (summary by Poole 1989; Hennekam et al. 2010) and exome sequencing has suggested the gene SF3B2 playing a role in some cases (Timberlake et al., 2021). The features of hemifacial microsomia include unilateral deformity of the external ear and a small ipsilateral half of the face with epibulbar dermoid and vertebral anomalies. Coloboma of the upper eyelid is frequent. The ear deformities range from pre-auricular tags of cartilaginous masses, to atresia of the external auditory canal, anomalies in the size and shape of the external auricle, and even to anotia.

1.4.14.6 Smith–Lemli–Opitz Syndrome

Four patients with moderate short stature, facial and genital anomalies were first described by Smith et al. in 1964. The craniofacial features included microcephaly, ptosis of eyelids, low-set ears, anteverted nostrils with a broad nasal tip and cleft palate in some cases. Limb abnormalities include syndactyly of the second and third toes and genital hypospadias and cryptorchidism. This disorder is inherited as an autosomal recessive trait owing to a severe defect in an enzyme involved in cholesterol metabolism, 7-dehydrocholesterol reductase, which results in elevated concentrations of the cholesterol precursor, 7-dehydrocholesterol. Cholesterol is necessary for maintenance of cell membranes, myelination of the nervous system, and steroid metabolism. More interesting is the effect of decreased levels of cholesterol on Sonic hedgehog (Shh) signalling. Shh is an extracellular signalling protein molecule that is involved in a developmental pathway, the Sonic hedgehog (Shh)-Patched (Ptch)-Gli pathway. Sequential biochemical defects along this vital signalling pathway result in a number of related disorders. This pathway has become the paradigm for the basis of the concept of the biochemical basis of development.

1.4.14.7 EEC3 Syndrome

Ectrodactyly, ectodermal dysplasia, and cleft lip/palate syndrome-3 (ECC3) is an autosomal dominant disorder comprising absence of the central parts of the hands and feet, resulting in split-hand/foot malformation, ectodermal dysplasia and cleft lip with or without cleft palate. EEC syndrome-3 is caused by heterozygous mutation in the gene encoding p63 on chromosome 3q28. CL/P occurs in 68% of cases. This disorder is illustrative of genetic heterogeneity in that Type 1 has been assigned to chromosome 7q11.2-q21.3.

1.4.15 Genetics of Speech and Language Disorders

Next-generation sequencing and GWAS studies are revolutionising our understanding of such neuro-developmental disorders as schizophrenia and autism. A genomic approach to understanding language development is revealing insights into the neural and molecular networks crucial for normal brain development and abnormal language-related phenotypes. The human capacity for language is unique among animals. A normal human infant is capable of mastering any spoken language. The infant's innate ability to do this suggests that there are neural mechanisms for language acquisition and subsequently these are probably hard-wired in our genome. Proof of the biological basis of language is the description of language-related genes. The first example of a specific gene implicated in language development was the discovery that heterozygous FOXP2 disruptions lead to severe speech and language defects.

Most cases of developmental language impairments are likely to involve genetic complexity, resulting from the inheritance of multiple risk factors with small individual effect sizes. Nonetheless, it has been established that disorders of speech and language sometimes occur in monogenic form. One relevant disorder that may be enriched for damaging gene variants of large effect size is childhood apraxia of speech (CAS), also known as developmental verbal dyspraxia. CAS is a rare severe developmental disorder characterised by difficulties with automatically and accurately sequencing speech sounds into syllables, syllables into words, and words into sentences with the correct prosody. In CAS it is thought that impairments in the neural planning or programming of spatio-temporal parameters of movement sequences result in errors in speech sound production and prosody. Diagnostic features of CAS include inconsistency in the types of speech error that are made, and greater problems such as the complexity and length of the utterance increase.

In 2001, studies of a large multi-generational pedigree named the KE family, along with an unrelated case with a chromosomal translocation, led to the discovery that disrupting one copy of the FOXP2 gene (on chromosome 7q31) is sufficient to cause CAS. Multiple different cases of FOXP2 disruption have since been identified, including missense and nonsense mutations, insertions/deletions and chromosomal rearrangements of various kinds; CAS is the most consistent phenotypic consequence in the affected people. More than 15 years after the identification of FOXP2, progress in identifying additional genetic risk factors has been slow, and mainly driven by studies of chromosomal rearrangements. For example, deletion of a ~ 600 kb region in human chromosomal band 16p11.2, encompassing >25 genes, significantly increases risk of CAS. The BCL11A and ERC1 genes have been found to be disrupted by deletions at 2p16.1 and 12p13.33, respectively, in children with CAS. Still, the majority of speech apraxia cases do not seem to carry causal mutations in FOXP2, BCL11A or ERC1.

Whole-genome sequencing (WGS) was used to identify additional genes that cause CAS. Eising et al. in 2019 studied 19 test subjects with a diagnosis of CAS to identify single nucleotide variants (SNVs) and small insertions and deletions (indels). It has been shown that genes involved in speech and language disruptions cluster in related functional pathways. The WGS findings in this study uncovered a neural co-expression module of functionally-related genes in addition to ERC1 and BCL11A. Some of the newly implicated candidate genes in CAS susceptibility have already been reported in connection with other neurodevelopment disorders. The WGS analyses revealed eight genes (CHD3, SETD1A, KAT6A, SETBP1, TNRC6B, ZHFX4, ARID1A and TRIO) linked to both CAS and neurodevelopmental phenotypes.

1.4.16 Genetics of Deafness

Hearing loss is relatively common, affecting approximately 1–3 per 1000 infants. It is heterogeneous in nature and can be characterised by the affected structures of the ear, age of onset, and whether other organ systems are implicated. The acquisition and transduction of sound by the human ear is a highly complex process involving numerous tissues and cell types. The complexity of the auditory process is reflected not only in the elaborate organ of Corti and its stereocilia but also in a host of other cell types that make up the cochlea. The onset of hearing loss may be pre-lingual, with occurrence before normal speech development, or post-lingual after normal speech development. There are three types of the hearing loss, conductive, sensorineural and mixed. Of these the most common is sensorineural, which is secondary to environmental factors in about 50% of cases and may be either syndromic or non-syndromic. The majority of sensorineural hearing loss (~70%) is non-syndromic. More than 400 genetic syndromes include hearing loss and there were 1095 OMIM entries when accessed in September 2020 that include deafness. Over 400 genes have been implicated in syndromic hearing loss, accounting for up to 30% of pre-lingual sensorineural hearing loss. Additionally, over 90 genes have been implicated in non-syndromic sensorineural hearing loss, with up to 80% of pre-lingual non-syndromic hearing loss inherited in an autosomal recessive fashion, followed by dominant and X-linked inheritance in terms of relative frequency. Dominant loci are denoted with the prefix DFNA, recessive loci with DFNB, X-linked loci with DFN and modifying loci with DFNM. In individuals with autosomal recessive non-syndromic hearing loss, approximately 50% have a variant associated with DFNB1, caused by pathogenic variants of the GJB2/GJB6 genes. Gene discovery in the auditory system has been rapid. Many of the encoded proteins are expressed within the cochlea and can be grouped into functional categories. These include hair cell structure (MYO7 an unconventional myosin gene is critical for the structural integrity of stereocilia), extracellular matrix (the tectorial membrane gene TECTA codes for the extracellular matrix of this membrane), ion homeostasis (GJB2 encodes a subunit of the gap junction protein that maintains the correct ion flux) and transcription factors (MITF,

PAX3 and SOX10 have been found to be mutated in different types of Waardenburg syndromes).

Genetic testing can be a very important and informative step in the diagnosis of hearing loss. Identification of one or more pathogenic variants in a specific gene or genes can provide the physician and family with important information regarding prognosis, treatment and recurrence. Hereditary deafness genetic test panels contain as many as 146 nuclear genes and 6 variants in 4 mitochondrial genes accounting mainly for non-syndromic forms of hearing loss and select genetic syndromes associated with hearing loss.

1.4.17 Future Directions

1.4.17.1 Craniofacial Defects and Tissue Engineering

Gene editing techniques utilise some type of nuclease that can cut DNA along with some sort of guide to direct the enzyme to the right place in the genome. They have been around for more than 20 years and include zinc finger nucleases (ZFN), transcription activator-like effector nucleases (TALENS), and the most recent, clustered regularly interspersed short palindromic repeats (CRISPR). CRISPR-Cas9 utilises the CRISPR-associated protein number 9 for gene editing by using a short RNA guide sequence to target a specific DNA sequence. The guide sequence can be introduced into a cell containing a mutant sequence, cut the abnormal DNA and then allow the cell's own DNA repair machinery to replace the defective gene copy with a normal sequence. Gene editing is being used in tissue engineering which depends upon the interplay of progenitor cells such as embryonic stem cells, regulatory signals and the biomaterials/scaffolds used to deliver them (the tissue engineering triad). Various tissue engineering efforts have been attempted to correct craniofacial defects. Stem cells can be easily modified by CRISPR technology. Mesenchymal stem cells (MSC) are being utilised in mouse models of oral and craniofacial diseases. Alveolar bone, periodontal ligament and dental pulp contain subsets of MSCs that can be edited by CRISPR/Cas9. MSCs could be a valuable tool in correcting oral, periodontal, and craniofacial defects (Yu et al. 2019).

1.4.17.2 Treacher Collins Syndrome (TCS)

This is a severe disorder of craniofacial development caused by mutations in the TCOF1 gene. The cellular basis for TCS is a deficiency of NCCs secondary to extensive p53-dependent neuroepithelial apoptosis (Dixon et al. 2006). Treatment of Tcof1 embryos (the mouse model of TCS) with a specific inhibitor of p53 results in the rescue of cranioskeletal development. Trainor (2010) describes the prevention of TCS craniofacial anomalies in mice as the first successful rescue of a congenital neurocristopathy that may provide a model for future research in craniofacial defects with a similar aetiology and pathogenesis.

1.4.17.3 Pierre Robin Sequence (Robin Sequence)

This is a craniofacial disorder characterised by micrognathia (small lower jaw), a wide U-shaped palatal cleft and glossoptosis (retracted tongue position) that can cause difficulty in swallowing and neonatal respiratory distress. The U-shaped cleft palate is thought to be secondary to a physical block of palatal shelf elevation or fusion by the abnormal tongue position. Med23 is a new candidate gene for Robin sequence. Mice in which Med23 is conditionally deleted in the cranial neural crest cell population produce a phenotype similar to PRS.

1.4.17.4 Matrix Metalloproteinase 2 (MMP2)

This has become a gene of interest in studies of CL/P after it was revealed that the gene was differentially expressed between wild-type zebrafish and crispld2 morphants (mutant fish produced by using a morpholino antisense oligonucleotide). Variants in human CRISPLD2, a novel non-syndromic cleft lip and palate candidate gene, had previously been shown to be significantly associated with susceptibility in multiple Caucasian and Hispanic cohorts. CRISPLD2 encodes a secreted protein suggested to have a role in regulating cranial neural crest migration. Morpholino-knockdown of zebrafish mmp2 results in embryos with smaller heads and an abnormal mandibular arch skeleton (Swindell et al. 2015). Furthermore, in a cohort of Hispanic families a significant association of a variant, rs243836, in MMP2 with human NS-CL/P was found (2021).

References

Ahlberg PE, Clack JA, Blom H (2005) The axial skeleton of the Devonian tetrapod Ichthyostega. Nature 437:137–140

Ballard JL, Auer CE, Khoury JC (2002) Ankyloglossia: assessment, incidence, and effect of frenuloplasty on the breastfeeding dyad. Pediatrics 110(5):e63. https://doi.org/10.1542/peds.110.5.e63

Birnbaum S, Reutter H, Lauster C et al (2008) Mutation screening in the IRF6-gene in patients with apparently nonsyndromic orofacial clefts and a positive family history suggestive of autosomal-dominant inheritance. Am J Med Genet 146A(6):787–790

Bluestone CD (1971) Eustachian tube obstruction in the infant with cleft palate. Ann Otol Rhinol Laryngol 80(Suppl 2):1–30

Böhme G (2003) In: Klinik (ed) Sprach-, Sprech-, Stimm- und Schluckstörungen (Speech, language, voice and swallowing disorders), vol 1, 4th edn. Urban und Fischer, Munich Jena, p 109

Boveri TH (1904) Ergebnisse über die Konstitution der chromatischen Substanz des Zelkerns. Fisher, Jena

Brown JS, Shaw RJ (2010) Reconstruction of the maxilla and midface: introducing a new classification. Lancet Oncol 11(10):1001–1008

Burg ML, Chai Y, Yao CA et al (2016) Epidemiology, etiology, and treatment of isolated cleft palate. Front Physiol 7:67. https://doi.org/10.3389/fphys.2016.00067

Busse T, Graham JM, Feldman G et al (2011) High-resolution genomic arrays identify CNVs that phenocopy the chromosome 22q11.2 deletion syndrome. Hum Mutat 32(1):91–97

Centers for Disease Control (2010) Birth Defects Research and Prevention. https://www.cdc.gov/ncbddd/birthdefects/research.html. Accessed 11 Nov 2021

Croft CB, Shprintzen RJ, Daniller AI et al (1978) The occult submucous cleft palate and the musculus uvuli. Cleft Palate J 15(2):150–154

Croft CB, Shprintzen RJ, Rakoff SJ (1981a) Patterns of velopharyngeal valving in normal and cleft palate subjects: a multi-view videofluoroscopic and nasendoscopic study. Laryngoscope 91(2):265–271

Croft CB, Shprintzen RJ, Ruben RJ (1981b) Hypernasal speech following adenotonsillectomy. Otolaryngol Head Neck Surg 89(2):179–188

Crouzon LEO (1912) Dysostose cranio-faciale héréditaire (hereditary craniofacial dysostosis). Bulletin de la Société des Médecins des Hôpitaux de Paris (Bulletin of the Society of Doctors of the Hospitals of Paris) 33:545–555

Dahm R (2008) Discovering DNA: Friedrich Miescher and the early years of nucleic acid research. Hum Genet 122(6):565–581

D'Antonio LL, Marsh JL, Province MA et al (1989) Reliability of flexible fiberoptic nasopharyngoscopy for evaluation of velopharyngeal function in a clinical population. Cleft Palate J 26(3):217–225

Darwin C (1859) The origin of species by means of natural selection. John Murray, London

Davidson TM (2003) The great leap forward: the anatomic basis for the acquisition of speech and obstructive sleep apnea. Sleep Med 4(3):185–194

Davidson TM, Sedgh J, Tran D et al (2005) The anatomic basis for the acquisition of speech and obstructive sleep apnea: evidence from cephalometric analysis supports the great leap forward hypothesis. Sleep Med 6(6):497–505

Dickson DR (1976) Anatomy of the normal and cleft palate Eustachian tube. Ann Otol Rhinol Laryngol 85(Suppl 25):25–29

Dickson DR, Dickson WM (1972) Velopharyngeal anatomy. J Speech Hear Res 15(2):372–381

Dixon J, Jones NC, Sandell LL et al (2006) Tcof1/Treacle is required for neural crest cell formation and proliferation deficiencies that cause craniofacial abnormalities. Proc Natl Acad Sci USA 103(36):13403–13408

Eising E, Carrion-Castillo A, Vino A et al (2019) A set of regulatory genes co-expressed in embryonic human brain is implicated in disrupted speech development. Mol Psychiatry 24(7):1065–1078

Friedrich G (2013) Dysglossien (Dysglossia). In: Bigenzahn W, Zorowka P (eds) Phoniatrie und Pädaudiologie (phoniatrics and pedaudiology), 5th edn. Huber Hogrefe, Bern, pp 135–139

Funato N (2020) New insights into cranial synchondrosis development: a mini review. Front Cell Dev Biol 8:706. https://doi.org/10.3389/fcell.2020.00706

Golding-Kushner KJ (1995) Treatment of articulation and resonance disorders associated with cleft palate and VPI. In: Shprintzen RJ, Bardach J (eds) Cleft palate speech management. Mosby, St Louis, MO, pp 327–351

Golding-Kushner KJ (2001a) Therapy techniques for cleft palate speech and related disorders. San Diego, CA, Singular, p 27

Golding-Kushner KJ (2001b) Therapy techniques for cleft palate speech and related disorders. Singular Publishing, San Diego, CA, p 175

Golding-Kushner KJ, Shprintzen RJ (2011) Velo-cardio-facial syndrome, vol 2. Plural Publishing, San Diego, CA, pp 14–15

Golding-Kushner KJ, Argamaso RV, Cotton RT et al (1990) Standardization for the reporting of nasopharyngoscopy and multiview videofluoroscopy: a report from an international working group. Cleft Palate J 27(4):337–347

Grati FR, Gomes DM, Ferreira JCPB et al (2015) Prevalence of recurrent pathogenic microdeletions and

microduplications in over 9500 pregnancies. Prenat Diagn 35(8):801–809
Guris DL, Fantes J, Tara D et al (2001) Mice lacking the homologue of the human 22q11.2 gene CRKL phenocopy neurocristopathies of DiGeorge syndrome. Nat Genet 27(3):293–298
Hennekam RCM, Krantz ID, Allanson JE (2010) Branchialarch and oral-acral disorders. In: Gorlin's syndromes of the head and neck, 5th edn. Oxford University Press, New York, NY, pp 879–887
Hilton W (1836) Case of a large bony tumor in the face completely removed by spontaneous separation. Guys Hosp Rep 1:493–506
Hong P (2013) Five things to know about…ankyloglossia (tongue-tie). CMAJ 185(2):E128. https://doi.org/10.1503/cmaj.120785
Jin W, Qin P, Lou H et al (2012) A systematic characterization of genes underlying both complex and Mendelian diseases. Hum Mol Genet 21(7):1611–1624
Kaplan EN (1975) The occult submucous cleft palate. Cleft Palate J 12(4):356–368
Koppetsch S, Dahlmeier K (2004) Funktionelle Störungen der Artikulation bei intra-oralen Tumoren-eine prä- und postoperative Langzeitstudie (functional disturbances of articulation in intra-oral tumors—a pre-and postoperative long-term study). Sprache-Stimme-Gehör 27(4):155–160
Leme M, Barbosa T, Castelo P et al (2014) Associations between psychological factors and the presence of deleterious oral habits in children and adolescents. J Clin Pediatr Dent 38(4):313–317
Leonard R, Goodrich S, McMenamin P et al (1992) Differentiation of speakers with glossectomies by acoustic and perceptual measures. Am J Speech Lang Pathol 1(4):56–63
Lewin ML, Croft CB, Shprintzen RJ (1980) Velopharyngeal insufficiency due to hypoplasia of the musculus uvulae and occult submucous cleft palate. Plast Reconstr Surg 65(5):585–591
Lin YS, Jen YM, Lin JC (2002) Radiation-related cranial nerve palsy in patients with nasopharyngeal carcinoma. Cancer 95(2):404–409
López-Barroso D, Catani M, Ripollés P et al (2013) Word learning is mediated by the left arcuate fasciculus. Proc Natl Acad Sci USA 110(32):13168–13173
MacKenzie-Stepner K, Witzel MA, Stringer DA et al (1987) Velopharyngeal insufficiency due to hypertrophic tonsils. A report of two cases. Int J Pediatr Otorhinolaryngol 14(1):57–63
Maue-Dickson W, Dickson DR, Rood SR (1976) Anatomy of the Eustachian tube and related structures in age-matched human fetuses with and without cleft palate. Acad Ophtalmol Otolaryngol 82(2):159–164
Mendel JG (1866) Versuche über Pflanzenhybriden (experiments on plant hybrids). Verhandlungen des naturforschenden Vereines in Brünn (deliberations of the nature research association in Brno) part 4 for 1865, Abhandlungen (treatises) 3–47
Mitchell LE, Risch N (1992) Mode of inheritance of nonsyndromic cleft lip with or without cleft palate: a reanalysis. Am J Hum Genet 51(2):323–332
Miyazaki T, Matsuya T, Yamaoka M (1975) Fiberscopic methods for assessment of velopharyngeal closure during various activities. Cleft Palate J 12:107–114
Moll KL (1965) A cinefluorographic study of velopharyngeal function in normals during various activities. Cleft Palate J 31:112–122
Morgan TH (1911) Chromosomes and associative inheritance. Science 34(880):636–638
Müller R, Gebelein K (2001) Sprache und Sprechen nach Therapie von Mundhöhlen-und Mundrachentumoren (2000/2001) (speech and language after therapy for oral cavity and oral pharyngeal tumors (2000/2001)). In: Gross M, Kruse E (eds) Aktuelle phoniatrisch-pädaudiologische Aspekte (current phoniatric-pediatric aspects), vol 8. Medianverlag, Heidelberg, pp 140–142
O'Shea JE, Foster JP, O'Donnell CPF et al (2017) Frenotomy for tongue-tie in newborn infants. Cochrane Database Syst Rev 3:CD011065. https://doi.org/10.1002/14651858.CD011065.pub2
OMIM®-Online Mendelian Inheritance in Man (2021). https://www.omim.org
Pigott RW (1969) Nasendoscopic appearance of the normal palatopharyngeal valve. Plast Reconstr Surg 43(1):19–24
Pigott RW, Bensen JF, White FD (1969) Nasendoscopy in the diagnosis of velopharyngeal incompetence. Plast Reconstr Surg 43(2):141–147
Poole MD (1989) Hemifacial microsomia. World J Surg 13(4):396–400
Rich AR (1920) Physiological study of the Eustachian tube and its related muscles. Bull Johns Hopkins Hosp 31:206–214
Scheier M (1909) Die Bedeutung des Röntgenverfahrens fur die Physiologie der Sprache und der Stimme. Archiv Laryngol Rhinol 22:175–179
Schönweiler R, Alternbernd C, Schmelzeisen R et al (1996) Artikulationsfähigkeit und Verständlichkeit der Sprache bei Patienten mit Mundhöhlenkarzinomen (articulatory ability and intelligibility of speech in patients with oral cavity carcinoma). HNO 44:634–639
Schröter-Morasch H, Ziegler W (2005) Rehabilitation of impaired speech function (dysarthria, dysglossia). GMS Curr Top Otorhinolaryngol Head Neck Surg 4:Doc15. PMID: 22073063
Sher AE, Shprintzen RJ, Thorpy MJ (1986) Endoscopic observations of obstructive sleep apnea in children with anomalous upper airways: predictive and therapeutic value. Int J Pediatr Otorhinolaryngol 11(2):135–146
Shprintzen RJ (1979) Hypernasal speech in the absence of overt or submucous cleft palate: the mystery solved. In: Ellis R, Flack R (eds) Diagnosis and treatment of Palato Glossal malfunction. College of Speech Therapists, London, pp 37–44
Shprintzen RJ (1982) Palatal and pharyngeal anomalies in craniofacial syndromes. Birth Defects Orig Artic Ser 18(1):53–78
Shprintzen RJ (1995) Instrumental assessment of velopharyngeal valving. In: Shprintzen RJ, Bardach J (eds)

Cleft palate speech management: a multidisciplinary approach. Mosby, St Louis, MO, pp 221–256
Shprintzen RJ (2003) The origin of speech ease: evolution of the human upper airway and its functional implications for obstructive sleep apnea. Sleep Med 4(3):171–173
Shprintzen RJ, Croft CB (1981) Abnormalities of the Eustachian tube orifice in individuals with cleft palate. Int J Pediatr Otorhinolaryngol 3:15–23
Shprintzen RJ, Golding Kushner K (1989) Evaluation of velopharyngeal insufficiency. Otolaryngol Clin N Am 22(2):519–536
Shprintzen RJ, Ysunza PA (2020) Endoscopic recording (or its absence): a disappointment. Sch J Oto 2(5):200–201
Shprintzen RJ, Lencione RM, McCall GN et al (1974) A three dimensional cinefluoroscopic analysis of velopharyngeal closure during speech and nonspeech activities in normals. Cleft Palate J 11(4):412–428
Shprintzen RJ, Croft CB, Berkman MD et al (1979a) Pharyngeal hypoplasia in the Treacher Collins syndrome. Arch Otolaryngol 105:127–131
Shprintzen RJ, Lewin ML, Croft CB et al (1979b) A comprehensive study of pharyngeal flap surgery: tailor made flaps. Cleft Palate J 16:46–55
Shprintzen RJ, Croft CB, Berkman MD et al (1980) Velopharyngeal insufficiency in the facio-auriculo-vertebral malformation complex. Cleft Palate J 17(2):132–137
Shprintzen RJ, Schwartz RH, Daniller A et al (1985a) Morphologic significance of bifid uvula. Pediatrics 75(3):553–561
Shprintzen RJ, Siegel-Sadewitz VL, Amato J et al (1985b) Anomalies associated with cleft lip, cleft palate, or both. Am J Med Genet 20(4):585–596
Shprintzen RJ, Sher AE, Croft CB (1987) Hypernasal speech caused by hypertrophic tonsils. Int J Pediatr Otorhinolaryngol 14:45–56
Sidoti EJ, Shprintzen RJ (1995) Pediatric care and feeding of the newborn with a cleft. In: Shprintzen RJ, Bardach J (eds) Cleft palate speech management. Mosby, St Louis, MO, pp 63–74
Siegel-Sadewitz VL, Shprintzen RJ (1982) Nasopharyngoscopy of the normal velopharyngeal sphincter: an experiment of biofeedback. Cleft Palate J 19(3):194–200
Siegel-Sadewitz VL, Shprintzen RJ (1986) Changes in velopharyngeal valving with age. Int J Pediatr Otorhinolaryngol 11:171–182
Skolnick ML (1969) Video velopharyngography in patients with nasal speech, with emphasis on lateral pharyngeal motion in velopharyngeal closure. Radiology 93(4):747–755
Skolnick ML (1970) Videofluoroscopic examination of the velopharyngeal portal during phonation in lateral and base projections—a new technique for studying the mechanics of closure. Cleft Palate J 7(4):803–816
Skolnick ML, McCall GN (1972) Velopharyngeal competence and incompetence following pharyngeal flap surgery: video-fluoroscopic study in multiple projections. Cleft Palate J 9(1):1–12
Skolnick ML, McCall GN, Barnes M (1973) The sphincteric mechanism of velopharyngeal closure. Cleft Palate J 10(3):286–305
Smith DW, Lemli L, Opitz JM (1964) A newly recognized syndrome of multiple congenital anomalies. J Pediatr 64:210–217
Stein MJ, Zhang Z, Fell M et al (2019) Determining postoperative outcomes after cleft palate repair: a systematic review and meta-analysis. J Plast Reconstr Aesthet Surg 72(1):85–91
Stranger BE, Forrest MS, Dunning M et al (2007) Relative impact of nucleotide and copy number variation on gene expression phenotypes. Science 315:848–853
Subtelny JD (1957) A cephalometric study of the growth of the soft palate. J Plast Reconstr Surg 19:49–62
Sutton WS (1902) On the morphology of the chromosome group in Brachystola magna. Biol Bull 4:24–39
Swindell EC, Yuan Q, Maili LE et al (2015) Crispld2 is required for neural crest cell migration and cell viability during zebrafish craniofacial development. Genesis 53(10):660–667
Tandon B (2021) Significant association of variant rs243836 in MMP2 with human NS-CL/P. University of Texas, Health Science Center at Houston. Personal Communication, Houston
Trainor PA (2010) Craniofacial birth defects: the role of neural crest cells in the etiology and pathogenesis of Treacher Collins syndrome and the potential for prevention. Am J Med Genet A 152A(12):2984–2994
Timberlake AT, Griffin C, Heike CL et al. (2021) Haploinsufficiency of SF3B2 causes craniofacial microsomia. Nat Commun 12(1):4680. https://doi.org/10.1038/s41467-021-24852-9. PMID: 34344887; PMCID: PMC8333351
van der Woude A (1954) Fistula labii inferioris congenita and its association with cleft lip and palate. Am J Hum Genet 6(2):244–256
Walsh J, McKenna BM (2019) Ankyloglossia and other oral ties. Otolaryngol Clin N Am 52(5):795–811
Watson JD, Crick FH (1953) Molecular structure of nucleic acids: a structure for deoxyribose nucleic acid. Nature 171(4356):737–738
Ysunza A, Vazquez MC (1993) Velopharyngeal sphincter physiology in deaf individuals. Cleft Palate Craniofac J 30(2):141–143
Ysunza A, Pamplona M, Femat T et al (1997) Videonasopharyngoscopy as an instrument for visual biofeedback during speech in cleft palate patients. Int J Pediatr Otorhinolaryngol 41(3):291–298
Ysunza PA, Bloom D, Chaiyasate K et al (2016) Velopharyngeal videofluoroscopy: providing useful clinical information in the era of reduced dose radiation and safety. Int J Pediatr Otorhinolaryngol 89:127–132
Ysunza PA, Chaiyasate K, Rontal M et al (2019) Comparison of three different surgical techniques for designing pharyngeal flaps according to findings of videonasopharyngoscopy and multiplanar videofluoroscopy. Int J Pediatr Otorhinolaryngol 20:123–129
Yu N, Yang J, Mishnia Y et al (2019) Genome editing: a new horizon for oral and craniofacial research. J Dent Res 98(1):36–45

2 Special Kinds of Dysglossia, Resonance Disorders and Velopharyngeal Insufficiency

Wolfgang Bigenzahn, Doris-Maria Denk-Linnert, and Ariane Hohoff

2.1 Orofacial Dysfunctions (Orofacial Myofunctional Disorders) with Special Focus on Paediatric Patients

Doris-Maria Denk-Linnert and Wolfgang Bigenzahn

2.1.1 Introduction

According to Hanson and Andrianopoulos (1982), orofacial dysfunctions (orofacial myofunctional disorders, OMD) refer to abnormal resting labial-lingual posture of the orofacial musculature, atypical chewing and swallowing patterns, dental malocclusions, blocked nasal airways and speech problems. OMDs occur in children as well as in adults and are found at every age.

At the end of the nineteenth century, the masticatory system, occlusion and orofacial functions started to be dealt with scientifically in Europe and Northern America. In 1912, Nadoleczny described, for the first time, a functional relationship between an anterior position of the tongue ('tongue thrust'), orofacial muscle imbalance, open lip and mouth posture and the development of tooth and jaw abnormalities (malocclusion) and the disturbed articulation (/s/formation) (Nadoleczny 1912). The Austro-American laryngologist and phoniatrician Emil Fröschels was concerned with the relationship between Stomatology and Speech-Language Pathology (Logopaedics) regarding the influence of the stomatognathic system on the abnormalities of the articulatory organs and speech production (Fröschels 1914).

In recent decades, the stomatognathic system has been increasingly recognised as a functional unit, and the form–function relationships are analysed interdisciplinarily (Fig. 2.1).

A physiological interplay between form and function results in normal oral functions and structures. Pathological relationships bring about skeletal, myoskeletal and myofunctional problems. On the one hand, the size and shape of the orofacial system influence the primary functions (i.e. breathing, sucking, biting, chewing, swallowing) and also affect the secondary functions (articulation, phonation, facial expression).

W. Bigenzahn (✉)
Private Practice, Formerly: Division of Phoniatrics and Speech Language Therapy, Department of Otorhinolaryngology, Medical University of Vienna, Vienna, Austria
e-mail: wolfgang.bigenzahn@chello.at

D.-M. Denk-Linnert
Division of Phoniatrics and Speech Language Therapy, Department of Otorhinolaryngology, Medical University of Vienna, Vienna, Austria
e-mail: doris-maria.denk-linnert@meduni.wien.ac.at

A. Hohoff
Department of Orthodontics, University Hospital of Münster, Münster, Germany
e-mail: hohoffa@uni-muenster.de

A. am Zehnhoff-Dinnesen et al. (eds.), *Phoniatrics II*, European Manual of Medicine,
https://doi.org/10.1007/978-3-031-25175-7_2

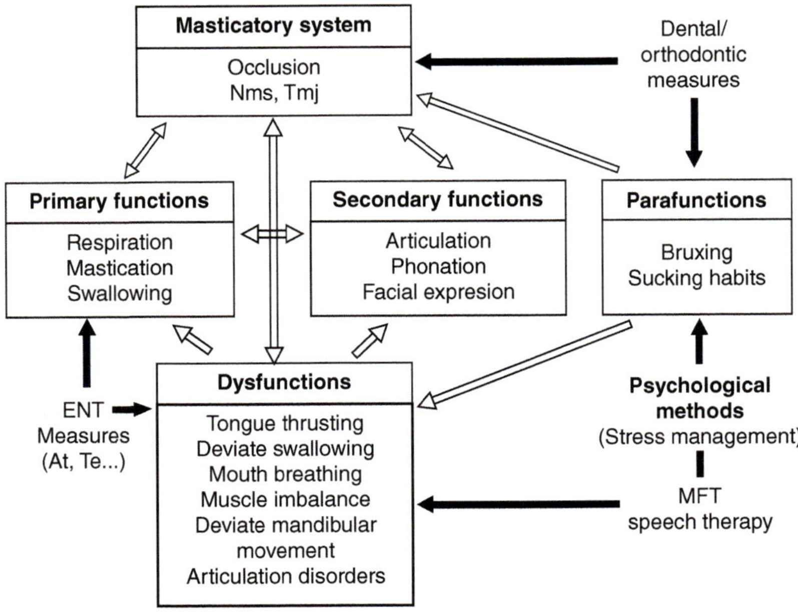

Fig. 2.1 Relation- and inter-relationships in the stomatognathic system between primary and secondary functions, dysfunctions, parafunctions and the masticatory system, as well as possible therapeutic measurements (from Bigenzahn and Fischman 1992) Copyright©1992 Karger Publishers, Basel, Switzerland. Abbreviations: *Nms* Neuromuscular system, *Tmj* temporomandibular joint, *ENT* ear-nose-throat, *At* Adenotomy, *Te* Tonsill-ectomy/-otomy

On the other, aberrant movement patterns of the masticatory muscles, the facial muscles and the tongue influence the shape of the mouth, the teeth (occlusion) and jaw position (Meilinger 1999). Therefore, in most cases, the treatment of malocclusions has not only to consist of orthodontic appliances, but also of myofunctional therapy (Saccomanno et al. 2012).

2.1.2 The Structures of the Orofacial System and the Infantile and Mature Swallowing Pattern

In general, the orofacial system consists of the anatomical structures of the vocal tract. According to their functions, the orofacial muscles can be divided into mimic muscles, muscles for mastication and swallowing. However, in the centre of the orofacial system is the tongue, which is not only responsible for articulation but also for the masticatory function, deglutition and the following four senses: taste, pain, temperature and touch.

In the resting position, the tip of the tongue contacts the front part of the hard palate (papilla incisiva), the lips are closed and the mentalis muscle is relaxed. In child development, with increasing age, the tongue has a tendency to change its position from a rather 'infantile' front to a more 'adult' (mature) back position (Condò et al. 2012). The tongue reaches its full size by the age of eight. Its size and shape can only be evaluated in relation to the size of the oral cavity.

Swallowing is necessary for:

- Ingestion and absorption of food and liquids.
- Transportation of saliva.
- Protection of the respiratory tract against aspiration.

The physiological swallowing process is initiated in the oral cavity and will be continued reflexively in the pharynx and the oesophagus. In reference to the anatomical and functional issues, four swallowing phases can be distinguished: oral preparatory (chewing phase), oral, pharyngeal and oesophageal.

2.1.3 Infantile Swallowing Pattern

This is defined as an interdental swallowing pattern persisting after the fourth year of life. Synonymous terms are 'tongue thrusting', 'tongue thrust' or 'tongue kick'. The main symptom is a slight protrusion of the tongue against or between the front teeth while swallowing or speaking. Tongue thrusting may be responsible for articulation disorders or incorrect sound production. Owing to an anterior tongue position, the alveolar sounds are produced more anteriorly, thus resulting in an interdental, addental or lateral articulation (/n/, /d/, /t/, /l/; /s/, /z/, /sch/). Articulation proficiency has to be judged with regard to age.

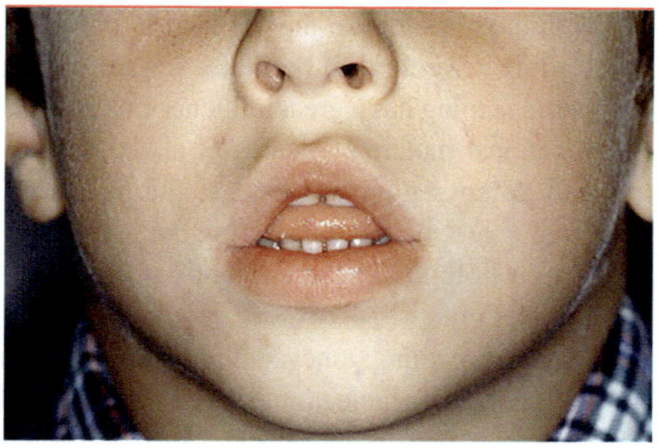

Fig. 2.2 Adenoid face: mouth breathing, incomplete lip closure, interdental tongue position (©Bigenzahn 2019)

2.1.4 Clinical Symptoms of Orofacial Dysfunction

From the perspective of the phoniatrician and speech-language pathologist, the most important signs of orofacial dysfunction include tongue thrust, infantile swallowing pattern, mouth breathing, orofacial muscle imbalance and abnormal jaw movements. Para-functional activities (e.g. oral habits, bruxism) may contribute to or aggravate dysfunctions and morphological changes. Anomalies in posture, perception or balance are often associated with orofacial dysfunctions (Clausnitzer 2001). The symptoms and their severity can vary considerably and have to be assessed age-dependently.

The following symptoms give a hint of the presence of a myofunctional disorder (Bigenzahn 1990):

- Orofacial muscle imbalance, hyperactivity of the mentalis muscle.
- Incomplete lip closure.
- Week lip structure.
- Mouth breathing: obstructed nasal breathing due to adenoid or tonsillar hyperplasia must be detected and treated!
- 'Adenoid face' (Fig. 2.2)
- Tongue protrusion: an anterior position of the tongue can be promoted by tonsillar hyperplasia!
- Interdental tongue position.
- Tongue thrust: according to Garliner (1974), tongue thrust is associated with orofacial muscle imbalance, aberrant tongue movements and abnormal lingual resting position.
- Hypersalivation, perioral dermatitis.
- Non-nutritive oral habits.
- Malocclusion (e.g. open bite).
- Articulation disorders: they are not developmentally or phonologically caused, but a result of poor oral placement and inappropriate muscle development.
- High narrow hard palate.
- Pronounced rugae palatinae (mucosal folds on the hard palate).

Moreover, in children and adults can be observed:

- Myoarthropathies.
- Orofacial pain.
- Paradontosis, tooth loss.

2.1.5 Aetiology

Various factors, e.g. genetic, structural, environmental and behavioural, are regarded as responsible for the development of orofacial dysfunctions (Hanson and Barrett 1988; Doshi and Bhad-Patil 2011; Elad et al. 2014).

A holistic multidisciplinary approach helps in identifying the following aetiological factors (Bigenzahn 2003;Friedrich et al. 2013):

1. Genetic influence.
2. Prematurity, birth weight under 1500 g.
3. Incorrectly learnt swallowing pattern: main reason is the early start of using a feeding bottle

with unphysiological nipples instead of breast-feeding or prolonged bottle feeding. Breast or bottle feeding has a great influence on orofacial functional patterns (Aizawa et al. 2010). Jaw and throat region movements during breast-feeding are smaller than during bottle feeding.

4. Unphysiological head and body posture during feeding.
5. Mouth breathing: one distinguishes between habitual and organic mouth breathing. Habitual oral breathing can be caused by a muscular dysfunction, an orofacial hypotonicity or oral (sucking) habits. Reasons for organic mouth breathing are adenoid hypertrophy, tonsillar hypertrophy, septal deviation, nasal polyps, vasomotoric or allergic rhinopathies. Recent studies reveal that the blockage of the nose with consequential abnormal airflow results in skeletal changes, such as anterior cross bite, maxillary overjet or an increase in anterior facial height (Guilleminault and Akhtar 2015). One has to keep in mind that there is a dependent relationship between appropriate nasal breathing and skeletal and soft-tissue growth and distribution. Any defect in nasal breathing may lead to sleep-disordered breathing.
6. Macroglossia: mostly a 'pseudo-macroglossia' mimics a large tongue owing to its abnormal anterior position and hypotonicity.
7. Short lingual frenulum/ankyloglossia (Acevedo et al. 2010; Defabianis 2000). A short lingual frenulum may also be associated with Obstructive Sleep Apnoea in Children (Huang et al. 2015).
8. Tonsil hypertrophy: hypertrophic tonsils may not only interfere with normal breathing, but can also add to an anterior position of the tongue in the resting position as well as during swallowing or speaking.
9. Skeletal anomalies of the jaw and palate (e.g. cleft lip palate, Malmenholt et al. 2019) or dental malocclusions: the tongue tends to adjust to the morphological conditions of the oral cavity. This leads to an abnormal resting position of the tongue with a consecutive orofacial muscle balance.
10. Bad oral habits: sucking habits, such as thumb, finger, lip or dummy sucking, but also dyskinesias, such as lip, nail or cheek biting, cause a shifting of the dental arches or the jaw. These may result in malocclusions, abnormal swallowing patterns or articulation disorders.
11. Not age-appropriate food (lack of solid food).
12. Disorders of the sensory-tactile control.
13. Central movement disorders.
14. Other diseases, such as cranial nerve paresis (facial, hypoglossus, velum paresis), myasthenia gravis, muscular hypotonia, minimal-cerebral dysfunctions, Moebius syndrome, Pierre–Robin syndrome.

2.1.6 Epidemiology

Myofunctional disorders are a common entity and have been increasingly recognised in recent decades. Higher rates of survival of very preterm infants lead to a higher incidence of neonatal feeding and swallowing disturbances (Kühn et al. 2014). Orofacial dysfunctions are observed in approximately one-third of the population.

In preschool children, the incidence of tongue thrust is reported to be 61.4%, that of complex myofunctional disorders 19.8% (Hanson and Barrett 1988). The prevalence is higher with malocclusion, e.g. with increased overjet, frontal open bite, lateral cross-bite and Class II with increased mandibular prognathism (Grabowski and Stahl 2008). Therefore, an early detection of the risk factors helps to establish preventive and treatment concepts.

2.2 Lip Frenulum, Ankyloglossia, Tongue-Tie

Ariane Hohoff

2.2.1 Oral Frenula

All told, there are seven oral frenula, which are attachments of the muscles of the lips, cheeks and tongue: the maxillary and mandibular midline frenulum (or upper lip and lower lip frenulum), the upper and lower buccal frenula, and the lower lingual frenulum (or tongue frenulum) (Fig. 2.3).

The primary function of these small folds of connective tissue, which are covered with a mucous membrane, is to keep the aforementioned muscles in harmony with the growing bones of the mouth during foetal development (Northcutt 2009). Absence, aplasia or hypoplasia of the oral frenula, and in particular of the lingual frenulum, may help in the diagnosis of Ehlers–Danlos syndrome in specific cases (Celletti et al. 2011). Infants with true umbilical cord knots show significantly higher proportions of mandibular frenulum agenesis than controls (De Felice et al. 2004).

2.2.2 Embryology of the Lingual Frenulum

Embryologically, the lingual frenulum is the part of the tongue that includes contributions from the first through the fourth pharyngeal arch, and starts its development at the fourth week of gestation (Walsh and Tunkel 2017). Tongue development begins with the growth of a medial swelling from the first pharyngeal arch, known as the tuberculum impar. Gradually, two lateral lingual swellings start to grow in the fifth week from the same arch. As the lateral swellings increase in size, they eventually merge and overlap the tuberculum impar. This merging leads to the formation of the anterior two-thirds of the tongue (Jain and Rathee 2019).

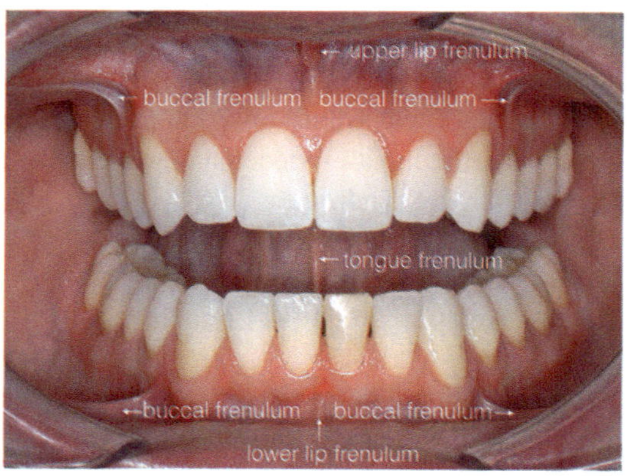

Fig. 2.3 Oral frenula (Hohoff©2021)

Although no exact embryological cause is known, in the event of, e.g. incomplete apoptosis anteriomedially of the lingual prominence, overfusion of the lateral lingual prominences or under-development of anterior tongue length, an attachment of mucosa and fibromuscular frenular tissue in the midline may occur, which may have a significant impact on tongue function, and is called ankyloglossia (Walsh and Tunkel 2017). The term originates etymologically from the Greek words **αγκύλος** (curved) and **γλώσσα** (tongue).

2.2.3 Ankyloglossia or Tongue-Tie: Definition

While in the normal sequence the lingual frenulum recedes during the first 6 months to 6 years of life, owing to growth and development (Ruffoli et al. 2005; Bai and Vaz 2014), ankyloglossia or tongue-tie is a congenital condition, defined as a remnant of tissue in the midline between the lower surface of the tongue and the floor of the mouth (IATP 2019) (Fig. 2.4a, 2.4b), resulting in limitation of tongue movement (partial ankyloglossia) or by the tongue appearing to be fused to the floor of the mouth (total ankyloglossia) (AAPD 2019).

The tongue-tie may contain some fibres of the genioglossus muscle and branches of the sublingual artery and veins (García Pola et al. 2002), and can be observed in neonates, children and adults (Suter and Bornstein 2009).

According to Becker and Mendez (2018), "there is no standard definition of ankyloglossia, and multiple classifications exist. When examined, the 'free tongue' length in newborns should be greater than 16 mm; measurements of less than 11 mm indicate moderate ankyloglossia and less than 7 mm indicates severe ankyloglossia".—Becker and Mendez (2018)

In contrast, the International Affiliation of Tongue-Tie Professionals recommends the following terminology:

1. Infant and mother dyads who have breastfeeding difficulties not solved by a lactation

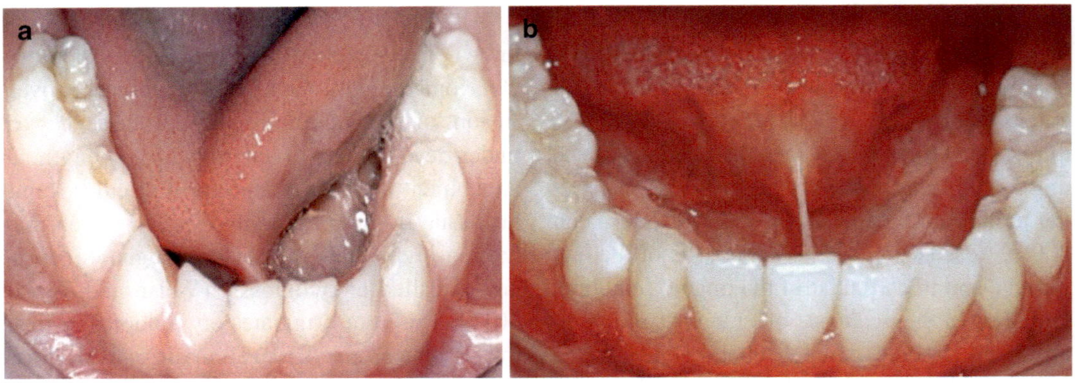

Fig. 2.4 (**a**) Ankyloglossia or tongue tie–deciduous dentition (Kleinheinz©2021). (**b**) Ankyloglossia or tongue tie–permanent dentition (Kleinheinz©2021)

consultation and judged as being due to the infant's lingual frenulum should be clinically diagnosed as having 'symptomatic tongue-tie' or 'symptomatic ankyloglossia'.

2. Infants with no breastfeeding difficulties and those with breastfeeding difficulties that are corrected after a lactation consultation should be considered as having an asymptomatic 'sublingual frenulum'.
3. The term 'short frenulum' should be abandoned, given that clinical measurement of the length of the lingual frenulum is impossible and can be based solely on subjective assessment (IATP 2020).

2.2.4 Ankyloglossia—Incidence and Prevalence

Definitive incidence and prevalence statistics are elusive because of an absence of a standard criterion or clinically practical diagnostic criteria (Francis et al. 2015). This lack of consistency in the definition and classification accounts for a wide variation in the reported prevalence of ankyloglossia (Patel et al. 2018); estimates range from 2.1% (Suter and Bornstein 2009) to 16.4% (Bai and Vaz 2014), with no racial (Suter and Bornstein 2009) but usually a mild (but insignificant) male predilection (ratio 1.5:1) (Srinivasan and Chitharanjan 2013) suggesting an X-linked inheritance (Klockars and Pitkäranta 2009; Han et al. 2012). Maternal cocaine use is reported to increase the risk of ankyloglossia to more than threefold when controlled for race and sex (Harris et al. 1992).

2.2.5 Ankyloglossia—Genetic Aspects

Most cases of ankyloglossia are sporadic (Becker and Mendez 2018), but familial ones can also occur (Walsh and Tunkel 2017); e.g. in X-linked cleft palate, a genetic developmental defect during embryogenesis which is characterised by a complete, partial or submucous cleft palate in association with ankyloglossia or short lingual frenulum, potentially abnormal uvula (e.g. absent, bifid, shortened or laterally deviated) and dental (e.g. buccal crossbite, absent or misshapen teeth) or digital abnormalities, such as mild clinodactyly or syndactyly or both (Orphanet 2019)). Autosomal dominant inheritance has also been described (Klockars 2007). Several syndromes include ankyloglossia association, such as Kindler (Suter and Bornstein 2009), Opitz, van der Woude, Beckwith–Wiedemann, Simosa and oro-facio-digital syndromes.

2.2.6 Ankyloglossia—Location

The lingual frenulum can be attached at various locations along the tongue that can be positioned either more anteriorly or more posteriorly (Walsh and Tunkel 2017).

Anterior ankyloglossia or **classic ankyloglossia** is often defined as a frenulum attachment at or near the tongue tip (Walsh and Tunkel 2017). Here, the frenulum connects the floor of the mouth with the anterior bottom of the tongue; in some instances, it can even be attached at the median part of the anterior lingual alveolar process. This classic ankyloglossia diagnostic criterion does not incorporate posterior ankyloglossia (Walsh and Tunkel 2017).

In **Posterior Ankyloglossia**, the frenulum attaches at the middle to posterior aspect of the lower surface of the tongue and connects it to the floor of the mouth (Walsh and Tunkel 2017). Posterior ankyloglossia is rarer and more difficult to assess, and a grooved instrument (a so-called 'tongue director') is mandatory for examination (Hentschel 2018) (Fig. 2.5).

The posterior ankyloglosson can be short, thickened or even submucosal; the identification can often only be achieved with palpation under the tongue; its diagnosis remains controversial, and it has been more frequently discussed in the literature only in the past decade (Walsh and Tunkel 2017).

The location of insertion is used in some of the classifications for ankyloglossia.

2.2.7 Ankyloglossia—Classification

Various classifications have been proposed (Suter and Bornstein 2009), which are based on expert opinion with respect to visual inspection and case series (Horton et al. 1969), anatomical or functional criteria or measurements (García Pola et al. 2002; Ruffoli et al. 2005; Bai and Vaz 2014). The Coryllos classification allows the distinction of four types of ankyloglossia based on the insertion point of the frenulum (Coryllos et al. 2004):

- Type 1 is the attachment of the frenulum to the tip of the tongue, usually in front of the alveolar ridge in the lower lip sulcus.

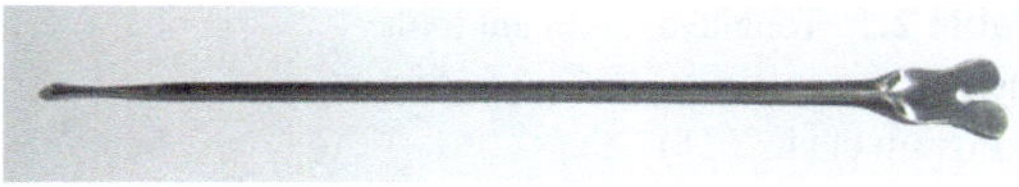

Fig. 2.5 Tongue director (Hohoff©2021)

- Type 2 is 2–4 mm behind the tongue tip and attaches on or just behind the alveolar ridge.
- Type 3 is the attachment to the mid-tongue and the middle of the floor of the mouth and is usually tighter and less elastic.
- Type 4 is essentially against the base of the tongue, and is thick, shiny and very inelastic. (N.B. according to Hentschel (2018), there is still a need for a definition of the consistency and thickness of the membrane.)

Types 1 and 2, considered 'classical', are the more common and obvious tongue-ties, and probably account for 75% of the incidence. Types 3 and 4 are less common, and since they are more difficult to visualise, are the most likely to go untreated. Type 4 is most likely to cause difficulty with bolus handling and swallowing, resulting in more significant symptoms for mother and infant (Coryllos et al. 2004).

The metrical classification according to Kotlow has been published in two versions (Kotlow 1999, 2011): Class 1 means insertion of the ankyloglosson at 0–3 mm, class 2 at 4–6 mm, class 3 at 7–9 mm and class 4 at 10–12 mm from the tip of tongue, or submucosal.

An example of a classification based on anatomical or functional criteria is the Hazelbaker score assessment (Hazelbaker 1993) (Table 2.1), with the main drawbacks of having a low inter-rater reliability, especially for the function items (Amir et al. 2006) and being time consuming (Walker et al. 2018).

Many classifications are difficult for routine clinical use (Walsh and Tunkel 2017), so the four-item Bristol Tongue Assessment Tool was developed on the basis of clinical practice, which cites the Hazelbaker Assessment Tool for Lingual Frenulum Function, but has an inter-rater reliability of 76% (Ingram et al. 2015) (Table 2.1).

Table 2.1 Tongue assessment tools

Bristol tongue assessment tool (BTAT) (Ingram et al. 2015)	Score 0	Score 1	Score 2
Tongue-tip appearance	Heart-shaped	Slight cleft/ notched	Rounded
Attachment of frenulum to lower gum ridge	At top of gum ridge	To inner aspect of gum	To floor of mouth
Lift of tongue with mouth wide (crying)	Minimal	Edges only to mid-mouth	Full to mid-mouth
Protrusion of tongue	Tip stays behind gum	Tip over gum	Tip can extend over lower lip

Assessment Tool for Lingual Frenulum Function (ATLFF) (according to Hazelbaker 1993; Drazin 1994; Forlenza et al. 2010)			
Appearance items			
Appearance of tongue when lifted	Heart-shaped	Slight cleft in tip apparent	Round or square
Attachment of lingual frenulum to tongue	Notched or under the mucosa at the tongue base	At tip	Posterior to tip
Attachment of lingual frenulum to inferior alveolar ridge	To ridge	Just below ridge	To floor of mouth or well below ridge
Elasticity of lingual frenulum	Little or no	Moderately elastic	Very elastic (excellent)
Length of lingual frenulum when tongue is lifted	Less than 1 cm	1 cm	More than 1 cm or absent frenulum
Function items			
Cupping of tongue	Poor or no cup	Side edges only, moderate cup	Entire edge, firm cup
Extension of tongue	Neither of the above or anterior or mid-tongue humps and/or dimples	Tip over lower gum only	Tip over lower lip
Lateralisation	None	Body of tongue but not tongue tip	Complete
Lift of tongue	Tip stays at alveolar ridge or tip rises only to mid-mouth with jaw closure and/or mid-tongue dimples	Only edges to mid mouth	Tip to mid-mouth
Peristalsis	None or reverse peristalsis	Partial: Originating posterior to tip	Complete anterior to posterior (originates at tip)
Snap back	Frequent or with each suck	Periodic	None
Spread of anterior tongue	Little or none	Moderate or partial	Complete

2.2.8 Ankyloglossia—Potential Sequelae in Newborns and Infants

An understanding of the relationship between tongue posture and growth and development of craniofacial structures is essential for anticipating sequelae (Jang et al. 2011).

Heated debates still persist on the clinical significance of ankyloglossia (Opara et al. 2012), e.g. with respect to breastfeeding problems in association with tongue tie (Billington et al. 2018), which had already been described in 1601 by Jean Héroard, the physician of the Dauphin of France, who became Louis XIII (Héroard 1868). Whereas the popularity of breastfeeding declined in the 1940s and 1950s, and the vast majority of infants with tongue-tie are able to bottle-feed successfully (Griffiths 2004), tongue-tie has come into the focus again owing to an increased commitment to breastfeeding in the last decade (Hentschel 2018). Nowadays, there is a reported incidence of breastfeeding problems in 25–80% of infants with ankyloglossia (Francis et al. 2015).

Mechanistically, infants with restrictive ankyloglossia cannot extend their tongues over the lower gum line to perform a proper seal and therefore use their jaws to keep the breast in their mouth (Francis et al. 2015) resulting in excessive jaw excursions, jaw tremor, pulling off the breast and hypersalivation (Henry and Hayman 2014), poor latching, frequent loss of latch, prolonged feeding, irritability with feeding, poor weight gain, inability to breastfeed (Walsh and Tunkel 2017), refusing the breast or engorgement (Francis et al. 2015), nipple pain (Dollberg and Botzer 2011), nipple ulceration, bleeding or infection, poor milk let-down or incomplete emptying owing to inadequate infant sucking and mastitis (Walsh and Tunkel 2017). Therefore, tongue-tie may result in a lower lactation rate or a shorter duration of breastfeeding, neither of which is desirable (Hentschel 2018).

According to Walker et al. (2018), mothers of newborns with a visible cord were 3.65 times more likely to report pain during breastfeeding, and the average tongue tip-frenulum length of these newborns was 5.1 mm, compared with a mean of 9.11 mm in the whole sample ($n = 100$, kappa coefficient 0.91, interrater reliability 0.82); for each millimetre decrease in tongue tip-frenulum length mothers were 22% more likely to report nipple pain (Walker et al. 2018). However, pain symptoms during breastfeeding are not unique to ankyloglossia; in the context of other problems that may affect feeding (e.g. maternal experience, milk production, breast and nipple anatomy) whether frenula are or are not symptomatic may be difficult to determine (Walsh and Tunkel 2017). Furthermore, psychological sequelae, including maternal stress, postpartum depression and mother-infant bonding are important next steps in the research on infants with ankyloglossia (Hill 2019).

Despite all the above mentioned reports, there is no clear association between tongue tie and breastfeeding problems, as some infants who undoubtedly have tongue-tie can be breastfed without any problems (Hentschel 2018). A recent review (Hatami et al. 2022) could not show a statistical correlation between tongue-tie severity, as measured by pre-treatment assessment tools, and post-operative outcome. Nevertheless, most authorities in the field of infant feeding and lactation agree that breastfeeding problems are common signs of a clinically significant tongue tie, while the sole presence of a visible lingual frenulum is not. In contrast, the lack of a visible frenulum does not rule out the diagnosis of clinically significant tongue-tie, since submucosal ties, also called posterior tongue-tie, may interfere with efficient breastfeeding (Dollberg and Botzer 2011).

A minority of surveyed paediatricians (10%) and otolaryngologists (30%) believes that ankyloglossia affects feeding, whereas 69% of lactation consultants feel that it frequently causes breastfeeding problems (Messner and Lalakea 2000). In infants, ankyloglossia accompanied by displacement of the epiglottis and larynx may lead to unstable and slightly low oxygen saturation, clinically shown by snoring, harsh respiratory sounds and dyspnoea (Mukai et al. 1991).

2.2.9 Ankyloglossia—Potential Sequelae in Later Life

Further functional problems of ankyloglossia, e.g. on speech, were described by Aristotle (350 BC) and Celsus (50 AD) (Patel et al. 2018). Speech alteration, speech impediments, articulation errors and problems with fluent speech are named (Hentschel 2018). Systematic reviews, however, found no significant data to suggest a causative association between ankyloglossia and speech articulation problems (Webb et al. 2013; Wang et al. 2022).

Sleep-disordered breathing (Yoon et al. 2017a), difficulties in smiling (Northcutt 2009), kissing, deglutition, moving food boluses or consumption of licking foods may occur in ankyloglossia; spilling, dribbling, drooling, choking, 'excess wind' (both, eructation and flatulence), spitting while talking or playing wind instruments can also be a consequence and lead to social concerns or difficulties with self-esteem and psychological stress (Chinnadurai et al. 2015).

The mechanical problems can also lead to a lack of oral clearance (ability to clean the teeth or to lick the lip with the tongue (Chinnadurai et al. 2015)), so the hypothesis arose that dental caries may occur (Chandrashekar et al. 2014). However, there remains no high-quality evidence to support a correlation between ankyloglossia or maxillary lip tie and an increased risk of early childhood caries (Patel et al. 2018), and the current recommendation in both kinds of tie is that when surgical release is considered owing to higher caries risk, anticipatory guidance and other preventive measures should be emphasised first (AAPD 2019).

Two elements of physiology are essential for understanding the influence of the lingual frenulum on the dentition and the development of malocclusions:

- First, muscles determine the shape of bone—if the lingual frenulum is too short, the tongue will not generate enough upward pressure to create a normal width of the palate or upper dentition, potentially resulting in gnathic uni- or bi-lateral crossbite or lingually tipped upper premolars and molars, and thus smaller upper dental arch circumferences, causing crowding of the anterior teeth.
- Second, food is swallowed by a vacuum force in the mouth, creating a seal and giving the palate a normal shape—if the frenulum is short, upward tongue movement is restricted, the tongue must thrust forward to create a seal at the front of the mouth, so cases of maxillary protrusion and anterior open bite might result (Northcutt 2009), with the latter potentially resulting in subsequent difficulty in chewing food (Seo et al. 2014).

The inability to raise the tongue to the top of the palate prevents a normal adult swallowing pattern and leads to an infantile pattern, where the tongue position is in between the teeth. The restriction of free upward and backward movement of the tongue may result in exaggerated anterior thrusting of the tongue against the mandible (Williams and Waldron 1985), producing maxillary hypo-development (Suter and Bornstein 2009) and mandibular prognathism (Horton et al. 1969; Suter and Bornstein 2009). Development of mandibular prognathism with maxillary hypo-development resolved after lingual frenectomy in a 7-year follow-up case report, owing to spontaneous upper arch expansion, thereby avoiding the need for orthognathic surgery (Defabianis 2000).

Localised gingival recession on the lingual aspect of the mandibular incisors has been associated with ankyloglossia in some cases where attachment of the frenulum causes gingival retraction (AAPD 2019). Separation of the lower incisors is also attributed to ankyloglossia (Chinnadurai et al. 2015; Patel et al. 2018), as is mandibular incisor irregularity (Walsh and Tunkel 2017).

In *deciduous dentition*, according to a study by Melink et al. (2010), short frenula linguae (defined as an inability of the lifted tongue to contact the maxillary central incisors) were only found in children with posterior crossbite and were found to be statistically significantly correlated with a narrower maxilla in the intercanine und intermolar regions. Confounders of this study, with 30 children with and 30 children without unilateral crossbite, however, could have been non-nutritive sucking habits, surplus, reliability of the method, i. e. inter–/intra-rater reliability has also not been described.

In *6-year-old children* ($n = 962$), according to a publication by García Pola et al. (2002), in contrast to the above mentioned study, no significant association was shown between crossbites, overbites or narrow palates and a short lingual frenulum. The latter was present in 2.4% of the children, and defined as lingual mobility of less than 51%, while proportioning the distance between homolateral canines at mouth opening when the tip of the tongue touches the palatal papilla, and the distance during maximum mouth opening at the same points of reference. However, the reliability of that method in this transversal epidemiological study with only one examiner was not tested.

In *6-to 12-year-old children* ($n = 200$), according to a study by Ruffoli et al. (2005), those with anterior or posterior open bite or crossbite showed mean values of frenulum length similar to or even longer than that of children with normal bite; in contrast, those with deep bite and Angle class III (Angle class I: the mesiobuccal cusp of the upper first permanent molar occludes with the mesiobuccal groove of the lower first permanent molar; Angle class II: the former occludes anterior to the latter; Angle class III: the former occludes distal to the latter (Angle 1899)) possessed the lowest mean value of frenulum length which was statistically significant. The authors discuss that low tongue posture due to ankyloglossia could result in mandibular hyperdevelopment (the frenulum length was determined directly by measurement of the length of the frenulum intraorally, but reliability of the method was not tested).

In *6-to 67-year-old subjects* ($n = 302$) of different ethnicities, an association between restricted tongue mobility, narrowing of the maxillary dental width and elongation of the soft palate could be shown within the frame of a cross-sectional study with reliability rates ≥98% (Yoon et al. 2017a).

In *7-to 12-year-old children* ($n = 80$), according to a study by Sepet et al. (2015), no significant differences between different types of ankyloglossia (mild to severe as assessed according to Kotlow 1999) and mandibular incisor irregularity or occlusion types were found. A significant positive correlation was determined between lingual frenulum length and mandibular incisor irregularity and age (reliability of the method and number of investigators not given).

In *9- to 17-year-old-children* ($n = 700$), the differences between groups from regular and from special schools (50% each) with respect to tongue-tie (as assessed by measurements of the free tongue according to Kotlow (1999)) were not significant; maxillary transverse deficiency constituted the greatest malocclusion trait (46%), followed by crowding (41%), spacing (21%) and anterior open bite (19%) (Vaz and Bai 2015). Interestingly, the lower grades of tongue-tie were associated with high lower incisor crowding, while the higher grades of tongue-tie showed lower grades of irregularity. Short, tight frenula were more associated with maxillary constriction, anterior open bite and spacing of the lower anterior teeth. Angle class II malocclusions were associated with grade I and II tongue-ties to a greater extent than grade III and IV tongue-ties, and Angle class III malocclusion was found to be highest (4%) in grade IV tongue-ties. Weaknesses of the study were the lacking calibration of an unknown number of raters.

In *adults*, according to a study by Srinivasan and Chitharanjan (2013), significantly reduced maxillary and mandibulary intercanine widths and maxillary intermolar widths were diagnosed in patients with ankyloglossia ($n = 57$) compared with patients without ($n = 60$). Ankyloglossia was assessed by measuring the distance between the tip of the tongue and the point of attachment of the lingual frenulum. The study was performed by one investigator, but the reliability of the method was not given.

In *adults with skeletal class III* (i.e. where the mandible is located more anteriorly than normal), according to a study by Jang et al. (2011), significantly longer median sagittal frenulum lengths (i.e. tongue-tie tendency) and significantly more reduction in maximum mouth opening were present than in age-matched peers with skeletal class II (i.e. where the mandible is located more distally than normal) and skeletal class I (i.e. where the mandible is located within the normal range). In this study, each of the skeletal groups consisted of 50 patients and the error of the method was given, but the number of investigators for intra-oral measurements remained unclear.

A prominent lingual frenulum may dislodge an individual's lower denture whenever the tongue tip is raised (Horton et al. 1969; Williams and Waldron 1985).

2.2.10 Ankyloglossia—Clinical Signs and Examination

As a tongue-tie can only be noticed if an infant lifts its tongue spontaneously (for instance during crying), apart from a meticulous inspection by an experienced person, the oral cavity should be routinely inspected in the first days of life, especially when the mother reports breastfeeding problems. For this purpose, the tongue should be lifted upwards with either a special, paddle-like instrument with a groove (Fig. 2.5), or with two spatulas held in parallel, with the midline of the tongue between them: then from a lateral view, a tongue-tie appears like a triangular sail with its base at the floor of the mouth and the top of the sail at the lower surface of the tongue close to the tip, and the three sides of the triangular sail can be measured with a graded periodontal probe (Hentschel 2018). The closer the above-mentioned sail is moved towards the alveolar ridge, the more the mobility of the tongue will be restricted, but the grade of restriction also depends on the distance between the mouth floor and the lower surface of the tongue and the elasticity of the membrane (Hentschel 2018).

In cases of posterior tongue-tie, the anterior part of the tongue often shows a normal mobility upwards and laterally, but the posterior part of the tongue is fixed downwards to the floor of the mouth and limits its protrusion. The rigid membrane infiltrating the posterior part of the lower surface of the tongue can sometimes only be identified by manual palpation (Hentschel 2018).

In addition to its attachment being more anterior or more posterior, the lingual frenulum may be abnormally short, thickened, tight (Chinnadurai et al. 2015), fibrosed (Patel et al. 2018), or cord-like, more like a planar tendon, but it can also be translucent, like parchment (Hentschel 2018). The diagnosis of a palpable cord can vary among examiners and should be interpreted with caution when evaluating newborns for posterior tongue tie (Walker et al. 2018). Recently, a nationally mandatory, Brazilian neonatal tongue screening test for detecting ankyloglossia in newborns has been proven to be neither reliable nor valid, including the danger that false positive results may lead to overtreatment and unnecessary health expenditures (Brandão et al. 2018).

Sometimes, the 'N point', which is where the tongue shifts from horizontal to vertical in the mouth upon extended opening or swallowing, thus creating the 'N angle', can also be indicative of ankyloglossia. Distal to the N point, the dorsum of the tongue lies flat, which indicates that it is tied to the floor of the mouth by the lingual frenulum, preventing the tongue from rising (Northcutt 2009). Further signs of symptomatic tongue-tie include tethering of the tongue, dimpling (Walsh and Tunkel 2017), a 'w-shaped' (Bowen 2019), 'heart shaped' (Walsh and Tunkel 2017; Walker et al. 2018) (Fig. 2.6) or 'notched' tongue on protrusion, inability to protrude the tongue beyond the lower gums (UNICEF 2019), beyond the mandibular alveolar ridge (Walker et al. 2018), beyond the edges of the lower incisors (Bowen 2019), to the maxillary alveolar ridge (behind the upper incisors) (Bowen 2019) or beyond the lip vermillion border (Walsh and Tunkel 2017).

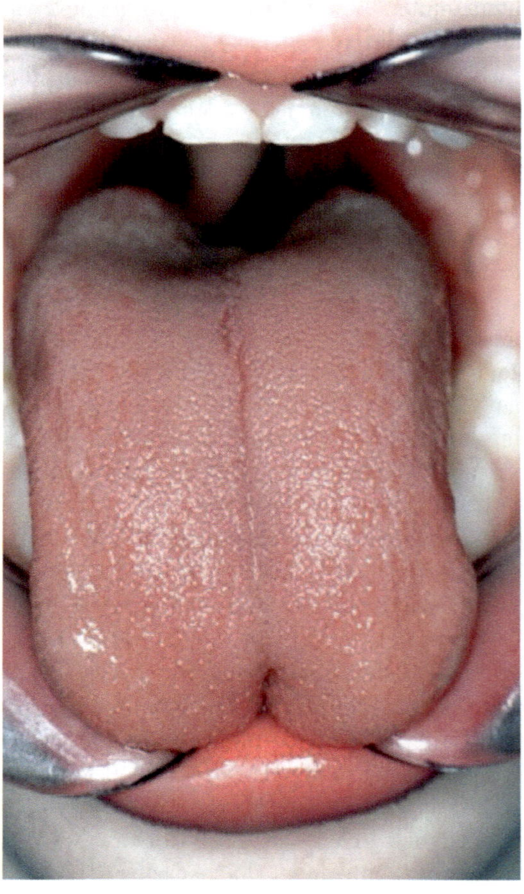

Fig. 2.6 Ankyloglossia or tongue tie leading to a w- or heart-shaped or notched form of the tongue on protrusion (Kleinheinz©2021)

The tongue tip can also be flattened or square when the tongue is extended, and there might be an inability to move the tongue sideways. The tongue's range of motion (i.e. the ratio of mouth opening with tongue tip to the maxillary incisive papilla and maximal inter-incisal mouth opening) could be an initial screening tool to assess for restrictions in tongue mobility (Yoon et al. 2017b).

Ulcerations of the lingual frenulum resulting from oral sex (Williams and Waldron 1985) can be falsely classified as tongue-tie.

2.2.11 Ankyloglossia—Treatment

Some propose that a short frenulum will elongate spontaneously with progressive stretching and thinning of the frenulum with age and use, making treatment unnecessary (Lalakea and Messner 2003).

Research is lacking in non-surgical treatments, which include complementary and alternative medicine approaches, e.g. craniosacral therapy, myofascial release and other chiropractic therapies, positioning techniques and lactation intervention, speech or oral motor therapy and stretching exercises (Francis et al. 2015) or case report-based options with tongue elevators. These are removable orthodontic plates for the lower jaw with occlusal rests and several retentive elements, where the acrylic base occupies the entire sublingual space, except for the lingual frenulum; the function of the tongue elevator is to keep the tongue in a higher position than usual, which is accomplished by the sheer volume of the acrylic base; the positional change induced by the tongue elevator is considered to induce dento-alveolar effects, e.g. intrusion of the lower posterior teeth and expansion of the upper arch (Seo et al. 2014).

In some instances, nipple shields, which are however not risk-free, may be helpful during breastfeeding of a child with ankyloglossia (Henry and Hayman 2014).

As with most periodontal conditions, elimination of plaque-induced gingival inflammation can minimise gingival recession without any surgical intervention; when recession continues even after oral hygiene management, surgical intervention of the ankyloglosson may be indicated (AAPD 2019).

Concerning surgical treatment, there is continuing controversy dating back many centuries (Opara et al. 2012). Documented midwifery practice guides published in 1487 recommended midwives to perform the release of tongue-ties, while in 1480 another cautions against midwives acting without a physician's advice (Henry and Hayman 2014). In 1742, Petit introduced a slit in the flat end of a grooved instrument by which he could protect the deep lingual artery during tongue-tie surgery (Horton et al. 1969). Up to the nineteenth century, midwives not only tore the frenulum with dirty fingernails (they used to keep one sharp), but in addition stripped it up to the tongue. The wound thus created often resulted in an infection, which spread to other intra-oral structures. Additionally, the stripped-up tongue occasionally fell backwards and caused asphyxia by 'tongue swallowing', and haemorrhage from the lingual artery too often proved fatal. An inevitable scar followed, and as a result, the tongue secondarily became fixed in a pathological condition of ankyloglossia (Horton et al. 1969). Complications of this procedure included bleeding and injury to the muscles (Opara et al. 2012).

According to the AAPD (2019), a complete orthodontic evaluation, diagnosis and treatment plan are necessary before any surgical intervention in the event of ankyloglossia, and surgical interventions for functional relief should be considered on an individual basis; dressing placement or the use of antibiotics is not necessary. Postoperative recommendations include maintaining a soft diet, regular oral hygiene, analgesics as needed, and exercises to prevent reattachment of the wound and relapse of the previous symptoms associated with the tongue or lip-tie (AAPD 2019). The use of electrosurgery or laser technology for frenotomies/frenectomies has demonstrated a shorter operative working time, a better ability to control bleeding, reduced intra- and post-operative pain and discomfort, fewer postoperative complications (e.g. swelling, infection), no need for suture removal, and increased patient acceptance—these procedures require extensive training as well as skilful technique and patient management (AAPD 2019).

Because of the limited evidence available to date, no specific surgical methods for treatment of tongue-tie can be favoured (Suter and Bornstein 2009), among which are frenotomy (also termed frenulotomie), frenuloplasty and frenectomy.

Frenotomy, i.e. simple cutting or incision of the frenulum (AAPD 2019), fell out of favour when the popularity of breastfeeding declined in the 1940s and 1950s (Griffiths 2004). Nowadays, private lactation consultants are the main persons recommending this surgical intervention (Muldoon et al. 2017). It is a minor procedure, often performed with scissors without anaesthetics (Patel et al. 2018). Some physicians choose to give sucrose before frenotomy, to minimise and help with the pain (Becker and Mendez 2018). In children older than 4 months, anaesthesia is usually required because of the infant's strength and awareness (Ballard et al. 2002). The infant is placed supine with the elbows held flexed securely close to the face and the assistant's index finger on the chin for stabilisation; the tongue is lifted gently with a sterile grooved retractor to expose the frenulum (Ballard et al. 2002). A frenotomy may be accomplished by incising 2–3 mm into the lingual frenulum (Opara et al. 2012), directly at the surface of the tongue (Hentschel 2018), at the thinnest portion of the frenulum (Ballard et al. 2002). The posterior limit of the frenulum incision is the anterior genioglossus muscle, and caution must be taken because orifices of submandibular and lingual salivary glands open under the tongue on the floor of the mouth (Steehler et al. 2012). Care must also be taken not to incise any vascular tissue, i.e. the base of the tongue, the genioglossus muscle or the gingival mucosa (Ballard et al. 2002). There should be minimal blood loss (not more than a drop or two), collected on sterile gauze (Ballard et al. 2002). Afterwards, pressure should be applied with gauze with or without oxymetazoline for immediate haemostasis, then post-procedure non-nutritive sucking or breastfeeding should be used for pain control; adequate breastfeeding dyad support services and follow-up to assess feeding improvement as well as possible complications should be available (Walsh and Tunkel 2017). Parents should understand that frenotomy does not guarantee improved breastfeeding (Henry and Hayman 2014).

One attempt to perform a meta-analysis was impossible because of the paucity and heterogeneity of research; thus, a systematic review of comparative studies was published instead; bottle feeding and social concerns, such as the ability to use the tongue to eat ice cream or to clean the mouth from leftovers after meals, improved more in groups treated with frenotomy; supplementary bottle feeding decreased over time in case series (Chinnadurai et al. 2015). Two cohort studies of poor quality reported improvement in articulation and intelligibility with treatment, but benefits in word, sentence and fluent speech were not demonstrated, so that given the lack of good-quality studies and limitations in the measurement of outcomes the authors concluded that the strength of the evidence for the effect of surgical tongue tie interventions to improve speech and articulation was insufficient (Chinnadurai et al. 2015). This is especially evident, as no standard definitions or established norms of tongue mobility exist, so further research is needed to determine such parameters (Chinnadurai et al. 2015).

According to a second systematic review, a small body of evidence suggests that frenotomy may be associated with mother-reported improvements in breastfeeding, and potentially in nipple pain (Francis et al. 2015). But with small, short-term studies with inconsistent methodology, the strength of evidence is low to insufficient, and there is a paucity of data on the durability of outcomes after frenotomy (Francis et al. 2015).

In a third systematic review on infants younger than 3 months of age with tongue-tie, the authors found five randomised clinical trials: two of them demonstrated no change, one study showed objective improvement of breastfeeding following frenotomy, four publications showed a reduction in maternal nipple pain; no adverse effects following frenotomy were reported (O'Shea et al. 2017). All trials, however, had serious methodological shortcomings with respect to sample size or blinding or both, and none was able to report whether frenotomy led to long-term successful breastfeeding (O'Shea et al. 2017).

Harm from (surgical) treatment of ankyloglossia is usually mild to non-existent (Chinnadurai et al. 2015). Among studies reporting harm, bleeding has been most frequently named and described as minor and limited, but the amount of posterior extension of the incision is not clearly defined and appears to be left up to the clinical expertise of the person executing the procedure (Francis et al. 2015). Nevertheless, rare but potentially life-threatening consequences of lingual frenotomies have been described in the scientific literature, such as profuse bleeding, respiratory distress, severe anaemia, hypovolaemic shock and neonatal sepsis (Opara et al. 2012), sublingual infected haematoma (Isaiah and Pereira 2013) and upper airway collapse (Suter and Bornstein 2009). Care must be taken not to damage the submandibular and sublingual ducts of the salivary glands, and not to touch the lingual artery or veins, which can become varicose with increasing age at the floor of the mouth; and it must be taken into account that, at a very young age, haemophilia might not yet have become apparent, which could lead to bleeding (Hentschel 2018). The need for surgical retreatment due to failure of the initial procedure is difficult to assess (Walsh and Tunkel 2017), but rates for revision have been reported to range from 2.6% (Steehler et al. 2012) to 6.5% (Argiris et al. 2011).

Until now, there is no international consensus on the appropriateness of frenotomy among newborns, and in some countries, the desire to increase rates of breastfeeding has resulted in runaway rates and huge regional variations in rates of ankyloglossia and frenotomy (Lisonek et al. 2017). As part of the decision-making process, a comprehensive head and neck evaluation for factors such as retrognathia and palatal abnormalities must be considered before proceeding with frenotomy (Ghaheri et al. 2017).

Frenectomy Fig. 2.7 is defined as complete excision, i.e. removal of the whole frenulum (Suter and Bornstein 2009) to heal by secondary intention (AAPD 2019). Frenectomy and frenuloplasty, both with complete release of the frenulum by scalpel, laser or electrocautery and with plastic closure, usually require the child to undergo general anaesthesia, but result in lower recurrence rates than in frenotomy (Patel et al. 2018).

Frenuloplasty refers to excisions involving sutures releasing the frenulum and correcting the anatomical situation (AAPD 2019) (Figs. 2.8).

Various methods have been described (Suter and Bornstein 2009). In the event of a need for additional length, in order to distribute tissue tensions in different directions, a Z-plasty can be performed (Horton et al. 1969) (Figs. 2.8a–g).

One poor-quality randomised controlled trial reported improved articulation after Z-frenuloplasty compared with horizontal-to-vertical frenuloplasty (Chinnadurai et al. 2015). Sometimes, post-operative management of tongue-tie surgery includes active kinaesthetic therapy and functional re-education for a month (Suter and Bornstein 2009). Multifaceted supportive educational programmes establishing consistent multi-disciplinary assessment and availability of online information for health professionals and consumers may help to reduce the rate of tongue-tie release (Dixon et al. 2018).

2.2.12 Maxillary Frenulum

The maxillary frenulum, also called the superior labial frenum, median labial frenum or maxillary labial frenum (Patel et al. 2018), is highly associated with a number of syndromes and developmental anomalies (Delli et al. 2013). Its attachment can be classified with respect to its anatomical insertion level as:

(a) Mucosal (frenal fibres are attached up to the mucogingival junction).
(b) Gingival (frenal fibres are inserted within the attached gingiva).
(c) Papillary (frenal fibres are extended into the interdental papilla).
(d) Penetrating papilla (frenal fibres cross the alveolar process and extend up to the palatine papilla).

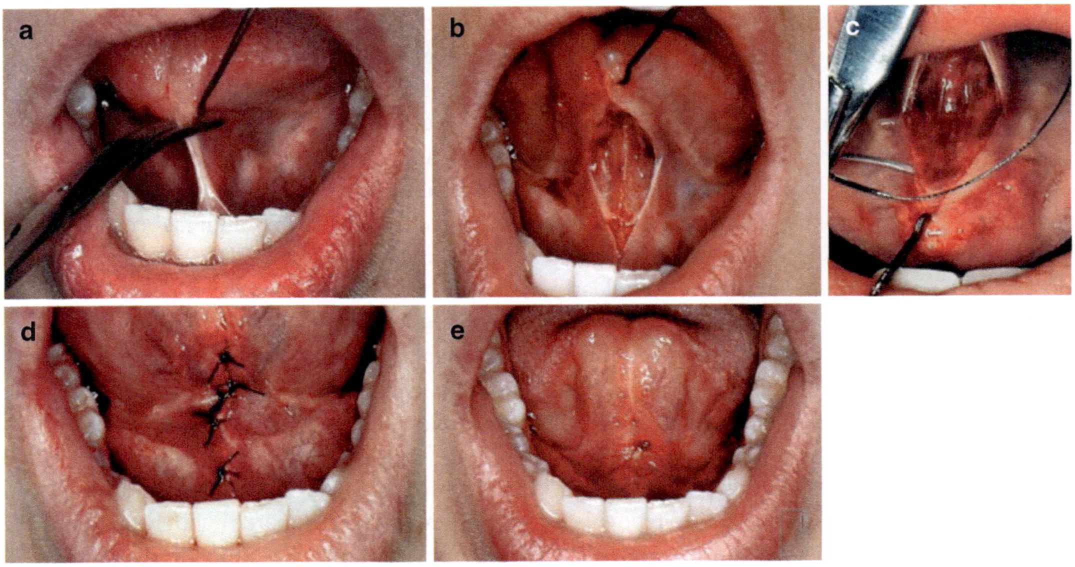

Figs. 2.7 (**a–e**) Frenectomy (Kleinheinz©2021)

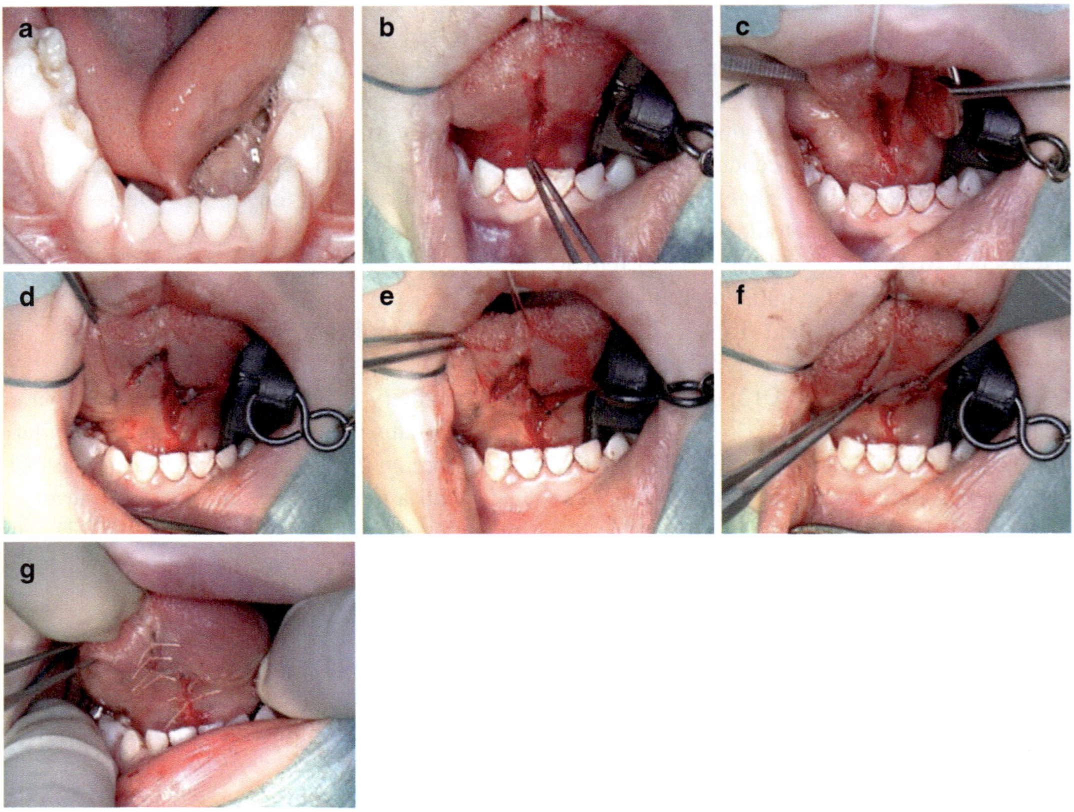

Figs. 2.8 (**a–g**) Z-plasty (Kleinheinz©2021)

(e) where a) and b) are the more common types (AAPD 2019).

If the attachment is tight, it may (like tongue-tie) interfere with lip flanging, resulting in poorer weight gain due to poorer latch and prolonged and frequent breastfeeding with poor milk transfer, with milk leaking from the baby's mouth, irritability from swallowing excessive air, clicking or smacking noises (AAPD 2019) due to tongue recoil, colic and reflux-like symptoms in the children and plugged ducts, pain during feeding, flattened, compressed and injured nipples and mastitis (Patel et al. 2018).

A hyperplastic labial frenulum that inserts into the free or marginal gingiva has been suggested to interfere with proper oral hygiene measures, potentially leading to labial cervical caries as well as initiation and progression of gingival/periodontal disease, but to date no evidence supports this conclusion although anecdotal speculation persists; further research is required to substantiate this cause-and-effect relationship (AAPD 2019).

A frenulum that attaches too close to the gingival margin can cause tooth rotations (Northcutt 2009). A hypertrophic, high-inserted frenulum may be involved in the aetiology of a diastema between the central incisors (Delli et al. 2013; Srinivasan and Chitharanjan 2013) (Fig. 2.9) and post-orthodontic relapse (AAPD 2019).

Diastema due to a hypertrophic frenulum is true in only 4% of the patients with that gap, a condition also found under the terms 'dents du bonheur' or 'lucky teeth'. To confirm the presence of a high labial frenulum insertion, a simple test of ischaemia can be performed, in which the location of alveolar insertion is observed while simultaneously lifting and stretching the upper lip. If this activity causes blanching and tension of the interdental papilla, a high frenulum insertion can be considered as the main cause for diastema, and frenectomy with or without gingivoplasty can be performed (Kapusevska et al. 2014). Treatment is also suggested when the attachment causes a diastema wider than two millimetres, which is rarely known to close spontaneously during further development (AAPD 2019) (N.B. before surgical treatment of the maxillary labial frenulum it must be ensured that the diastema is not caused by a- or hypo-plasia of the lateral incisors (the so called 'false diastema') or by a mesiodens (the latter can only be detected radiologically)!). There is general agreement between paediatric dentists and orthodontists that a frenectomy should not be performed before the permanent canines erupt and that the operation should follow orthodontic closure of the space (AAPD 2019), as closure of the maxillary midline diastema with a prominent frenulum is more predictable with frenectomy and concomitant orthodontic treatment than with frenectomy alone (Suter et al. 2014).

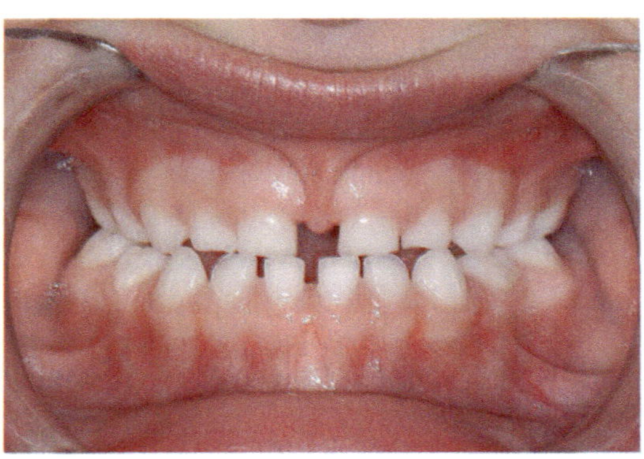

Fig. 2.9 Maxillary frenulum and diastema (Hohoff©2021)

A multicausal nature of diastema should always be considered, as in 49% of cases hereditary factors, in 14% disproportions and discrepancies in the dental arch (e.g. ectopic canines), in 11% inborn or acquired missing teeth, in 10% harmful habits, in 6% pathological objects between the central incisors, in 3% iatrogenic factors and in another 3% periodontal diseases are causative (Kapusevska et al. 2014). Orthodontically a midline diastema in the deciduous dentition is physiological and usually a good prognostic sign that there might be sufficient room in the dental arch for the placement of the permanent teeth.

When the permanent central incisors first erupt their crowns may incline distally (a condition also leading to a usually transitory diastema and named as 'ugly duckling stage' (Elhag and Abdulghani 2015) as permanent canines, which erupt much later, use the roots of the permanent lateral incisors as a guidance for eruption and displace them. By that—as in a chain reaction—the roots of the permanent central incisors also become displaced and the condition of root crowding occurs. With the eruption of the permanent lateral incisors and canines, the transitory diastema may reduce or even close, making active treatment of that condition unnecessary. Thus, when treating patients with diastema, dental and not chronological age should be considered, as an incorrect determination of high frenulum insertion as a reason for diastema, and its subsequent removal, can lead to the appearance of gummy smile (Kapusevska et al. 2014).

Torn upper labial frenula have been reported as a result of both non-accidental (a direct blow to the face (Maguire et al. 2007)) and accidental trauma (instrumental delivery (Gurung and Cohn 2015), oral intubation (Price et al. 2000), motor vehicle accidents with airbag deployment (Morrison et al. 1988) and children who fall while in early stages of ambulation (Gurung and Cohn 2015)). They can be associated with profuse bleeding, but heal spontaneously without long-term consequences (AAP 2009). An injured frenulum in combination with other traumas and doubtful history might point to child abuse (Delli et al. 2013).

The involvement of a hyperplastic upper labial frenulum in the pathogenesis of peri-implant diseases remains uncertain, and the superiority of laser treatment in relation to conventional surgical methods has not yet been demonstrated in literature (Delli et al. 2013).

2.2.13 Lower Labial Frenulum

Mixed reddish and whitish, partially ulcerated plaques at a markedly thickened lower labial frenulum with ulcerations covered by fibrin may be a sign of oral syphilis (Hertel et al. 2014). In 1003 15-year-old subjects, 1% had true gingival recession; frenal pull was the second more highly associated factor (Stoner and Mazdyasna 1980).

2.2.14 Conclusion

Inspection of all oral frenula and their function should be a part of the routine neonatal examination, whether the infant is breastfeed or not. Oral frenula can provide hints towards maternal cocaine abuse, syndromes, child abuse, sexual practices and sexually transmitted diseases. Oral frenula represent a typical interdisciplinary problem and should also be a part of the first examination of each lactation consultant, logopaedist, dentist, dental specialist, maxillofacial surgeon, paediatrician, speech pathologist and otolaryngologist. Accurate diagnosis requires a comprehensive understanding of the anatomical range of normal and abnormal tongue, lip and cheek movement, lip closure, (neonatal) swallow function, nasal airway, jaw size, growth and development.

Surgical treatment of ankyloglossia should only be considered after the following combination of signs:

(a) Poor breastfeeding symptoms, such as poor latch and increased duration of feeding, are still present after a lactation consultation.
(b) The infant meets the criteria for poor breastfeeding (hunger, long feeds, restlessness, poor weight gain).
(c) Clinical evidence of a tongue tie is present (Hentschel 2018).

The ability to make definitive practice guidelines is limited by our current understanding of ankyloglossia and the lack of a uniform, reliable—but urgently needed—classification, and this is why to date there are differences in treatment recommendations among paediatricians, otolaryngologists, lactation consultants, speech pathologists, surgeons and dental specialists (AAPD 2019). Additional research is needed for better understanding of the complexity of infant feeding and the role of ankyloglossia (Walsh and Tunkel 2017). Furthermore, as there is a great confusion over terminology ('frenum', 'fraenum', 'fraenum', 'phrenum', 'frenulum' (Maguire et al. 2007), 'frenums', 'frenulums', 'frenulae', 'frena'), an internationally uniform nomenclature is urgently needed, too.

There is evidence that surgical treatment of ankyloglossia in order to treat a lingual gingival recession is not an effective therapy without initial thorough plaque control (Suter and Bornstein 2009). Elimination of gingival inflammation often stops recessions without any additional invasive treatment.

Currently, there is only limited evidence that tongue-tie might represent a (co)factor in the development of malocclusions, as most of the studies have not given the reliability of their method of determining it. Until further research has clarified this issue, a clinician, however, should not overlook potential associations and should closely follow children with ankyloglossia (Póvoa-Santos et al., 2024).

Frenotomy, frenectomy and frenuloplasty are the main surgical treatment options to release or remove an ankyloglosson. While plotting a decision-tree to decide between these different interventions and also their timing would be desirable, because of the limited evidence available no specific surgical method can be favoured. More controlled clinical trials and a uniform classification system for 'ankyloglossia' are needed, and furthermore, clear outcome parameters to justify surgery need to be standardised (Suter and Bornstein 2009).

If there is the suspicion that the maxillary or mandibular frenulum could lead to a diastema, surgical intervention should be performed only after the permanent canines have erupted, after a radiological control has been performed to exclude that the diastema is due to other reasons (e.g. aplasia of the lateral incisors or foreign objects, e. g. mesiodens), after a consultation with an orthodontist and in conjunction with an orthodontic treatment to close the diastema.

References

AAP (American Academy of Pediatrics) (2009) A pediatric guide to children's oral health. AAP (American Academy of Pediatrics), Elk Grove Village IL

AAPD (American Academy of Pediatric Dentistry) (2019) Policy on Management of the Frenulum in Pediatric Dental Patients. https://www.aapd.org/globalassets/media/policies_guidelines/p_mgmt_frenulum.pdf. Accessed 12 Dec 2019

Acevedo AC, da Fonseca JAC, Grinham J et al (2010) Autosomal-dominant ankyloglossia and tooth number anomalies. J Dent Res 89(2):128–132

Aizawa M, Mizuno K, Tamura M (2010) Neonatal sucking behavior: comparison of perioral movement during breast-feeding and bottle feeding. Pediatr Int 52(1):104–108

Amir LH, James JP, Donath SM (2006) Reliability of the Hazelbaker assessment tool for lingual frenulum function. Int Breastfeed J 1(1):3. https://doi.org/10.1186/1746-4358-1-3

Angle EH (1899) Classification of malocclusion. Dental Cosmos 41:248–264

Argiris K, Vasani S, Wong G et al (2011) Audit of tongue-tie division in neonates with breastfeeding difficulties: how we do it. Clin Otolaryngol 36(3):256–260

Bai PM, Vaz AC (2014) Ankyloglossia among children of regular and special schools in Karnataka, India: a prevalence study. J Clin Diagn Res 8(6):ZC36–ZC38

Ballard J, Auer C, Khoury J (2002) Ankyloglossia: assessment, incidence, and effect of frenuloplasty on the breastfeeding dyad. Pediatrics 110(5):1–6

Becker S, Mendez MD (2018) Ankyloglossia. In: StatPearls [Internet]. StatPearls Publishing, Treasure Island, FL. https://www.ncbi.nlm.nih.gov/books/NBK482295/. Accessed 24 June 2020

Bigenzahn W (1990) Myofunktionelle Störungen der Orofazialregion im Kindesalter. Klinik-Ätiologie-Therapie (Myofunctional disorders of the orofacial region in childhood clinical etiology therapy). Laryngol Rhinol Otol 69(5):231–236

Bigenzahn W (2003) Orofaziale Dysfunktionen im Kindesalter: Grundlagen, Klinik, Ätiologie, Diagnostik und Therapie (orofacial dysfunctions in childhood: basics, clinic, aetiology, diagnostics and therapy). In: Springer L, Schrey-Dern D (eds) Forum Logopädie, end edition. Thieme, Stuttgart, New York, NY

Bigenzahn W, Fischman L, Mayerhofer-Kramme lU (1992) Myofunctional therapy in patients with orofacial dysfunctions affecting speech. Folia Phoniatr 44(5):238–244

Billington J, Yardley I, Upadhyaya M (2018) Long-term efficacy of a tongue tie service in improving breast feeding rates: a prospective study. J Pediatr Surg 53(2):286–288

Bowen C (2019) Information for families: tongue-tie (ankyloglossia). http://www.speech-language-therapy.com. Accessed 13 Mar 2019

Brandão CA, de Marsillac MWS, Barja-Fidalgo F et al (2018) Is the neonatal tongue screening test a valid and reliable tool for detecting ankyloglossia in newborns? Int J Paediatr Dent 28(4):380–389

Celletti C, Castori M, La Torre G et al (2011) Reassessment of oral frenula in Ehlers-Danlos syndrome: a study of 32 patients with the hypermobility type. Am J Med Genet 155A(12):3157–3159

Chandrashekar L, Kashinath KR, Suhas S (2014) Labial ankyloglossia associated with oligodontia: a case report. J Dent (Tehran) 11(4):481–484

Chinnadurai S, Francis DO, Epstein RA et al (2015) Treatment of ankyloglossia for reasons other than breastfeeding: a systematic review. Pediatrics 135(6):e1467–e1474

Clausnitzer V (2001) Orofaziale Muskelfunktionstherapie (OMF). Ein myofunktionelles Übungsbuch (orofacial muscle function therapy (OMF). A myofunctional exercise book). Modernes Lernen, Dortmund

Condò R, Costacurta M, Perugia C et al (2012) Atypical deglutition: diagnosis and interceptive treatment. A clinical study. Eur J Paediatr Dent 13(3):209–214

Coryllos E, Genna CW, Salloum AC (2004) Congenital tongue-tie and its impact on breastfeeding. In: breastfeeding: best for baby and mother. American Academy of Pediatrics._Section on breastfeeding newsletter summer 2004 1-6. https://www.researchgate.net/publication/301346077_Congenital_tongue-tie_and_its_impact_on_breastfeeding. Accessed 16 Nov 2021

De Felice C, Bianciardi G, Parrini S et al (2004) Congenital oral mucosal abnormalities in true umbilical cord knots. Biol Neonate 86(1):34–38

Defabianis P (2000) Ankyloglossia and its influence on maxillary and mandibular development. (a seven year follow-up case report). Funct Orthod 17(4):25–33

Delli K, Livas C, Sculean A et al (2013) Facts and myths regarding the maxillary midline frenum and its treatment: a systematic review of the literature. Quintessence Int 44(2):177–187

Dixon B, Gray J, Elliot N et al (2018) A multifaceted programme to reduce the rate of tongue-tie release surgery in newborn infants: observational study. Int J Pediatr Otorhinolaryngol 113:156–163

Dollberg S, Botzer E (2011) Neonatal tongue-tie: myths and science (article in Hebrew). Harefauh 150(46–49):67

Doshi UH, Bhad-Patil WA (2011) Speech defect and orthodontics: a contemporary review. Orthodontics (Chic) 12(4):340–353

Drazin P (1994) The assessment tool for lingual frenulum function (ATLFF): use in a lactation consultant private practice. https://www.semanticscholar.org/paper/The-Assessment-Tool-for-Lingual-Frenulum-Function-a-Drazin/c9db2cbee4a8e4194cdd2526dc-9f13ac49ab0591. Accessed 16 Nov 2021

Elad D, Kozlovsky P, Blum O et al (2014) Biomechanics of milk extraction during breast-feeding. Proc Natl Acad Sci USA 111(14):5230–5235

Elhag SB, Abdulghani AS (2015) Bilateral double mesiodentes in the ugly duckling stage. Int J Oral Health Sci 5(1):45–48

Forlenza GP, Paradise Black NM, McNamara EG et al (2010) Ankyloglossia, exclusive breastfeeding, and failure to thrive. Pediatrics 125:e1500–e1504

Francis DO, Krishnaswami S, McPheeters M (2015) Treatment of ankyloglossia and breastfeeding outcomes: a systematic review. Pediatrics 135(6):e1458–e1466

Friedrich G, Bigenzahn W, Zorowka P (2013) Phoniatrie und Pädaudiologie. Einführung in die medizinischen, psychologischen und linguistischen Grundlagen von Stimme, Sprache und Gehör (Phoniatrics and pedaudiology. Introduction to the medical, psychological and linguistic basics of voice, speech and hearing). In: 5. überarbeitete Auflage, 5th edn. Verlag Hans Huber, Bern

Fröschels E (1914) Über die Beziehung der Stomatologie zur Logopädie (about the relationship between stomatology and speech therapy). Z Stomatol 12:241–262

García Pola MJ, González García M, García Martín JM et al (2002) A study of pathology associated with short lingual frenum. ASDC J Dent Child 69(1):59–62, 12

Garliner D (1974) Myofunctional therapy in dental practice. Bartel, New York, NY

Ghaheri BA, Cole M, Fausel SC et al (2017) Breastfeeding improvement following tongue-tie and lip-tie release: a prospective cohort study. Laryngoscope 127(5):1217–1223

Grabowski R, Stahl F (2008) Open mouth posture in children—frequency and effects. Inf Orthod Kieferorthop 40(2):101–109

Griffiths DM (2004) Do tongue-ties affect breast-feeding? J Hum Lact 20(4):409–414

Guilleminault C, Akhtar F (2015) Pediatric sleep-disordered breathing: new evidence on its development. Sleep Med Rev 24:46–56

Gurung H, Cohn A (2015) Labial frenum tear from instrumental delivery. Arch Dis Child 100(8):773. https://doi.org/10.1136/archdischild-2014-307733

Han SH, Kim MC, Choi YS et al (2012) A study on the genetic inheritance of ankyloglossia based on pedigree analysis. Arch Plast Surg 39(4):329–332

Hanson ML, Andrianopoulos MV (1982) Tongue thrust and malocclusion: a longitudinal study. Int J Orthod 20(2):9–18

Hanson M, Barrett RH (1988) Fundamentals of orofacial myology. Thomas, Springfield IL

Harris EF, Friend GW, Tolley EA (1992) Enhanced prevalence of ankyloglossia with maternal cocaine use. Cleft Palate Craniofac J 29(1):72–76

Hatami A, Dreyer CW, Meade MJ, Kaur S (2022) Effectiveness of tongue-tie assessment tools in diagnosing and fulfilling lingual frenectomy criteria: a systematic review. Aust Dent J 67(3):212–219. https://doi.org/10.1111/adj.12921. Epub 2022 Jul 4. PMID: 35689515; PMCID: PMC9796854

Hazelbaker AK (1993) The assessment tool for lingual frenulum function (ATLFF): use in a lactation consultant private practice. Pacific Oaks College, Pasadena CA

Henry L, Hayman R (2014) Ankyloglossia its impact breastfeeding. Nurs Womens Health 18(2):122–129

Hentschel R (2018) Breastfeeding problems should be the only relevant criteria for deciding whether to carry out a frenotomy in infancy. Acta Paediatr 107(10):1697–1701

Héroard J (1868) Journal de Jean Héroard Sur l'enfance et al jeunesse de Louis XIII (1601–1628). Librairie de Firmin Didot Frères, Fils et C^{ixe}, Paris 1868 (Journal of Jean Héroard on the childhood and youth of Louis XIII (1601–1628). Firmin Didot Frères, Fils et Cie bookshop, Paris 1868). p7. https://reader.digitale-sammlungen.de/de/fs1/object/display/bsb10414530_00007.html. Accessed 16 Nov 2021

Hertel M, Matter D, Schmidt-Westhausen AM et al (2014) Oral syphilis: a series of 5 cases. J Oral Maxillofac Surg 72(2):338–345

Hill R (2019) Implications of ankyloglossia on breastfeeding. MCN Am J Matern Child Nurs 44(2):73–79

Horton CE, Crawford HH, Adamson JE et al (1969) Tongue-tie. Cleft Palate J 6:8–23

Huang YS, Quo S, Berkowski JA et al (2015) Short lingual frenulum and obstructive sleep apnea in children. Int J Pediatr Res 1:1–4

IATP (International Affiliation of Tongue tie Professionals) (2019). https://tonguetieprofessionals.org. Accessed 3 Mar 2019

IATP (International Affiliation of Tongue tie Professionals) (2020). https://tonguetieprofessionals.org/about-tongue-tie/. Accessed 24 June 2020

Ingram J, Johnson D, Copeland M et al (2015) The development of a tongue assessment tool to assist with tongue-tie identification. Arch Dis Child Fetal Neonatal Ed 100(4):F344–F348

Isaiah A, Pereira KD (2013) Infected sublingual hematoma: a rare complication of frenulectomy. Ear Nose Throat J 92(7):296–297

Jain P, Rathee M (2019) Embryology, tongue. [Updated 2019 Sep 26]. In: Stat Pearls [Internet]. StatPearls Publishing, Treasure Island FL. https://www.ncbi.nlm.nih.gov/books/NBK547697/. Accessed 12 Dec 2019

Jang SJ, Cha BK, Ngan P (2011) Relationship between the lingual frenulum and craniofacial morphology in adults. Am J Orthod Dentofacial Orthop 139(4 Suppl):e361–e367

Kapusevska B, Dereban N, Zabokova-Bilbilova E et al (2014) The influence of etiological factors in the occurence of diastema mediana. Prilozi 35(2):169–178

Klockars T (2007) Familial ankyloglossia (tongue-tie). Int J Pediatr Otorhinolaryngol 71(8):1321–1324

Klockars T, Pitkäranta A (2009) Inheritance of ankyloglossia (tongue-tie). Clin Genet 75(1):98–99

Kotlow LA (1999) Ankyloglossia (tongue-tie): a diagnostic and treatment quandary. Quintessence Int 30(4):259–262

Kotlow L (2011) Diagnosis and treatment of ankyloglossia and tied maxillary fraenum in infants using Er: YAG and 1064 diode lasers. Eur Arch Paediatr Dent 12(2):106–112

Kühn D, Miller S, Schwemmle C et al (2014) Frühkindliches Schlucken (Infantile swallowing). Laryngorhinootologie 93(4):231–236

Lalakea ML, Messner AH (2003) Ankyloglossia: does it matter? Pediatr Clin N Am 50(2):381–397

Lisonek M, Liu S, Dzakpasu S et al (2017) Canadian perinatal surveillance system (Public Health Agency of Canada). Changes in the incidence and surgical treatment of ankyloglossia in Canada. Paediatr Child Health 22(7):382–386

Maguire S, Hunter B, Hunter L et al (2007) Welsh child protection systematic review group. Diagnosing abuse: a systematic review of torn frenum and other intra-oral injuries. Arch Dis Child 92(12):1113–1117

Malmenholt A, McAllister A, Lohmander A (2019) Orofacial function, articulation proficiency, and intelligibility in 5-year-old children born with cleft lip and palate. Cleft Palate Craniofac J 56(3):321–330

Meilinger M (1999) Untersuchung ausgewählter Aspekte myofunktioneller Störungen im Vorschulalter (investigation of selected aspects of myofunctional disorders in pre-school age). Herbert Utz Verlag, Munich

Melink S, Vagner MV, Hocevar-Boltezar I et al (2010) Posterior crossbite in the deciduous dentition period, its relation with sucking habits, irregular orofacial functions, and otolaryngological findings. Am J Orthod Dentofacial Orthop 138(1):32–40

Messner AH, Lalakea ML (2000) Ankyloglossia: controversies in management. Int J Pediatr Otorhinolaryngol 54(2–3):123–131

Morrison AL, Chute D, Radentz S et al (1988) Air bag-associated injury to a child in the front passenger seat. Am J Forensic Med Pathol 19(3):218–222

Mukai S, Mukai C, Asaoka K (1991) Ankyloglossia with deviation of the epiglottis and larynx. Ann Otol Rhinol Laryngol Suppl 153:3–20

Muldoon K, Gallagher L, McGuinness D et al (2017) Effect of frenotomy on breastfeeding variables in infants with ankyloglossia (tongue-tie): a prospective before and after cohort study. BMC Pregnancy Childbirth 17(1):373. https://doi.org/10.1186/s12884-017-1561-8

Nadoleczny M (1912) Die Sprach-und Stimmstörungen im Kindesalter (Speech and voice disorders in childhood). In: Pfaundler M, Schlossmann A (eds) Handbuch der Kinderheilkunde (handbook of pediatrics). Vogel, Leipzig

Northcutt ME (2009) The lingual frenum. J Clin Orthod 43(9):557–565

Opara PI, Gabriel-Job N, Opara KO (2012) Neonates presenting with severe complications of frenotomy: a case series. J Med Case Rep 6:77

Orphanet (2019) X-linked cleft palate and ankyloglossia. https//www.orpha.net/consor/cgi-bin/OC_Exp.php?lng=EN&Expert=324601. Accessed 2 Dec 2019

O'Shea JE, Foster JP, O'Donnell CP et al (2017) Frenotomy for tongue-tie in newborn infants. Cochrane Database Syst Rev 3:CD011065

Patel J, Anthonappa RP, King NM (2018) All tied up! Influences of oral frenulae on breastfeeding and their recommended management strategies. J Clin Pediatr Dent 42(6):407–413

Póvoa-Santos L, Lacerda-Santos R, Alvarenga-Brant R et al. (2024) Ankyloglossia and malocclusion: A systematic review and meta-analysis. J Am Dent Assoc 155(1):59–73.e9. https://doi.org/10.1016/j.adaj.2023.09.014. Epub 2023 Nov 22. PMID: 37999659

Price EA, Rush LR, Perper JA et al (2000) Cardiopulmonary resuscitation-related injuries and homicidal blunt abdominal trauma in children. Am J Forensic Med Pathol 21(4):307–310

Ruffoli R, Giambelluca MA, Scavuzzo MC et al (2005) Ankyloglossia: a morphofunctional investigation in children. Oral Dis 11(3):170–174

Saccomanno S, Antonini G, D'Alatri L et al (2012) Causal relationship between malocclusion and oral muscles dysfunction: a model of approach. Eur J Paediatr Dent 13(4):321–323

Seo YJ, Kim SJ, Munkhshur J et al (2014) Treatment and retention of relapsed anterior open-bite with low tongue posture and tongue-tie: a 10-year follow-up. Korean J Orthod 44(4):203–216

Sepet E, Yildiz C, Erdem AP et al (2015) Relationship between mandibular incisor irregularity and type of occlusion in ankyloglossia. Oral Health Prev Dent 13(1):59–63

Srinivasan B, Chitharanjan AB (2013) Skeletal and dental characteristics in subjects with ankyloglossia. Prog Orthod 14:44. https://doi.org/10.1186/2196-1042-14-44

Steehler MW, Steehler MK, Harley EH (2012) A retrospective review of frenotomy in neonates and infants with feeding difficulties. Int J Pediatr Otorhinolaryngol 76(9):1236–1240

Stoner JE, Mazdyasna S (1980) Gingival recession in the lower region of 15-year-old subjects. J Periodontol 51(2):74–76

Suter VG, Bornstein MM (2009) Ankyloglossia: facts and myths in diagnosis and treatment. J Periodontol 80(8):1204–1219

Suter VGA, Heinzmann AE, Grossen J et al (2014) Does the maxillary midline diastema close after frenectomy? Quintessence Int 45(1):57–66

UNICEF (United Nations International Children's Emergency Fund) (2019) Overcoming breastfeeding problems: tongue tie. https://www.unicef.org.uk/baby-friendly/support-for-parents/tongue-tie/. Accessed 28 Mar 2019

Vaz AC, Bai PM (2015) Lingual frenulum and malocclusion: an overlooked tissue or a minor issue. Indian J Dent Res 26(5):488–492

Walker RD, Messing S, Rosen-Carole C et al (2018) Defining tip-frenulum length for ankyloglossia and its impact on breastfeeding: a prospective cohort study. Breastfeed Med 13(3):204–210

Walsh J, Tunkel D (2017) Diagnosis and treatment of ankyloglossia in newborns and infants: a review. JAMA Otolaryngol Head Neck Surg 143(10):1032–1039

Wang J, Yang X, Hao S, Wang Y (2022) The effect of ankyloglossia and tongue-tie division on speech articulation: A systematic review. Int J Paediatr Dent 32(2):144-156. https://doi.org/10.1111/ipd.12802. Epub 2021 May 22. PMID: 33964037

Webb AN, Hao W, Hong P (2013) The effect of tongue-tie division on breastfeeding and speech articulation: a systematic review. Int J Pediatr Otorhinolaryngol 77(5):635–646

Williams WN, Waldron CM (1985) Assessment of lingual function when ankyloglossia (tongue-tie) is suspected. J Am Dent Assoc 110(3):353–356

Yoon AJ, Zaghi S, Ha S et al (2017a) Ankyloglossia as a risk factor for maxillary hypoplasia and soft palate elongation: a functional—morphological study. Orthod Craniofac Res 20(4):237–244

Yoon A, Zaghi S, Weitzman R et al (2017b) Toward a functional definition of ankyloglossia: validating current grading scales for lingual frenulum length and tongue mobility in 1052 subjects. Sleep Breath 21(3):767–775

Diagnosis and Differential Diagnosis of Dysglossia, Resonance Disorders and Velopharyngeal Insufficiency

3

Fatemeh Abnavi, Wolfgang Angerstein, Ana Martínez Arellano, Wolfgang Bigenzahn, Tim Bressmann, María Bielsa Corrochano, Philippe H. Dejonckere, Doris-Maria Denk-Linnert, Tanja Fuhr, Uta Hanning, Alexander Hemprich, Florian Lasse Lefarth, Igor Leuchter, Barbara Maciejewska, Katrin Neumann, Thomas Niederstadt, Ute Pröschel, Karen J. Reichmuth, Saskia Rohrbach-Volland, Martina Scharitzer, Melanie Vauth-Weidig, and Pablo Antonio Ysunza

Saskia Rohrbach-Volland and Philippe H. Dejonckere have shared first authorship.

Supplementary Information The online version contains supplementary material available at https://doi.org/10.1007/978-3-031-25175-7_3.

F. Abnavi (✉)
Audiology and Speech-Language Pathology Program, University of Ottawa, Ottawa, ON, Canada
e-mail: fabna054@uottawa.ca

W. Angerstein
Phoniatrie und Paedaudiologie, Uni-klinikum Düsseldorf, Düsseldorf, Germany
e-mail: angerstein@uni-duesseldorf.de

A. M. Arellano
Clinica Foniatria Y Logopedia, Pamplona, Spain
e-mail: anamarellano@medena.es

W. Bigenzahn
Private Practice: Lazarettgasse 25/1. Stock A-1090 Vienna, Formerly Medical University of Vienna, Vienna, Austria
e-mail: wolfgang.bigenzahn@chello.at

T. Bressmann
Department of Speech-Language Pathology, University of Toronto, Toronto, ON, Canada
e-mail: tim.bressmann@utoronto.ca

M. B. Corrochano
Clinica Foniatria Y Logopedia Bielsa, Talavera de la Reina, Spain
e-mail: info@foniatriabielsa.com

P. H. Dejonckere
Federal Agency for Occupational Risks, Brussels, Belgium

D.-M. Denk-Linnert
Division of Phoniatrics and Speech Language Therapy, Department of Otorhinolaryngology, Medical University of Vienna, Vienna, Austria
e-mail: doris-maria.denk-linnert@meduni.wien.ac.at

T. Fuhr
Fresenius University of Applied Sciences, Idstein, Germany
e-mail: anja.fuhr@hs-fresenius.de

U. Hanning
Centre for Radiology and Endoscopy, University Clinic Hamburg-Eppendorf, Hamburg, Germany
e-mail: u.hanning@uke.de

A. am Zehnhoff-Dinnesen et al. (eds.), *Phoniatrics II*, European Manual of Medicine,
https://doi.org/10.1007/978-3-031-25175-7_3

3.1 History Taking in Dysglossia, Resonance Disorders and Velopharyngeal Dysfunction (VPD)

Philippe H. Dejonckere
and Saskia Rohrbach-Volland

The diagnostic interview or history-taking is a central, well-structured component of the decision-making process during which health professionals explore, identify and document a patient's problems, complaints and needs. The aim of the diagnostic interview is to work out a diagnostic and therapeutic path (APA 2020; ASLHA 2004; Tylor and Tolbert 2002). It should consider functioning, disability and health (ICF, WHO) (WHO 2001):

1. Impairments in body structure and function, including underlying strengths and weaknesses in speech sound production and verbal/non-verbal communication.
2. Co-morbid deficits or conditions, such as developmental disabilities or syndromes.
3. Limitations in activity and participation, including functional communication, interpersonal interactions with family and peers, and learning.
4. Contextual (environmental and personal) factors that serve as barriers to or facilitators of successful communication and life participation.
5. The impact of communication impairments on quality of life and family.

Neumann and Romonath (2012) applied the ICF to children with cleft lip and palate.

Owing to its manifold underlying causes and depending on the examiners´ qualification, the diagnostic interview in dysglossia/resonance disorders/velopharyngeal dysfunction (VPD) focuses on different topics. Thus, at best, a multiprofessional team contributes to it. A standardised interview for dysglossia/resonance disorders/VPD for all professionals´ requirements does not exist (John et al. 2006).

Basically, it should consider some special aspects: information about possible genetic and environmental factors and the prenatal, perinatal and postnatal history, as well as the overall health

A. Hemprich
Dept. of Maxillofacial and Facial Plastic Surgery, University Hospital of Leipzig, Leipzig, Germany
e-mail: hemprich@medizin.uni-leipzig.de

F. L. Lefarth
Phoniatrics and Pedaudiology, Univ.-Klinik für Hals-Nasen-Ohren-Heilkunde, Oldenburg, Germany
e-mail: florian.lefarth@hhu.de

I. Leuchter
Division of Phoniatrics, Geneva University Hospitals, Geneva, Switzerland
e-mail: igor.leuchter@hug.ch

B. Maciejewska
Department and Clinic of Phoniatrics and Audiology, Poznan University of Medical Sciences, Poznan, Poland
e-mail: barbaramaciejewska@ump.edu.pl

K. Neumann
Department of Phoniatrics and Pedaudiology, University Hospital Münster, Münster, Germany
e-mail: Katrin.Neumann@uni-muenster.de

T. Niederstadt
Retired, Institute of Clinical Radiology, University Hospital of Münster, Münster, Germany
e-mail: niederstadt@web.de

U. Pröschel
Clinic of Phoniatrics and Pedaudiology, Univ.-HNO-Klinik Erlangen, Erlangen, Germany
e-mail: u.proeschel@kinderklinik-datteln.de

K. J. Reichmuth · M. Vauth-Weidig
Clinic of Phoniatrics and Pedaudiology, University Hospital Münster, Münster, Germany
e-mail: karen.reichmuth@ukmuenster.de; melanie-jasmin.vauth-weidig@ukmuenster.de

S. Rohrbach-Volland
Praxis für Neurologie, Psychiatrie, Psychotherapie und Nervenheilkunde, HNO Paxis, Berlin, Germany

M. Scharitzer
Department of Biomedical Imaging and Image-Guided Therapy, Medical University of Vienna, Vienna, Austria
e-mail: martina.scharitzer@meduniwien.ac.at

P. A. Ysunza
Ian Jackson Craniofacial and Cleft Palate Clinic of Beaumont Hospital, William Beaumont School of Medicine, Oakland University, Royal Oak, MI, USA
e-mail: antonio.ysunza@beaumont.edu

status and ability to differentiate syndromic from non-syndromic patients. The history of conservative and operative therapy (i.e. the amount of resection of the tongue after tumour, operation on cleft palate) gives a hint on the preliminary health course and special characteristics and sources of malfunctions (Ünal-Logacev et al. 2018). Questionnaires for parents and teachers have also been elaborated (Dunaway 2004), which cover several points.

First, because of its frequency of occurrence and irrespective of the pathogenesis, such topics as articulation, language, resonance, feeding, respiration, hearing, dental and skeletal (mal)position, cognition, aesthetic, psychosocial and academic or vocational aspects should be taken into account.

Second, the prenatal history, provided by caregivers and by medical reports, gives information on family members with dysglossia/resonance disorders/VPD or consanguineous marriages; both conditions are related to the high incidence of e.g. cleft lip and palate. Advanced maternal age, miscarriages or abortions can also be predictors, as are exposure to alcohol, smoking, teratogenic radiation, poor nutrition, viral infections, drugs, severe stress, geographical factors and race, which should be taken into account (Litin 2009; Adetayo and Martin 2012).

Third, postnatal history should focus on feeding and respiratory difficulties, cardiological problems, as well as other organic dysfunction.

Concrete questions could include the following topics, provided by Kummer (2011b):

- Current concerns
  - What concerns you about your child's speech?
  - When did you first become concerned?
  - Who referred your child for the evaluation, and what was that person's concern?
- Speech production
  - What types of sound does your child use during vocal play: vowels only or some consonants?
  - If the child uses consonants, what are some of the consonants that you hear?
  - Are they produced individually or over and over again?
  - Does your child "jabber" or use jargon?
  - Does your child leave out sounds in words?
  - Do you understand your child's speech all of the time, most of the time, some of the time, or hardly at all?
  - How well do strangers understand your child's speech?
  - Are there any particular speech sounds that are difficult for your child to produce?
- Resonance
  - Does your child sound nasal? If so, does it sound as if your child is talking through the nose, or does it sound as if he or she has a cold?
  - Do you ever hear air coming through his or her nose during speech?
  - Do you ever hear a bubbling sound or snorting during the speech?
  - When did you first notice the problem with nasality?
  - If the onset was sudden, what event preceded it?
  - Has your child had an adenoidectomy? If so, did it change his or her speech?
  - Does your child's speech vary with the weather, allergies, fatigue or any other factors?
- Language
  - Does your child communicate with gestures, single words, short phrases, incomplete sentences?
  - How many words does your child usually put together in an utterance?
  - Does your child leave out little words (e.g. "of, "to", "the" or "is") in the sentence?
  - Is your child communicating as well as other children of his or her age?
  - Have you ever had a concern about how well your child understands the speech of others or follows directions?
- Medical history
  - Was your child born with any congenital problems? If so, what were they? How and when were they treated?
  - Does your child have any medical problems, medical diagnoses or medical conditions?
  - What surgeries has your child undergone?
  - Does your child take any medication on a regular basis?

  - Does your child hear normally? When was the last hearing test?
  - Has your child had many ear infections? If so, how were they treated?
  - Does your child have any problems with vision?
  - Where is your child on the growth chart?
- Developmental history
  - Was your child quiet, about average, or very vocal as an infant?
  - Did you have any concerns about his or her initial speech development?
  - Did your child begin to use words before or after his or her first birthday?
  - When your child was learning to sit up, stand, and walk, did he or she seem normal or behind that of other children?
  - Did your child walk before or after his or her first birthday?
  - Does your child have any difficulty learning in preschool or school?
- Feeding and oral-motor skills
  - Does your child have any difficulty chewing, sucking or swallowing?
  - Is there a history of feeding problems?
  - Does your child drool or keep his or her mouth open during the day?
- Airway
  - Does your child snore at night?
  - Does your child ever gasp for breath at night or sleep restlessly?
  - Is your child's breathing ever noisy during the day?
  - Does your child have allergies, asthma or chronic congestion?
- Treatment history
  - Has your child ever had a speech or language evaluation or speech or language therapy?
  - Is your child currently receiving therapy? If yes, what are the goals?
  - Has your child's speech improved in the last 6 months? If so, in what way?

3.2 Clinical Examination in Dysglossia, Resonance Disorders and Velopharyngeal Dysfunction (VPD)

Saskia Rohrbach-Volland
and Philippe H. Dejonckere

3.2.1 Introduction

The lips, the tongue and the velopharyngeal valve are responsible for the production of oral speech sounds (Kummer 2011a). Hence, malformation (anatomical aberrances), malfunction (physiological aberrances) and mislearning can cause dysfunction. The latter cause is often forgotten, but the tongue, the lips and also the velopharyngeal valve all are articulators and as such have a learned component (Kummer 2011a; Peterson-Falzone et al. 2006). Since no direct correlation between speech problems and the size of the anatomical defect exists, the *examination of functions* is essential for the decision-making process on further diagnostics and therapy. The examiner should have a profound knowledge of the physiology and pathophysiology of oral posture and movements, including nasal and velopharyngeal function, orthodontics (dysgnathia), neurology (peripheral and central paralysis of the cranial nerves), other forms of malfunction (i.e. apraxia of speech) as well as common craniofacial and associated genetic sequences or syndromes. Prompt diagnosis and individual effective therapy (speech therapy alone or medical intervention (i.e. surgical or prosthetic) can then be effective. A collaborative team that may include family members or caregivers and other professionals serves the best.

Screenings for suspected dysglossia/resonance disorders/velopharyngeal dysfunction (VPD) do not result in a diagnosis, but rather identify the necessity for additional comprehensive assessment (ASLHA 2021a). A screening should include a limited speech sample to register articulation errors, resonance disorders and presence of nasal emission. Hearing must be tested and should include otoscopic examination, immittance testing to assess middle ear function, pure-tone air and bone conduction, otoacoustic emission testing to register outer hair cell function and the speech detection threshold.

Several *assessments* exist that focus on resonance disorders and VPD in cleft lip and palate, fewer on dysglossia (Peterson-Falzone et al. 2006; Ünal-Logacev et al. 2018; Schröter-Morasch and Ziegler 2005; Rudnick and Sie 2008; Shprintzen and Marrinan 2009). Assessments give a deeper diagnostic insight and can differ between obligatory, compensatory and learned articulation errors and nasal emission (see below).

The following steps illustrate a path for the clinical examination of dysglossia/resonance disorders/VPD.

3.2.2 Perceptual Examination Tests

These register the effect on respiration, articulation, phonation and prosody and give a first insight into the quality of articulation of phones and phonemes, nasality and the intelligibility of speech (Henningsson et al. 2008). They precede and determine the need for further instrumental examination (Trost-Cardamone 2013).

Speech sound production must differentiate between obligatory articulation errors (those that are physically based due to VPD or dental/occlusal/lingual problems), compensatory articulation errors (including retracted oral productions and learned nasal fricative patterns) and developmental articulation errors with phonological errors. Dysglossia, according to the localisation of the impairment or lesion, can additionally be classified as labial, dental, lingual, palatal, velopharyngeal or nasal, with also possible impairments of phonation.

Resonance-testing assesses hypernasality (pronounced nasal resonance enhancement on vowels, glides, liquids and voiced oral consonants) and hyponasality (less or no resonance enhancement on nasal consonants and adjacent vowels, especially /i/ and /u/ due to nasal cavity obstruction). Mixed resonance includes elements of both hypernasality and hyponasality. Cul-de-sac resonance is a variation of hyponasality with sounds resonating in the nasal, oral or pharyngeal cavity and caught by additional obstruction: nasals /m/, /n/, and /ng/ and nasalised sounds are "muffled" (owing to anterior nasal obstruction), speech seems "mumbled" (ASLHA 2021a).

Stops, fricatives and affricates should be assessed for examination of nasal airflow. Nasal emission can show nasal fricative substitutions or nasal emission that exits with the target sound. Nasal emission may be phoneme-specific (phoneme-specific nasal emission PSNE) or persist after surgical intervention (Peterson-Falzone et al. 2006, 2016; Golding-Kushner 2015; Morgan and O'Gara 2014).

3.2.3 Inspection and Palpation of Speech Organs

The *functional endoscopy* of the nasopharynx, the velopharyngeal valve, the larynx, in some cases of feeding problems and dysphagia or nasal regurgitation, functional swallowing testing, are essential in diagnostics. Conditions such as central or peripheral nerve paralysis, cleft lip and palate, submucosal cleft, adenoid and tonsillar hypertrophy, as well as adenoid atrophy or adenoidectomy, irregular adenoids (mostly when the tissue has regrown after adenoidectomy), tonsillectomy, deep pharynx, maxillary malposition (maxillary advancement or midface retrusion and class III malocclusion) and oral cavity tumours are underlying conditions that have to be distinguished.

Clinical examination includes the following aspects (ASLHA 2021b):

- Structural differences/abnormalities of proportion and symmetry including face, nose, eyes, ears, skull and profile including inflammation, defects, scars, changes in the mucosa.

- The oral cavity has to be examined for:
  - Symmetry and movement of oral structures (lips, jaw, tongue, velum).
  - Abnormalities of the tongue (i.e. macroglossia, ankyloglossia, asymmetry).
  - Presence and size of tonsils (large tonsils can play a role in airway and resonance problems).
  - Dentition and occlusal status.
  - Fistulae in the hard or soft palate.
  - Prior surgery (scars, position of velopharyngeal valve or pharyngeal flap).
  - Signs of possible submucous cleft palate (bony notch at the junction of the hard and soft palate, (bluish line or translucent appearance down the midline of the palate (zona pellucida); midline furrow or V-shaped elevation during phonation; and bifid uvula.
- Nasal congestion.
- Characterisation of the sensorimotor disorders reflecting changes in muscle tone, reduction in amplitude and speed of movement, signs of hyperkinesia and apraxia, muscular atrophy, presence of fasciculations or myoclonus.
- Impairment of sensibility and reflectory reaction.
- Voice problems may include laryngeal hyperfunction when trying to compensate for the loss of pressure at the velopharyngeal valve through muscle tension dysphonia. In contrast, the voice may sound soft owing to non-compensated loss of pressure through the velopharyngeal valve or as a compensatory strategy to minimise hypernasality, nasal emission or hoarseness (Peterson-Falzone et al. 2010). Hence, laryngoscopy, video-laryngo-stroboscopy and glottography are useful methods to investigate concomitant malfunctions and differential diagnoses. Videorecording permits the analysis in a slow-motion modus.

Specific forms and checklists can be used (e.g. Paul 1995).

A special focus has to be laid on (childhood) apraxia of speech, a neurological condition with oral-motor dysfunction, characterised by difficulty in executing and sequencing speech movements. Characteristics are, among others, a great variability in articulation, perseverance movements (persistence in effort to articulate despite difficulty or delay in achieving success) and the lack of progress in therapy.

3.2.4 Instrumental Tests

Instrumental tests help to make objective perceptual speech findings and may improve planning surgical or prosthetic interventions.

3.2.4.1 Low-Technique Procedures

To distinguish hypernasality from nasal emission and turbulence, resonance testing can be easily performed by using a straw with repeat high-pressure phonemes: at the nostril entrance and the other end to the examiner's ear during production of oral consonants. Listen for sound or airflow exiting the nostril. Nasal emission has to be verified by instrumental testing before diagnosis.

Aerodynamic testing can be carried out with *nasal auscultation*: a stethoscope with a nasal olive can be used for nasal auscultation during the production of oral consonants (Fig. 3.1) and a simple commercial device comprising a styrofoam piston inside a clear vertical tube, the probe tip placed in the nostril visualises nasal airflow by a rising piston (Fig. 3.2).

Transnasal *(video-)nasopharyngoscopy* with a velopharyngeal functional examination should be carried out in *all patients* with age-suitable endoscopes. It is a minimally invasive, effective method to evaluate adenoids and the pattern of

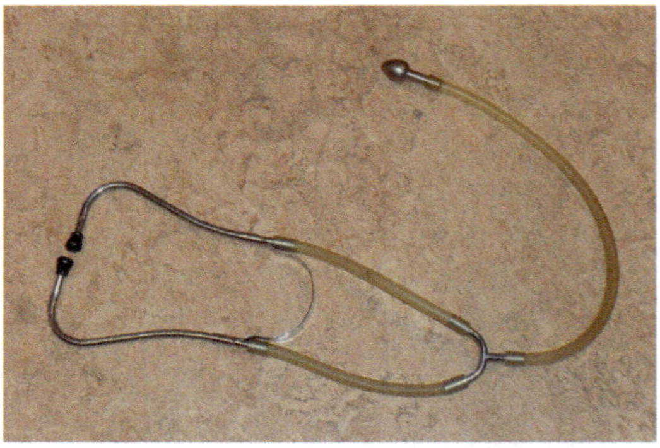

Fig. 3.1 Stethoscope with a nasal olive for nasal auscultation during production of oral consonants

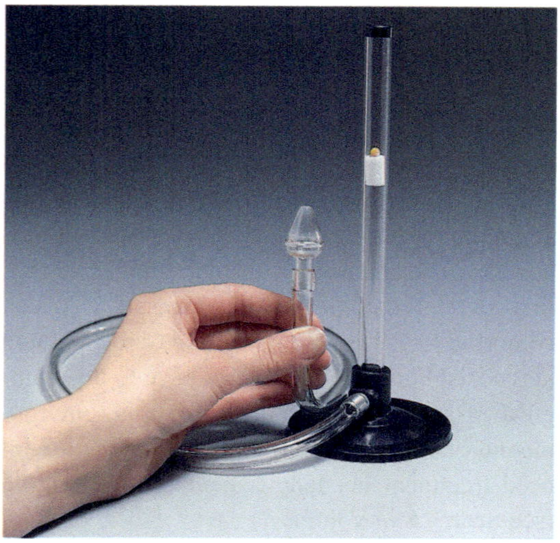

Fig. 3.2 Device See-Scape to detect nasal emission of air during speech. (Image used with permission of PRO-ED, Inc)

closure of the velopharyngeal valve and cannot be replaced by the auditive impression of nasality. The sound /i/ shows the movements of the soft palate, words such as 'coca-cola' or 'marmalade' are able to show if the valve closes in a coronar, a saggital, a circular or a circular manner with the Passavant's ridge (Skolnick et al. 1973; Croft et al. 1981). Depending on the pattern of closure, a surgical approach might be suitable to reduce hypernasality (velopharyngoplasty). Examination with the Czermak-mirror which is held under the nares to detect nasal air emission (fogging during production of phrases containing oral pressure consonants and no nasal consonants; Czermak 1860), the Gutzmann A-I-test (Gutzmann 1913), the head-turning symptom after Nadoleczny, the test after Schlesinger (1906) are old but nevertheless easy visual and perceptual tests.

3.2.4.2 Indirect Measures

These comprise nasometry and measure nasalance, a ratio of acoustic energy from the speaker's oral and nasal cavities (Fletcher 1970). The advanced technique (NasalView®) indicates the digital change of only acoustic energy to sound (Awan 1997). Standard values exist for several languages and can serve as pre- to post-operative comparison and biofeedback-therapy (Shin et al. 2017; Sinko et al. 2017).

Pressure-flow studies measure oral and nasal pressure and nasal airflow. Since nasality and nasal air flow are directly correlated, rhinomanometry can objectively show velopharyngeal insufficiency and status before and after surgical therapy (Finck et al. 1987; Trindade et al. 2014).

Electromyography of the levator and tensor veli palatini muscles is mostly used in a scientific context or as biofeedback-therapy in patients with dysarthria or dysphagia (Hammer et al. 2014).

Direct observation via imaging such as multiview videofluoroscopy (real-time X-ray video with imaging of velopharyngeal function during speech) and lateral cephalograms (static X-ray of the palate at rest and during phonation of /i/, /u/ or sustained oral /s/) play a role in special questions but do expose patients to radiation (Golding-Kushner et al. 1990). If suitable, examination with imaging (ultrasound and real-time speech MRI) might additionally be helpful, i.e. in dysglossia (Preston et al. 2017; Lingala et al. 2016).

3.2.5 Essential Activities for the Individual

According to the WHO ICF, communication participation and activity (i.e. difficulty being understood; reduced participation in classroom activities), facilitators (i.e. desire to interact with peers; supportive family and teachers) and barriers (i.e. aversion to initiate conversation with peers) should be identified and overcome (ASLHA 2021a; Neumann and Romonath 2012).

3.3 Evaluation of Speech

3.3.1 Assessment of the Developmental Speech and Language Status of Children

Katrin Neumann

3.3.1.1 Normal Language Development: The Concept of Milestones and Border Stones

For the proper evaluation of the language status of a child, knowledge of the distinct age-appropriate developmental targets of the acquisition of a specific language is necessary. As for other domains of infant and child development, the concept of milestones and borderline stones is useful for characterizing important steps in the acquisition of the native language for each linguistic domain (Kliegman et al. 2011). As demonstrated in Table 3.1 for the example of German language acquisition, milestones indicate at which average age a child has reached domain-specific levels of competence. Border stones are distinct developmental targets that are reached by 90% of all normally developed children by a certain age (Michaelis 2004).

3.3.1.2 Diagnostics of Developmental Disorders of Speech and Language

For the diagnosis of developmental disorders of speech and language (DDSL), the separation of specific developmental disorders of speech and language (SDDSL) and DDSL with comorbidities has to be taken into consideration. Hence the first step of the diagnostic process is to seek comorbidities, because SDDSL is an exclusion diagnosis. Furthermore, DDSL have to be distinguished from socioculturally caused environmental language abnormalities, which do not need treatment but language input and training (see Sect. 9.8 in Volume 1).

3.3.1.3 Analysis of Spontaneous Speech

The analysis of spontaneous speech is an important tool in the diagnostics of developmental language deficits, and it complements language tests. It is based on the observation of the child during a guided game or a dialogue, mostly with adults (parents or examiner). It is important to create situations that stimulate the child to communicate. Speech and language-related behaviour and utterances of the child have to be documented. Video recordings may be helpful for language and interaction analyses and may also provide information

Table 3.1 Time course of the normal German language acquisition (modified according to de Langen-Müller et al. 2012, with kind permission from Peter Lang GmbH, Internationaler Verlag der Wissenschaften)

Domain	Stage of development	Milestone (average age)	Borderline stone (age at 90th percentile)
Early language perception	Interest in human language ('eavesdropping')	Prenatally, first weeks of life	
	Perception of rhythmic and prosodic features of mother tongue	Prenatally, first weeks of life	
Development of vocalization	Crying	Birth	
	Cooing	Sixth to eighth week	
	Marginal babbling (testing of sound production)	Fourth month	
	Canonic babbling (syllables of consonants and vowels, e.g. *ba*)	Sixth month	Eighth to tenth month
	Reduplicated babbling (doubling of syllables, e.g. *baba*)	Eighth to tenth month	11th to 15th month
	Varying babbling (e.g. *bada*)	Eighth to tenth month	

(continued)

Table 3.1 (continued)

Domain	Stage of development	Milestone (average age)	Borderline stone (age at 90th percentile)
Acquisition of the phonological system	Elementary sound inventory Simple syllable structures (mostly open syllables)	12th month	
	Starting organization of the phonological system (use of sounds of the target language)	18th month	
	Starting to overcome phonological processes (systematic developmental changes of pronunciation of the target language)	2.5–4.5 year of life	
	Development of phonological awareness: detect syllables; 'clap' syllables; detect rhymes; detect initial sounds	About third year of life	
	Development of phonological awareness: detect and localize phonemes (smallest contrasting unit regarding meaning in the sound system), segmentation, analysis and synthesis of sounds into words	About fifth year of life	
Acquisition of vocabulary	Starting to understand words	Ninth month	
	Understanding approximately 50 words	16th month	
	Pre-forms of naming (situation-dependent proto-words)	Tenth month	
	Purposeful usage of *mama* and *papa*	Tenth to 15th month	18th to 20th month
	Production of the first words (one-word utterances)	13th to 20th month at latest	18th to 20th month
	Production of at least 50 words	18th to 24th month at latest	24th month
	Vocabulary spurt	18th to 21th month	
	Stage 1: personal/social words (*yes*, *hello*), relational words (*there*, *on*), onomatopoeia, proper names, some nouns	12th to 18th month	
	Stage 2: noun growth, start of verb acquisition	19th to 30th month	
	Stage 3: verb growth, function words (*because)*, pronouns	30th to 36th month	
	Overextensions and underextensions (e.g. *dog*/*bow-wow* for naming all animals)	Second year of life	
	Acquisition of the hierarchical organization of the mental lexicon; understanding semantic relations	Third year of life till school age	
	Acquisition of word formation: compounding (composition, e.g. *front door*) + derivation (e.g. *heat* → *heater*; *sun* → *sunny*)	Second to fifth year of life	

(continued)

Table 3.1 (continued)

Domain	Stage of development	Milestone (average age)	Borderline stone (age at 90th percentile)
Acquisition of grammar	Production of word combinations (two- or more-word utterances)	18th to 24th month at latest	25th to 26th month
	Increase of utterance length: at the age of 3 years, approximately 3 words per utterance on average	Third year of life	
	Production of simple syntactic structures	Third year of life	
	Decrease of omissions of obligatory constituents (e.g. subject)	Third year of life	
	Decrease of omissions of function words	Third to fourth year of life	
	Verbs in second position (*Lisa cake eat* → *Lisa eats cake* or *What eats Lisa?*)	30th to 36th month	
	Use of variable sentence types: declarative sentence, interrogative sentence, exclamatory sentence	30th to 36th month	
	Occurrence of subordinate clauses	36th month	
	Use of the definite article (*the*)	30th to 36th month	
	Correct subject-verb congruency (*I eat—she eats*)	Second to third year of life	
	Acquisition of the German case system, accusative at first, dative later	36th month to school entry age	
	Acquisition of the plural system	Second to sixth year of life	
	Acquisition of tempus markers	Third year of life	
	Temporary grammatical overextensions (*I runned away.*)	Third to fourth year of life	
Development of conversational and narrative abilities	Eye contact with primary attachment figure	Third month	
	Early expression of communicative intentions via looking, gestures and vocalizations	First year of life	
	Triangular eye contact Establishing shared focus of attention	Ninth month	
	Adherence to turn-taking rules	Second year of life	
	Child relates to conversation partner in dialogue	18th month	
	Organization of topics in dialogue	Third year of life	
	Development of narrative competence; increasing coherence (content-related) and cohesion (formal connection of text elements) in narration	36th month to early school age	
	Understanding irony and metaphors	Sixth year of life	
Literary language acquisition	Logographic stage (recognition of frequent words)	Preschool age, early elementary school age	
	Alphabetic stage (linkage between sounds and letters)	Early elementary school age	
	Orthographic stage (learning of orthographic rules)	Elementary school age	

on the parental communicative behaviour and style. From such informal observations, important information about phonetic-phonological, semantic-lexical, morphologic-syntactical and pragmatic-communicative abilities of a child can be gained. Furthermore, prosody, speech fluency and motivation to speak and to communicate as well as joyfulness of speaking may be analysed. For the evaluation of the spoken utterances, speech competence (the mastery of the speech-language systems) has to be distinguished from performance (the demonstration of the competence while communicating). Speech-language diagnostics aims to elicit as much as possible competence via performance within a short time (Neumann et al. 2009).

For a more thorough analysis of spontaneous speech, a detailed transcription, coding and analysis of language samples can be gained from audio or video recordings. Computer programs may be useful here, such as the Systematic Analysis of Language Transcripts (SALT) (Miller et al. 2011; SALT Software 2014) and the Computerized Language Analysis (CLAN) Program (MacWhinney 1995), which is a part of the Child Language Data Exchange System (CHILDES 2014), a database of speech audio files and text transcriptions in more than 20 languages serving as a central repository for first-language acquisition data (CHILDES 2014). Transcripts are necessary to calculate, for example, the mean length of utterances (MLU). This is a measure of linguistic productivity and language proficiency in children. It is the average number of morphemes per utterance contained in a sample of 100 utterances. The MLU is a benchmark of language acquisition, a good marker of DDSL, and may predict the further reading abilities of children (Bishop and Adams 1990; Rice et al. 2010). However, because the usefulness of MLU is questioned, it should not be used as the only diagnostic measure of language proficiency in children.

3.3.1.4 Examination of the Developmental Speech and Language Status with Informal and Nonstandardized Procedures

For a rough, informal evaluation of the phonetic-phonological, semantic-lexical and pragmatic competence of a child, simple test tools such as picture cards are suitable. Grammatical abilities might also be judged by using pictures that stimulate the production of specific grammatical structures, such as 'Brush your teeth!' to elicit the imperative or 'This is one apple, and these are two…?' for eliciting information on plural production (Neumann et al. 2011). The informal judgement of the types of language-related competence of a child requires the knowledge from professionals on the age-appropriate developmental targets (milestones) for each tested linguistic level (see Table 3.1).

3.3.1.5 Language Tests

The assessment of language skills should be performed with valid and normed tests, in order to get, as far as possible, examiner-independent, reproducible and reliable results. The use of only such tests enables the comparison of an individual test result with normal values, its interpretation and a differentiated evaluation of a child's language developmental status compared with the age norm. Comprehensive language tests that examine all or at least some linguistic levels have to be distinguished from tests that analyse only one type of competence, for example, vocabulary. The scores of single subtests of comprehensive tests ought not to be interpreted separately for different linguistic domains (grammar, vocabulary, etc.); otherwise such tests would reveal more children suspected of a DDSL than its prevalence (Neumann et al. 2011). In other words, if many subtests are performed, the probability is high by chance alone that at least one of them would indicate a deficit, which may lead to overdiagnosis. Therefore, a weighting system is required that evaluates test results according to the severity and prognosis of the specific deficiency.

Principles of the Interpretation of Test Values

Test results may be available as raw values or standardized values. Raw values are related to scores that result from an assignment prescription of a test. This could be, for example, the number of correct results in a language test or a sum score in a questionnaire test based on Likert scales ranging from 0 (does not fit at all) to 5 (fits perfectly). Raw values are useful (a) when related to reaching a cut-off value and as a base for (b) different categories (e.g. below average, average, above average) and (c) further transformations, e.g. in standardized values. Standardized values, on the other hand, are easier to interpret than raw values.

> *Example*: A child has performed a speech perception test and has solved 6 of 10 items correctly. At first glance this suggests a quite good test result, which, however, may be oversimplified and wrong, because from the reference values it is clear that in the normative sample all children are able to solve five items correctly, and the majority of subjects even at least six items. A transformation of the raw value '6' into a standardized value, for example into the tenth percentile (to be interpreted roughly as: 90% of the subjects of the normative sample have solved more items) or a value that is even more related to the distribution of the normative values, such as the intelligence quotient, indicate a rather 'below average' result in this example—(Petermann and Macha 2005).

A classical test construction is based on standard scales. For the tests applied during the assessment of DDSL/SDDSL, percentile scales, *z* scales, *T* scales, *C* scales and intelligence scales are used most frequently (Fig. 3.3). Standard scales enable the identification of the position of an examined child relative to a control sample. This requires an empirically gained reference frame from a sufficiently large, representative control sample. The named scales relate a test value to the average of the standard distribution and to the variance of the latter in order to answer the question: Is, or by how much is, the test score above or below the average?

The standardized values shown in Fig. 3.3 follow this sequence: (a) The average value of a distribution is identified. (b) A numerical value according to the chosen scale is attributed to the average. The percentile scale attributes the percentage of 50 to the average of the scale; the IQ scale, the IQ value 100; the *z* scale, the *z* value 0; the *T* scale, the *T* value 50; and the *C* scale, the value 5. (c) In order to interpret a test score, the spread of the distribution is of interest, in particular the distance between the average and the standard deviation (SD), because the test values on a specific scale are related to the SD. For example, the IQ scale subdivides the distance between the average and one standard deviation into 15 scale units (an IQ value of 85 represents an intelligence that deviates 1 SD from the average downwards; an IQ of 70 indicates a deviation of 2 SD from the

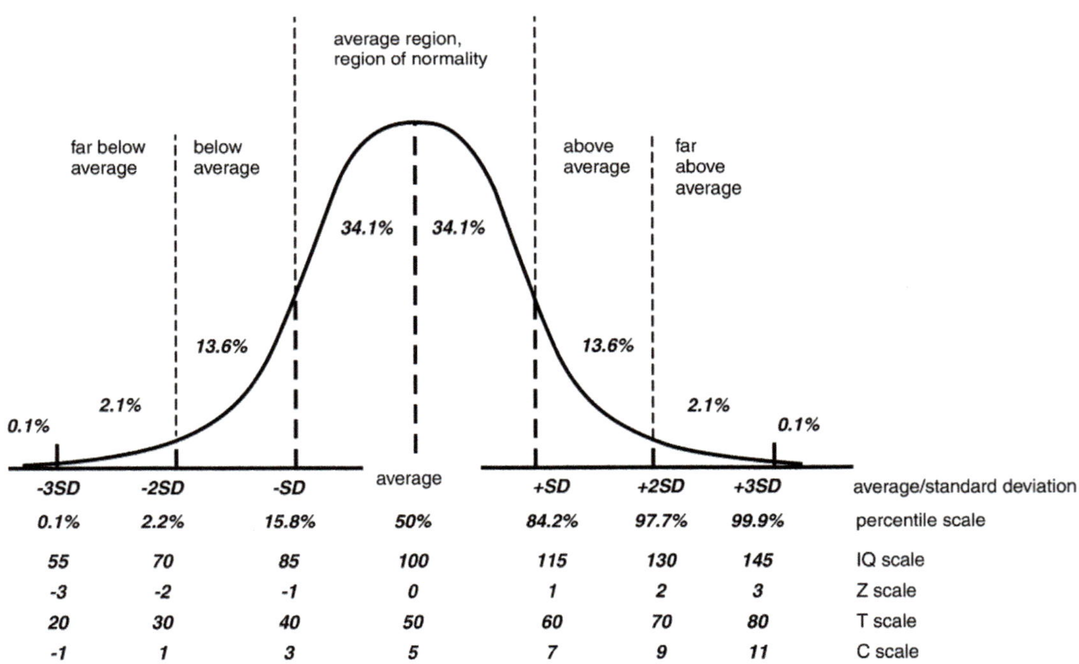

Fig. 3.3 Principles of generation of standard values and frequently used standard scales for the assessment of DDSL/SDDSL. Percentile, *z*-, *T*-, *C*- and intelligence (IQ) scales: selected standard values in a normal distribution (Gaussian curve) and convention of their interpretation. (Modified according to Petermann and Macha (2005) with kind permission from the authors)

average downwards). The *T* scale attributes 10 points to the distance of the SD from the average. In this way each of the scales enables the quantification of direction and extent of a deviation from the average by a scale value.

The percentages given on the Gaussian bell curve of a normal distribution are useful for orientation. They indicate the proportion of subjects of a sample (e.g. the norming sample) which is in the respective performance range. Between −1 and +1 SD lie about 68.2% of all subjects, i.e. more than two thirds. Below −1 SD are located the worst 15.8% of the subjects of the normative sample related to the values of a specific test; below −2 SD, the worst 2.2%; and below −3 SD, the worst 0.1%.

Related to those reference values, the performance in a certain test can be interpreted. The region between −1 and +1 SD from the average is regarded as the average or normal region (~68.2% of all subjects), i.e. a *T* value of 43 or an IQ of 91 is 'average'. The deviation of a test value of more than one but not more than two SD from the average may be interpreted as 'below average' or 'above average' (13.6% of subjects are located on each side of the average distribution). The 'below average' region is often considered as a region of risk. Thus, a *T* value of 35 or the 12th percentile is 'below average' and an IQ value of 125 'above average'. Deviations of more than ±2 SD from the average may be named 'far below/above average' (2.2% on each side). A *T* value of 26 or the second percentile is thus 'far below average' and an IQ < 70 as well (regarded an intellectual disability), and an IQ > 130 is 'far above average' (intellectual giftedness) (Petermann and Macha 2005).

Diagnostic Criteria for Specific Developmental Disorders of Speech and Language

Four diagnostic criteria are defined for the diagnosis of an SDDSL (F80.1 and F80.2) according to the International Statistical Classification of Diseases and Related Health Problems, the ICD-10 of the World Health Organization (2011), slightly modified by Dilling et al. (2008) and de Langen-Müller et al. (2012). They are based on the discrepancy between the language skills of a child and the age-related normative values and on the assumption of normality. According to this assumption, neurological, sensory, emotional, social or physical disorders, which could explain the language problems, are lacking. There is no reduced intelligence (IQ < 85, as measured with a nonverbal intelligence test).

- Perceptive and expressive language skills, as assessed from standardized and normed tests, are 1.5–2 SD below the age-dependent normative values at one or more than one language/communicative level.
- The expressive and receptive language skills, as assessed by structured behavioural and linguistic analyses, are considerably below the average abilities of the age norm.
- The use and understanding of nonverbal communication are within the age norm.
- The assumption of normality is justified.

Additionally, the ICD-10 defines a double discrepancy criterion between cognitive and language competence: for an SDDSL diagnosis, language perception or language production of a child is below the level appropriate for his or her age. Additionally, the receptive/expressive language competence is 1–1.5 SD below the nonverbal IQ that is at least average (IQ ≥ 85) (see criteria 1 and 4). This criterion is, however, under debate.

A diagnostic algorithm as shown in Fig. 3.4 demonstrates the steps of an interdisciplinary diagnostics of a (S)DDSL and the subsequent interventions. If there is suspicion of an age-inappropriate language development, audiological assessment of the hearing of a child is inevitable. Thereafter, the language competence is assessed. A subsequent differential diagnostics does not follow a fixed scheme but depends on the specific symptoms (de Langen-Müller et al. 2012). If there is suspicion of an SDDSL, possible comorbidities have to be excluded.

3.3.1.6 Screening Tests for the Developmental Speech and Language Status

Parent questionnaires have been shown to be a useful screening for the language development status of young children (Dale 1991). Universal

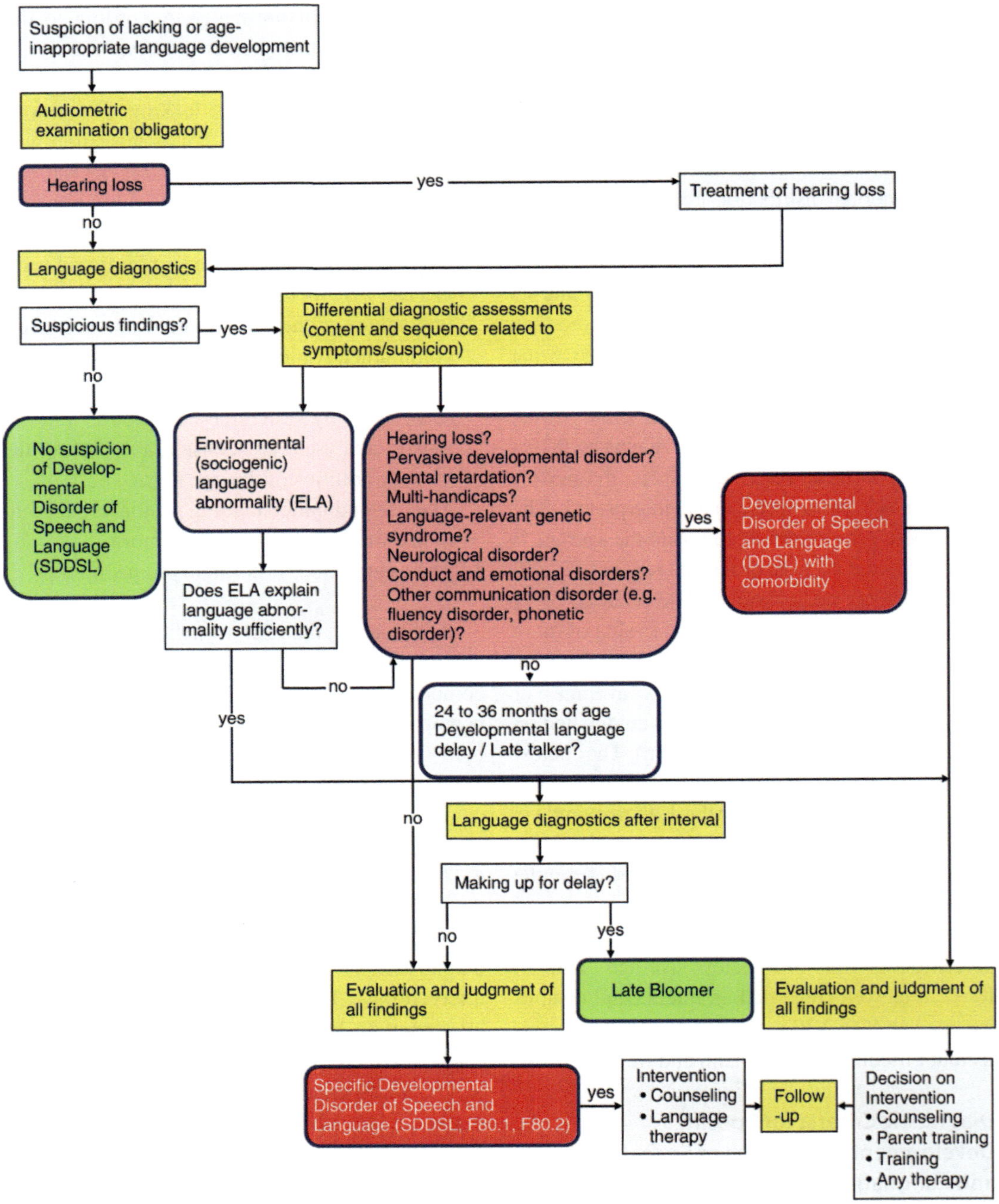

Fig. 3.4 Diagnostic algorithm for developmental disorders of speech and language. (Modified according to de Langen-Müller et al. 2012, with kind permission from Peter Lang GmbH, Internationaler Verlag der Wissenschaften)

or regional screening tests at kindergarten or preschool ages, i.e. short and easy to perform and to analyze language tests, have been implemented in some European regions. They aim at the detection and support of children with language abnormalities by either language therapy or training, in order to ensure sufficient language competence at school entry. In most cases such screening can distinguish between children who have language abnormalities and those who do not. Only a few screening tests, such as the German Kindersprachscreening (KiSS.2), trichotomize between (a) normally developed children, (b) children who have sociogenically caused language abnormalities and who require language training and (c) those who are suspect for having a DDSL and need therapy (Neumann and Euler 2013).

In order to evaluate the validity of a screening, the proportion of children who fail it (REFER, screening-positive) and of those who pass it (PASS, screening-negative) have to be evaluated by comparing the results of the screening and those of reference language tests (gold standard) in a sufficient large, unselected sample of screened children. Furthermore, the proportion of false and correct positives (REFER rate) and false and correct negatives (PASS rate) have to be calculated (Table 3.2). From these values, sensitivity and specificity of the screening may be calculated, the most important validity criteria. Specificity measures the ability of language screening to detect children with normal language development correctly, and the sensitivity indicates the ability to identify children with language abnormalities correctly.

Sensitivity and specificity of screening are related to each other. This can be demonstrated by a receiver operating characteristic (ROC) curve, which shows the ability of screening to distinguish between two conditions such as PASS and REFER (Fig. 3.5).

For a PASS/REFER decision, a cut-off criterion has to be defined. Cut-off values may be derived from the prevalence of a disease. If the prevalence of SDDSL is given as 4–7% and that of DDSL with comorbidity estimates at least 3%, then diagnostic testing for DDSL should not reveal much more than 10% of children in a normal population who fail it, which is between −1 and −2 SD (see 'Diagnostic Criteria' in Sect. 3.3.1.5). For screening the borderlines have to be extended, because a certain number of false positives (children who do not pass the test but have no DDSL) have to be accepted in order to minimize the number of false negatives (children who pass the test despite a DDSL). The cut-off value of a screening depends on a trade-off between the

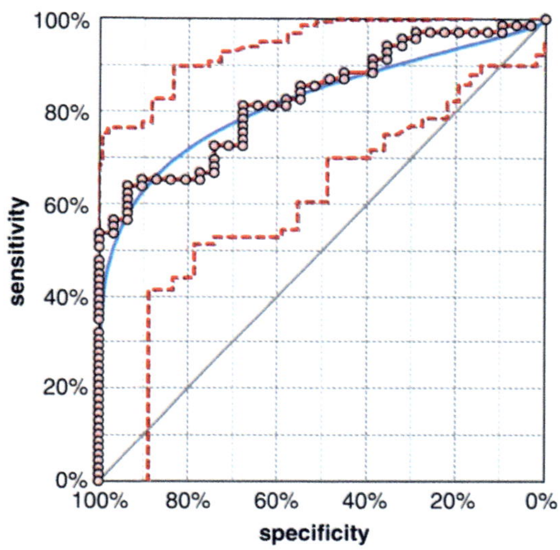

Fig. 3.5 Hypothetical ROC curve of a screening procedure. Because for ROC analyses the original proportions of false positives have been used, which are 1-specificity, the *x*-axis values descend from 100. The figure demonstrates an ROC curve (circles), a trend curve assuming a normal distribution of the data (blue curve), the upper and lower 95% confidence limits (dashed red lines) and the diagonal (grey line). The predictive power of a screening starts above the diagonal. The larger the AUC, the higher the validity of the screening. An increase in specificity in the decision algorithm of the screening results in a decrease of the sensitivity. An ideal curve would run rectangularly along the *y*-axis and the upper borderline of the diagram. (Image adapted from Keller (2014) with kind permission of Dr. Thomas Keller)

Table 3.2 Agreement between the results of language screening and diagnostic language assessment with language tests

		Diagnostic tests		
		DDSL (D+)	No DDSL (D−)	Total
Screening	REFER (S+)	**cp**	fp	cp + fp
	PASS (S−)	**fn**	rn	fn + cn
	Total	cp + fn	fp + rn	cp + fp + cn + fn

S+ screening-positive, *S−* screening-negative, *D+* diagnostics-positive, *D−* diagnostics-negative, *cp* correct positive, *cn* correct negative, *fp* false positive, *fn* false negative proportion of false negatives that is acceptable and that of false positives, which would increase the number of children who have to undergo follow-up diagnostics. It seems reasonable that screening should reveal about 15% of children who do not pass it in order to get the (at maximum) 10% of children who really have a DDSL from subsequent diagnostics.

The real language status of a child and the screening result for a given cut-off point can be compared in a contingency table (Table 3.2). In ROC curves the value pairs of specificity and sensitivity of a screening are drawn for all possible cut-off values. The area under the curve (AUC) indicates the validity of a screening. The more it approaches 1, the higher the validity.

Language screening programs are crucial because (a) children without language abnormalities are easier to detect than those with abnormalities (Law et al. 2000), (b) the language development for each specific linguistic competence has large variance and (c) there is often only poor evidence for a sufficient validity of a reference tests. Therefore, sensitivities and specificities of language screening that do not lie below 80% are assumed by convention to be acceptable (Petermann and Macha 2005; Plante and Vance 1994).

Examples of Language Screening, General and Specific Speech-Language Tests and Developmental Tests that Include Language Subtests

Tables 3.3, 3.4, and 3.5 show examples of valid and standardized language screening and general speech, language and developmental tests, which also include language subtests, for German- and English-speaking Europe.

Table 3.3 Register of examples of language screening tests, general and specific language tests and language-covering developmental tests for German- and English-speaking Europe

Test	Language	References
AVAK	German	Hacker D, Wilgermein H (2001) AVAK-Test mit CD-ROM Analyseverfahren zu Aussprachestörungen bei Kindern, 2nd edn CD-ROM 2006) Reinhardt, München
AWMA	English	Alloway TP (2007) Automated working memory assessment (AWMA). Pearson, Oxford. Available via www.psychcorp.co.uk/product.aspx?n=1343&s=1492&cat=1356&skey=3909. Accessed 7 June 2014
AWST-R	German	Kiese-Himmel C (2005) Aktiver Wortschatztest für 3-bis 5-jährige Kinder—Revision. Beltz, Göttingen
BISC	German	Jansen H, Mannhaupt G, Marx H et al. (2002) Bielefelder Screening zur Früherkennung von Lese-Rechtschreibschwierigkeiten. 2nd revised edn. Hogrefe, Göttingen
BISD III	English	Bayley N (2006) Bayley scales of infant and toddler development, 3rd edn. Harcourt Assessment Inc., San Antonio
BLDT	German	Niemeyer W (1976) Bremer Lautdiskriminationstest 2. Klasse BLDT, Herbig, Bremen
BUEVA	German	Esser G, Wyschkon A (2002) BUEVA—Basisdiagnostik umschriebener Entwicklungsstörungen im Vorschulalter. Hogrefe, Göttingen
CDI	English	Ireton H (1992) Child Development Inventory. Behavior Science Systems, Inc., Minneapolis Ireton H, Glascoe FP (1995) Assessing children's development using parents' reports: the Child Development Inventory. Clin Pediatr (Phila) 34(5):248–255
CELF	English	Semel E, Wiig E, Secord W (1995) Clinical evaluation of language fundamentals, 3rd edn. The psychological corporation, Harcourt Brace & Company, San Antonio
CELF-P	English	Wiig EH, Secord W, Semel E (1998) Clinical evaluation of language fundamentals —preschool (CELF-preschool). The psychological corporation, Harcourt Brace Jovanovich, San Antonio
CREFT-3	English	Wallace G, Hammill DD (1994) Comprehensive receptive and expressive vocabulary test, 3rd edn (CREFT-3). Pro-Ed, Austin
Das Pragmatische Profil	German	Dohmen A, Dewart H, Summers S (2009) Das Pragmatische Profil—Analyse kommunikativer Fähigkeiten von Kindern. Elsevier, München

(continued)

Table 3.3 (continued)

Test	Language	References
ELAN	German	Bockmann AK, Kiese-Himmel C (2006) ELAN—Eltern Antworten. Beltz, Göttingen
ELFRA	German	Grimm H, Doil H (2006) ELFRA—Elternfragebögen für die Früherkennung von Risikokindern, 2nd revised edn. Hogrefe, Göttingen
EOWPVT-R	English	Gardner MF (2000) Expressive one-word picture vocabulary test—revised (EOWPVT). Academic Therapy, Novato
ESGRAF-R	German	Motsch HJ (2018) ESGRAF-R Testmanual: Evozierte Sprachdiagnose grammatischer Fähigkeiten, 2nd revised edn. Reinhardt, München
ETS 4–8	German	Angermaier M (2007) Entwicklungstest Sprache 4 bis 8 Jahre (ETS 4–8). Pearson Assessment, Frankfurt
FRAKIS	German	Szagun G, Stumper B, Schramm SA (2007) Fragebogen zur frühkindlichen Sprachentwicklung und FRAKIS-K (Kurzform). Pearson, Frankfurt
GFTA-2	English	Goldman R, Fristoe M (2000) Goldman-Fristoe Test of Articulation-2 (GFTA-2). American Guidance Service, Circle Pines
HASE	German	Schöler H, Brunner M (2008) HASE—Heidelberger Auditives Screening in der Einschulungsdiagnostik, 2nd revised edn. Westra, Wertingen
HSET	German	Grimm H, Schöler H (1991) Heidelberger Sprachentwicklungstest (HSET), 2nd revised edn. Hogrefe, Göttingen
ITPA-3	English	Hammill DD, Mather N, Roberts R (2001) Illinois test of psycholinguistic abilities, 3rd edn (ITPA-3). Pro-Ed, Austin
KISS.2	German	Euler HA, Holler-Zittlau I, van Minnen S et al (2010) Psychometrische Gütekriterien eines Kurztests zur Erfassung des Sprachstandes vierjähriger Kinder. HNO 58(11):1116–1123 Neumann K, Holler-Zittlau I, Euler HA (2011) Kinder-Sprach-Screening “KiSS”. Available via https://soziales.hessen.de/gesundheit/kinder-sprachscreening-kiss. Accessed 7 June 2014
LDS	English	Rescorla L (1989) The language development survey: a screening tool for delayed language in toddlers. J Speech Hear Disord 54:(4)587–599
LiSe-DaZ	German	Schulz P, Tracy R (2012) LiSe-DaZ. Linguistische Sprachstandserhebung—Deutsch als Zweitsprache. Hogrefe, Göttingen
LSV	German	Götte R (1976) Landauer Sprachentwicklungstest für Vorschulkinder LSV. Beltz, Weinheim
LTB-J	German	Barwitzki K, Hofbauer C, Huber M et al. (2008) LTB-J - Leipziger Testbatterie zur Messung des formal-sprachlichen Entwicklungsstandes bei Jugendlichen. BBW, Leipzig
MBCDI	English	Fenson L, Marchman VA, Thal DJ et al. (2007) MacArthur-Bates communicative development inventories: user’s guide and technical manual, 2nd edn. Paul H. Brookes Publishing, Baltimore
Mottier	German	Kiese-Himmel C, Risse T (2009) Normen für den Mottier-Test bei 4- bis 6-jährigen Kindern. HNO 57(9):943–948 Risse T, Kiese-Himmel C (2009) Der Mottier-test. Teststatistische Überprüfung an 4- bis 6-jährigen Kindern. HNO 57(5):523–528
MSVK	German	Elben CE, Lohaus A (2000) Marburger Sprachverständnistest für Kinder MSVK. Hogrefe, Göttingen
MÜSC	German	Mannhaupt G (2006) Das Münsteraner Screening zur Früherkennung von Lese- und Rechtschreibschwierigkeiten (MÜSC). Cornelsen, Berlin
NRDLS	English	Edwards S, Letts C, Sinka I (2011) The New Reynell Developmental Language Scales (NRDLS). GL Assessment, London
NSST	English	Lee, Lee LL (1969) Northwestern syntax screening test. Northwestern University Press, Evanston
NSST S	English	Ratusnik DL, Klee TM, Ratusnik CM (1980) Northwestern syntax screening test: a short form. J Speech Hear Disord 45(2):200–208
PDSS	German	Kauschke C, Siegmüller J (2009) Patholinguistische Diagnostik bei Sprachentwicklungsstörungen, 2nd edn. Elsevier, Heidelberg

(continued)

Table 3.3 (continued)

Test	Language	References
PAT	English	Pendergast K, Dickey SE, Selmar JW et al. (1984) Photo articulation test. Stoelting, Chicago
PPVT III	English	Dunn LM, Dunn LM (1997) Examiner's manual for the Peabody Picture Vocabulary Test-third edition (PPVT-III). American Guidance Service, Circle Pines
	German	Bulheller S, Dunn LM, Dunn LM et al. (German edition) (2003) Peabody Picture Vocabulary Test: (PPVT); Manual. Swets Test Services, Frankfurt
P-ITPA	German	Ballaschk K, Hänsch S, Esser G (2010) P-ITPA. Potsdam-Illinois Test für Psycholinguistische Fähigkeiten. Hogrefe, Göttingen
PLAKSS-II	German	Fox A (2014) PLAKSS-II Psycholinguistische Analyse kindlicher Sprechstörungen-II, 1st edn. Pearson, Frankfurt
PLS-5	English	Zimmerman IL, Steiner VG, Pond RE (2011) PLS-5 Preschool Language Scales, 5th edn. Pearson, San Antonio
PLS-5 ST	English	Zimmerman, IL, Steiner VG, Pond RE (2011) Preschool Language Scale-5 Screening Test, 5th edn. (PLS-5 Screening Test). Pearson, San Antonio
Prüfbögen zur Mundmotorik	German	Garliner D (1989) Myofunktionelle Therapie in der Praxis - Gestörtes Schluckverhalten, gestörte Gesichtsmuskulatur und die Folgen - Diagnose, Planung und Durchführung der Behandlung. Hütig, Heidelberg Giel B, Tillmanns-Karus M (2004) Kölner Diagnostikbogen für Myofunktionelle Störungen. Modernes lernen, Dortmund Kittel AM (2009) Myofunktionelle Therapie, 9th revised edn. Schulz-Kirchner, Idstein
SBE-2-KT	German	Suchodoletz Wv, Sachse S (2009) Sprachbeurteilung durch Eltern, Kurztest für die U7 (SBE-2-KT). Available via http://www.kjp.med.uni-muenchen.de/download/SBE-2-KT.pdf. Accessed 7 June 2014
		Suchodoletz Wv, Sachse S (2009) Sprachbeurteilung durch Eltern, Kurztest für die U7 (SBE-2-KT), non-normalized translation in 33 languages. Available via https://www.kjp.med.uni-muenchen.de/download/SBE-2-KT.pdf. Accessed 13 April 2018
SBE-3-KT	German	Suchodoletz Wv, Kademann S, Tippelt S (2009) Sprachbeurteilung durch Eltern, Kurztest für die U7a (SBE-3-KT). Available via http://www.kjp.med.uni-muenchen.de/download/SBE-3-KT.pdf. Accessed 7 June 2014
SET 5–10	German	Petermann F, Metz D, Fröhlich LP (2010) SES 5–10. Sprachstandserhebungstest für Kinder im Alter zwischen 5 und 10 Jahren. Hogrefe, Göttingen
SETK-2	German	Grimm H, Aktas M, Frevert S (2000) Sprachentwicklungstest für zweijährige Kinder SETK-2. Hogrefe, Göttingen
	German	Grimm H, Aktas M, Frevert S (2010) Sprachentwicklungstest für drei- bis fünfjährige Kinder SETK 3-5, 2nd revised edn. Hogrefe, Göttingen
SSV	German	Grimm H, Aktas M, Kießig U (2003) Sprachscreening für das Vorschulalter SSV. Kurzform des SETK 3–5. Hogrefe, Göttingen
Teddy-test	German	Friedrich G (1998) Teddy-Test. Hogrefe, Göttingen
TDA	English	Templin MC, Darley FL (1969) The Templin-Darley tests of articulation; a manual and discussion of articulation testing, 2nd edn. Bureau of Educational Research and Service, Division of Extension and University Services, University of Iowa, Iowa City
TELD, TELD-2, TELD-3	English	Hresko WP, Reid DK, Hammill DD (1981) Test of early language development. Pro-Ed, Austin, TX
TTFC-2	English	McGhee RL, Ehrler DJ, DiSimoni F (2007) Token test for children-second edition (TTFC-2). Pro-Ed, Austin, TX
TOLD-P:4	English	Newcomer PL, Hammill DD (2008) Test of Language Development-Primary, 4th edn (TOLD-P:4). Pro-Ed, Austin
TOLD-I:4	English	Hammill DD, Newcomer PL (2008) Test of Language Development-Intermediate, 4th edn (TOLD-I:4). Pro-Ed, Austin
TPB	German	Fricke S, Schäfer B (2011) Test phonologischer Bewusstheitsfähigkeiten, 2nd edn. Schulz-Kirchner, Idstein

(continued)

Table 3.3 (continued)

Test	Language	References
TROG-D	German	Fox AV (2008) TROG-D - Test zur Überprüfung des Grammatik-Verständnisses, 3rd edn. Schulz-Kirchner, Idstein
TSVK	German	Siegmüller J, Kauschke C, van Minnen S et al (2010) Test des Satzverständnisses bei Kindern. Eine profilorientierte Diagnostik der Syntax. Elsevier, Heidelberg
Vineland-II	English	Sparrow SS, Balla DA Cicchetti DV (2005) Vineland Adaptive Behaviors Scales, 2nd edn (Vineland-II). American Guidance Service, Circle Pines
WJ-III	English	Woodcock RW, McGrew KS, Mather N (2001) Woodcock-Johnson-III Tests of achievement. Riverside Publishing, Itasca
WRAT-4	English	Wilkinson GS, Robertson GJ (2006) Wide Range Achievement Test - fourth edition (WRAT-4) professional manual. Psychological Assessment Resources, Lutz
WWT 6–10	German	Glück CW (2007) WWT 6–10. Wortschatz- und Wortfindungstest für 6- bis 10-Jährige. Urban & Schwarzenberg, München

3.3.2 Oral-Motor Examination Protocol

Ana Martínez Arellano
and María Bielsa Corrochano

3.3.2.1 Introduction

The orofacial system consists of bony, nervous and muscular components. As in all mammals, the primary functions of this orofacial system are food intake (sucking, eating, drinking, biting, swallowing) and breathing. Furthermore, its potential for mimicry is an important communication means. In humans it additionally serves a secondary function: speech sound production. For children, the structural and functional adequacy of the oral-motor system provides the basis for the development of all the named functions.

An oral-motor examination, as part of the phoniatric assessment in cases of developmental speech, language and swallowing abnormalities, helps to verify normal patterns as well as organic or functional deficits underlying *phonetic* (mechanical and acoustical forming of speech sounds) speech sound disorders and swallowing problems in childhood. This examination together with an assessment of the status of speech sound development as described in Sect. 3.3.6 should be used systematically in order to enable a distinction between *phonetic* and *phonological* (linguistic) components of speech sound abnormality or disorder.

After a parental interview on the clinical history of their child, focusing on the development of the primary functions and oral perception, oral-motor examination includes the exploration of the following orofacial components and their interplay, in order to

> determine their structural and functional adequacy for speech
> —Nicolosi et al. (2003)

and swallowing: lips, jaws, teeth, tongue, hard palate, soft palate and pharynx. It should comprise the following aspects:

- Inspection of the structure and muscle tone at rest, assessing size, symmetry, shape and possible presence of scars, clefts or other anomalies of the specific orofacial components.
- Examination of oral functions during the performance of specific oral movements, observing muscle tone, coordination and extent of mobility.

The results of the above-named examinations provide relevant information about the possible causes of speech sound disorders and swallowing problems of the children examined. With respect to differential diagnoses, this examination also serves as a decision-making ('pass/fail') procedure (ASHA 2004) to initiate further comprehensive assessments if cardinal symptoms of specific disorders are found, such as dysglossia, central speech motor processing disorders (dyspraxia, dysarthria) or peripheral or central swallowing disorders (ASHA 2004). In the following key aspects of an oral-motor examination, potential methods and possible observations are listed.

Table 3.4 Screenings, general developmental language tests and (The spelling *x*; *y* years in the table means *x* years and *y* months of age.) language-covering general developmental tests for German- and English-speaking Europe for the evaluation of a risk for a DDSL and other developmental disorders or delays

Method	Aim	Age-related test (year; month)					
		≤12 months	12–24 months	25–36 months	3–5 years	6–10 years	≥11 years
Screenings Parent questionnaires	Evaluation of a risk	ELFRA 1 (1;0) PLS-5 ST (0–7;11) MBCDI (0;8–3;1)	ELFRA 2 (2;0) ELAN (1; 4–2;2) FRAKIS (1;6–2;5) SBE-2-KT (1;9–2;0)[a,b] CDI (1;3–5;11) PLS-5 ST (0–7;11) LDS (1;6–2;11) MBCDI (0;8–3;1)	ELAN (1;4–2;2) SBE-3-KT (2;8–3;4) CDI (1;3–5;11) PLS-5 ST (0–7;11) LDS (1;6–2;11) MBCDI (0;8–3;1)	KiSS.2 (4;0–4;5)[b] SSV (3;0–5;0) LSV (4;0–6;5) BISC (preschool age) HASE (4;0–6;11) ETS 4–8 (4;0–8;11) CDI (1;3–5;11) PLS-5 ST (0;0–7;11) NSST S (3;0–7;11) LiSe-DaZ (3;0–6;11)[b]	ETS 4–8 (4;0–8;11) NSST S (3;0–7;11) LiSe-DaZ (3;0–6;11)[b]	
General developmental language tests and language-covering general developmental tests	Evaluation of a deviation from the age norm	PLS-5 (0;0–7;11) BISD III (0;1–3;6)	BISD III (0;1–3;6)	SETK-2 (2;0–2;11) PDSS (2;0–6;11) TELD, −2, −3 (2;0–7;11) NRDLS (2;0–7;5) WJ-III (2;0–90;0) BISD III (0;1–3;6) Vineland-II (0;0–90;0)	SETK 3–5 (3;0–5;11) PDSS (2;0–6;11) P-ITPA (4;0–11;0) BUEVA (4;0–5;11) HSET (3;0–9;0) TELD, −2, −3 (2;0–7;11) TOLD (4;0–17;11) NRDLS (2;0–7;5) CELF (5;0–21;0) CELF-P (3;0–6;11) WJ-III (2;0–90;0) BISD III (0;1–3;6) ITPA-3 (5;0–12;11) LiSe-DaZ (3;0–6;11)[b] TOLD-P:4 (4;0–8;11) Vineland-II (0;0–90;0) WRAT-4 (5;0–94;0)	PDSS (2;0–6;11) P-ITPA (4;0–11;0) BUEVA (4;0–5;11) SET 5–10 (5;0–10;11) HSET (3;0–9;0) TELD, −2, −3 (2;0–7;11) TOLD (4;0–17;11) NRDLS (2;0–7;5) CELF (5;0–21;0) CELF-P (3;0–6;11) WJ-III (2;0–90;0) ITPA-3 (5;0–12;11) LiSe-DaZ (3;0–6;11)[b] TOLD-P:4 (4;0–8;11) TOLD-I:4 (8;0–17;11) Vineland-II (0;0–90;0) WRAT-4 (5;0–94;0)	LTB-J (grade 9–10) TOLD (4;0–17;11) CELF (5;0–21;0) WJ-III (2;0–90;0) ITPA-3 (5;0–12;11) TOLD-I:4 (8;0–17;11) Vineland-II (0;0–90;0) WRAT-4 (5;0–94;0)

[a]Available in 34 languages
[b]Also suited for bi- and multilingual children

Table 3.5 Examples of specific language tests examining distinct linguistic skills for German- and English-speaking Europe

Diagnostic fields	Competence	Age-related test (year; month)					
		≤12 months	12–24 months	25–36 months	3–5 years	6–10 years	≥11 years
Basal or precursor functions							
	Verbal/phonological working memory				HASE (4;0–6;11) BISC (preschool age) Mottier (4;0–16;0) KiSS.2 (4;0–4;5) ETS 4–8 (4;0–8;11) AWMA (4;0–22;0) SSV (3;0–5;11)	HASE (4;0–6;11) BISC (preschool age) Mottier (4;0–16;0) AWMA (4;0–22;0) ETS 4–8 (4;0–8;11) MÜSC (first 5 school weeks)	AWMA (4;0–22;0) Mottier (4;0–16;0)
	Oral-motor skills			Check lists (e.g. Garliner; Giel & Tillmanns-Karus; Kittel)	Check lists (e.g. Garliner; Giel & Tillmanns-Karus; Kittel)	Check lists (e.g. Garliner; Giel & Tillmanns-Karus; Kittel)	
	Phonological awareness				TPB (4 to about 7 years) BISC (preschool age) ETS 4–8 (4;0–8;11	TPB (4 to about 7 years) MÜSC (first 5 school weeks) ETS 4–8 (4;0–8;11)	
Language competence							
Phonetics/ phonology	Articulation		PLAKKS-II (1;6–5;11)	PLAKKS-II (1;6–5;11) PDSS (2;0–6;11) GFTA-2 (2;0–21;11)	AVAK (children) PLAKKS-II (1;6–5;11) PDSS (2;0–6;11) KiSS.2 (4;0–4;5) TDA (3;0–8;0) GFTA-2 (2;0–21;11) PAT (3;0–8;11)	PDSS (2;0–6;11) TDA (3;0–8;0) GFTA-2 (2;0–21;11) PAT (3;0–8;11)	GFTA-2 (2;0–21;11)
	Phoneme discrimination			PDSS (2;0–6;11)	PDSS (2;0–6;11) KiSS.2 (4;0–4;5) Mottier (4;0–16;0)	PDSS (2;0–6;11) Mottier (4;0–16;0) BLDT (end of second grade)	

(continued)

Table 3.5 (continued)

Diagnostic fields	Competence	Age-related test (year; month)					
		≤12 months	12–24 months	25–36 months	3–5 years	6–10 years	≥11 years
Grammar	Morphology Perception			PDSS (2;0–6;11)	SETK 3–5 (3;0–5;11) PDSS (2;0–6;11) TROG-D (3;0–10;11) KiSS.2 (4;0–4;5) NSST (3; 0–7; 11 years) NRDLS (2; 0–7; 5) TTFC-2 (3;0–12;11) TOLD-P:4 (4;0–8;11)	PDSS (2;0–6;11) NSST (3;0–7;11) TROG-D (3;0–10;11) TTFC-2 (3;0–12;11) TOLD-I:4 (8;0–17;11) TOLD-P:4 (4;0–8;11)	TTFC-2 (3;0–12;11) TOLD-I:4 (8;0–17;11)
	Production		FRAKIS (1;6–2;5)	PDSS (2;0–6;11)	SETK 3–5 (3;0–5;11) ESGRAF-R (4–16 years) PDSS (2;0–6;11) KiSS.2 (4;0–4;5) NSST (3;0–7;11) TOLD-P:4 (4;0–8;11)	ESGRAF-R (4–16 years) PDSS (2;0–6;11) NSST (3;0–7;11) TOLD-I:4 (8;0–17;11) TOLD-P:4 (4;0–8;11)	ESGRAF-R (4;0–16;0) TOLD-I:4 (8;0–17;11)
	Syntax Perception			TSVK (2–8 years) PDSS (2;0–6;11) NRDLS (2;0–7;5)	TSVK (2;0–8;0) TROG-D (3;0–10;11) MSVK (5 year-end of first grade) SETK 3–5 (3;0–5;11) PDSS (2;0–6;11) KiSS.2 (4;0–4;5) NSST (3;0–7;11) NRDLS (2;0–7;5) TTFC-2 (3;0–12;11) TOLD-P:4 (4;0–8;11)	TSVK (2;0–8;0) TROG-D (3;0–10;11) MSVK (5 year-end of first grade) PDSS (2;0–6;11) NSST (3;0–7;11) NRDLS (2;0–7;5) TTFC-2 (3;0–12;11) TOLD-I:4 (8;0–17;11) TOLD-P:4 (4;0–8;11)	TTFC-2 (3;0–12;11) TOLD-I:4 (8;0–17;11)
	Production		ELFRA 2 (2;0) FRAKIS (1;6–2;5)	PDSS (2;0–6;11) NRDLS (2;0–7;5)	SETK 3–5 (3;0–5;11) PDSS (2;0–6;11) KiSS.2 (4;0–4;5) NSST (3;0–7;11) NRDLS (2;0–7;5) TOLD-P:4 (4;0–8;11)	PDSS (2;0–6;11) NSST (3;0–7;11) NRDLS (2;0–7;5) TOLD-I:4 (8;0–17;11) TOLD-P:4 (4;0–8;11)	TOLD-I:4 (8;0–17;11)

(continued)

Table 3.5 (continued)

Diagnostic fields	Competence	Age-related test (year; month) ≤12 months	12–24 months	25–36 months	3–5 years	6–10 years	≥11 years
Semantics and vocabulary	Semantics	ELFRA 1 (1;0)		PDSS (2;0–6;11) NRDLS (2;0–7;5) PPVT III (2;6–90;0)	Teddy-test (3;0–8;6) MSVK (5 year-end of first grade) PDSS (2;0–6;11) KiSS.2 (4;0–4;5) NRDLS (2;0–7;5) PPVT III (2;6–90;0)	Teddy-test (3;0–8;6) MSVK (5 year-end of first grade) NRDLS (2;0–7;5) PPVT III (2;6–90;0) TOLD-I:4 (8;0–17;11)	PPVT III (2;6–90;0) TOLD-I:4 (8;0–17;11)
	Vocabulary Perception (passive)	ELFRA 1 (1;0)		PDSS (2;0–6;11) PPVT III (2;6–90 years) NRDLS (2;0–7;5)	PDSS (2;0–6;11) KiSS.2 (4;0–4;5) TTFC-2 (3;0–12;11) CREFT-3 (5;0–89;11) PPVT III (2;6–90;0) NRDLS (2;0–7;5)	PDSS (2;0–6;11) CREFT-3 (5;0–89;11) TTFC-2 (3;0–12;11) TOLD-I:4 (8;0–17;11) NRDLS (2;0–7;5)	PPVT (14;0–60;0) CREFT-3 (5;0–89;11) TOLD-I:4 (8;0–17;11) TTFC-2 (3;0 = 12;11) PPVT III (2;6 = 90;0) PPVT German version (13;0–90;0)
	Production (active)	ELFRA 1 (1;0)	ELFRA 2 (2:0) ELAN (1;4–2;2) FRAKIS (1;6–2;5)	PDSS (2;0–6;11) NRDLS (2;0–7;5)	AWST-R (3;0–5;6) PDSS (2;0–6;11) KiSS.2 (4;0–4;5) CREFT-3 (5;0–89;11) NRDLS (2;0–7;5)	WWT 6–10 (6;0–10;0) PDSS (2;0–6;11) CREFT-3 (5;0–89;11) NRDLS (2;0–7;5) TOLD-I:4 (8;0–17;11)	CREFT-3 (5;0–89;11) TOLD-I:4 (8;0–17;11)
Pragmatics/ communication			Vineland-II (0;0–90;0) Das pragmatische Profil (0;0–10;0)	Vineland-II (0;0–90;0) Das pragmatische Profil (0;0–10;0)	MSVK (5 year-end of first grade) KiSS.2 (4;0–4;5) Vineland-II (0;0–90;0) Das pragmatische Profil (0;0–10;0)	MSVK (5 year-end of first grade) Vineland-II (0;0–90;0) Das pragmatische Profil (0;0–10;0)	Vineland-II (0;0–90;0)

Constituents of an oral-motor examination protocol:

- Clinical history.
- Test instruments and materials.
- Inspection of the orofacial structures and evaluation of muscle tone at rest.
- Examination of oral function in motion.
- Interpretation.

3.3.2.2 Clinical History

Clinical history should include questions regarding:

- Pregnancy and birth: foetal distress, natural or assisted childbirth, prematurity, damaging or deleterious factors.
- Age of acquisition of developmental skills (walking, early speech, micturition/faecal control). If these functions are delayed, a potential developmental retardation has to be taken into consideration.
- Feeding, diet and food intake: natural, artificial (e.g. tube feeding), type of bottle nipple, difficulties in sucking, mastication, age of weaning, coughing or choking while or after eating/drinking, aspiration of food or liquid into the lungs (chronic respiratory failure, pneumonia).
- Development of oral perception: intensity of oral exploration in the first year of life; tolerance/acceptance of varying food consistencies and food tastes/flavours.
- Diseases of ear, nose and throat.
- Parafunctions: dummy/pacifier (type, frequency, age of weaning), digit or object sucking, labial or lingual sucking, nail biting, bruxism, snoring, dribbling.

3.3.2.3 Test Instruments and Materials

In order to carry out the examination, a source of frontal light and basic examination materials are needed: gloves, tongue depressors, small mirror for mirror-fogging test and nasal speculum or nasal fibrescope. For the evaluation of swallowing and chewing, solid, semisolid and liquid aliments are used.

3.3.2.4 Inspection of the Orofacial Structure and Muscle Tone at Rest

Assess the size, symmetry, shape and possible presence of scars, clefts or other anomalies of each orofacial structure as below.

External Orofacial Examination

Facies:

- Facial malformations or other anomalies, e.g. hypo–/hypertelorism, epicanthus.

Lips:

- Structure: size, symmetry, lingual frenulum, scars, clefts.
- Function:
  - Resting position: lips open or closed, hypo- or hypertonus.
  - Closure: complete, incomplete.

Nose/Nostrils:

- Examination using the nasal speculum or nasal fibrescope and a small mirror for:
  - Structure: size, form variants, malformations, deviation of nose or nose septum, hyper- or hypoplasia of nasal conchae, width of nostrils, nasal entrance and ducts.
  - Function: nasal airway obstruction, mucus, mucosal swallowing.

Temporomandibular Joint:

- Structure: symmetry of the mandibular branches, protrusion or retraction/hypoplasia of mandibula.
- Function: degrees of freedom and extent of movement.

Intraoral Examination

Tongue:

- Structure: form and size such as macroglossia, microglossia, scars, symmetry.
- Function: muscular tone, position at rest (protrusion, support on the palate, support on incisors interdental), motility, fasciculation, deviation.

Cavum Oris and Pharynx:

- Structure: dental status, status of palate and pharyngeal tonsils (hypertrophy, status after adeno–/tonsillectomy or tonsillotomy, scars), status of mucosa (mucus, swelling, infections), salivary cysts.
- Function: closure of mouth, muscular tone, hypersalivation, velopharyngeal insufficiency.

Hard Palate:

- Structure: malformations or abnormalities such as clefts or fissures, scars, fistulae, form deviations (flat or 'Gothic').
- Function: closure between the mouth and nose, mouth closure.

Soft Palate:

- Structure: malformations or abnormalities such as clefts, bifid uvula, short, long or deviating uvula.
- Function: velopharyngeal insufficiency, hypernasal speech, nasal regurgitation during swallowing.

Teeth and Occlusion:

- Structure: dental status (decayed, missing or filled teeth, dental diastema, malposition) for the primary dentition (deciduous teeth) and for the permanent dentition.
- Function: occlusion. The child is requested to bite and to show her or his teeth.
  - Anteroposterior match: Class I (normocclusion), Class II (distocclusion), Class III (mesiocclusion).
  - Vertical match: normal bite, open bite (anterior, lateral), overbite.
  - Transversal match: crossbite (uni- or bilateral), lateral deviation.

3.3.2.5 Examination of Functionality

Lips:

- In order to examine mobility, the child is requested to make the following movements: lifting, stretching, lateralization, vibration (lip flapping) and kissing. The child's ability to perform these movements and the muscular tone and strength with which they are performed are assessed for:
  - Tone and strength: hypotonus, hypertonus.
  - Mobility: normal, difficult/restricted in a certain direction, very limited, impossible.
  - Closing: complete, incomplete, impossible.

Tongue:

- For examining mobility the child is requested to stretch his or her tongue out; to raise, lower and lateralize it; and to press it against the cheeks from inside the mouth. The tone is examined by using a tongue depressor, asking the child to press against it. In babies and young children, the examination is completed by tactile stimulation of the mouth mucosa and the tongue:
  - Mobility: stretching out, upwards (touching nose), downwards, right, left, rotation.
  - Tone and strength: hypotonus, hypertonus.
  - Lingual frenulum: normal, shortened (ankyloglossia).

Temporomandibular Joint:

- For examining mobility the child is requested to open and close his or her mouth and to complete lateral motions. Muscle tone is evaluated by palpating the joints bimanually:
  - Mobility: opening (normal, difficult/restricted in certain directions, very limited, impossible), symmetry of closure.
  - Dysfunctions: cracking, bruxism, clicks, blockage.

Soft Palate:

- In order to evaluate sufficient velopharyngeal closure of the soft palate, the child is requested to vocalize a word with the plosive /c/ (e.g. cuckoo, Coca-Cola). Breath noise (rhinophonia aperta) indicates lacking or incomplete velopharyngeal closure. Furthermore, vowel sounds are examined, for example, of /u:/ or /a:/. A nasal component (airy noise) indicates a functional rhinophonia aperta.

Chewing and Swallowing:

- The child's myofunctional maturity is evaluated according to her or his age. Food intake (chewing and drinking), oral preparation and swallowing should be observed. Possible findings are:
  - Chewing with open mouth.
  - Gathering of saliva at the corners of the mouth or on the lips.
  - Food remaining in the mouth after swallowing.
  - Drooling, dribbling of saliva or food.
  - Movement forward of the tongue while speaking, chewing and swallowing (tongue thrust), tongue pressure on teeth, lateral tongue pressure, lingual interposition between teeth.
  - Head movements, effort in perioral muscles.
  - For babies: adaptation to the bottle nipple.
  - For infants and young children: licking a spoon.

3.3.2.6 Interpretation

By interpreting the results of the examination for an individual child, the causes for developmental speech sound and swallowing disorder as named in the following can be differentiated. Other disorders, which should either be excluded or considered as potential diagnoses that need further assessment, are listed below:

Phonological Speech Sound Disorder

In the case of a speech sound disorder or abnormality, a phonological cause or at least a component has to be assumed, if the organic and myofunctional adequacy of the orofacial system is given and other potential comorbidities (including hearing loss) are excluded. In this case, the phonological developmental status must be examined closely as described in Sect. 3.3.6.

Phonetic Speech Sound Disorder

Orofunctional causes: immaturity or imbalance of orofacial functions and oral senses without organic abnormalities (including normal hearing); functional inadequacy such as hypotonus of orofacial muscles, poor coordination of oral-motor sequences, often associated with abnormal development of food intake or oral perception (e.g. limited acceptance of a sufficient variety of food flavours or consistencies).

Mechanical causes: for example, a missing tooth, diastema, velopharyngeal insufficiency.

In cases of insufficient velopharyngeal closure and excessive nasal component of speech sounds (rhinophonia aperta), careful differential diagnosis is essential because several underlying causes are possible (e.g. neurological; organic; functional) (Grunwell 1993); see also Part I, Speech Disorders (Dysglossia/Nasality/Velopharyngeal Insufficiency), this Volume.

In the following, differential diagnoses of speech sound and swallowing disorders that may involve orofacial muscle dysfunctions are listed with respect to organic and functional as well as peripheral and central causes:

- *Speech sound disorders* due to hearing impairment (see Part IV, Disorders of Hearing Development).
- *Dysglossia*: a speech sound disorder due to an organic affection of articulation organs (lips, tongue, palate, teeth, jaw, vocal folds) caused by oro- or craniofacial malformations, paralyses, injuries, tumours, muscle disorders or surgery (e.g. cleft lip or palate, macroglossia, scars); see Part I, Speech Disorders (Dysglossia/Nasality/Velopharyngeal Insufficiency), this Volume.
- There is evidence that a shortened lingual frenulum (ankylogossia) may affect breastfeeding and can be treated by surgical procedures. However, there is insufficient evidence that it affects speech sound development or that surgery improves articulatory development of a child. Therefore, frenulotomy or frenuloplasty is not recommended for improvement of speech sound disorders in cases of ankyloglossia (Francis et al. 2015).
- *Speech-language-relevant syndromes*: oro- or craniofacial malformations or abnormalities are often symptoms of a syndrome and should be diagnosed comprehensively (see Sect. 9.10 in Volume 1).

- *Functional (peripheral) swallowing disorders*: orofacial dysfunctions/myofunctional disorders with orofacial muscle imbalance and difficulties in motor coordination and sequencing lead to insufficient oral preparation of swallowing, tongue thrust, malocclusion, mouth breathing, retardation in the development of oral perception and oral hyper−/hypo-sensibility; see Part I, Speech Disorders (Dysglossia/Nasality/Velopharyngeal Insufficiency), this Volume.
- *Central swallowing disorders*: coughing or choking during or after eating/drinking; penetration or aspiration of food or liquid into the lungs; recurrent episodes of pneumonia; raised temperature (as early sign of subclinical pneumonia); substantial/rapid weight loss with no clear cause (Nicolosi et al. 2003); see Part VI, Swallowing Disorders including Rehabilitation of Tumour Patients, this Volume.
- *Oral dyspraxia*: inability to plan and perform an oral-motor task on purpose; symptoms:

> groping, trial-and-error behaviour; purposeful programming of muscular movement while involuntary movements remain intact.
> —Nicolosi et al. (2003)

- *Childhood apraxia of speech* (CAS), also termed developmental verbal dyspraxia, is regarded as a special form of oral dyspraxia and needs diligent assessment (see Sect. 10.2 in Volume 1).
- *Dysarthria*: a

> motor speech disorder due to impairment originating in the central or peripheral nervous system... Usually part of a more generalised neurological impairment...

- (e.g. cerebral palsy)

> Respiration, articulation, phonation, resonation and/or prosody may be affected; volitional and automatic actions, such as chewing and swallowing and movements of the jaw and tongue may also be deviant.
> —Nicolosi et al. (2003)

See Part IV, Acquired Motor Speech Disorders (Dysarthria, Dyspraxia), this Volume.

3.3.3 Assessment of Speech Sound Development

Karen Reichmuth and Melanie Vauth-Weidig

3.3.3.1 Speech Sound Disorders (SSDs) in Children

The assessment of speech sound development is obligatory for comprehensive speech and language evaluation of a child with communication concerns or whenever an SSD is suspected (ASHA 2016).

> Speech sound disorders (SSD) is an umbrella term...
> —(introduced by the ASHA in 2004)...
> referring to any combination of difficulties with perception, motor production and/or the phonological representation of speech sounds and speech segments...that impact speech intelligibility.
> —ASHA (2016)

SSDs constitute the largest group of communication difficulties amongst young children. In English-speaking countries, the prevalence of SSDs in childhood (3–11 years) varies from 3 to 15% (for an overview see McLeod et al. 2013). SSDs in children can be of known (e.g. organic) or unknown aetiology (McLeod et al. 2013); those of unclear origin represent the largest portion (Fox-Boyer et al. 2016). Organic causes of an SSD are hearing impairment, orofacial dysfunction (myofunctional disorder), craniofacial anomalies such as cleft palate or other dysglossia, genetic or non-genetic syndromes and neurological impairment or diseases (e.g. cerebral palsy leading to dysarthria or apraxia) (ASHA 2016). Genetically based SSDs identified by familial clustering of SSDs are also included. For SSDs with unknown causes, several risk factors are discussed (e.g. repeated otitis media, deficits in phonological working memory, delayed phonological development) (Fox-Boyer et al. 2016). Childhood apraxia of speech (CAS) depicts an outlier in the field of SSD (for details see Sect. 10.2 in Volume 1). Neurological causes are hypothesized without the evidence of neurological findings associated with the disorder (Fox-Boyer et al. 2016).

Following aetiology and psycholinguistics, the classification of SSDs in children with developmental speech and language disorders should broadly distinguish three subgroups: phonetic disorders, phonological disorders and neurological motor-speech disorders (see Fig. 3.6 for overview and Table 3.6 for closer definitions). Speech sound abnormalities due to dysphonia, psychogenic speech disorders that mimic other speech disorders (Duffy 2016), speech fluency disorders such as stuttering and cluttering and prosodic abnormalities are excluded from the classification outlined here. For a critical review on various classification and more details of SDDs, see Dodd (2014).

Children with speech sound disorders can have difficulties with perception, articulation/motor production, phonological representation of speech segments (consonants and vowels), phonotactics (syllable and word shapes) and prosody (lexical and grammatical tones, rhythm, stress, and intonation) that may affect speech intelligibility and acceptability.
—International Expert Panel on Multilingual Children's Speech (2012)

Differential diagnosis is needed but often difficult to provide, owing to the large heterogeneity of speech sound disorders. Mixed profiles (phonetic and phonological abnormalities) are also common (Strand and McCauley 2008; Namasivayam et al. 2013). Mandatorily, organic causes should ini-

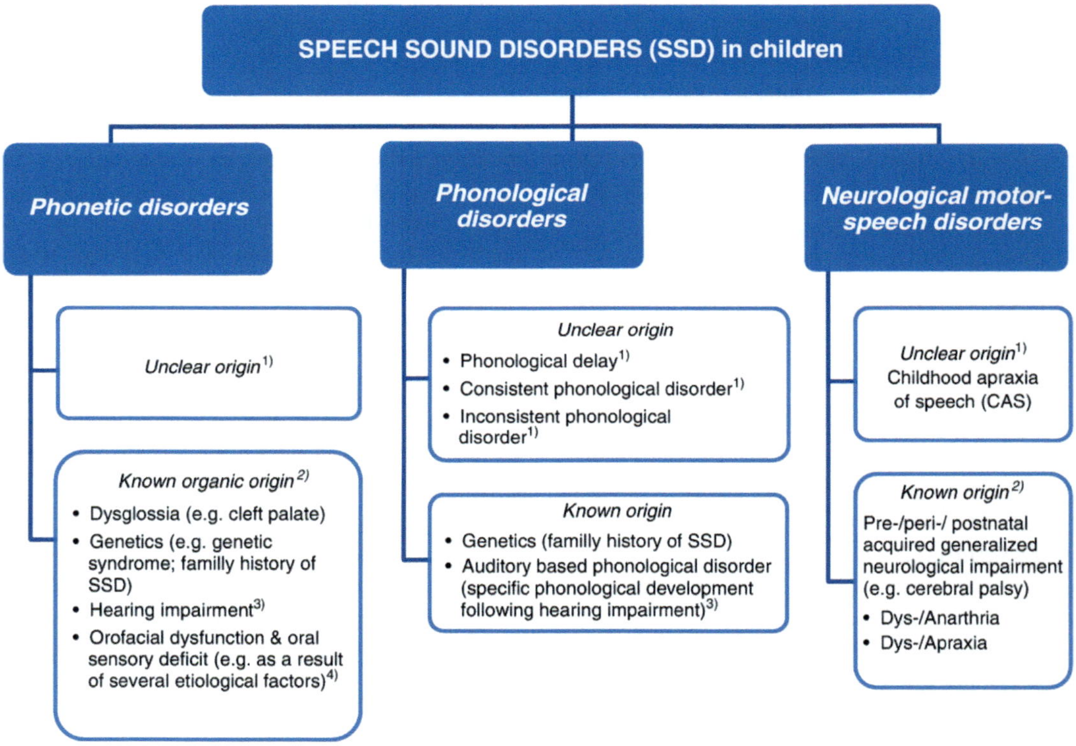

Fig. 3.6 Classification of speech sound disorders (SSD) in children based on etiology and psycholinguistics developed by Reichmuth and Vauth. (1) The five subgroups from the classification of speech sound disorders of unclear origins are from Dodd (2005), Fox-Boyer et al. (2016). (2) Excluding functional dysphonia and speech fluency disorders. (3) For diagnostic and treatment reasons, Reichmuth (2018) underlines the necessity to classify speech sound disorders in hearing-impaired children as a both phonetic and phonological disorder. (4) Several aetiological factors are known to foster the emergence of orofacial dysfunction and sensory deficits: e.g. preterm birth, organic reasons for persisting mouth breathing, oral habits and tongue thrust (Bigenzahn 2003); see also Part I, Speech Disorders (Dysglossia/Nasality/Velopharyngeal Insufficiency), this Volume. The organic origin does not always become obvious. So orofacial dysfunction and sensory deficits can be subsequent or co-occurring symptom as long as the origin is not known

Table 3.6 Characteristics of SSD subtypes (Overview developed by Reichmuth and Vauth)

Subgroup	Definition
Phonetic disorder	General inability to perform correctly the articulatory movements required to produce a certain phone (isolated or in word); maintained ability to realize phonological information correctly if a hearing impairment is excluded
Of unknown origin	
– (without evident organic reason)	• Substitutions or distortions of the same sounds in isolation and in all phonetic contexts during imitation, elicitation and spontaneous speech tasks (e.g. lateral lisp) (Dodd 2014); affects around 12% of all children with SSDs of unknown origin (Dodd 2014)
Of known origin	
– orofacial dysfunction	• Oral sensory deficits; orofacial dysbalance; orofacial hypotonus: for example, tongue thrust, an oral myofunctional phenomenon that can affect production of some sounds, e.g. /s/, /z/, /sh/, /ch/ and /j/ (ASHA 2016), and may cause multiple interdentality of other alveolar sounds (e.g. t, l, n) (see Part I, Speech Disorders (Dysglossia/Nasality/Velopharyngeal Insufficiency), this Volume)
– Dysglossia	• Structural causes: e.g. craniofacial malformations such as cleft palate or macroglossia influence the ability to perform correct articulatory movements; both articulation and resonance (e.g. nasal component, hypernasality) may be affected; maintained ability to realize phonological information correctly if a hearing impairment is excluded (see Part I, Speech Disorders (Dysglossia/Nasality/Velopharyngeal Insufficiency), this Volume)
– Hearing impairment	• Peripheral hearing loss; sensory-input-caused limitations in speech sound development, which can be reduced by early identification (e.g. by newborn hearing screening) and treatment (hearing devices) of the hearing loss (see also 'phonetic-phonological disorder in hearing-impaired children' in this table)
– Genetic (e.g. syndromes)	• Genetic causes lead to diverse aspects of organic origins of SSDs (e.g. dysglossia, hearing loss, orofunctional deficits); syndrome-specific SSD expression, e.g. in Down syndrome, Pierre Robin syndrome, Franceschetti syndrome
Phonological disorder	Defined as failure of the correct use of the linguistic component of a speech sound (phoneme); inability to process or deficiency in processing phonological information correctly and to use a phoneme linguistically correctly in words, even though the isolated performance of the phone is possible
Of unknown origin	
– Phonological delay	• Prolonged use (at least 6 months) of at least one (formerly) physiological phonological process of normal speech sound development (see Table 3.7) (Fox-Boyer et al. 2016; Dodd 2014); isolated performance of the phone is (often) possible
– Consistent phonological disorder	• Consequent use of at least one pathological phonological process (Fox-Boyer et al. 2016; see also Dodd 2014); isolated performance of the phone is (often) possible
– Inconsistent phonological disorder	• Inability to pronounce repeatedly a specific word identically; a high rate of inconsistency >40% (in a given wordlist of 25–30 words) (see also Dodd 2005, 2014; Fox-Boyer 2014); isolated performance of the phone is (often) possible
Of known origin	
– Genetic	Family history of SSD
– Phonetic-phonological disorder in hearing-impaired children	• Overall influence of the hearing loss on the phonological acquisition often leads to specific, mostly consistent, phonological processes (even when hearing devices are fitted): structural simplification such as deletion of (weak) syllables and final consonants, nasalization of vowels and vowel shift; structural simplification such as deletion of speech sounds or weak syllables and assimilation as well as systemic simplifications such as stopping of fricatives (see Table 3.7)

(continued)

Table 3.6 (continued)

Subgroup	Definition
Neurological motor-speech disorders	
Of unknown origin	
– Childhood apraxia of speech (CAS; synonym: verbal developmental dyspraxia)	• Failure of central oral or verbal motor planning functions are assumed (see Sect. 10.2 in Volume 1 for details) without obvious neurological impairment; inadequate intonation (e.g. word stress and prosody); speech characterized by inconsistency, oromotor symptoms (e.g. difficulty in sequencing of articulatory movements), slow speech rate, disturbed prosody, short length of utterance, poorer performance in imitation than in spontaneous speech production (Dodd 2014); predominant use of vowels; reduced use of consonants; adiadochokinesis (inability to execute repetitions of rapidly changing articulatory movements)
Of known origin	
– Dysarthria	• Motor-speech disorder due to impairment of the central or peripheral nervous system; respiration, articulation, phonation, resonation or prosody may be affected; volitional and automatized motor actions such as jaw and tongue movements in chewing and swallowing may also be deviant; usually part of a neurological impairment, e.g. cerebral palsy (Nicolosi et al. 2003); see Part IV Acquired Motor Speech Disorders (Dysarthria, Dyspraxia), this Volume
– Dyspraxia	• Impaired capacity to programme the position of speech musculature and the sequencing of muscle movements (respiratory, laryngeal and oral) for the volitional production of phones as part of a neurological impairment, e.g. cerebral palsy; involuntary production of the same phone or movement is possible, e.g. cerebral palsy (Nicolosi et al. 2003; see Part II)

tially be detected or excluded (including hearing tests and oral-motor examination). Especially in cases of excessive nasal components of speech (hypernasality), differential diagnosis is essential because several underlying serious causes are possible for insufficient velopharyngeal closure (e.g. neurological, organic, functional, sensory). In case of uncertainty, a referral to a neuro-pediatrician for excluding a neurological cause is obligatory.

3.3.3.2 About Speech Sounds: Linguistic Fundamentals for Assessment

Every language has its specific inventory of speech sounds (for details on 57 languages, see Speech Accent Archive, Weinberger 2015). The way children develop the proper articulation of speech sounds (phonetics) and their correct linguistic use in language (phonology) follows physiological processes.

Accordingly, speech sounds in a certain language are determined by these two components:

- The *phonetic component* emphasizes the specific physical and articulatory characteristics of each speech sound.
- In this sense speech sounds are called *phones*. The regular development of a child's phonetic inventory depends on normally developed speech organs, as well as normal hearing and oral-motor control. In this context the acquisition of the correct use of phones is an *aspect of speech development*. Speech sounds are usually subclassified into two broad groups: consonants and vowels. See Fig. 3.7 for an example of the phonetic inventory of consonants in English from the Speech Accent Archive (Weinberger 2015). See Fig. 3.8a, b for vowel charts of Jones (1972, adapted) and the International Phonetic Association (IPA 1999).
- The *phonological component* emphasizes the linguistic aspect speech sounds have in language as *phonemes*. A phoneme is the.

> shortest arbitrary unit of sound in a given language.
> —Nicolosi et al. (2003)

It distinguishes the meaning of one word from another in the particular language: e.g. the use of the phonemes /t/ or /p/ distinguishes between the word *cut* and *cup*. So the acquisition of the cor-

Consonants (Pulmonic)

	Bilabial	Labiodental	Dental	Alveolar	Postalveolar	Retroflex	Palatal	Velar	Uvular	Pharyngeal	Glottal
Plosive	p b			t d				k g			
Nasal	m			n				ŋ			
Trill											
Tap or Flap											
Fricative		f v	θ ð	s z	ʃ ʒ						h
Affricate					tʃ dʒ						
Lateral fricative											
Approximant				ɹ			j				
Lateral approximant				l							

Where symbols appear in pairs, the one to the right represents a voiced consonant. Shaded areas denote articulations judged impossible.

Fig. 3.7 Native phonetic inventory—English: the consonants found in most native English dialects are demonstrated. Source: Speech Accent Archive, Weinberger (2015) Speech Accent Archive, for English, adapted from Ladefoged (2006). Matrix of consonants: consonants are determined by three parameters according to the manner of formation—(**a**) place of articulation (*x*-axis), (**b**) mode of articulation (*y*-axis) and (**c**) use of voice (voiced/voiceless), e.g. [t] vs. [d] (definition adapted from Nicolosi et al. 2003). The worldwide convention is to transcribe phones according to the International Phonetic Alphabet (IPA). (Republished with permission of South-Western College Publishing, a division of Cengage Learning, from A Course in Phonetics. Ladefoged P. 5th edition. Thomson Wadsworth, Boston © 2006)

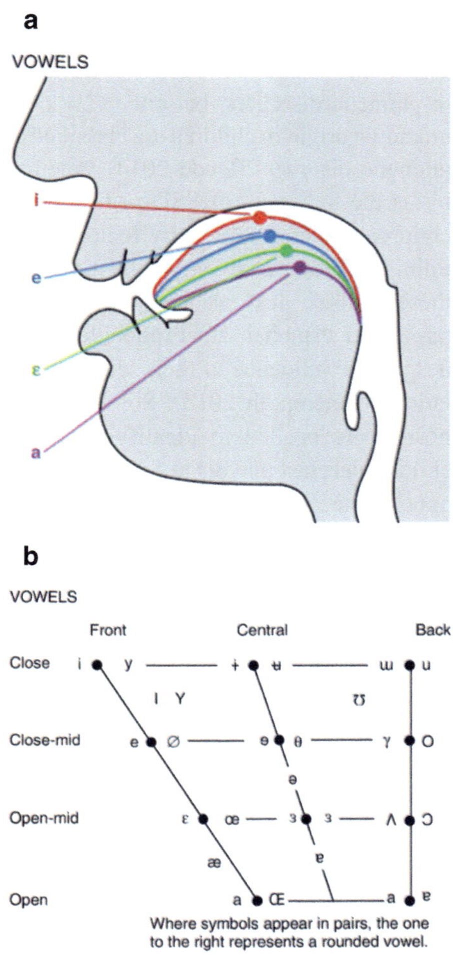

Fig. 3.8 (**a**) Cardinal tongue position regarding tongue height (vertical dimension) and tongue backness (horizontal dimension) for different vowels (i, e, ɛ, **a**; see **b**). (Adapted by Ishwar and LadyofHats, based on Jones (1972). Image URL: https://de.wikipedia.org/wiki/Datei:Cardinal_vowel_tongue_position-back(png).svg. Covered by Creative Commons Attribution-ShareAlike 3.0 licence) (**b**) Schematic vowel diagram from the International Phonetic Alphabet representing the three main features to describe vowels: (1) In the vertical dimension vowels are arranged according to the degree of *aperture of the mouth and jaw* (from open to closed vowels) and the tongue *height* relative to the roof of the mouth. (2) In the horizontal dimension, vowels are arranged according to the position of the tongue in the mouth during the articulation (tongue *backness*: front, central, back). (3) The rounding of the lips during articulation determinates rounded from unrounded vowels (*roundedness*). The worldwide convention is to transcribe vowels according to the International Phonetic Alphabet (IPA) (definition adapted from IPA 1999, IPA Chart 2015; Nicolosi et al. 2003; Ladefoged 2006)

rect linguistic use of phonemes is an *aspect of language development.*

3.3.3.3 Considering the Framework for Assessing Speech Sound Development

Traditionally, immature speech motor skills were considered to cause SSD. As a consequence, investigating oral and speech motor movements with informal protocols is still one of the standard methods in assessing speech sound disorders. This traditional reduction of phonetic analysis only provides a gross quantitative measure of speech sound development (Dodd 2014; Fox-Boyer et al. 2016). For treatment recommendations this procedure does not provide a sufficient classification. It is, for example, well documented that phonological SSD nonverbal oral-motor training does not lead to an improved competence in speech sound use or to better sound intelligibility (e.g. Dodd 2014; Powell 2008). Specific phonological treatment is necessary. By contrast, traditional articulation therapy is most successful in phonetic disorders, but only 12% of SSDs of unknown origin in children are classified as purely phonetic disorders (Dodd 2014). Another example is the treatment of SSD in hearing-impaired children, which traditionally focuses on auditory training. From a psycholinguistic perspective, these children also need phonological treatment targets to establish their phonological system, despite the influence of their sensory-based limitations (Reichmuth 2018). So, differential diagnostics are needed to identify the nature of a child's speech sound disorder in order to select an appropriate treatment approach (Strand and McCauley 2008; Namasivayam et al. 2013; Dodd 2014). The structure of the diagnostic process for identifying SSDs should provide a well-based diagnosis enabling recommendations for efficient and evidence-based treatment. It has to be based on the best available evidence of therapy efficiency and effectiveness.

The contemporary theoretical framework coming from psycholinguistic research on SSD permits a broader look at children's developing speech sound processing with regard to phonological aspects of speech sounds, input and output difficulties or deficits in memory functioning. The two most noted psycholinguistic models are those of Stackhouse and Wells (1997) and Dodd (2005, 2014). Following Dodd (2005, 2014) and others (Fox-Boyer et al. 2016), cross-linguistic research on SSDs of unclear origin (i.e. excluding hearing impairment, dysglossia, dysarthria) are classified into five subgroups (marked in Fig. 3.6). Reasons for phonological disorders are delayed phonological development, e.g. due to repeated otitis media, and deficits in perceiving phonological information correctly, leading to consequent phonological disorders or severe deficits in phonological working memory, causing inconsequent phonological disorders (Dodd 2014; Fox-Boyer et al. 2016).

3.3.3.4 Cross-Linguistic Features in Normal Speech Sound Acquisition

Summarizing cross-linguistic studies on normal speech sound acquisition in 24 languages, McLeod (2012b) described the following cross-linguistic features in normal speech sound acquisition:

- Vowels, nasals, and plosives appear to be the *earliest sounds* to be produced by children. Children produce more sounds and greater articulatory variation as they grow older (McLeod 2012b).
- *Intelligibility* of speech rises continuously during the first 5 years of age. A guideline of Coplan and Gleason (1988) for expected conversational intelligibility levels of typically developing children is recommended by the ASHA (2016): 1 year, 25% intelligible; 2 years, 50% intelligible; 3 years, 75% intelligible; and 4 years, 100% intelligible.
- The *age of acquisition of consonants*, defined by the age when most children (90% or 75% by convention) are able to pronounce a consonant as does an adult and shows a wide diversity across languages. Nevertheless the 90% criterion of correct consonant production is reached in 5-year-olds cross-linguistically, whereas 2-year-olds produce consonants correctly at least 70% of the time (McLeod 2012b).
- *Common mismatches* are.

sounds children typically produce before they achieve the adult target.—McLeod (2012b).

Some similarities are found across such sounds, but generally they differ between languages. For example, common mismatches for /s/ are (examples from McLeod 2012b):

- /s/—plosive consonant, e.g. [t] in many languages such as in English, Dutch, Finnish, Hungarian and Portuguese
- /s/—lateralized fricative, e.g. [ɮ] in Greek
- /s/—palatal consonant, e.g. palatalization in Japanese and [ʃ] in Israeli Hebrew.

Typically, children's sound changes during speech development follow certain phonological error patterns, defined as *physiological phonological processes*. See Table 3.7 for these systemic and structural simplifications, which can be observed cross-linguistically in preschool children attempting to produce adultlike utterances (McLeod 2012b).

- In cases of *systematic simplifications*, the error pattern is conditioned by one phonological feature of the speech sound itself or its phoneme category, regardless of its position in the word. So fricatives are systematically replaced by a stop consonant, for example, and therefore the phonological error pattern is called *stopping* (see Table 3.7).
- In cases of *structural simplifications*, the error pattern is conditioned by word structure, phoneme surrounding and intonation. With the tendency to delete final consonants, even though they can be correctly pronounced in another position of the word, for example, the phonological error pattern is called 'final consonant deletion' (see Table 3.7).

Table 3.7 Physiological phonological processes in speech development (cross-linguistic)

Physiological phonological processes in speech development (cross-linguistic)[a]		
	Description of the phonological processes[b]	Example[b]
Systemic simplifications		
– Backing	Substitution of any nonvelar consonant by a velar	For example, tub = tʌg
– Fronting	Tendency to replace velar or palatal consonants by alveolar, bilabial or labiodental consonants	For example, velar fronting: cot = tot For example, palatal fronting: mash = mæs
– Stopping	Replacement of fricatives […] with a stop consonant	For example, soup = dup
– Devoicing	Substitution of a voiced consonant by a voiceless consonant	For example, big = bɪk
– Voicing	Voicing of voiceless consonants	For example, pen = bɛn
Structural simplifications		
– Assimilation/ consonant harmony	Tendency to create internal symmetry within words; a process whereby a child changes one or more phonemes to match production features of other sounds or characteristics of an utterance	For example, velar assimilation: duck = gək For example, labial assimilation: top = bop
– Cluster reduction	Reduction of a consonant cluster to a single consonant	For example, spoon = pun
– Initial consonant deletion	Deletion of the initial consonant of a syllable or word	For example, house = aʊs
– Final consonant deletion	Reduction of consonant-vowel-consonant (CVC) words or syllables to a consonant-vowel (CV) form	For example, pig = pɪ
– Reduplication	Syllable duplication, doubling	For example, kitty = tɪ tɪ
– (Weak) syllable deletion	Dropping of unstressed syllables	For example, telephon = təfon

[a]McLeod (2012b)
[b]Description and examples from Nicolosi et al. (2003)

3.3.3.5 Assessment Procedure of Speech Sound Disorders

A screening procedure of the developmental speech sound status for detecting an SSD has to fulfil the usual validity criteria for a screening, such as appropriate sensitivity and specificity. If a screening has failed or in cases of suspicion of an SSD, a comprehensive assessment should follow, examining the speech sound disorder in depth in order to classify the SSD subgroup (ASHA 2016).

Following international guidelines (ASHA 2004, 2016), the diagnostic procedure of a child with SSD should include the following assessments:

- History.
- Oral-motor examination (see Sect. 3.3.2).
- Observation and documentation of spontaneous speech.
- Judgement of intelligibility.
- Examination with a naming test.
- Stimulability of isolated phones.
- Examination of speech perception.
- Proving of phonological consequence in words.
- Conclusion of assessment.

3.3.3.6 History

Following the ASHA (2016), the case history typically includes gathering information about the:

- Family's concerns about the child's speech.
- History of middle ear infections.
- History of speech, language or literacy difficulties in the family.
- Languages used in the home.
- Primary language spoken by the child.

Further information such as on oral sensory and functional development is gathered by the clinical history, e.g. on the birth, feeding, etc., which is part of the oral-motor examination (see Sect. 3.3.2).

3.3.3.7 Oral-Motor Examination

The oral-motor examination assesses the structural and functional adequacy of the speech movements (Nicolosi et al. 2003). The recommended procedure is outlined in Sect. 3.3.2. It should be applied regularly in order to supplement the assessment of the speech sound developmental status, to detect organic causes of an SSD and to enable distinctions between *phonetic* (articulatory movements) and *phonological* (linguistic) components of a speech sound disorder.

3.3.3.8 Observation and Documentation of Spontaneous Speech

The observation of spontaneous speech constitutes a relevant part of speech sound assessment. Spontaneous speech samples of the child during a dialogue or play activity provide an impression of the error patterns and the intelligibility of the child's speech. Moreover, the severity of the SSD and its influence on communicational behaviour and success can be observed. Severe to profound SSDs may lead to frequent conversational breakdown. Following the framework of the International Classification of Disability and Functioning in its children and youth version (ICF-CY; WHO 2007), the ASHA (2004) recommends appreciating the limitations of a child's activity and participation in social life caused by the SSD. Regarding this, parental concerns and burdens have also to be considered in the assessment.

3.3.3.9 Intelligibility

A judgement of a child's intelligibility is a useful indicator of the severity of its speech problem. It should be done by the examiner and may be supported by the impression of family members or other related persons. It is a subjective, perceptual judgement, based on how much of the child's spontaneous speech is understood by the listener. In order to guarantee comparability, it should be assessed from a Likert scale. Intelligibility is often used to determine the need for intervention and to evaluate the progress of a therapy (ASHA 2016).

> A child of 3 years of age or older who is unintelligible is generally recognized as a candidate for treatment.
> —Bernthal et al. (2013)

The *Intelligibility in Context Scale (ICS)* (McLeod 2012a, b) is recommended as a seven-item screening measure of children's speech intelligibility. It is designed for parents who rate the child's speech intelligibility for a range of communicative partners on a Likert scale (0–5). It is available free online in 60 languages, thus also enabling an assessment of speech intelligibility in multilingual children. In preschool children aged 4–5 years and 5 months, for example, the application of the ICS revealed significant differences between children whose parents had concerns about their child's speech and those who did not (McLeod et al. 2015). First data on bilingual children show that the ICS scores are robust across languages (McLeod et al. 2015).

3.3.3.10 Examination with a Naming Test

Single-word picture elicitation by the use of naming tests is standard for speech assessments in many languages. However, the use of well-validated, reliable and normed naming tests is still not established (McLeod and Verdon 2014). Besides single-word testing, the ASHA (2016) recommends the analysis of an additional speech sample of connected speech (e.g. story telling). The error analysis is aimed at determining whether the individual displays primarily phonetic speech production deficits or deficits associated with phonological constraints (ASHA 2004; Dodd 2005).

The construction of naming tests follows segment-orientated or process-orientated criteria (Fox-Boyer et al. 2016):

- *Segment-orientated assessment*. This focuses exclusively on the phonetic aspects of speech sound development by testing the correct articulation of every phone in single words. The result reveals a child's phonetic inventory and an independent analysis of speech sound error types (e.g. deletions, omissions, substitutions, distortions, additions or a description of atypical articulation). For assessing the *phonetic inventory* of children, the language-specific construction of the inventory (see Speech Accent Archive (online) for 57 languages, Weinberger 2015) and the language-specific course of phone development (normative data) should build the diagnostic basis for distinguishing age-adequate errors in the test performance from age-inadequate errors.

  For a more comprehensive assessment, a relational analysis process-orientated testing is needed.
- *Process-orientated assessment*. This enables the analysis of the underlying phonological system of the child's speech sound development to explain the observed error pattern from a phonological perspective. Phonological error patterns are systemic or structural simplifications (see Table 3.6 for an overview) (McLeod 2012b; ASHA 2004). For assessing the correct or incorrect linguistic use of phonemes in children, the language-specific course of phoneme development (normative data) should establish the basis for distinguishing age-adequate errors and phonological processes (see Table 3.6) from the prolonged use of age-inadequate phonological processes and problems to overcome them.

Relying only on segment-orientated testing does not fulfil contemporary requirements for classifying SSDs, especially for the deduction of specific treatment recommendations (Fox-Boyer et al. 2016; Dodd 2014).

As to quality assurance of tests, McLeod and Verdon (2014) included 98 instruments designed to assess children's speech sound production in languages other than English in a review (62 had been commercially published, 17 had been published in journal articles and 19 were informal assessments). Thirty of the commercially published assessment tests were available for in-depth analysis. These tests encompass the assessment of speech sounds for 17 languages other than English (Cantonese, Danish, Finnish, German, Greek, Japanese, Korean, Maltese-English, Norwegian,

Pakistani-heritage languages, Portuguese, Putonghua (Mandarin), Romanian, Slovenian, Spanish, Swedish, Turkish). According to the review, about half (53%) of these assessment tests are norm-referenced with large variability in the size of the normative sample. These norm-referenced tests are listed in Table 3.8. The other assessments are criterion-referenced.

McLeod (2012c) further offers an unevaluated online collection of speech sound assessment instruments, templates and tests for 36 languages. It includes

> published tests and word lists that can be used to assess children's articulation and phonology in languages other than English.
> —McLeod (2012c)

But a critical evaluation of test quality should be done by the professionals before they are used. As for all psychometric tests, adequate psychometric properties (e.g. validity, objectivity, reliability, norming) of tests to assess articulation (speech motor performance) and phonology (phonological error patterns) need to be fulfilled and documented. However, test construction and quality often do not fulfil these requirements (e.g. McCauley and Strand 2008; Kirk and Vigeland 2014; McLeod and Verdon 2014).

For high standards of assessment, normative data for each language regarding phonetic and phonological speech sound development are indispensable. Aiming at this target, test developers and researchers in the field need to improve the quality of available tests in order to increase the reliability and validity of speech sound assessment, because many tests do not fulfil classical criteria of test construction (see review of Flipsen and Ogiela (2015) for psychometric criteria for good test construction).

3.3.3.11 Stimulability of Isolated Phones

Eliciting isolated phones enables the examiner to evaluate the degree of a child's ability to produce or imitate a previously misarticulated phone correctly. This procedure provides information about the speech motor skills of the child and the level of cueing that seems to be necessary to achieve the best speech sound production (e.g. auditory model; auditory and visual model; tactile cues) (ASHA 2016). Standards for the testing procedures are given by Glaspey and Stoel-Gammon (2007). Some test batteries include stimulability subtests (see Table 3.8) (ASHA 2016).

It is assumed that a good ability of sound imitation predicts the acquisition of a sound with or without intervention; this may help the selection of appropriate cues and therapy targets and may predict the improvement by an SSD therapy (ASHA 2016). This holds true at least for phonetic disorders and childhood apraxia of speech (CAS), but for phonological disorders, testing the speech sound stimulability is of questionable predictive value with respect to treatment necessity and success.

3.3.3.12 Speech Perception Testing

A child's fundamental linguistic and auditory perceptual abilities or limitations for acquiring correct phoneme use is examined by testing its speech sound discrimination (another part of auditory speech perception is tested by speech audiometry).

The following test constituents are recommended (ASHA 2016; Nicolosi et al. 2003):

- Auditory speech sound discrimination: the basic auditory ability to differentiate paired speech sounds with minimal contrasts in syllables or words without lip reading; assessment requires a same-different response (e.g. /jam/ vs. /jam/; /cam/ vs. /jam/).
- Phoneme discrimination by picture identification: the auditory and linguistic ability to discriminate slight phonemic contrast of phonemes in minimal word pairs without lip reading; assessment requires the identification of one picture out of two to four by pointing (e.g. house/mouse/louse).

Children with phonetic SSD and normal hearing should perform properly in these tasks, whereas children with phonological SSD and healthy hearing often show difficulties. In cases of abnormal test results, further examinations are used to determine if errors are related to a generalized perceptual problem (Bernthal et al. 2013).

Table 3.8 Norm-referenced assessment tools of the speech sound developmental status of children for different languages

Assessed language	Name of assessment	Age range (years; months)	Areas assessed		
			Phones *(segmental-oriented)*	Phonological processes *(process-orientated)*	Other areas relevant for SSD
Cantonese[a]	Hong Kong Cantonese Articulation Test (Cheung et al. 2006)	2;6–5;6	+	–	–
English[a,b]	*Diagnostic evaluation of Articulation & Phonology (DEAP)* (Dodd et al., UK-edition, 2016 and US-edition, 2006)	3;0–6;11/8;11	+	+	Inconsistency of phonological processes; oromotor assessment
English[a,b]	*Toddler Phonology Tests (TPT)* (McIntosh and Dodd 2011)	2;0–2;11	+	+	–
Finnish	*Fonologiatesti* (Kunnari et al. 2012)	2;0–6;11	+	–	–
German	*Patholinguistische Diagnostik von Sprachentwicklungsstörungen* (Kauschke and Siegmüller 2009, 2nd ed.)	2;0–6;11	+	+	Perception; prosody; oromotor assessment
German[b] (incl. Austrian & Swiss-German)	*Psycholinguistische Analyse kindlicher Aussprachestörungen-II PLAKKS-II* (Fox-Boyer 2014)	2;6–8;0	+	+	Inconsistency of phonological processes
Greek	*Assessment of Phonetic & Phonological development* (Panhellenic Association of Logopedists 1995)	2;6–6;0	+	–	–
Korean	*Assessment of Phonology & Articulation for children* (Kim et al. 2007)	2;6–6;5	+	+	–
Korean	*Urimal Test of Articulation & Phonology* (Kim and Shin 2004)	2;0–6;11	+	+	–
Maltese-English[a]	*Maltese-English Speech Assessment* (Grech et al. 2011)	2;0–6;0	+	+	Stimulability, inconsistency of phonological processes; oromotor assessment
Pakistani[a] heritage languages: Mirpuri, Punjabi, Urdu	*Bilingual Speech Sound Screen: Pakistan heritage Languages* (Stow and Pert 2006)	1;4–7;11	+	+	
Putonghua	*Putonghua Segmental Phonology Test* (So and Jing 2000)	2;0–6;11	+	–	–
Spanish[a]	*Bilingual English-Spanish Assessment* (Peña et al. 2014)	4;0–6;11	+	–	–

(continued)

Table 3.8 (continued)

Assessed language	Name of assessment	Age range (years; months)	Areas assessed: Phones *(segmental-oriented)*	Phonological processes *(process-orientated)*	Other areas relevant for SSD
Spanish[a]	*Contextual Probes of Articulation Competence: Spanish* (Goldstein and Iglesias 2006)	3;0–8;11	+	+	–
Spanish[a]	*Spanish Preschool Articulation Test* (Tsugawa 2002)	Not specified	+	–	–
Swedish	*Svenskt Artikulations-och Nasalittets Test* (Lohmander et al. 2005)	2;8–10;2	+	+	Oromotor assessment
Turkish	*Ankara Artikülasyon Testi* (Ege et al. 2004)	2;6–12;11	+	–	–
Turkish	*Türkçe* Sesletim-Sesbilgisi Testi (Topbaş 2004, 2005)	1;3–14;3	+	+	Perception; oromotor assessment

Modified according to McLeod and Verdon (2014)
[a]Manual in English included
[b]Two English and one German assessment tools added by the section authors

Children with hearing impairment often have limitations in speech sound perception. Diagnostic procedures of these children should allow the examiner to determine which speech sounds are properly understood and whether hearing devices are well-fitted and functioning. Auditory discrimination tasks may help to evaluate which phonemic contrasts are audible for the child and which speech sounds must be cued visually throughout therapy.

3.3.3.13 Proving of Phonological Consistency in Words

This examination is needed in cases of a phonological disorder. To identify whether a phonological error occurs consistently (in all naming trials of a word the same phonological process is used) or inconsistently (the use of phonological processes in a word differs in the repeated naming procedure), certain criteria for test material are needed. Fox-Boyer et al. (2016) summarize the following international criteria for designing a speech test that focuses on phonological process analysis including the assessment of consistency:

- The test includes about 100 items.
- All phonemes are tested in different positions in the word up to four times.
- Items vary in number of syllables, structure of syllables and word stress.
- Normative data allow the differentiation of a developmental delay of speech sound acquisition and a speech sound disorder.

3.3.3.14 Conclusion of Assessment

The assessment of the speech sound developmental status of a child should result in:

- Diagnosis and subclassification (see Figs. 3.6 and Table 3.6) of a speech sound disorder.
- Description of the characteristics and severity of the disorder (mild-severe-profound).
- Identification of factors that might contribute to the speech sound disorder.
- Referral to other professionals or further comprehensive assessment as needed.
- Parental guidance by giving information and advice about the SSD of their child.
- Recommendations for specific intervention targets based on the classified SSD.

Planning follow-up assessments in order to control the outcome of an SSD intervention (see Dodd 2005 for treatment targets of phonological disorders).

3.4 Phonological Evaluation of Speech

See mainly in 3.3.1 and 3.3.3 and in Volume 1, Chap. 11.

3.5 Evaluation of Speech, Prosodic Level

See mainly in 3.3.1 and in Volume 1, Chap. 11.

3.6 Evaluation of Speech Intelligibility

See mainly in 3.3.3 and in Volume 1, Chap. 11.

3.7 Orofacial Dysfunctions (Orofacial Myofunctional Disorders) with Special Focus on Paediatric Patients: Diagnostics

Doris-Maria Denk-Linnert and
Wolfgang Bigenzahn

3.7.1 Introduction

The otorhinolaryngological/phoniatric-logopaedic examination identifies orofacial myofunctional disorders (OMD), reveals aetiological factors and establishes a treatment regimen. The contribution of the otolaryngologist/phoniatrician is of utmost importance for evaluating and treating airway interference (Mason and Franklin 2014). Orofacial myofunctional therapy will not be successful without the resolution of airway problems.

3.7.2 Screening Tests

For the identification of OMDs the following screening tests are used:

NOT-S (Nordic Orofacial Test-Screening) (Bakke et al. 2007). This reliable and valid screening instrument can be easily performed on children aged three and over by different health professionals without special equipment. It comprises a structured interview (six domains: (I) Sensory function, (II) Breathing, (III) Habits, (IV) Chewing and swallowing, (V) Drooling and (VI) Dryness of the mouth) and a clinical examination (six domains: (1) The face at rest, and tasks regarding (2) Nose breathing, (3) Facial expression, (4) Masticatory muscle and jaw function, (5) Oral motor function and (6) Speech).

"Airway and Myofunctional Screening in the Dental Office" This is another screening form (Gatto et al. 2018), which is published on the homepage of the International Association of Orofacial Myology (https://www.iaom.com).

3.7.3 History Taking, Diagnostics and Documentation

The History taking with parents/caregivers includes information regarding:

- Birth and developmental history/milestones.
- Maternal health during pregnancy.
- Early infancy.
- Early nursing and feeding history: duration of breastfeeding, onset of solid food, feeding and swallowing problems.
- Eating habits, daily diet.
- Oral habits: thumb/digit/pacifier/object sucking.
- Occlusal anomalies, dental/orthodontic history, e.g. tooth eruption patterns, oral hygiene, orthodontic appliances and treatment plan.
- Speech-language history, speech problems.
- Hearing history.
- Medical history: illnesses that possibly affect oral function, e.g. upper respiratory infections, allergies, snoring and sleep habits, previous oral surgery (frenectomy, tonsillectomy or adenoidectomy).
- Breathing history (nasal/mouth breathing).
- Neurological illnesses, also of parents and siblings.

The **Phoniatric-Logopaedic Examination** includes the inspection of the oral structures and their assessment, with reference to the primary and secondary functions; in addition, an audiological test and a thorough documentation (e.g. photo and sound documentation, sonographic evaluation of the tonsils, etc.) are performed.

The **Myofunctional Status** comprises evaluation of body-head-neck posture, the facial symmetry, shape of the lips and the rugae palatinae. The functional tests include examining the orofacial muscles (m. orbicularis oris, m. mentalis, m. masseter), mimic muscles, as well as the mobility of the tongue and velum. The chewing and swallowing processes are tested with and without oral food intake. Furthermore, the perioral and oral sensitivity are examined, including the senses of taste and temperature, as well as the oral stereognosis (i.e. perception of shape, texture and consistency) (Bigenzahn 2003). In detail, the examination pays attention to Bigenzahn (2003) and Billings et al. (2018):

- **Body Posture** (Orth and Block 1987).
- **Breathing Mechanism**: disturbed nose breathing/mouth breathing? *The most commonly noted aetiology of OMD is a lack of nasal breathing!* Long-term mouth breathing disturbs the natural resting position of the jaw, tongue and lips and interferes with growth patterns of the jaw and maxilla, resulting in the development of a malocclusion. The importance of physiological nose breathing has been underestimated. Its influence on facial morphology (Al Ali et al. 2015) and interrelations with paediatric obstructive sleep apnoea (Huang and Guilleminault 2013; Guilleminault and Sullivan 2014) are increasingly discussed.
- **Phonatory Function.**
- **Resonance Function.**
- **External Appearance of the Head/Face.**
- **Cranial Nerve Function**, especially **V** (jaw opening/closing and side-to-side jaw movements, palpation of masseter muscle), **VII, X, XII** (tongue mobility and strength).
- **Jaw Function and Temporomandibular Joint** (TMJ).
- **Lip Structure and Function**, presence of maxillary or mandibular lip-ties (Pransky et al. 2015).
- **Tactile Intra- / Peri-oral Sensitivity.**
- **Dentition** (primary, mixed and permanent), **Occlusion** (normal, open bite, overjet, overbite, underbite, crossbite), dental or orthodontic appliance.
- **Lingual Structure and Function** (resting posture, mobility, identification of lingual restriction / anterior or posterior tongue-tie (short lingual frenulum/**Ankyloglossia**)).
- **Hard Palate—Structure and Function**: shape, exclusion of clefting or fistulas, rugae palatinae.
- **Soft Palate—Structure and Function**: velopharyngeal closure.
- **Palatal Tonsils**: hypertrophy?
- **Eating and Swallowing** (type of feeding, saliva management, drinking, biting, chewing).
- **Tongue Thrust** (e.g. anterior, unilateral, bilateral) (Fig. 3.9, malocclusion, anterior tongue thrust).
- **Non-nutritive Sucking or Chewing Habits** (de Arruda Telles et al. 2009). Extended use of a pacifier or long-term use of sippy cups have to be inquired about.
- **Articulation Tests.**

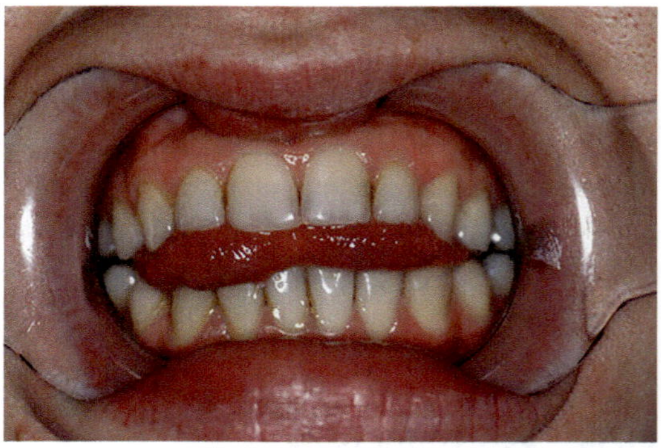

Fig. 3.9 Malocclusion, anterior tongue thrust. (©Bigenzahn 2019)

During the exam, the (little) patient's cooperation capability and the patient's/caregiver's ability for treatment purposes are estimated. If necessary, referrals to other medical or therapeutic disciplines are arranged.

3.7.4 Further Examinations

Measurement of Lip Strength Lip strength is measured with the Force Scale as described by Garliner (1974): a button 1 in. in diameter is placed between the lips with a protruding string, which is put into the hook of the force scale. The force scale is pulled until the patient is forced to release the button. The exam is carried out three times. A lip strength between 1.5 and 2.5 pounds (pound force, corresponds to 6.67–11.12 Newton) is considered normal.

Measurement of Tongue Pressure Tongue (and also lip) pressure measurement can be performed with the IOPI System (Iowa Oral Performance Instrument). In children, it has been shown that the average tongue pressure in a mouth-breathing group is lower than that in a nasal-breathing group (Azevedo et al. 2018).

Payne Technique A fluorochemical substance is placed on the tip and lateral borders of the tongue. After the patient swallows, the substance adheres to the area that the tongue touches. This can be clearly seen with 'Black Light'. In normal swallowing, the anterior marking should appear in the area of the incisive papilla and the lateral markings should be against the alveolar ridge.

Oral Stereognosis Oral stereognosis is tested with differently shaped acrylic test plates (1 mm thick and 12 mm in diameter) (Hahn 1997).

Sonography of the Tongue and Tonsils In the case of tonsillar hyperplasia, the sonographic evaluation of the tonsils assesses the size and the topography of the tonsils and the base of the tongue. Large tonsils favour a forward position of the body of the tongue and an interdental tongue posture. In some cases, this sonographic evaluation of function helps to decide upon the indication for tonsillotomy or tonsillectomy (Bigenzahn et al. 1991, 1992).

Articulography and Axiography Electronic articulography (Piehslinger et al. 1994) and axiography (Piehslinger et al. 1991; Bigenzahn et al. 1991) enable early differential diagnostics of disturbances in the stomatognathic system. In our own axiographic studies, dynamic movement asymmetries in the form of asymmetric mandibular movements and muscular dyscoordination were determined by orofacial dysfunctions. Patients with parafunctional habits showed a high proportion of muscular dyscoordination and morphological changes in the temporomandibular joint (TMJ) (Bigenzahn et al. 1991; Bigenzahn 2003).

3.8 Examination of Cranial Nerve Function

Barbara Maciejewska

3.8.1 Introduction

There are 12 pairs of cranial nerves (CNs) connected to the under surface of the brain, with most coming from the brainstem (Felten et al. 2015). They belong to the peripheral nervous system and are essentially equivalent to the spinal nerves. CNs can be motor alone or sensory (e.g. smelling, tasting) or both (mixed). Therefore sensory as well as motor functions are used in combination in their evaluation. Some CNs are responsible for innervation of muscles associated with the oral, pharyngeal and laryngeal phases of speech. Moreover, they supply the skin of the face as well as the mucosa of the nasal cavity, the oral cavity, the pharynx and the larynx. Some CNs build reflexes—automatic responses mediated by the nervous system and transmitted via the spinal cord. Examination of the reflexes can test the reflex arc and the integrity of the nervous system (Binder et al. 2010; Wilson-Pauwels et al. 2001). To sum up, CNs V, VII, IX, X and XII supply the organs involved in phonation and articulation. They should therefore be obligatorily tested when speech disorders are observed.

3.8.2 Cranial Nerve V (Trigeminal Nerve)

The fifth CN is a mixed nerve, with both sensory and motor components. As a result, it is responsible for proper chewing, facial and mouth sensation and the corneal reflex (Wilkinson and Lennox 2005).

3.8.2.1 Innervation

The nerve has three branches: the optic (V1), maxillary (V2) and mandibular (V3). They all supply the skin of the face (except the skin over the angle of the jaw). The nerve innervates:

- The mucosa of the oral cavity (the cheek, gums, upper and lower teeth, palate).
- The anterior 2/3 of the tongue.
- The nasal cavity and paranasal sinuses.
- The cornea (corneal reflex).

The motor fibres supply the muscles of mastication (the masseter, temporal, medial and lateral pterygoid muscle) (Wilson-Pauwels et al. 2001; Davenport and Manji 2018).

3.8.2.2 Assessment and Tests

- When the patient's eyes are closed, touch her or his face with cotton or something soft, and ask about the feeling, ask to identify the irritated area, remember to check the sensation symmetrically. Pain, touch and temperature should be tested in the three branches of the nerve.
- Ask the patient to clench their teeth and palpate the tension of the masseters on both sides; compare the symmetry of the muscle tone.
- Ask the patient to open their mouth and try to close it, then ask them to close the jaw against resistance.
- Ask the patient to move their chin and the jaw side-to-side against resistance.
- Evoke the corneal reflex—gently touch the cornea with a cotton applicator or tissue paper and observe rapid blinking movements (the correct reaction).
- Evoke the jaw reflex by gently tapping the chin, observe the closure of the jaw.

3.8.3 Cranial Nerve VII (Facial Nerve)

The seventh CN is a mixed nerve and is responsible for facial expression, taste, corneal reflex (motor branch).

3.8.3.1 Innervation

The facial nerve provides motor innervation to the muscles of facial expression and taste to the anterior two-thirds of the tongue. Most of the nerve is motor and supplies the facial muscles, so emotional expression is possible as well as articulatory movements. The chorda tympani branch contains taste fibres from the anterior 2/3 of the tongue. The secretomotor (parasympathetic) fibres to the salivary glands and lacrimal glands also pass via the seventh nerves (Wilkinson and Lennox 2005; Davenport and Manji 2018).

3.8.3.2 Assessment and Tests

- Ask the patient to smile, purse the lips, show the teeth, raise the eyebrows, wrinkle the forehead, keep eyes closed and try to open them. In each case assess the symmetry of the face. Further testing can involve testing the strength of facial muscles by overcoming them (by trying to open the closed eyes or to pull the closed lips apart manually). From the examination an observed lesion of facial nerve should be categorised into central facial palsy (due to damage above the facial nucleus) or peripheral (due to damage at or below the facial nucleus).
- Assess articulation. Labial sounds can be tested by asking the patient to say "pa. … pa. … pa." Notice dysarthria, which can result from weakness of the orbicularis oris.
- Ask the patient to protrude their tongue, then have the patient identify some flavour placed on one side of the tongue (e.g. sugar, salt), but only on the anterior 2/3 of the tongue. The patient must identify the substance before putting the tongue back in the mouth. Remember about dysgeusia/hypogeusia/ageusia.
- Evoke the corneal reflex (see below).
- Observe saliva production and the moistness of the mouth.

Subtle facial asymmetries are common and not necessarily pathological. It is helpful to have a family member or an old photo (e.g. a driver's license) to verify the long-standing nature of a subtle asymmetry.

3.8.4 Cranial Nerve IX (Glossopharyngeal Nerve)

The glossopharyngeal nerve is a mixed motor but predominantly a sensory nerve. Isolated lesions of that nerve are rare.

3.8.4.1 Innervation

The IX CN provides sensory innervation to the mucosa of the oropharynx, palatine tonsils, palate, fauces. It is responsible for taste on the posterior 1/3 of the tongue; it sends secretomotor fibres to the salivary glands and lacrimal gland (Wilson-Pauwels et al. 2001).

3.8.4.2 Assessment and Tests

- Touch the posterior wall of the pharynx with a tongue depressor and evoke the gag (pharyngeal) reflex. The gag reflex is usually brisk. In the case of the pharyngeal reflex:
  - The sensory limb is mediated predominantly by CN IX.
  - The motor limb by CN X.
- The gag reflex involves a brisk and brief elevation of the soft palate and bilateral contraction of the pharyngeal muscles evoked by touching the posterior pharyngeal wall. Touching the soft palate can lead to a similar reflex response. However, in that case, the sensory limb of the reflex is the CN V (trigeminal nerve). An absent gag reflex suggests a lesion of the brainstem, cranial nerves IX or X, neuromuscular junction or pharyngeal muscles.
- Have the patient swallow some saliva, some water (5–15 mL), semi-solid (jelly) and solid food (bread). Being unable to swallow, having pain while swallowing (odynophagia), any difficulties in *swallowing saliva/water/food, having to cough after swallowing,* bringing food back up (regurgitation), *drooling or* being hoarse are pathological symptoms.
- Afterwards, assess the sensation in the oral cavity over the posterior third of the tongue, soft palate, uvula, and larynx by touching the mucosa of the mentioned structures.
- Notice if the speech has a nasal sound, if does—make tests for nasality.
- Ask the patient to say 'aaah' and watch for the degree of palate elevation and symmetry. Palatal speech dysfunction can be assessed by evaluating the clarity and speed of palatal sounds such as "ga. … ga. … ga." Labial, lingual, and palatal sounds can be tested together by having the patient repeat: 'pa. … ta. … ka'.

3.8.5 Cranial Nerve X (Vagus Nerve)

This is a mixed motor sensory and autonomous nerve. Its influence exceeds the head and neck region. Besides many effects on the cardiac and gastrointestinal systems, it controls gagging, phonation and swallowing and even has fibres for taste in the epiglottis.

3.8.5.1 Innervation

Sensory fibres of the vagus nerve supply the mucosa of the soft palate, laryngopharynx, larynx and posterior tongue. The X nerve provides motor innervation to the muscles of the palate, the pharynx and the larynx. It provides proper phonation and mobility of the vocal folds.

3.8.5.2 Assessment and Tests (Wilson-Pauwels et al. 2001)

- Check the gag reflex. Symmetry of the response on each side should be noted.
- Assess swallowing (together with nerve IX). An inability to swallow secretions can lead to drooling.
- Assess the palatal function (together with nerve IX). Observe the soft palate when patient says "ah".
- Assess the phonation vocal quality. Speech may be hoarse, weak.
- Perform indirect or direct laryngoscopy, the examination can help confirm ipsilateral vocal cord palsy.

The glossopharyngeal and vagus nerves are usually assessed together, because of their intimately related functions (Davenport and Manji 2018). These nerves serve the motor and sensory functions of the palate and vocal cords. A patient with IX or X injury or both might experience:

- Weak, breathy or nasal speech, and nasal regurgitation of food—nasality.
- Weak sucking, drooling, inability to handle secretions, depressed gag reflex, or ipsilateral palatal palsy—dysphagia.
- A motor speech disorder resulting from neurological injury of the motor component of the motor-speech system—poor phonation or articulation of phonemes or both—dysphonia, dysarthria.

3.8.6 Cranial Nerve XII (Hypoglossal Nerve)

The hypoglossal nerve provides motor innervation to the tongue. It includes only motor fibres. The hypoglossal nerve is involved in speech production as are CNs VII, IX and X. Patients with a hypoglossal nerve injury can experience speech alteration and also have difficulty in moving the food bolus in the mouth.

3.8.6.1 Innervation

CN XII supplies the tongue muscles, both extrinsic and intrinsic, and is responsible for tongue movements (Wilson-Pauwels et al. 2001).

3.8.6.2 Assessment and Tests

- Ask the patient to protrude the tongue straight out, and move it to the left and to the right, up and down, look at the symmetry of the movements and deviation of the tongue (always observed toward the side of lesion).
- Compare the bulk of the muscle on both sides of the tongue, notice muscle atrophy, wasting, fasciculation of the tongue.
- Assess articulation; lingual speech dysfunction can be evaluated by assessing the speed and clarity of lingual sounds, such as 'la. … la. … la'.

3.8.6.3 It Is Worth Remembering

- The same cranial nerves take part in speech production as well as control the stages of deglutition.
- The gag reflex depends on more than one CN (IX and X).
- The feeling sensation of the tongue is enabled by V, IX, X; taste is controlled by CN VII, IX and X, while CN XII is responsible for motor innervation.
- Three cranial nerves, glossopharyngeal (IX), vagal (X) and hypoglossal (XII), should be examined and considered together for the following reasons:
  - Together they innervate the mouth, the throat and the larynx for normal speech and swallowing.
  - They are usually involved in disease processes together leading to bulbar palsy (Wilkinson and Lennox 2005).
- Because many of the nerves to be tested need the patient's cooperation, the assessment of a comatose patient is incomplete.
- Because CNs never cross, except for CN IV, clinical abnormalities found on clinical examination always exist on the same side as the injured CN's roots/fibres.

The characteristic neurological consequences of the injury of the CNs in speech follow.

Nasality: As a result of the velopharyngeal insufficiency; it causes a leak of sound or air into the nose during speech. It can cause several speech problems, including:

- Hypernasality, where there is too much sound in the nose during speech.
- Nasal emission of air when making certain speech sounds.
- Weak consonants because of the leak of air through the nose.
- Making speech sounds in the throat owing to the lack of air in the mouth.

Dysarthria: As an impairment of central nervous system function this causes speech impairment due to a motor speech disorder, related to dysfunction of the nerves and disruption of the neuromuscular pathways to the tongue, lips, palate or mouth. In turn, this leads to abnormal articulation of sounds or phonemes, or more precisely, abnormal neuromuscular activation of the speech muscles, affecting the speed, strength, timing, range or accuracy of movements involving speech.

Bulbar Palsy: Lower motor neuron lesions affect the group of cranial nerves within the brainstem (IX-XIII) or along the course of the nerves. Weakness of the tongue results in difficulty with lingual sounds, while palatal weakness gives a nasal quality to the speech (Wilkinson and Lennox 2005; Felten et al. 2015).

3.9 Diagnosis and Differential Diagnosis of Speech Disorders: Oral Motor Examination Protocol

Tanja Fuhr

3.9.1 Introduction

The human orofacial complex consists of bony, muscular and nervous structures of the head and neck, and provides primary and secondary functions: the primary functions of the orofacial system are the mechanisms for breathing and food ingestion (e.g. biting, chewing, swallowing) as well as for controlling facial expressions (and therefore supporting communication); the secondary functions of the orofacial complex are the mechanisms for speech sound production (Miller and Lowit 2014). This section focuses on the examination of the primary functions of the orofacial complex, i.e. the orofacial functions that do not affect speech sound production. Section 3.10 covers the assessment of the secondary functions, related to speech sound production.

According to the American Speech-Language-Hearing Association (2004) and the World Health Organization (2001), the oral motor examination is the primary tool to assess the bony, muscular and nervous functioning of the orofacial complex, including the identification of structural and functional impairments, the limitations in activities, and restrictions in participation as well as the contextual, environmental and personal factors that are barriers to or enablers of achieving the patient's demands and goals.

The oral motor examination protocol and its interpretation, which are presented below, conform to the above-mentioned international guidelines by evaluating limitations and restrictions of activities, social participation, as well as corresponding factors, as part of the medical history. The structural impairments are identified during the oral motor examination from two aspects: examination of the facial appearance at rest provides information about motor tone and symmetry; during the assessment of orofacial functions, the movement of the articulators, the range of motions and precision of movements, as well as their symmetry and coordination, are evaluated. Additional instrumental or imaging tests can be conducted if necessary.

Finally, the interpretation of the protocol is aligned with the "International Classification of Diseases" (ICD) system of the World Health Organization (2019). The results of the assessments are evaluated to identify the goals for therapy by examining the above-mentioned strengths and weaknesses of the orofacial system from an expert's point of view, as well as the effects of structural and functional impairments on the patient's activities and participation from the patient's point of view.

The oral motor examination protocol provides a decision-making procedure (a decision of pass or fail) to identify oral motor disorders such as (components of) dysglossia or velopharyngeal insufficiency, or it may hint at disorders of adjacent medical disciplines such as speech sound or swallowing disorders (Clark 2005); in the latter case, further diagnostics are required. In addition, the protocol documents the patient's clinical picture and can lead to recommendations for intervention consistent with the patient's goals, for further support, as well as for referrals to additional assessments or treatments.

The following aspects are part of the oral motor examination protocol:

- The medical history of the patients, including limitations and restrictions in activities and social participation, their personal goals and contextual factors of the impairments.
- A description of appropriate test instruments and material.
- A procedure to inspect the orofacial structures at rest.
- A procedure to examine the orofacial functions in motion.
- A guideline to interpret the findings and to identify possible diagnoses.

3.9.2 Medical History

When assessing the medical history of patients, clinical, contextual, personal and environmental factors are evaluated, as well as the demands, strengths and weaknesses regarding the patients' activities and participation (Schröter-Morasch and Ziegler 2005). In particular, the medical assessment should include questions regarding the following aspects:

- Information about possible underlying diseases.
  - Existing diagnoses.
  - Onset, progression and duration of the disease.
  - Medication.
- Information about former treatments.
- Types of former treatments.
- Beginning and end of former treatments.
- Progression during the treatments.
- Limitations of the orofacial complex that existed before an underlying disease.
- Abnormalities in oral motor movement development.
- Medical history of conditions that might affect oral functions.
- Current limitations of the orofacial complex.
- Impairments of eating, chewing or swallowing, alteration of taste.
- Sensory disturbance or disturbed motor function or pain in the orofacial complex.
- Abnormal salivation or dryness of the mouth.
- Hoarseness or getting tired of the voice, feeling that something is stuck in the throat, pressure to clear one's throat, foreign-body sensations in the throat.
- Effects of the disorder on daily life.
- Limitations of activities.
- Restrictions in participation (social contacts, work, leisure, family and social environment).
- Contextual factors.
- Personal factors such as those that influence how a disability is experienced by the patient (coping style, social background, education, profession, past and current experience, behaviour patterns).
- Environmental factors (physical, social, and attitudinal environment in which the patient lives and conducts his or her life).
- Demands and goals.
- Subjective goals of the patient.
- Prioritisation of the patient's goals.

3.9.3 Test Instruments and Materials

For the examination of oral motor functions, visual observation of structures and movements, and palpation of the tissues of the orofacial components are the main assessment tools. Basic examination materials such as gloves, a penlight, a ruler, a spatula, and if necessary, a nasal fiberscope, are required. Solid, semi-solid and liquid aliments are used when assessing chewing and swallowing functions.

3.9.4 Perceptual Structural Assessment of the Orofacial Complex

The oral motor examination includes an evaluation of the orofacial system, especially that of the peripheral orofacial structures at rest. The speech-language pathologist inspects and palpates the patient's orofacial structures at rest to identify abnormalities in proportions or symmetry or in muscle tone. The assessment includes the observation of the extra- und intra-oral structures of the orofacial complex such as the face, nose, jaw, lips, tongue, teeth, hard palate, soft palate and pharynx. The following aspects are assessed through observation of:

- Face
  - Signs of facial weakness in rest.
  - Asymmetry of the eyes' or mouth's angles.
  - Flattening of the naso-labial fold on one side.
- Nose
  - Structural abnormalities of the nose (size and form).
  - Abnormal width of the nostrils.
  - Malformations of the nasal conchae.
  - Breathing through only one of the nostrils or only through the mouth.
  - Increased effort in breathing.
  - Breathing sounds.
  - Mixed or oral respiration in rest and during speech.
- Jaw
  - Mandibular weakness (the mandible hangs lower than normal in a resting position).
  - Abnormal interocclusal distance at rest.
- Lips
  - Resting position of the lips without contact.
  - Visual abnormalities of the lips (size or structure).
  - Dry or chapped lips.
- Tongue
  - Abnormal resting position of the tongue (weakness on one or both sides; for a unilateral weakness, the tongue deviates towards the side of the weakness).
  - Visual abnormalities of the tongue (e.g. macroglossia, microglossia, ankyloglossia, fasciculations).
  - Abnormal impressions of the teeth.
- Teeth
  - Bad health status of teeth, missing teeth.
  - Badly fitting dentures.
  - Anterior or lateral gaps between the teeth.
- Hard and Soft Palate
  - Abnormal palatal arch (high palatal arch or narrow maxillary arch).
  - Bad health status of the palatal tissues.
  - Asymmetry of the palatal structures.
  - Velum: position and form, especially the uvula; asymmetry at rest with the mouth wide open (bilateral weakness: both sides of the soft palate rest near the posterior part of the tongue; unilateral weakness: the weak side appears lower than normal).
- Pharynx
  - Structural abnormalities of the pharyngeal tissues by simple examination with a front light (for the visible part).
  - Structural abnormalities of the pharyngeal tissues by nasal fibrescope.

3.9.5 Examination and Instrumental Assessment of the Orofacial Functions

In addition to the structural assessment at rest, the orofacial functions (e.g. movement, strength, coordination, accuracy of movement, range of motion, tiring of movement) in non-speech activities are examined. Instructions for the examination procedure as well as possible pathological findings are provided below:

3.9.5.1 Face

- Movement of the facial muscles (disability or asymmetry of movement) (Adunka and Buchman 2011). For a detailed testing of the facial movements and synkinesis, various grading scales are available, e.g. the 'Sydney', 'Sunnybrook' or 'House Brackmann' facial grading system[1] (Fattah et al. 2015). The following main facial functions should especially be assessed to obtain the basic status of the core rami of the n. facialis (tested cranially to caudally). The ability to move the muscles, symmetry of the movement of the muscles as

[1]The House Brackman grade categorises patients on the basis of their degree of facial function, the Sydney system evaluates the relevant anatomical branch of the facial nerve that supplies each movement, and the Sunnybrook system rates the movements made when producing five defined standard expressions.

well as the range of motions and precision of movements of the muscles are evaluated:
 - rr. temporales: movement of the eyebrows, wrinkling of the forehead. To examine the mobility of the facial muscles of the rr. temporales, the patient is requested to make the following movements: looking amazed, looking angry,
 - rr. zygomatici: movement of the upper lip during smiling, eye closure (upper and lower lids). To examine the mobility of the facial muscles of the rr. zygomatici, the patient is requested to make the following movements: close the eyes, smile with open lips,
 - rr. buccales: movement of the corners of the mouth during smiling. To examine the mobility of the facial muscles of the rr. buccales, the patient is requested to make the following movements: smiling with a closed mouth, pursing the lips,
 - r. marginalis mandibulae: movement of the corners of the mouth during sulkiness. To examine the mobility of the facial muscles of the r. marginalis, the patient is requested to make the following movements: looking disappointed,
 - r. digastricus: tensing the skin of the neck (e.g. for shaving). To examine the mobility of the facial muscles of the r. digastricus, the patient is requested to make the following movements: pretend to shave the neck on the one side of the neck and afterwards on the other side of the neck. The ability to move the muscles, and the range of motions and precision of movements of the muscles are evaluated.

3.9.5.2 Jaw

- To examine the opening of the mandibles, the patient is requested to open the mouth slowly as far as possible and afterwards to close the mouth slowly. The following observations should be made from a position directly in front of the patient:
  - Ability and symmetry in opening the mandibles, lateral differences during opening and closing of the jaw. Possible sideways aberrations of the top of the chin during opening and closing the mouth are evaluated (Stelzenmüller 2010).
  - Grade of opening of the mandibles. The distance between the incisal edges of the upper and lower anterior teeth is measured, as is the degree of mandibular opening. Opening of less than 35 mm is defined as abnormal in an adult (Walker et al. 1990). The distance can be measured with a ruler.
  - Ability to control the speed of opening (slow and fast opening, constancy of the movement). By evaluating how the closing and opening muscles of the jaw act together, the control of speed and constancy is evaluated.

3.9.5.3 Lips

- To examine the movements of the lips, patients are requested to:
  - Actively close the lips.
  - Smack and blow with the lips.
  - Show their teeth.
  - Smile and pout.
  - Close their lips around a spoon.
  - Close their lips when chewing and when sucking on a straw.
  - Close their lips against lateral pressure on the m. buccinator (lip power is evaluated).
- For all activities of the lips, the tone and strength of the lip movement are evaluated with a view to determining hypotonus or hypertonus. The mobility is estimated as normal, limited or impossible.

3.9.5.4 Tongue

- For examining the mobility of the tongue, patients are asked to:
  - Push out the tongue, lick the upper and lower lip, and move the tongue between the corners of the mouth. The motility of the tongue is evaluated here.
  - Press the tongue against a spatula (downwards, upwards, sideways). The strength of the tongue is evaluated here.
  - Repeated movements of the tongue. Aspects such as the tongue getting tired, the quality or range of the movement get-

ting worse, and compensatory co-movements of the mimic muscles, jaw or head are evaluated.
  - Lift the lateral lingual edges for visual assessment of the frenulum.

3.9.5.5 Velopharyngeal System

- Movement of the velum and posterior pharynx; when problems in the velopharyngeal system are assumed, endoscopic or videofluoroscopic diagnostics can provide additional information about:
  - Velopharyngeal insufficiencies during swallowing.
  - Sufficiency of velopharyngeal closure.

3.9.5.6 Chewing and Swallowing

- For the evaluation of swallowing and chewing, solid, semi-solid and liquid aliments are used when the patient is requested to take in food. The oral preparation and swallowing are evaluated. Possible findings are:
  - Difficulties achieving lip closure when chewing.
  - Anterior or posterior leaking while chewing.
  - Excessive or abnormal movement of the mouth when chewing.
  - Salivation.
  - Food residuals on the tongue or in the cheek pouches.
  - Nasal regurgitation.
  - Insufficient clearing of the throat after swallowing.
- Evidence or hints of aspiration should be evaluated by additional endoscopic or videofluoroscopic diagnostics.

3.9.6 Interpretation

To identify possible diagnoses for the patient's disorders, the oral motor examination protocol is interpreted by an expert. Impairments of oral motor functions are classified into components of the primary functions of the orofacial system: biting, chewing, oral control of food intake, swallowing and facial expression.

Every impairment, whether functional or structural, should be evaluated and addressed by therapy whether the limitations affect the daily activities of the patient and are perceived as disturbing, or the limitations of the primary functions influence the secondary functions of speech sound production. Hereby, the subjective demands and goals of the patient affect the prioritisation in the treatment of the impairments.

Impairments of the primary function of the orofacial system can also result in a speech-motor disorder, e.g. dysglossia, dysarthria or rhinophonia (hypernasal speech). If limitations of the orofacial system's primary functions exist, the secondary function of the orofacial system should be examined in more detail. A speech motor examination protocol and possible diagnoses related to speech motor disorders are described in Sect. 3.10.

Possible diagnoses of oral motor disorders are described and adjacent disorders (which should either be excluded or considered as potential diagnoses that need further assessment) are listed below with the corresponding ICD-10 codes.

3.9.6.1 Facial Palsy (ICD-10: G51.0)

Functional or structural impairment of the facial muscles (facial palsy) is mainly characterised by restrictions in the control mechanisms of the orofacial muscles.

Indicative signs are weaknesses of the orofacial muscles, restrictions or decelerations of muscle movements, and incoordination of muscle control. Additional symptoms may be a loss of food from the mouth when chewing or swallowing, biting on one's cheek, uncontrollable salivation, or food residues on the tongue or in the cheek pouches after swallowing. To determine the degree of facial palsy, a standardised facial grading system (e.g. the 'Sydney', 'Sunnybrook' or 'House Brackmann' system) should be used (Fattah et al. 2015; Ortega et al. 2009).

3.9.6.2 Buccofacial Apraxia (ICD-10: R48.2)

Buccofacial or orofacial apraxia is defined as the inability to programme the position of orofacial muscles and the sequence of muscle movements upon request. The indicative sign is that patients are unable to perform muscle movements such as smiling, coughing or winking on command, but can do so spontaneously.

3.9.6.3 Dysphagia (ICD-10: R13.1)

The indicating sign of dysphagia is difficulty in swallowing in any of the swallowing phases. Additional symptoms are coughing or gagging when swallowing, hoarseness directly after swallowing, drooling, leaking or having painful swallowing (Bonilha et al. 2013). Impairments of orofacial structures, such as the tongue or the velopharyngeal system (Bettens et al. 2018), as well as disturbances in oral motor functions such as chewing and swallowing, can give additional hints at dysphagia. When such irregularities are identified by this oral motor examination protocol, a full dysphagia assessment should be considered, and imaging diagnostics should be used to exclude the possibility of aspiration. Besides raising the suspicion of dysphagia, nasal regurgitation might also be a hint for velopharyngeal insufficiency. Further symptoms such as speech motor limitations of velopharyngeal insufficiency are found in Sect. 3.10.

3.9.6.4 Speech Motor Disorders (ICD-10: R47)

Although speech motor disorders are not primarily targeted by the oral motor examination protocol, various impairments of the orofacial complex may be related to speech motor disorders and should therefore trigger a more detailed assessment as described in Sect. 3.10. Symptoms related to speech motor disorders are especially abnormalities of the tongue or velopharyngeal insufficiencies, but also impairments of the jaw, lips, teeth or palatal structures (Beals et al. 2015).

3.10 Diagnosis and Differential Diagnosis of Speech Disorders: Speech Motor Examination Protocol

Tanja Fuhr

3.10.1 Introduction

The speech motor system is a complex network of structures that organises and executes speech movements. For speech production, the articulating organs must meet high demands of fast sequences of sound production during speaking. All muscles involved in the speech production process must provide a complex pattern of movement (Schröter-Morasch and Ziegler 2005). Speech disorders, caused by limitations of movement or control of the articulating organs, are characterised by such symptoms as weakness, incoordination, reduction in speech and altered muscle tone (Duffy 2012).

In this context, ‘speech’ is seen as a medium that conveys a message and not primarily its content. The speech motor examination protocol focuses on the execution of speech motor functions and will not determine if speech motor performance belongs to so-called high or low levels of speech production or if limitations of speech performance are caused by planning or execution functions. The outcome of the speech performance is examined.

In patients suffering from dysglossia or velopharyngeal insufficiency, speech intelligibility is often reduced because of structural changes in the speech organs (Maier et al. 2010). The decrease in intelligibility and manner of speech, as well as the reduction of verbal emotional expressiveness, can influence a patient’s quality of life, confine social contacts and can have negative effects on a job and career (Schröter-Morasch and Ziegler 2005).

The examination of such speech motor difficulties as dysglossia should be performed under two main aspects:

- The assessment of the primary orofacial functions and therefore aberrations of physiological parameters of the orofacial complex, such as the evaluation of the movement of single components of the orofacial tract or of strength. This allows the identification of existing pathomechanisms and leads to conclusions about the type, dimension or localisation of the disease (described in detail in Sect. 3.9). Assessing oral motor functions is an integral part of a speech motor examination protocol; the results of the oral motor examination protocol described in Sect. 3.9 should be considered together with the results of the speech motor examination protocol described in this section for a comprehensive assessment.
- The evaluation of acoustic and auditory-perceptual components to assess the impact on speech motor limitation and disturbance of communication (described in this section).

Both components, the primary functions (non-speech movements of the articulating organs) and secondary functions (speech movements of the articulating organs) of the orofacial system are necessary for a comprehensive diagnosis.

The major goals of the speech motor evaluation are to:

- Identify deficits in speech production.
- Attribute the deficits to the speech production subsystems (respiration, articulation, voicing, resonance, and prosody).
- Estimate the severity of the limitations imposed by the affected subsystems, as well as the impact on intelligibility, activity limitations and participation restrictions (Hartelius et al. 2000).

For analysing speech motor performance, several approaches are available: auditory-perceptual evaluation, acoustic analysis or automatic speech recognition systems of speech performance, and imaging procedures are examples (Guyton et al. 2018). Single speech segments as well as suprasegmental aspects should be the content of the examination (Miller and Lowit 2014). In this section, assessment procedures focus on the auditory-perceptual assessment of speech motor functions.

The following aspects are part of the speech motor examination protocol:

- The medical history of the patients, including limitations and restrictions on activities and participation, their personal goals and contextual factors of the impairments.
- A description of appropriate test instruments and material.
- Procedures to assess the speech motor functions.
- Guidelines for interpreting the findings and identifying possible diagnoses.

Results of the assessment of speech motor functions from the use of auditory-perceptual methods can be appended, and supported, for example by using acoustic analyses (Sect. 3.16) or imaging procedures (Sects. 3.19 and 3.20); these methods are described in their own Sections in detail.

3.10.2 Medical History

When assessing the medical history of the patients, clinical, contextual, personal and environmental factors are evaluated, as well as the demands, limitations of intelligibility, strengths and weaknesses regarding the patients' activities and participation (American Speech-Language-Hearing Association 2004). In particular, the medical assessment should include questions about the following aspects:

- Subjective patient's report, containing:
  - A description of the symptoms of speech activities.
  - A description of how the speech and voice actually sound.

  - A sense of the effort associated with speaking.
  - Signs of getting tired during speech.
  - Signs of reduced breath.
  - Pain during speaking.
  - Voice capacity and possible length of utterances.
  - The physical ability to manage conversation.
  - The impact of the symptoms on intelligibility.
  - Signs of misapprehension by listeners as signs of lack of motivation, cognitive incapacity or depression.
  - The patient's own perspective of their speech performance.
- Medical diagnoses:
  - Medical diagnosis directly related to speech and date of onset of speech impairment.
  - Other medical diagnoses or surgery, especially concerning the hearing and vision status.
  - Medical history, occurrences of tracheostomy or mechanical ventilation.
  - Medications and allergies.
  - Methods that patients have already applied to manage speech impairment.
- Contextual, personal and environmental factors:
  - Primary languages spoken.
  - Educational history.
  - Family background.
  - Current life situation.
  - Occupation.
  - Mental status, especially responsiveness, compliance and motivation.
- Limitations in activities and restrictions in participation caused by impairments of speech motor functioning, especially:
  - Limitations on the patient's interpersonal interactions, such as in face-to-face situations, over the phone, or in a group conversation.
  - Activity limitations and participation restrictions in the following or other situations; general tasks and demands, household tasks, education, employment or community.
- Demands and subjective goals of the patient and prioritisation of the patient's goals.

3.10.3 Test Instruments and Materials

For assessing speech motor performance, the examiner should, if possible, record on tape or film the examination, to allow more reliable decisions through repeated viewing and to facilitate the auditory perceptual observations necessary for differential diagnosis. Furthermore, a standardised diagnostic tool for intelligibility testing should be used, for the spoken language of the patient if one is available.

3.10.4 Auditory-Perceptual Assessment of Speech Motor Function

The perceptual evaluation of speech motor movement is a common method for evaluating the attributes of speech performance. The goal of the auditory perceptual assessment is to evaluate all relevant characteristics of speech performance (Duffy 2012).

The auditory-perceptual assessment should systematically test each subsystem of speech sound production: respiration, articulation, voicing, resonance and prosody (Barkmeier-Kraemer and Clark 2017). For testing each subsystem, knowledge of the neurophysiology of speech sound production is required for identifying aberrations from physiological speech sound production. In the following, the theory and testing procedures for each subsystem are described.

3.10.4.1 Respiration/Phonation

Speech breathing is a complex process requiring precise coordination of the subglottal, glottal and supraglottal components of the speech-producing system. Physiological speech breathing produces the steady and constant airflow to the vocal tract that is necessary for normal speech production. The limitations and impairment of speech breathing are difficult to capture in detail on the basis of perceptual analysis only (Murdoch et al. 1993).

The evaluation of information on the physiological basis, as well as the respiratory disturbance, can be confirmed in a more valid way by using aerodynamic analyses. A loss of control of speech breathing can lead to a reduced intonation for example.

Respiration and phonation are evaluated on the criteria 'quality', 'duration', 'loudness' and 'steadiness' at three levels of difficulty ('phone', 'oral reading', 'conversation'). The quality is rated on (partial) aphonia, breathiness, hoarseness, harshness and strained voice/strangled voice. For rating the duration, the maximum time of a phonation at the phone level is captured and the duration is classified into categories (i.e. not impaired, mildly impaired, moderately impaired, severely impaired). The loudness can be assessed as mono-loudness, reduced or excessive loudness or variable loudness. Finally, the steadiness of the tests, especially the voice getting tired when speaking, is observed at all levels of difficulty.

The quality criteria are evaluated on three increasing levels of difficulty: for testing at the phone level, the vowel [a] is often used (Yokonishi et al. 2016). Oral reading and conversation each test the patient's strengths and weaknesses/impairments in longer sequences of respiration and phonation.

3.10.4.2 Articulation and Intelligibility

For evaluating articulation, there are two common ways of assessment: analysing single components of speech and analysing connected speech. Both types of assessment should be part of a speech motor examination protocol to evaluate all relevant aspects. Single component assessment includes testing single phones and testing the production of single words. For connected speech assessment, full sentences and paragraphs are test subjects, as is the evaluation of conversation. Test results at each level can be documented by using such categories as 'not impaired'/'mildly impaired'/'moderately impaired'/'severely impaired'.

Single Component Testing: Phone Inventory

Every language has a specific inventory of speech sounds. The auditory perceptual assessment of speech sound must be adapted to the phone inventory of the patients' languages. To identify pathological speech sound production, the examiner must know the physiological place of articulation for all phones (i.e. consonants and vowels). In the following, the English phone inventory is used as an exemplary language to describe the single steps of evaluating the phone inventory and to provide an overview of important aspects that should be considered when testing. English contains 14 vowels and 24 consonants.

Vowels: The examiner should be aware of the aspects that influence physiological vowel production. For a systematic description of vowel production, the following characteristics are relevant knowledge, as impairments in vowel production can hint at the physical systems that cause the impairment:

- The part of the tongue that reaches the highest point ('direction of tongue advancement': front/central/back).
- Degree of tongue elevation (low/medium/high).
- Degree of jaw opening (open/mid-open/mid/mid-close/close).
- Muscle strength (tense/lax).
- Position of the lips (rounded/neutral/spread).
- Vowel quantity (the duration a vowel is kept: long/short).

The physiological direction of tongue advancement, degree of tongue elevation and degree of jaw opening when producing the IPA vowels are presented in the vowel chart in Fig. 3.10 Vowels are tested at the single phone level for aberrations from the physiological production. Any deficit in one of the mentioned characteristics of vowel production may lead to low contrasts between different vowels and therefore may influence the speaker's intelligibility.

Consonants: The production of English constants (found in most native English dialects) is characterised by three aspects: the place of articulation, the manner of the phone and the voicing. The place of articulation is the point of contact where obstructions exist in the vocal tract between active articulators (mainly, some part of the tongue) and passive articulators (mainly, some part of the palate). Figure 3.11 shows the places of articulation.

The manner describes the type of shutter sound forming the phone. Shutter sounds in English are plosives (explosion), fricatives (friction), affricates (a combination of explosion and friction), nasals (nasal passage), laterals (sideways passage) and approximants (approaching articulators to each other).

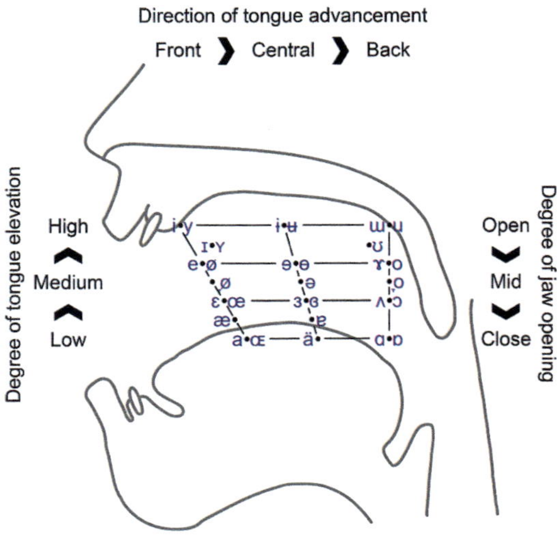

Fig. 3.10 IPA vowel chart (©Fuhr 2021)

Voicing describes the differences between the two conditions 'voiced' or 'unvoiced' sounds. For example, voicing is a meaningful unit to differentiate between the two sounds [b] and [p]. The manner and the place of articulation are the same in the two sounds [b] and [p]. A limitation of voicing of sounds can impair the meaningful unit of words such as /bass/ and /pass/.

Table 3.9 shows the physiological characteristics of English consonants. The place of articulation within the vocal tract is shown in the columns and the manner of phones, as well as the voicing, are shown in the rows.

To examine the speech motor performance of consonants at the single phone level, the place of articulation, the manner and the voicing are evaluated. Identifying which of these aspects are affected in pathological consonant sound production can give hints on the underlying pathomechanism. For example, dysglossia can influence the place of articulation of consonants (Miller and Lowit 2014).

For a precise localisation of impairments, Table 3.10 provides a more detailed view of

Fig. 3.11 Places of articulation for consonants (©Fuhr 2021)

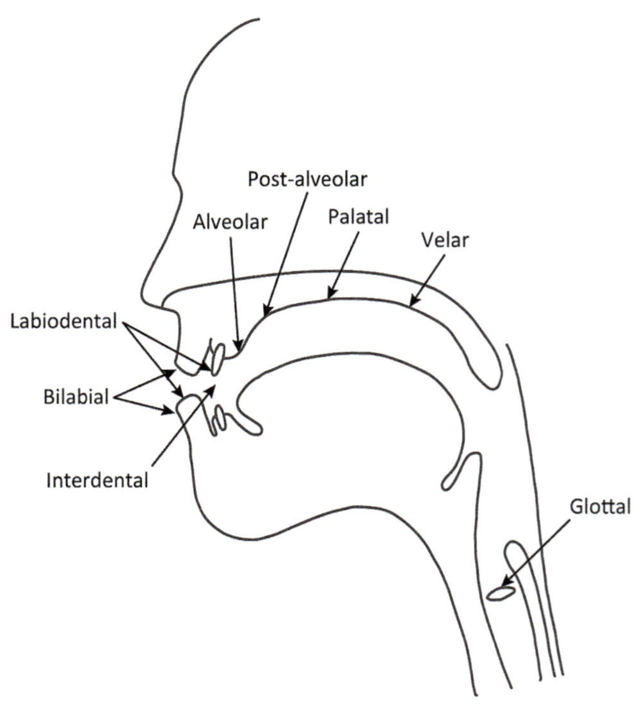

Table 3.9 Feature matrix of consonants (© Fuhr 2021)

		Place of articulation							
Manner	Voicing	Bilabial	Labio-dental	Inter-dental	Alveolar	Post-alveolar	Palatal	Velar	Glottal
Plosive	Voiceless	P			t			k	
	Voiced	B			d			g	ʔ
Fricative	Voiceless		f	θ	s	ʃ			H
	Voiced		v	ð	z	ʒ			
Affricate	Voiceless					tʃ			
	Voiced					dʒ			
Nasal	Voiced	M			n			ŋ	
Lateral	Voiced				l				
Approximant	Voiced					R	j		

Table 3.10 Characteristics of English consonants (©Fuhr 2021)

	p	b	t	d	k	g	ʔ	f	v	θ	ð	s	z	ʃ	ʒ	h	m	n	ŋ	l	r	j
Tip	–	–	+	+	–	–	–	–	–	–	–	–	–	–	–	–	–	+	–	+	–	–
Front	–	–	–	–	–	–	–	–	–	+	+	+	+	–	–	–	–	+	–	+	–	–
Coronal	–	–	+	+	–	–	–	–	–	–	–	+	+	+	+	–	–	+	–	+	+	–
Back	–	–	–	–	+	+	–	–	–	–	–	–	–	–	–	–	–	–	+	–	–	–
Nasal	–	–	–	–	–	–		–	–	–	–	–	–	–	–	–	+	+	+	–	–	–
High	–	–	–	–	+	+	–	–	–	–	–	–	–	+	+	–	–	–	+	–	+	+
Labial	+	+	–	–	–	–	–	+	+	–	–	–	–	–	–	–	+	–	–	–	–	–

places of articulation (single segments of the tongue: tip/front/coronal/back), velopharyngeal involvement (nasal), involvement of the palate (high) or the lips (labial). Certain diagnoses such as a (semi-)resection of the tongue may require an exact localisation of the impairments in speech sound production. Distinct segments of the tongue that are affected can be identified by testing and evaluating these consonants. For velopharyngeal insufficiency, the rate of nasality—i.e. the involvement and degree of elusion of airflow through the nose—is of importance.

Single Component Testing: Single Words

Single-word intelligibility testing is a main part of speech assessment. The test execution is based on word lists. The patient is asked to produce single words in the form of reading, picture naming or repeating. The correctly produced words are rated and counted by the examiner. If the ability of the patient to produce a contrast of sounds is impaired, a limitation of intelligibility may exist. For testing, items are used that differ in their manner of articulation, place of articulation, prosody (i.e. stress pattern), voicing or syllable structure. For example, test items only differ in (a) single components such as voicing (e.g. vine/fine), (b) tongue tip, or dorsum as a place of articulation (e.g. tea/key), (c) manner of articulation (e.g. die/lie) and (d) syllable structure and word length.

Counting the correctly produced words during single-word intelligibility testing often achieves greater inter-rater reliability than the scaling methods or percentage judgments of connected speech testing, and therefore is seen as a valid method for measuring intelligibility (Miller 2013). However, the method of counting the intelligible single words may not identify those aspects of speech production impairment that led to limitations of intelligibility in detail. Furthermore, the examiner must evaluate which phonetic contrast is impaired. Thus, the aim of single-word testing should be to examine contrasts that functionally imitate the intelligibility of the speaker.

For the English language, word lists for testing can be found in the Dysarthria Profile (Robertson 1982), the Assessment of Intelligibility of Dysarthria Speech (Yorkston and Beukelman 1981) and the Frenchay Dysarthria Assessment (Enderby 1983).

Similar single-word testing procedures exist for various languages. All tests follow the same principles and provide different sets of phonetic contrasts in single words. Single-word testing lists exist for example for German (Ziegler and Hartmann 1993), French (Gentil 1992) and Danish (Petersen 1997).

When using such single-word lists, the examiner should ensure that the validity of those lists has been demonstrated by research studies.

Connected Speech Assessment: Full Sentences and Spontaneous Speech

Connected speech assessment evaluates speech performance during reading sample sentences, reading passages and spontaneous speech. The analysis of spontaneous speech is especially important for general judgment because it consists of everyday speech production and allows the examiner to get an impression of routine motor speech performance. However, it is difficult to evaluate connected speech reliably and to determine improvement of the speech performance over time, by using perceptual methods. In addition, evaluating spontaneous speech does not lead in detail to answers about which speech impairments lead to a reduction of communication capabilities (Miller and Lowit 2014).

For reading single sentences or passages, the examiner is more aware of the target production than in spontaneous speech. However, there are many influencing factors, both segmental and non-segmental, in passage reading that differ from those in spontaneous speech, making it difficult for the examiner to evaluate the exact impact on intelligibility.

Therefore, standardised diagnostic tools for intelligibility testing should mainly focus on single words, as well as on well-controlled sentences, for the identification of which components of speech impairment exist and which are responsible for a reduction of communication efficiency.

3.10.4.3 Voicing

Voicing, especially the voice onset time (VOT, i.e. the interval between stop release and vowel voicing) can give important clues to the distinction of plosives in English such as [b] and [p], or [t] and [d], or [k] and [g]. For such fricatives as [f] and [w], or [s] and [z], the manner of voicing also plays an important role in perceptive discrimination. The existence of contrasts between voiced and unvoiced sounds should be evaluated. The examiner must assess if single sounds such as [p] and [b] are auditorily distinguishable, as well as if words (these can be minimal pairs such as buy and pie) can be distinguished through voicing. In addition, connected speech contains perceptive attributes to distinguish voiced and unvoiced sounds. For patients suffering from difficulties in using voicing in speech production, assimilation of voicing is often presented in spontaneous speech (Miller and Lowit 2014).

3.10.4.4 Resonance/Velopharyngeal Insufficiency

Signs and symptoms of resonance disorders depend on several factors, including the type and severity of the resonance disorder, as well as the consistency of symptoms (Cahill et al. 2004). The activity of the velum in regulating the degree of nasality, and therefore the presence of nasal emission, as well as the type of articulation error, need to be evaluated.

Excessive nasal resonance (hypernasality) can mostly be recognised in vowels, liquids and glides. The high vowels (i.e. [i] and [u]) are especially prone to hypernasality (American Speech-Language-Hearing Association 2020).

Reduced nasal resonance on vowels, sonorants or nasal consonants is called hyponasality. It can be recognised best on nasal consonants. These nasal consonants will stand out with more oral sound quality; for example, the [m] sounds like a [b], the [n] sounds similar to a [d], and a [ŋ] sounds similar to a [g].

An obstruction of one of the cavities of the vocal tract (i.e. the oral, pharyngeal or nasal cavity of the vocal tract) leads to 'muffled' speech production. Mixed forms of resonance limitation can also occur simultaneously or at different times when speaking.

To identify limitations of resonance, the examiner must evaluate oral, nasal and velopharyngeal functions of speech production. The examiner must identify if the patient would benefit from speech therapy or if surgical or prosthetic intervention might be useful, or if both components, speech therapy and medical intervention, are necessary to achieve an improvement in resonance.

One diagnostic tool that includes the analysis of resonance as one of the speech-relevant dimensions is the Bogenhausen Dysarthria Scales (Ziegler et al. 2015) and the Asahi Speech Assessment Test (Nishio 2004).

3.10.4.5 Prosody

Prosodic functions are expressed differently in various languages through specific variations of the fundamental frequency, intensity, pauses and speech segment duration (Miller and Lowit 2014).

For the English language, specific components of stress levels characterise prosody. According to Hayes (1995), the English language shows three stress levels: primary, secondary and unstressed. These specific characteristics must be integrated into the estimation of prosodic limitations. For the English language, stressed syllables can be identified by characteristics of longer duration, a higher fundamental frequency as well as a higher intensity compared to physiological non-stressed syllables. The manner and degree of reduction of intonation must be estimated for single words and sentences. For sentences, the ability to mark the intonation of questions is also of interest to evaluate.

The examiner evaluates to what extent changes or limitations of prosody have an impact on the ability of the patient to be understood. For example, the components of prosody constitute one of the main impairments of Chinese patients with dysarthria (Ciocca et al. 2002). An impairment in intonation will have a great impact on intelligibility—depending on the influence of prosody in a language (Tani et al. 2002). Prosody can be evaluated through producing words with contrasting intonation and stress. The patient is asked to produce speech with different stress and intonation, such as ‘small cat’ vs. ‘small cat’ (the underlined word will be produced with intonation) or producing ‘no’ with rising vs. falling intonation, or using heteronyms that vary in their stress pattern, such as abstract (adjective: existing in thought but not having a concrete existence) in contrast to abstract (verb: extracting the general from something concrete).

A language-specific diagnostic tool for estimating the impact of the impairment of prosodic function on intelligibility should be used. Knuijt and de Swart (2007) developed for example a diagnostic instrument for the Dutch to evaluate, amongst other things, the prosody of speech. The diagnostic tool is used as a preferred method of reading standardised texts and performs an additional diadochokinetic test.

3.10.4.6 Oral Agility: Diadochokinetic Rates

Some diagnostic tools such as the DYVA test for assessing speech motor performance determine the oral diadochokinetic rate (syllables per second) and performance (Dharmaperwira-Prins 2009). Assessing the capability of oral diadochokinesis involves testing the ability to repeat a segment of speech at high speed (Padovani et al. 2009).

Depret (2005) confirmed that the rate of oral diadochokinesis is a sensitive measure for distinguishing between healthy and non-healthy speech motor performance. For testing the diadochokinetic and syllable repetition rate, sequencing and alternating items are used. The level of complexity should increase during this test (Knuijt and de Swart 2007): in general, tests begin with producing single CVs (consonant-vocal clusters such as [pa]) at various places of articulation, e.g. [pa], [ta], [ka]. The level of complexity is then increased by using CV-CV clusters such as [pa-ta] or CV-CV-CV clusters such as [pa-ta-ka]. Finally, tests are completed with CCVCC structures such as [drʌŋk] and [drɪŋk].

3.10.5 Awareness/Strategy Use

In addition to identifying speech motor impairments, the patient’s awareness of these impairments and applied strategies should be evaluated during the assessment. The examiner evaluates if patients recognise their impairments and if they use or would be able to use strategies to cope with them. It is also evaluated if applied strategies are effective and consistent, i.e. if patients use them permanently or if they are used only intermittently.

3.10.6 Interpretation

The speech motor examination protocol should provide detailed information on which features of speech motor performance contribute to the reduction of intelligibility and which should be given priority for treatment. If available, a standardised diagnostic tool for intelligibility and naturalness of speech should be chosen to confirm a potential diagnosis identified by a speech motor examination protocol. Single components that are listed in the speech motor protocol but not included in a chosen diagnostic tool should be tested by auditory perception to determine possible diagnoses. Potential diagnoses are described in the following.

3.10.6.1 Dysarthria (ICD-10: R47.1)

Sensorimotor impairments of the central or peripheral nervous system (of parts of the respiratory system, the phonatory and articulatory system, as well as parts of the resonance system or the prosody system) cause dysarthria. The causes and location of the brain damage within the nervous system led to different types of dysarthria. Forms such as spastic dysarthria, rigid hypokinetic dysarthria, ataxic dysarthria, dyskinetic and dystonic types of dysarthria, flaccid dysarthria and mixed dysarthria can be differentiated (Enderby 2013). Hence, the limitation of naturalness and intelligibility of speech performances is caused by limitations of the nervous system.

3.10.6.2 Dysglossia (ICD-10: R47.89)

Reduction in intelligibility can have structural causes, especially after surgical and radiochemical treatment of tumours. Because of structural changes in the speech organs, the ability to perform and coordinate precise articulatory movements with natural speech components and adequate intelligibility is impaired (Schröter-Morasch and Ziegler 2005). Hence, dysglossia is a speech motor disorder caused by structural alterations.

3.10.6.3 Apraxia of Speech (ICD-10: R48.2)

Signs of apraxia of speech may also be signs of limitations in intelligibility. The latter are caused by a failure in the oral and verbal motor planning function. Symptoms of apraxia of speech are more far-reaching than having only limitations of naturalness and intelligibility of speech. Such symptoms as semantic and phonological aberrations may exist. Patients suffering from apraxia of speech may have trouble imitating and saying sounds on their own. They might produce sounds wrongly, add new sounds or leave sounds out during speaking. They often show a variability in intelligibility: at one time, they can produce sounds phonetically correctly and at the other times they produce sounds phonetically incorrectly (Utianski et al. 2018). A variation in the intelligibility of some articulatory complexity may give hints of apraxia of speech.

3.10.6.4 Velopharyngeal Insufficiency (ICD-10: K13.79)

Signs of hyper- or hypo-nasal speech may hint at velopharyngeal insufficiency. Further symptoms such as regurgitation of solid and fluid food through the nose (evaluated through medical history in the oral motor protocol, see Sect. 3.9), may confirm the suspicion of velopharyngeal insufficiency. An inspection of the oral and nasal cavity during phonation with instruments, e.g. a fibreoptic naso-endoscope, can be used to confirm velopharyngeal insufficiency.

3.10.6.5 Voice Disorders (ICD-10: R49)

Voice impairments may influence the voice quality, loudness and pitch. These result from possible alterations caused by structural aberrations in respiratory, laryngeal or vocal tract mechanisms. When such irregularities of voice production are identified by this oral motor examination protocol, a full auditory-perceptual, instrumental and aerodynamic assessment should be considered. If necessary, an objective acoustic assessment of vocal function related to parameters such as loudness, quality and pitch should be applied.

3.11 Ultrasound of the Lips

Florian Lasse Lefarth and Wolfgang Angerstein

3.11.1 Introduction

Medical ultrasound devices are increasingly used and can be powerful tools for phoniatricians. Using high-resolution ultrasound provides the opportunity to take a look inside the lips. Functional aspects especially can be examined, such as physiological actions or such pathological findings as scars of the orbicularis oris muscle (OOM).

> 'Functional diagnostics during tension and relaxation facilitate the detection of muscular dysfunction and thus contribute to the diagnosis of dystonic or hypotonic diseases'.
> —Lefarth (2019)

Unfortunately, many clinicians are unsure of how to perform a reliable and thorough sonographic lip examination. In this section, a systematic overview of the specific labial ultrasound examination techniques is given.

3.11.2 Basic Ultrasound Equipment

3.11.2.1 Requirements

An ultrasound device with a resolution of at least 10 MHz, the possibility to create and store video clips and a linear probe (minimum 10 MHz; currently 18 MHz probes are state-of-the-art) should be available. Common ultrasound gel can be used. For good comfort of the patient—as well as for the examiner—an examination couch with adjustable backrest should be used.

3.11.2.2 Specific Adjustments

Before starting the examination, the relevant software of the ultrasound system should be adjusted and documented. A precise record of the ultrasound device's settings especially is highly recommended—otherwise future examiners will be unable to repeat the examination. Useful settings for beginners are often pre-adjusted by the manufacturers (the settings are mostly called 'small-parts' settings). Once selected, the chosen setting should be used for all of the examinations.

3.11.2.3 Starting the Examination

The patient or test person (TP) should be instructed to keep the mouth closed so that the ultrasound gel cannot penetrate into the oral cavity. Closing the mouth should be done with the least possible effort in order to avoid contraction of the OOM (while contracted the OOM becomes thicker and changes shape).

3.11.2.4 Examining Via B-Mode Using Predefined Scan Planes

Ultrasound examinations of the OOM should include scans of both the whole upper lip (UL) and the whole lower lip (LL). Furthermore, it is important to scan the UL and LL in sagittal and transverse planes. This allows a three-dimensional (3D) reconstruction of the peri-oral structures. We introduce below an exemplary examination procedure that can be reproduced easily. If combined with video scans, it can be stored and revisited on demand.

The sagittal dynamic B-mode investigation starts in the middle of the UL and LL (Fig. 3.12a, plane 1 in Fig. 3.13).

Then the transducer is moved slowly to the right about 2 cm beyond the angle of the mouth, then back to the median starting position and analogously to the left side (Fig. 3.12a). During execution, targeted short breaks for a few seconds in the median position, the paramedian position (corresponding to the philtrum ridges; planes 2 and 3 in Fig. 3.13), the lateral position (in the area of the modiolus) and again by reaching the starting position are important because this facilitates the orientation on the video recordings for later evaluation.

If no recording function is available, still (frozen) images should be taken. Regardless of the vertical plane (median, paramedian or lateral), the sagittal images of UL and LL are very similar

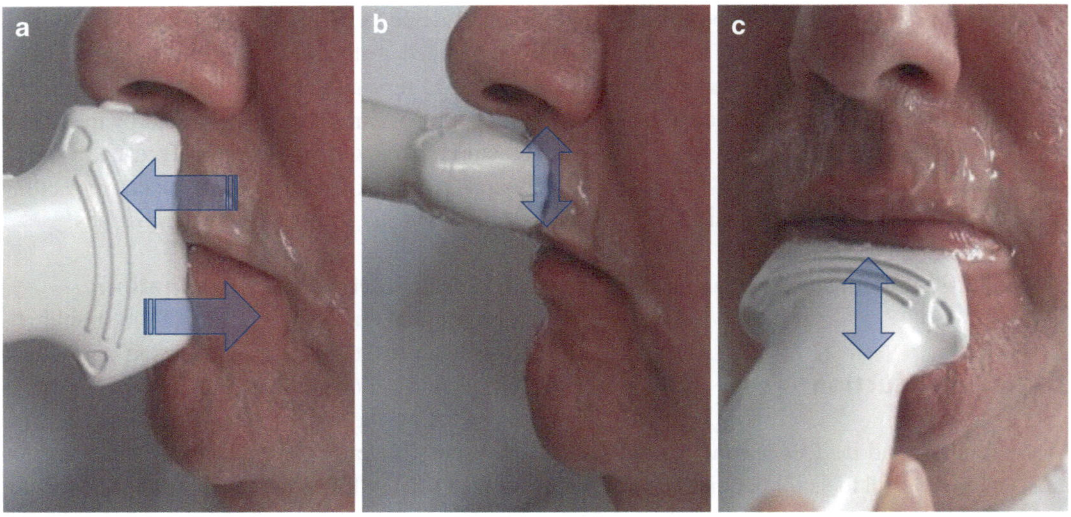

Fig. 3.12 Transducer positions for labial sonography. (**a**) upper and lower lip sagittal position. (**b**) upper lip transverse position. (**c**) lower lip transverse position. (©Lefarth 2021)

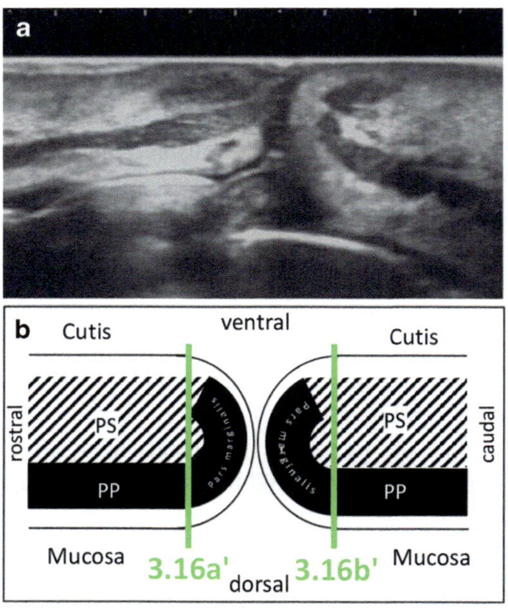

Fig. 3.14 Sono-anatomy of the OOM in median-sagittal sectional scans. (**a**) Median-Sagittal Section of UL and LL. The shape of the OOM looks like a 'hockey stick' or 'hook'. (**b**) Schematic Median-sagittal Section of UL and LL. The green lines mark the cutting height and the spatial course of the transverse cuts of UL and LL shown in Fig. 3.16 (PS = Pars superficialis [superficial part], PP = Pars peripheralis [peripheral part], Pars marginalis [marginal part]). (©Lefarth 2021)

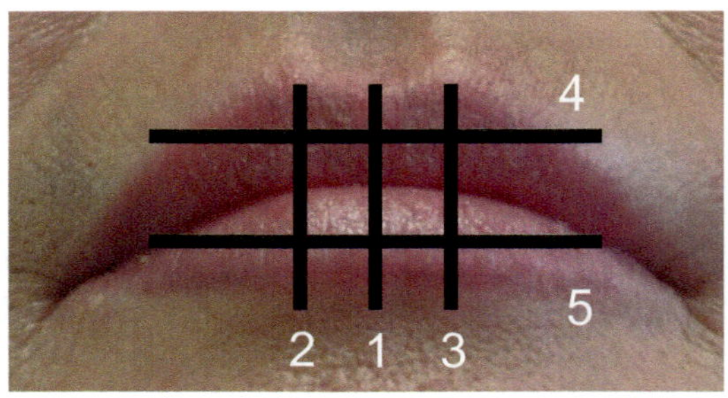

Fig. 3.13 Scan planes for labial sonography. The black lines mark the different scanning planes. The examination sequence is numbered from 1 to 5. (©Lefarth 2021)

(Figs. 3.14 and 3.15), and often both lips can be seen in one image (Fig. 3.14).

The transverse images should be created separately for UL and LL (planes 4 and 5 in Figs. 3.13, 3.16 and 3.17). The UL is first examined medially (Fig. 3.12b, plane 4 in Figs. 3.13, 3.16, and 3.17a): the transducer is placed on the largest curvature in the middle of the lip at the vermilion zone.

Starting from this position, the probe can be moved slightly downwards towards the mouth opening, depending on the individual thickness of the TP's lips. Swivelling movements of the transducer can be useful to prevent decoupling artifacts in the area of the mouth opening. The LL

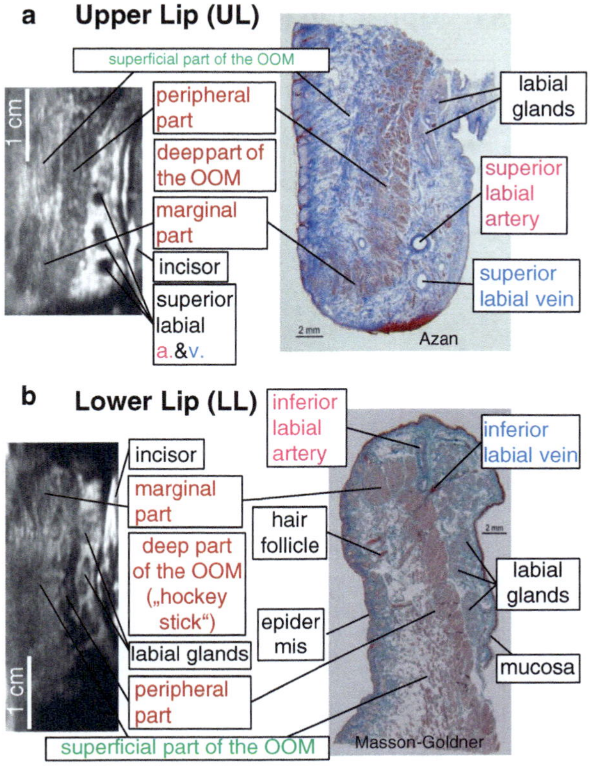

Fig. 3.15 Comparative anatomy of the OOM in sagittal views. Left: Native Ultrasound Images. Right: Corresponding Histological Sections. (©Lefarth 2021)

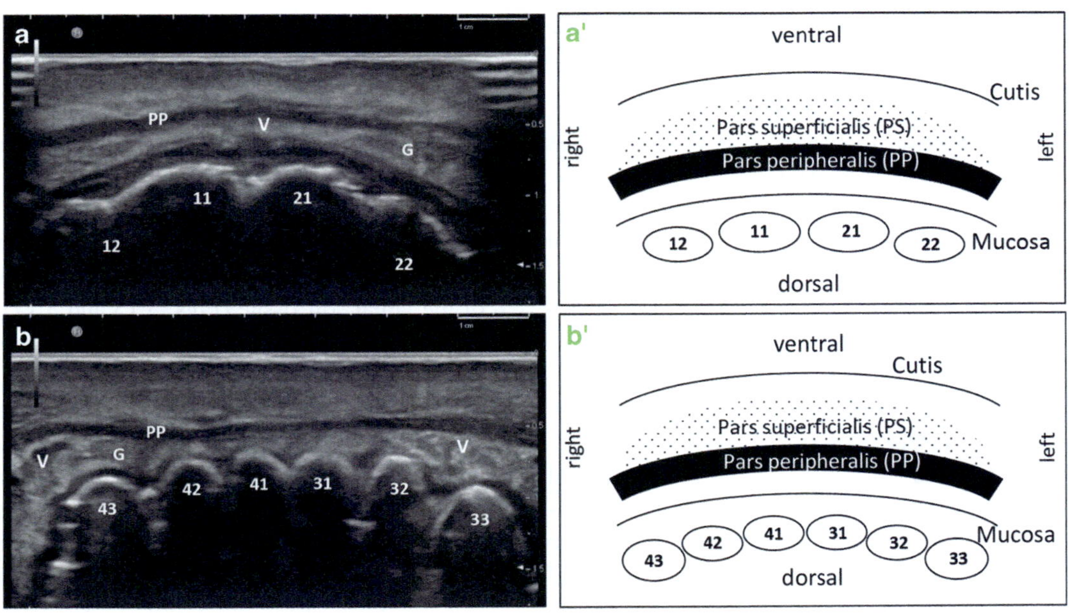

Fig. 3.16 Sono-anatomy of the OOM in transverse sectional scans. (**a**) Transverse Cut of the Upper Lip (UL) in Relaxed Condition. The peripheral part of the OOM (Pars peripheralis = PP) appears as a thin hypoechogenic line. Also marked are the dentes incisivi (12, 11, 21, 22), a lip vessel (V) and a labial gland (G). (**b**) Transverse Cut of the Lower Lip (LL). Similar to a but with dentes incisivi (42, 41, 31, 32) and dentes canini (43, 33). **a′** Schematic Transverse Cut of the UL. Both Parts of the OOM and Dentes Incisivi are shown. **b′** Schematic Transverse Cut of the LL. Similar to **a′** but with visibility of dentes incisivi and dentes canini. (©Lefarth 2021)

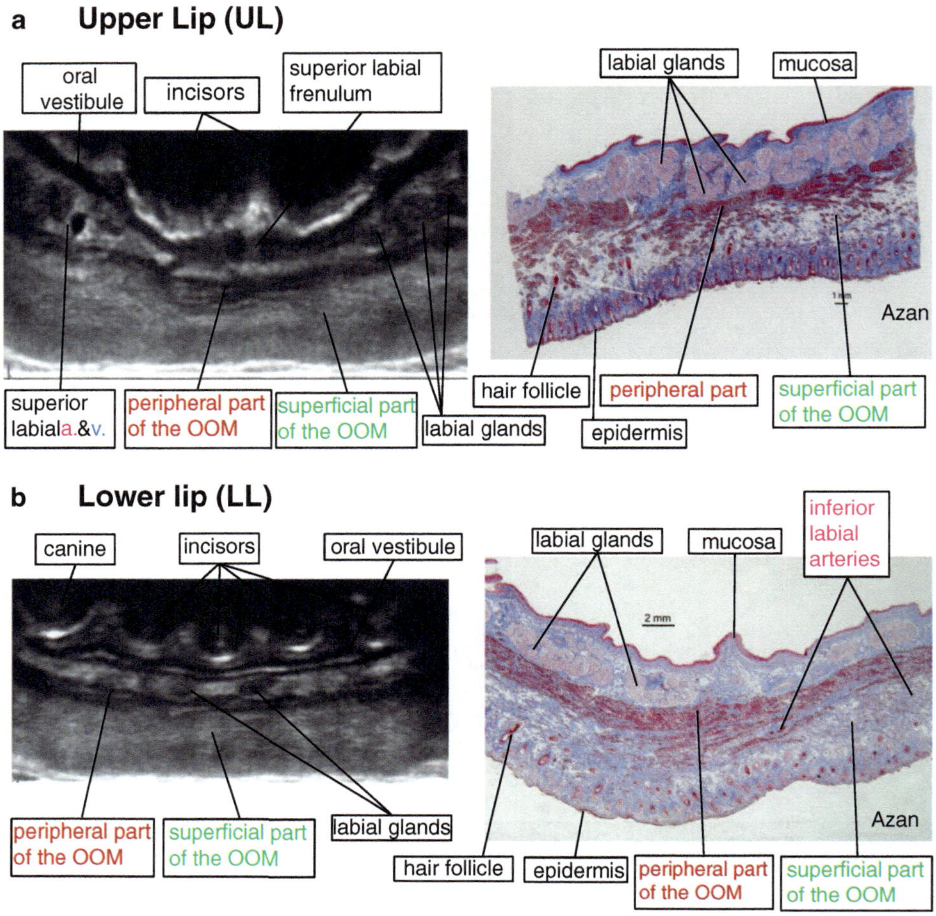

Fig. 3.17 Comparative anatomy of the OOM in transverse views. Left: native ultrasound images; right: corresponding histological sections. (©Lefarth 2021)

is examined analogously (Fig. 3.12c, plane 5 in Figs. 3.13 and 3.17b).

3.11.2.5 Sonographic and Corresponding Histological Sectional Images of the Lips

- During the ultrasound investigation several labial structures can be identified from comparison with histological sectional images: according to Park and Ha (1995), histological examination of the lips reveals a superficial layer (superficial part) and a deep layer (marginal and peripheral parts) of the OOM (Figs. 3.14, 3.15 and 3.17).
- The superficial part sometimes cannot be precisely distinguished sonographically in conventional B-mode sequences and proves to be slightly hypoechoic compared with the rest of the labial soft tissue (Figs. 3.15 and 3.17). This is because the superficial musculature consists of many small mimic facial muscles, whose thin fibres radiate into the OOM from different directions (Park and Ha 1995).
- Owing to its compact structure, the deep layer of the OOM can usually be identified in all cut planes, because it is much more echo-poor than the rest of the lips (Figs. 3.14, 3.15, 3.16 and 3.17). The teeth are visible most of the time both in sagittal and horizontal planes, thus they can be used as landmarks (Figs. 3.15, 3.16 and 3.17).
- In sagittal planes the deep part of the OOM has the shape of a hook or a hockey stick (Figs. 3.14,

3.15 and 3.18a, b), and the superficial muscle fibres can hardly be distinguished from the surrounding connective tissue. The labial vessels and glands are located in the submucosa (Figs. 3.15, 3.16a, b and 3.17). The arteries and veins may easily be detected in the colour duplex mode (Fig. 3.18). They are mainly found at the inner edge of the lips (Fig. 3.18a, b) and have a meandering course (Fig. 3.18c, d).

- While swivelling through the lips, functional ultrasound examinations of the OOM during contraction and relaxation are possible. By starting the ultrasonic investigation, the TP should be asked to relax the lips as much as possible to gain a 'native' view of the OOM with no thickening. A contracted lip in tension shows a considerable thickening of the peripheral part (PP) of the OOM compared with the relaxed state (Fig. 3.19).
- For contraction, it can be useful to give a predefined motion command aiming to obtain a facial expression with a lip movement that is more or less uniform among different individuals regardless of their ethnic or cultural background. The command should thus create a commonly known facial expression—according to Charles Darwin 'the same state of mind is expressed throughout the world with remarkable uniformity' (Darwin et al. 1872). Suitable commands proven in clinical practice might be 'please pucker up your lips as if kissing' or 'please purse your lips'.
- While contracting, the lips change their shape multi-directionally depending on the individual action of the TP. Therefore, the probe should always try to follow the changing lip contour in order to have good contact with the

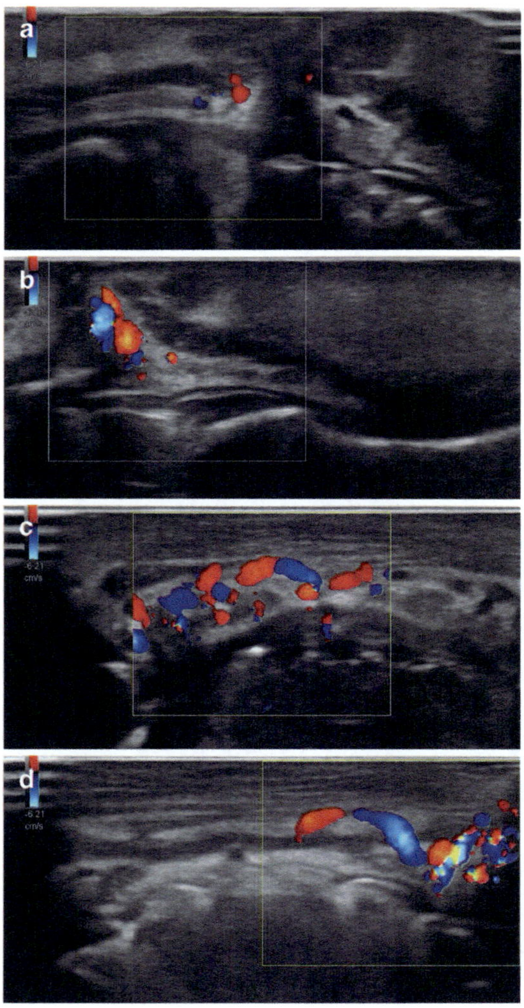

Fig. 3.18 Colour duplex sonography of UL and LL. (**a**, **b**) Median (or paramedian) Sagittal Sectional Images of the UL/LL. Characteristic position of the labial vessels at the inner edge of the lips. (**c**, **d**) Transverse Sectional Images of the UL/LL. Typical meandering course of the vessels in the area of the PM. (©Lefarth 2021)

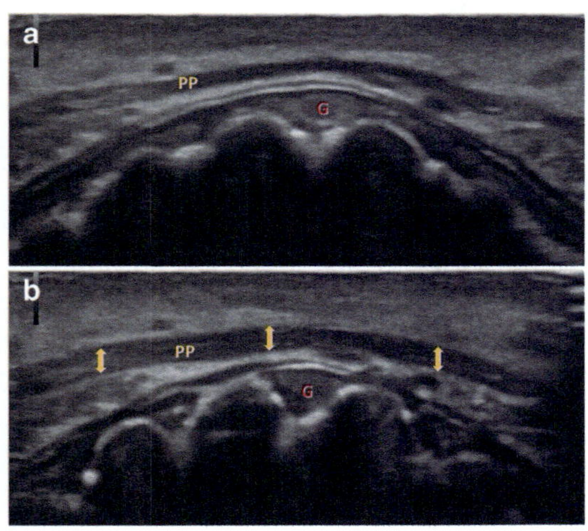

Fig. 3.19 Thickening of the OOM during contraction. (**a**) Transverse Section of the UL. The image shows a transverse cut of the peripheral part (PP) of the OOM in the area of the tooth necks. The gingiva (G) is also visible. (**b**) Transverse Section of the UL in Tension. The PP under tension is significantly thicker (↔) in comparison to a. (©Lefarth 2021)

lips irrespective of the actual state of contraction.

3.11.3 Indications for Labial Sonography

3.11.3.1 Subepithelial Cleft Lip (SCL)

These patients have clinically inconspicuous lips, but ultrasound examination reveals discontinuities of the OOM due to a genetic predisposition (Neiswanger et al. 2007; Weinberg et al. 2006). The muscular defects are hidden by intact submucous tissue and an unobtrusive mucosa of the lips.

3.11.3.2 Intrauterine 3D Sonography

In Europe, nowadays most human lips are scanned in 3D by gynaecologists during prenatal ultrasound screening for orofacial clefts (Maarse et al. 2010, 2011).

3.11.3.3 Wind Instrument Players

Patients with extensive use or overuse of the lip musculature, such as brass players, may suffer from morphological disorders of the OOM.

Brass players are at high risk of damage to the OOM owing to overuse provoked by excessive playing. According to Planas (1982), the most famous patient who probably suffered from rupture of the OOM was the trumpet player Louis 'Satchmo' Armstrong (1901–1971). Consequently, this pathology was named 'Satchmo-Syndrome' (Planas 1982). Unfortunately, in the early 1980s, Planas had no ultrasound available—his investigations were made non-invasively by clinical observation and digital palpation, or invasively by surgical exposure of the OOM. He thus found ruptured labial muscle fibres. Today, (partial) ruptures of the OOM can be detected non-invasively by transverse ultrasonic B-mode images (Arcier and Vernay 1994; Llobet 2005).

Even if no severe pathology is found, most musicians are grateful for sono-morphological investigations of the OOM. Ultrasound is also useful for evaluating the position of the front teeth, which is highly important for musicians (Methfessel 1995; Clemente et al. 2021; Czech and Alt 2024).

3.11.3.4 Detection of Scars in the OOM

Sonography may detect all kinds of scars in the OOM—regardless of whether they result from overuse (Satchmo-Syndrome), trauma, tumour excision or cleft lip repair (Lefarth 2019; Lefarth and Angerstein 2013). Scars appear as discontinuities and hyper-echoic areas of the OOM (Fig. 3.20a), which are normally identified as a homogeneous hypoechoic line in transverse B-mode scans.

Post-operative scans of the lip may help to evaluate the healing process. The scar zone can be compared with unaffected parts of the OOM.

Another sonographic examination tool, which is still relatively new and therefore often not available in common ultrasound devices, is elastography. Elastography uses the measured contact pressure of the transducer and the tissue-specific echogenicity to enable conclusions about the elasticity of an examined tissue to be drawn; it emphasises the differences in elasticity by colour-coding. Similar to colour-duplex, the elasto-mode is visible as an overlay in common B-mode images. Thus, scars are highlighted in B-mode scans (Fig. 3.20b).

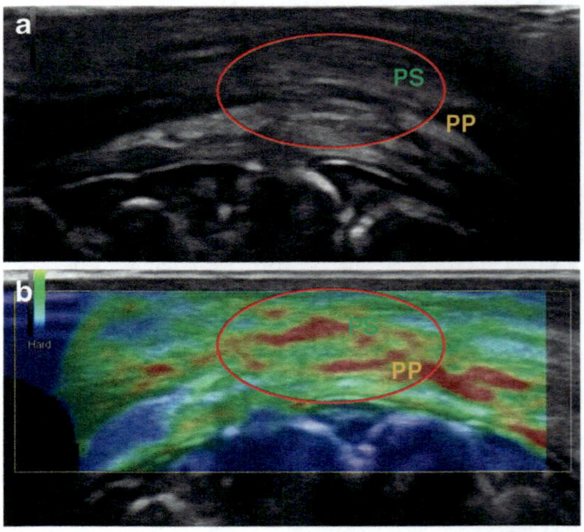

Fig. 3.20 Elastography of scars in the OOM. (**a**) Transverse B-mode-Image of the UL. The **scar** is marked by a **red circle** in the middle of the OOM. The peripheral part (**PP**) is disrupted after cleft lip surgery (m., 35 y.). In the superficial part (**PS**) muscle fibres and scar strands have similar echogenity and can hardly be distinguished in B-mode. (**b**) Transverse Image of the UL using the Elasto-mode. The scar region which was poorly visible in B-mode is highlighted in yellow-orange to red. (©Lefarth 2021)

3.11.3.5 Evaluation of Labial Muscle Training

Ultrasound examination gives the opportunity to assess the training status of the OOM by measuring the muscle thickness after facial exercises in (a) children with dental malocclusion (Kumar and Kuriakose 2004; Munshi et al. 2000; Prabhu and Munshi 1995; Rasheed and Munshi 1996) and (b) patients with facial palsy (Volk et al. 2014). Training effects of brass playing can also be documented sonographically by measuring the thickness of the OOM (Lefarth 2019).

3.12 Auditory-Perceptual Evaluation of Velopharyngeal Function

Igor Leuchter

3.12.1 General Aspects

As well as vocal fold pathologies, auditory-perceptual evaluation of voice quality and speech is one of the primary outcome measures of velopharyngeal insufficiency (VPI): most patients consult because of a perception (by themselves or their social circle) of changes in their voice and speech, and therapists (phoniatricians or speech therapists) judge the therapeutic results on the basis of an improvement in the sound of the voice (Leuchter 2015). Auditory-perceptual methods carry strong advantages: they are easy to use, economical and robust. However, it is also clear that these methods are susceptible to a variety of biases and subjectivity as with any human judgements (Kent 1996). In an extensive literature review of 57 articles dealing with the perceptual evaluation of voice quality, Kreiman et al. (1993) demonstrated that both intra-rater and inter-rater reliability fluctuated greatly from study to study.

The methodology used for the perceptual assessment of hypernasality in the literature differs with respect to the type of speech samples, the expertise of judges, and the grading scales used (Keuning et al. 2002). Major issues in acoustic-perceptual assessment are the choice of speech samples and the listener's jury. Concerning the speech samples, Sell (2005) insisted on the necessity to construct standardised samples for perceptual assessment. These samples should include words loaded with high-pressure consonants and non-nasal words, thus making them sensitive to resonance disorders (Kummer and Lee 1996). Kuehn and Moller (2000) state that conversational speech samples provide important information about articulation and resonance characteristics. However, standardised words or sentences allow evaluation of specific phonetic content and have the advantage of allowing a comparison between centres. In a review of 88 articles investigating the methodology for perceptual assessment in patients with cleft palate (CP), Lohmander and Olsson (2004) reported that only one type of speech sample was used in more than one-third of articles, the most common being spontaneous speech. Twenty percent of articles reported having used two different types of speech samples, the most frequent combination being single words and spontaneous speech. The text was used in four articles. Concerning the method of sentence elicitation, Keuning et al. (1999) found no difference when sentences were read or repeated. Repetition has the advantage of being usable in small children, and not interacting with literacy skills. Kuehn and Moller (2000) recommend the use of a standard reading passage for older patients. Sell (2005) recommends that each language should have a nationally agreed speech sample. In English, the usual standard text is the 'Rainbow' passage, a phonetically balanced passage where the ratios of the various phonemes reflect their ratios in English (Fairbanks 1960). The rainbow passage contains 35% of nasal phonemes. The 'Zoo' passage is devoid of nasal phonemes and broadly used in speech evaluation (Fletcher 1972).

The question of the most appropriate listener jury is a subject of debate. In the review published by Lohmander and Olsson (2004), one-third of articles reported only one listener; 23% reported more than four listeners. Most listeners (80%) were speech-language pathologists. Only 4% used exclusively other professionals or naive listeners. The argument to support the non-use of expert listeners is that the speech therapist may be too critical, while naive listeners may add real-life significance (Sell 2005). For this reason, several authors (Witt et al. 1996; Kuehn and Moller 2000) have recommended the inclusion of both professional and peer or lay judges in perceptual evaluation. Audio recordings are necessary to store and compare speech samples and to allow listener jury testing. It has been demonstrated that ratings for hypernasality made from audio recordings are consistent with clinical evaluation (Williams et al. 2024). Appropriate recording conditions are mandatory: a professional quality microphone, a sound-recording device that records frequencies between 60 and 10,000 Hz, minimal room noise, constant mouth-to-microphone distance and adjusted recording levels (Karnell 2011).

3.12.2 Resonance Evaluation

The evaluation of a patient with suspected VPI must begin with a global language evaluation, especially in children, and then continue with a specific speech and resonance evaluation. The perceptual assessment should first determine whether resonance is normal or not. Resonance problems can be qualified as hypernasality, hyponasality or mixed, depending on whether the transmission of acoustic energy in the vocal tract is affected. The literature dealing with speech evaluation in VPI is essentially in the field of CP repair.

The assessment of nasality, particularly *hypernasality*, is the key task and the most challenging aspect of the evaluation of VPI patients. The major controversy concerns the type of hypernasality rating scale used (Sweeney and Sell 2008). The Thurstone scale with an equal-appearing interval (EAI) method was originally developed as a means of measuring people's attitudes. EAI scales are very easy to use and intuitive, and thus is a widespread method for resonance assessment (Keuning et al. 2002, 2004). However, the validity of EAI for measuring phenomena such as voice or speech disorders has been questioned (Zraick and Liss 2000; Metz et al. 1992). The validity of a rating system depends on the psychological nature of the dimension to be scaled. Stevens (1975) has described two classes of dimensions to be scaled: metathetic and prothetic. Metathetic dimensions are considered qualitative and vary in terms of a change in quality. Pitch is an example of a metathetic stimulus. By contrast, prothetic dimensions are considered quantitative and thus vary in terms of a change in degree of magnitude. Loudness and hypernasality are examples of prothetic stimuli. Stevens (1975) also demonstrated that prothetic stimuli were not amenable to linear partition, such as EAI scaling. The reason behind this is that when a listener attempts to partition a prothetic stimulus (hypernasality) into equal intervals, there is a systematic bias to partition the lower end of the continuum into smaller intervals than the upper end. Therefore Zraick and Liss (2000) concluded that EAI scaling is not appropriate for the measurement of hypernasality, and suggested the use of direct magnitude estimation (DME) to measure nasal voice quality. In DME scaling, judges are asked to estimate the magnitude of a perceptual stimulus by assigning a number to it, in a Likert-like fashion. Brancamp et al. (2010) compared nasality grades in 39 subjects by using both EAI and DME with an instrumental measurement of nasality (nasometry), and observed no significant difference between scales.

The width of the grading scale remains controversial. Most authors use a 5-point scale for hypernasality (0 for normal, 1 for slight, 2 for mild, 3 for moderate and 4 for severe (Brunnegård et al. 2012; Watterson et al. 1993, 1996; Lewis et al. 2003; Vallino-Napoli and Montgomery 1997; John et al. 2006; Hirschberg and Van Demark 1997). Others report a 4- and a 6-point scale and define a clinically important nasality if rated greater than 2 on each scale (Dalston et al. 1993). Hardin et al. (1992) and Counihan and Cullinan (1970) use a 7-point scale. Sweeney and Sell (2008) report a 6-point scale, giving a more precise definition for each point scale (1 for mild, evident but acceptable; 2 for mild/moderate, evident on high vowels; 3 for moderate, evident on high and low vowels; 4 for moderate, evident on high and low vowels; 5 for moderate/severe, evident on all vowels and some consonants; and 6 for severe, evident on all vowels and most voiced consonants). A major limitation of any classification system, especially in large-ranging scales, is the difficulty of discriminating between intermediate ranges. This was demonstrated particularly in ranges of dysphonia scores. The French literature uses a specific grading system, the Borel-Maisonny classification, initially not developed specifically to describe resonance disorders types, but rather different groups of cleft patients according to their global functional results (Veau and Borel-Maisonny 1931). This classification includes three main grades (I for normal, II for hypernasality, III for compensatory articulation). For each grade, a sub-grade may be added, i.e. "B" for good intelligibility and "M" for bad intelligibility (Vernel-Bonneau and Thibault 1999).

Although many clinical assessments report rating scales for nasality, few have been rigorously evaluated for reliability and validity. On a 5-point scale, Sweeney and Sell (2008) reported good intra-rater reliability with 88% agreement and 0.7 kappa for rating nasality and a less good inter-rater reliability with 77% agreement and 0.4 kappa. Hayden and Klimacka (2000) evaluated a 4-point scale and reported good inter-rater correlations for experienced listeners, ranging from 88% to 97%. The fact that the hypernasality grading system seems to be resistant to consensus may be due to the variable nature of nasality. Many factors may influence the nasality judgements: speech stimulus, intelligibility, articulation errors, vocal intensity and quality (recorded or live), and judge training (Lewis et al. 2003).

In addition to hypernasality, which is perceived essentially on vowels, *nasal air emission* can be perceived during speech. Some authors have added this item to their grading system. Brunnegård et al. (2012) grade nasal air emission into 5 levels: 0 for normal, 1 for slight or mild but intermittent, 2 for mild but consistent, 3 for moderate, and 4 for severe. In the Temple Street Scale devised by Sweeney and Sell (2008) to describe nasality, nasal emission is graded as weak/strong, frequent/infrequent, consistent/inconsistent and phoneme-specific. Keuning et al. (2002, 2004) use a 100-mm visual analogue scale from normal to extremely deviant for nasal air emission. In the Cleft Audit Protocol for Speech, John et al. (2006) make a distinction between nasal emission and turbulence. They have also added a specific item for the presence or absence of *facial grimace* during speech, similar to that of other groups (Hirschberg and Van Demark 1997; Subtelny et al. 1972). Concerning *hyponasality*, most protocols (Sweeney and Sell 2008; John et al. 2006) report a 3-point scale for hyponasality (1 for evident, 2 for moderate, and 3 for severe). Hirschberg and Van Demark (1997) specify in their protocol the presence or absence of mixed resonance disorders (hyper- and hypo-nasality).

Interestingly, although it is known that high-pitch phonation may be a compensatory mechanism of phonation in VPI, only very rarely do authors add a pitch evaluation. Subtelny et al. (1972) propose a 5-point scale where 1 signifies much below optimum pitch level and 5 for much above.

3.12.3 Speech Evaluation

The investigator also evaluates speech production, including articulation and speech intelligibility. All *articulation errors* that are not age-appropriate are inventoried. These errors mainly concern consonants and may be classified as pre- and post-uvular according to the place of production errors (Henningsson et al. 2008). Among the post-uvular errors, pharyngeal or nasal fricatives and glottal stops have been described as the most common compensatory errors in VPI speakers. These misarticulations may impair the velopharyngeal movements (Henningsson and Isberg 1991a; Zajac 2015). Consequently, the resonance evaluations of speech samples containing glottal or pharyngeal articulations may be erroneously skewed. Several articulation tests have been developed containing all the phonemes and loaded with high-pressure consonants, thus making these sensitive to resonance disorders (Templin and Darley 1960; Morris et al. 1961). Other tests have included speech symptoms specific to VPI, such as compensatory articulation production, i.e. the Bzoch Error Pattern Diagnostic Articulation Test (Bzoch 1989), the Temple Street Scale (Sweeney and Sell 2008) and the Categorical System of Articulation Problems in Cleft Palate (Ainoda and Okazaki

1996). The Great Ormond Speech Assessment (Sell and Grunwell 1994) was developed as a comprehensive and standardised assessment for speech in UK cleft centres. More recently, the Scandinavian Scandcleft Group (Lohmander et al. 2009) and the Eurocleft Speech Group (Grunwell et al. 2000) have proposed an international and cross-linguistic assessment of speech assessment for CL and CP patients. Lohmander et al. (2009) concluded that speech assessment comparison is possible across different languages if the assessment concerns speech units that are phonetically similar across languages.

Intelligibility is a measure of how comprehensible speech is, or the degree to which speech can be understood, and thus is one of the primary goals of therapeutic intervention, especially in the field of CP repair. Intelligibility may be influenced by many factors, including the severity of the speech disorder (e.g. articulation errors, hypernasality) and the speech stimuli used, but also by many variables other than the speech characteristics under assessment, such as developmental speech and language immaturities, listening conditions and the listener's experience with the disorder under investigation (Whitehill 2002; Starr et al. 1984; Witt et al. 1996; Moller and Starr 1984). The difficulty in isolating intelligibility from other aspects of speech and methodological complications explains the disagreement in the literature, particularly in the cleft groups, regarding the necessity of evaluating intelligibility, and how it should be performed. Whitehill published an exhaustive review of the literature on intelligibility assessment in CP speakers. Fifty-seven articles were selected over a 40-year period. Only about half used a rating scale for intelligibility assessment, and most did not include a report of reliability. When assessed, intelligibility is usually rated by expert listeners by means of an EAI scale differing by their grading approach: 4- (Maegawa et al. 1998; Copeland 1990), 5- (Subtelny et al. 1972) or 7- (Forner 1983; Moore and Sommers 1975) -point scales or a 100-mm visual analogue scale (Keuning et al. 2004). The intelligibility 5-point scale described by John et al. (2006) in their multicentre Cleft Audit Protocol by contrast is based on the questioning of parents or the social circle: 0, normal; 1, different from other children's speech, but not enough to cause comment; 2, different enough to provoke comment, but possible to understand most speech; 3, only just intelligible to strangers; and 4, impossible to understand. Independently of the choice of the rating scale and the difficulty in isolating this feature of the speech from the others, intelligibility should be always assessed as an essential indicator of outcome.

3.12.4 Conclusion

VPI is a complex phenomenon with important repercussions on communication ability, identity, social representation and quality of life (Barr et al. 2007; Boseley and Hartnick 2004; Skirko et al. 2013). Its evaluation remains challenging: the heterogeneity of the aetiologies, the patient's condition and the environment led to a great variety of clinical manifestations. Therapists have the task of identifying all these clinical characteristics through a comprehensive and rigorous evaluation. Besides the instrumental evaluation (acoustic and aerodynamic), perceptual evaluation remains the central axis around which the individualised and appropriate treatment is proposed. Perceptual evaluation of VPI should always include a global language and a specific speech evaluation. Hypernasality, nasal air emission and turbulence, facial grimacing and intelligibility are parameters to be evaluated. The choice of rating scales is widely discussed in the literature and is specific to each centre.

3.13 Aerodynamic Evaluation of Velopharyngeal Function

Igor Leuchter

3.13.1 General Aspects

The phonatory process occurs when air is expelled from the lungs through the vocal folds, thus producing a sound. This airflow (and sound) is then modulated and redirected into the resonators, including the nasal cavity. Thus, the assessment of nasal airflow during speech is crucial. This evaluation may be perceptual, by an auditory-perceptual evaluation of nasal air emission during speech (see Sect. 3.12), or instrumental, acoustic (see Sect. 3.16) and aerodynamic. The oldest and certainly the most widespread instrumental aerodynamic assessment of VPI is the Glatzel mirror test described in 1910 (Foy 1910): a mirror is placed between the nose and the mouth and the patient is asked to pronounce oral phonemes, words or sentences. Nasal air emission is evaluated according to the presence of mist on the nasal surface of the mirror. This method of evaluation is qualitative; for a quantitative assessment more sophisticated instrumental devices are used. The two measures applicable in clinical practice are *airflow*, which records separate volumes of air flowing through the nose and mouth, and *airway pressure*.

3.13.2 Airflow Measurements

3.13.2.1 Nasal Airflow Measurement

This requires a heated pneumotachograph, which consists of a flowmeter and a differential pressure transducer. When airflow encounters a resistance, the resultant pressure drops linearly as the volume rate of airflow. The resistance is a wire-mesh screen heated to avoid condensation. During the production of oral sounds, nasal air emission usually denotes incompetence of velopharyngeal closure. Nasal airflow increases with VPI, but a number of confounding factors may influence the outcome, particularly nasal airway resistance and respiratory effort. For example, a VPI subject with a high nasal resistance and using a low respiratory effort will generate less nasal airflow. Nevertheless, previous findings have demonstrated a positive correlation between increased nasal air emission during the production of oral phonemes and insufficient closure of the velopharyngeal port (Warren et al. 1994). Furthermore, Laine et al. (1988) demonstrated a good correlation between nasal airflow rates (above 125 cc/s) and velopharyngeal orifice size, estimated by the pressure-flow technique (Warren and Dubois 1964) (see below). More recently, Dotevall et al. (2001) conducted a study on nasal airflow patterns in children with and without cleft palate (CP). They clearly demonstrated differences in the duration, declinations and rates of airflow. The same authors (Dotevall et al. 2002) studied the relationship between the perceptual evaluation of speech and nasal airflow in 14 children with CP and 15 controls. They found a strong association between the nasality rating (5-point EAI scale) and the nasal airflow rates with high sensitivity (1.0) and specificity (0.96). Rousteau et al. (1995) described an ingenious instrument, named an Aerophonoscope, composed of two heated pneumotachographs, oral and nasal, associated with a microphone, and allowing an objective measurement of both nasal and oral airflow while recording the voice. It can be used to assess nasal air loss during the production of oral phonemes and to observe the different characteristics of velopharyngeal closure during speech. In summary, nasal airflow assessment presents a number of advantages: it is easy to perform, even in small children, related to physiology, reliable and a good predictor of velopharyngeal function.

3.13.2.2 Air Pressure Measurements

Another aerodynamic measure used to evaluate the velopharyngeal function is the *pressure-flow technique* described by Warren and Dubois (1964). This inventive technique allows objective evaluation of the parameters related to velopharyngeal closure, i.e. nasal and oral pressure levels, the rate of nasal airflow and estimates of the velopharyngeal opening area (Dotevall et al. 1998). This method is derived from the theoretical hydraulic principle of Bernoulli and assumes that the area of an orifice can be determined if the differential pressures (in this case oral and nasal pressures) across the orifice (velopharyngeal opening area) are measured simultaneously with airflow through it (nasal airflow) (Warren and Dubois 1964). Practically, two pressure catheters are used, one placed in the mouth, and the other in one nostril. Nasal airflow is measured by a heated pneumotachograph connected to a tube placed in the other nostril.

The area of velopharyngeal opening is calculated from the Warren and Dubois equation

$$A = \frac{V}{\sqrt{2\frac{(P1 - P2)}{D}}}$$

where A = area of opening, V = nasal airflow, P_1 = oral pressure, P_2 n= asal pressure and D = density of air (0.001 g/cm^3). The subject is asked to produce a series of bilabial plosive consonants /p/. Velopharyngeal opening size calculation derived from aerodynamic measurement has been validated both in a bench model (Smith and Weinberg 1982; Guyette and Carpenter 1988), in normal subjects (Zajac 2000) and patients with VPI (Guyette et al. 1994; Lohmander-Agerskov et al. 1996).

Concerning the correlation between the perceptual evaluation and the aerodynamic measurement, the data are limited. Warren et al. (1994) evaluated the relationship between the perceptual judgment of hypernasality by using a 6-point scale and the aerodynamic measurement assessed by the pressure-flow technique in 124 subjects. The results indicated a significant but moderate correlation between hypernasality rating and the velopharyngeal area (0.66), nasal airflow (0.61), and nasal airflow duration (0.53).

3.13.3 Conclusion

Aerodynamic evaluation of velopharyngeal function brings precious information about the physiological events occurring in the velopharyngeal port during speech and should be part of any VPI evaluation. The different instrumental assessments (acoustic vs aerodynamic) or perceptual judgement are not equivalent, but rather complementary. They all allow an appreciation of the same phenomenon through different perspectives. Ultimately, every instrumental score should always be interpreted cautiously in the light of the clinical expertise but not as a substitute for the perceptual rating (Leuchter 2015).

3.14 Fibre-Optic Evaluation of Velopharyngeal Function

Alexander Hemprich

3.14.1 Introduction

In the case of a suspected velopharyngeal insufficiency, it is of utmost importance to determine the underlying cause of the pathology. A thorough clinical examination has to be performed first, in order to detect structural or functional deficiencies in the velopharyngeal closure. There may be neurological, inborn or acquired anatomical problems such as a cleft palate or the sequelae of some kind of trauma or tumour surgery.

In cleft patients, the results of the reconstructive (palatal) reconstruction have to be evaluated by the surgeon together with an experienced well-trained speech pathologist. If the routine examination detects some persisting speech problems (open rhinophonia or even a rhinolalia) without severe anatomical problems up to the third year of life, usually special speech training should be instigated. If this proves not to be successful after several repeated therapy sessions, other methods for an objective assessment of the patient's speech should be undertaken; first of all, nasometry (the least invasive method) (Dalston et al. 1991) and nasopharyngoscopy.

In the 1980s video-(cine-) fluoroscopy was highly valued since it provided much real-time information on the velopharyngeal closure mechanism. Bearing in mind the relatively high radiation exposure of very young patients, this method can no longer be justified; especially since cine-MRI has become available for clinical use since the 2010s (Raol et al. 2015) and has proven its usefulness in difficult cases of submucous clefts (Schenck et al. 2021).

3.14.2 Nasopharyngoscopy

This method was introduced by Pigott (1969) for the postoperative evaluation of a velopharyngeal flap, then still using a rigid endoscope. This instrument guaranteed high-resolution pictures but could not always be guided to the desired position and caused pain to the patients in many cases.

As early as 1975 Sommerlad was so enthusiastic about this new tool that he declared:

> Pharyngoplasty without prior pharyngoscopy is similar to an operation on the bladder without cystoscopy
> —Sommerlad et al. (1975)

In the 1980s, several research groups switched to small flexible endoscopes which made it possible to examine children beginning from age 5 without any kind of anaesthesia. Since then, nasopharyngoscopy has contributed markedly to the understanding of the anatomy and physiology of the velopharyngeal sphincter (Shprintzen et al. 1979; Karnell et al. 1983).

Nevertheless, some problems still remain:

1. Even in children *a minimum diameter of the scope* is necessary to obtain a good overview of the velopharyngeal sphincter. 3.5 mm straightforward flexible optic systems have proven to be sufficient in the author's own hands (Hemprich et al. 1984).

   They have the advantage of being accepted by children from 5–6 years of age (only two out of 168 consecutively examined patients refused the endoscopy, but they were somewhat mentally handicapped). The disadvantage of such a small system is the lack of a suction canal.

   This can usually be solved by giving decongesting nose drops 5 minutes before the examination. In older children, larger endoscopes with suction canals can be used.
2. *The image on the screen is 2-dimensional.* Thus, the examiner has to move the optic system forwards-downwards and back in order to be able to evaluate the movements of the velum and pharyngeal walls under function (swallowing, speech) as a 3D unit. There is a certain learning curve but experience will come soon.

   Cine MRI is a wonderful solution for this problem but is still very costly so far and more difficult to handle with the patients. Thus, it has not come to routine use in cleft clinics.

3.14.3 Endoscopic Findings and Therapeutic Consequences

The main purpose of nasopharyngoscopy is the distinction between anatomical disorders after veloplasty and persisting functional problems. The correct form of treatment cannot be derived from clinical findings alone in many cases but should finally be based on the results of nasoendoscopy.

Even a velar closure with a seemingly long soft palate can prove to be unsuccessful owing to inactive muscles so a gap in the velopharyngeal valve remains. This problem may probably be solved by a consequent speech training/muscle activation. A speech-improving procedure is not indicated here in the first place.

On the other hand, a very mobile velum may not be able to reach the dorsal pharyngeal wall. The muscles can be very well united but the velum is just too short. This is a classical indication for a re-veloplasty or some kind of velopharyngoplasty. Speech training would very soon become frustrating for the patient and the speech pathologist in these cases.

Croft et al. (1981) identified four main patterns of velopharyngeal valving 'coronal', 'sagittal', 'circular', and 'circular with Passavant's ridge', which have distinct importance for speech-improving surgery. Interestingly enough, however, none of these can only be found in cleft cases but also in unaffected persons.

The most common pattern is the *coronal* (about 47%) where the closure is achieved mainly by the movement of the velum and some support from the dorsal pharyngeal wall (Fig. 3.21a, b).

A favourable closure for cleft patients is the *sagittal* (16%), mainly achieved by the lateral pharyngeal walls, since the possibly problematic movement of the velum is of lesser importance (Fig. 3.22).

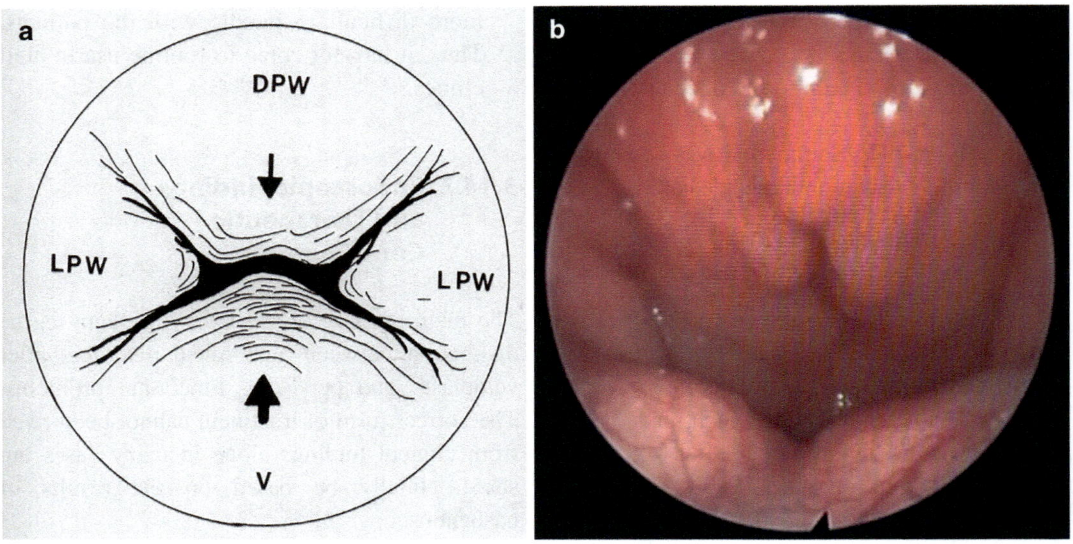

Fig. 3.21 (**a**) Coronal velopharyngeal closure (schematic drawing: V = velum, LPW = lateral pharyngeal wall, DPW = dorsal pharyngeal wall). (With generous permission of Dr. Almut Hemprich) (**b**) Coronal velopharyngeal closure with a central groove in the velum (clinical endoscopic view). (With permission of Professor Siegmar Reinert, Department of Oral and Maxillofacial Surgery, Tübingen, Germany)

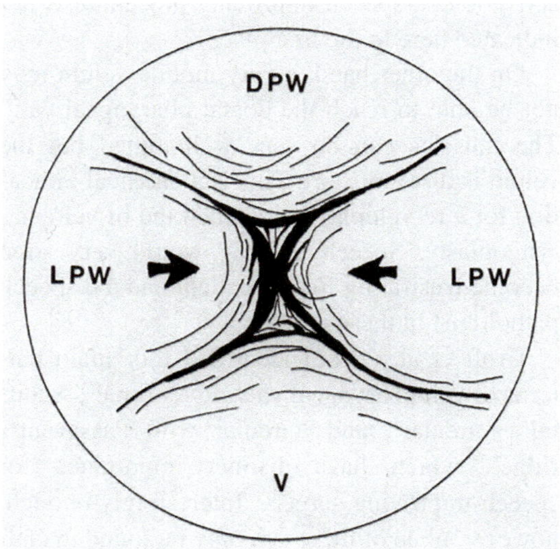

Fig. 3.22 Sagittal velopharyngeal closure (schematic drawing: V = velum, LPW = lateral pharyngeal wall, DPW = dorsal pharyngeal wall). (With generous permission of Dr. Almut Hemprich)

In 22% there is a *circular* closure of the velopharyngeal valve by almost all surrounding structures alike (Fig. 3.23a, b).

Finally, 14% of all cleft patients show a prominent Passavant's ridge in addition to the circular valving (Fig. 3.24).

When the individual velopharyngeal closure of the patient is known to the phoniatrician, the right form of speech training can be prescribed.

Finally, endoscopy is able to reveal the place and size of the leak in the velopharyngeal valve. If it is situated in the middle there is a very good chance for a successful velopharyngoplasty, the width of which can be adjusted to the endoscopic finding ('tailor made flap') (Fig. 3.25a, b) (Shprintzen et al. 1979).

The results can be verified about 3–6 months postoperatively when the shrinking process of the flap has come to an end (Fig. 3.26a, b).

An unfavourable closure pattern is a narrow velum that just reaches the dorsal pharyngeal wall but leaves wide lateral openings (Fig. 3.27). There is no form of speech-improving surgery that can completely solve this problem.

3.14.4 Conclusion

Fibre-optic evaluation of velopharyngeal function plays an important role for all medical specialties that deal with speech problems due to difficulties in the velopharyngeal closure, no

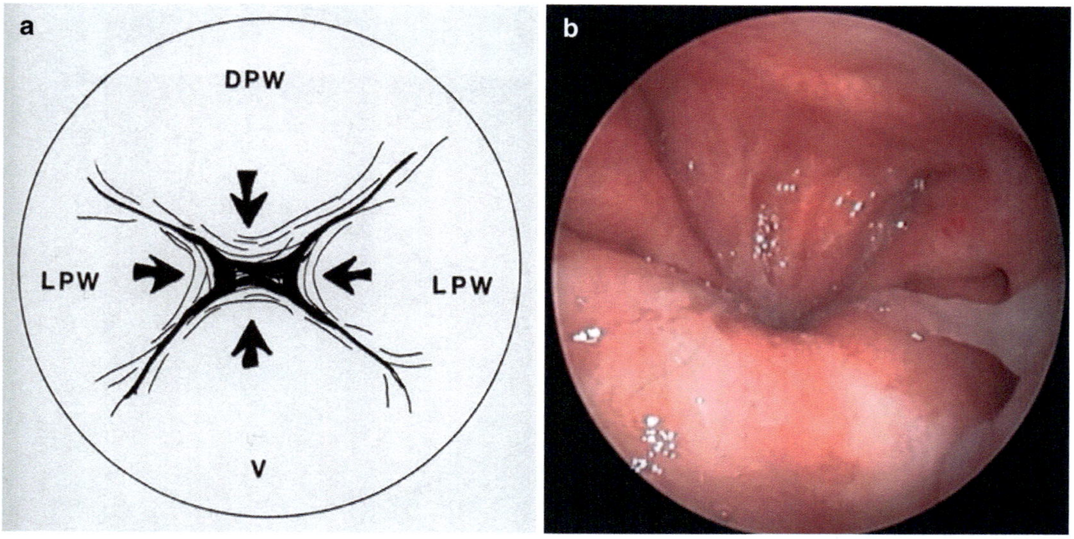

Fig. 3.23 (**a**) Circular velopharyngeal closure (schematic drawing: V = velum, LPW = lateral pharyngeal wall, DPW = dorsal pharyngeal wall). (With generous permission of Dr. Almut Hemprich) (**b**) Circular velopharyngeal closure (endoscopic view). (With permission of Professor Siegmar Reinert, Department of Oral and Maxillofacial Surgery, Tübingen, Germany)

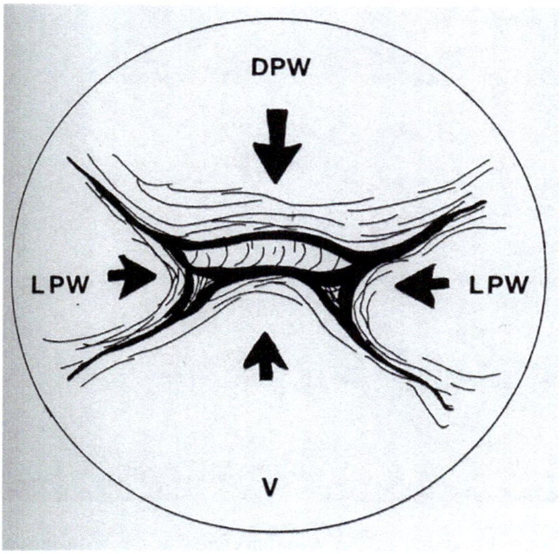

Fig. 3.24 Circular velopharyngeal closure with Passavant's ridge (schematic drawing: V = velum, LPW = lateral pharyngeal wall, DPW = dorsal pharyngeal wall). (With generous permission of Dr. Almut Hemprich)

matter whether they are inborn or acquired later. It will support the clinical findings and contribute very much to the choice of the right form of therapy, especially in borderline cases. The equipment is available in most cleft centres and phoniatric units, and the handling can be learned rather quickly. Thus, it will probably keep its importance in the future even though cine-MRI may play a greater role for special scientific questions.

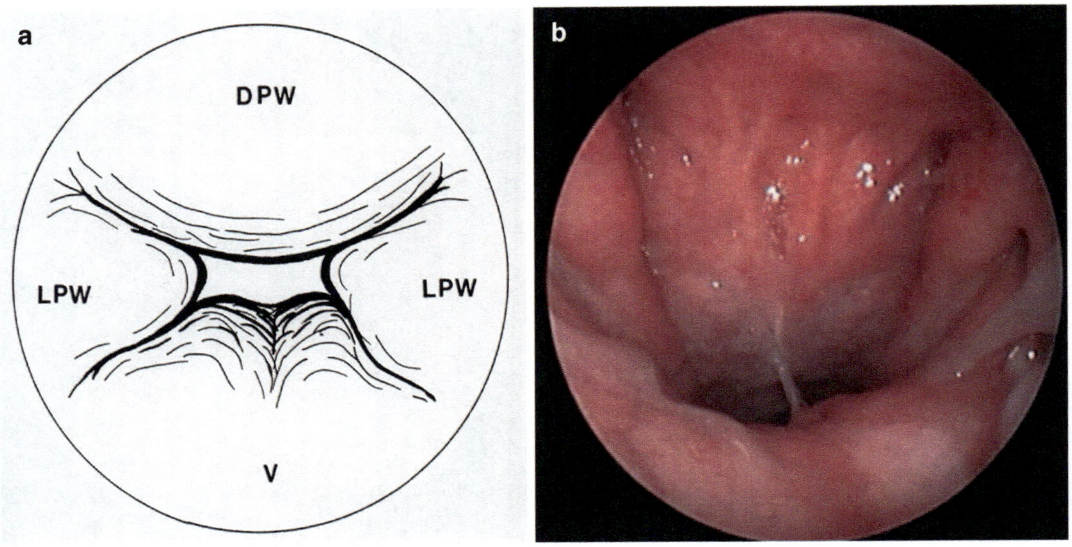

Fig. 3.25 (**a**) Central opening in the velopharyngeal valve (schematic drawing: V = velum, LPW = lateral pharyngeal wall, DPW = dorsal pharyngeal wall). (With generous permission of Dr. Almut Hemprich) (**b**) Central opening in the velopharyngeal valve under function (clinical endoscopic view). (With permission of Professor Siegmar Reinert, Department of Oral and Maxillofacial Surgery, Tübingen, Germany)

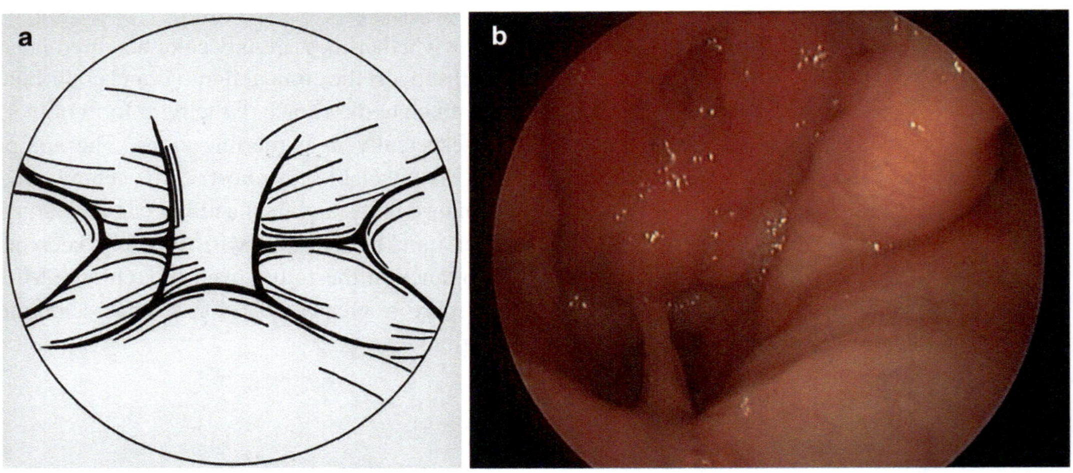

Fig. 3.26 (**a**) Velopharyngeal flap covering the central opening in the velopharyngeal valve (schematic drawing: V = velum, LPW = lateral pharyngeal wall, DPW = dorsal pharyngeal wall). (With generous permission of Dr. Almut Hemprich) (**b**) Narrow velopharyngeal flap covering the central opening in the velopharyngeal valve with movement of the lateral and pharyngeal walls towards the velopharyngeal flap (clinical endoscopic view). (With permission of Professor Siegmar Reinert, Department of Oral and Maxillofacial Surgery, Tübingen, Germany)

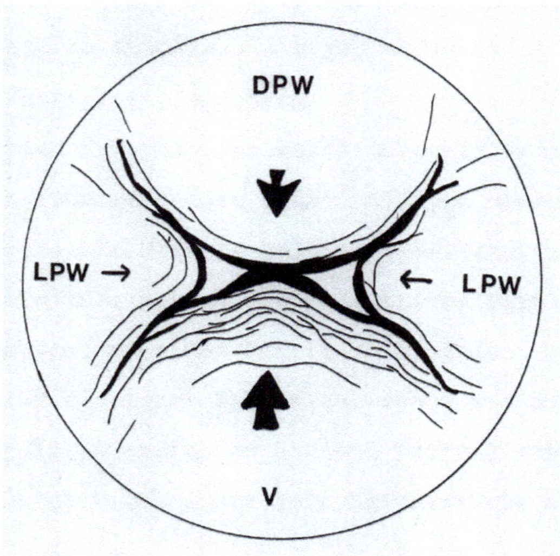

Fig. 3.27 Lateral openings in the velopharyngeal valve (schematic drawing: V = velum, LPW = lateral pharyngeal wall, DPW = dorsal pharyngeal wall). (With generous permission of Dr. Almut Hemprich)

3.15 Classification of Cleft (Lip and) Palate

Alexander Hemprich and Ute Pröschel

3.15.1 Introduction

The classification of cleft (lip and) palate is necessary to describe and categorise the phenotypes of this malformation in order to compare the various forms of clefts, the results of surgery and the functional outcome according to the measures taken.

During the last 100 years, many classifications have been suggested. Some of them are described briefly below to portray the historical development of the different systems up to the present-day ICD classification of the WHO (ICD-10-GM 2020).

3.15.2 From Anatomically to Embryologically Based Systems

As early as 1922, at the meeting of the American Medical Association in St. Louis, Davis and Ritchie suggested abandoning the old (derogatory) zoomorphism 'harelip' and replacing it with the term 'congenital cleft of the lip'. Moreover, they proposed a three-group classification of clefts, based on the alveolar process as a dividing line for their categories:

- Group I: Pre-alveolar process clefts (clefts affecting the lip).
- Group II: Post-alveolar process clefts (clefts affecting the palate).
  - Soft palate.
  - Hard palate.
- Group III: Alveolar process cleft (any cleft involving the alveolar process).

Whenever the alveolar process is involved in overlapping cases; however, the cleft should be categorised as group III.

> Blair criticised this system as being not detailed enough and based on 'contemporary surgical perspectives (that were subject to change) rather than on anatomy alone (which is immutable)'.
>
> —Personal Communication documented in Davis and Ritchie (1922) and cited in Allori et al. (2017)

In his great book 'Division Palatine' Veau, together with Mme Borel (1931), describes a large number of different anatomical findings in about 1000 cases but finally proposes a minimalistic classification on a morphological basis with good clinical relevance. Palatal clefts are divided into four morphological categories:

I. Clefts of the soft palate.
II. Clefts of the soft and hard palate, up to the incisive foramen.
III. Clefts of the soft and hard palate extending unilaterally through the alveolus.
IV. Clefts of the soft and hard palate extending bilaterally through the alveolus (Fig. 3.28).

Stark and Kernahan introduced their classification in 1958, using an embryological approach for their system: the primary and the secondary palate. The primary palate includes a small area of the hard palate anterior to the foramen incisivum, the alveolus and the lip. The secondary palate consists of the hard palate dorsal to the

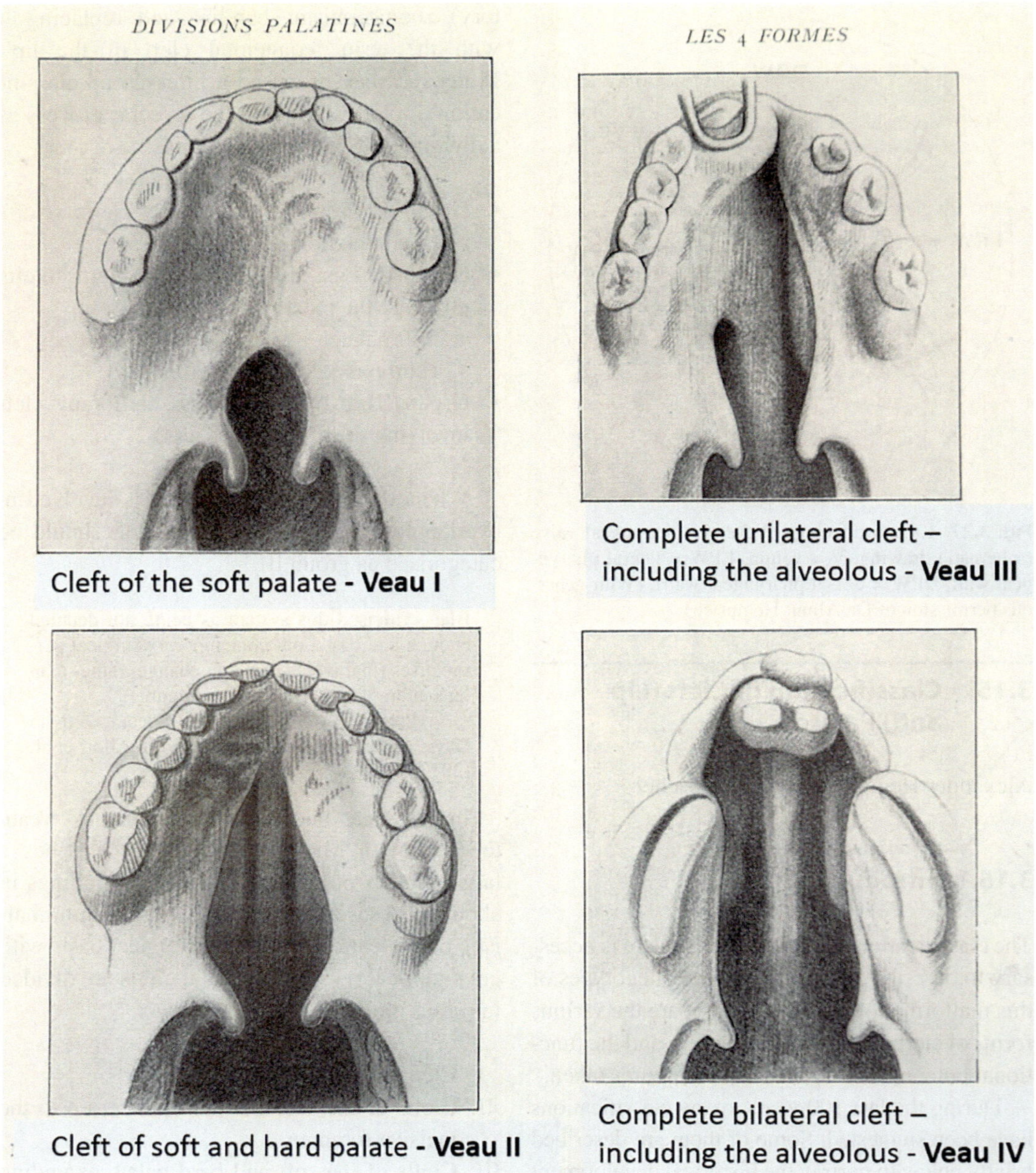

Fig. 3.28 Veau's classification (Veau and Borel 1931)

foramen incisivum and the soft palate. Kernahan and Stark (1958) stated that either the primary palate or the secondary palate, or both, could be affected by the cleft. Their classification resulted in the striped Y-logo (Fig. 3.29).

Areas 1 and 4 represent the lip; areas 2 and 5, the alveolus; areas 3 and 6, the hard palate between the alveolus and the incisive foramen; areas 7 and 8, the hard palate (posterior to the foramen incisivum) and areas 9 the soft palate.

The classification of Davis and Ritchie (1922) only acknowledges two major groups, which are then subdivided on the extent of the cleft. Group 1 consists of cleft lips (unilateral, median or bilateral). Group 2 includes all clefts dorsal of the

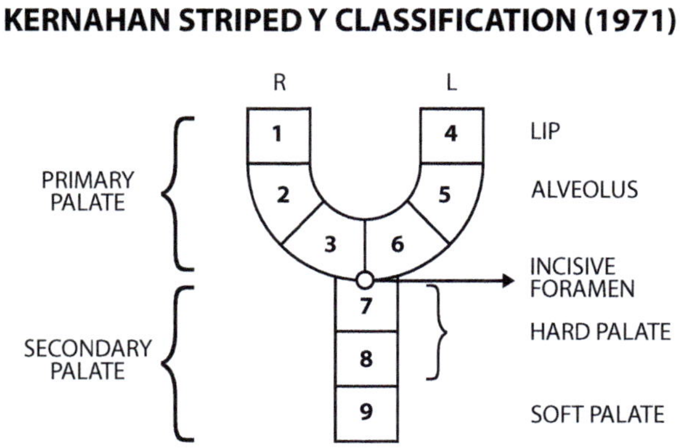

Fig. 3.29 The striped Y-logo. (Modified from Kernahan (1971))

alveolus: soft palate, soft and hard palate and submucous clefts.

3.15.3 Cleft Congress in Rome 1967

In order to be able to record all forms of clefts of lip, alveolus and palate in the daily routine, Kriens and Koch at the Cleft Palate Congress in Rome 1967 suggested an alphanumeric classification for the affected areas with the relevant abbreviations: L, lip; A, alveolus; H, hard palate; and S, soft palate) (Subcommittee, Rome 1967).

Since the lip, alveolus and hard palate may be affected unilaterally or bilaterally, but the soft palate only medially, the complete classification results in LAHSHAL (naming the structures from right to left when looking at the patient (Fig. 3.30). Additionally, the authors classified the grade of the cleft by using numbers from 1–3: 1, minor form; 2, incomplete cleft; 3, complete cleft. A second digit stands for 1, submucous (covered) clefts; 2, partially open; and 3, open clefts (Koch et al. 1995). This allows accurate, comparable computer-based documentation of the type and grade of any form of cleft (Subcommittee, Rome 1967).

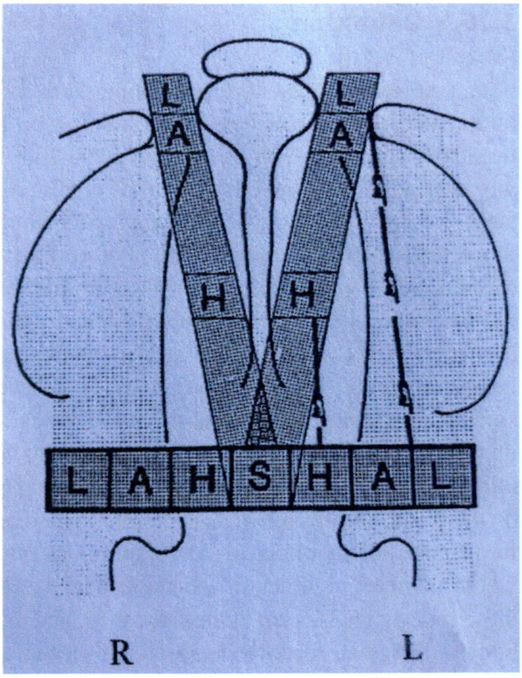

Fig. 3.30 LAHSHAL code. (Republished with permission of Georg Thieme Verlag KG, Stuttgart, from Kriens (1989) LAHSHAL—a concise documentation system for cleft lip, alveolus and palate diagnoses. In: Kriens O (ed) What is a cleft lip and palate? A multidisciplinary update. Workshop, Bremen 1987; permission conveyed through Copyright Clearance Center, Inc.)

Later Kriens (1989) suggested a simpler modification using upper case letters to describe complete forms of a cleft, lower case letters for incomplete forms and an asterisk (*) to represent microforms (e.g. LAHS-l for a complete unilateral cleft on the right side with an incomplete cleft lip on the left). This classification was finally adopted, but using only LAHSHAL, by the World Health Organization (WHO) in their classification of diseases (ICD-10-GM 2020). It has become the basis for the 'Minimal Documentation System of Clefts of Lip, Alveolus and Palate' by the German Cleft Palate Craniofacial Association in 2002 (Nolting et al. 2002).

In Anglo-American publications, however, the less precise abbreviations UCLP and BCLP (uni- or bi-lateral cleft palate) are still widely used. The alveolus is not named since it may be looked upon as part of the primary palate.

3.16 Spectral Speech Analysis of Hypernasality

Tim Bressmann and Fatemeh Abnavi

3.16.1 Definition

Sound waves propagate through compression and rarefaction of air molecules. When a string on a musical instrument such as a guitar is struck, it vibrates and produces audible sound by displacing air molecules. The string vibrates at a fundamental frequency, which we hear as the pitch of the musical note that is played. However, the vibration of the string is not uniform along its length: the excursion of the centre of the string will be the largest while the vibrations towards the ends have smaller amplitudes. This means that the surrounding air molecules will be excited at different amplitudes and frequencies of vibration along the length of the string. Acoustically, this results in partial frequencies or harmonics. The harmonics are whole number multiples of the fundamental. All these sound signals occur at the same time, and the body of the guitar serves to amplify and shape the sound (resonance). The whole adds up to a complex sound wave that radiates from the instrument (Behrman 2007; Hixon et al. 2008).

First described by Joseph Fourier (1808), spectral analysis decomposes complex patterns such as sounds into a set of sinusoidal waves. These represent the fundamentals and harmonics, so it becomes possible to understand the frequency components that make up a signal. Going back to the example of the guitar string in the paragraph above, the listener perceives the musical pitch (the fundamental) but also the instrument's timbre (the harmonics and resonance) from the complex sound wave. When spectral analysis is applied to speech signals, it describes the distribution of energy over different frequency ranges and over time, which helps in the identification of acoustic features that correspond to the auditory perception of speech (Behrman 2007; Hixon et al. 2008).

The sound spectrograph (sometimes also called sonagraph) divides the acoustic signal into short segments of equal length (time windows). The width of the spectral bands must also be set. The spectrogram (or sonagram) is then calculated on the basis of a Fast Fourier Transform algorithm. Time window and frequency bandwidth function as complementary variables according to the uncertainty principle described by Werner Heisenberg (1927). This means that an increase in time measurement accuracy requires a tradeoff in frequency resolution, and vice versa. If abrupt spectral events over time are of interest, a wide-band spectrogram with high temporal resolution is preferable (Fig. 3.31).

To show the harmonic content of a signal that has less variation over time, such as a sustained vowel, a narrow-band spectrogram has a better frequency resolution (Fig. 3.32).

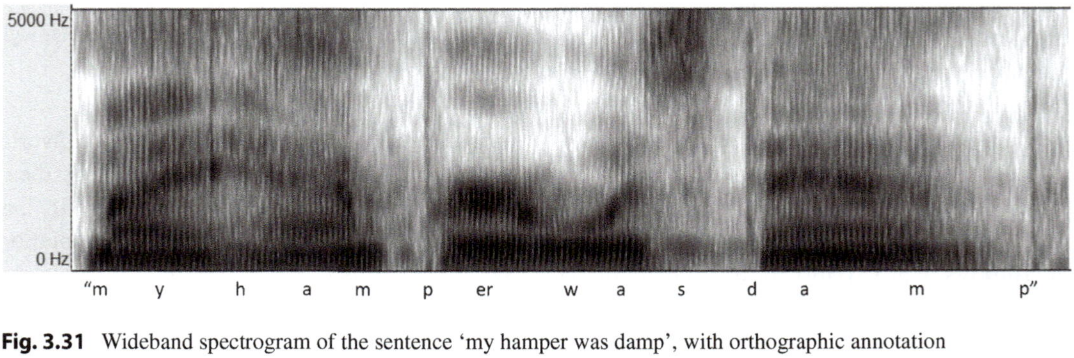

Fig. 3.31 Wideband spectrogram of the sentence 'my hamper was damp', with orthographic annotation

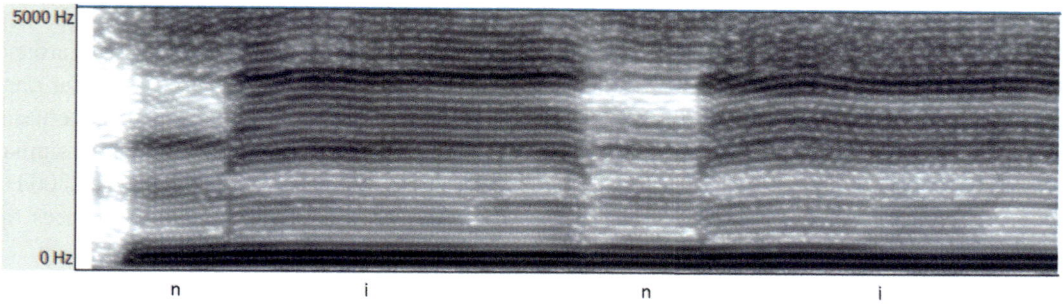

Fig. 3.32 Narrowband spectrogram of 'nee nee'. Note the improved visibility of the harmonic frequencies compared with the wideband spectrogram in Fig. 3.31

The spectrograms in Figs. 3.31 and 3.32 show time along the horizontal axis, frequency along the vertical axis, and higher intensity as darker grey-scale shading. Another way of displaying spectrographic information without the time dimension is to calculate the average energy in different energy bands and display them in a long-term average spectrogram (Fig. 3.33).

Finally, it can sometimes be difficult to find the energy maxima for vowels (formants) in a spectrogram. Linear predictive coefficients serve to smooth the spectrogram peaks and valleys, which facilitates the visual identification and statistical analysis of vowel formants (Behrman 2007).

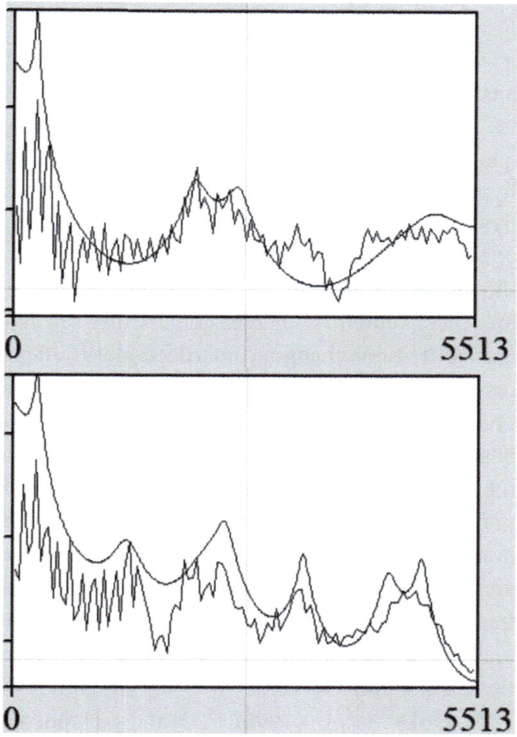

Fig. 3.33 Long-term average spectra (jagged line) and linear predictive coefficients (smooth line) of typical (top) and nasalised /i/ (bottom)

3.16.2 Spectrographic Features of Nasality

Typical nasal consonant sounds are produced with a lowered velum and an occlusion in the oral cavity, such as bilabial closure for /m/ or linguoalveolar contact for /n/. As a result, sound and airflow are redirected through the nasal passages. Once a threshold of velopharyngeal opening is surpassed, listeners start perceiving the sound as nasal or nasalized (Story and Bunton 2023). The nasal cavities are relatively large and have a complex anatomy. Intranasal structures, such as the nasal turbinates, and acoustic blind pouches, such as the paranasal sinuses, serve to divert and attenuate the sound energy travelling through the nasal passages, much like the exhaust muffler on a car reduces the engine noise coming from the tailpipe (Hixon et al. 2008). In adults, the spectral energy maxima of nasal sounds have been described as 250–300 Hz and 800–1000 Hz (Stevens 1985, 1997). These low-frequency energy peaks are also known as the nasal murmur. The harmonic frequencies above this murmur drop off relatively steeply, and the resulting energy minima are referred to as anti-resonances. For /m/ and /n/, Johnson (2012) described the anti-resonances centred around 750 Hz and 1400 Hz.

When a vowel is nasalised, the oral cavity has lower flow resistance than the nasal cavity, so the latter functions as a side-branch resonator. Depending on the vowel, the nasalisation may show in the spectrogram as a first formant peak with a wider bandwidth and lower amplitude or, in the case of a high vowel such as /i/, as an extra resonance between the first and second vowel formants (Chen 1997).

3.16.3 Spectrographic Analysis of Hypernasal Speech

From the above information about the effects of nasality on the spectrogram, one might expect it to be reasonably straightforward to develop quantitative acoustic indicators of pathological hypernasality in speakers with velopharyngeal dysfunction related to cleft palate as well as other conditions. However, the acoustic correlates of the auditory-perceptual impression of nasality are inconveniently inconsistent. Curtis (1970) argued that the changing interdependence of the resonating cavities in the vocal tract during the production of different speech sounds caused nasalisation to have variable acoustic effects on the spectrum. He concluded that while listeners may perceive hypernasality as a constant phenomenon in a speaker, this should not be taken as an indication of physical constancy in the vocal tract. The following paragraphs provide an overview of selected attempts to assess hypernasality from the sound spectrum.

Kataoka et al. (1996, 2001) used spectrographic analysis with one-third-octave bands to identify frequency bands that corresponded to perceived characteristics of hypernasality. These bands were spaced so that for every three spectral bands, the frequency doubled (a musical octave), which aligns well with the way humans perceive pitch. Graphic equalisers on music equipment or in audio software typically use this spacing of frequency bands. Kataoka et al. (2001) analysed the sustained vowel [i], produced by typical speakers and hypernasal children with cleft palate. The children with moderate to severe hypernasality had nasal extra-resonances between F1 and F2 (in the bands 1000 Hz and 1600 Hz) and anti-resonances in the region of F2 (around 2500 Hz). Lee et al. (2003) used a similar one-third-octave analysis on adults with hypernasal speech of varying aetiologies and found a similar pattern of extra-resonances at the 630 Hz, 800 Hz and 1000 Hz bands and anti-resonances at 2500 Hz.

At this point, the reader may have noted that the studies summarised above all identified slightly different frequency bands as indicative of nasality. In general, nasality results in increased spectral energy in low-frequency bands and decreased energy in the higher bands. Rather than trying to pinpoint specific frequencies, which may vary between participants and speech stimuli, some researchers suggested simply splitting the spectrum into low and high-frequency components. Lee et al. (2009) used a 'voice low tone to high tone ratio' for hypernasality detection in six sustained vowels produced by hypernasal patients. The authors experimented with various split points for a power spectrum from 65 to 8000 Hz and found that the frequency range of 600 to 800 Hz gave the best results for all vowels.

Apart from a pronounced nasal murmur in the sound frequency distribution, hypernasal speech is also characterised by the speaker's inability to differentiate oral and nasal speech sounds sufficiently. Phoniatricians and speech-language pathologists sometimes use the i-a or cul-de-sac test (Gutzmann 1913) to confirm an auditory-perceptual impression of hypernasality. The patient repeats the vowels /i/ and /a/ while blocking and unblocking the nares with their fingers. In a speaker with good velopharyngeal function, the sound of the blocked and unblocked nose will not be different. A hypernasal speaker will demonstrate a noticeable muffled cul-de-sac quality on /i/ when the nose is blocked. Haapanen et al. (1996) took advantage of the cul-de-sac test to identify changes in individual speakers' spectra as they produced /i/, /a/ and /u/ vowels with plugged and unplugged noses. The authors used pattern recognition with a self-organising neural network to differentiate the sustained /i/ and /u/ vowels of six hypernasal and nine typical speakers.

The above studies all used sustained vowels to facilitate the spectral analysis. In contrast, Golabbakhsh et al. (2017) used support vector analysis to classify hypernasal speakers automatically, on the basis of a combination of different acoustic measures that were extracted from connected speech samples. The authors used different combinations of spectral measures (cepstral coefficients in Mel, bionic wavelet transform measures) as well as voice stability measures (jitter, shimmer) to optimise the classification algorithm up to an accuracy of 85%.

Most available research has focused on hypernasality, and less is known about the acoustic characteristics of hyponasality (Lee et al. 2005). De Boer & Bressmann (2015) argued that hyper- and hypo-nasality can occur in the same patient (e.g. a patient with unilateral cleft lip and palate who has velopharyngeal dysfunction as well as a septum deviation) and that these features need to be assessed together. In de Boer and Bressmann (2016) typical speakers simulated hyper-, hypo- and mixed-nasality in connected speech, and the authors used linear discriminant analysis to distinguish the long-term average spectra of the simulations, on a selection of frequency bands.

3.16.4 Discussion

In recent decades, research about the spectrographic classification of hypernasality has often yielded interesting and promising results. However, while some of the methods described in this section have been used in subsequent research projects (Yoshida et al. 2000; Ferreira et al. 2020), it is unclear if any of them have found their way into routine clinical practice. Fifty years after Curtis's (1970) review of the literature available at his time, we have not moved very far past his conclusions that inter-individual differences in vocal tract morphology, acoustic interactions of vocal tract settings for different sounds, and inadequate signal resolution of spectrography all contribute to the variability of acoustic measures of hypernasality.

> An adequate theoretical model for vocal resonance gives little reason to predict that nasalization will lead to invariant changes in the acoustic spectra of speech. On the contrary, the spectral changes which are to be expected will depend very considerably on what is happening in other portions of the vocal cavity system. If one accepts this conclusion, the apparent inconsistency and lack of invariance in the data concerning the acoustic effects of nasalization are not mystifying (Curtis 1970, p. 392).

Nevertheless, the research summarised here offers a few different perspectives for increasing the robustness of spectrographic measures of nasality in future research, such as the ideas to compare patients with themselves on different tasks (Haapanen et al. 1996), to assess aspects of hyper- and hypo-nasality simultaneously (de Boer and Bressmann, 2016) and to use pattern recognition and automatic classification to develop multi-dimensional diagnostic algorithms (Golabbakhsh et al. 2017; Haapanen et al. 1996).

3.17 Acoustic Evaluation of Velopharyngeal Function

Philippe H. Dejonckere and Igor Leuchter

3.17.1 Pathophysiological Background of Acoustic Evaluation of Velopharyngeal Function: Principle of Nasometry

During speech or singing, the passage connecting the oral pharynx with the nasal pharynx needs to be frequently opened and closed, depending on the specific speech sounds to be produced. This is mainly accomplished by lowering and raising, respectively, the soft palate. This velopharyngeal passage is open when producing nasal consonants (such as /m/ or /n/), and is generally closed when producing consonants that require a pressure build-up in the oral cavity, as for occlusives (such as /p/ and /b/) and fricatives (as /s/ and /z/). During the production of vowels and sonorant consonants (such as /l/ or /r/ in English), the oro-nasal passage must be closed or almost closed for a clear sound to be produced, though in some languages there are nasal vowels (such as /ɑ̃/, /ɛ̃/, /œ̃/, /ɔ̃/) requiring an appreciable oronasal opening for proper pronunciation.

Disorders such as a cleft palate, severe prelingual hearing loss and some neurological and developmental disorders may cause velopharyngeal insufficiency (VPI), giving rise to an abnormal, hypernasalised voice. The assessment of hypernasality is the key task and most challenging aspect of the evaluation of VPI patients. As with voice disorders, auditory-perceptual assessment is essential (see Sect. 3.12). However, perceptual assessment has its limitations and may be a source of error, e.g. the expertise of the listeners, confounding effects such as misarticulations, or delayed language development (Keuning et al. 2002). It has therefore been necessary to develop objective tools for velopharyngeal function assessment, by aerodynamic (see Sect. 3.13) and acoustic measurements (e.g. Nasometry).

Practically, the nasometer is a combination of headgear, computer and analysing software. During speech, the nasal and oral sound productions are measured by two transducers (microphones) separated by a horizontal plate at the level of the upper lip of the subject (Fig. 3.34).

The nasalance score represents the nasal proportion of the total sound energy (after filtering). The procedure is easy and non-invasive, and provides—when applied accurately—objective and reproducible data. Furthermore, the method has a pathophysiological basis.

3.17.2 Nasalance Measurements

Fletcher and Bishop (1970) developed the first commercially available instrumentation for automatic derivation of the ratio of nasal to oral sound pressure: the TONAR ('The Oral Nasal Acoustic Ratio'). The term nasalance was proposed for the first time by Fletcher and Frost (1974) for an acoustic measure of velopharyngeal closure during voiced speech in which nasally emitted acoustic energy is compared with the orally emitted energy (both after filtering). Horii (1980) proposed an accelerometric approach. Later, Kay Elemetrics Corp. marketed the Nasometer™, which has become particularly popular among speech clinicians. Currently, more systems are available (e.g. NasalView® by Tiger DRS Inc.) (Fig. 3.35).

Other devices or systems, based on the same principle and with applications for specific languages, are in development (e.g. Kiliç 2019). An example is illustrated in Fig. 3.36.

3.17.3 Speech Material and Normative Values

Nasalance is influenced by the speaker's native language and may be affected by regional dialects (Baken and Orlikoff 2000; Mishima et al. 2008; Putnam Rochet et al. 1998) since the proportion of nasal and non-nasal sounds in each differs: the 'Rainbow passage' is phonetically balanced to

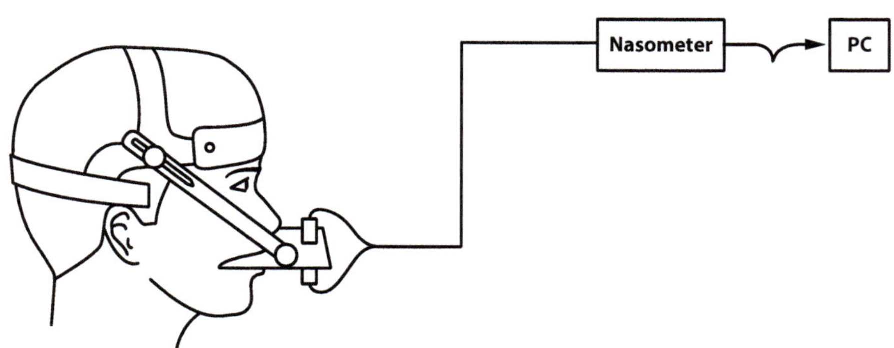

Fig. 3.34 Concept of Nasometer in principle: the nasal and oral sound productions are measured by two transductors (microphones) separated by a horizontal plate at the level of the upper lip of the subject. (Modified from Dalston (2004))

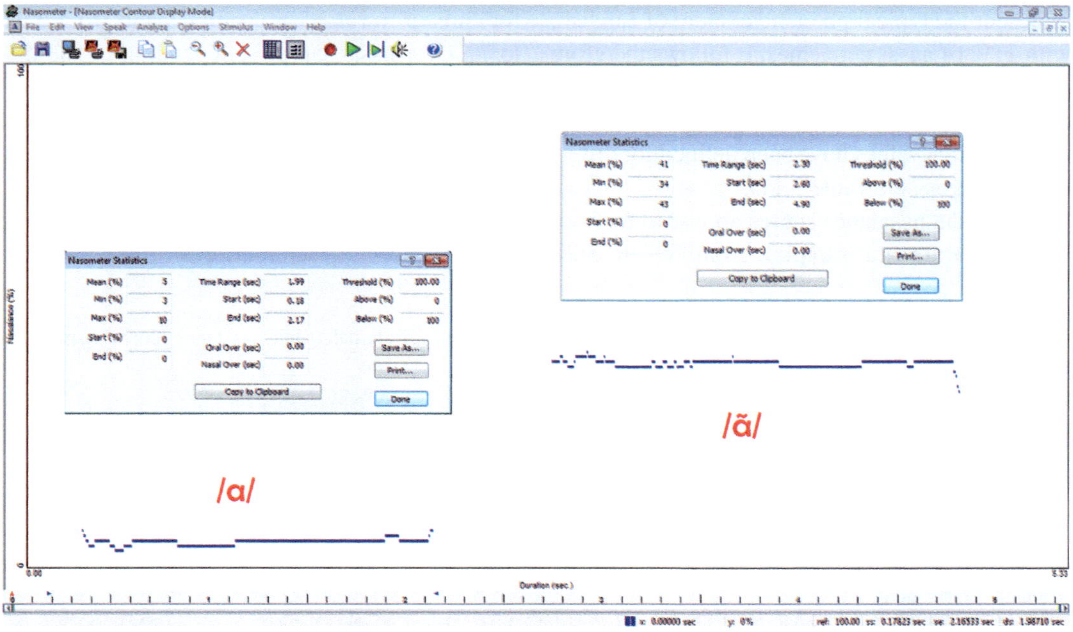

Fig. 3.35 Screenshot of the NasalView showing nasalance curves and statistics recorded in real-time for two phonemes: sustained/a/ with a mean nasalance of 5% and sustained /ã/ with a mean nasalance of 41%. (With kind permission from Tiger DRS, Inc., Seattle)

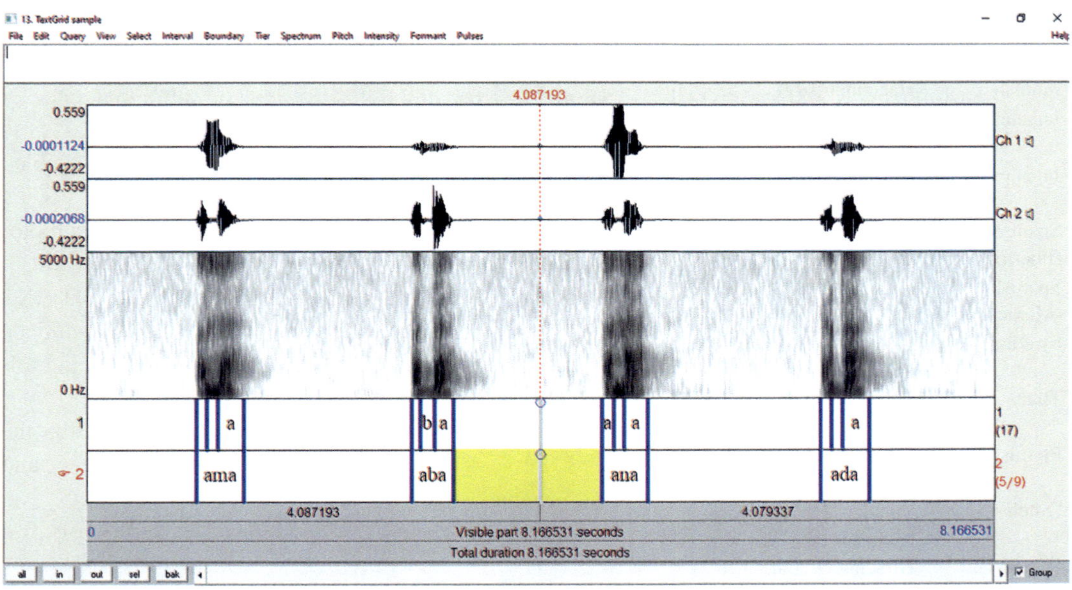

Fig. 3.36 Nasal-oral dual-channel waveform, spectrogram, segmentation and labelling image obtained in Praat program of Turkish [ama], [aba], [ana] and [ada] words. The sound file used here (sample.wav) has been recorded via a PANM (Praat-Assisted Nasalance Meter) device developed by Kılıç; this file and the related TextGrid file can be accessed at https://goo.gl/rNgnyQ. The nasalance value of the segments can be measured using the 'nasalance.praat' script in the same address. (With kind permission from Professor Mehmet Akif Kilic, Istanbul. Referenced to Boersma and Weenink (2021))

represent the typical phonetic content of English, with 11% of nasal phonemes. It follows therefore that standard passages should be developed for each language.

Normative values have been defined for different languages (see Table 3.11).

The mean nasalance scores appear to be from 9% to 30% for oral samples, from 16% to 36% for 'mixed' (oral–nasal) samples and from 35% to 77% for nasal samples, depending on the different languages.

There is some controversy regarding sex effects on nasalance scores in normal speakers. Most authors have observed no effect of sex (Litzaw and Dalston 1992; Kavanagh et al. 1994; Mayo et al. 1996; Tachimura et al. 2000; Sweeney

Table 3.11 Means for nasalance scores in different languages, M: male; F: female when nasalance scores are reported separately by sex

Language	Author	Number of subjects	Age (y)	Nasalance of oral phonemes (%)	Nasalance of mixed phonemes (%)	Nasalance of nasal phonemes (%)
American	Seaver et al. 1991	148	16–63	16	36	62
English Canada	Kavanagh et al. 1994	52	18–33	13	37	65
English Canada	Putnam Rochet et al. 1998	315	9–85	11(M)/12 (F)	33(M)/35(F)	62(M)/63(F)
French Canada	Putnam Rochet et al. 1998	153	9–85	12(M)/12(F)	26(M)/28(F)	36(M)/39(F)
English Ireland	Sweeney et al. 2004	70	4–13	14	16	51
English Ireland	Lee and Browne 2013	60	18–28	12	30	48
Australian	van Doorn and Purcell 1998	245	4–9	13	–	60
Cantonese	Whitehill 2001	141	21	17	36	56
Finnish	Haapanen 1991	58	21	14	–	69
Japanese	Tachimura et al. 2000	100	24	9	–	–
Japanese	Mishima et al. 2008	68	23.5	10(M)/16(F)	–	–
Spanish (Puerto Rican)	Anderson 1996	40	21–43	22	36	62
Spanish (Mexican)	Nichols 1999	152	8–40	17	–	55
Swedish	Brunnegård and van Doorn 2009	220	9	13	30	57
Thai	Prathanee et al. 2003	188	9.5	14	36	51
Flemish	Van Lierde et al. 2001	58	19–27	11	34	56
Dutch	Van der Heijden et al. 2011a	55	4–6	11	27	–
Hungarian	Hirschberg et al. 2006	30	5–25	11	32	–
Portuguese	Falé and Hub Faria 2008	25	19–27	10	–	44
Arabic	Abou-Elsaad et al. 2012	300	3–54	29(M)/33(F)	–	77(M)/75(F)
Greek	Okalidou et al. 2011	80	18–34	12	26	42
French	Leuchter 2017	107	9	13	26	63

et al. 2004; Brunnegård and van Doorn 2009; Okalidou et al. 2011), while some have reported higher nasalance scores in females reading passages containing nasal consonants (Seaver et al. 1991; Van Lierde et al. 2007).

Both nasal congestion (rhinitis) and the effects of nasal decongestants may influence nasometric results (Pegoraro-Krook et al. 2006), although Ziade et al. (2017) found no significant effect of nasal obstruction. It is, however, not exactly known to what extent turbulent nasal or oral flow may affect nasalance.

3.17.4 Clinical Applications of Nasometry

If the speech material is adapted, nasometry is suitable for young children from the age of about 5 (Hogen Esch and Dejonckere 2004; Van der Heijden et al. 2011b). Young children can repeat the sentences: recent systems have an editing possibility for skipping the mother's voice signals. Acoustic nasometry has been successfully used for quantitative short- and long-term functional assessment of surgical procedures (Dejonckere and van Wijngaarden 2001; Van Lierde et al. 2004). This tool can also be used in speech therapy to provide feedback during exercises.

The usefulness of this instrumental assessment primarily depends on its positive correlation with the auditory-perceptual evaluation of nasality. Most authors report a good correlation (Hirschberg et al. 2006; Dalston et al. 1991; Sweeney and Sell 2008; Brunnegård et al. 2012; Hardin et al. 1992), others moderate (Watterson et al. 1993), yet others low (Keuning et al. 2002) or no significant correlation (Nellis et al. 1992).

Nasometry has been recommended by the Cleft Palate Committee (IALP) within the standard assessment of speech in individuals with cleft palate and VPI (Hirschberg and Van Demark 1997; van der Heijden et al. 2011b). Specific normative data from the different systems for standardised voicing/speech tasks have to be considered.

In conclusion, nasometry as an acoustic evaluation of a velopharyngeal function is a very useful method. However, any treatment decision should be always based upon cumulated evidence from various sources, including auditory-perceptual evaluation, instrumental assessment and clinical evaluation.

3.18 Velopharyngeal Muscle Electromyography

Philippe H. Dejonckere

Electromyography (EMG) can be defined as the recording of the electrical phenomena that are associated with the first stage in the sequence of events that link muscle excitation with muscle contraction (Aidley 1989).

Electromyographic investigations of velopharyngeal muscles have been performed since the late 50s (Li and Lundervold 1958), but the pioneering work in this specific field was achieved by Fritzell (1969). By using hooked-wire electrodes inserted into the velopharyngeal muscles (levator veli palatini, tensor veli palatini, constrictor pharyngeus superior, palatopharyngeus and palatoglossus) Fritzell found that (1) the levator veli palatini is the primary muscle used in achieving velopharyngeal closure and that the strength of its contraction varies directly with velar height, (2) the activity of the constrictor pharyngeus superior parallels that of the levator, (3) the palatopharyngeus activity for speech is inconsistent, (4) the tensor veli palatini is not active for speech, and (5) the palatoglossus activity occurs for nasal segments. Bell-Berti (1976) confirmed that the levator veli palatini is the primary muscle of velopharyngeal closure in speech. However, besides speech, the velopharyngeal muscles are also involved in swallowing and tubal functions. Swallowing disorders have elicited a regain of interest in pharyngeal EMG (Perlman 2006).

Different types of electrodes can be used for exploring velopharyngeal muscles: surface electrodes are best suited for kinesiological studies, while traditional EMG-needle electrodes allow the identification of abnormal motor unit potentials, as observed in peripheral neurogenic damage (paresis) and myopathies, such as the oculopharyngeal muscular dystrophy. Picciotti et al. (2005) have designed a surface electrode to be applied transnasally under endoscopic control, in order to evaluate the function of the tuba auditiva. This electrode records the activity of the tensor veli palatini, involved in the active opening of the tuba, during swallowing. Su et al. (1993) used a concentric needle electrode introduced transnasally in the levator and tensor veli palatini under endoscopic guidance to investigate tubal dysfunction. Guindi et al. (1981) recorded EMG activity of the levator veli palatini muscle during swallowing by means of a non-invasive surface electrode applied to the soft palate. Honjo et al. (1979) used a monopolar needle electrode inserted into the levator and tensor veli palatini (tubal function) transnasally through a ventilation catheter. Bipolar wire-hooked electrodes were inserted transorally by Hairston and Sauerland (1981) to explore the tensor and levator veli palatini, whereas Kamere (1978) used the same approach with a unipolar needle electrode. However, for speech tasks, EMG is often disruptive of normal speech behaviour (Baken and Orlikoff 2000). Swallowing and suction have been investigated transorally with a thin needle electrode, even in very young children (Renault and Raimbault 1992). More recently, Freitas et al. (2015) explored the use of surface EMG electrodes positioned in the face and neck regions to obtain useful information about velar movement. Giannantoni et al. (2016) used a nasopharyngeal surface electrode in patients with acute ischaemic stroke patients for demonstrating reduced pharyngeal motility. Electromyography was used by Morice et al. (2018) to investigate the levator veli palatini muscles in children with syndromic Pierre Robin Syndrome and isolated Pierre Robin Syndrome. They concluded that soft palate muscle deficiency is not a predictor of speech prognosis.

Diagnostic EMG of velopharyngeal muscles can be used in the objective diagnosis of neuromuscular diseases, particularly muscle paralysis secondary to lower motor neuron injury or disease: for example, amyotrophic lateral sclerosis, medullary infarct, Wallenberg's syndrome (Perlman 2006) (Fig. 3.37).

The clinical applications for assessing velopharyngeal function are actually quite limited, owing to the invasive nature of the procedure when using hooked-wire or needle electrodes, the difficulty with surface electrode placement, and the interference with articulatory movements during speech (Murdoch and Theodoros 2001).

Wan et al. (2013) reported about EMG-guided injection of botulinum toxin type A (Botox; Allergan, Irvine, CA, USA) into the salpingopharyngeus and tensor veli palatini for palatal myoclonus with objective clicking tinnitus.

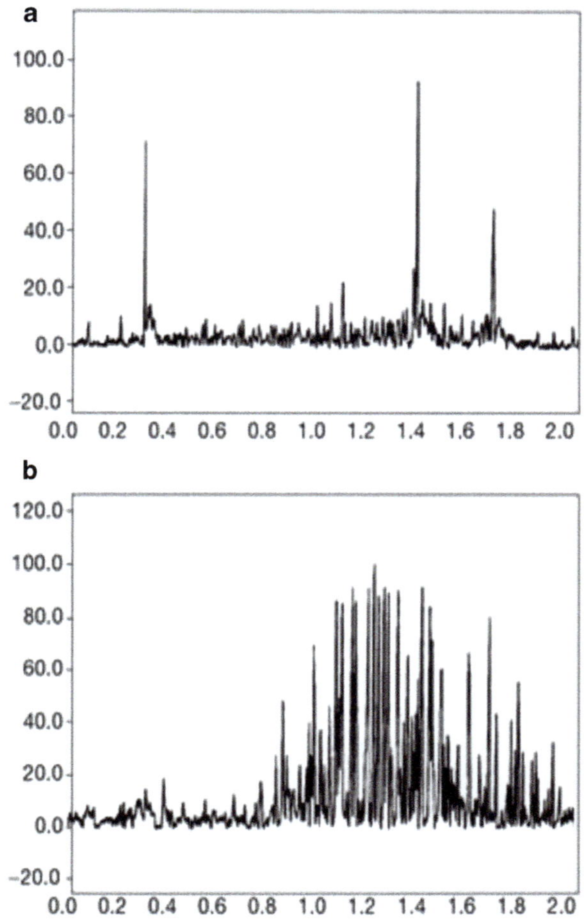

Fig. 3.37 Rectified EMG recording (all negative values are squared and brought to the positive side of baseline) from the superior pharyngeal constrictor. The top image is representative of the recording from the paralysed side, whereas the bottom image is from the healthy contralateral side (*x*-axis is time in sec, *y*-axis is μV). (Reprinted by permission from Springer Nature provided by Springer Nature and Copyright Clearance Center from Perlman (2006) Electromyography in oral and pharyngeal motor disorders. GI Motility online. Doi: 10.1038/gimo32)

3.19 Imaging Procedures for Assessing the Velopharyngeal Sphincter During Speech

Pablo Antonio Ysunza

3.19.1 Introduction

The earliest recorded examination of the velopharyngeal mechanism in motion during speech was reported by Hilton in 1836. Williams published his book about Roentgen rays in medicine and surgery in 1901. He described the use of radiographs as an aid in diagnosis and also as a therapeutic agent. The earliest radiographic assessment of the velopharyngeal valve appeared in 1909 (Scheier 1909) and the first application of motion pictures was probably in 1930 as reported by Barclay (1930). From the advent of radiographic studies until 1969, the assessment of velopharyngeal function by using imaging procedures was almost exclusively a lateral (midsagittal) view of the head and neck by still or motion picture radiographic procedures. Reducing a three-dimensional function to a two-dimensional view led to a broad assumption that velopharyngeal valving was exclusively an upward and backward elevation of the soft palate to the posterior pharyngeal wall or adenoid mass.

In 1969, the first reports of the use of nasal endoscopy and fluoroscopic assessment of the pharynx in multiple projections (lateral, midsagittal and submentovertical) provided three-dimensional views of the velopharyngeal mechanism that revealed much more than had been known before. For example, reports describe that the function of the velopharyngeal valve during the production of non-nasal speech is highly variable from individual to individual (Croft et al. 1981; Golding-Kushner et al. 1990; Shprintzen et al. 1979; Shprintzen and Golding-Kushner 1989). Therefore, in order to perform an adequate assessment of the velopharyngeal valve, it is necessary to assess each case carefully by using procedures that will describe every aspect of how the mechanism is working in that individual. An intra-oral examination cannot provide useful clinical information on the physiology of velopharyngeal closure. The anatomy of the hard and soft palate can be examined intra-orally, but these observations are not only insufficient for a reliable clinical assessment, they are completely invalid. For one thing, the movements of the lateral pharyngeal walls cannot be visualised by intra-oral examination and only on rare occasions can the posterior pharyngeal wall be seen. Moreover, the speech sounds or phonemes in which the velopharyngeal sphincter has to seal the communication between the oral and nasal cavities are plosive and fricative phonemes. For the articulation of these sounds the lips have to be partially or completely closed, precluding any observation of velopharyngeal function. Moreover, the only sounds that can be made with the mouth open are vowels. Vowels produced in isolation do not require velopharyngeal closure so any observation would be invalid (Moll 1962).

It is with good reason that the last update of the parameters of the American Cleft Palate Association for the evaluation and treatment of patients with cleft lip/palate and other craniofacial anomalies specify that secondary surgery for VPI should be performed only after imaging of the velopharyngeal mechanism during speech and after input from speech-language specialists and other disciplines is obtained (American Cleft Palate Association 2017).

3.19.2 Video-Nasopharyngoscopy and Videofluoroscopy of the Velopharyngeal Sphincter

Combining flexible video-nasopharyngoscopy (FVNP) and multi-view videofluoroscopy (MVF) has been reported as the best approach for obtaining accurate imaging data of the VPS during speech (Golding-Kushner et al. 1990; Shprintzen and Golding-Kushner 1989; Ysunza and Pamplona 2008). FVNP provides dynamic direct visualisation and in-vivo imaging of the vocal tract during articulation. MVF uses ionising radiation during fluoroscopy to show the movements of the velopharyngeal valve from above, as well as the entire upper airway from the nose to the larynx.

The main advantage of FVNP is that it provides imaging of the entire vocal tract from the glottis to the nasal cavity. However, FVNP cannot provide a three-dimensional assessment. The images are two-dimensional, lacking an adequate assessment of depth. It is also not possible to perform true size measurements of the structures and spaces. MVF can provide true size measurements of the structures and movements of the velopharyngeal valve during speech. It also provides dynamic visualisation of the entire area of both lateral pharyngeal walls. MVF also provides information about the precise location of velopharyngeal closure during speech in all three dimensions (height, width, depth) (Ysunza et al. 2016). The use of nasopharyngoscopy for assessing velopharyngeal closure was first reported in 1969 (Pigott et al. 1969), almost simultaneously with the first report of multi-view videofluoroscopy (Skolnick 1970). Although these two procedures are distinctly different in terms of technology and the type of view obtained (solid tissue versus fluoroscopic shadow), it has been found that the information obtained from both studies on the same patient is the only method for complete information valuable to the treatment of VPI (Golding-Kushner et al. 1990; Shprintzen et al. 1979; Ysunza and Pamplona 2008; Ysunza et al. 2008).

Ten years after the introduction of nasopharyngoscopy and multi-view videofluoroscopy, the routine use of FVNP for nasopharyngeal exams and a comprehensive study of velopharyngeal surgery in children were reported in detail (Shprintzen et al. 1979). When first introduced, nasopharyngoscopy was often done with rigid side-viewing endoscopes (Pigott et al. 1969). It should be pointed out that when first introduced, FVNP was described with video recording including sound. As an imaging procedure of a complex task involving movement and sound such as speech, recording of imaging and sound is essential for an accurate assessment (Shprintzen and Ysunza 2019).

In 1990, an international working group was formed consisting of 27 international experts from around the world who were well-published scientists from the USA, Canada, Mexico, the United Kingdom and Sweden. These experts represented frequent authors of research and clinical papers describing differing aspects of velopharyngeal insufficiency and assessment procedures, and included the past and present Editor of the Cleft Palate-Craniofacial Journal and several past presidents of the American Cleft Palate-Craniofacial Association, the Past President of the Society for Ear Nose and Throat Advances in Children, and the Past President of the Society for Craniofacial Genetics. Among the disciplines represented were paediatricians, speech pathologists, plastic surgeons, otolaryngologists, radiologists and dental specialists. Karen Golding-Kushner Ph.D. served as the recorder and arbitrator of the proceedings, which were written up for publication in the Cleft Palate-Craniofacial Journal (Golding-Kushner et al. 1990) after circulation to the Working Group and unanimous agreement to the group's recommendations. The results were a standardisation of reporting of FVNP and MVF.

According to these guidelines, the movements of the structures of the velopharyngeal valve during speech should be analysed separately and completely. Velum movement from its position at rest up to the maximum point of displacement towards the posterior pharyngeal wall should be assessed as a proportion from 0 to 1.00. The full extent indicates full contact of the velum and posterior wall. By the same token, the movement of the posterior wall, if a Passavant's ridge is detected, is assessed as a percentage in the opposite direction. The level of the ridge has also to be described as at, above or below the level of velum movement. It should be noted that in most cases the ridge moves slightly below velar movement. The movements of the lateral pharyngeal walls are also assessed as a percentage from their position at rest up to the maximum displacement towards the midline. Each wall has a maximum displacement of 50 percent (0.50) if reaching the midline. The symmetry of the movement of the walls should be described too. It should be mentioned that all these assessments are estimates, which although clinically useful, may not be statistically reliable. Because of this situation, it is recommended that the displacement of the different structures be given in no less than 10% intervals. The closure pattern should also be included in the description.

The size of the gap if present has also to be described as a percentage. One hundred percent would be the total space of the velopharyngeal at rest, and the gap during the best closure is estimated in proportion to the total space. If no gap is discernible but consistent bubbling is observed during speech the gap would be conventionally considered as 10%. The shape of the gap is also important. The shape can be classified according to the closure pattern in each case: circular, coronal, sagittal and hourglass (Figs. 3.38, 3.39, 3.40 and 3.41).

The size of the adenoid pad at rest during nasal inspiration should be assessed on a 1–4 category scale. Category one is when the adenoid pad does not cover 50 percent of the space. Category four is when the adenoid pad contacts the velum at rest.

Assessment of the pharyngeal tonsils is extremely important. For the palatine tonsils, most clinicians use a 1–4 category scale, with assessment from peroral examination. Observation of the tonsils confined within the faucial pillars is classified as category 1. If the tonsils contact each other at the midline they are classified as category 4. However, this type of

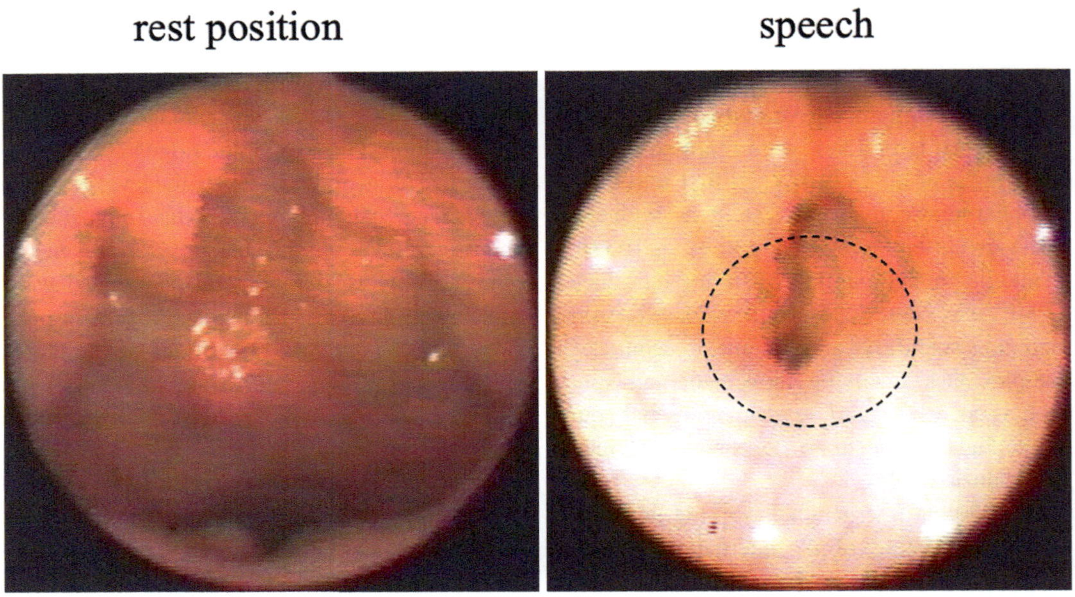

Fig. 3.38 Videonasopharyngoscopy views of the velopharyngeal sphincter at rest and during speech. On the bottom of the view at rest, a central submucous cleft can be discerned. During speech, there is a circular closure pattern. A central gap is observed. The size of the gap is approximately 20%

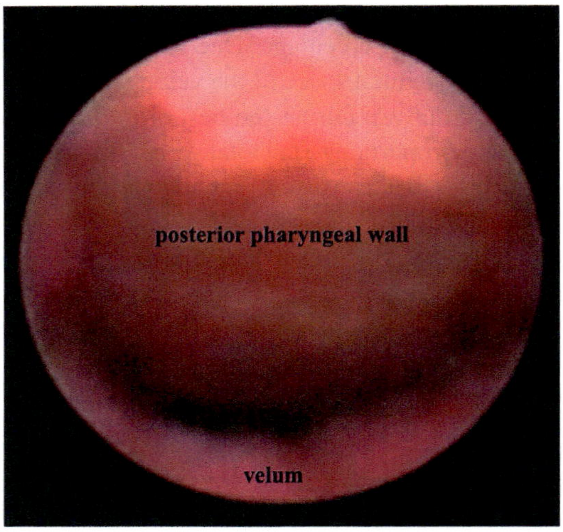

Fig. 3.39 Videonasopharyngoscopy view of the velopharyngeal sphincter during speech. The posterior pharyngeal wall and the velum can be identified. A large velopharyngeal closure gap is observed. The shape of the gap is coronal

oral examination presumes that the tonsils always remain within the confines of the faucial pillars. However, as has been reported (Shprintzen et al. 1987) from endoscopic examination, the tonsils can grow posteriorly into the pharyngeal airway with the upper poles sometimes extruding into the nasopharynx, and the lower poles growing downward into close approximation with the epiglottis and blocking the hypopharyngeal airway and pyriform sinuses (Fig. 3.42).

FVNP should include examination of the vocal tract from the nasal cavities down to the glottis, including the pharyngeal tonsils laterally, the lingual tonsil, epiglottis, and false and true vocal cords.

For a useful imaging assessment of the VPS during speech, including FVNP and MVF, it is essential to use an adequate speech sample. This should include isolated words and sentences with plosive and fricative sounds in combination with high and low vowels. It should be adapted to the native language of the patient. Repetition of vowel sounds in isolation is not necessary and could be misleading because velopharyngeal closure is not achieved for most isolated vowels.

The movements of the VPS during speech should be analysed as many times as necessary for a complete and reliable examination. The movements can be assessed in slow motion or even frame-by-frame when necessary. The best

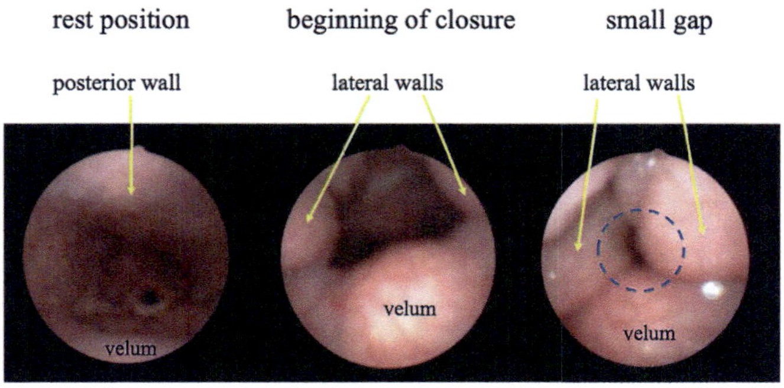

Fig. 3.40 Videopharyngoscopy view of the velopharyngeal sphincter during speech. Minimal movement of lateral pharyngeal walls is observed. There is a closure gap with an hourglass shape

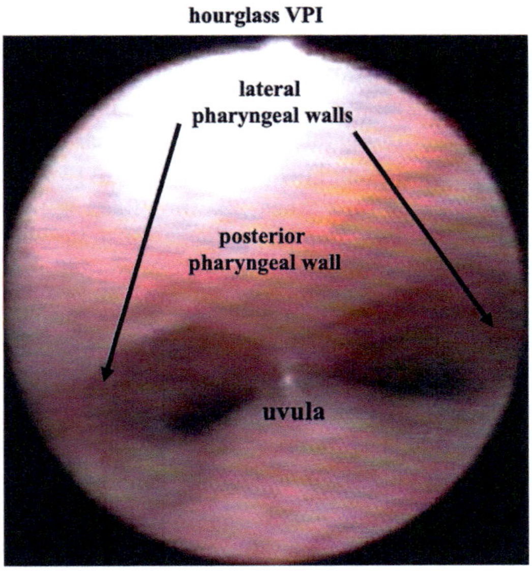

Fig. 3.41 Videonasopharyngoscopy views of the velopharyngeal sphincter at rest, at the beginning of closure during speech and at the end of closure. A sagittal pattern can be observed with predominant movement of the lateral pharyngeal walls. It should be noted that velum does not reach the posterior pharyngeal wall because of the interposition of the lateral walls during speech. There is a central gap with a sagittal shape

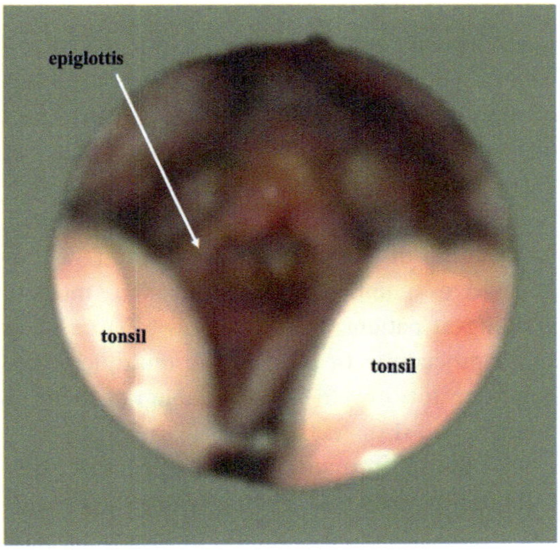

Fig. 3.42 Videonasopharyngoscopy view of the vocal tract below the velopharyngeal sphincter. Enlarged tonsils on both sides can be observed. The lower poles have grown downwards into a close approximation to the epiglottis

examinations are achieved by a panel of clinicians including the speech-language specialist, the surgeon, the radiologist and the otolaryngologist/phoniatrist.

In recent years, the use of MVF for assessing VPI has become somewhat controversial because the medical literature has suggested theoretical risks of excess cancers, including fatal ones, from ionising radiation, especially in young children (who constitute the population in which MVF is more frequently used as a diagnostic tool). Yet MVF remains an integral component in the assessment and treatment planning of patients with VPI. At the present time, medical sources of radiation affecting the population are increasing. This is of particular concern in children whose tissues are more radiosensitive, whose organs receive a larger effective dose for a given level of ionising radiation, and who potentially have an increased time to develop cancers as a result of radiation exposure. Moreover, it has been suggested that the risk is cumulative with repeated radiation exposure (Frush 2014). Therefore, all studies that expose a child to ionising radiation should be carefully evaluated as to the potential risk versus the likely benefit.

When an imaging procedure is being considered for use as a diagnostic marker, it is necessary to determine if the exam is essential and if no other study, without ionising radiation, can provide the same information. MVF meets these criteria. When an MVF is performed, it should be considered that the amount of radiation resulting from these fluoroscopic procedures is highly variable, depending upon the individual radiologist's skill and fluoroscopic parameters, which in turn depend upon several factors, including patient size and desired image detail. The details of the procedure performed have a great impact on patient dose. The final unit of importance is the effective dose, which is measured in milliSieverts (mSv). Recently, the American Association of Physicists in Medicine (AAPM) released a statement that the risks of medical imaging at patient dosages below <50 mSv for single procedures or 100 mSv for multiple procedures are too low to be detectable and may be non-existent (Frush 2014).

For the performance of a reliable and clinically useful MVF with minimal radiation dosage, the following methods should be followed: adequate compliance for reducing procedure time. All patients, but especially patients younger than 10 years of age, should be carefully informed about how the procedure will be performed. The use of pictures or a video can be useful for showing the actions and equipment. The patient should be familiar with the speech sample, and an experienced speech pathologist or phoniatrist should verify that the patient is truly able to repeat the speech sample with adequate articulation placement, regardless of hypernasality and nasal emission. The patient and the parents or accompanying persons should be allowed in the videofluoroscopy room. Lead aprons should be provided. Nectar-thick barium should be instilled through both nasal cavities with a 5-cc syringe, dropper or pipette. Coating of the pharynx can be confirmed through intra-oral examination or is evident on the first moment of fluoroscopic exposure. Additional barium can be instilled if the structures are not well coated. Adequate fluoroscopic images can be obtained by using pulsed fluoroscopy thereby decreasing radiation dosage. Magnification is not necessary because the actual assessment should not be performed during the procedure but afterward from the recording. It is essential that the recording includes sound. As in the case of FVNP, a panel of clinicians can provide the best evaluations. The tower should be kept as close to the patient as possible. Coning should be used to avoid radiosensitive structures such as the lens and thyroid.

Posterior-Anterior, lateral and submentovertical views (Fig. 3.43) should be obtained in all cases (Golding-Kushner et al. 1990).

Oblique views may be used in selected cases if asymmetry of lateral wall motion or velar movement is evident in lateral or frontal (P-A) views. In our experience when a well-defined speech sample is used, which includes all consonant sounds native to the patient's language in short speech phrases, the examination time (exposure to ionising radiation) should not exceed approximately 40 seconds. Total radiation dosage would therefore not exceed 10 mSv.

For greater accuracy in describing the volume of the VPI, we use moveable radio-opaque markers for performing measurements on the recorded images. The markers can be placed with a 10-mm distance between them. At least two marks should be clearly visible in all views. For true size measurements, the number of pixels between two marks is used as a reference for obtaining a ratio and measuring distances in mm. The distances between lateral pharyngeal walls at rest and during articulation are measured. These can provide important information for the tailoring of pharyngeal flaps or other types of pharyngoplasties.

With a good barium coat of the tissues in the upper airway, the lymphoid tissue, including the adenoid, pharyngeal tonsils and lingual tonsil, can be assessed with the same category scale used for FVNP. The location and size of these tissues is particularly important for determining the post-operative risk of obstructive airway disorders, including obstructive sleep apnoea or even

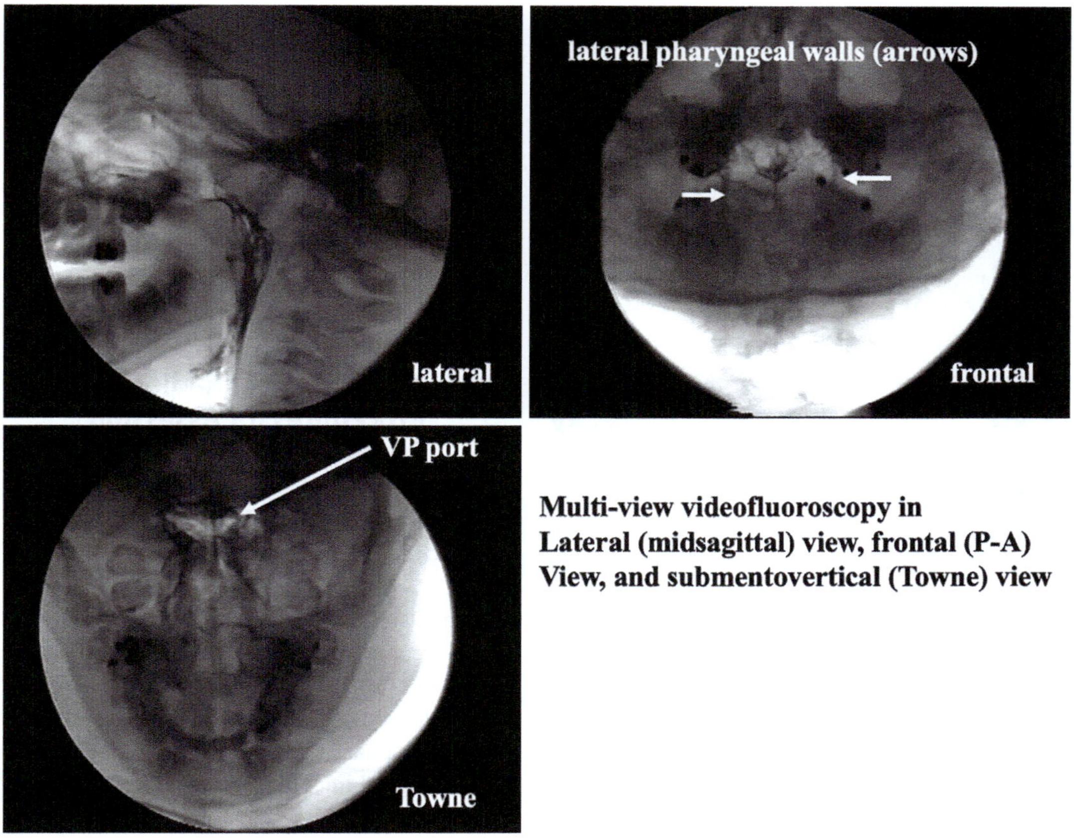

Fig. 3.43 Videofluoroscopy views of the velopharyngeal sphincter parallel to the sagittal plane (lateral view), coronal plane (frontal view), and axial plane (Towne view). The structures of the velopharyngeal sphincter can be identified. An assessment of the velopharyngeal sphincter in three dimensions can be performed by analysing these views

compromise of respiration when awake, related to reduced airway size, resulting in decreased vitality and poor cognitive functioning. It is our practice to reduce postoperative airway obstruction by removing the tonsils and adenoids completely before reconstructive surgery, on the basis of the significantly improved outcomes related to complications in large cohorts of cases (Chegar et al. 2007; Shprintzen et al. 1992).

It should be pointed out that the best assessment of the lateral pharyngeal wall movements during speech is provided by the frontal and submentovertex views. During FVNP, it is often difficult to visualise the lateral walls during speech because of velar interposition between the movement of the lateral pharyngeal walls and the elevation of the velum. Velar elevation is often above the plane of the hard palate, while lateral pharyngeal wall motion is almost always below the plane of the hard palate (Shprintzen 1995). It is for this reason that the combination of both nasopharyngoscopy and multi-view videofluoroscopy is used in all cases. The lateral view can provide the best assessment of pharyngeal tonsil hypertrophy interfering with velum movements during speech (Fig. 3.44).

The imaging provided by this view is better than that of FVNP. Intra-oral examination seems to be the gold standard for evaluating tonsil hypertrophy, but there are some cases in which tonsil tissue growths are in a superior direction behind the anterior pillar when the interaction of this hypertrophy and the velum can be clearly visualised by the lateral view of MVF.

Besides the usefulness of the data provided by MVF, another issue to be considered is tolerance

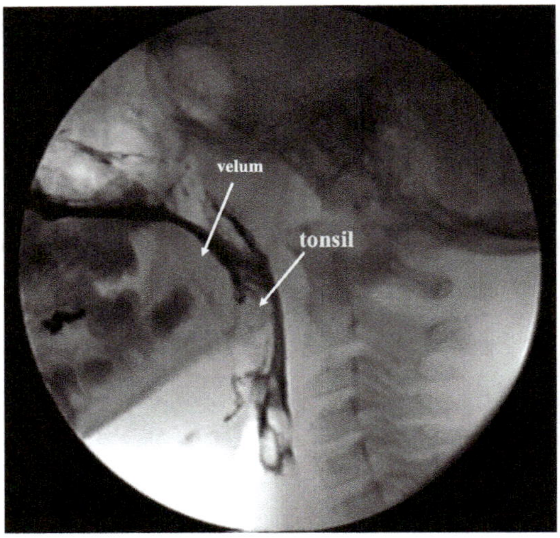

Fig. 3.44 Lateral view of a videofluoroscopy. An enlarged tonsil can be identified. Tonsil hypertrophy can hinder velum movement during speech causing VPI even in cases of a normal velopharyngeal sphincter

and compliance during MVF and FVNP, especially in young children. One of the more important factors for performing useful imaging procedures of the velopharyngeal valve during speech is improving the patient's compliance for achieving complete and accurate evaluations. It has been reported that MVF is significantly better tolerated than FVNP (Ysunza et al. 2008). Although both procedures (MVF and FVNP) are necessary for adequate planning of the surgical treatment of VPI, in some cases is reasonable to perform MVF as a first imaging diagnostic procedure. Barium coating during FNVP usually does not affect the evaluation.

Shprintzen et al. (1979) were the first to use the term tailor-made flaps. The rationale behind customising the surgical procedure according to the findings of MVF and FVNP is that it has been extensively demonstrated that VPS anatomy and physiology is highly variable between individuals. Thus, performing the same surgical procedure in every case of VPI has a low probability of successfully restoring velopharyngeal closure during speech. Imaging procedures provide the specific features of velopharyngeal anatomy and velopharyngeal closure during a speech in each case and it has been demonstrated that these data are useful for planning an individualised surgery and improving the post-operative outcome (Chegar et al. 2007; Shprintzen et al. 1979; Ysunza et al. 2004, 2015, 2019; Ysunza and Pamplona 2008).

The combination MVF and FVNP, as advocated by the International Working Group (Golding-Kushner et al. 1990) has proven to be the best approach for planning surgical procedures aimed at correcting VPI.

3.20 MRI and Other Radiological Procedures for Assessing Speech Disorders

Uta HanningUte Pröschel, Thomas Niederstadt and Martina Scharitzer

Speech disorders are assessed in a multidisciplinary approach with a combination of dynamic diagnostic tests, including videofluoroscopy, naso-endoscopy, MRI and CT. This section will focus on resonance disorders and their evaluation by radiological imaging.

3.20.1 Radiological Imaging Modalities

3.20.1.1 Videofluoroscopy

Basic Principles

Videofluoroscopy is a radiographic imaging technique that uses X-rays to produce real-time movies of the deep structures in the body. This technique enables visualisation of the velopharyngeal sphincter during speech and swallowing by using several standard views. It offers an overview of the pharynx's posterior and lateral wall and the length and motion of the soft palate (Lam et al. 2006). Most of the studies describe the first step in diagnosing speech disorders as videofluoroscopy combined with naso-endoscopy (Havstam et al. 2005). In a few studies, naso-endoscopy is preferred (Henningsson and Isberg 1991b). Videofluoroscopy is significantly better tolerated than naso-endoscopy, although it should be applied in a targeted manner, especially in the

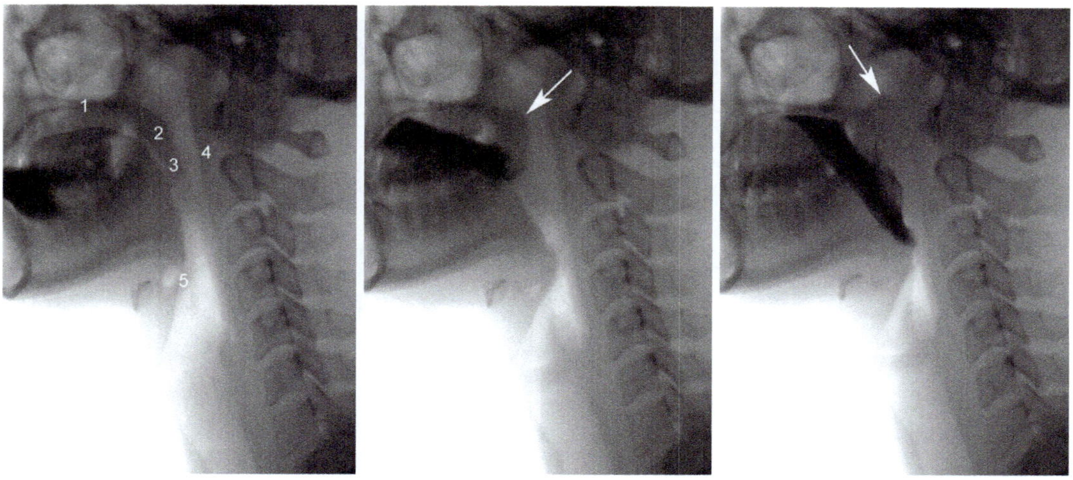

Fig. 3.45 Videofluoroscopic images illustrating the anatomy of the velopharynx. Left panel: (1) hard palate; (2) velum; (3) uvula; (4) posterior pharyngeal wall; (5) epiglottis. When initiating swallowing, the velum starts elevating (middle panel, arrow). After elevation and retraction of the velum (right panel, arrow), complete contact against the posterior pharyngeal wall can be seen

paediatric population owing to its use of radiation (Ruda et al. 2012). Besides evaluating the velum during speech, it enables testing of swallowing in a regular sitting or standing position (Fig. 3.45). In paediatric patients with genetic syndromes resulting in hypernasality (such as DiGeorge syndrome, Treacher Collins syndrome, Turner syndrome, Robin sequence and others: Kobrynski and Sullivan 2007), videofluoroscopy reveals nasopharyngeal regurgitation and can detect concomitant penetration or aspiration.

3.20.1.2 Magnetic Resonance Imaging (MRI)

MRI is a new application in evaluating velopharyngeal insufficiency and so far, only applied in specialised centres.

Basic Principles

MRI is based on nuclear magnetic resonance imaging of atomic nuclei inside the body (see physical basics in Sect. 11.16 from Volume 1).

Advantages

MRI is a non-ionising, non-invasive diagnostic imaging modality capable of producing high-contrast soft-tissue images. It enables visualisation of the velopharyngeal sphincter in various planes without the need for the patient's repositioning. Owing to the superior soft-tissue contrast, evaluating the levator veli palatini muscle (LVP, the dominant muscle of the soft palate) is feasible. Pre-operative evaluation in suspected submucosal or occult clefts is another indication of this non-invasive imaging methodology. However, it often requires sedation of young children (Ruda et al. 2012). Studies comparing MRI with videofluoroscopy demonstrated that MRI could illustrate the pattern of velopharyngeal closure (Beer et al. 2004) and persistent or recurrent inadequate velum closure in patients following surgical correction of velopharyngeal dysfunction (Arendt et al. 2021).

Disadvantages

Artifacts occur when the patient moves while imaging.

3.20.1.3 Dynamic Imaging (MRI)

Recent dynamic MRI studies have been used to attempt quantitative measurements of the velopharynx and to assess the levator veli palatine muscle during rest and phonation (Fig. 3.46) (Sagar and Nimkin 2014; Drissi et al. 2011).

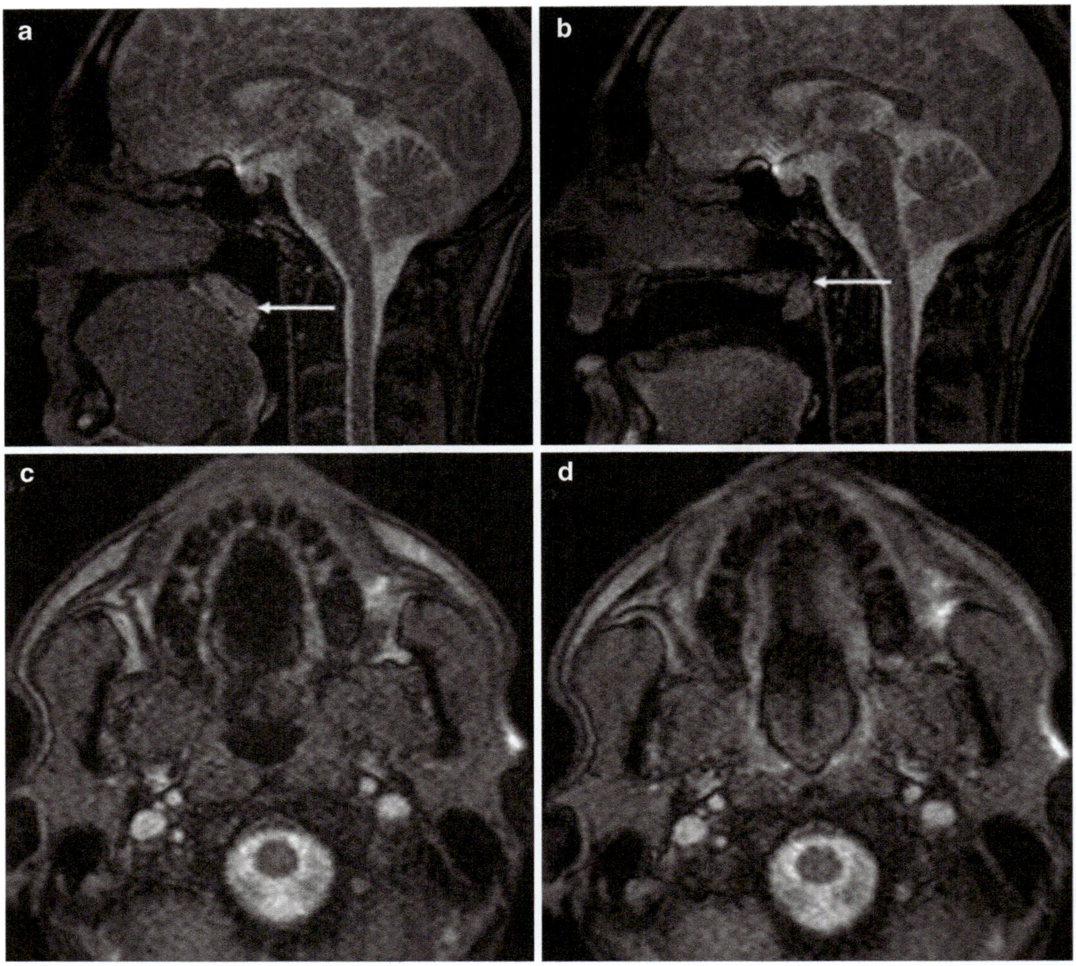

Fig. 3.46 Normal dynamic pattern of speech; sagittal and axial TrueFISP images at rest (**a**, **c**) and during speech (**b**, **d**). (Reproduced from Drissi C, Mitrofanoff M, Talandier C et al. (2011) Feasibility of dynamic MRI for evaluating velopharyngeal insufficiency in children. Eur Radiol 21(7):1462–1469 with permission of Springer Nature Customer Service Centre GmbH)

Basic Principles

Dynamic MRI imaging is based on the application of T2-weighted high-temporal-resolution real-time imaging-sequences in mid-sagittal and axial planes during rest, during phonation (e.g. phonation of "e") and repeated articulation (e.g. consonant "k") (Kulinna-Cosentini et al. 2016). However, there might be changes in the pattern of the movement due to the patient's position, as the MRI usually is performed in a horizontal, and not in the normal vertical, position of the patient.

3.20.1.4 Computed Tomography (CT)

Attempts have been made to use continuous computed tomography during vowel phonation and swallowing for the kinematic analysis of velopharyngeal function (Sakamoto et al. 2015; Kobayashi et al. 2019). Nevertheless, the significant radiation exposure cannot be ignored, especially in the paediatric patient population. Before the cleft palate operation with maxillary growth restriction, CT imaging may be used to stratify the risk for postoperative velopharyngeal insufficiency, by measuring the ratio of the soft palate and the airway depth at the level of the hard palate (McComb et al. 2011; Abramson et al. 2015), (Fig. 3.47). In patients with overt, submucous or occult submucous cleft palate, computed tomography is particularly useful for demonstrating osseous and dental structural abnormalities resulting in velopharyngeal insufficiency and resonance disorders.

3.20.1.5 Lateral Radiography

The advent of ionising radiation has significantly contributed to the understanding of velopharyngeal function. The first published report of a lateral neck radiograph evaluating velopharyngeal function dates from 1909 (Scheier 1909). Its use was replaced by the introduction of videofluoroscopy in the late 1960s (Skolnick 1969).

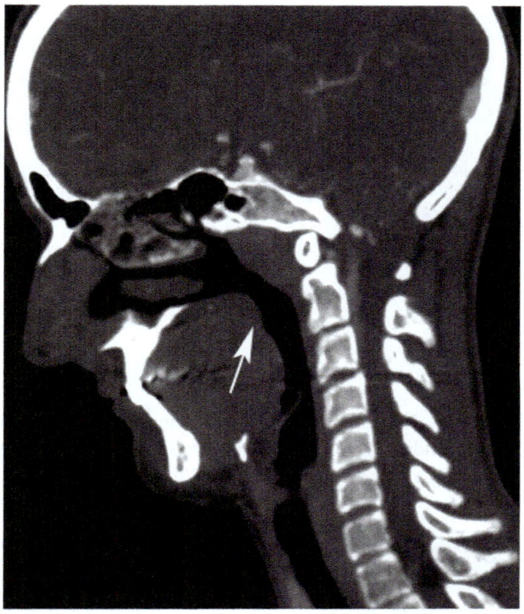

Fig. 3.47 Midline sagittal CT image in a 16-year-old girl with velopharyngeal insufficiency following surgical cleft palate repair. For planning pharyngoplasty CT was performed, showing a short soft palate (arrow). (Courtesy of Medical University of Vienna)

3.20.2 Resonance Disorders

3.20.2.1 Hypernasality

Pathological deviations of nasality can be distinguished as hypernasality (excessive resonance in the nasal cavity, open nasalisation) or hyponasality (insufficient nasal resonance during speech, closed nasalisation). Hypernasality is clinically observed in cases of soft palate dysfunction with velopharyngeal insufficiency and skeletal malformations (especially in cleft palate).

Normal Velopharyngeal Anatomy

Anatomically, the velopharyngeal port is defined anteriorly by the soft palate (velum) and laterally and posteriorly by the lateral and posterior pharyngeal walls. It is the distance that the velum and pharyngeal walls have to overcome to enable complete closure during speech and swallowing. Swallowing is a complex mechanism and primarily consists of three phases, an oral, a pharyngeal and an oesophageal phase (Fig. 3.48). Additionally, velopharyngeal closure is required for the articulation of non-nasal consonants. There are different patterns of velopharyngeal closure depending on the different contributions of velum or lateral pharyngeal walls for closure (Perry 2011). During breathing, the velum rests against the surface of the tongue. During the production of oral speech sounds or swallowing, the velum elevates and retracts with complete contact with the posterior pharyngeal wall, creating an eminence (Fig. 3.45).

Velopharyngeal Insufficiency

Velopharyngeal insufficiency (VPI) is a disorder of speech and swallowing induced by the incomplete closure of the velopharyngeal gap, which normally separates the naso- from the oropharynx. The reasons for VPI are either functional or structural disorders of the velum (Drissi et al. 2011). Figure 3.49 illustrates a patient's swallowing pattern after oropharyngeal tumour resection, showing the resulting swallowing disorders.

Other structural reasons for the failure of the velopharyngeal closure and articulation difficulties are overt or submucous cleft palate or a repaired cleft palate resulting in a deficiency of palatal tissue in up to 30% of patients following cleft palate surgery (Phua and de Chalain 2008) (Fig. 3.47). Neuromuscular disorders such as stroke, myopathy or cerebral palsy may also lead to incomplete closure of a regular structured velopharyngeal sphincter (Hillarp et al. 1994) (Fig. 3.50). The most common radiological tests

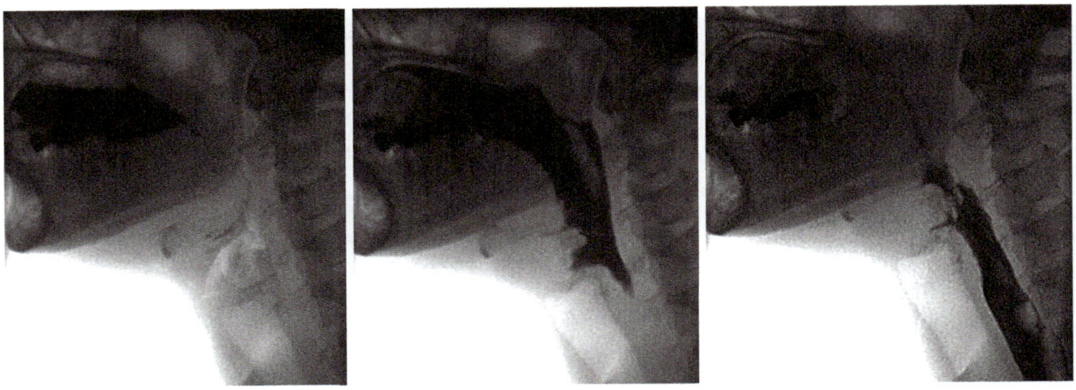

Fig. 3.48 Normal pattern of swallowing (left panel) oral phase, (middle panel) pharyngeal phase and (right panel) oesophageal phase. (Courtesy of Clinic for Radiology, University and University Hospital Muenster (Chair: Univ.-Prof. Dr. med. Walter Heindel))

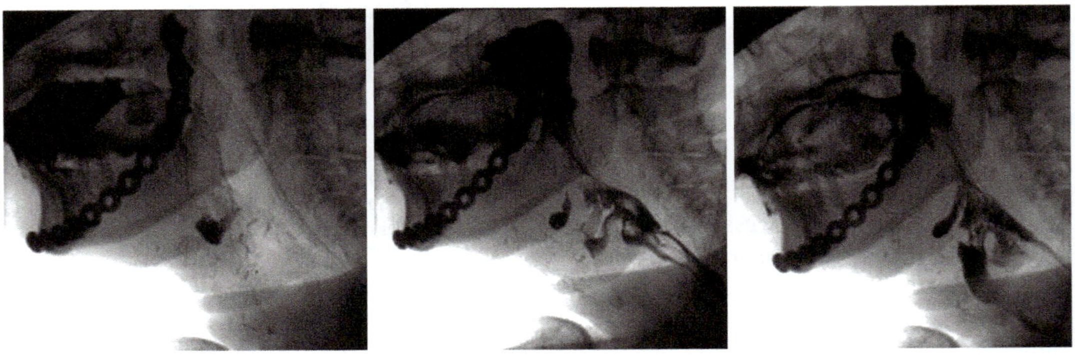

Fig. 3.49 A pattern of swallowing after oropharyngeal tumour resection. (Left panel) oral phase: dorsal leakage due to impaired oral bolus control; (middle panel) pharyngeal phase with nasal regurgitation and simultaneous penetration of contrast material into the laryngeal vestibulum; (right panel) lack of epiglottalal tilting and incomplete closure of the laryngeal vestibule with subsequent intratracheal aspiration. (Courtesy of Clinic for Radiology, University and University Hospital Muenster (Chair: Univ.-Prof. Dr. med. Walter Heindel))

for evaluating the degree of velopharyngeal insufficiency are naso-endoscopy and videofluoroscopy (Lam et al. 2006). Naso-endoscopy is an invasive method with reduced ability to assess the anatomical information of the velopharyngeal port. Videofluoroscopy has the disadvantage of using ionising radiation, making dynamic magnetic resonance imaging a promising radiological method for assessing velopharyngeal insufficiency.

3.20.2.2 Hyponasality

In most cases, hyponasality is caused by an organic blockage of the resonance cavities of the nasopharynx, nasal cavity or sinus. Functional causes are rare. Often the direct inspection of the nose and nasopharynx will provide some information about the underlying reason. However, before an operation, the structure and the extent of the process have to be evaluated. The possible destruction of bone or neighbouring soft tissues especially has to be considered. MRI or CT illustrates the expansion of the underlying process. In some cases, such as juvenile nasopharyngeal fibroma, angiography should also be used to display the number of blood vessels supplying the tumour (Fig. 3.51). A radiographically controlled embolisation of the tumour might be reasonable before any surgical procedure.

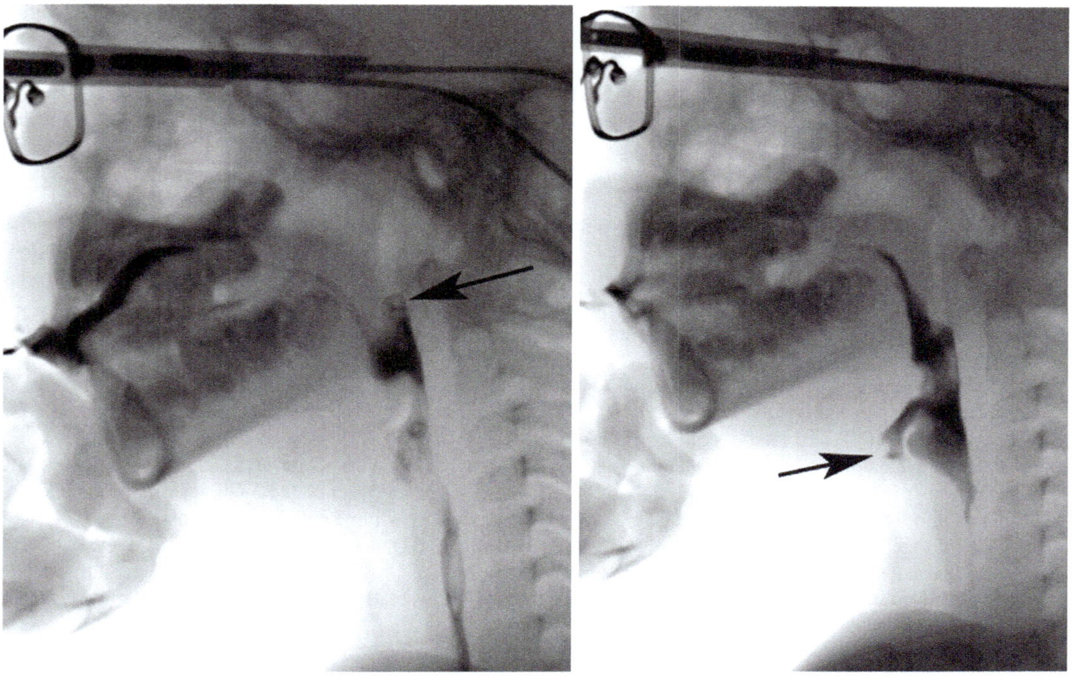

Fig. 3.50 Nine-year-old boy with juvenile dermatomyositis resulting in incomplete velopharyngeal closure (left panel, arrow) and concomitant intra-deglutitive deep penetration of contrast material (right panel, arrow)

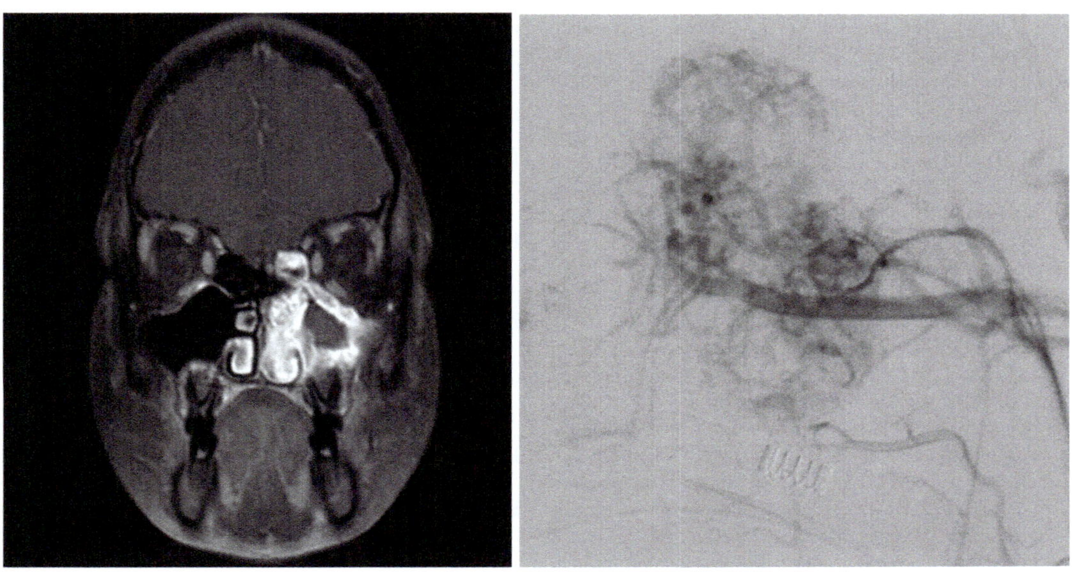

Fig. 3.51 Juvenile nasopharyngeal fibroma; MRI Gadolinium-enhanced fat-suppressed axial T1-weighted image (left panel) and angiography (right panel). (Courtesy of Clinic for Radiology, University and University Hospital Muenster (Chair: Univ.-Prof. Dr. med. Walter Heindel) 93:747–755)

References

Abou-Elsaad T, Quriba A, Baz H et al (2012) Standardization of nasometry for normal Egyptian Arabic speakers. Folia Phoniatr Logop 64(6):271–277

Abramson ZR, Peacock ZS, Cohen HL et al (2015) Radiology of cleft lip and palate: imaging for the prenatal period and throughout life. Radiographics 35(7):2053–2063

Adetayo OA, Martin MC (2012) Demographics of cleft care providers in Africa and reported experience in training and practice: direct analysis of continent-based practitioners. Cleft Palate Craniofac J 49(3):286–290

Adunka OF, Buchman CA (2011) Evaluation of the facial nerve. In: Adunka OF, Buchman CA (eds) Otology, neurotology, and lateral skull-base surgery: an illustrated handbook. (1st edn) Thieme, Stuttgart, New York, NY

Aidley D (1989) The physiology of excitable cells, 3rd edn. Cambridge University Press, Cambridge

Ainoda N, Okazaki K (1996) Results of systematic speech sound monitoring in children with cleft palate. Folia Phoniatr Logop 48(2):86–91

Al Ali A, Richmond S, Popat H et al (2015) The influence of snoring, mouth breathing and apnoea on facial morphology in late childhood: a three-dimensional study. BMJ Open 5(9):e009027

Allori AC, Mulliken JB, Meara JG et al (2017) Classification of cleft lip/palate: then and now. Cleft Palate Craniofac J 54(2):175–188

American Cleft Palate Association (2017) Parameters for evaluation and treatment of patients with cleft lip/palate or other craniofacial differences. Cleft Palate Craniofac J 55(1):137–156

American Psychological Association (APA) (2020) Dictionary of psychology. https://dictionary.apa.org/. Accessed 21 Dec 2020

American Speech-Language-Hearing Association (ASHA) (2004) Preferred practice patterns for the profession of speech-language pathology. www.asha.org/policy. Accessed 27 Aug 2020

American Speech-Language-Hearing Association (2020) Resonance disorders. https://www.asha.org/practice--portal/clinical-topics/. Accessed 25 May 2020

American Speech-Language-Hearing Association (ASHA) (2016) Practice portal for clinical topics: speech sound disorders: articulation and phonology. www.asha.org/Practice-Portal/Clinical-Topics/Articulation-and-Phonology. Accessed 3 Sept 2016

American Speech-Language-Hearing Association (ASLHA) (2004) Preferred practice patterns for the profession of speech-language pathology [preferred practice patterns]. https://www.asha.org/policy/pp2004-00191/ Accessed 21 Dec 2020

American Speech-Language-Hearing Association (ASLHA) (2021a) Resonance disorders. https://www.asha.org/practice-portal/clinical-topics/resonance--disorders. Accessed 13 Feb 2021

American Speech-Language-Hearing Association (ASLHA) (2021b) Comprehensive assessment for cleft lip and palate: typical components. https://www.asha.org/practice-portal/clinical-topics/cleft-lip-and--palate/comprehensive-assessment-for-cleft-lip-and-palate. Accessed 13th Feb 2021

Anderson RT (1996) Nasometric values for normal Spanish-speaking females: a preliminary report. Cleft Palate Craniofac J 33(4):333–336

Arcier AF, Vernay A (1994) Observation clinique: lésions musculaires labiales liées au jeu des cuivres. Médecine des Arts 8:14–19

Arendt CT, Eichler K, Mack MG et al (2021) Comparison of contrast-enhanced videofluoroscopy to unenhanced dynamic MRI in minor patients following surgical correction of velopharyngeal dysfunction. Eur Radiol 31:76–84

Awan S (1997) Analysis of nasalance: nasal view. In: Ziegler K, Deger K (eds) Clinical phonetics and linguistics. Whurr Publishers, London

Azevedo ND, Lima JC, Furlan RMMM et al (2018) Tongue pressure measurement in children with mouth-breathing behaviour. J Oral Rehabil 45(8):612–617

Baken RJ, Orlikoff RF (2000) Clinical measurement of speech and voice. Singular Publishing Group, San Diego, CA

Bakke M, Bergendal B, McAllister A et al (2007) Development and evaluation of a comprehensive screening for orofacial dysfunction. Swed Dent J 31(2):75–84

Barclay AE (1930) The normal mechanism of swallowing. Br J Radiol 3(36):534–546

Barkmeier-Kraemer JM, Clark HM (2017) Speech–language pathology evaluation and management of hyperkinetic disorders affecting speech and swallowing function. Tremor Other Hyperkinet Mov 7:489. https://doi.org/10.7916/D8Z32B30

Barr L, Thibeault SL, Muntz H et al (2007) Quality of life in children with velopharyngeal insufficiency. Arch Otolaryngol Head Neck Surg 133(3):224–229

Beals K, Dahl D, Fink R et al (2015) Speech and language technology for language disorders. De Gruyter, Berlin, Boston, MA

Beer AJ, Hellerhoff P, Zimmermann A et al (2004) Dynamic near-real-time magnetic resonance imaging for analyzing the velopharyngeal closure in comparison with videofluoroscopy. J Magn Reson Imaging 20(5):791–797

Behrman A (2007) Speech and voice science. Plural, San Diego, CA

Bell-Berti F (1976) An electromyographic study of velopharyngeal function in speech. J Speech Hear Res 19:225–240

Bernthal J, Bankson NW, Flipsen P (2013) Articulation and phonological disorders. Pearson Higher Education, New York

Bettens K, Bruneel L, Maryn Y et al (2018) Perceptual evaluation of hypernasality, audible nasal airflow and speech understandability using ordinal and visual ana-

logue scaling and their relation with nasalance scores. J Commun Disord 76:11–20
Bigenzahn W (2003) Orofaziale Dysfunktionen im Kindesalter: Grundlagen, Klinik, Ätiologie, Diagnostik und Therapie (orofacial dysfunctions in childhood: basics, clinic, aetiology, diagnostics and therapy). In: Springer L, Schrey-Dern D (eds) Forum Logopädie, 2nd edn. Thieme, Stuttgart, New York NY
Bigenzahn W, Piehslinger E, Slavicek R (1991) Computerized axiography for functional diagnosis of orofacial dysfunctions. Folia Phoniatr 43(6):275–281
Bigenzahn W, Fischman L, Mayerhofer-Kramme U (1992) Myofunctional therapy in patients with orofacial dysfunctions affecting speech. Folia Phoniatr 44(5):238–244
Billings M, Gatto K, D'Onofrio L et al (2018) Orofacial myofunctional disorders. http://iaom.com/wp--content/uploads/2018/10/OMD-Overview-IAOM.pdf. Accessed 3 Jul 2020
Binder DK, Sonne CD, Fischbein NJ (2010) Cranial nerves: anatomy, pathology, imaging, 1st edn. Thieme, New York, NY
Bishop DV, Adams C (1990) A prospective study of the relationship between specific language impairment, phonological disorders and reading retardation. J Child Psychol Psychiatry 31(7):1027–1050
Boersma P, Weenink D(2021) Praat, doing phonetics by computer. Computer program, version 6.1.40, downloaded from praat.org
Bonilha HS, Humphries K, Blair J et al (2013) Radiation exposure time during MBSS: influence of swallowing impairment severity, medical diagnosis, clinician experience, and standardized protocol use. Dysphagia 28:77–85
Boseley ME, Hartnick CJ (2004) Assessing the outcome of surgery to correct velopharyngeal insufficiency with the pediatric voice outcomes survey. Int J Pediatr Otorhinolaryngol 68(11):1429–1433
Brancamp TU, Lewis KE, Watterson T (2010) The relationship between nasalance scores and nasality ratings obtained with equal appearing interval and direct magnitude estimation scaling methods. Cleft Palate Craniofac J 47(6):631–637
Brunnegård K, van Doorn J (2009) Normative data on nasalance scores for Swedish as measured on the Nasometer: influence of dialect, gender, and age. Clin Linguist Phon 23(1):58–69
Brunnegård K, Lohmander A, van Doorn J (2012) Comparison between perceptual assessments of nasality and nasalance scores. Int J Lang Commun Disord 47(5):556–566
Bzoch KR (1989) Measurements and assessment of categorical aspects of cleft palate language, voice and speech disorders. In: Bzoch KR (ed) Communicative disorders related to cleft lip and palate. College-Hill Press, Boston, MA
Cahill LM, Turner AB, Stabler PA et al (2004) An evaluation of continuous positive airway pressure (CPAP) therapy in the treatment of hypernasality following traumatic brain injury: a report of 3 cases. J Head Trauma Rehabil 19(3):241–253
Chegar BE, Shprintzen RJ, Curtis MS et al (2007) Pharyngeal flap and obstructive apnea: maximizing speech outcome while limiting complications. Arch Facial Plast Surg 9(4):252–259
Chen MY (1997) Acoustic correlates of English and French nasalized vowels. J Acoust Soc Am 102:2360–2370
Cheung PSP, Ng A, To CKS (2006) Hong Kong Cantonese articulation test. Language Information Sciences Research Centre, City University of Hong Kong, Hong Kong
CHILDES (2014) Child language data exchange system. http://childes.talkbank.org/. Accessed 1 June 2014
Ciocca V, Whitehill TL, Ng SS (2002) Contour tone production by Cantonese speakers with cerebral palsy. J Med Speech Lang Pathol 10(4):243–248
Clark HM (2005) Clinical decision making and oral motor treatments. ASHA Leader 10(8):8–35
Clemente MP, Moreira A, Morais C, Amarante JM, Ferreira AP, Mendes J (2021) Tooth Position in Wind Instrument Players: Dentofacial Cephalometric Analysis. Int J Environ Res Public Health. 18(8):4306. https://doi.org/10.3390/ijerph18084306. PMID: 33921609 ; PMCID: PMC8073265
Copeland M (1990) The effects of very early palatal repair on speech. Br J Plast Surg 43(6):676–682
Coplan J, Gleason JR (1988) Unclear speech: recognition and significance of unintelligible speech in preschool children. Pediatrics 82(3):447–452
Counihan DT, Cullinan WL (1970) Reliability and dispersion of nasality ratings. Cleft Palate J 7(1):261–270
Croft CB, Shprintzen RJ, Rakoff SJ (1981) Patterns of velopharyngeal valving in normal and cleft palate subjects: a multi-view videofluoroscopic and nasendoscopic study. Laryngoscope 91(2):265–271
Curtis JF (1970) The acoustics of nasalized speech. Cleft Palate J 7:480–496
Czermak JN (1860) Der Kehllkopfspiegel und seine Verwertung in Physiologie und Medizin (the laryngeal mirror and its utilization in physiology and medicine). Engelmann, Leipzig
Czech NP, Alt KW (2024) Wind Instruments and Oral Health: Challenges Faced by Professional Wind Musicians. Dent J (Basel). 12(10):306. https://doi.org/10.3390/dj12100306.PMID:39452434; PMCID: PMC11505960.
Dale PS (1991) The validity of a parent report measure of vocabulary and syntax at 24 months. J Speech Hear Res 34(3):565–571
Dalston RM (2004) The use of nasometry in the assessment and remediation of velopharyngeal inadequacy. In: Bzoch KR (ed) Communicative disorders related to cleft lip and palate. Pro-Ed, Boston, pp 493–516
Dalston RM, Warren DW, Dalston ET (1991) Use of nasometry as a diagnostic tool for identifying patients with velopharyngeal impairment. Cleft Palate Craniofac J 28(2):184–188

Dalston RM, Neiman GS, Gonzalez-Landa G (1993) Nasometric sensitivity and specificity: a cross-dialect and cross-culture study. Cleft Palate Craniofac J 30(3):285–291

Darwin C, de Beer G, Wright MA (1872) The expression of the emotions in man and animals. John Murray, London

Davenport R, Manji H (2018) The nervous system. In: Innes JA, Dover AR, Fairhurst K (eds) Macleod's clinical examination, 14th edn. Elsevier, Amsterdam, pp 119–150

Davis JS, Ritchie HP (1922) Classification of congenital clefts of the lip and palate. JAMA 79(16):1323–1327

de Arruda B, Telles F, Ferreira RI, Magalhaes L et al (2009) Effects of breast-and bottle-feeding duration on the age of pacifier use persistence. Braz Oral Res 23(4):432–438

de Boer G, Bressmann T (2015) Application of linear discriminant analysis to the nasometric assessment of resonance disorders: a pilot study. Cleft Palate Craniofac J 52:73–82

de Boer G, Bressmann T (2016) Application of linear discriminant analysis to the long-term averaged spectra of simulated disorders of oral-nasal balance. Cleft Palate Craniofac J 53(5):e163–e171

de Langen-Müller U, Kiese-Himmel C, Neumann K et al (equal authorship) (2012) Diagnostik von (umschriebenen) Sprachentwicklungsstörungen, 1st edn. Peter Lang, Frankfurt am Main

Dejonckere PH, van Wijngaarden HA (2001) Retropharyngeal autologous fat transplantation for congenital short palate: a nasometric assessment of functional results. Ann Otol Rhinol Laryngol 110(2):168–172

Depret MMP (2005) Articulatory and glottal alternative motion rate (AMR) in subjects with or without neurological disorders. Dissertation, Universidade Federal de São Paulo (UNIFESP)

Dharmaperwira-Prins R (2009) Dysartrie en verbale apraxie; Dyva-onderzoek: Beschrijving, onderzoek, behandeling; dysartrie en verbale apraxie onderzoek, 4e ongew. In: Dr Dysarthria and verbal apraxia; Dyva examination: description, examination, treatment; dysarthria and verbal apraxia examination, 4th edn. Harcourt, Amsterdam

Dilling H, Mombour W, Schmidt MH (2008) Internationale Klassifikation psychischer Störungen, 6th edn. Hans Huber, Bern

Dodd B (2005) Differential diagnosis and treatment of children with speech disorder, 2nd edn. Whurr, London

Dodd B (2014) Differential diagnosis of pediatric speech sound disorder. Curr Dev Disord Rep 1(3):189–196

Dotevall H, Lohmander-Agerskov A, Almquist SA et al (1998) Aerodynamic assessment of velopharyngeal function during normal speech containing different places of articulation. Folia Phoniatr Logop 50(2):53–63

Dotevall H, Ejnell H, Bake B (2001) Nasal airflow patterns during the velopharyngeal closing phase in speech in children with and without cleft palate. Cleft Palate Craniofac J 38(4):358–373

Dotevall H, Lohmander-Agerskov A, Ejnell H et al (2002) Perceptual evaluation of speech and velopharyngeal function in children with and without cleft palate and the relationship to nasal airflow patterns. Cleft Palate Craniofac J 39(4):409–424

Drissi C, Mitrofanoff M, Talandier C et al (2011) Feasibility of dynamic MRI for evaluating velopharyngeal insufficiency in children. Eur Radiol 21(7):1462–1469

Duffy JR (2012) Motor speech disorders: substrates, differential diagnosis, and management, 3rd edn. Mosby, St. Louis, MO

Duffy JR (2016) Functional speech disorders: clinical manifestations, diagnosis, and management. Handb Clin Neurol 139:379–388

Dunaway C (2004) Articulation differences and disorders manual. Claudia Dunaway Consulting. San Diego, CA. http://www.thinkspeaksuccess.com/wp-content/uploads/2012/10/Articulation-Differences-and-Disorders-Manual.pdf. Accessed 21 Dec 2020

Enderby PM (1983) Frenchay dysarthria assessment. College-Hill Press, San Diego, CA

Enderby PM (2013) Disorders of communication: Dysarthria. Handb Clin Neurol 110:273–281

Ege P, Acarlar F, Turan F (2004) Ankara Artikülasyon Testi. Key Tasarim, Ankara

Fairbanks G (1960) Voice and articulation drillbook, 2nd edn. Harper & Row, New York, NY, pp 124–139

Falé I, Hub Faria I (2008) Nasometric values for European Portuguese: preliminary results. ISCA Workshop on Experimental Linguistics, Athens, Greece

Fattah AY, Gurusinghe ADR, Gavilan J et al (2015) Facial nerve grading instruments: systematic review of the literature and suggestion for uniformity. Plast Reconstr Surg 135(2):569–579

Felten DL, O'Banion MK, Maida ME (2015) Brain stem and cerebellum. In: Felten DL, O'Banion MK, Maida ME (eds) Netter's atlas of neuroscience, 3rd edn. Elsevier, Amsterdam, pp 71–75

Ferreira GZ, Bressmann T, de Cássia Rillo Dutka J et al (2020) Analysis of oral-nasal balance after intensive speech therapy combined with speech bulb in speakers with cleft palate and hypernasality. J Commun Disord 85:105945. https://doi.org/10.1016/j.jcomdis.2019.105945

Finck C, Gaspard M, Melon J (1987) Evaluation fonctionelle d'une insuffisance velaire par rhinomanometrie anterieure (functional assessment of velar insufficiency by anterior rhinomanometry). Folia Phoniatr 39:192–195

Fletcher S (1970) Theory and instrumentation for quantitative measurement of nasality. Cleft Palate J 7(2):601–609

Fletcher SG (1972) Contingencies for bioelectronic modification of nasality. J Speech Hear Disord 37(3):329–346

Fletcher SG, Bishop ME (1970) Measurement of nasality with tonar. Cleft Palate J 7(2):610–621

Fletcher SG, Frost SD (1974) Quantitative and graphic analysis of prosthetic treatment for "nasalance" in speech. J Prosthet Dent 32(3):284–291
Flipsen P Jr, Ogiela DA (2015) Psychometric characteristics of single-word tests of children's speech sound production. Lang Speech Hear Serv Sch 46(2):166–178
Forner LL (1983) Speech segment durations produced by five and six year old speakers with and without cleft palates. Cleft Palate J 20(3):185–198
Fourier J (1808) Mémoire sur la propagation de la chaleur dans les corps solides, présenté le 21 Décembre 1807 à l'Institut national—Nouveau Bulletin des sciences par la Société philomatique de Paris. I. (Dissertation on the propagation of heat in solid bodies, presented on December 21, 1807 to the National Institute—Nouveau Bulletin des sciences by the Philomatic Society of Paris. I) Bernard, Paris
Fox-Boyer A (2014) Psycholinguistische Analyse kindlicher Aussprachestörungen (PLAKKS-II) (revised edition of PLAKKS, 2002). Pearson Assessment, Frankfurt
Fox-Boyer A, Salgert K, Clausen MC (2016) Diagnostik von kindlichen Aussprachestörungen unklarer Genese. Sprache Stimme Gehör 40(02):61–67
Foy R (1910) Contribution rhinométrique à l'étude de la respiration nasale (Rhinometric contribution to the study of nasal breathing). Annales des maladies de l'oreille, du larynx, du nez et du pharynx 36:130–149
Francis DO, Chinnadurai S, Morad A et al (2015) Treatments for ankyloglossia and ankyloglossia with concomitant lip-tie. Rockville: Agency for Healthcare Research and Quality (US). Comparative Effectiveness Reviews, No. 149. https://www.effectivehealthcare.ahrq.gov/ehc/products/558/2074/ankyloglossia-report-150504.pdf. Accessed 7 May 2017
Freitas J, Teixeira A, Silva S et al (2015) Velar movement assessment for speech interfaces: an exploratory study using surface electromyography. In: Plantier G, Schultz T, Fred A et al (eds) Biomedical engineering systems and technologies. Springer International, Cham, pp 246–260
Fritzell B (1969) The velopharyngeal muscles in speech: an electromyographic and cineradiographic study. Acta Otolaryngol Suppl 250:1
Frush D (2014) Radiation risks to children from medical imaging. Rev Med Clin Condes 24:15–20
Garliner D (1974) Myofunctional therapy in dental practice. Bartel, New York, NY
Gatto K, Chastain A, Frey L et al (2018) Airway and myofunctional screening in the dental office. www.iaom.com/wp-content/uploads/2019/04/Airway-and-myofunctional-screening-in-the-dental-office.pdf. Accessed 3 Jul 2020
Gentil M (1992) Phonetic intelligibility testing in dysarthria for the use of French language clinicians. Clin Linguist Phon 6(3):179–189
Giannantoni NM, Minisci M, Brunetti V et al (2016) Evaluation of pharyngeal muscle activity through nasopharyngeal surface electromyography in a cohort of dysphagic patients with acute ischaemic stroke. Acta Otorhinolaryngol Ital 36(4):295–299
Glaspey AM, Stoel-Gammon C (2007) A dynamic approach to phonological assessment. Adv Speech Lang Pathol 9(4):286–296
Golabbakhsh M, Abnavi F, Kadkhodaei Elyaderani M et al (2017) Automatic identification of hypernasality in normal and cleft lip and palate patients with acoustic analysis of speech. J Acoust Soc Am 141:929–935
Golding-Kushner KJ (2015) Issues in speech development and management of children with craniofacial disorders, cleft palate and velopharyngeal dysfunction. In: Bowen C (ed) Children's speech sound disorders. Wiley-Blackwell, Oxford, pp 137–142
Golding-Kushner KJ, Argamaso RV, Cotton RT et al (1990) Standardization for the reporting of nasopharyngoscopy and multiview videofluoroscopy: a report from an international working group. Cleft Palate J 27(4):337–347. discussion 347-348
Goldstein B, Iglesias A (2006) CPACS: contextual probes of articulation competence: Spanish. Super Duper, Greenville
Grech H, Dodd B, Franklin S (2011) Maltese-English Speech Assessment (MESA). University of Malta, Guardamangia
Grunwell P (1993) Analysing cleft palate speech. Whurr Publishers, London
Grunwell P, Brondsted K, Henningsson G et al (2000) A six-centre international study of the outcome of treatment in patients with clefts of the lip and palate: the results of a cross-linguistic investigation of cleft palate speech. Scand J Plast Reconstr Surg Hand Surg 34(3):219–229
Guilleminault C, Sullivan SS (2014) Towards restoration of continuous nasal breathing as the ultimate treatment goal in pediatric obstructive sleep apnea. Enliven 1(1):1–5
Guindi GM, Payne JK, Higenbottam TW (1981) Clinical electromyography in ear, nose and throat practice. J Laryngol Otol 95:407–413
Gutzmann H (1913) Untersuchungen über das Wesen der Nasalität. (studies on the nature of nasality.). Archiv Laryngol Rhinol 27:59–128
Guyette TW, Carpenter MA (1988) Accuracy of pressure-flow estimates of velopharyngeal orifice size in an analog model and human subjects. J Speech Hear Res 31(4):537–548
Guyette TW, Smith BE, Reisberg DJ (1994) Aerodynamic estimates of induced anterior orifice openings in human subjects. Cleft Palate Craniofac J 31(3):185–192
Guyton KB, Sandage MJ, Bailey D et al (2018) Acquired velopharyngeal dysfunction: survey, literature review, and clinical recommendations. Am J Speech Lang Pathol 27(4):1572–1597
Haapanen ML (1991) Nasalance scores in normal Finnish speech. Folia Phoniatr (Basel) 43(4):197–203
Haapanen ML, Liu L, Hiltunen T et al (1996) Cul-de-sac hypernasality test with pattern recognition of LPC indices. Folia Phoniatr Logop 48:35–43

Hahn V (1997) Untersuchung zur oralstereognostischen Leistung bei orofazialen Dyskinesien (investigation of oral stereostatic performance in orofacial dyskinesias). Sprache-Stimme-Gehör 21:185–191

Hairston LE, Sauerland EK (1981) Electromyography of the human palate: discharge patterns of the levator and tensor velipalatini. Electromyogr Clin Neurophysiol 21:287–297

Hammer MJ, Jones CA, Mielens JD et al (2014) Evaluating the tongue-hold maneuver using high-resolution manometry and electromyography. Dysphagia 29(5):564–570

Hardin MA, Van Demark DR, Morris HL et al (1992) Correspondence between nasalance scores and listener judgments of hypernasality and hyponasality. Cleft Palate Craniofac J 29(4):346–351

Hartelius L, Runmarker B, Andersen O (2000) Prevalence and characteristics of dysarthria in a multiple-sclerosis incidence cohort: relation to neurological data. Folia Phoniatr Logop 52(4):160–177

Havstam C, Lohmander A, Persson C et al (2005) Evaluation of VPI-assessment with videofluoroscopy and nasoendoscopy. Br J Plast Surg 58(7):922–931

Hayden C, Klimacka L (2000) Inter-rater reliability in cleft palate speech assessment. J Clin Excel 2:169–173

Hayes B (1995) Metrical stress theory: principles and case studies. University of Chicago Press, Chicago, IL

Heisenberg W (1927) Über den anschaulichen Inhalt der quantentheoretischen Kinematik und Mechanik (about the descriptive content of quantum theoretical kinematics and mechanics.). Z Phys 43(3–4):172–198

Hemprich A, Eggeling V, Becker R (1984) Die Nasoendoskopie—eine Methode zur objektiven Beurteilung des velopharyngealen Abschlusses (Nasal endoscopy—a method for objective assessment of velopharyngeal closure). Dtsch Z Mund Kiefer Gesichtschir 8:461–464

Henningsson GE, Isberg AM (1991a) A cineradiographic study of velopharyngeal movements for deviant versus non-deviant articulation. Cleft Palate Craniofac J 28(1):115–118

Henningsson G, Isberg A (1991b) Comparison between multiview videofluoroscopy and nasendoscopy of velopharyngeal movements. Cleft Palate Craniofac J 28(4):413–417. discussion 417-418

Henningsson GE, Kuehn DP, Sell D et al (2008) Universal parameters for reporting speech outcomes in individuals with cleft palate. Cleft Palate Craniofac J 45(1):2–17

Hillarp B, Ekberg O, Jacobsson S et al (1994) Myotonic dystrophy revealed at videoradiography of deglutition and speech in adult patients with velopharyngeal insufficiency: presentation of four cases. Cleft Palate Craniofac J 31:125–133

Hilton W (1836) Case of a large bony tumour in the face completely removed by spontaneous separation. Observations upon some of the functions of the soft palate and pharynx. Guys Hosp Rep 1:493–506

Hirschberg J, Van Demark DR (1997) A proposal for standardization of speech and hearing evaluations to assess velopharyngeal function. Folia Phoniatr Logop 49(3–4):158–167

Hirschberg J, Bok S, Juhasz M et al (2006) Adaptation of nasometry to Hungarian language and experiences with its clinical application. Int J Pediatr Otorhinolaryngol 70(5):785–798

Hixon TJ, Weismer G, Hoit JD (2008) Preclinical speech science. Plural, San Diego, CA

Hogen Esch TT, Dejonckere PH (2004) Objectivating nasality in healthy and velopharyngeal insufficient children with the Nasalance acquisition system (NasalView). Defining minimal required speech tasks assessing normative values for Dutch language. Int J Pediatr Otorhinolaryngol 68(8):1039–1046

Honjo I, Kumazawa T, Honda K et al (1979) Electromyographic study of patients with dysfunction of the Eustachian tube. Arch Otolaryngol 222:47–51

Horii Y (1980) An accelerometric approach to nasality measurement: a preliminary report. Cleft Palate J 17(3):254–261

Huang YS, Guilleminault C (2013) Pediatric obstructive sleep apnea and the critical role of oral-facial growth: evidences. Front Neurol 3:184. https://doi.org/10.3389/fneur.2012.00184

ICD-10-GM (2020) Deutsches Institut für Medizinische Dokumentation und Information DIMDI (German Institute of Medical Documentation and Information). https://www.dimdi.de/static/de/klassifikationen/icd/icd-10-gm/kode-suche/htmlgm2020/. Accessed 30 Dec 2021

International Phonetic Association (IPA) (1999) Handbook of the International Phonetic Association: a guide to the use of the International Phonetic Alphabet. Cambridge University Press, Cambridge

IPA (2015) IPA Chart. http://www.internationalphoneticassociation.org/content/ipa-chart, available under a Creative Commons Attribution-Sharealike 3.0 Unported License. Copyright © 2015 International Phonetic Association

Jones D (1972) An outline of English phonetics, 9th edn. W. Heffer & Sons, Cambridge

John A, Sell D, Sweeney T et al (2006) The cleft audit protocol for speech-augmented: a validated and reliable measure for auditing cleft speech. Cleft Palate Craniofac J 43(3):272–288

Johnson K (2012) Acoustic and auditory phonetics, 2nd edn. Blackwell, Oxford

Kamere DB (1978) Electromyographic correlation of tensor tympani and tensor velipalatini muscles in man. Laryngoscope 88:651–662

Karnell MP (2011) Instrumental assessment of velopharyngeal closure for speech. Semin Speech Lang 32(2):168–178

Karnell MP, Ibuki K, Morris HL et al (1983) Reliability of the nasopharyngeal fiberscope (NPF) for assessing velopharyngeal function: analysis by judgment. Cleft Palate J 20:199–208

Kataoka R, Michi K, Okabe K et al (1996) Spectral properties and quantitative evaluation of hypernasality in vowels. Cleft Palate Craniofac J 33:43–50

Kataoka R, Warren DW, Zajac DJ et al (2001) The relationship between spectral characteristics and perceived hypernasality in children. J Acoust Soc Am 109:2181–2189
Kauschke C, Siegmüller J (2009) Patholinguistische Diagnostik bei Sprachentwicklungsstörungen (PDSS), 2nd edn. Elsevier, Amsterdam
Kavanagh JL, Fee EJ, Kalinoswki J et al (1994) Nasometric value for three dialectal groups within the Atlantic provinces of Canada. J Speech Lang Pathol Audiol 18(1):7–13
Keller T (2014) ROC-Analysen. http://www.acomed-statistik.de/roc-kurve.html. Accessed 1 June 2014
Kent RD (1996) Hearing and believing: some limits to the auditory-perceptual assessment of speech and voice disorders. Am J Speech Lang Pathol 5(3):7–23
Kernahan DA (1971) The striped Y—a symbolic classification for cleft lip and palate. Plast Reconstr Surg 47(5):469–470
Kernahan DA, Stark RB (1958) A new classification for cleft lip and cleft palate. Plast Reconstr Surg Transplant Bull 22(5):435–441
Keuning KH, Wieneke GH, Dejonckere PH (1999) The intrajudge reliability of the perceptual rating of cleft palate speech before and after pharyngeal flap surgery: the effect of judges and speech samples. Cleft Palate Craniofac J 36(4):328–333
Keuning KH, Wieneke GH, van Wijngaarden HA et al (2002) The correlation between nasalance and a differentiated perceptual rating of speech in Dutch patients with velopharyngeal insufficiency. Cleft Palate Craniofac J 39(3):277–284
Keuning KH, Wieneke GH, Dejonckere PH (2004) Correlation between the perceptual rating of speech in Dutch patients with velopharyngeal insufficiency and composite measures derived from mean nasalance scores. Folia Phoniatr Logop 56(3):157–164
Kiliç (2019) Nazal ve oro-farengeal rezonans bozuklukları (nasal and oro-pharyngeal resonance disorders). In: Yiğit Ö, Kara CÖ, Alkan Z (eds) Kulak burun boğaz ve baş boyun cerrahisi uzmanlık eğitimi: Kaynak kitap—2. (Ear, nose throat and head and neck surgery specialty training: Source book—2.). Logos Yayıncılık Tic. A.Ş, Istanbul, pp 617–621
Kim Y, Shin M (2004) Urimal Test of Articulation and Phonology (U-TAP). Hakjisa Publisher, Seoul
Kim M, Pae S, Bak C (2007) Assessment of Phonology and Articulation for Children (APAC). Human Brain Research and Consulting Company, Inchon
Kirk C, Vigeland L (2014) A psychometric review of norm-referenced tests used to assess phonological error patterns. Lang Speech Hear Serv Sch 45(4):365–377
Kliegman RM, Stanton BF, St. Geme JW et al (eds) (2011) Nelson textbook of pediatrics, 19th edn. Elsevier, Philadelphia
Kunnari S, Savinainen-Makkonen T, Saaristo-Helin K (2012) Fonologiatesti. Niilo Mäki Instituutti, Jyväskylä
Knuijt S, de Swart BJM (2007) Handleiding 'Radboud Dysartrieonderzoek' (Manual 'Radboud Dysarthria Examination'). www.umcn.nl/logopedie. Accessed 27 May 2020
Kobayashi Y, Kanamori D, Fujii N et al (2019) Velopharyngeal closure analysis using four-dimensional computed tomography: a pilot study of healthy volunteers and adult patients with cleft palate. BMC Med Imaging 19(1):54. https://doi.org/10.1186/s12880-019-0350-4
Kobrynski LJ, Sullivan KE (2007) Velocardiofacial syndrome, DiGeorge syndrome: the chromosome 22q11.2 deletion syndromes. Lancet 370(9596):1443–1452
Koch H, Grzonka M, Koch J (1995) Cleft malformation of lip, alveolus, hard and soft palate, and nose (LAHSN)—a critical view of the terminology, the diagnosis and gradation as a basis for documentation and therapy. Br J Oral Maxillofac Surg 33(1):51–58
Kreiman J, Gerratt BR, Kempster GB et al (1993) Perceptual evaluation of voice quality: review, tutorial, and a framework for future research. J Speech Hear Res 36(1):21–40
Kriens O (1989) LAHSHAL—a concise documentation system for cleft lip, alveolus and palate diagnoses. In: Kriens O (ed) What is a cleft lip and palate? A multidisciplinary update. Workshop, Bremen 1987. Thieme, Stuttgart
Kuehn DP, Moller KT (2000) Speech and language issues in the cleft palate population: the state of the art. Cleft Palate Craniofac J 37(4):348–348
Kulinna-Cosentini C, Czerny C, Baumann A et al (2016) TrueFisp versus HASTE sequences in 3T cine MRI: evaluation of image quality during phonation in patients with velopharyngeal insufficiency. Eur Radiol 26(9):2892–2898
Kumar TVA, Kuriakose S (2004) Ultrasonographic evaluation of effectiveness of circumoral muscle exercises in adenotonsillectomized children. J Clin Pediatr Dent 29(1):49–55
Kummer AW (2011a) Disorders of resonance and airflow secondary to cleft palate and/or velopharyngeal dysfunction. Semin Speech Lang 32(2):141–149
Kummer AW (2011b) Types and causes of velopharyngeal dysfunction. Semin Speech Lang 32(2):150–158
Kummer AW, Lee L (1996) Evaluation and treatment of resonance disorders. Lang Speech Hear Serv Sch 27:271–281
Ladefoged P (2006) A course in phonetics, 5th edn. Thomson Wadsworth, Boston
Laine T, Warren DW, Dalston RM et al (1988) Screening of velopharyngeal closure based on nasal airflow rate measurements. Cleft Palate J 25(3):220–225
Lam DJ, Starr JR, Perkins JA et al (2006) A comparison of nasendoscopy and multiview videofluoroscopy in assessing velopharyngeal insufficiency. Otolaryngol Head Neck Surg 134(3):394–402
Law J, Boyle J, Harris F et al (2000) The feasibility of universal screening for primary speech and language delay: findings from a systematic review of the literature. Dev Med Child Neurol 42(3):190–200
Lee A, Browne U (2013) Nasalance scores for typical Irish English-speaking adults. Logoped Phoniatr Vocol 38(4):167–172

Lee ASY, Ciocca V, Whitehill TL (2003) Acoustic correlates of hypernasality. Clin Linguist Phon 17(4–5):259–264
Lee GS, Yang CC, Wang CP et al (2005) Effect of nasal decongestion on voice spectrum of a nasal consonant-vowel. J Voice 19(1):71–77
Lee GS, Wang CP, Fu S (2009) Evaluation of hypernasality in vowels using voice low tone to high tone ratio. Cleft Palate Craniofac J 46(1):47–52
Lefarth FL (2019) Sonographische Untersuchungen der Mundlippen. Inaugural dissertation, Heinrich-Heine-Universität, Düsseldorf
Lefarth F, Angerstein W (2013) Sonografische Diagnostik von Narbengewebe im Musculus orbicularis oris. forum. HNO 15(5):187–192
Leuchter I (2015) Clinical aspects of velopharyngeal insufficiency (privat-docent). University of Geneva, Geneva
Leuchter I (2017) Normative nasalance values in a population of French-speaking children. In: Paper presented at the Annual Congress of the French Society of Phoniatry, Nice, France, 24-25 November 2017
Lewis KE, Watterson TL, Houghton SM (2003) The influence of listener experience and academic training on ratings of nasality. J Commun Disord 36(1):49–58
Li C, Lundervold A (1958) Electromyographic study of cleft palate. J Plast Reconstr Surg 21:427–432
Lingala SG, Sutton BP, Miquel ME et al (2016) Recommendations for real-time speech MRI. J Magn Reson Imaging 43(1):28–44
Litin S (2009) Mayo Clinic family health book, 4th edn. Simon & Schuster, New York, NY
Litzaw LL, Dalston RM (1992) The effect of gender upon nasalance scores among normal adult speakers. J Commun Disord 25(1):55–64
Llobet JRI (2005) New tools for the assessment of the embouchure's biomechanics. ITG J 29(5):51–53. 81
Lohmander A, Borell E, Henningsson G et al (2005) SVANTE- Svenskt artikulations- och Nasalittets Test: Pedagogisk Design. Skivarp, Sweden
Lohmander A, Olsson M (2004) Methodology for perceptual assessment of speech in patients with cleft palate: a critical review of the literature. Cleft Palate Craniofac J 41(1):64–70
Lohmander A, Willadsen E, Persson C et al (2009) Methodology for speech assessment in the Scandcleft project—an international randomized clinical trial on palatal surgery: experiences from a pilot study. Cleft Palate Craniofac J 46(4):347–362
Lohmander-Agerskov A, Dotevall H, Lith A et al (1996) Speech and velopharyngeal function in children with an open residual cleft in the hard palate, and the influence of temporary covering. Cleft Palate Craniofac J 33(4):324–332
Maarse W, Bergé SJ, Pistorius L et al (2010) Diagnostic accuracy of transabdominal ultrasound in detecting prenatal cleft lip and palate: a systematic review. Ultrasound Obstet Gynecol 35(4):495–502
Maarse W, Pistorius LR, van Eeten WK et al (2011) Prenatal ultrasound screening for orofacial clefts. Ultrasound Obstet Gynecol 38(4):434–439
MacWhinney B (1995) The CHILDES project: tools for analyzing talk, 2nd edn. Erlbaum, Mahwah
Maegawa J, Sells RK, David DJ (1998) Speech changes after maxillary advancement in 40 cleft lip and palate patients. J Craniofac Surg 9(2):177–182. discussion 183-174
Maier A, Haderlein T, Stelzle F et al (2010) Automatic speech recognition systems for the evaluation of voice and speech disorders in head and neck cancer. Eurasip J Audio Speech Music Process 2010:1–7
Mason RM, Franklin H (2014) Orofacial myofunctional disorders and otolaryngologists. Otolaryngology 4(4):1–3
Mayo R, Floyd LA, Warren DW et al (1996) Nasalance and nasal area values: cross-racial study. Cleft Palate Craniofac J 33(2):143–149
McComb RW, Marrinan EM, Nuss RC et al (2011) Predictors of velopharyngeal insufficiency after Le fort I maxillary advancement in patients with cleft palate. J Oral Maxillofac Surg 69(8):2226–2232
McIntosh B, Dodd B (2011) Toddler Phonology Test (TPT). Pearson Education, London
McLeod S (2012a) Multilingual children's speech. http://www.csu.edu.au/research/multilingual-speech/. Accessed 28 May 2016
McLeod S (2012b) Summary of 250 cross-linguistic studies of speech acquisition. http://www.csu.edu.au/research/multilingual-speech/speech-acquisition. Accessed 28 May 2016
McLeod S (2012c) Multilingual speech assessments. http://www.csu.edu.au/research/multilingual-speech/speech-assessments. Accessed 28 May 2016
McLeod S, Verdon S (2014) A review of 30 speech assessments in 19 languages other than English. Am J Speech Lang Pathol 23(4):708–723
McLeod S, Verdon S, Bowen C (2013) International aspirations for speech-language pathologists' practice with multilingual children with speech sound disorders: development of a position paper. J Commun Disord 46(4):375–387
McLeod S, Crowe K, Shahaeian A (2015) Intelligibility in Context Scale: normative and validation data for English-speaking preschoolers. Lang Speech Hear Serv Sch 46(3):266–276
Methfessel G (1995) Die Bedeutung von Form und Funktion im Kiefer- Gesichtsbereich für das Blasinstrument. In: Wagner C (ed) Medizinische Probleme bei Instrumentalisten. Laaber-Verlag, Laaber, pp 209–221
Metz DE, Schiavetti N, Knight SD (1992) The use of artificial neural networks to estimate speech intelligibility from acoustic variables: a preliminary analysis. J Commun Disord 25(1):43–53
Michaelis R (2004) Das Grenzsteinprinzip als Orientierungshilfe für die pädiatrische Entwicklungsbetrachtung. In: Schlack HG (ed) Entwicklungspädiatrie. Marseille, München, pp 123–129
Miller J, Andriacchi K, Nockerts A (2011) Assessing language production using SALT software: a clinician's guide to language sample analysis. SALT Software LLC, Middleton

Miller N (2013) Measuring up to speech intelligibility. Int J Lang Commun Disord 48(6):601–612
Miller N, Lowit A (2014) Motor speech disorders. Multilingual Matters, Bristol, Blue Ridge Summit, PA
Mishima K, Sugii A, Yamada T et al (2008) Dialectal and gender differences in nasalance scores in a Japanese population. J Craniomaxillofac Surg 36(1):8–10
Moll KL (1962) Velopharyngeal closure on vowels. J Speech Hear Res 5(1):30–37
Moller KT, Starr CD (1984) The effects of listening conditions on speech rating obtained in a clinical setting. Cleft Palate J 21(2):65–69
Moore WH, Sommers RK (1975) Phonetic contexts: their effects on perceived intelligibility in clef-palate speakers. Folia Phoniatr (Basel) 27(06):410–422
Morgan A, O'Gara M (2014) Therapy principles for children with cleft palate. In: Paper presented at the Annual Convention of the American Speech-Language-Hearing Association, Orlando, FL
Morice A, Renault F, Soupre V et al (2018) Predictors of speech outcomes in children with Pierre Robin sequence. J Craniomaxillofac Surg 46(3):479–484
Morris HL, Spriestersbach DC, Darley FL (1961) An articulation test for assessing competency of velopharyngeal closure. J Speech Hear Res 4(1):48–55
Munshi AK, Hegde AM, Srinath SK (2000) Ultrasonographic and electromyographic evaluation of the labial musculature in children with repaired cleft lips. J Clin Pediatr Dent 24(2):123–128
Murdoch BE, Theodoros DG (2001) Traumatic brain injury: associated speech language and swallowing disorders. Singular Publishing Group, San Diego, CA
Murdoch BE, Theodoros DG, Stokes PD et al (1993) Abnormal patterns of speech breathing in dysarthric speakers following severe closed head injury. Brain Inj 7(4):295–308
Namasivayam AK, Pukonen M, Goshulak D et al (2013) Relationship between speech motor control and speech intelligibility in children with speech sound disorders. J Commun Disord 46(3):264–280
Neiswanger K, Weinberg SM, Rogers CR et al (2007) Orbicularis oris muscle defects as an expanded phenotypic feature in nonsyndromic cleft lip with or without cleft palate. Am J Med Genet A 143A(11):1143–1149
Nellis JL, Neiman GS, Lehman JA (1992) Comparison of Nasometer and listener judgments of nasality in the assessment of velopharyngeal function after pharyngeal flap surgery. Cleft Palate Craniofac J 29(2):157–163
Neumann K, Euler HA (2013) Kann ein Sprachstandsscreening zwischen Sprachförder- und Sprachtherapiebedarf trennen? In: Redder A, Weinert S (eds) Sprachförderung und Sprachdiagnostik - interdisziplinäre Perspektiven. Waxmann, Münster, pp 297–321
Neumann K, Keilmann A, Rosenfeld J et al (2009) Leitlinien der Deutschen Gesellschaft für Phoniatrie und Pädaudiologie zu Sprachentwicklungsstörungen bei Kindern (gekürzte Fassung). Kindh Entwickl 18(4):222–231
Neumann K, Holler-Zittlau I, van Minnen S et al (2011) Katzengoldstandards in der Sprachstandserfassung. Sensitivität-Spezifität des Kindersprachscreenings (KiSS). HNO 59(1):97–109
Neumann S, Romonath R (2012) Application of the international classification of functioning, disability and health—children and youth version (ICF-CY) to cleft lip and palate. Cleft Palate Craniofac J 49(3):325–346
Nichols AC (1999) Nasalance statistics for two Mexican populations. Cleft Palate Craniofac J 36(1):57–63
Nicolosi L, Harryman E, Kresheck J (2003) Terminology of communication disorders. Speech-language-hearing, 5th edn. Lippincott Williams & Wilkins, Philadelphia
Nishio M (2004) Assessment of motor speech for dysarthria (AMSD). Interuna, Tokyo
Nolting PT, Koch R, Werkmeister R et al (2002) Cleft data—Programm zur minimal Dokumentation der LKG-Spalten (cleft data. Programme for minimal documentation of lip-jaw-palate clefts). Mund Kiefer Gesichtschir 6(3):140–145
Okalidou A, Karathanasi A, Grigoraki E (2011) Nasalance norms in Greek adults. Clin Linguist Phon 25(8):671–688
Ortega ADOL, Ciamponi AL, Mendes FM et al (2009) Assessment scale of the oral motor performance of children and adolescents with neurological damages. J Oral Rehabil 36(9):653–659
Orth H, Block R (1987) Die Beeinflussung orofazialer Funktionen durch die Wirbelsäulenhaltung (the influencing of orofacial functions by spine posture). Kinderarzt 18(9):1174–1177
Padovani M, Gielow I, Behlau M (2009) Phonarticulatory diadochokinesis in young and elderly individuals. Arq Neuropsiquiatr 67(1):58–61
Park CG, Ha B (1995) The importance of accurate repair of the orbicularis oris muscle in the correction of unilateral cleft lip. Plast Reconstr Surg 96(4): 780–788
Paul R (1995) Language disorders from infancy through adolescence: assessment and intervention. Mosby, St. Louis, MO
Peña ED, Gutiérrez-Clellen VF, Iglesias A et al (2014) BESA: Bilingual English-Spanish Assessment. AR-Clinical Publications, San Rafael
Pegoraro-Krook MI, Dutka-Souza JC, Williams WN et al (2006) Effect of nasal decongestion on nasalance measures. Cleft Palate Craniofac J 43(3):289–294
Perlman AL (2006) Electromyography in oral and pharyngeal motor disorders. GI Motility online. https://doi.org/10.1038/gimo32
Perry JL (2011) Anatomy and physiology of the velopharyngeal mechanism. Semin Speech Lang 32(2):83–92
Petersen EF (1997) Phonetic intelligibility testing in dysarthria. Validity and reliability of listeners' perceptions. Logoped Phoniatr Vocol 22(3):105–117
Petermann F, Macha T (2005) Psychologische Tests für Kinderärzte. Hogrefe, Göttingen

Peterson-Falzone S, Trost-Cardamone J, Karnell M et al (2006) The Clinician's guide to treating cleft palate speech, 2nd edn. Elsevier, St. Louis, MO
Peterson-Falzone SJ, Hardin-Jones MA, Karnell MP (2010) Cleft palate speech. Mosby, St. Louis, MO
Peterson-Falzone SJ, Trost-Cardamone JE, Karnell MP et al (2016) The Clinician's guide to treating cleft palate speech. Mosby, St. Louis, MO
Phua YS, de Chalain T (2008) Incidence of oronasal fistulae and velopharyngeal insufficiency after cleft palate repair: an audidt of 211 children born between 1990 and 2004. Cleft Palate Craniofac J 45:172–178
Picciotti PM, Della Marca G, Restuccia D et al (2005) Tensor velipalatini electromyography with surface electrodes applied transnasally. Acta Otorhinolaryngol Ital 25:120–124
Piehslinger E, Celar A, Celar E et al (1991) Computerized axiography: principles and methods. Cranio 9(4):344–355
Piehslinger E, Bigenzahn W, Celar R et al (1994) Diagnostik orofazialer Dysfunktionen mit Hilfe der elektromagnetischen Artikulographie (diagnostics of orofacial dysfunction with the help of electromagnetic artulography). Z Stomatol Suppl 6:49–51
Pigott RW (1969) The nasendoscopic appearance of the normal palato-pharyngeal valve. Plast Reconstr Surg 43:19–24
Pigott RW, Bensen JF, White FD (1969) Nasoendoscopy in the diagnosis of velopharyngeal incompetence. Plast Reconstr Surg 43(2):141–147
Planas J (1982) Rupture of the orbicularis oris in trumpet players (Satchmo's syndrome). Plast Reconstr Surg 69(4):690–693
Plante E, Vance R (1994) Selection of preschool language tests: a data-based approach. Lang Speech Hear Serv Sch 25(1):15–24
Powell TW (2008) An integrated evaluation of non-speech oral motor treatments. Lang Speech Hear Serv Sch 39:422–227
Prabhu NT, Munshi AK (1995) Ultrasonographic observation of the circumoral musculature: an in-vivo study. J Clin Pediatr Dent 19(3):195–203
Pransky SM, Lago D, Hong P (2015) Breastfeeding difficulties and oral cavity anomalies: the influence of posterior ankyloglossia and upper-lip ties. Int J Pediatr Otorhinolaryngol 79(10):1714–1717
Prathanee B, Thanaviratananich S, Pongjunyakul A et al (2003) Nasalance scores for speech in normal Thai children. Scand J Plast Reconstr Surg Hand Surg 37(6):351–355
Preston JL, McAllister Byun T, Boyce SE et al (2017) Ultrasound images of the tongue: a tutorial for assessment and remediation of speech sound errors. J Vis Exp 119:55123. https://doi.org/10.3791/5512329
Putnam Rochet A, Rochet BL, Sovis EA et al (1998) Characteristics of nasalance in speakers of Western Canadian English and French. J Speech Lang Pathol Audiol 22(2):94–102
Raol N, Sagar P, Nimkin K et al (2015) New technology: use of cine MRI for velopharyngeal insufficiency. Adv Otorhinolaryngol 76:27–32
Rasheed SA, Munshi AK (1996) Electromyographic and ultrasonographic evaluation of the circum-oral musculature in children. J Clin Pediatr Dent 20(4):305–311
Renault F, Raimbault J (1992) Electromyographie faciale, linguale et pharyngée chez l'enfant: Une méthode d'étude des troubles de succion-déglutition et de leur physiopathologie (facial, lingual and pharyngeal electromyography in children: a method of studying sucking-swallowing disorders and their pathophysiology). Neurophysiol Clin 22:249–260
Reichmuth K (2018) Kommunikationsorientierte-sprachspezifische Therapie nach Reichmuth [German]. In: Wachtlin B, Bohnert A (eds) Kindliche Hörstörungen in der Logopädie. Thieme, Stuttgart
Rice ML, Smolik F, Perpich D et al (2010) Mean length of utterance levels in 6-month intervals for children 3 to 9 years with and without language impairments. J Speech Lang Hear Res 53(2):333–349
Robertson SJ (1982) Dysarthria profile. Communication skill builders, Tucson, AZ
Rousteau G, Bouric JM, Rineau (1995) L'aérophonoscope: principe-intérêts (The aerophonoscope: principle-interests). Bulletin d'audiophonologie, Ann scientifiques univ Franche-Comté 11(6):571–603
Ruda JM, Krakovitz P, Rose AS (2012) A review of the evaluation and management of velopharyngeal insufficiency in children. Otolaryngol Clin North Am 45(3):653–669
Rudnick EF, Sie KC (2008) Velopharyngeal insufficiency: current concepts in diagnosis and management. Curr Opin Otolaryngol Head Neck Surg 16(6):530–535
Sagar P, Nimkin K (2014) Feasibility study to assess clinical applications of 3-T cine MRI coupled with synchronous audio recording during speech in evaluation of velopharyngeal insufficiency in children. Pediatr Radiol 45(2):217–227
Sakamoto Y, Soga S, Jinzaki M et al (2015) Evaluation of velopharyngeal closure by 4D imaging using 320-detector-row computed tomography. J Plast Reconstr Aesthet Surg 68(4):479–484
SALT Software (2014) Computerized language sample analysis. http://www.saltsoftware.com/. Accessed 1 June 2014
Scheier M (1909) Die Bedeutung des Röntgenverfahrens fur die Physiologie der Sprach und der Stimme (the importance of the X-ray procedure for the physiology of speech and voice). Archiv Laryngol Rhinol 22:175–179
Schenck GC, Perry JL, O'Gara MM et al (2021) Velopharyngeal muscle morphology in children with unrepaired submucous cleft palate: an imaging study. Cleft Palate Craniofac J 58:313–323
Schlesinger H (1906) Ein nicht bekanntes symptom der Gaumensegellähmung (an unknown symptom of palatal paralysis). Neurol Zbl 25:50
Schröter-Morasch H, Ziegler W (2005) Rehabilitation of impaired speech function (dysarthria, dysglossia). GMS Curr Top Otorhinolaryngol Head Neck Surg 4:Doc 15
Seaver EJ, Dalston RM, Leeper HA et al (1991) A study of nasometric values for normal nasal resonance. J Speech Hear Res 34(4):715–721

Sell D (2005) Issues in perceptual speech analysis in cleft palate and related disorders: a review. Int J Lang Commun Disord 40(2):103–121
Sell D, Grunwell P (1994) Speech studies and the unoperated cleft palate subject. Eur J Disord Commun 29(2):151–164
Shin YJ, Kim Y, Kim HG (2017) The comparative study of resonance disorders for Vietnamese and Korean cleft palate speakers using nasometer. Maxillofac Plast Reconstr Surg 39(1):9. https://doi.org/10.1186/s40902-017-0108-2
Shprintzen RJ (1995) Instrumental assessment of velopharyngeal valving. In: Shprintzen RJ, Bardach J (eds) Cleft palate speech management: a multidisciplinary approach. Mosby, St. Louis, MO, pp 221–276
Shprintzen RJ, Golding-Kushner K (1989) Evaluation of velopharyngeal insufficiency. Otolaryngol Clin North Am 22(3):519–536
Shprintzen RJ, Marrinan E (2009) Velopharyngeal insufficiency: diagnosis and management. Curr Opin Otolaryngol Head Neck Surg 17(4):302–307
Shprintzen RJ, Ysunza PA (2019) Endoscopic recording (or its absence): a disappointment. Sch J Otolaryngol 2(5):200–201
Shprintzen RJ, Lewin ML, Croft CB et al (1979) A comprehensive study of pharyngeal flap surgery: tailor made flaps. Cleft Palate J 16(1):46–55
Shprintzen RJ, Sher AE, Croft CB (1987) Hypernasal speech caused by tonsillar hypertrophy. Int J Pediatr Otorhinolaryngol 14(1):45–46
Shprintzen RJ, Singer L, Sidoti EJ et al (1992) Pharyngeal flap surgery: postoperative complications. Int Anesthesiol Clin 30(4):115–124
Sinko K, Gruber M, Jagsch R et al (2017) Assessment of nasalance and nasality in patients with a repaired cleft palate. Eur Arch Otorhinolaryngol 274(7):2845–2854
Skirko JR, Weaver EM, Perkins JA et al (2013) Validity and responsiveness of VELO: a velopharyngeal insufficiency quality of life measure. Otolaryngol Head Neck Surg 149(2):304–311
Skolnick ML (1969) Video velopharyngography in patients with nasal speech, with emphasis on lateral pharyngeal motion in velopharyngeal closure. Radiology 93:747–755
Skolnick L (1970) Videofluoroscopic examination of the velopharyngeal portal during phonation in lateral and base projections—a new technique for studying mechanism of closure. Cleft Palate J 7:803–816
Skolnick ML, McCall GN, Barnes M (1973) The sphincteric mechanism of velopharyngeal closure. Cleft Palate J 10:286–305
Smith BE, Weinberg B (1982) Prediction of modeled velopharyngeal orifice areas during steady flow conditions and during aerodynamic simulation of voiceless stop consonants. Cleft Palate J 19(3):172–180
So LKH, Jing Z (2000) Putonghua Segmental PhonologyTest (PSPT). Nanjing Normal University Press, Nanjing
Sommerlad BC, Hackett ME, Watson J (1975) A simplified method of recording in nasal pharyngoscopy. Br J Plast Surg 28:34–36
Stackhouse J, Wells BW (1997) Children's speech and literacy difficulties. A psycholinguistic model. Whurr, London
Starr CD, Moller KT, Dawson W et al (1984) Speech ratings by speech clinicians, parents and children. Cleft Palate J 21(4):286–292
Stelzenmüller W (ed) (2010) Therapie von Kiefergelenkschmerzen: Ein Behandlungskonzept für Zahnärzte, Kieferorthopäden und Physiotherapeuten (therapy of temporomandibular joint pain: a treatment concept for dentists, orthodontists and physiotherapists), 2nd edn. ZMK Praxis, Thieme, Stuttgart
Stevens SS (1975) Psychophysics: introduction to its perceptual, neural, and social prospects. Transaction Publishers, New York, NY
Stevens KN (1985) Spectral prominences and phonetic distinctions in language. Speech Commun 4:137–144
Stevens KN (1997) Articulatory-acoustic-auditory relationships. In: Hardcastle WJ, Laver J (eds) The handbook of phonetic sciences. Blackwell Publishing, Oxford, pp 462–506
Story BH, Bunton K (2023) The relation of velopharyngeal coupling area and vocal tract scaling to identification of stop-nasal cognates. J Acoust Soc Am. 154(6):3741–3759. https://doi.org/10.1121/10.0023958
Stow C, Pert S (2006) BiSSS: bilingual speech sound screen: Pakistani heritage languages. Speechmark, Winslow
Strand EA, McCauley RJ (2008) Differential diagnosis of severe speech impairment in young children. AHSA Leader 13:10–13
Su C-Y, Hsu S-P, Chee EC-Y (1993) Electromyographic recording of tensor and levatorvelipalatini muscles: a modified transnasal insertion method. Laryngoscope 103:459–462
Subcommittee for approach by the delegates of the 4th Congress for Plastic Surgery, Rome (1967) Classification of clefts of lip, alveolus and palate. In: Transactions of the 4th Congress for Plastic and Reconstructive Surgery. Excerpta Medica, Amsterdam
Subtelny JD, Van Hattum RJ, Myers BB (1972) Ratings and measures of cleft palate speech. Cleft Palate J 9(1):18–27
Sweeney T, Sell D (2008) Relationship between perceptual ratings of nasality and nasometry in children/adolescents with cleft palate and/or velopharyngeal dysfunction. Int J Lang Commun Disord 43(3):265–282
Sweeney T, Sell D, O'Regan M (2004) Nasalance scores for normal-speaking Irish children. Cleft Palate Craniofac J 41(2):168–174
Tachimura T, Mori C, Hirata SI et al (2000) Nasalance score variation in normal adult Japanese speakers of mid-west Japanese dialect. Cleft Palate Craniofac J 37(5):463–467
Tani T, Izuka Y, Araki R (2002) Analysis of articulation errors and change of prosody in a case of apraxia of speech. High Brain Funct Res 22(4):280–291

Templin M, Darley FL (1960) Templin-Darley tests of articulation. Bureau of Educational Research and Service, University of Iowa, Iowa City, IA

Topbaş S (2004/2005) Türkçe Sesletim-Sesbilgisi Testi (SST). TC Milli Eğitim Yayınevi, Ankara, p 4. Akşam Sanat Okulu Matbaası. Test Bataryası

Trindade IE, Araújo BM, Teixeira AC et al (2014) Velar activity in individuals with velopharyngeal insufficiency assessed by acoustic rhinometry. J Appl Oral Sci 22(4):323–330

Trost-Cardamone J (2013) Cleft palate speech: a comprehensive 2-part set. American Speech-Language-Hearing Association, Rockville, MD

Tsugawa L (2002) Spanish Preschool Articulation Test: SPAT. Lexicon Press, Billings

Tylor AA, Tolbert LC (2002) Speech-language assessment in the clinical setting. Am J Speech Lang Pathol 11(3):215–220

Ünal-Logacev Ö, Kazanoglu D, Balo E et al (2018) Cleft lip and palate assessment form: medical history, oral-peripheral characteristics, speech problems. Turk J Plast Surg 26(4):156–168

Utianski RL, Duffy JR, Clark HM et al (2018) Prosodic and phonetic subtypes of primary progressive apraxia of speech. Brain Lang 184:54–65

Vallino-Napoli LD, Montgomery AA (1997) Examination of the standard deviation of mean nasalance scores in subjects with cleft palate: implications for clinical use. Cleft Palate Craniofac J 34(6):512–519

van der Heijden P, Hobbel HHF, Van der Laan BFAM et al (2011a) Nasometry normative data for young Dutch children. Int J Pediatr Otorhinolaryngol 75(3):420–424

van der Heijden P, Hobbel HH, van der Laan BF et al (2011b) Nasometry cooperation in children 4-6 years of age. Int J Pediatr Otorhinolaryngol 75(5):627–630

van Doorn J, Purcell A (1998) Nasalance levels in the speech of normal Australian children. Cleft Palate Craniofac J 35(4):287–292

Van Lierde KM, Wuyts FL, De Bodt M et al (2001) Nasometric values for normal nasal resonance in the speech of young Flemish adults. Cleft Palate Craniofac J 38(2):112–118

Van Lierde KM, Monstrey S, Bonte K et al (2004) The long-term speech outcome in Flemish young adults after two different types of palatoplasty. Int J Pediatr Otorhinolaryngol 68(7):865–875

Van Lierde KM, Wuyts FL, Bonte K et al (2007) The nasality severity index: an objective measure of hypernasality based on a multiparameter approach. A pilot study. Folia Phoniatr Logop 59(1):31–38

Veau V, Borel S (1931) Division Palatine: Anatomie, Chirurgie, Phonétique (Palatal division: anatomy, surgery, phonetics). Masson, Paris

Veau V, Borel-Maisonny S (1931) La phonation après les opérations pour division palatine (Phonation after surgery for cleft palate). Revue Française de Pédiatrie 7:333–342

Vernel-Bonneau F, Thibault C (1999) Les fentes faciales. In: Embryologie, rééducation, accompagnement parental (Facial clefts. Embryology, rehab, parenting support). Masson, Paris

Volk GF, Pohlmann M, Sauer M et al (2014) Quantitative ultrasonography of facial muscles in patients with chronic facial palsy. Muscle Nerve 50(3):358–365

Walker HK, Hall WD, Hurst JW (1990) Clinical methods: the history, physical, and laboratory examinations, 3rd edn. Butterworths, Boston, MA

Wan TK, Chen JT, Wang PC (2013) EMG-guided salpingopharyngeus Botox® injection for palatal myoclonus. B-ENT 9:67–69

Warren DW, Dubois AB (1964) A pressure-flow technique for measuring velopharyngeal orifice area during continuous speech. Cleft Palate J 16:52–71

Warren DW, Dalston RM, Mayo R (1994) Hypernasality and velopharyngeal impairment. Cleft Palate Craniofac J 31(4):257–262

Watterson T, McFarlane SC, Wright DS (1993) The relationship between nasalance and nasality in children with cleft palate. J Commun Disord 26(1):13–28

Watterson T, Hinton J, McFarlane S (1996) Novel stimuli for obtaining nasalance measures from young children. Cleft Palate Craniofac J 33(1):67–73

Weinberg SM, Neiswanger K, Martin RA et al (2006) The Pittsburgh Oral-facial cleft study: expanding the cleft phenotype. Background and justification. Cleft Palate Craniofac J 43(1):7–20

Weinberger S (2015) Speech accent archive. George Mason University. http://accent.gmu.edu. Accessed 28 May 2016

Whitehill TL (2001) Nasalance measures in Cantonese-speaking women. Cleft Palate Craniofac J 38(2):119–125

Whitehill TL (2002) Assessing intelligibility in speakers with cleft palate: a critical review of the literature. Cleft Palate Craniofac J 39(1):50–58

Wilkinson I, Lennox G (2005) Cranial nerve disorders. In: Wilkinson I (ed) Essential neurology, 4th edn. Oxford University Press, Oxford, pp 111–136

Williams FH (1901) The roentgen rays in medicine and surgery as an aid in diagnosis and as a therapeutic agent: designed for the use of practitioners and students. Macmillan, New York, NY

Williams JL, Cordero KN, Sitzman TJ (2024) Assessing the Agreement of Hypernasality and Audible Nasal Emission Ratings Between Audio-Recordings and a Clinic Setting. Cleft Palate Craniofac J. 61(11):1901–1906

Wilson-Pauwels L, Akesson E, Stewart P et al (2001) Cranial nerves in health and disease, 2nd edn. McGraw-Hill Medical, New York, NY

Witt PD, Berry LA, Marsh JL et al (1996) Speech outcome following palatoplasty in primary school children: do lay peer observers agree with speech pathologists? Plast Reconstr Surg 98(6):958–965. discussion 966-970

World Health Organization (WHO) (2007) International classification of disability and functioning. Children and youth version (ICF-CY). http://apps.who.int/iris/bitstream/10665/43737/1/9789241547321_eng.pdf. Accessed 28 May 2016

World Health Organization (2001) International classification of functioning, disability, and health: ICF. WHO, Geneva

World Health Organization (2019) International statistical classification of diseases and related health problems 10th revision: ICD-10. WHO, Geneva

World Health Organization (2011) International statistical classification of diseases and related health problems, 10th revision, edition 2010. http://www.who.int/classifications/icd/en/. Accessed 1 June 2014

Yokonishi H, Imagawa H, Sakakibara KI et al (2016) Relationship of various open quotients with acoustic property, phonation types, fundamental frequency, and intensity. J Voice 30(2):145–157

Yorkston K, Beukelman D (1981) Assessment of intelligibility of dysarthric speech. CC Publications, Tigard, OR

Yoshida H, Furuya Y, Shimodaira K et al (2000) Spectral characteristics of hypernasality in maxillectomy patients. J Oral Rehabil 27(8):723–730

Ysunza A, Pamplona M (2008) Velopharyngeal dysfunction: diagnosis and management. J Maxillofac Oral Surg 7(1):168–173

Ysunza A, Pamplona M, Molina F et al (2004) Surgery for speech in cleft palate patients. Int J Pediatr Otorhinolaryngol 68(12):1499–1505

Ysunza A, Pamplona M, Ortega J et al (2008) Videofluoroscopy for evaluating adenoid hypertrophy in children. Int J Pediatr Otorhinolaryngol 72(8):1159–1172

Ysunza PA, Repetto G, Pamplona M et al (2015) Current controversies in diagnosis and management of cleft palate and velopharyngeal insufficiency. Biomed Res Int 2015:196240. https://doi.org/10.1155/2015/196240

Ysunza PA, Bloom D, Chaiyasate K et al (2016) Velopharyngeal videofluoroscopy: providing useful clinical information in the era of reduced radiation and safety. Int J Pediatr Otorhinolaryngol 89:127–132

Ysunza PA, Chaiyasate KC, Rontal M et al (2019) Comparison of three different surgical techniques for designing pharyngeal flaps according to findings of videonasopharyngoscopy and multiplanar videofluoroscopy. Int J Pediatr Otorhinolaryngol 120:123–129

Zajac DJ (2000) Pressure-flow characteristics of /m/ and /p/ production in speakers without cleft palate: developmental findings. Cleft Palate Craniofac J 37(5):468–477

Zajac DJ (2015) The nature of nasal fricatives: articulatory-perceptual characteristics and etiologic considerations. Perspect Speech Sci Orofac Disord 25:17–28

Ziade G, Kasti M, Sarieddine D et al (2017) Clinical application of nasometry in patients with nasal obstruction. Ear Nose Throat J 96(10–11):E13–E16

Ziegler W, Hartmann E (1993) Das Münchner Verständlichkeits-Profil (MVP): Untersuchungen zur Reliabilität und Validität (The Munich Intelligibility Profile (Mvp)—Reliability and validity). Nervenarzt 64:653–658

Ziegler W, Schölderle T, Staiger A et al (2015) Die Bogenhausener Dysarthrieskalen (BoDyS): Ein standardisierter test für die Dysarthriediagnostik bei Erwachsenen (the Bogenhausen dysarthria scales (BoDyS): a standardised test for the diagnosis of dysarthria in adults). Sprache Stimme Gehör 39:171–175

Zraick RI, Liss JM (2000) A comparison of equal-appearing interval scaling and direct magnitude estimation of nasal voice quality. J Speech Lang Hear Res 43(4):979–988

Prevention of Dysglossia, Resonance Disorders and Velopharyngeal Insufficiency

4

Ahmet Atas, Songul Aksoy, Antoinette am Zehnhoff-Dinnesen, Doris-Eva Bamiou, Sylva Bartel-Friedrich, Claire Benton, Hanno J. Bolz, Nicole G. Campbell, Frans Coninx, Jakub Dršata, Mona Hegazi, Ariane Hohoff, Armagan Incesulu, Kristin Kerkhofs, Christiane Kiese-Himmel, Arne Knief, Sabrina Kösling, Jill Massey, Peter Matulat, David R. Moore, Dirk Mürbe, Katrin Neumann, Emmanuelle Noirrit-Esclassan, Haldun Oguz, Levent N. Ozluoglu, Waheeda Pagarkar, Ross Parfitt, Simona Poisson-Markova, Ewa Raglan, Charlotte Rogers, Maxime Rotenberg, Mustafa Asim Safak, Pavel Seeman, Eva Seemanova, Tony Sirimanna, Martine de Smit, Ad Snik, Piotr Swidzinski, Monika Tigges, Carole Vargas, and Thomas Wiesner

Eva Seemanova was deceased at the time of publication.

Supplementary Information The online version contains supplementary material available at https://doi.org/10.1007/978-3-031-25175-7_4.

A. Atas (✉)
Department of Audiology, Faculty of Health Science, Istanbul University Cerrahpasa, İstanbul, Turkey

Department of ENT–Audiology and Speech Pathology, Faculty of Medicine, İstanbul University Cerrahpasa, İstanbul, Turkey

S. Aksoy
Department of Audiology, Hacettepe University, Sıhhiye-Ankara, Turkey

A. am Zehnhoff-Dinnesen · A. Knief · P. Matulat
R. Parfitt
Clinic of Phoniatrics and Pedaudiology, University Hospital Münster, Münster, Germany
e-mail: am.zehnhoff@uni-muenster.de; knief@uni-muenster.de; matulat@uni-muenster.de; ross.parfitt@ukmuenster.de

D.-E. Bamiou
National Hospital for Neurology and Neurosurgery, University College London, London, UK
e-mail: d.bamiou@ucl.ac.uk

S. Bartel-Friedrich
Department of Otorhinolaryngology—Head and Neck Surgery, University Hospital Martin Luther University Halle-Wittenberg, Halle (Saale), Germany
e-mail: sylva.bartel-friedrich@uk-halle.de

C. Benton
Nottingham Audiology Services, Ropewalk House, Nottingham, UK
e-mail: claire.benton@nuh.nhs.uk

H. J. Bolz
Senckenberg Centre for Human Genetics, Frankfurt am Main, Germany
e-mail: h.bolz@senckenberg-humangenetik.de

A. am Zehnhoff-Dinnesen et al. (eds.), *Phoniatrics II*, European Manual of Medicine,
https://doi.org/10.1007/978-3-031-25175-7_4

N. G. Campbell
University of Southampton, Southampton, UK
e-mail: N.G.Campbell@soton.ac.uk

F. Coninx
Institut für Audiopädagogik, University of Cologne, Solingen-Ohligs, Germany
e-mail: f.coninx@ifap.info

J. Dršata
Department of Otorhinolaryngology and Head and Neck Surgery, University Hospital Hradec Kralove, Hradec Kralove, Czech Republic
e-mail: drsata@fnhk.cz

M. Hegazi
ENT Department, Ain Shams University, Cairo, Egypt

A. Hohoff
Department of Orthodontics, University Hospital of Münster, Muenster, Germany
e-mail: hohoffa@uni-muenster.de

A. Incesulu
Department of Otolaryngology-Head and Neck Surgery, Faculty of Medicine, Eskisehir Osmangazi University, Eskişehir, Turkey
e-mail: saincesulu@ogu.edu.tr

K. Kerkhofs
Rehabilitationcentre De Poolster, Brussels, Belgium
e-mail: Kristin.kerkhofs@vgc.be

C. Kiese-Himmel
Phoniatrics/Pediatric Audiological Psychology, University Medical Center, Goettingen, Germany
e-mail: c.kiese@med.uni-goettingen.de

S. Kösling
Department of Diagnostic Radiology, Martin-Luther University Halle-Wittenberg, Halle (Saale), Germany
e-mail: sabrina.kosling@medizin.uni-halle.de

J. Massey
Evelina London Children's Hospital, Guys and St Thomas' NHS Foundation Trust, London, UK

D. R. Moore
Cincinnati Children's Hospital Medical Center, Cincinnati, OH, USA
e-mail: david.moore2@cchmc.org

D. Mürbe
Department of Audiology and Phoniatrics, Charité—University Medicine Berlin, Berlin, Germany
e-mail: dirk.muerbe@uniklinikum-dresden.de

K. Neumann
Department of Phoniatrics and Pedaudiology, University Hospital Münster, Münster, Germany
e-mail: Katrin.Neumann@uni-muenster.de

E. Noirrit-Esclassan
Paediatric Dentistry, School of Dental Medicine, Marseille, France
e-mail: emmanuelle.noirrit@univ-amu.fr

H. Oguz
Fonomer, Ankara, Turkey

L. N. Ozluoglu
Department of Otolaryngology, Baskent University, Etimesgut/Ankara, Turkey
e-mail: leventozluoglu@baskent-ank.edu.tr

W. Pagarkar
Royal National Throat Nose & Ear Hospital, Nuffield Hearing and Speech Centre, London, UK
e-mail: wpagarkar@nhs.net

S. Poisson-Markova · P. Seeman · E. Seemanova
Department of Child Neurology, 2nd Medical School of Charles University Prague, Prague, Czech Republic
e-mail: Pavel.seeman@lfmotol.cuni.cz; Eva.seemanova@lfmotol.cuni.cz

E. Raglan
Department of Audiology and Audiovestibular Medicine, Great Ormond Street Hospital for Children NHS Foundation Trust, London, UK
e-mail: eraglan@doctors.org.uk

C. Rogers
Leicester School of Allied Health Sciences, De Montfort University, Hawthorn Building, Leicester, UK
e-mail: charlotte.rogers@dmu.ac.uk

M. Rotenberg
UFR Odontology, Toulouse, France
e-mail: maxime.rotenberg@univ-tlse3.fr

M. A. Safak
Department of Otolaryngology, Near East University, Lefkosa, Turkey

T. Sirimanna
Audiological Medicine and Cochlear Implant Department, Great Ormond Street Hospital, London, UK
e-mail: Tonysirimanna@yahoo.co.uk

M. de Smit
Artevelde University College, Ghent, Belgium
e-mail: martine.desmit@arteveldehs.be

A. Snik
Audiologisch Centrum, KNO Klinik, Radboud University Medical Center, Nijmegen, The Netherlands

P. Swidzinski
Department of Phoniatrics and Audiology, Poznan University of Medical Sciences, Poznan, Poland

M. Tigges
Städt. Klinikum Karlsruhe GmbH, ENT Clinic, Phoniatrics and Pedaudiology, Karlsruhe, Germany
e-mail: monika.tigges@klinikum-karlsruhe.de

C. Vargas
Private Practice, Labarthe-sur-Leze, Occitanie, France
e-mail: contact@carole-vargas-orthodontiste.fr

T. Wiesner
Department of Phoniatrics and Pediatric Audiology, Werner Otto Institut gGmbH, Hamburg, Germany
e-mail: twiesner@werner-otto-institut.de

4.1 Concise Overview of the Physiology of Hearing

Ad Snik

4.1.1 Anatomy and Physiology of the Hearing Organ

The hearing organ, schematically presented in Fig. 1.37 taken from Sect. 1.2 (Vol 1), can be subdivided into four parts:

- The external part, comprising the auricle and external auditory canal. This part of the ear collects the airborne sounds and transports these sounds to the entrance of the middle ear, the tympanic membrane.
- The middle ear is an air-filled cavity that comprises the tympanic membrane and (coupled) the middle ear ossicles. The middle ear system transforms the sound waves into mechanical vibrations that are led to the entrance of the inner ear, the oval window.
- The inner ear or cochlea, a fluid-filled, spiral-formed organ that comprises the sensory cells. The mechanical vibrations of the middle ear system are propagated as vibrations through the cochlear fluids. These vibrations activate the sensory cells in the cochlea. In fact, the vestibular system and the cochlea form one organ often referred to as the audiovestibular system. The vestibular system is addressed in Sects. 1.2 and 4.2.6.
- The auditory neural system that transports the action potentials generated by the activated sensory cells to the brainstem and (sub)cortical auditory areas.

If we look in more detail (Fig. 1.37 from Sect. 1.2 Vol 1), first of all at the outer ear, the auricle or pinna is characterised by certain folds, which play an important part in the processing of high frequencies that we use for localisation of sound sources, in particular in the vertical plane. Furthermore, the auricle is important for separating frontal and rear sources because its shape causes sounds from the front or rear to be diffracted differently, resulting in slight but detectable differences in the frequency spectrum. The tympanic membrane at the end of the external canal has relatively low impedance, comparable to the acoustic impedance of sound in air. As a result, airborne sound waves efficiently vibrate the tympanic membrane. Its low-power but relatively high-amplitude vibrations are transformed into more powerful vibrations with low amplitude, by the ossicular chain system. Thus this system works as an 'impedance' match that effectively transforms the acoustic energy of the airborne sound wave into mechanical energy of the fluid wave in the cochlea, a mechanical amplification procedure that requires no additional energy to perform. The ossicular system is connected to the tympanic membrane via the malleus at one end and to the cochlea at the other. The last ossicle, the stapes, moves piston-wise in the oval window of the cochlea (Slis and Snik 1997a).

The cochlea comprises a spiral-formed twisted canal with approximately 2.5 turns. Fig. 4.1 presents schematically the unrolled cochlea. In fact, three different parallel canals can be distinguished, called the scala, the scala media and the scala vestibuli (see Fig. 4.1). Stapes-induced vibrations of the oval window, at the base of the cochlea, cause the fluid in the scala vestibuli to be set into motion, resulting in a longitudinal fluid wave. That motion reaches the top of the cochlea, or the apex, where the scala vestibuli and the scala tympani are connected (illustrated in Fig. 4.1). The longitudinal wave reverses its direction through the scala tympani, towards the second window in the base of the cochlea, the round window. At the round window, the energy of the fluid wave is dissipated at the round window. The third scala is a separated canal in the middle, not connected to the other two scalae. It contains fluid, endolymph, with different ion concentrations than the fluid in the other two scalae, the perilymph. The scala vestibuli is separated from the scala media by a thin, highly mobile membrane, the membrane of Reissner. For the longitudinal waves in the scala vestibuli, mechanically, this membrane does not exist. This means that the longitudinal wave on either side of the (stiffer) membrane between the scala media

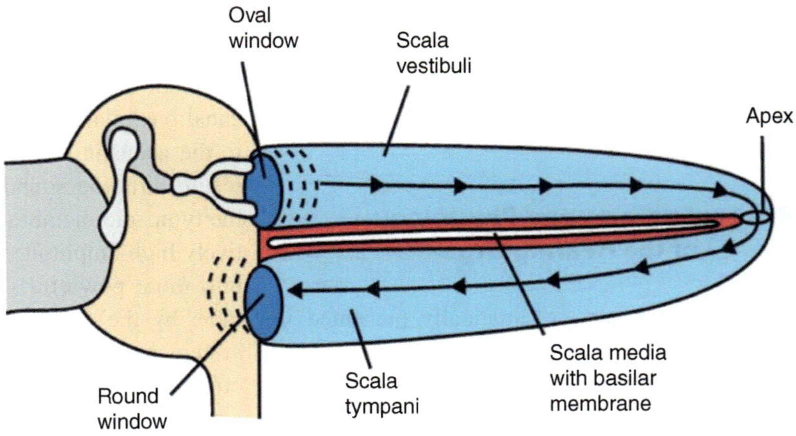

Fig. 4.1 The unravelled cochlea comprising three compartments, the scala vestibuli, the scala tympani and, in between, the scala media with the sensory elements

and scala tympani, the basilar membrane, creates pressure differences over this membrane, causing up-down movements of that membrane. These movements look like a transversal travelling wave. The basilar membrane comprises the sensory elements that are activated by the transversal movements of the membrane. These elements are called the organ of Corti (Slis and Snik 1997b).

At the base of the cochlea, the basilar membrane is relatively thick and narrow. At the apex, the basilar membrane is relatively thin and broad. Between these two extremes, the width of the membrane and its thickness change rather linearly. As a result, the stiffness of the membrane is much higher at the base than at the apex. For high frequencies, the basilar membrane is highly mobile near the base, while for low frequencies, the highest mobility is found near the apex. As a consequence, the mobility of the basilar membrane is frequency-dependent from the base to the apex; when stimulated, the amplitude of the travelling wave will peak at a certain distance from the base, where the distance is determined by the frequency of the sound. This is referred to as tonotopic organisation of the basilar membrane.

The organ of Corti is situated on top of the basilar membrane (see Fig. 1.44 taken from Sect. 1.2 Vol 1), close to the modiolus. Along the full length of the basilar membrane, this organ contains four parallel rows of hair cells, one row of inner hair cells (closest to the modiolus) and three rows of outer hair cells.

Inner and outer hair cells are situated on either side of a rather solid ridge, the tunnel of Corti. Each hair cell is connected to neurons; the inner hair cells mainly to afferent neurons and the outer hair cells mainly to efferent neurons. The differences in anatomy and neural connections suggest that inner hair cells and outer hair cells have different functions. Above the hair cells, the tectorial membrane is situated, which is (only) connected to the cochlear wall near the modiolus. The tips of the cilia of the hair cells are connected to the tectorial membrane, such that they bend when the basilar membrane moves relative to the stiff tectorial membrane. The connection of the cilia to the tectorial membrane is tighter for the outer hair cells than for the inner hair cells (Green 1976).

The endolymph, in the scala media, and the perilymph, in the other two scalae, have different ion concentrations. This causes a potential difference of about 80 mV over the membranes that separate the scala media from the other two scalae, the basilar membrane and membrane of Reissner. This difference in potential is kept constant by ion pumps in the stria vascularis, which covers the outer wall of the scala media. Positively charged ions are pumped from the perilymph to the endolymph. When the cilia of hair cells bend, an influx of positive ions causes depolarisation of the hair cell, which subsequently leads to an action potential in the afferent neuron connected to that hair cell. Inner hair cells are the main sensors. However, only loud sounds stimulate the cilia of the inner hair cells forcefully enough to cause depolarisation. Outer hair cells have another function; apart from sensory properties, they also have motor properties. These cells can amplify the relatively small movements of the basilar membrane caused by soft sounds (the 'active mechanism' or 'cochlear amplifier', which requires the input of additional energy via the efferent neurons), with subsequent sufficiently strong movements of the inner hair cells for depolarisation. These motoric actions of the outer hair cells are controlled by neural feedback loops (Moore 2008) (see Sect. 1.4.3.2) and are the main loci of the non-linearity of the cochlear response.

4.1.2 Perception of Sounds

4.1.2.1 Fundamental Concepts

Our perception of sound is based on logarithmic scales. Concerning loudness, this has led to the introduction of the decibel scale, which is a logarithmic measure of physical sound pressure levels. In pitch perception, we use the octave scale, which is a logarithmic measure of frequency.

Our 'hearing range' is often visualised in a graph of sound pressure levels in decibels (dB) versus frequency in Hertz (Hz) organised into octaves (the interval of one octave represents a doubling of frequency, so that 250 Hz, 500 Hz, 1 kHz and 2 kHz, e.g. are octave steps). Sect. 1.3 Fig. 1.50 (vol 1) shows the hearing range of a normal-hearing subject, which is determined by the frequency-dependent threshold of hearing (in dB SPL, dB sound level pressure; lower limit) and the loudness discomfort level (also in dB SPL; the blue line marked 100). Adolescents have the best hearing, in a frequency range from 20 Hz to 20 kHz, with a hearing range at 1 kHz from approximately 0 to 110–125 dB SPL. Normal thresholds of hearing differ at each frequency and are worse at the low and high frequencies, as displayed in Sect. 1.3 Fig. 1.50 (Vol 1), which shows the standardised normal threshold (the lower red line). For this reason, the hearing thresholds of an individual subject are usually not plotted in dB SPL but in dB HL, or dB Hearing Level, which is relative to the standardised normal-hearing threshold. This standardised normal threshold is 0 dB HL at all frequencies. Thus, hearing thresholds in dB HL are 0 for a normal-hearing person. In clinical practice, however, a normal range of <20 dB HL is typically used. A further decibel scale, dB SL, or dB Sensation Level, is sometimes used, especially in research, to present sounds at a set level above each subject's threshold. Any individual's threshold (in dB SPL or dB HL) can be represented as 0 dB SL. 20 dB SL is therefore 20 dB above the individual's threshold. The loudness discomfort level now equals approximately 100 dB HL for all frequencies. For diagnostic purposes, hearing thresholds and loudness discomfort levels are only measured in the frequency range from 0.25 to 8 kHz. The resulting graph, called an audiogram, is displayed in Fig. 4.2. Note that in an audiogram, hearing levels are presented upside-down. For counselling purposes, the speech dynamic range is indicated, which is the mean sound pressure level of normal conversational speech as a function of frequency, together with its range of 30 dB, expressed in dB HL. During normal running speech, the speech sound levels will be within this area 90% of the time.

4.1.2.2 Air-and Bone-Conduction Stimulation

Normal hearing is based on the perception of airborne sounds via the outer, middle and inner ear routes. However, a vibrating head (e.g. in an environment with loud sound) also leads to sound perception. The 'normal' route is called air-conduction stimulation, whereas the latter route is bone-conduction stimulation. Stimulation by bone conduction can be demonstrated by placing a vibrating tuning fork anywhere on the skull. The vibrations of the tuning fork induce vibrations of the skull, which are transmitted to the cochlea where they are perceived as sounds. Self-perception of our own voices comes via the 'normal' air-conduction route as well as via bone-conduction (from the vibration of our vocal folds on phonation). Measurements in the cochlea of animals have shown that air-conduction stimulation and bone-conduction stimulation lead to similar movements of the basilar membrane. The mechanism by which the vibrating skull results

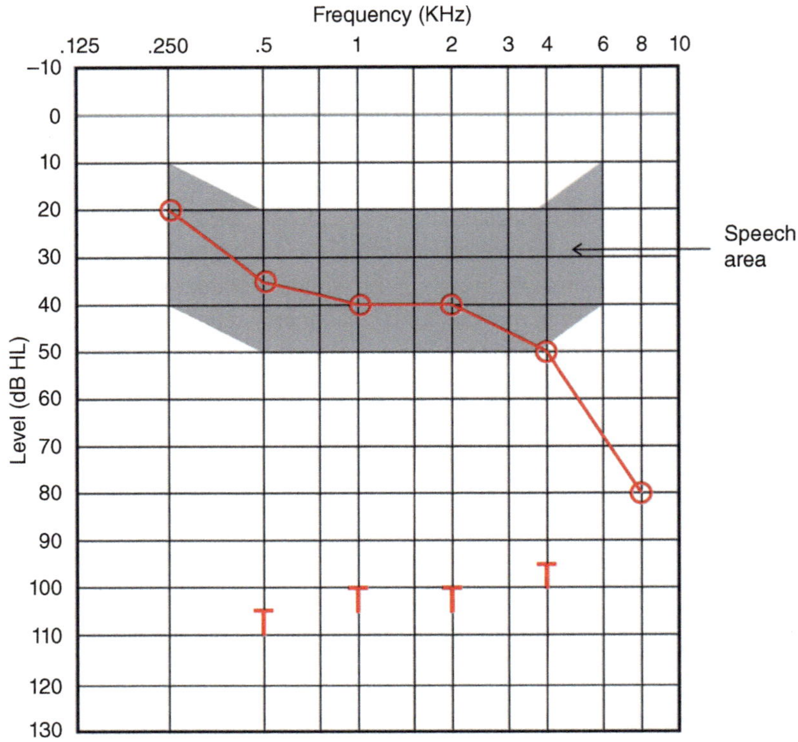

Fig. 4.2 Audiogram format with the speech area indicated in grey (according to Mueller and Killion 1990). The red symbols (open dots) are hearing thresholds of a hearing-impaired patient; the T symbols refer to his loudness discomfort levels

in fluid waves in the cochlea is complicated. Several factors play a role, such as inertia of the cochlear fluid, compression of the cochlear walls upon the fluid and inertia of the middle ear ossicles, to name the most important ones (Stenfelt and Goode 2005). The relative importance of these factors depends on frequency. Bone conduction can be as much as 50 dB less efficient than air-conduction stimulation. Bone-conduction is more efficient at lower frequencies, explaining why we perceive our own voices to be lower in pitch than others perceive them. During clinical hearing tests in hearing-impaired patients, both stimulation routes are tested, using headphones for the air-conduction route and a bone-conduction vibrator, placed on the head, to test the bone-conduction route. Owing to calibration, these two routes will show similar hearing thresholds in most hearing-impaired subjects; however, this is no longer the case in patients with an obstructed air-conduction route (e.g. because of absent or fixated middle ear ossicles).

Figure 4.2 shows a patient's hearing thresholds, measured via the air-conduction route. If the cause of the hearing loss is situated in the cochlea (e.g. loss of outer hair cells), then soft sounds are no longer properly detected; however, loud sounds are well perceived by a normal functioning cochlea. This results in a reduced hearing range (or 'dynamic range'). In this case, at 1 kHz, the dynamic range extends from 40 to 100 dB HL. Such a hearing loss is called a sensorineural hearing loss (SNHL). The reduced dynamic range found in SNHL leads to the perceived loudness of a sound growing more rapidly as the level of the sound increases than in normal hearing. This process is called recruitment. If the hearing loss is situated in the middle ear, while the cochlea is functioning normally, then the thresholds and loudness discomfort level will be shifted equally and the hearing range remains unchanged. Such a hearing loss is referred to as a conductive hearing loss.

4.1.3 Temporal-Spectral Processing

4.1.3.1 Frequency Resolution

Owing to the tonotopic organisation of the basilar membrane, this membrane works as a frequency analyser. A longitudinal wave of a certain frequency leads to maximal membrane motion at a characteristic distance from the oval window. In principle, this enables the separation of simultaneous sounds based on frequency. However, frequency resolution is not perfect. A pure tone will not only excite the basilar membrane at its characteristic point but a certain area around it, the excitation area. The width of excitation areas determines frequency resolution; within such an area, frequency resolution is low; however, between nonoverlapping excitation regions, frequency resolution is optimal (Moore 2008). The 'mechanical' filtering of the basilar membrane seems to be a good explanation for the frequency resolution, as has been reported for loud sounds. Then, typically, excitation areas are approximately one octave. Note that loud sounds, above 60 dB HL, stimulate the inner hair cells directly. For softer sounds, better frequency resolution has been measured. To explain this, a second filter, just for soft sounds, has been postulated, which is based on the (controlled) motoric actions of the outer hair cells.

4.1.3.2 Tuning Curve or Critical Bands and Temporal Resolution

The frequency selectivity of a single auditory neuron, connected to a specific inner hair cell, thus frequency tuned, is quantified by its 'tuning curve'. A tuning curve presents the threshold of activation by sounds of different frequencies. The lowest sound level (threshold) that evokes an action potential occurs at the specific frequency of the inner hair cell, the characteristic frequency (Moore 2008). For frequencies close to that frequency, activation occurs at higher stimulation levels, caused by spread of excitation. Fig. 4.3 shows an example. In principle this is a sensitivity curve for that neuron/hair cell. Such a curve can also be determined behaviourally (Slis and Snik 1997b), for example, a psychophysical tuning curve can be obtained by presenting a pure tone at a specific frequency and measuring the levels required to 'mask' it (i.e. to make the pure tone inaudible) by narrow bandwidth noise centred on that same frequency and then on other surrounding frequencies. The outcome represents the response of the 'auditory filter', a functional conceptualisation of neural tuning curves (Moore 2008). The inverted tuning curve is the critical band for that characteristic frequency and is much more 'sharply tuned' than that reported for loud sounds. The outer hair cells play a role: as previously stated, for soft sounds these cells enable perception of the sound via the inner hair cells by amplification of the movements of the basilar membrane. Inhibition of the motor actions of the outer hair cells occurs, controlled by neural loops; outer hair cells above and below the hair cell with the characteristic frequency are inhibited. This sharpens up the tuning curves.

When outer hair cells are not functional, soft sounds are not perceived, and the louder sounds

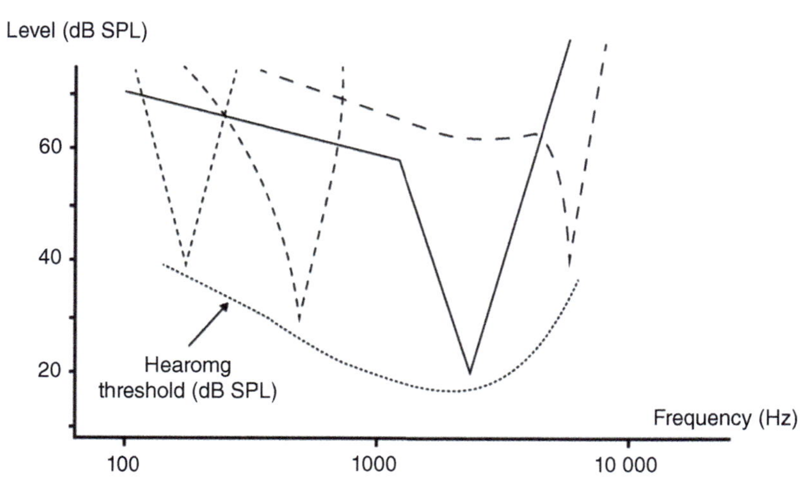

Fig. 4.3 Schematic representation of tuning curves (four) obtained from four different nerves. The lines connect the measured sound pressure levels (in dB SPL) that just resulted in stimulation of the nerve under study (adapted figure from Slis and Snik, 1997b)

that are perceived directly by the inner hair cells have poor spectral resolution. This affects speech perception in patients with sensorineural hearing loss to a degree that depends on the severity of the hearing loss. Perception of speech relies on spectral resolution and also on temporal resolution; the shortest perceptible time interval between sounds ('gap detection') is a measure of interest here, indicating, as it does, the listener's ability to distinguish, and therefore more easily process separate speech sounds. For normal-hearing subjects, the gap detection threshold is in the order of a few milliseconds. Temporal resolution varies according to the spectral content and level and duration of the particular sound stimuli, but no single theory adequately explains how temporal processing occurs (Moore 2008). Temporal resolution plays a role not only in speech processing but also in our ability to localise sounds in space (the inter-aural time difference component of Lord Rayleigh's Duplex theory (Rayleigh 1907)) and our perception of the intensity of sounds shorter than 200 ms (Moore 2008).

See Part IV (from Vol 1) for further information on the pathology of hearing.

4.2 Diagnostics of Hearing Impairment

4.2.1 Diagnostic Interview, Recording of Family Tree and Clinical Examination

Monika Tigges

4.2.1.1 Diagnostic Interview

The evaluation of a suspected hearing disorder begins with a detailed medical anamnesis. The history is usually obtained from the parents or caregivers. Clinical signs of hearing disorders are often unspecific. The purpose of the history is to obtain information regarding the onset, duration and degree of the hearing disorder, possible risk factors and cause of the disease.

The child should also be spoken to in an age-appropriate manner. In this way, information regarding the speech development of the child can be obtained, and a basis of trust can be established for the subsequent physical examination. Observing the child is also important. A thorough history is essential for a fruitful relationship between the physician and the child/family, and it additionally affects the choice and specification of further tests.

The history should include the following topics:

Reactions to Sound

The interview begins with questions regarding the child's reactions to acoustic signals. Reactions should be appropriate to their age (being startled by very loud noises, attentive listening for low noises, reactions to speech and music). Results of previous hearing tests and possible newborn hearing screening should be requested. Relevant information regarding speech development, including the age at which first words were spoken, the number of words spoken, the length of sentences, the child's understanding of speech and bilingualism, should be gathered.

Risk Factors

In the following paragraphs, risk factors are presented.

Questions regarding risk factors during the pre-and perinatal periods should include:

- Prematurity.
- Low birth weight.
- Complications of delivery.
- Perinatal distress, delivery by Caesarean section and the indications for this.
- Asphyxia.
- Treatment in a neonatal intensive care unit.
- Hyperbilirubinaemia, ABO and rhesus incompatibility.
- Sepsis.
- Maternal endocrine disorders (diabetes, hyperthyroidism).
- Maternal infections (CMV, rubella, toxoplasmosis, syphilis, HIV).
- Maternal drug abuse.

The following postnatal risk factors should be assessed:

- Meningitis.
- Viral infection (rubella, mumps, CMV).
- Ototoxic drugs.
- Recurrent otitis media.
- Head injury.
- Noise exposure.

General Development

In order to establish a picture of general developmental progress, the dates of the main milestones of motor development should be asked for (crawling, ability to walk, gross motor skills, fine motor skills, interest in play). Bear in mind that behavioural disorders may occur as a result of a hearing problem.

Vestibular Symptoms

Vestibular involvement can lead to delay in milestones. Direct questions regarding possible tinnitus or vertigo can be asked of older children, in order to indicate a possible vestibular problem.

Illnesses Possibly Connected with Hearing Problems

Disorders of the kidneys, heart and eyes, among many others, may be linked to certain diseases or syndromes with associated hearing abnormalities.

4.2.1.2 Family History and Recording of Family Tree

The family history may suggest a hearing disorder of genetic origin. As genetic factors are a major cause of hearing disorders, a family history of possible hearing loss and speech disorders should be taken. Number, gender, ages and state of health of siblings should be provided. In families with hearing disorders, a family tree of at least three generations should be constructed. The possibility of consanguinity should be inquired into, as the risk for an autosomal recessive hearing disorder is higher in these cases.

An example of a family with an autosomal recessive hearing disorder is given in Fig. 4.4.

4.2.1.3 Clinical Examination

During the examination neonates and smaller children will usually sit on the lap of the caregiver. Older children may sit alone on the examination chair.

Examination begins with an assessment of the head and neck. Any craniofacial abnormality is to be regarded as suspicious when found in relation with a hearing disorder. For exam-

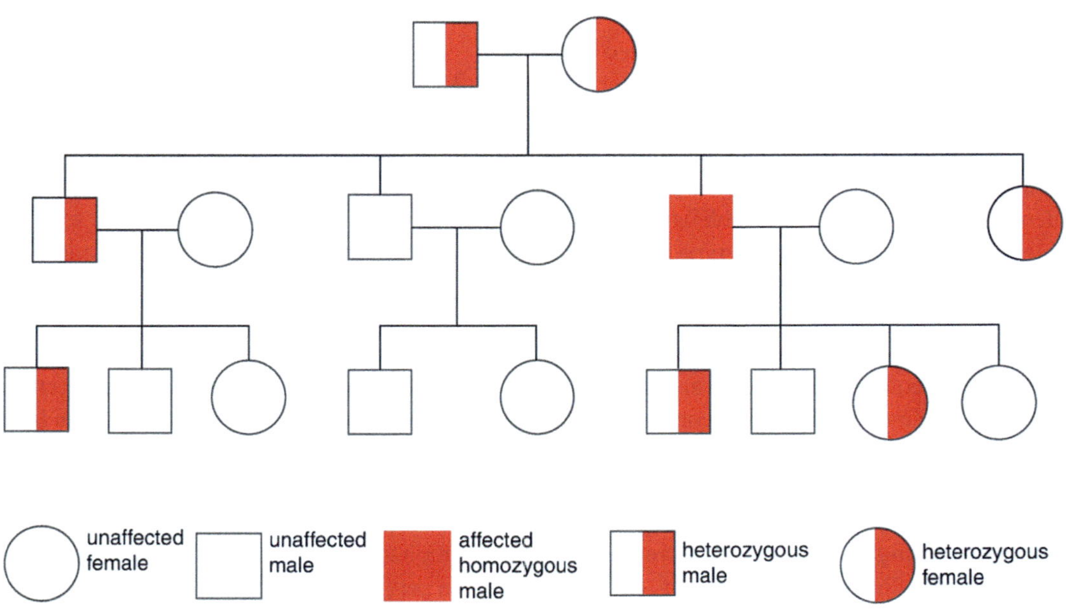

Fig. 4.4 Family tree of an autosomal recessive hearing disorder

ple, heterochromia of the iris and a patch of white hair are observed in Waardenburg syndrome. An enlarged thyroid gland may be a sign of hypothyroidism (Pendred syndrome). Microgenia is related to Pierre Robin sequence. Malformations of the jaw occur in syndromes such as Franceschetti or Goldenhar. Branchiogene developmental disorders such as cervical cysts or fistulas may be related to hearing disorders as well.

The pinnae and their surrounding area should be examined for malformations such as pre-auricular pits or pre-auricular tags, atresia or microtia.

Pre-auricular pits may be connected with a fistula and an epidermal cyst at its end. Some authors recommend surgery before superinfection (Shoman et al. 2014).

Microtia is classified in Grades I–IV:

- I: malformation of the external ear with identifiable structures and a small but present external ear canal.
- II: partially developed ear with a closed or stenotic external ear canal.
- III: absence of the external ear with a small tissue structure, absence of the external ear canal.
- IV: absence of the total ear.

These abnormalities may be associated with middle ear malformation and congenital or progressive hearing loss (Germiller 2007).

A binocular inspection with the microscope is essential to assess the ear canal and the tympanic membrane. The width or possible atresia of the external canal should be examined. Cerumen should be removed until at least a part of the tympanic membrane is visible—if tolerated.

The tympanic membrane is judged for decline, translucency, colour, integrity and morphology of manubrium of malleus. The most common pathological findings are effusions and acute or chronic otitis media.

By inspection of the nose and nasopharynx, mucosal swelling, erythema and secretion may give hints to allergies, inflammation or reflux (Alexiades and Hoffmann 2008).

A nasal pit may be associated with a fistula and an epidermal cyst at its end extending into the nasal cavity or even intracranially. Because of the risk of infection, surgery should be performed; preoperative MRI is strongly recommended (Rizzi and Dunham 2014).

The size of the adenoids should be assessed. Choanal opening can be judged indirectly by strained expiration through the nose on a Link mirror. If necessary flexible or rigid endoscopes can be used. Examination of the oral area should include the teeth, tongue and tonsils. Additional attention should be paid to the soft and hard palate (high palate, short velum, cleft palate). Cleft or bifid uvula may hint to submucous cleft palate. Palpation and inspection of the velum during phonation are useful to exclude submucous cleft palate. Submucous cleft palate may affect the soft or the bony palate.

If a hearing disorder has been diagnosed, a full clinical examination is recommended to look for signs of syndromal disease, for example, café au lait spots in neurofibromatosis (Ruben 2001; Potsic and Lando 2012; Gibbin 2007).

During the examination every care should be taken to ensure that the child remains as comfortable as possible. In this way the cooperation of the child is maintained for the further audiological evaluations.

4.2.2 Basics of Technical Standards and Calibration

Arne Knief

In clinical audiometry there are many sources of error. The patient may vary in his or her answers and may not be cooperative; the audiometric technician may misinterpret the responses of the patient. Therefore it is important to reduce errors with well-maintained equipment. The standards provide good instructions for purchasing and assuring error-free operation. A huge spectrum is covered from the properties of microphones for calibration to word lists for speech audiometry as well as service for hearing aids. A rough list of standards is shown in Table 4.1.

Table 4.1 Selection of standards important in audiometry

ISO 266	Preferred frequencies
ISO 389	Standard reference zero for the calibration of audiometric equipment (all kinds of signals and sound sources)
ISO 7029	Statistical distribution of hearing thresholds as a function of age
ISO 8253	Audiometric test methods (pure tones, narrowband tones, frequency-modulated tones with air and bone conduction and one or more loudspeakers; minimum requirements of precision and comparability between different test procedures; basic methods of speech recognition tests and requirements for the composition, validation and evaluation (not the content) of speech material; noise for masking and as competing sound)
EN 15927	Services offered by hearing aid professionals
ISO 16832	Loudness scaling by means of categories
EN 60118	Hearing aids
EN 60318	Simulators of human head and ear (ear simulator for the measurement of earphones, acoustic coupler for the calibration of earphones, occluded-ear simulators, coupler for the measurement of hearing aids and earphones coupled to the ear by means of ear inserts, mechanical coupler for the measurement of bone vibrators, head and torso simulator for the measurement of hearing aids)
EN 60645	Equipment for audiometry: Pure-tone audiometry, speech audiometry, test signals, high-frequency audiometry (8–16 kHz), instruments for the measurement of aural acoustic impedance/admittance, otoacoustic emissions and auditory brainstem responses
EN 60942	Sound calibrators
EN 61094	Specification for measurement microphones
EN 62489	Audio-frequency induction loop systems for assisted hearing

More about standards are on the worldwide web:

- European Committee for Standardization www.cen.eu.
- International Organization for Standardization www.iso.org.
- Sound and Vibration Standards acoustic-standards.co.uk/index.htm.
- Freestd Standards Worldwide www.freestd.us.

For detailed overview see Wilber (2002). It is important to implement good calibration practice into the daily performance of audiometry. Various guidelines and protocols for audiometry mention calibration as part of essential practice (e.g. British Society of Audiology 2011a).

4.2.3 Pure-Tone Audiometry

Piotr Swidzinski and Ross Parfitt

4.2.3.1 Introduction

Pure-tone audiometry (PTA) is the most common test within audiology, apart from newborn hearing screening tests, and forms the backbone of audiological diagnosis and management. PTA is a behavioural test (i.e. responses require the conscious cooperation of the patient) of the threshold of hearing (the lowest level of an acoustic signal that the patient can hear). It is appropriate for patients of approximately 3–5 years of developmental age and older.

Various protocols and guidelines for PTA have been created by different international organisations, such as the American Speech-Language-Hearing Association (1978), British Society of Audiology (2011a), US National Health and Nutrition Examination Survey (National Centre for Health Statistics 2003), Ireland's Health and Safety Authority (2007) and World Health Organization (2013). A well-structured PTA protocol, if correctly followed, has high test-retest reliability (Stuart et al. 1991), and intra-subject deviation of less than 10 dB is expected in >94% of subjects (Schmuziger et al. 2004). This article gives an overview of the core concepts of PTA which underlie most modern pure-tone audiometry protocols.

4.2.3.2 Resources

PTA is performed with an audiometer (which generates the sound stimuli), transducers (which deliver the stimuli to the patient) and a patient response but-

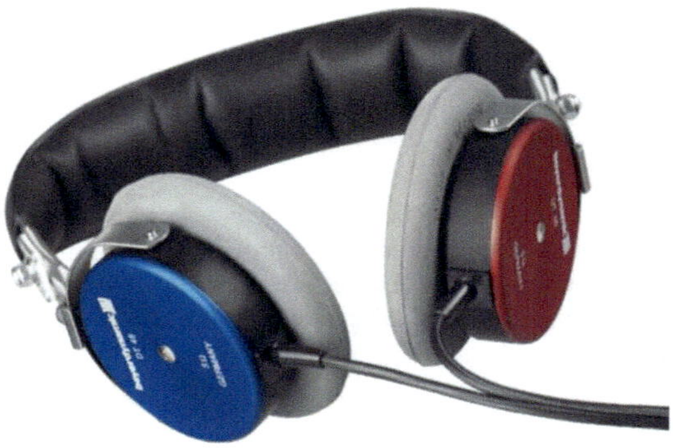

Fig. 4.5 Beyerdynamic DT 48 headphones. Image copyright and with permission from Beyerdynamic

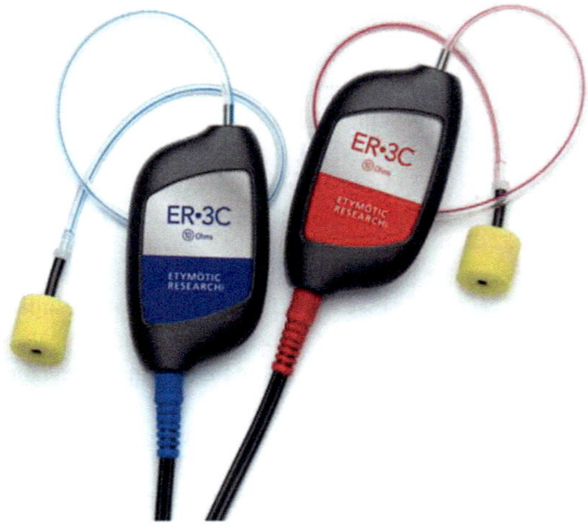

Fig. 4.6 Etymotics ER-3C insert earphone. Image copyright and with permission from Etymotic Research, Inc.

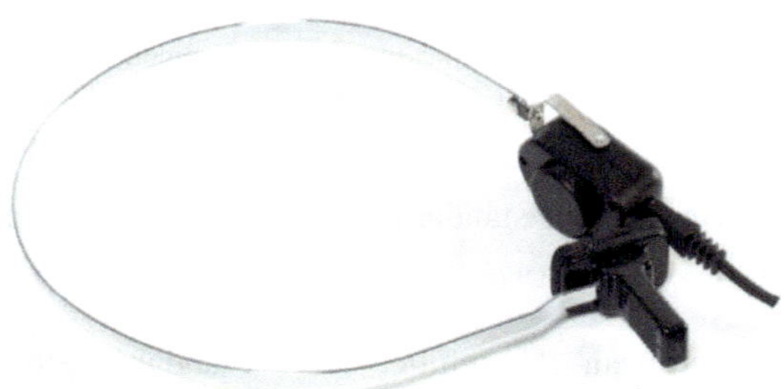

Fig. 4.7 Radioear B71 bone-conduction transducer. Image copyright and with permission from Radioear

ton (which the patient presses to indicate that they have heard the sound stimulus). Audiometers can be stand-alone devices but are these days often attached to conventional computers and controlled by software, allowing results to be digitally recorded and connected with patient medical systems.

Air-conduction transducers include supra-aural headphones, typically Telephonics TDH 39 or Beyerdynamic DT 48 (Fig. 4.5), and (occasionally) insert earphones, such as Etymotics ER-3C (Fig. 4.6). Bone-conduction signals are delivered through a dedicated transducer such as Radioear B71 (Fig. 4.7).

Calibration of each audiometer (together with its dedicated transducers) must be performed at least annually (Stage B calibration, defined in ISO 8253-1 (2010)) in order to ensure the accuracy of the stimuli delivered to the patient. Simple checks (also known as Stage A checks) ought to be performed before each session of use to flag any technical issues or drift in the calibration.

PTA is typically performed within a sound-treated room, which reduces both background noise from outside the room and resonance within it. Soundfield audiometry is not covered in this article (see Sect. 4.2.4 for more details).

4.2.3.3 Key Principles of PTA

Stimulus Type

The stimuli (also known as 'signals' or 'tones') used in PTA are pure tones (i.e. sine waves) (see Sect. 4.1.1), which are the most frequency-specific stimuli possible.

Frequency and Level of Stimulus

PTA is typically performed over the frequency range 250 Hz to 8 kHz and includes frequencies at each octave (250, 500, 1000, 2000, 4000 and 8000 Hz). Additional testing at intermediate frequencies, such as 1.5, 3 and 6 kHz, is sometimes done for specific purposes, such as to enable the gain of hearing aids to be set more accurately. Air-conduction testing can be performed at all of the above standard frequencies and is occasionally performed at higher frequencies (known as extended high-frequency audiometry), for example, in younger patients at risk of sensorineural hearing loss, such as those receiving ototoxic medication. Specific headphones are required for high-frequency audiometry, such as the Sennheiser HDA 200.

Bone-conduction testing is typically only performed between 500 Hz and 4 kHz, though some centres test up to 6 kHz. Bone-conduction signals can lead to vibrotactile sensation at lower frequencies (Boothroyd and Cawkwell 1970) and be airborne at higher frequencies (Lightfoot 1979) because of poor distortion performance of bone-conduction transducers at both low and high frequencies (Lightfoot 2000; Lightfoot and Hughes 1993). For this reason, precautions should be taken when using bone conduction above 2 kHz, such as covering the test ear with a supra-aural headphone (BSA 2011a). Both air-and bone-conduction stimulations are limited in their maximum output levels (air conduction is limited to approx. 120–130 dB HL output and bone conduction to approx. 60 dB HL output (both varying at different frequencies and dependent on audiometer manufacturer).

4.2.3.4 Test Procedure

Before Testing

Otoscopy before PTA is recommended. PTA is not advised in cases of obstructed ear canal (owing to a risk of falsely raised air-conduction thresholds) or ear infection (owing to a risk of discomfort and cross infection). See more detailed protocols, such as those named in the introduction, for other specific contraindications.

The patient should be clearly instructed to press the response button every time he hears a sound, even if the sound is very quiet. Other responses, such as the patient's raising their hand or saying 'yes', are reasonable if the patient is physically unable to push the button. Adaptations for patients who do not understand their task (e.g. younger children or people with cognitive difficulties) are covered in Sects. 4.2.4 and 4.2.27.

Care should be taken to position the transducers accurately in order to avoid artificially lowering the level of the signal delivered to the ear. Supra-aural headphones should rest on the pinnae with the centre of each headphone-loudspeaker in line with the auditory meatus. The bone-conduction transducer should be placed on the mastoid behind the 'test' ear (i.e. the ear which is being tested at the time), not touching any part of the ear and with as little hair between the transducer and the skin as possible.

Test Protocol

Most PTA test protocols are based on the modified Hughson-Westlake procedure (Carhart and Jerger 1959), which establishes the 'ascending' psychometric threshold by presenting a stimulus to the test ear at a suprathreshold level and reducing the level in 10 or 20 dB steps until no response is present (i.e. the signal level is too low for the patient to hear). The level is then increased in 5 dB steps until a response is obtained (i.e. until the patient can again hear the signal). From this level the '10 down, 5 up' procedure is repeated until more than 50% of these ascending responses occur at the same level, with a minimum of two ascending trials. As soon as 2/2, 2/3, 3/5, etc., responses have been obtained at the same level, that level can be accepted as the threshold of hearing at that frequency (see, e.g. Fig. 4.8a–d). In practice, it is unwise to pursue individual thresholds for a great number of ascending trials because the patient can become tired and the reliability of their responses can suffer. If no threshold is identified within approx. 5 ascending trials, either start again at a clearly suprathreshold level, move on to another frequency and come back later or take a short break. Different protocols for measuring threshold exist, and results obtained will be slightly different for each one. Consistency of test protocol used is essential in order for results to be truly comparable (Franks 2001).

Presentation of the test tones should be arrhythmic with silences in between; otherwise the patient could (consciously or not) predict the presence of a tone which they cannot actually hear, thus resulting in falsely lowered thresholds. The tones should vary in length, and the patient should be instructed to hold the response button for as long as the sound is present, rather than just pressing it when they first hear the sound. This enables the tester to check the response to both the onset and offset of the tone, thereby increasing the certainty of the response.

This procedure is typically carried out beginning with air-conduction stimuli (starting at 1 kHz) on the suspected better ear. All desired air-conduction frequencies are usually tested on the same ear and then moving to the other ear and then finally using bone conduction.

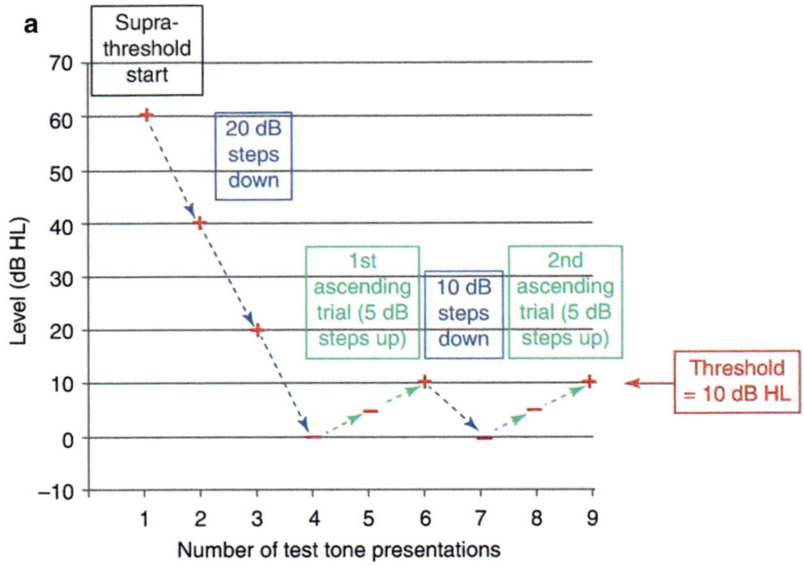

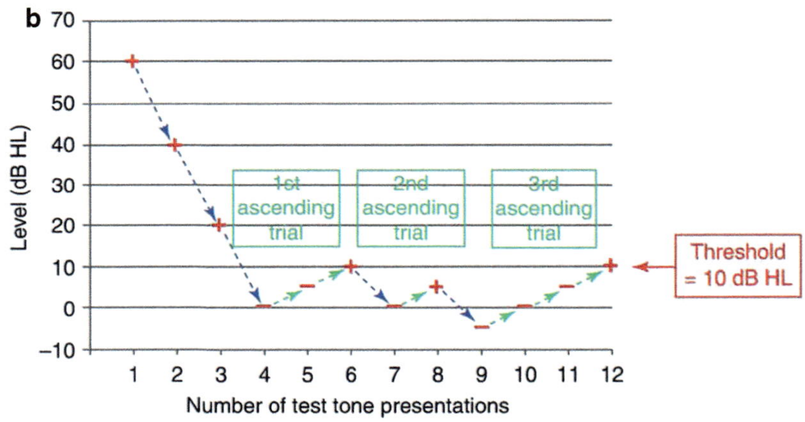

Fig. 4.8 (**a**–**d**) Four examples of tone presentations, ascending trials and responses in pure-tone audiometry, in the search for the auditory threshold, based on the modified Hughson-Westlake procedure (Carhart and Jerger 1959). The + symbol indicates a patient response; the – symbol indicates no patient response. (**a**) Two positive responses at 10 dB HL out of two ascending trials: threshold = 10 dB HL. (**b**) Two positive responses at 10 dB HL out of three ascending trials: threshold = 10 dB HL. (**c**) Two positive responses at 5 dB HL out of three ascending trials: threshold = 5 dB HL. (**d**) Three positive responses at 10 dB HL out of five ascending trials: threshold = 10 dB HL

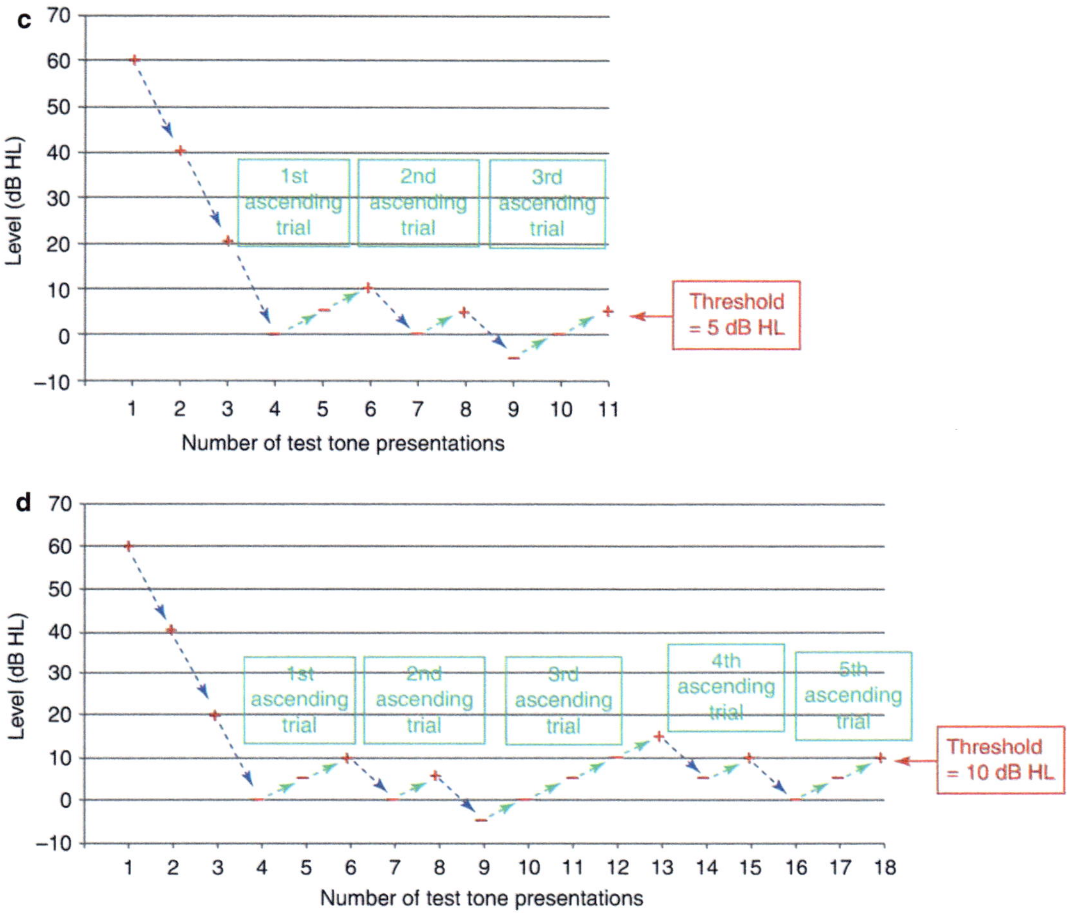

Fig. 4.8 (continued)

If air-conduction thresholds are within the normal range (usually accepted as <20–25 dB HL; see Sect. 4.1.1 and the 'Interpretation' subsection), bone-conduction testing is usually not clinically indicated.

Masking

Munro and Agnew (1999) measured inter-aural attenuation levels (i.e. the level at which a signal played from a transducer to one ear could be 'cross-heard' by the other ear) of 40 dB for Telephonics TDH 39 supra-aural headphones and 55 dB for Etymotics ER-3A insert earphones. In clinical terms, this means that a large asymmetry in air-conduction thresholds between the two ears may mistakenly appear to be no greater than 40 dB (using supra-aural headphones) or 55 dB (using insert earphones). Masking is the essential process by which we can measure the 'true' threshold in these cases.

In masking, a noise (usually 1/3-octave narrowband noise, though white noise or others are used in some clinics) is played to the non-test ear at the 'effective masking level' (the lowest level of masking noise required to prevent the threshold-level pure-tone signal from being heard). The patient is asked to ignore the noise and only respond when they hear the pure-tone signals (played to the test ear). Using the common 'plateau' technique, the levels of noise and signal are increased to the point at which responses occur consistently at a particular signal level despite the noise level increasing further. This is taken as the true threshold.

Masking as part of bone-conduction testing is somewhat more problematic because the interaural attenuation of bone-conduction signals can be as low as 0 dB. Bone-conduction masking (in which a bone-conduction signal is masked by noise via an air-conduction transducer) is therefore essential in cases of asymmetrical air-conduction thresholds and where bone-conduction thresholds appear significantly better than air-conduction thresholds (the 'air-bone gap'). It is, however, clinically inefficient to mask all incidences of an air-bone gap because they are actually more likely than not to occur (Studebaker 1967). Small air-bone gaps should not necessarily be taken as evidence of middle ear pathology (Margolis 2015). The BSA protocol therefore recommends bone-conduction masking only where there is a ≥ 10 dB gap between the not-masked bone-conduction threshold and the air-conduction threshold of either ear (BSA 2011a).

The tester must be careful not to play uncomfortably loud sound into the non-test ear and must be aware of the risks of central masking and cross-masking. In central masking the patient is unable to identify a tone when masking noise is present. In cross-masking the masking noise is itself cross-heard, with the effect of masking the test ear. In cases such as this, masking to find the true threshold may not be possible.

A more comprehensive guideline for masking is beyond the scope of this article. See specific protocols (e.g. BSA 2011a) for further detail.

4.2.3.5 Recording the Results of PTA

The Audiogram

The results of PTA are typically displayed on an audiogram (see Fig. 4.9), which is a graph showing auditory thresholds with frequency (Hz) on the X-axis and level (dB HL) on the Y-axis. Different countries and clinics use different symbols, though the circle and cross (representing right-and left-sided air-conduction thresholds, respectively), the use of red and blue (for right and left sides) and results for the right side being displayed on the left side of the page, and vice versa, are universal. Not-masked bone-conduction thresholds are represented by triangles in Fig. 4.9 and masked bone-conduction thresholds by square brackets.

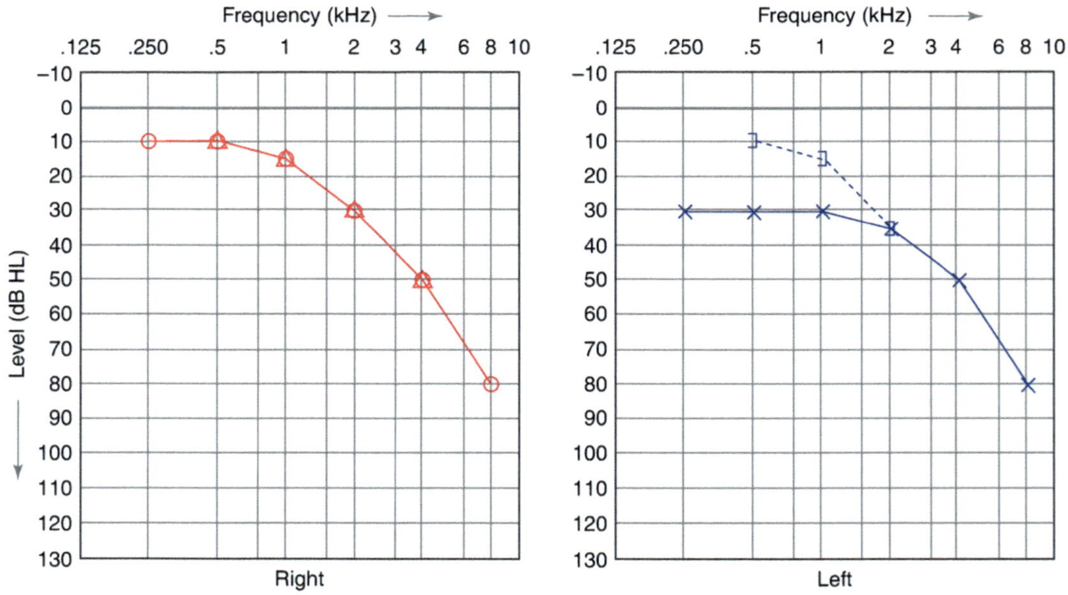

Fig. 4.9 An audiogram showing hearing thresholds for a hypothetical bilateral high-frequency sensorineural hearing loss with a low-frequency conductive component on the left. Results for the right ear are shown in red on the left side and results for the left ear in blue on the right side. The circles and crosses represent air-conduction thresholds; triangles represent not-masked bone-conduction thresholds; square brackets represent masked bone-conduction thresholds. These symbols are standard in the UK. Different symbols are used in different countries and clinics

Interpretation of Normal Range of Hearing

Various descriptions of the 'normal range' of hearing can be found (see Sect. 14.1) and are generally accepted as being hearing thresholds better than 20–25 dB HL.

Interpretation of Conductive Hearing Loss

Where bone-conduction thresholds are within the normal range and air-conduction thresholds are outside of the normal range, a conductive hearing loss is indicated (see Fig. 4.10).

Interpretation of Sensorineural Hearing Loss

Where air-and bone-conduction thresholds are outside of the normal range to the same degree, a sensorineural hearing loss is indicated (see Fig. 4.9, right ear).

Interpretation of Mixed Hearing Loss

Where air-and bone-conduction thresholds are both outside of the normal range but there is a difference between them (an air-bone gap) and bone-conduction thresholds are better than air-conduction thresholds, a mixed hearing loss is indicated (see Fig. 4.11).

Different threshold levels are typically found at different frequencies. For example, otitis media with effusion is typically characterised by conductive hearing loss in the lower frequencies and normal thresholds in the higher frequencies (see Fig. 4.10). Presbyacusis (age-related sensorineural hearing loss) is characterised by normal or near-normal-hearing thresholds in the low frequencies and a sensorineural hearing loss affecting higher frequencies (see Fig. 4.9, right ear).

4.2.3.6 Limitations of PTA

As with all audiological tests, the cross-check principle (Jerger and Hayes 1976), which encourages the use of other tests (such as tympanometry; see Sect. 4.2.10) and the subjective impression made by the patient to corroborate the result, is worth following. As the test results rely on behavioural responses, falsely raised thresholds (whether conscious or not) could be obtained. See Sect. 15.5 for insight into nonorganic hearing loss (NOHL) and Lightfoot and Kennedy (2006) on the use of cortical electric response audiometry (which measures the electrical response to auditory stimulation within the auditory cortex) as 'objective pure-tone audiometry'. Expectation bias can lead to inaccu-

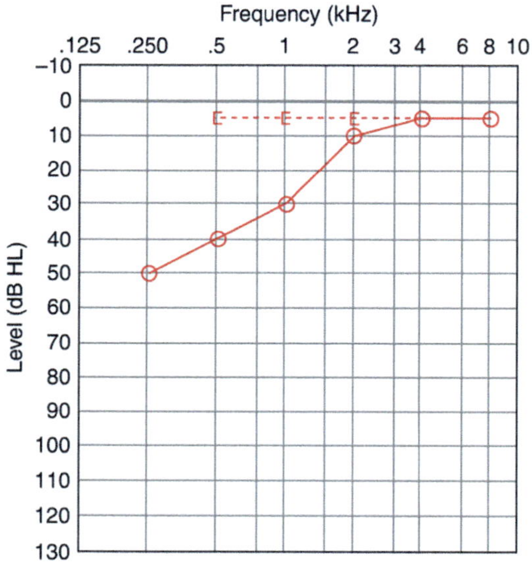

Fig. 4.10 Audiogram showing typical hearing thresholds found in conductive hearing loss caused by otitis media with effusion. This audiogram shows right-sided air-conduction thresholds (circles) and masked bone-conduction thresholds (square brackets)

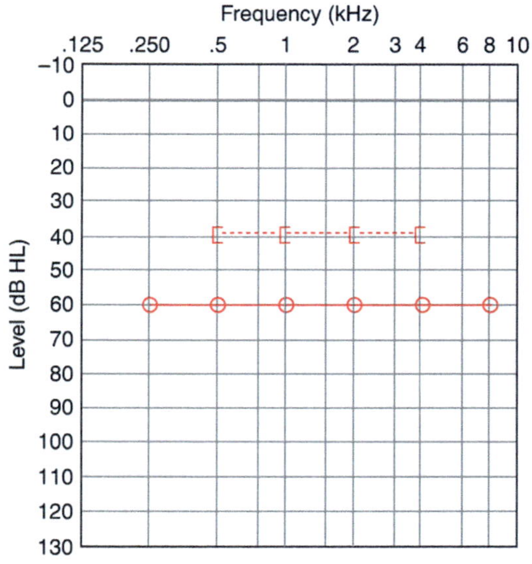

Fig. 4.11 Audiogram showing possible hearing thresholds found in mixed hearing loss. This audiogram shows right-sided air-conduction thresholds (circles) and masked bone-conduction thresholds (square brackets)

racy during testing (Margolis et al. 2015), and there is a risk of responses being falsely interpreted by the tester (especially where time pressure and insufficient training are factors).

Classic pure-tone audiometry only tests the threshold of hearing in response to pure tones. Although this is sufficient for the diagnosis of many audiological conditions, it does not provide full evidence about the patient's functional hearing (e.g. his/her ability to process suprathreshold speech and other functional sounds or their tolerance of loud sound). See Sect. 4.2.8 for information on speech audiometry. Loudness investigations are outlined in the following subsection.

4.2.3.7 Loudness Tests

'Loudness' refers to the subjective perception of a sound, whereas 'sound level' is an objective measure (see Sects. 1.3 and 1.4 (Vol 1)). Uncomfortable loudness level (ULL) (also known as 'loudness discomfort level' (LDL)) testing measures the lowest level at which a sound becomes uncomfortable for the subject. This can be useful in providing additional accuracy regarding the patient's degree of loudness recruitment (in which a small increase in sound intensity is perceived as a large increase, as is typically found in sensorineural hearing loss) (see Sect. 4.1.1), thereby informing hearing aid gain settings, and is also often used in cases of suspected hyperacusis (see Sect. 15.3).

The basic procedure of ULL testing is to increase the level of a sound stimulus gradually until it just becomes uncomfortably loud for the patient (BSA 2011b). It is important to remember that the ULL is not the same as the threshold of pain. Agreeing an appropriate response method with the patient and issuing clear instructions are obviously crucial. ULLs are usually shown on the audiogram using the └ and ┘ symbols for right and left ears, respectively. Sherlock and Formby (2005) surveyed previous literature and proposed a normal ULL of around of 100 dB HL, but they noted considerable variance in normal ULLs reported between different studies across different signals, frequencies and transducers.

Loudness scaling seeks to investigate the subjective loudness of sound in more detail. Various scales exist, and most use verbal descriptors, e.g. very soft, soft, OK, loud, very loud and too loud (Loudness Growth in 1/2-Octave Bands, LGOB scale) (Allen et al. 1990), and specific test procedures to measure the subjective perception of loudness. The highly subjective and non-linear nature of (loudness) sensation can lead to potentially significant interindividual and inter-scale differences, e.g. Elberling (1999); however the international standard ISO 16832 (2006), based on Brand and Hohmann's Adaptive Categorical Loudness Scaling (ACALOS) (Brand and Hohmann 2002), has sought to increase reliability. The 'Würzburger Hörfeld' and 'Oldenburger Hörfeld' loudness scaling tests are well established within German clinics (Lehnhardt and Laszig 2009).

4.2.3.8 Dead-Region Testing

A cochlear dead region is an area of the cochlea in which the inner hair cells or auditory neurons are damaged to the extent that none are functional (Moore 2001). Given the tonotopic nature of the cochlea and the spread of acoustic sensation over the basilar membrane (see Sect. 4.1.1), stimulation of a cochlear dead region by using a signal of a frequency to which the non-functioning hair cells/neurons were tuned results in 'off-frequency listening', in which functional hair cells/neurons of a neighbouring region of the cochlea respond. Off-frequency listening is not detected on classic PTA, so specific tests are required. The threshold-equalising noise (TEN) test is one such test (Moore et al. 2000).

In the TEN test, a pure tone is played at the frequency of the suspected dead region, and a specifically designed TEN stimulus is played at 10 dB above the notional threshold of the suspected dead region. If the pure-tone threshold in the presence of TEN stimulus is <10 dB above the level of the TEN stimulus, then no dead region is judged to be present; if the pure-tone threshold is >10 dB above the level of the TEN stimulus, then a dead region is present. If a dead region is identified in a hearing aid user, the gain of the hearing aid could be adjusted to avoid stimulation at the affected frequencies, thus avoiding the distorted perceptual effects of off-frequency listening which can include impaired speech perception (Moore et al. 2000).

4.2.4 Paediatric Behavioural Audiometry (0–6 Years)

Kristin Kerkhofs and Martine de Smit

4.2.4.1 Introduction

Behavioural audiometry is an essential part of the diagnosis of hearing loss in very young children, even those younger than 6 months of age. Physiological measures (i.e. tympanometry, otoacoustic emissions, ABR and ASSR) should be complemented with behavioural measures to be able to determine the type and degree of hearing loss. The purpose of behavioural audiometry is to obtain air-and bone-conduction thresholds for the whole frequency range. Cross-checking of all measurements is needed before starting hearing aid fitting. This cross-check principle was described 40 years ago by Jerger and Hayes (1976) and is still up to date.

Behavioural audiometry needs well-experienced audiologists and is a time-consuming measurement that has to be done in optimal conditions. The test protocol will vary with the chronological age of the child. In case of retardation, it follows the developmental age of the child. Therefore you have to know the level of development and physical status (i.e. visual, motor abilities) before starting testing.

Testing can be done in a single or double soundproof booth. In a single soundproof booth, the examiner(s) and the child are in the same room. In a double soundproof booth, two examiners are needed, one with the child and one outside with the audiometer. The choice depends on personal preference. It may be useful to have both options.

General test strategy:

- To select the appropriate test method and setup, look into the *developmental status* of the child, especially in case of prematurity and mental or motor retardation.
- Try to *collect the results of all previous measurements*. This information helps you to find the optimal starting level.
- Always start with *bone conduction* if possible. It gives you the opportunity to use a vibrotactile stimulus (65 dBHL at 500 Hz or 45 dBHL at 250 Hz) (Cole and Flexer 2011), which you can use for conditioning the child when testing visual reinforcement audiometry (VRA) or conditioned play audiometry (CPA) (both outlined below). Even deaf children can feel these stimuli. At the same time, you obtain the result of the best inner ear, which you can compare with air-conduction results. Middle ear problems are very common in this age group. Moreover keep in mind that not every conductive hearing loss can be excluded with tympanometry.
- Continue with *air conduction*. Always try to obtain ear-specific thresholds. Insert earphones are recommended for this population to avoid a collapsed ear. A higher inter-aural attenuation makes masking less necessary. Using the child's earmould instead of the foam tip is even better.
- Use warble tones, narrowband noise or fresh noise (a more frequency-specific stimulus than typical narrowband noise (which usually has a 1/3-octave range)) instead of pure tones. Sometimes it will be necessary to find other more interesting frequency-specific stimuli to get the child's attention.
- Be very *flexible* during the test. The proposed flowcharts can be a support for those who are not used to working in this way. It will be important to maximise the child's attention span.
- Sometimes it will be necessary to *repeat* the test. Some children need more time, are not in the best condition or ask for a different way of working. Tests may need to be conducted over several sessions in order to obtain appropriate diagnostic information.

4.2.4.2 Behavioural Observation Audiometry (BOA): 0–5 Months

Leading-In

Since universal hearing screening has been introduced in many countries, diagnosis will often happen before the age of 3 months. At this age behavioural observation audiometry can be an added value with the results of objective measurement, not only as an essential part of the cross-checking but also in counselling and supporting parents.

Although BOA is not generally accepted as an integral part of the paediatric audiometry test protocol, some paediatric audiologists provided evidence of BOA in this target group many years ago (e.g. Delaroche 2001; Delaroche et al. 2004, 2005; Madell and Flexer 2008).

BOA's purpose is to obtain air-and bone-conduction data as close as possible to the hearing threshold for a broader frequency range of at least 500–4000 Hz.

This can only be performed in optimal conditions and by following a strict protocol.

Developmental Milestones

In the first 3 months of life, auditory reactions are unisensory and are based on reflexes. The most common reflexes are the cochleo-palpebral reflex, rudimentary head spin, changes in sucking, breathing, etc.

Between 3 and 5 months of age, unisensorial development becomes intersensory (i.e. the child becomes more able to combine input from more than one sensory system) (Piaget and Inhelder 1969). Most babies are already able to make a head turn to the sound, which can be reinforced by multimodal communication and personalised relationships. This has been described in the Delaroche protocol (Delaroche et al. 2011) as 'congratulating with smiles, signs, caresses and speech'.

In the following paragraphs, test equipment and setup are explained:

Conditions

It is not the purpose of behavioural audiometry to search for strong reflexes as a reaction to loud sounds, but to look for minimal changes in behaviour as a reaction to soft sounds. These reactions are called the minimal response levels (MRLs). They can only be obtained in optimal conditions, as in a light sleep or while feeding or sucking (awake but peaceful). If the child is in a deep sleep, it will not respond, so its sleep state should be confirmed, by touching the eyelashes (the eyelids will move slightly when the child is not in a deep sleep).

When the child is hungry or does not feel comfortable, it may be too distracted to respond to the quietest sounds it can hear.

Testing has to be done in a soundproof booth with minimal distraction. Minimise tactile or visual impulses; no people other than the parents are allowed. When the mother is feeding, ideally the test can start from the moment the sucking becomes effortless and regular.

Transducers

It is preferable to use the vibrator for bone conduction on an adapted diadem or softband. Air conduction with insert earphones gives ear-specific information with a great inter-aural difference. Therefore soundfield is not recommended. Furthermore, soundfield stimulation is less reactive (i.e. clear responses are more difficult to observe) and limited in loudness for finding the minimal response level (MRL) at this age.

Start with bone conduction to obtain the MRL of the better-functioning cochlea without influence of middle ear problems. The vibrator has to be placed only at the mastoid. The diadem of the vibrator has to be adjusted to the size of the child's head. Continue with insert earphones and be aware that the foam tip is not blocked with earwax (Fig. 4.12). In a later stage, one can use the customised earmould of the hearing aid instead of the foam tip.

Stimuli

To obtain a proper response of the child, use warble tone, fresh noise or narrowband noise. At this age pure tones are not attractive enough. It may be necessary to change the nature of the stimulus while testing.

Procedure

To obtain the minimal response level of the child, it is necessary to start below the expected threshold. A proper reaction can only be obtained when reaching the minimal response level for the first time for each frequency.

Start with *bone conduction*. Place the vibrator on the mastoid (Fig. 4.12 left), and observe the child's behaviour for a few minutes before presenting any sound in order to know the behaviour without auditory stimulation. If a bone-conduction hearing loss can be expected, start at the MRL of a normal-hearing child at this age, which will be 30–40 dBHL (Delaroche et al. 2011).

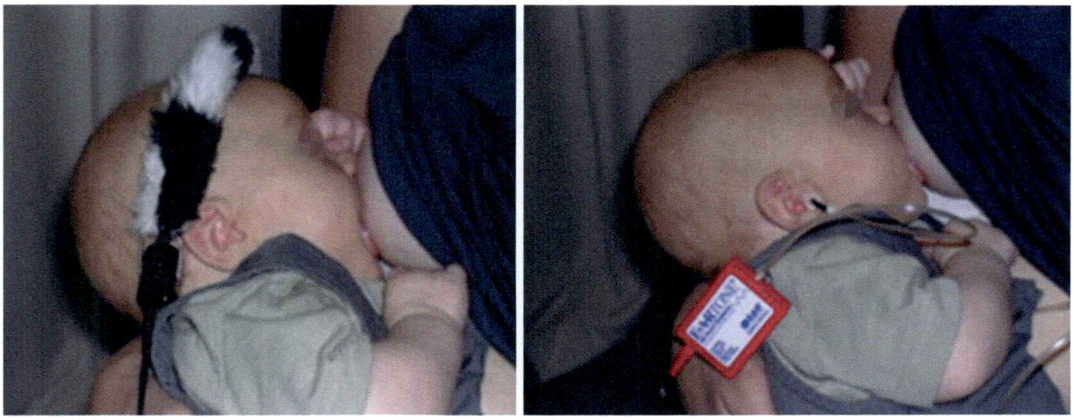

Fig. 4.12 BOA with vibrator (left) and insert earphones with foam tip (right). Photo with kind permission of the parents

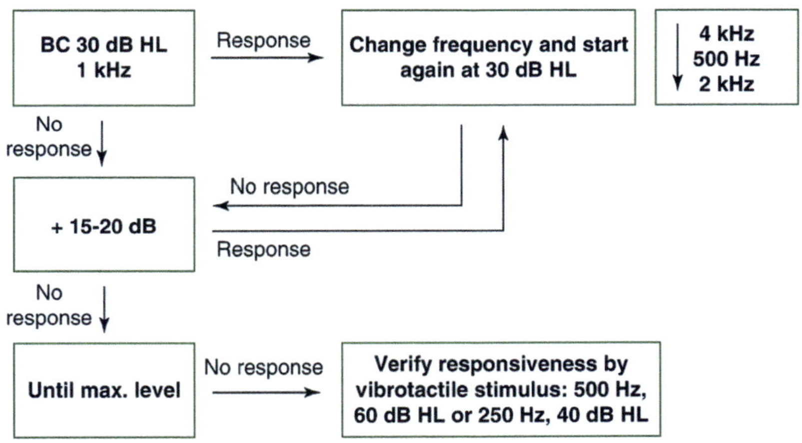

Fig. 4.13 Flowchart BOA bone conduction

Follow the steps as indicated in the flowchart (Fig. 4.13).

Continue with *air conduction* using insert earphones (Fig. 4.12 right) on the basis of information from objective measurements, if available, or start from the bone-conduction thresholds you have just measured.

If click ABR testing was performed, start at 2 kHz, 20 dB below the ABR threshold level, and choose the better ear. Preferably it is necessary to obtain ear-specific information as soon as possible. Eventually binaural stimulation by insert phones can be used to have an initial idea about the type of hearing loss and the responsiveness of the better inner ear.

Follow the steps as indicated in the flowchart (Fig. 4.14).

Characteristics of Responses

Most common responses are opening eyes, moving eyelashes and starting or stopping sucking.

The stimulation and response delay are different for each child. Make sure that this delay remains the same for the same child.

The number of observable responses is limited because of the problem of habituation. With BOA it is not possible to confirm each response as with conditioned behavioural audiometry with older children.

Minimal Response Level (MRL)

In threshold estimation with BOA, a clear distinction has to be made between neonates with normal hearing and neonates with a sensorineural hearing loss. While normal-hearing babies have higher

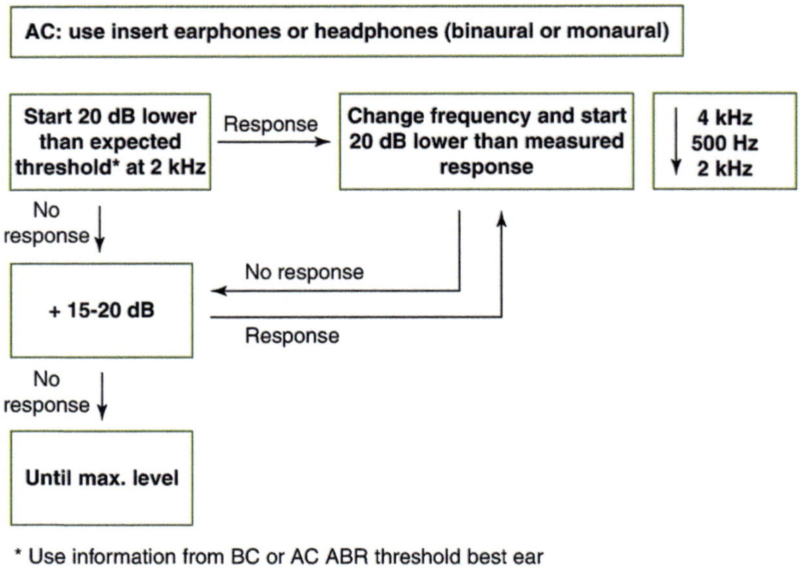

Fig. 4.14 Flowchart BOA air conduction

response levels, hearing-impaired babies with a loss of 50 dBHL or more react closer to their real hearing threshold. These findings are well described by Delaroche (Delaroche et al. 2011). One possible cause is the phenomenon of recruitment, which results in faster loudness scaling in case of sensorineural hearing loss. Another cause is the effect of surprise, which makes babies with a hearing loss respond faster and clearer to a sound that is right on or just above their threshold level.

4.2.4.3 Visual Reinforcement Audiometry (VRA): 5–24 Months

Leading-In

From the age of 5–6 months, most children can be conditioned to make a head turn response towards an auditory stimulus (Northern and Downs 2001). This will be the start of visual reinforcement audiometry (VRA) and conditioned orientation reflex audiometry (COR). In both cases a child's turning response is rewarded with a visual incentive. In VRA we use one reward. COR, using two rewards, requires adequate ability to localise a sound source. In this chapter we only discuss VRA.

Developmental Milestones

In a normal developing child of 5–6 months of age, the intersensory phase is expanding rapidly. Every time an audible sound is presented, we use the natural strong interest in coloured and illuminated animation to condition the child to look at a visual reward as reinforcer.

This will not be possible in children with intersensory problems such as autism spectrum disorders.

Conditions

VRA can be performed in a single or double soundproof booth where the lights can be dimmed. The younger the child, the more we prefer to work in a single booth. The test room should not be cluttered because, as in BOA testing, it is important to have fewer potential distractions. The examiner and test assistant keep the child attentive by being relatively quiet and not interfering while presenting the test stimuli. The presence of one parent, without interfering with the process of testing, can keep the child calm. The child needs to be seated in such a way that a head turn can easily be carried out in the direction of the visual reward.

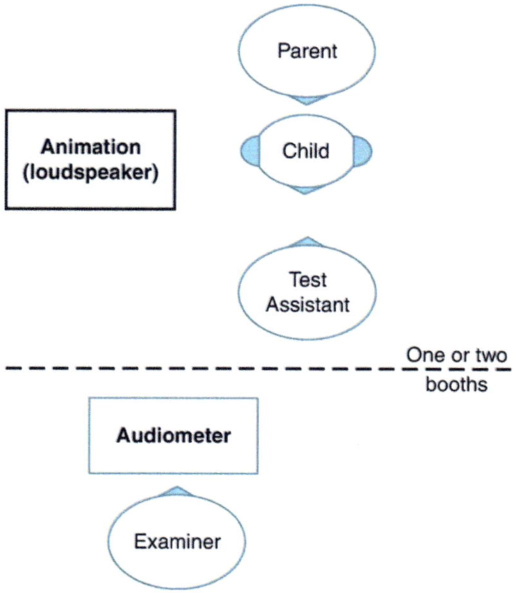

Fig. 4.15 The VRA test setup

Transducers

All transducers can be used.

Stimuli

Do not use pure tones but more reactive stimuli such as warble tone, frequency-specific fresh noise or narrowband noise. With hard-to-test children, it can be necessary to change the nature of sound during the test or even use familiar sounds (i.e. barking dog, melody, crying baby, etc.).

Setup (Fig. 4.15)

Animation and Distractors

A variety of visual animations and moving toys can be used as reinforcement. Moore et al. (1975) investigated in the effect of different kinds of visual animation. They demonstrated that auditory localisation behaviour of infants is influenced by the type of reinforcement. At the youngest age, three-dimensional animations are preferable, such as a flashing lamp and brightly illuminated mechanical toys (i.e. clown playing drums, dancing bear).

These toys have to be enclosed in a cloudy Lucite box so the child cannot easily see the animation until it is turned on. Older children, who are no longer interested in moving toys, can be reinforced with two-dimensional reinforcements such as a video or animation on a screen.

The test assistant keeps the child attentive, often by quietly playing with (interesting, but not fascinating) toys in front of the child. The tester and assistant should be relatively quiet, making sure not to interfere while the test stimuli are being presented. If the child finds the visual reinforcement very interesting, they might keep 'checking' (i.e. looking at the reinforcer even when there is no sound stimulus). In this case, the test assistant can help to distract the child from the visual animation, perhaps by temporarily increasing their level of play.

Procedure

The test procedure consists of two phases: the conditioning and the testing. It is recommended to start with *bone conduction on a vibrotactile level (500 Hz at 65 dBHL or 250 Hz at 45 dBHL)* in order to condition the child to respond by consistently turning the head to the auditory stimulus and to determine the bone-conduction thresholds.

Continue with *insert earphones* or *headphones* to determine ear-specific and air-conduction thresholds.

Follow the steps as indicated in the flowchart (Fig. 4.16).

In case of uncooperative behaviour when the vibrator or headphones cannot be used, it is better to work in free field in the first contact. In a second stage, ear-specific information should be obtained.

Free-field measurements are also useful for looking for the functional gain with hearing aids or cochlear implants. Soundfield can also be necessary to give the parents insight into the level of hearing impairment.

In cases where any contact with a vibrator or headphones is refused, it will be necessary to start in a soundfield setting.

Follow the steps as indicated in the flowchart (Fig. 4.17).

Minimal Response Level

Normal and hearing-impaired children can respond close to their hearing threshold at this age. Madell and Flexer (2008) refer to several studies

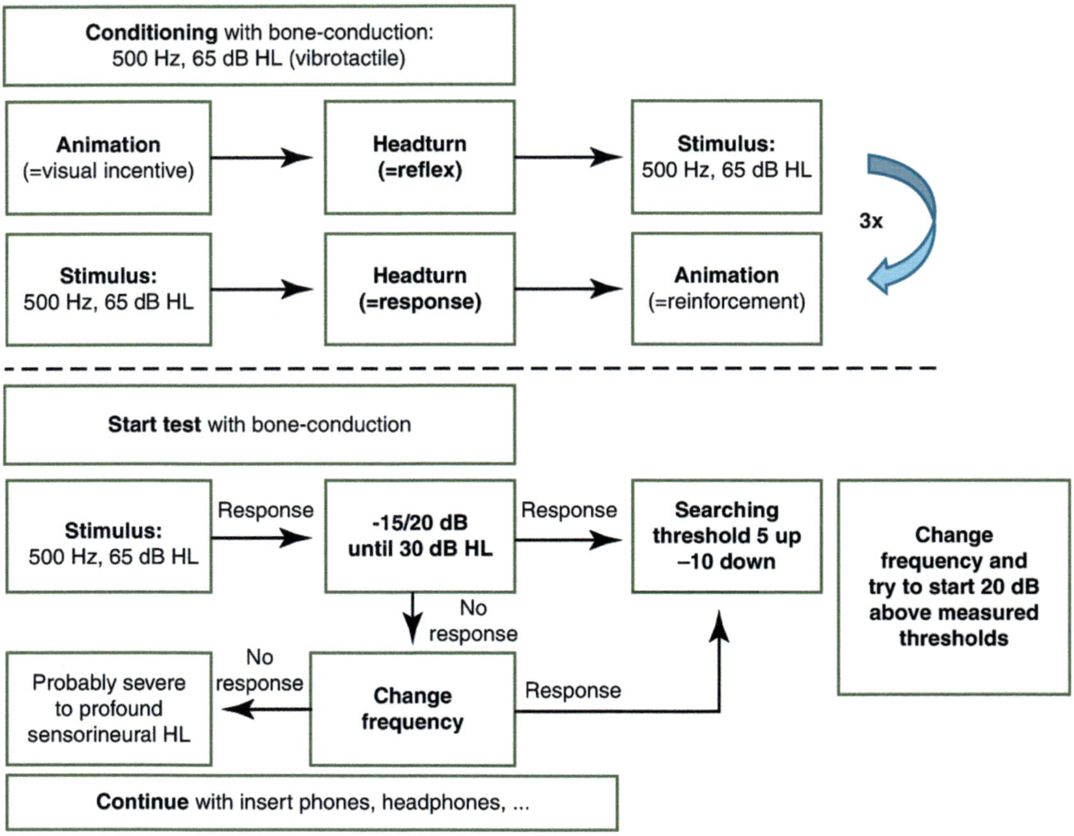

Fig. 4.16 Flowchart VRA starting with bone conduction

that demonstrate that infants with normal hearing respond to sound no higher than 15–20 dBHL and children at the age of 1 respond at an adult level. But it is still advisable to consider MRL because of the variability between the children. The responses in normal-hearing infants should not be higher than 20 dBHL for all frequencies.

4.2.4.4 Conditioned Play Audiometry (CPA): 2–5 Years

Leading-In

CPA demands the child's active cooperation by the need to perform an action after hearing an audible sound. This is a conditioned response. The 'listen and drop' task is the simplest level. The child may drop a block in a box or put a ring on a ring bar. The 'button-pushing response' to activate a rewarding animation requires a higher cognitive level, so is reserved for older children. Nowadays an interesting PowerPoint programme can be used on a laptop that is controlled by a remote mouse operated by the audiologist. Madell (Madell and Flexer 2008) called this special technique a 'computer-assisted reinforcement' procedure.

Developmental Level

Most normally developing children are near 2 or 2.5 years of age before they are able to participate in play audiometry. Children with hearing loss, who frequently have hearing tests, are able to learn the 'listen and drop' task earlier.

Infants at this age are not always cooperative. The paedaudiologist will have to be creative and flexible to obtain enough testing information. Good paedaudiologists should be able to swap quickly between a repertoire of games with different levels of engagement aimed at children with different attention and cooperation. More complex games can be reserved for older or more mature

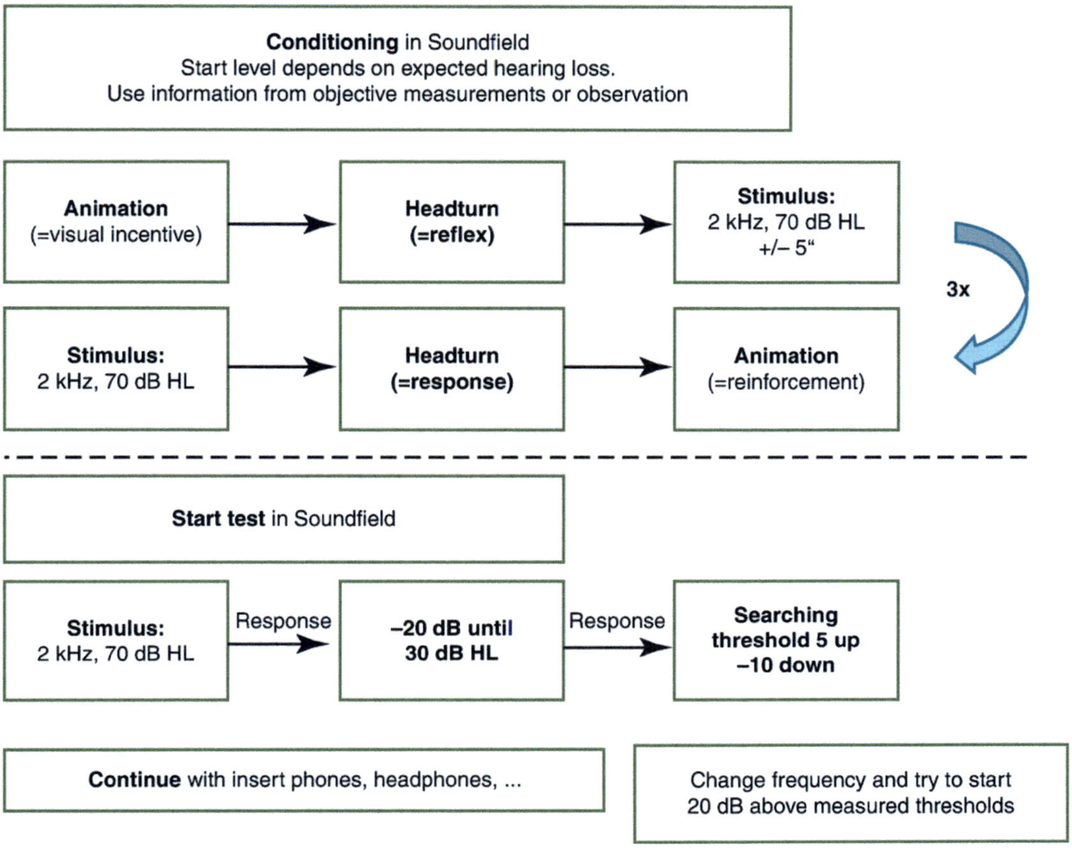

Fig. 4.17 Flowchart VRA starting in free field

children. Similarly, different types and levels of reward are appropriate. Even CPA may need to be conducted over several sessions in order to obtain appropriate diagnostic information.

Conditions
If one audiologist is performing the test, it will be necessary to work in a single soundproof booth. The test room should be orderly to avoid distraction. Parents can be involved during the training.

Transducer
Air-and bone-conduction transducers can be used in order to determine the type and the degree of hearing loss.

Stimuli
Use warble, fresh noise, speech sounds or familiar sounds.

Setup
The infant can sit at a children's table or in a highchair.

There are several possible test setups for CPA (example in Fig. 4.18). The examiner, preferably, has to sit close (next or in front of) the child in order to control their play quickly and provide social reinforcement.

Material
A variety of toys is needed, according to the interest and developmental age of the child, to be able to maintain the child's attention.

The 'listen and drop' task is the simplest level.

When using 'computer-assisted reinforcement', the child uses a push button that is not actually connected to the computer. The button-pushing responses of the child will only be

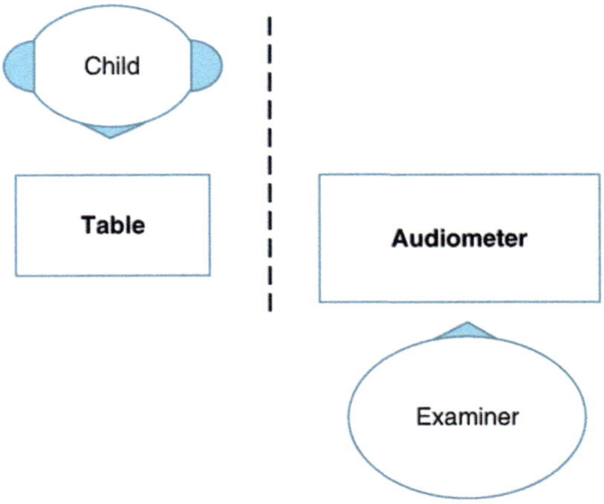

Fig. 4.18 An example of CPA test setup

rewarded if there was a preceding stimulus. Even a simple PowerPoint presentation with popular characters can maintain the child's interest.

Procedure

The test procedure consists of two phases: conditioning and testing. To start the conditioning session, it is important to use a test stimulus that the child is expected to hear. In case of doubt, bone conduction on a vibrotactile level (e.g. 500 Hz, 65 dBHL) can be used.

Conditioning

- Demonstrate the task: the audiologist and the child hold a toy to the ear to highlight the listening task. When sound (for at least 5 s) is presented, the audiologist clearly shows the presence of sound by dropping the toy. The child has to do the same. Parents can be involved as model in this process.
- After a few presentations, the child should hold the toy to the ear alone. When the sound is presented, the child must drop the toy on his/her own. Encouragement is important in this stage.
- When the child is able to do the task without assistance, the test can start.
- Remark: conditioning should be repeated at any point during the test if the child's responses seem to indicate that it is no longer cooperating.

Testing

- Rapidly decrease the level of the sound that you used for the conditioning task and continue with the '5-up-10-down method' (Hughson-Westlake method) to find the threshold.
- Change frequency and start approximately 20 dBHL above the measured response.
- If the child gets bored, the toys may need to be changed.
- When testing with insert earphones or headphones and the attention span seems to be very short, it may be necessary to change to the left or right ear after each frequency.

Response Behaviour

At this age the child may respond at an adult level, so the term 'minimal response level' is no longer appropriate.

4.2.4.5 Hard-to-Test Populations

Testing children with special needs follows the same principles as testing children without additional problems. Some adaptations and specific knowledge may be necessary.

The test procedure should be chosen according to the developmental age of the child.

- For children with an intellectual disability, the response can be significantly delayed because of the time needed to recognise the sound. Therefore it can be necessary to hold the stimulus for a longer time.
- For children with motor problems, modifications of the child's position may be necessary in order to enable clearly visible responses (i.e. when a child does not have a good trunk control, an adapted chair is needed).
- Children with visual impairment can benefit from dimming the room light in order to make the reinforcers more visible.
- For blind children, tested with VRA, air-puff reinforcement can be used instead of a visible reinforcer.
- A special technique for this population is TROCA (tangible reinforced operant conditioning audiometry), where food or tokens are used as reinforcers instead of flashing lights or mechanical toys.

With disabled children, it will be important to keep the carers involved in behavioural tests to be able to choose the right procedure and material and interpret the child's responses.

4.2.5 Assessment of Tinnitus: A Specialist Otorhinolaryngology Perspective

Armagan Incesulu, Haldun Oguz, Mustafa Asim Safak, Ahmet Atas, Songul Aksoy, Levent N. Ozluoglu and Ross Parfitt

4.2.5.1 Introduction

Tinnitus evaluation may differ according to the time of onset (acute vs chronic), classification (objective vs subjective) and accompanying symptoms; however the following steps are important and performed for almost all cases.

4.2.5.2 Medical History

An adequate, detailed medical history should gather information about possible causes (such as hearing loss, use of ototoxic drugs including salicylates, quinine and aminoglycosides), otological diseases (sensation of aural fullness, sporadic rotatory vertigo lasting hours or temporarily reduced hearing may give a hint towards Meniére's disease), non-otological diseases (head trauma, noise exposure and the presence of metabolic diseases symptoms) and the tinnitus percept: date of onset (sudden or gradual), localisation (unilateral, bilateral, in the head), subjective loudness, type of sound (ringing, buzzing, hissing, pulsating), temporal aspects (continuous, intermittent), anything that improves or worsens the tinnitus and impact upon the patient (depression, anxiety, concentration, disrupted sleep). Questionnaires to evaluate the psychological influence of the tinnitus (e.g. the Tinnitus Handicap Inventory (Newman et al. 1996)) are useful.

4.2.5.3 Clinical Examination

Ear, nose, throat and neck examination is essential for each patient in order to investigate possible objective causes. During this assessment, a temporomandibular joint examination, evaluation of the cranial nerves as well as auscultation of the neck and pressure on the ipsilateral internal jugular vein are very important. If the tinnitus percept is reduced during these manoeuvres, venous aetiology may be indicated (Baguley et al. 2013). In a very small percentage of tinnitus patients, the vascular aetiology may be due to a serious underlying disease such as carotid artery dissection or aneurysm.

4.2.5.4 Audiological Examination

Audiological Tests

Given that subjective tinnitus results primarily from dysfunction within the auditory system, an age-appropriate assessment of hearing thresholds and middle ear status may be worthwhile, both to investigate the aetiology and to guide later treatment. Such audiological investigation may include pure-tone audiometry, speech discrimination testing and tympanometry; however, uncomfortable loudness-level measurements and acoustic reflexes should be treated with caution as high-level sound may exacerbate the symptoms. Some evidence suggests that a causative auditory system change may not be detected by standard audiological tests (e.g. Fabijańska et al. 2012); therefore testing in an extended high-frequency range and the use of otoacoustic emissions may be useful. Electrocochleography (e.g. to diagnose Meniére's disease), auditory brainstem response audiometry (e.g. as one diagnostic element in detecting a cerebellopontine tumour) and videonystagmography (to find vestibular system dysfunction) (Jozefowicz-Korczynska et al. 2005) may be performed if needed.

Psychophysical and Other Tinnitus Assessment Procedures

Audiological tests, such as pitch and loudness matching, are often performed in order to define the parameters of the tinnitus percept. Note that these tests can only be carried out when the patient's tinnitus is audible to them during testing.

The basic procedure of pitch matching involves presenting low-level pure tones or narrowband noise of various frequencies and asking the patient to indicate when the pitch is similar to that of their tinnitus. As tinnitus may be a spectrum of sounds, spectral matching is recommendable (Henry 2016).

Loudness matching involves increasing the level of the pitch-matched signal (usually in 1 dB steps) from threshold until the patient indicates that the loudness of the signal and tinnitus are equal. Both procedures should be performed separately for each affected ear if possible.

It is important that the patient understands the difference between pitch and loudness during these matching procedures and that they are informed that slightly inexact responses will not hinder their treatment. The matched frequency and level are often indicated by a '*T*' sign on the audiogram.

Minimum masking level (MML) procedures are sometimes carried out with the aim of determining the patient's ability to suppress the tinnitus signal in the presence of competing noise. The level of white noise (a random broadband signal that includes energy at all audible frequencies) is gradually increased until the patient reports any change in the tinnitus (such as it becoming louder, softer or entirely suppressed). Tinnitus matching and MML testing are, however, much less simple than one might expect. For example, many different matching procedures have been tested since the 1940s, and this area is rife with methodological difficulties (see Henry and Meikle 2000).

Tinnitus can be inhibited for up to approx. 1 min in some patients following some types of auditory stimulation. This is known as residual inhibition. According to Henry (2016), studies should be performed to develop optimal stimuli for extending this effect as basis for a new therapeutic approach.

Given that parameters of the tinnitus percept, such as loudness, pitch and quality, do not correlate with the perceived severity of tinnitus (Meikle et al. 1984), tinnitus severity may be better assessed from questionnaires (such as the Tinnitus Handicap Inventory) which address the patient's perception of their tinnitus and its impact on their lives, rather than psychophysical investigation.

The Tinnitus Handicap Inventory (THI) (Newman et al. 1996) contains 25 self-reporting closed questions related to personal and social situations as well as feelings about tinnitus, designed to assess the severity of the patient's tinnitus (slight, mild, moderate, severe or catastrophic). Other tinnitus questionnaires exist, such as the Iowa Tinnitus Handicap Questionnaire (Kuk et al. 1990), the Tinnitus Reaction Questionnaire (Wilson et al. 1991) and the Tinnitus Functional Index (TFI) (Henry et al. 2014). But as to our knowledge, there are no standardised questionnaires for children (BSA 2014).

In patients with hearing impairment, the ten-item Tinnitus and Hearing Survey (THS) (Henry et al. 2015) separates complaints caused by hearing loss from self-perceived problems induced by tinnitus by two specific subscales.

Given the strong connection between tinnitus and anxiety/depression, some clinics also use tools such as the Hospital Anxiety and Depression Scale (Zigmond and Snaith 1983) to assess the psychological impact on the patient.

4.2.5.5 Other Investigations

If, e.g. chronic otitis media or otosclerosis is suspected, high-resolution computed tomography may be useful. Magnetic resonance imaging is usually the preferred method in patients with asymmetric hearing loss or asymmetric tinnitus to rule out a cerebellopontine angle tumour, such as vestibular schwannoma. Magnetic resonance angiography or venography may be necessary in cases with suspected cerebral ischemia, dural sinus thrombosis or neoplastic lesion (Sismanis 2011). Doppler ultrasonography may be useful for exploring the vascular structures in the neck. Blood tests for haemodynamic and metabolic diseases are also important.

4.2.6 Assessment of Tinnitus in Children and Teenagers: A Specialist Paediatric Audiology and Hearing Therapy Perspective[1]

Claire Benton and Charlotte Rogers

Prevalence figures for tinnitus in children in studies vary from 12 to 36% for normally hearing children and go up to 66% for children with

[1]Article written on behalf of the British Society of Audiology Paediatric Tinnitus Working Party. Supported by the British Tinnitus Association.

known hearing loss (Shetye and Kennedy 2010). The impact of tinnitus in children is in many ways similar to that in adults, affecting sleep, concentration and listening skills (Kentish et al. 2000).

4.2.6.1 History

A comprehensive history is necessary to get a full picture of the impact of a child's tinnitus, ensuring the child's views are fully included. The history should cover the following points:

- Description of tinnitus sounds: children can use very descriptive language to describe what they hear such as 'buzzing bees', 'swishing' and 'like a train'. Younger children may find it helpful to draw a picture of their tinnitus. Where possible details of onset, duration and how often it is heard are useful.
- Impact of tinnitus: there are currently no standardised tinnitus questionnaires for children. The impact and concerns of both the parents and the child should be investigated. Finding out about the effects of the tinnitus on school and home life is important. Standardised measures of anxiety and depression in children do exist and these can be helpful.
- Hearing difficulties and other audiovestibular symptoms: it is important to rule out any physiological reason for the tinnitus. Asking about their history of otitis media with effusion is also useful.
- Medical and neurological factors: any history of head trauma or noise trauma should be noted. Other general medical problems may also be relevant, for example, migraine can be associated with auditory sensitivity and tinnitus.
- Factors affecting their tinnitus: some children or families may have noticed factors that make the tinnitus better or worse, such as tiredness, school situations or stress. It is very important to find out about the child's whole life and potential areas of stress for him or her, such as bereavement or family breakdowns.

4.2.6.2 Clinical Assessment

Children with tinnitus can find audiometry particularly stressful; they may have a history of being difficult to assess or have variable results on previous tests. The testing environment should be child-friendly and the children given time to do the test at their own pace. It is important to establish accurate, ear-specific thresholds by using age-appropriate testing techniques. Observing the child closely throughout the test allows any signs of anxiety to be seen and reassurance given. Otoscopy and middle ear admittance measurements are always needed to rule out any pathology that requires further medical treatment. At the moment, loudness discomfort measures or any tinnitus-matching tests are not recommended, as there is very limited evidence for either the diagnostic or therapeutic benefit of such tests (see Henry and Meikle 2000 for a review of such psychoacoustic measures).

4.2.7 Speech Audiometry at the Phoneme and Word Level

Frans Coninx

4.2.7.1 Introduction

The assessment of auditory processing and recognition of speech in infants and children is important and complex: the child's performance in a speech recognition test does not only depend on the auditory skills themselves but also on factors such as language, cognition, articulation and speech, visual cognition, attention and concentration. Typically, these factors are dynamic and changing over time.

On the basis of the Erber (1982) level scheme for auditory functions (see Table 4.2), auditory speech tasks may be at the detection, discrimination or identification/recognition level. Comprehension is not included here, as such tasks (certainly in an open-set format) depend not only on hearing but are also determined to a major extent by central linguistic and cognitive skills.

4.2.7.2 Phoneme/Syllable Level

The Ling 6 sound test contains the phonemes for [m], [ah], [oo], [ee], [sh] and [s], being familiar speech sounds that cover the relevant speech range from 250 to 8000 Hz (Ling 1989). It can be

Table 4.2 Structured overview of auditory tests at four functional levels

Level	Phonemes/syllables	Words
Detection	• Ling 6 sound test • Ling sounds-based 'PTA' (pure-tone audiometry)	
Discrimination	• A§E (auditory speech sounds evaluation; Govaerts et al. 2006) • H-LAD (Heidelberger Lautdifferenzierungstest; Brunner et al. 1998) • WADT (Wepman auditory discrimination test; Ross 1979)	
Identification/ recognition		Pictures tasks • MTS (Monosyllable-Trochee-Spondee test; Erber and Alencewicz 1976) • AAST (adaptive auditory speech test; Coninx 2005)
Comprehension		

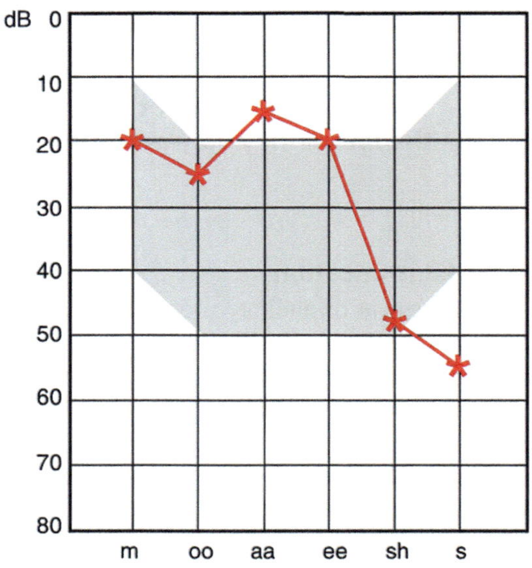

Fig. 4.19 The Ling Audiogram shows the detection thresholds of the six Ling sounds. In this example, the detection of the two fricatives is most likely not good enough for them to be heard in normal running speech

used with children who are conditioned for and familiar with this task, by professionals as well as by parents. The aim is to assess or verify the detection or identification of the six speech sounds. With the purpose of assessing detection thresholds, a Ling sounds-based PTA paradigm can be used. The 'Ling Audiogram' result (see Fig. 4.19) will show the six thresholds for detection-identification of Ling sounds and allows a quick and easy judgement of whether or not the six phonemes will be audible in normal running speech.

The Ling test uses isolated phonemes. A phoneme-based test, supplying useful information on the basic listening level, can also be based on a syllable form or even by using words.

As an example, in the A§E test (Govaerts et al. 2006), syllables are used to assess detection and discrimination skills in the child. For both skills, an operant conditioning protocol is used: visual reinforcement audiometry (VRA). The response of the child to the detection of a stimulus or the discrimination of a stimulus change has to be reliably observed by using paradigms that are adapted to the developmental level of the child. For the difficult-to-test younger children, VRA (Coninx and Moore 1997) might be the only successful procedure; for older children the usual techniques of play audiometry can be used. With the VRA paradigm, not only phoneme detection but also phoneme discrimination can be investigated. In case of discrimination testing, the visual reinforcer is presented in relation to a sudden change in a sequence of 'stable' phonemes or syllables (e.g. da-da-da…) to another sequence of 'stable' stimuli (e.g. ta-ta-ta…). A response of the child to the sudden phoneme change is visually reinforced.

For older children, easier and faster 'same-different'-based tasks can be used instead. The stimuli would be two isolated phonemes (/s/–/f/

or /a/–/e/), two consonant-vowel syllables (/sa/–/fa/ or /ba/–/be/) or a minimal word pair, differing only in the same phoneme contrast (seat-feet or ball-bell). Various responses from the child can be used: verbal feedback ('same' versus 'different') or pointing to a picture representing same or different. Isolated phonemes or consonant-vowel syllables are considered to be better than words, because the test result for word pairs might depend on the vocabulary of the child. This is caused by lexical neighbourhood processes (Janse and Newman 2013). Examples of word-pair tests are H-LAD (German, Brunner et al. 1998) and WADT (English, Ross 1979).

4.2.7.3 Word Level

The most frequently used form of speech audiometry in children is based on words. Children develop skills to identify or recognise words earlier than full sentences, as well as earlier than isolated phonemes (a subskill of phonological awareness). For test applications, the words have to be chosen carefully in order to be within the vocabulary of children in the target group age. The words can be presented as stimuli in a quiet or noisy environment. The response of the child can be different: repeating the spoken word or pointing (or comparable action) to a picture or object that represents the spoken word.

A well-known version of such a test is the MTS test (Erber and Alencewicz 1976). Each of the 12 words used as stimulus is in one of three prosodic categories: monosyllables, trochees and spondees. Within each of the categories, the child can identify the words only on phoneme-based information. A picture table is shown (see Fig. 4.20) and the child has to point; as a consequence, the MTP test is a closed-set test. Results can be analysed and differentiated at the prosodic and segmental levels. These closed-set tests are available in many languages.

Open-set tests are similar to many tests used for adult listeners. This choice has to be carefully considered, as interference with the speech and articulation skills and the vocabulary of the child will interfere with the auditory skills as such. A gold standard for an open-set test—for English—is the PB-K test (Haskins 1949), which uses a

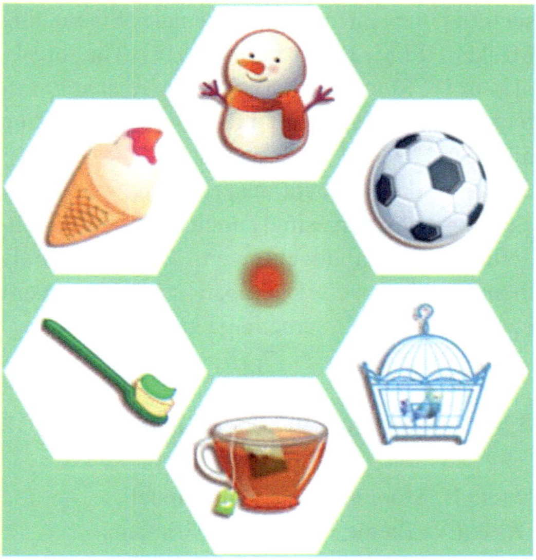

Fig. 4.20 The six spondee words of the AAST UK version. The red dot in the centre cell is a visual prompt during stimulus presentation

phonetically balanced word list for children in kindergarten.

Closed tests as described above are used to assess a word recognition score at a selected fixed intensity, at 65 dB SPL or at the individually different most comfortable level (MC).

In order to find a speech recognition threshold (SRT), the test has to be repeated several times; alternatively, adaptive paradigms have to be used. A typical example is the adaptive auditory speech test (AAST) for children aged 3–4 years and above (Coninx 2005). Only six spondee words are used, requiring little vocabulary and minimised influence of working memory and visual cognition when the child is searching for the correct picture to click. When using touchscreen technology, even young children 3–4 years old can do the test and are highly motivated and concentrated. After typically 1–1.5 min, the SRT measurement is completed. The result of a test has to be interpreted by taking the age-dependent normal values into account. An important advantage of AAST is the multi-lingual applicability with nearly language-independent normal values.

For tests in noise, steady-state noise can be used (more likely related to cochlear dysfunctions) (Smits et al. 2013) or fluctuating noises, such as the International Female Fluctuating Masker (IFFM, Holube et al. 2011). The thresholds in IFFM are more likely to be related to retrocochlear dysfunctions, i.e. auditory processing disorders.

Future development in speech audiometry for children will increasingly include modern technology with a touchscreen. This not only increases the level of motivation but also opens options for remote screening and testing.

4.2.8 Auditory Processing Tests

David R. Moore, Nicole G. Campbell, Doris-Eva Bamiou, and Tony Sirimanna

4.2.8.1 Diagnosis

There is no universally agreed diagnostic procedure for auditory processing disorder (APD). Diagnostic recommendations have been made by the American Speech-Language-Hearing Association (ASHA 2005a, b) and by the American Academy of Audiology (AAA 2010) on the basis of several distinct forms of impaired auditory processing outlined below. These recommendations are a quasi-international standard, but in practice the recommendations are adhered to only loosely in the USA (Emanuel et al. 2011) and even less so in other countries (Hind et al. 2011). In Germany, the diagnosis of 'auditory processing and perception disorder' (APPD) (German: auditive Verarbeitungs-und Wahrnehmungsstörung (AVWS)) includes auditory-specific cognitive impairment as a designated form of APPD (GSPP 2014), but only if that impairment is judged not to be described by other, more widely accepted terms (e.g. attention deficit disorder, language impairment). Some countries have issued practice guidelines in recent years, rather than stipulating comprehensive diagnostic measures and criteria. For example, Australian Hearing has implemented standard procedures for the diagnosis, assessment and management of some aspects of APD (Hearing 2013), and the British Society of Audiology (BSA APD SIG 2011a; 2018) has provided an evidence-based commentary to guide practice.

An attempt to reach a consensus on APD definition, diagnosis and management was the principal aim of two ASHA Technical Reports (ASHA 1996; 2005b). Auditory processing was determined to be the neural mechanisms underlying auditory discrimination and pattern recognition; temporal, spatial and binaural aspects of hearing; and perception of competing and degraded auditory signals. APD was defined as a disorder of one or more of these processes, which were noted to be necessary for both non-verbal and verbal perception. Impairments should be diagnosed by using a variety of non-standard indices (e.g. case history, observation of behaviour, questionnaires) and standardised auditory measures that use both non-verbal and verbal stimuli. Electrophysiological testing (e.g. auditory brainstem response, cortical event-related potentials) was also suggested, but details were not provided. Performance of at least two standard deviations (s.d.) below the (standardised) mean on two auditory processing tests, or 3 s.d. on one test, is 'generally required for diagnosis'. However, both the ASHA Reports and the AAA (2010) Guidelines suggest that the number and specific type of tests used should depend on individual cases. There is no specification of the number of tests that are to be used, and the criteria, like those proposed by other groups, are arbitrary. Statistically, the more tests performed, the more likely an individual will fail two of them. Wilson and Arnott (2013) showed in a large sample of children ($n = 150$) that diagnosis rates of APD can range from 7 to 93% depending upon which criteria are applied, even using the same test battery.

4.2.8.2 Differential Diagnosis

Because APD typically presents as problems involving speech perception, most guidelines recommend verbal (speech-based) testing. For example, the commonly used SCAN test battery (Keith 2009) has four core tests that all use verbal stimuli. Verbal stimuli used in APD diagnosis vary from nonmeaningful phonemes (e.g. 'da') or vowel-consonant-vowel (VCV) syllables (e.g. 'ata') through commonly used short words (e.g. 'dog') to longer words and whole sentences. These stimuli all involve a lesser or greater degree of memory and linguistic processing that strong neurological evidence suggests occurs beyond the central auditory nervous system, primarily in the anterior temporal and frontal brain lobes. An ongoing debate concerns whether APD should be diagnosed when only 'unimodal' auditory deficits (i.e. deficits specific to hearing) are found (Cacace and McFarland 2013).

To segregate distinctly auditory deficits, non-verbal testing for APD diagnosis is also recommended. Non-verbal tests attempt to isolate those aspects of auditory processing, as listed above (discrimination, pattern recognition, etc.), that are the building blocks of everyday listening. However, there is scant evidence that either these tests or those involving verbal stimuli are very good predictors of the listening problems that people being assessed for APD typically report (Moore et al. 2010; Watson and Kidd 2009). The most common of those problems are, for children, academic difficulties and attentive listening to speech, especially in challenging environments (AAA 2010; Campbell et al. 2012). In addition, listening to both speech in everyday life, and to verbal or non-verbal tests in the clinic, necessarily accesses cognitive resources that are mostly 'supra-modal' (not specific to hearing). These resources include attention, memory, fluid intelligence, motivation and emotion. Professional guidelines urge the clinician to ensure that the person being tested is attentive, but clinicians cannot adequately control or measure cognitive influences on perception with current test procedures.

4.2.8.3 Occurrence of APD (Not ADP!) with Other Learning Problems

Only a small proportion of children referred to audiology clinics are assessed for APD, and only a fraction of them receive a diagnosis of APD (Hind et al. 2011; Moore and Hunter 2013). However, around 20% of all children have speech, language, attention, behaviour, reading or intellectual difficulties. A substantial proportion of them perform poorly on tests of auditory processing (Amitay et al. 2002; Ferguson et al. 2011; Miller and Wagstaff 2011; Sharma et al. 2009) or have behaviour that overlaps extensively with that seen in children with APD (Chermak et al. 1999, 2002). Conversely, most children diagnosed with APD have multiple difficulties. Do those children all have APD? The relation between perception and cognition has been debated for well over 100 years, i.e. whether hearing or vision determines intelligence or vice versa (Spearman 1904). Surprisingly, this is still a current debate, for example, in the extensive literature on language and reading difficulties (Ziegler et al. 2005, 2009). The problem faced by hearing specialists is whether to diagnose APD, recognising the non-specific nature of the diagnosis, or to refer a child for a more broadly based assessment. In either case, identifying individual difficulties is the first step towards appropriate treatment.

4.2.8.4 How Should APD Be Diagnosed?

It has recently been suggested (Dillon et al. 2012) that specific treatment for APD may be an appropriate form of management for some children. These children may be identified by specific tests, for each of which there is a specific treatment, delivered in a hierarchical fashion. A scheme that builds on this model is shown in Fig. 4.21. The aim here is to provide a specific strategy for clinicians, so that a more rational and uniform approach to management may be delivered and the outcome may better describe a more specific problem that the child has.

4.2.8.5 Current Situation and Way Forward

Several groups around the world have now issued APD statements, guidelines or white papers, including the American Speech-Language-Hearing Association (ASHA 2005a, b), the American Academy of Audiology (AAA 2010), the British Society of Audiology (BSA APD SIG 2011a, b, 2018; Moore et al. 2013), the Canadian Interorganizational Steering Group for Speech-Language Pathology and Audiology (2012), the German Society of Phoniatrics and Paediatric Audiology (Nickisch et al. 2015), the Australian National Acoustics Laboratory (NAL 2015), the Dutch Position Statement (De Wit et al. 2017)

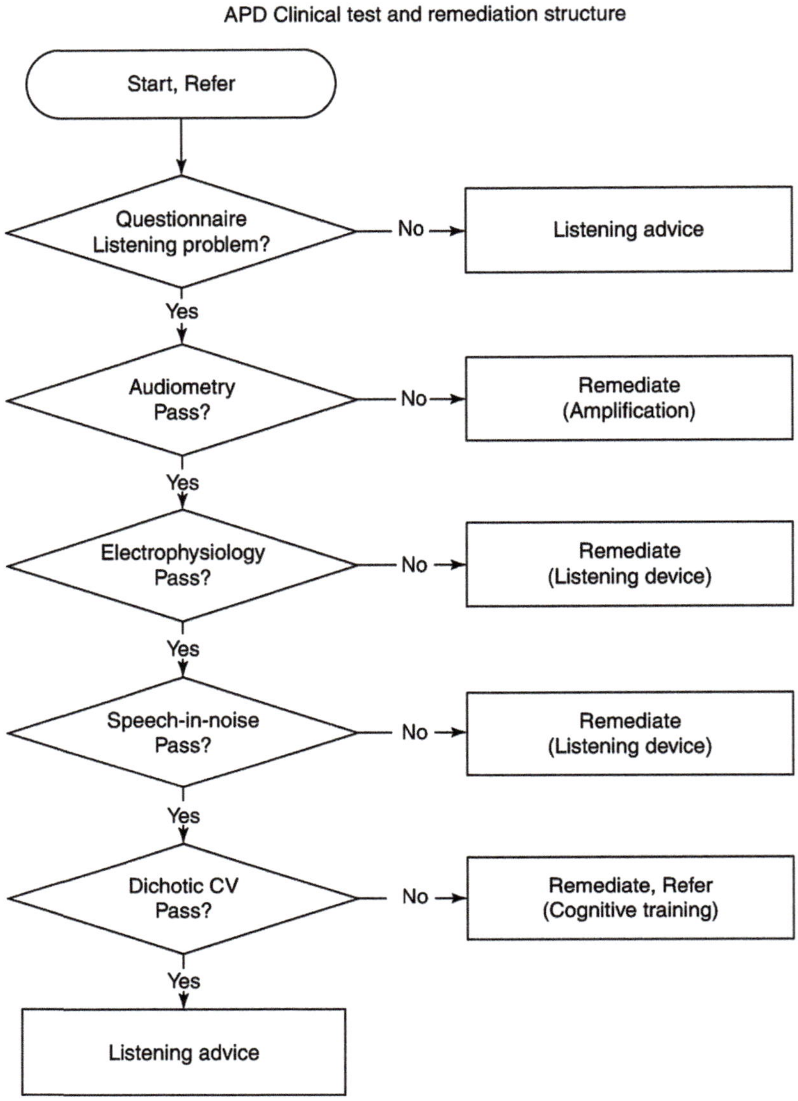

Fig. 4.21 Draft hierarchical scheme for the diagnosis and rehabilitation of APD by using specific assessments that incorporate a problem-orientated approach and differential and adaptive testing (Moore 2012; Dillon et al. 2012). The scheme includes conventional (audiometry) and research procedures. A validated questionnaire (e.g. ECLiPS (Barry and Moore 2014, Barry et al. 2015)) assesses everyday listening skills which, if deficient, lead to further objective assessments. Electrophysiological testing (auditory brainstem and frequency-following response) determines ear and brainstem function objectively. Speech-in-noise testing (e.g. LiSN-S) and 'forced attention' dichotic CV syllables (Hugdahl et al. 2009) differentiate 'bottom-up' and 'top-down' processing difficulties

and more recently a group in Europe which has published its perspective on APD (Iliadou et al. 2017). As outlined at the beginning of this section, there is no universally agreed diagnostic procedure for APD, but all of the above documents contribute to international debate and better understanding. High-calibre research, alongside international and interdisciplinary dialogue, is imperative for informing future evidence-based practice. The APD MESHGuide, a new evidence based online resource, offers practical guidance (Campbell et al. 2019).

Remediation is considered in Sect. 18.14.

4.2.9 Acoustic Immittance Measurements

Piotr Świdziński and Ross Parfitt

4.2.9.1 Introduction

The ability of the tympanic membrane and ossicular chain to transfer sound waves from the outer ear canal through the middle ear is known by a variety of related terms that have specific technical differences but are often used interchangeably in common practice: admittance, compliance, conductance, immittance and susceptance. The opposite (i.e. the ability of the mechanism to resist the transfer of sound) is typically known as impedance or reflectance.

The stiffer the tympanic membrane, the smaller the amount of sound energy admitted through it (low admittance) and the greater the amount of sound energy reflected by it (high impedance). Sound energy is optimally transferred across the tympanic membrane when the air pressure within the middle ear is equal to that in the outer ear canal, which is typically an atmospheric pressure of 0 daPa (decapascals). Most common disorders of the middle ear, such as middle ear effusion or Eustachian tube dysfunction, affect the air pressure within it, thus stiffening the tympanic membrane.

Tympanometry measures admittance at various external air pressures in order to assess the presence of middle ear disorders. Acoustic reflex testing assesses the basic function of cochlear and retrocochlear structures involved in the acoustic reflex arc by measuring the lowest sound level that triggers contraction of the stapedius muscle (a response that stiffens the ossicular chain and tympanic membrane, resulting in measurably reduced admittance).

While tympanometry and acoustic reflex testing are not direct measures of hearing sensitivity, tympanometry especially plays a crucial role in audiological diagnostics, providing further information in cases of conductive hearing loss and functioning as a cross-check to support the findings of other tests. Other acoustic immittance tests exist (e.g. acoustic reflectometry and tests of Eustachian tube function) but are not common in clinical audiology and are not discussed in this article.

The patient does not need to respond actively during acoustic immittance tests and should ideally be still and quiet.

A tympanometer is used for both tympanometry and acoustic reflex testing. Modern tympanometers are often hand-held, wireless devices linked to a computer, but older, larger stand-alone models are still common. The core mechanism is a probe consisting of three tubes: one attached to an air pump, another to deliver a pure tone (the 'probe tone') generated by a miniature loudspeaker in the main body of the device and the third a microphone (Fig. 4.22). The probe is inserted into the outer ear canal with an appropriately sized disposable silicone tip to create an airtight seal with the wall of the ear canal.

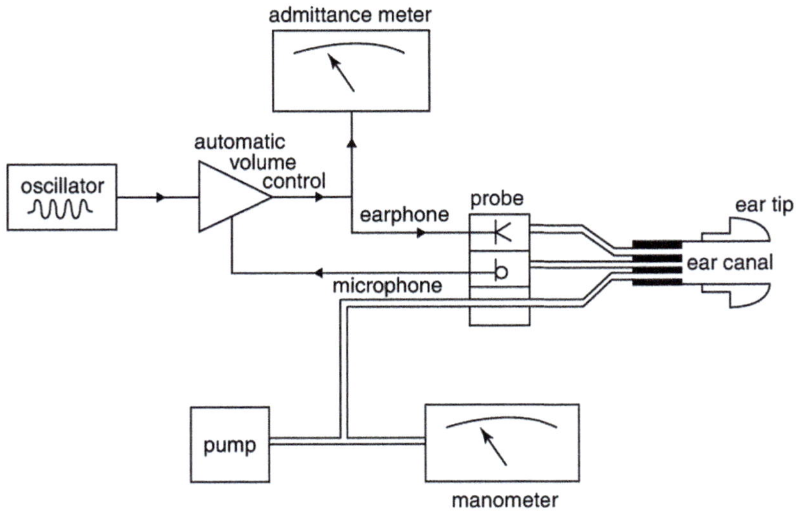

Fig. 4.22 Block diagram showing key components of an audiometer, the probe and ear tip and an air pump and manometer, to change and monitor air pressure in the outer ear canal; the probe tone is generated by the oscillator and conducted to the ear canal via the earphone; the microphone measures the level (dB SPL) of the probe tone in the opening of the outer ear canal and admittance is calculated. Image from Benton et al. (2004), with kind permission from Wiley © (2004)

International standards for the calibration of tympanometers (ISO 60645-5 2005) must be adhered to.

4.2.9.2 Tympanometry

In tympanometry, the air pressure in the outer ear canal is varied over the course of a few seconds, usually from a positive pressure of approximately 200 daPa to a negative pressure of approximately −400 daPa at a rate of 50 daPa/s (e.g. British Society of Audiology (BSA) 2013. The rate and direction of pressure change can be varied in many tympanometers, but variations in these parameters play little role in typical clinical testing. During this pressure change, the probe tone (usually 226 Hz) is played constantly into the outer ear canal, and the sound that is reflected from the tympanic membrane is detected by the microphone.

Results and Interpretation

A real-time trace of the inverse of the amount of reflected sound across the gradually changing air pressure is shown on the tympanometer display (admittance or compliance on the Y-axis and pressure on the X-axis) (Fig. 4.23). This graph is known as a tympanogram. The peak of the trace (i.e. the point at which compliance is highest)

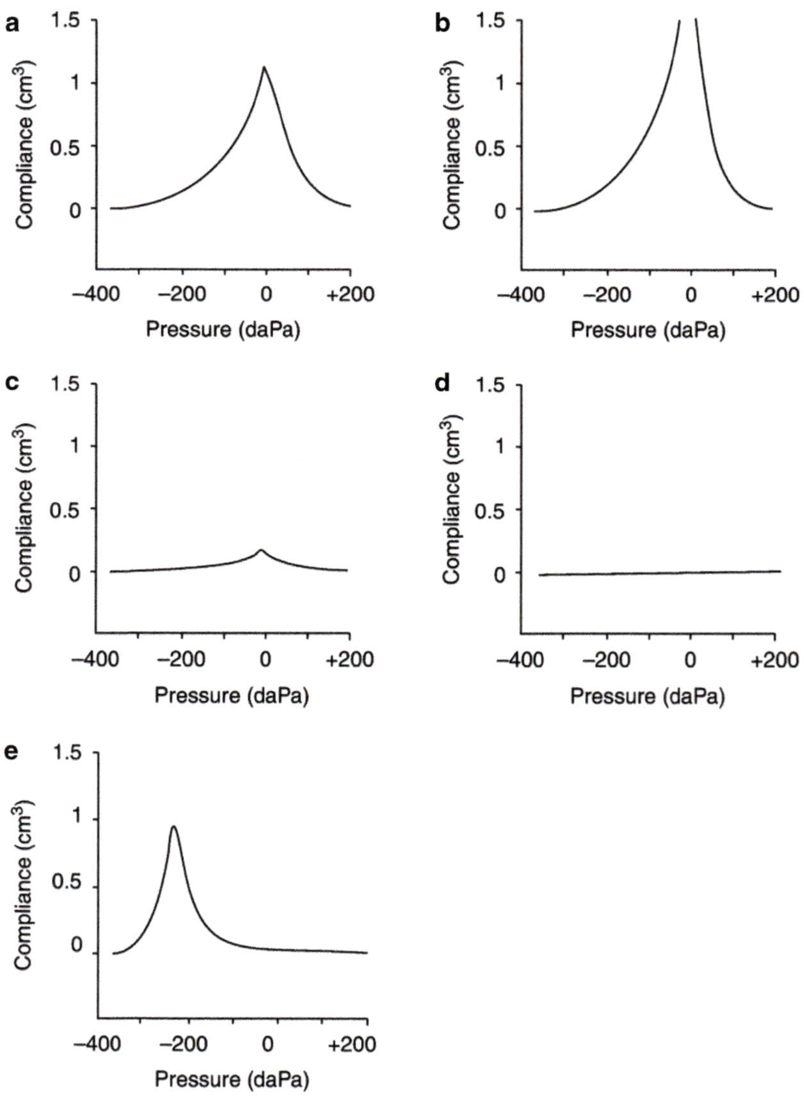

Fig. 4.23 Classic tympanogram shapes: (**a**) normal, (**b**) hypermobile, (**c**) reduced compliance, (**d**) flat, (**e**) negative

reflects the point at which air pressure is equal in the outer and middle ear. This can be compared with established normal values (Table 4.3). The volume of air required to fill the ear canal (known as the equivalent ear canal volume (EECV) or just the ear canal volume) is also recorded and can be compared with norms (Table 4.3). The norms shown in Table 4.3 are from the British Society of Audiology (2013). Other norms exist but the principle of interpretation is the same.

A classification system is sometimes used when reporting tympanometric results (e.g. Jerger 1970, Table 4.3), but it is preferable to report the actual values obtained. Some commonly used terms for reporting audiogram shape are also indicated in Table 4.3 (Fig. 4.23a–e showing common results of tympanometry).

Many tympanometers also show gradient, which essentially reports the sharpness or roundedness of the peak, but different manufacturers use different algorithms to calculate this (BSA 2013) so interpretation is not always clear. Gradient does not play an important role in typical clinical interpretation guidelines.

Contraindications

Tympanometry should be preceded by otoscopy or microscopy in order to check for occluding wax (which should be removed before testing), inflammation or infection of the outer ear (which would contraindicate the test owing to the risk of pain or cross infection) and to provide a visual check of the status of the tympanic membrane. Previous tympanic membrane surgery may con-

Table 4.3 Tympanogram interpretation when using a 226 Hz probe tone

Result				Description	
Peak compliance (mL, mmho/L or cm^3)	Peak pressure (daPa)	Ear canal volume (cm^3)	Interpretation	Commonly used term	Audiogram type (Jerger 1970)
Adults: 0.3–1.6 Children (6 m–6y): ≥0.2 (BSA 2013)	Adults: −50 to +50 Children: −200 to +50 (BSA 2013)	Adults: 0.6–1.5 Children: 0.4–1.0 (BSA 2013)	Middle ear function within the normal range	Normal	A
Higher than normal range	Normal range	Normal range	Hypermobile tympanic membrane or ossicular discontinuity	Hypermobile	A_D
Lower than normal range	Normal range	Normal range	Reduced tympanic membrane mobility or ossicular fixation	Reduced compliance	A_S
Flat	Flat	Normal range	Middle ear effusion	Flat	B
Normal range	Higher than normal range	Normal range	Possible acute middle ear pathology	Positive	–
Normal range	Lower than normal range	Normal range	Eustachian tube dysfunction	Negative	C
Flat	Flat	Higher than normal range	Grommet in situ and patent or perforated tympanic membrane	Large ECV	–
Flat	Flat	Lower than normal range	Occluding wax or incorrectly placed probe	–	–

traindicate tympanometry because of the risk of the change in air pressure damaging the TM.

The change in air pressure should not be painful or uncomfortable for the patient in the absence of infection or inflammation. Subjects with pressure-related vertigo, such as that resulting from a perilymph fistula in the vestibular system, may feel some dizziness, but other patients typically do not.

Tympanometry can be performed on compliant patients of any age, with a small but crucial change in probe tone frequency for younger patients (see below).

Probe Tone Frequency

For children younger than 6 months corrected age (BSA 2013) or with an ear canal volume less than 0.9 mL (Limberger et al. 2007), a probe tone frequency of 1000 Hz provides a better measure than the typical 226 Hz. This is because the walls of the infant ear canal are more flexible than those of older children and adults, and a large contribution to the tympanometry results can come from the compliance of the outer ear canal itself, rather than just the middle ear. This effect is reduced when using a higher-frequency probe tone.

Tympanogram interpretation is different when using the 1 kHz probe tone. The BSA recommends the following steps (see BSA 2013 for more details): first, drawing a straight line between the compliance levels at the positive and negative pressure endpoints of the trace (−400 and + 200 daPa) and then determining if the peak is above this line ('positive peak'), when middle ear function is essentially normal, or below this line ('negative peak') or there is no peak, when ear function should be considered abnormal (Fig. 4.24).

Wideband Tympanometry

Wideband tympanometry (also known as 3D or multi-frequency tympanometry) is a comparatively new development in the clinic. A broadband click is used instead of a single-frequency probe tone, allowing the response of the middle ear at many frequencies (typically 226–8000 Hz) to be measured simultaneously. The results are plotted on a 3D tympanogram (Fig. 4.25). The main measure is no longer compliance or admittance (in mmho/L, mL or cm^3) but absorption or absorbance, which is the percentage of the incoming sound energy absorbed by the middle ear (i.e. the percentage which is not reflected back to the probe microphone). Wideband tympanometry has potential benefits, such as measuring multiple different-frequency tympanograms simultaneously, the ability to measure without changing air pressure (therefore safer for postop-

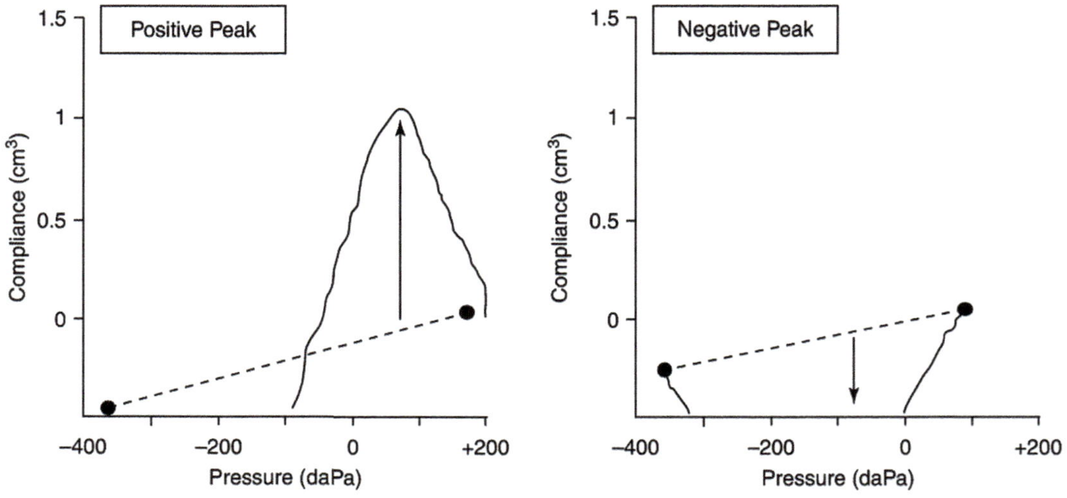

Fig. 4.24 Interpretation of tympanometry when using a 1 kHz probe tone. Image adapted with kind permission of the British Society of Audiology (2013)

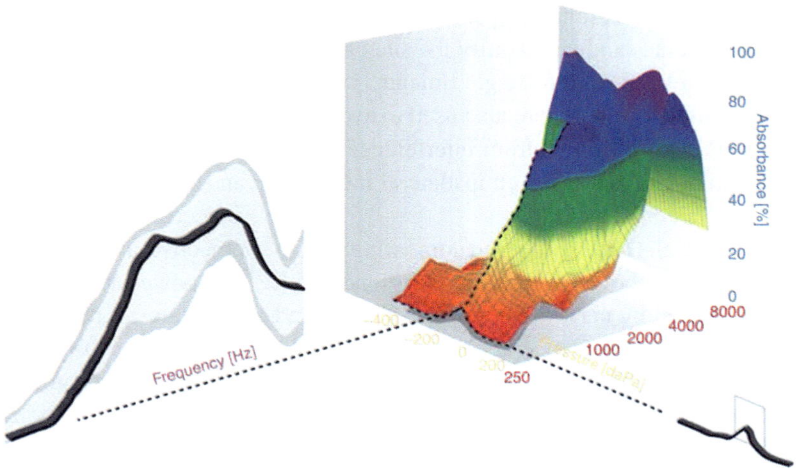

Fig. 4.25 A hypothetical 3D tympanogram on which frequency (in red), pressure (in orange) and absorbance (in blue) are shown. Image copyright and with kind permission of Interacoustics

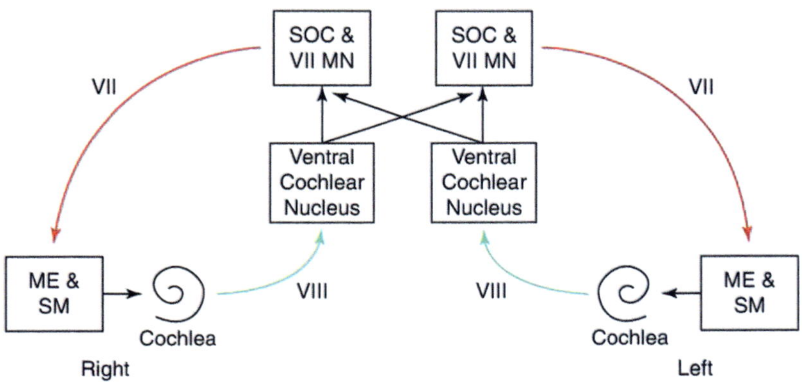

Fig. 4.26 Schematic diagram of the acoustic reflex arc. *ME* middle ear; *SM* stapedius muscle; *VIII* vestibulocochlear (8th) nerve; *SOC* superior olivary complex; *VII MN* medial nucleus of seventh nerve; *VII* facial (7th) nerve

erative ears) and potentially higher diagnostic power for specific pathologies such as otosclerosis (Shahnaz et al. 2009).

4.2.9.3 Acoustic Reflex Testing

Significantly suprathreshold acoustic stimulation triggers the acoustic reflex, by which the stapedius muscle contracts. The acoustic reflex arc involves acoustic stimulation of the inner hair cells of one cochlea, followed by afferent innervation of the vestibulocochlear (8th) nerve and the ventral cochlear nucleus, where it is sent to both superior olivary complexes and medial nuclei of the facial (7th) nerve, leading to bilateral efferent innervation of the seventh nerve terminating at the stapedius muscles of both ears (Fig. 4.26). The contraction of these muscles stiffens the ossicular chain and therefore stiffens the tympanic membrane, a movement that is measurable using a tympanometer.

The acoustic reflex threshold (ART) is the lowest signal level (dB SPL) from which the acoustic reflex is triggered. This is usually performed at the pressure level of peak compliance for the individual subject, in order that the response obtained is as large as possible. Various stimuli can be used, typically pure tones (500, 1000, 2000 and 4000 Hz) and broadband noise. Normal values are 90–95 dB SPL for tones and 70–75 dB SPL for broadband noise (Margolis 1993). Pathology affecting any of the structures of the reflex arc can lead to an increase in the threshold or obliterate the response. The acoustic reflex can also be used as an objective measure of recruitment in sensorineural hearing loss (Metz recruitment) (e.g. Thomsen 1955).

Ipsilateral measurements involve stimulating and measuring the response in the same ear; contralateral measurements involve stimulating one ear and measuring the response in the other.

Combining the results of ipsi-and contralateral measurements can help identify the site of lesion within the reflex arc (e.g. Emanuel 2009). Contralateral measures are also used to avoid test artefacts that can result from interference of the probe and stimulus tones on ipsilateral measurements (Benton et al. 2004).

Esser et al. (1987) proposed comparing acoustic reflex thresholds elicited by pure tones with those elicited by narrowband noises. They found a 10 dB higher pure-tone acoustic reflex threshold in children with auditory processing disorder (APD). Kunze et al. (2016) could not find such differences in children with or without APD. Another test paradigm in occasional use is the reflex decay. In this test, an acoustic reflex is evoked by a sound signal sustained over a longer duration, usually 10 s. The reflex decay is the amount of time during this acoustic stimulation by which the reflex is sustained at a level above 50%. The normal value is ≥5 s. A shorter duration (i.e. a quicker decay) may indicate retrocochlear or other central pathology, such as myasthenia gravis (e.g. Bischoff et al. 1989). This test is, however, not used very often these days because of the prevalence of imaging techniques such as MRI.

Acoustic reflex testing can be performed on patients of any age; however, given that high signal levels are required to evoke a response even in normal-hearing patients, caution should be used, especially in patients reporting sensitivity to loud sounds, such as suspected hyperacusis, patients with lowered uncomfortable loudness levels or patients with tinnitus. Contraindications are otherwise the same as for tympanometry.

4.2.10 Otoacoustic Emissions

Jakub Dršata and Ross Parfitt

4.2.10.1 Nature and History of Otoacoustic Emissions

Otoacoustic emissions (OAEs) are very low-level sounds that arise during active contraction of the outer hair cells in the organ of Corti. OAEs can emerge spontaneously or be evoked intentionally. The principle of OAE measurement is the detection of these sounds.

OAEs result from the active mechanism of cochlear amplification (see Sect. 4.1.1), a function that plays a significant role in the sensitivity and discrimination of hearing (Heinz et al. 2001). Detection of the OAE is therefore an important objective indicator of inner ear function. It does not, however, provide information about the general status of the auditory system.

The history of OAE measurement dates back to 1978, when David Kemp first demonstrated their existence and utility. Since then, several types of OAE, which can be used in the investigation of inner ear function, have been discovered. The most important clinical applications of OAEs are the transient-evoked OAE (TEOAE) and distortion product OAE (DPOAE). The most common use of TEOAEs these days is in newborn hearing screening programmes (see Sect. 17.1) and of DPOAEs is in audiological monitoring during therapy with ototoxic drugs (see Sect. 14.9).

4.2.10.2 Measurement of OAEs

All forms of OAE are based on the same principle: the detection of sounds produced by the cochlea by using a microphone placed in the outer ear canal. The difference between the various OAE methods lies essentially in the stimuli presented and the processing of results.

OAE measurements are widely used in audiological examination. Various pieces of OAE test equipment can be used, from basic screening devices to more sophisticated clinical equipment, depending on the purpose of the investigation. Screening devices are most common in routine practice and are typically user-friendly, to the extent that they can be operated by trained staff with a secondary school level of education. These devices report results simply as 'positive' (OAEs are present) or 'negative' (OAEs are absent and further audiological investigation is necessary) (Fig. 4.27).

In all OAE tests, the response must be distinguished from the presence of noise. Various strategies are used to aid this process, such as filtering of the response to focus only on the frequency range of interest. Averaging strategies work on

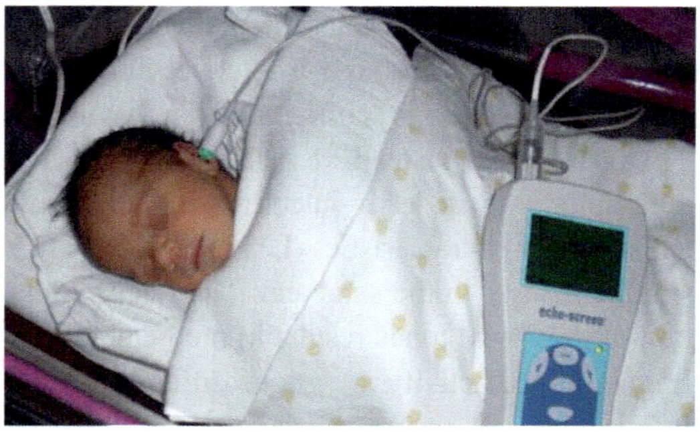

Fig. 4.27 Automated transient-evoked otoacoustic emission (TEOAE) testing in a neonate. Photograph with kind permission of the parents

the principle that the response occurs within a particular time window following the stimulus but that noise is essentially random. The results of repeated stimulation and measurement ('sweeps') can therefore be averaged to reduce the effects of noise. Artefact rejection is also employed in order to reject sweeps that feature recorded sound higher than a particular sound pressure level, thereby omitting transient background noise.

Measurement Conditions

The main conditions for acquiring reliable OAE results are:

- Proper sealing of the probe in the outer ear canal (i.e. no gap between the probe and the ear canal, orientation of the probe towards the tympanic membrane, no blockage of the ear canal (e.g. by earwax).
- Use of fully functional equipment (appropriate calibration, probe patency).
- Minimal environmental/background noise and subject movement during testing.
- Absence of middle ear pathology (see below).

Because OAEs are produced in the cochlea but measured by a microphone in the outer ear canal, the ability to measure them is hindered by the presence of any obstruction in the middle or outer ear. Such obstructions may include amniotic fluid and debris present in the ears of neonates on the first day of life, possibly until the second day of life.

OAEs do not measure the status of the entire auditory system: they may still be present in retrocochlear pathology (e.g. auditory neuropathy).

The reproducibility of OAEs decreases with age, and they are almost never present in any cochlear pathology. The correspondence of age-related 'normal' hearing with OAE presence in older age is, therefore, not reliable.

4.2.10.3 Spontaneous OAEs

Definition and Principle

Spontaneous otoacoustic emissions (SOAEs) are typically stable pure tones that are measurable at low intensity (10–15 dB SPL) in the outer ear canal (Hall 1999) and that occur without external stimulation. Current models of SOAE genesis suggest that SOAEs arise as a consequence of a complex sustained motion of the outer hair cells in the organ of Corti (Kemp 2002).

Importance, Interpretation and Limitations

SOAEs are measurable in 30–40% of healthy young people (Burns et al. 1992). SOAEs can occur at a broad range of frequencies, but the specific frequency measured is not particularly important, as it does not relate to the outer hair cell function at a particular tonotopic area of the cochlea. The detectability of the SOAE is critically dependent on the health of the cochlea; therefore the presence of an SOAE is a particularly sensitive indicator of the integrity of cochlear function. However, the absence of measurable SOAE should not necessarily be taken to indicate pathology or hearing loss.

4.2.10.4 Transient-Evoked OAEs

Definition and Principle

Transient-evoked otoacoustic emissions (TEOAEs) are very brief sounds, emitted over a 0.5–4 kHz frequency range as a response to transient (i.e. very brief) acoustic stimuli (usually click stimuli) presented at intensities of 80–85 dB SPL. A series of transient stimuli with very short pauses in between is used during stimulation.

Importance and Limitations

TEOAE testing is quick (usually lasting just a few seconds for each ear), non-invasive and technically simple and requires no active participation by the patient, and the result is very reliable. These features make TEOAE testing particularly useful for neonatal hearing screening, applied in an automated version.

The presence of amniotic fluid or debris in the ears of neonates may mean that the TEOAE cannot be recorded shortly after delivery.

Newborns at risk of retrocochlear pathology, such as auditory neuropathy, should not be tested solely with TEOAEs. Automated auditory brainstem response (AABR) audiometry should be used in these cases.

Interpretation

High-level click stimuli reliably evoke a response if the hearing threshold is 20 dB HL or better across frequencies (Kemp 1978). TEOAEs can also be evoked (though less reliably) where mild sensorineural hearing loss is present (Robinette et al. 2007). The presence of TEOAE indicates healthy cochlear function (Kemp 2002) or, at worst, mild hearing loss (Ramos et al. 2013). A positive response is indicated where the signal-to-noise ratio (SNR) is 3–6 dB (i.e. the level of the response is 3–6 dB higher than that of the noise), depending on the protocol and equipment used. Modern screening devices typically include automated data analysis, with positive result (TEOAE present) indicated as 'pass' or similar. A negative response ('refer') indicates that normal hearing cannot be confirmed and the patient requires further investigation (such as rescreening or AABR testing if within a newborn hearing screening programme).

Clinical devices enable more detailed analysis of the test data for scientific and research purposes. First studies are performed in the clinical application of high-frequency TEOAEs (Goodman 2011).

4.2.10.5 Distortion Product OAEs

Definition and Principle

DPOAEs are responses from non-linear elements in the cochlea to stimulation by the travelling wave of basilar membrane displacement that is the physical manifestation of sound as it moves through the cochlea. The stimulus is different from that used in TEOAE testing: instead of a click stimulus, two pure tones with closely related frequencies (f1, f2) and intensity characteristics (L1, L2) are presented simultaneously to the same ear. The intermodulation of these two tones results in predictable basilar membrane activity at various different relative frequencies (known as distortion products). Clinical DPOAE testing measures the amplitude of the response at one of these frequencies, usually 2f1-f2, which has the largest amplitude.

Importance, Interpretation and Limitations

DPOAEs complement TEOAEs in clinical practice. DPOAEs seem to be less sensitive to minor and subclinical conditions of the hearing system (e.g. Kemp 2002). They allow the measurement of a wider frequency range than do TEOAEs (Kemp 2002). The response corresponds to the hearing threshold near the f2 frequency (Robinette and Glattke 2007). Furthermore, the DPOAE can be detected at higher frequencies (up to 8 or 10 kHz), and the measurement of DPOAE amplitudes seems to be a promising method for the early detection of high-frequency cochlear damage (e.g. ototoxicity, noise). DPOAEs can be detected up to a cochlear hearing loss of 50 dB HL, so they cannot be used to identify lower degree hearing impairments.

The examination is usually performed and interpreted for individually tested frequencies, though many OAE devices run through a standard battery of tested frequencies. The frequency-specific characteristic of DPOAEs means that manufacturers have been able to place on the market devices with DPOAE-based hearing threshold estimation (DP audiogram) capability. The extrapolation of DPOAE input/output function can be used to estimate pure-tone thresholds up to 8 kHz (Stavroulaki et al. 2001). The clinical importance of DPOAE is nonetheless a subject of further research.

4.2.10.6 Other Applications of OAEs

Sustained-frequency otoacoustic emissions are acoustic responses to the presentation of an ongoing tonal stimulus. The wide frequency range

(0.5–8 kHz) of these emissions enables the study of inner ear function at specific frequencies, whereas TEOAEs and DPOAEs rely on the combined response or interaction of various areas of the basilar membrane. Because they are identifiable even in cases of severe hearing loss, sustained-frequency otoacoustic emissions may be useful as an objective tool for the quantification of hearing loss. Nevertheless, the method is still an object of study and is not routinely used in practice.

The bibliography includes some articles in which other applications of OAE have been studied, such as synchronised SOAE (Jedrzejczak et al. 2008), stimulus-frequency OAE (Ellison and Keefe 2008) and others. The utility of these methods is under study, and their clinical use in routine practice is currently marginal.

4.2.11 Evoked Response Audiometry

Arne Knief and Jakub Dršata

4.2.11.1 Impact of Evoked Response Audiometry on Objective Threshold Audiometry

The gold standard for hearing threshold assessment is pure-tone audiometry (PTA). This subjective examination requires active cooperation of the investigated subject. On the basis of this principle, a significant number of subjects (infants, psychically and mentally diseased persons, malingerers) cannot pass the examination. Objective threshold audiometry is aimed at covering this gap. Among its methods, evoked response audiometry (ERA) plays a most prominent role in newborn hearing screening and in auditory diagnostics of children and their hearing rehabilitation (Dršata et al. 2015). Optimising these methods has been a subject of intensive research, the essential goal of which is finding a method with the best correlation to the behavioural threshold (Stapells 2011).

Different stages of the auditory pathways can be studied with ERA signals. Early latency responses originate from the brainstem (the auditory brainstem response, ABR). Auditory steady-state responses (ASSR) have generators in the brainstem as well as in more central areas (Picton et al. 2003). Middle latency responses come from the primary auditory cortex and long latency response from the non-primary cortex (cortical ERA, CERA).

The more centrally the source of activity can be found, the more the activity is dependent on the arousal of the patient. Nonetheless, we are in a favourable position to measure responses from the brainstem in sleep as well as in narcosis.

4.2.11.2 Broadband and Frequency-Specific ABR

There are two kinds of ABR measurements: one with broadband stimuli such as clicks, to test the integrity of the auditory pathway and to determine an overall hearing threshold, and the other with frequency-specific stimuli, to estimate the hearing thresholds at these frequencies.

Jewett (1970) and Jewett et al. (1970) first described evoked responses from the brainstem. Therefore, the potentials from the brainstem were named after him, Jewett waves, enumerated I to V or J1 to J5. The sources of these waves were analysed by dipole analysis of the EEG (Scherg 1991). Scherg (1991) showed that wave I is identical with the compound action potential of the auditory nerve. Wave II is generated at the opening of the internal acoustic meatus, the porus acusticus internus. Scherg (1991) found the source of wave III in the efferent part of the ventral cochlear nucleus, still in the ipsilateral hemisphere. Waves IV and V were thought to originate from the nucleus olivaris superior and lemniscus lateralis, on the ipsi-and contralateral sides, respectively.

Nevertheless, Picton (2011) argued:

> At any point in time after … 2.5 ms, activities in many different places in the pathway overlap.

The conventional click stimulus (Fig. 4.28) excites the whole cochlea, which results in a clear identification of Jewett's waves. The intensities used in air-conduction ERA reach from threshold up to 100 dB HL and above. A healthy auditory pathway is characterised by latencies of Jewett's waves that fall within standard ranges. These

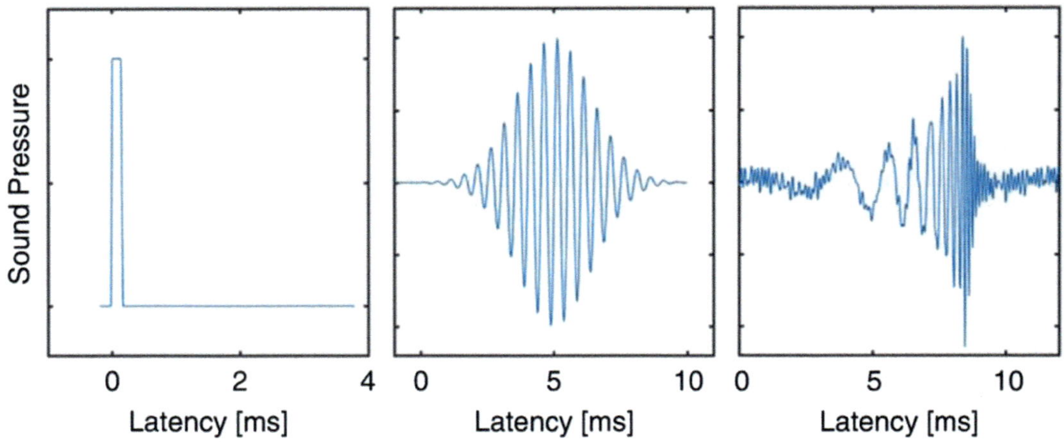

Fig. 4.28 Time courses of different stimuli are shown: left click, middle tone burst and right chirp stimulus

latency ranges are age-specific. Jewett's waves appear delayed and altered or can vanish in cases of conductive, sensorineural or retrocochlear neural hearing loss. An increase of the synchrony of neural activation is reached with the use of chirp stimuli (Fig. 4.28), which compensates for the frequency-dependent time delay of sensory perception in the cochlea (Dau et al. 2000; Elberling et al. 2007). The sound of a broadband chirp starts at low frequency and ascends to high frequency. These stimuli evoke higher amplitudes near threshold and therefore a higher signal-to-noise ratio than clicks.

Although the click and broadband chirp stimuli excite the whole cochlea and generate relatively well-synchronised neural responses, these stimuli are not frequency-specific, and so these methods cannot assess the hearing levels at individual frequencies.

Tone bursts (Fig. 4.28) compared with clicks are referred to as providing more frequency-specific results with good correlation with pure-tone behavioural thresholds (Gorga et al. 2006). In a clinical setting, the tone bursts are usually presented at 500, 1000, 2000 and 4000 Hz. To enhance the frequency specificity, the tonal stimuli are masked with notched-noise (so-called notched-noise ABR, Picton et al. 1979). The effect of masking is to prevent neighbouring regions of the cochlear from contributing to the response (Fig. 4.29, review: Stapells and Oates 1997).

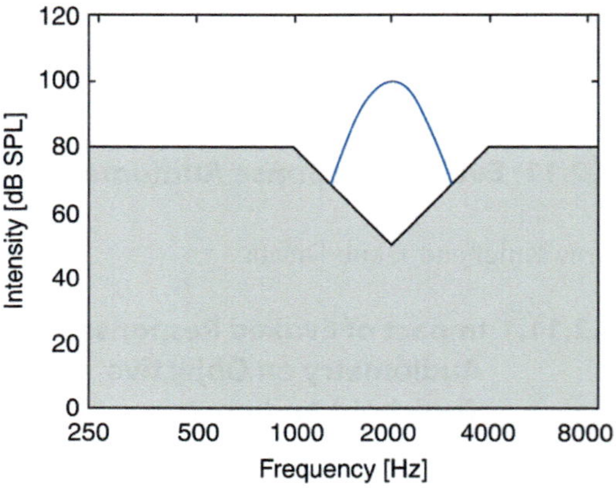

Fig. 4.29 Schematic spectrum of a frequency-specific notched-noise stimulus. The noise (in grey) is notched at the stimulus frequency and masks the possible side bands of the tone burst (blue line)

Comparable to the application of broadband chirps for overall threshold ABR measurements, narrowband chirps can also be used for frequency specificity, for which a part of the whole chirp is cut out and covers, for example, only one octave (Wegner and Dau 2002). Especially at low frequency, this narrowband chirp is more efficient than tone bursts (Mühlenberg and Schade 2012). Narrowband chirps have been proven to generate a frequency-specific response, with a reduction in the test time in newborns (Ferm et al. 2013).

The reliability and technical mastering of the described methods have resulted in commercially available ABR systems that offer different kinds of stimulation.

4.2.11.3 Auditory Steady-State Responses

Auditory steady-state responses (ASSR; steady-state evoked potentials, SSEP; amplitude-modulation following response, AMFR) are auditory evoked potentials from the brainstem and more central structures (Beck et al. 2007). The stimuli are usually continuous pure tones, modulated mostly with modulation frequency around 80 Hz in the amplitude alone or both the amplitude and frequency domains (see Sect. 4.2.13).

4.2.11.4 Cortical ERA

Cortical ERA (CERA), also called measurement of late auditory evoked potentials (LAEP), is much less sensitive to muscle activity than ABR, with the drawback that it is more dependent upon vigilance and attention. Different kinds of stimuli come into consideration: clicks, tone bursts (frequency-specific with a length of ≥50 ms) or speech signals (consonant-vowel or vowel-consonant-vowel). The examination requires the patient's alertness or at the most video sedation.

The reliance of CERA on the patient's mental vigilance makes the method suitable mostly for calm but awake children and adults (Stapells 2002). The observed response pattern is in a time window between 50 ms and 1000 ms and in a frequency range from near 0 Hz up to 600 Hz.

The CERA has its diagnostic value in the examination of the auditory pathway beyond the brainstem up to the cortical areas. The clinical application of CERA is not widespread and is at its beginnings. It can be useful in questions of maturation (after hearing aid use or cochlear implant), auditory neuropathy, auditory processing disorders, psychogenic hearing disorders, autism, lesions of the central pathway or aggravation and simulation (Walger et al. 2014).

4.2.11.5 Specific Issues of ERA

Patient Preparation and Test Implementation

For measurement of ERA—broadband and frequency-specific—the patient has to be relaxed and quiet. This means in the case of small children that they have at least to sleep. In the case of well-collaborating parents of children without neuropsychological disorders, the examination can be performed in a deep natural sleep following previous sleep deprivation. However, sedation or general anaesthesia is often to be considered for infants. Among sedatives and anaesthetics, different drugs are used (e.g. chloral hydrate, midazolam, ketamine and others), with variable pharmacokinetics, side effects and brain activity influences. Anaesthesia is accompanied by risks and a high logistic effort and therefore to be avoided if possible. The alternative is natural sleep. Sleep can be induced by oral administration of melatonin, a naturally produced hormone adjusting the circadian rhythm (Schmidt et al. 2007).

The measurement is comparable to that of electroencephalography. Four electrodes are fixed: at the vertex (or forehead), both mastoids and a ground electrode at the forehead, cheek, clavicle or neck (Fig. 4.30). The stimuli are pre-

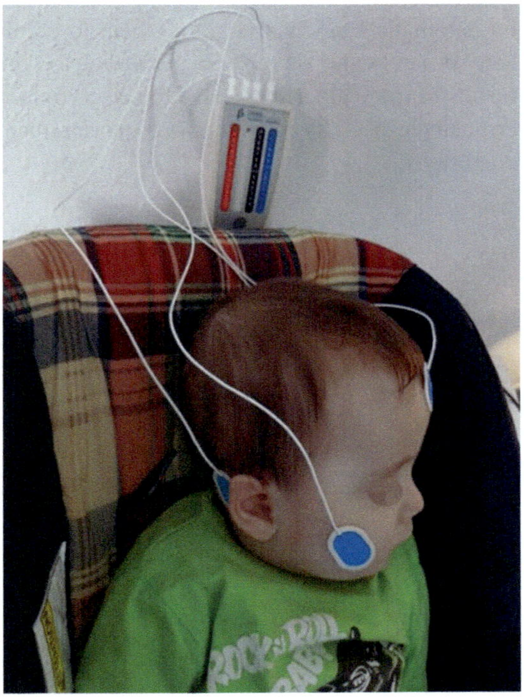

Fig. 4.30 Electrode positions are shown for ERA measurement. Photo from electrodes with kind permission from Ambu GmbH, photo from preamplifier of the BERA system Corona with kind permission from Pilot Blankenfelde medizinisch elektronische Geräte GmbH, photo of child with kind permission of the parents

sented via headphone, insert earphones or bone-conduction transducer (Fig. 4.31).

Frequency-specific ERA examination is carried out principally in an identical way as for conventional click-evoked ABR. Obviously, the estimation of hearing thresholds at individual frequencies takes a significantly longer time, and feeble responses to the specific stimuli are more sensitive to the ambient noise and measurement conditions than with a conventional click-evoked ABR.

Estimated Audiogram (EA)

The ABR objective threshold audiometry is based on detection of the most prominent Jewett V wave. The key point for the correct hearing level estimation is a faultless identification of the Jewett's wave complex. An expert audiologist takes the pattern of waves, their latencies and intensities and the age of the patient and measurement conditions into account when identifying Jewett waves and the thresholds. Evaluation algorithms specified by the manufacturers, based on automatic ERA analysis, may help to eliminate possible human errors. Nevertheless, the results of these algorithms have to be scrutinised critically, especially in nonoptimal measurement conditions.

ASSR measurements generally follow a complete automatic protocol. Thresholds at different frequencies as well as in both ears can be measured simultaneously (Korczak et al. 2012). This possibility leads to a shorter measurement time for a complete threshold estimation. Nevertheless, the major advantage of ABR (controlled by an audiologist) over ASSR remains the traceability of the results and the information about the auditory pathway given by the wave pattern above thresholds.

Level-Latency Curves

With the correct identification of the Jewett waves, especially wave V and in addition wave I, information is gained for differential diagnosis. The latencies of the waves t_V and t_I are a function of stimulus intensity: they increase with decreasing intensity. The comparison of these functions with normal ranges helps to identify different pathologies (Fig. 4.32). The latency difference $\Delta t = t_V - t_I$ is also taken into account.

In conductive hearing loss, the stimulus reaches the cochlea quieter than normal. Therefore, the curves are parallel but shifted to higher intensities. The difference Δt remains normal.

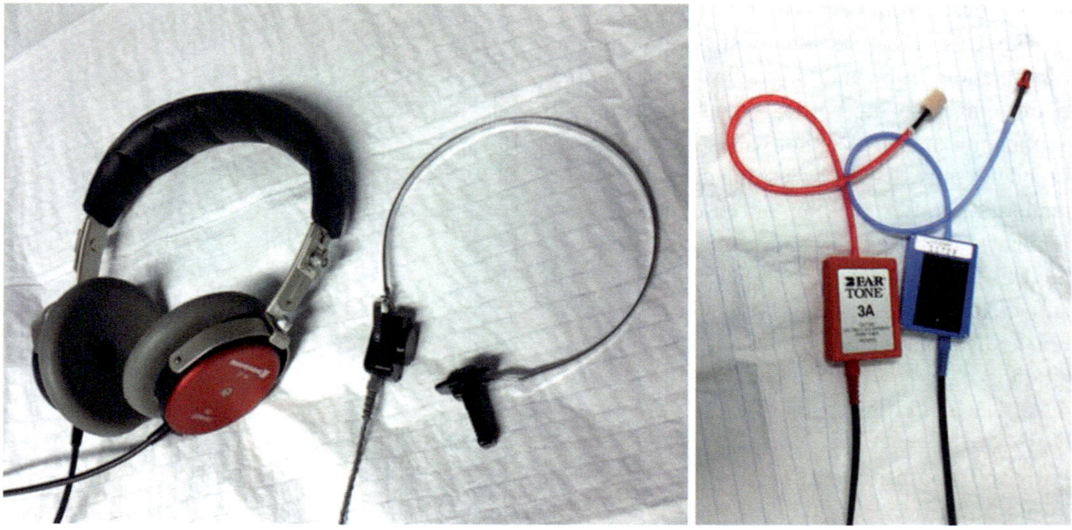

Fig. 4.31 For stimulation in ERA measurement, a headphone (left, type DT 48 with kind permission from Beyerdynamic), a transducer for bone-conduction ERA (middle, type B-71 with kind permission of Radioear) and insert earphones (right, with kind permission from 3 M) can be used. The earphones are shown with different ear tips for different sizes of the ear canal

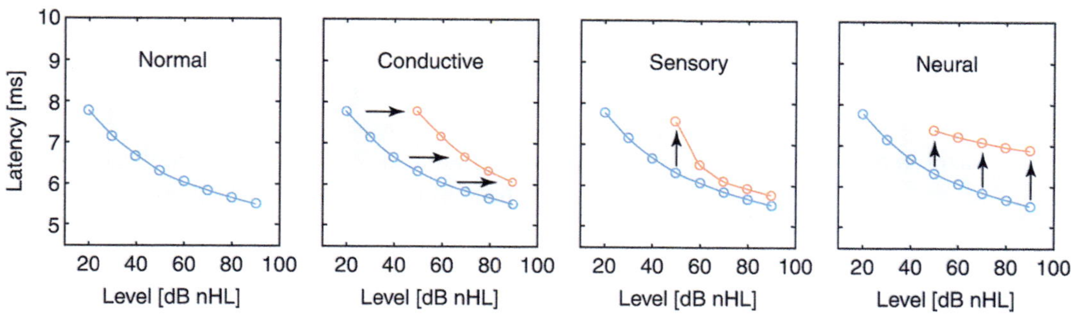

Fig. 4.32 Level-latency curves are shown for different pathologies. In grey is the normal range of latencies for wave V shown, in blue their mean. In red the divergent latencies for the noted pathologies are shown

In sensory hearing loss, the curves at high levels are almost normal and prolonged only at levels near threshold. In the case of low-frequency loss, t_V can even be shortened because of the lacking later low-frequency portion of the signal. The curve shape conforms to a defect of the outer hair cells and normal neuronal processing.

In contrast, in retrocochlear hearing loss latency, t_I is normal but t_V is severely prolonged. The wave pattern can also be irregular, e.g. in auditory neuropathy (Schmidt et al. 2012).

The interpretation of the level-latency graphs provides important hints for diagnostics. But be aware: in infants it is more difficult because of maturation of the auditory pathway, so additional diagnostics should be taken into account.

Bone Conduction in ABR

If conductive hearing loss is suspected, measurement of bone-conduction ABR is indicated. Unlike in (the normal) air-conduction ABR, the stimulus is presented by a transducer (Fig. 4.31) as similarly used for bone-conduction behavioural thresholds. The transducer ideally is held by an elastic band or clamp. The intensities used reach a maximal of 50 dB, which is sufficient for diagnostics of conductive problems. A large early artefact may occur owing to the vibrating mass, but the ABR response to frequency-specific stimuli appears after that artefact (Stapells and Oates 1997). In cases of threshold differences between ears, masking comparable to that for behavioural measurement is necessary. To identify conductive or mixed hearing loss, ear microscopy, tympanometry, stapedius reflex measurement and otoacoustic emissions should be taken into account.

Hearing Rehabilitation Based on ERA Results

The estimated audiogram is not identical to the behavioural threshold of hearing examined with PTA. The correlation of estimated audiogram and the behavioural threshold is strongly influenced by the chosen method and measurement conditions, individual hearing loss and condition (maturation) of the auditory pathways as well as experience of the audiologist. Nevertheless, in preschool children, infants and non-cooperating young patients, threshold estimation by physiological measurements is the best that can be achieved. In group means, the thresholds are within 10–15 dB of the behavioural threshold. In cases of steep hearing loss, the difference may be larger (~20 dB) in the range of the steep slope. The hearing loss is rather underestimated (Johnson and Brown 2005). The results of the electrophysiological measurements have to be checked for plausibility in synopsis with otoacoustic emissions, middle ear status, stapedius reflex measurements, sound field behavioural audiometry and language development of the child. The estimated thresholds are suitable for establishing the basal hearing aid settings. It is necessary to control the fitting, the development of hearing and language of the children regularly.

The results of objective threshold audiometry in the hearing rehabilitation process must be continually monitored, also with the help of behavioural methods, as soon as their achievement is possible.

4.2.12 Indication and Interpretation of Auditory Steady-State Responses

Piotr Swidzinski and Arne Knief

4.2.12.1 Characteristics of Auditory Steady-State Responses (ASSR)

Registration of the auditory evoked potentials (AEP) of specific frequencies, from the point of view of response correctness, has been and still is inconvenient (long time of stimulus duration—short time of response latency of auditory potentials). Towards the end of the twentieth century (1998), auditory steady-state responses (ASSR) were developed and introduced to the techniques of electrophysiological auditory investigations (Kuwada et al. 1986, Tlumak et al. 2012; review and tutorial: Korczak et al. 2012, Pruszewicz and Obrębowski 2010). The advantage of this method is the possibility of automatic assessment by statistical processing algorithms. Frequency specificity is obtained by the use of pure tones (sine waves) or 'chirp'-type auditory stimuli (Stürzebecher et al. 2006) as 'carrier signal' with frequencies of 500, 1000, 2000 and 4000 Hz, which are modulated by a signal with frequency around 80 Hz. It is possible to use multiple carriers in parallel by modulation with different frequencies around 80 Hz (Lins and Picton 1995; John et al. 1998). This enables time-saving acquisition setups. The sites where the potentials are generated are the brainstem and the thalamus—thus the test is a combination of two registrations: ABR (auditory brainstem responses) and MLR (middle latency responses). In the auditory system, a steady-state response is evoked at the frequency of the modulation. Names for this method are auditory steady-state response (ASSR) or amplitude-modulation following response (AMFR). Fig. 4.33 presents a simple diagram of the ASSR production.

4.2.12.2 Aim of the ASSR Production

The ASSR test is aimed first at producing a simple objective measurement of hearing whose result correlates directly with the audiogram; it is an instrument complying with the principle of audiological diagnostics, the 'cross-check principle' according to Jerger and Hayes (1976), in particular in the diagnostics of young children. The automatic analysis of the ASSR is based on a transformation into frequency space, e.g. by a fast Fourier transform (FFT). In the next step, it is evaluated by statistical testing to determine if there is a response to the stimuli at the modulation frequency or not. The methods used can be the calculation of phase coherence values or the F-test (Dobie and Wilson 1996). Phase coherence is calculated if the measured signal has random phases: then there is no response; if in each repetition the phase is the same and related to the stimulus, there is a valid response. In the F-test the energy at the modulation frequency is compared with that of neighbouring frequencies. Different variations and flavours of these algorithms are possible (Picton et al. 2003). Each device manufacturer uses its own estimation algorithm, and usually they do not disclose their methods.

The result of the measurement is not demonstrated as a typical wave form with assessment of registered wave latency, but evaluated as a graph resembling an audiogram. An example of the ASSR test result is presented in Fig. 4.34.

4.2.12.3 Indication and Interpretation of ASSR

The indication for the ASSR test is the need to obtain an objective audiogram, besides its use in newborn hearing screening. As the ASSR method makes use of tonal, frequency-specific stimuli (similar to that in the audiometric test), the test result can be compared with the behaviourally obtained audiogram. It can be a perfect instrument for objective hearing tests in children and uncooperative patients through earphones and in a free acoustic field through loudspeakers. The problem of this method is the need for a correction to estimate the hearing threshold. In normal-hearing adults and older children, this correction is averaged at 11 dB for 2 kHz up to 17 dB for 500 Hz (Tlumak et al. 2007). In hearing-impaired adults, it varies from 8 to 14 dB. Despite this correction the

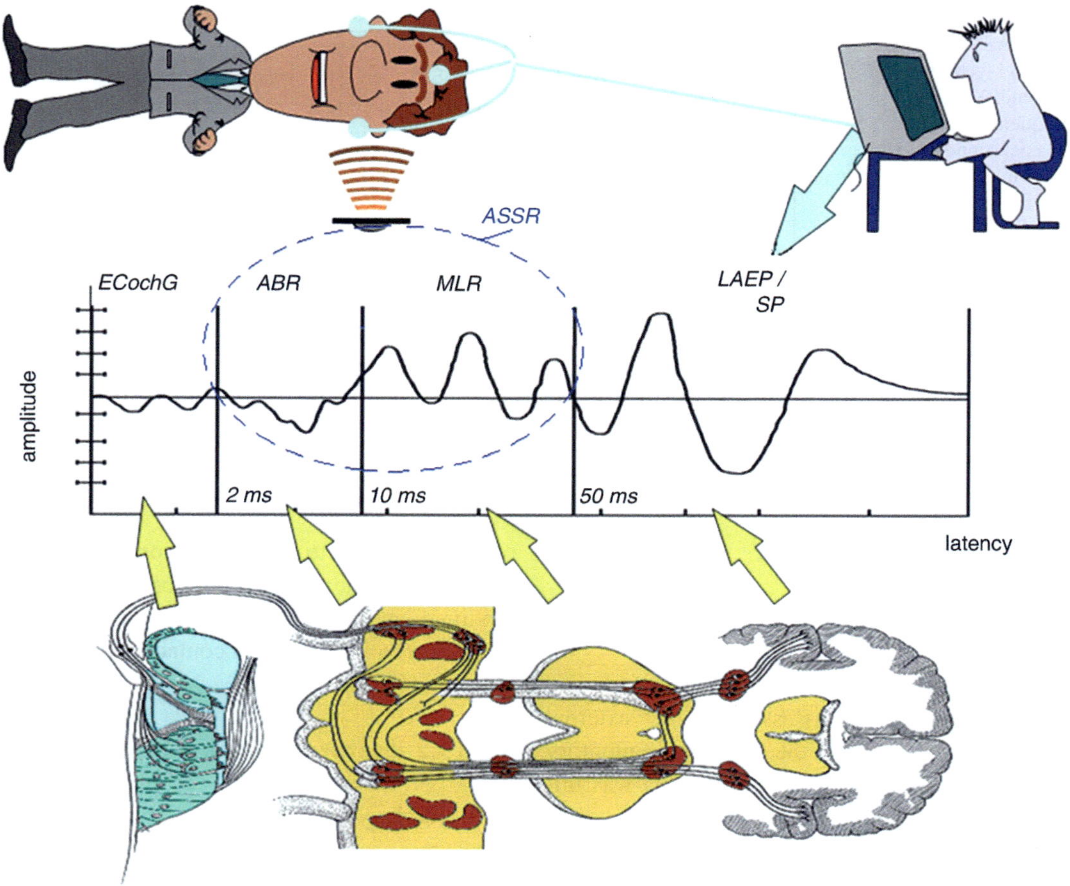

Fig. 4.33 The site of the ASSR response production (the author's own study based on the materials from the Department of Phoniatrics and Audiology, University of Medical Sciences in Poznań). *ECochG* electrocochleography; *ABR* auditory brainstem response; *MLR* middle latency response; *SP* sustained potential; *LAEP* late auditory evoked potential

method is considered to give a good estimate of hearing threshold. In children <6 years and infants, compared with ABR thresholds—which may lie 10 dB above behavioural thresholds—the ASSR for normal hearing is 17 dB, 13 dB, 13 dB and 9 dB worse than ABR in normal hearing and 9 dB, 9 dB, 9 dB and 6 dB worse in patients with hearing loss at 500 Hz, 1000 Hz, 2000 Hz and 4000 Hz, respectively (Van Maanen and Stapells 2010). These corrections vary in different publications (e.g. Chou et al. 2012; Luts et al. 2006; Rance et al. 2005) because of different study groups, stimuli, measurement time, noise floor and other parameters. Considerable variability in interpersonal and intrapersonal results is noticed. A large number of audiologists seem to indicate that so far the method represents poor diagnostic value (Pruszewicz and Obrębowski 2010; Tlumak et al. 2012). Owing to the good correlation of the ABR and ASSR thresholds, the method is quite usable. In commercial ASSR systems, an automatic correction is normally included; therefore the result of measurement is an estimated audiogram. The audiological assistant or semi-skilled examiner does not need to know much about the interpretation of the response, as in click or notched-noise ABR, as the measurement system delivers an audiogram. But this audiogram should be interpreted with caution depending on the degree of hearing loss, age and measurement conditions.

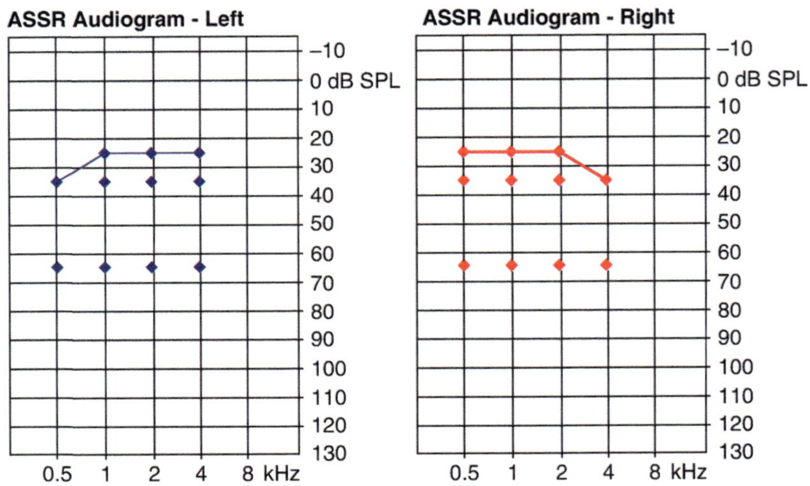

Fig. 4.34 An example of the ASSR registration in an 11-year-old child (legend: X-axis, frequency in kHz; Y-axis, sound pressure level in dB)

4.2.13 Promontory Test

Dirk Mürbe

4.2.13.1 Aim and Method

The promontory test assesses whether external electrical stimulation at the cochlear promontory generates an auditory percept. The test was initially introduced to ascertain deaf patients' candidacy for cochlear implantation, since conductivity of the auditory nerve is an essential prerequisite for a successful outcome after implantation.

The subjective test aims to assess thresholds and dynamic ranges of hearing sensation and can be performed in an outpatient procedure, in which the patient is seated and the external ear canal is under local anaesthesia. Under microscopic control, a needle electrode is then transtympanically positioned at the cochlear promontory, via the external ear canal. Different stimulation paradigms have been introduced to determine whether a patient will benefit from electrical stimulation. Commonly used stimulation rates include 50, 100 and 200 Hz. During stimulus application, the patient is asked to describe the hearing sensation associated with the different stimuli. For each stimulation rate, the patient indicates if there is an increase in perceptual loudness as stimulant current is increased. Further, the discrimination between the different stimulation rates is assessed. Thresholds and dynamic ranges can then be documented for the different stimulation rates.

Alternatively, to avoid the application of a needle electrode, the promontory test can be modified, and a ball electrode can be positioned in the external ear canal in contact with the tympanic membrane.

4.2.13.2 Interpretation and Diagnostic Value

In the early years of cochlear implantation, in which most patients scheduled for implantation suffered from complete deafness, the promontory test was an essential part of candidacy assessment. Since then, the indications for cochlear implantation have expanded to include patients with profound sensorineural hearing loss and residual hearing. In these cases, the promontory test is usually postponed, because reliable thresholds in pure-tone audiometry describe the basic conductivity of the auditory nerve. The promontory test has, however, been suggested to be a useful tool in predicting postoperative speech perception in patients at risk of poor auditory nerve functioning (neuropathies), especially in postinflammatory conditions such as meningitis, or after long auditory deprivation (Alfelasi et al. 2013).

4.2.14 Electro-Audiometry

Arne Knief

In deaf or nearly deaf patients, the only possibility of evoking an impression of hearing is the electrical stimulation of the auditory system.

Electrical stimulation can be used to measure the capability of the auditory pathway, as does acoustic brainstem audiometry. This examination can provide information about the status of the auditory pathway as well as thresholds for electrical stimulation to be used in cochlear implants.

Electro-audiometry may be used before cochlear implantation to examine if the post-cochlear system is adequate for electrical stimulation via a cochlear implant. There are two possibilities of measurement: the patients report their subjective impression of the stimulation (the so-called promontory test; see Sect. 4.2.14), or, perhaps more reliable, the nerve response is recorded with synchronous averaging by auditory brainstem response acquisition equipment. Nevertheless, its predictive value is low and the method has disappeared from medical guidelines (Lesinski et al. 1997).

After cochlear implantation, the electrically evoked compound action potentials can be measured by using the implanted electrodes (Fig. 4.35).

The test is controlled by proprietary software of the implant producer. As result of the measurement, threshold values are obtained that can be used for adjusting the speech processor programme of the implant recipient (Smoorenburg et al. 2002). This measurement is useful in non-cooperative patients such as small children, but it also enables adequate fitting of the speech processor in patients with intense tinnitus.

An electrically evoked brainstem response can also be measured in special cases, for example, if there is doubt that the auditory pathway is functioning well. The stimulation is executed with intra-cochlear electrodes and acquisition of the response with surface electrodes as in normal brainstem response measurement (Brown 2003).

4.2.15 Balance/Vestibular Assessment in Children

Waheeda Pagarkar and Ewa Raglan

4.2.15.1 Developmental Balance Assessment in Children: Development of Balance, History and Observation

Development of Balance

Balance is a complex modality that develops with input from the visual, proprioceptive/somatosensory and vestibular systems. This sensory information is integrated and processed within the central nervous system and results in outputs that help stabilise our eyes and body in space through the vestibulo-ocular (VOR) and vestibulospinal (VSR) reflexes, respectively, and help in perception and awareness of our posture and movement in space through cortical connections. Development of balance depends on the development of each of these sensory systems and on the development of the integrating pathways.

The vestibular labyrinth and receptors are developed to an adultlike form by 32-week gestation. The vestibular nerve is the first cranial nerve to complete myelinisation. The slow (reflexive) component of VOR can be seen at birth, but the fast (saccadic or central) component is immature and continues to develop until the age of 2 years. Absence of the VOR by the age of 10 months is an abnormal finding (Eviatar and Eviatar 1979; Fife et al. 2000). Infants prefer visual inputs to maintain balance, whereas adults rely more on somatosensory information. Infants perform better under conditions of sensory loss [e.g. visual difficulties] than conditions of sensory conflict, indicating that the central vestibular integrative pathways are immature. The role of the vestibular system in postural control depends on these integrative

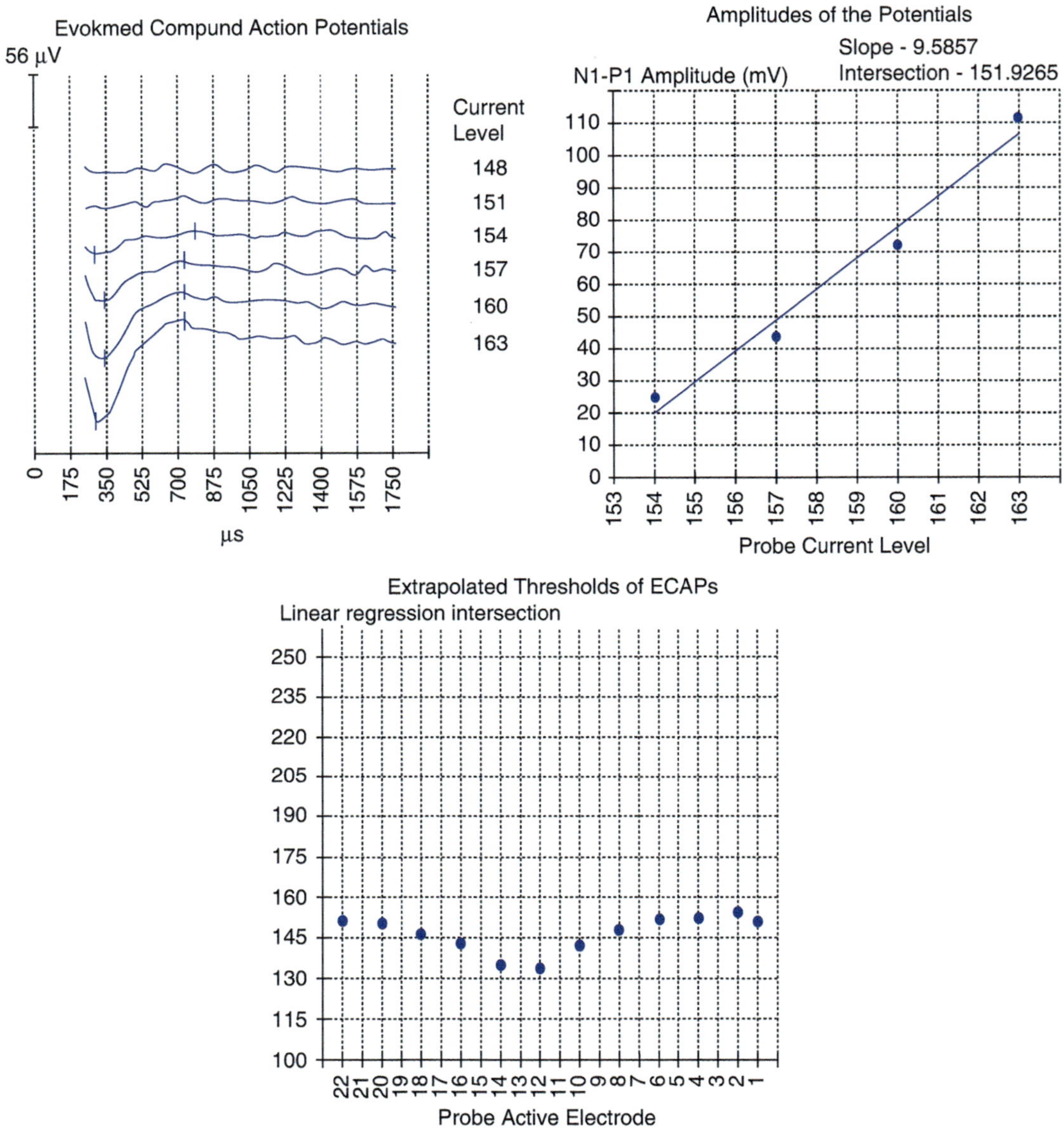

Fig. 4.35 Measurement of evoked compound action potentials with a cochlear implant (Software Custom Sound EP ver. 5.0, Cochlear Ltd., Australia). In the left panel, compound action potentials are shown for one electrode (no. 6) at increasing current levels (current levels are arbitrary units of the manufacturer and can be translated to currents in microampere range). In the middle panel, the amplitude differences of the marked positive and negative peaks are drawn over the current levels. The linearity of the amplitudes enables the extrapolation of a threshold. In the right panel, the extrapolated amplitude thresholds of the evoked compound action potentials are drawn for different electrodes. They generate a profile for speech processor fitting

pathways, and the ability to resolve intersensory conflict is mature approximately at the age of 15 years (Steindl et al. 2006; Shinjo et al. 2007).

Balance difficulties in children may present as delayed motor milestones, poor tone and floppy posture, frequent falls and unusual gait. They may be related to visual, neurological or vestibular pathology or psychological factors. Cardiac pathology and metabolic disturbances such as hypoglycaemia should also be considered. A comprehensive balance evaluation should include a clinical assessment of all the above conditions.

The vestibular aspects of a child's balance can be assessed from history, examination and selected investigations.

History

The onset and progress of the balance difficulty is often a pointer to its cause. In combination with deafness, poor tone and delayed walking in a neonate are likely to be due to a congenital vestibular hypofunction. Sudden vertigo, resolving in days, preceded by a viral infection and followed by fluctuating imbalance is likely to be related to vestibular neuritis. Associated conditions should be noted, as balance difficulties occur in Pendred's syndrome (with deafness and goitre), Usher syndrome (with deafness and retinitis pigmentosa), CHARGE syndrome (with deafness and dysmorphism) and migraine (often with headaches and vertigo). Family history is a pointer to inherited conditions (i.e. affected parents/siblings in branchio-oto-renal syndrome). Perinatal history is important, as deafness and cerebral palsy can be related to neonatal jaundice and perinatal hypoxia.

Observation and Examination

The key to successful examination of balance in a child, particularly the young toddler, involves knowledge of normal development, a keen eye for observing the child during natural activity and the ability to engage children in play. The general examination must include looking for dysmorphism, otoscopy, examination of the nose and throat, looking for neurocutaneous markers and a complete systemic examination to look for associated conditions and syndromes. A detailed neurological examination is mandatory. Clinical vestibular examination includes assessing the VOR, the vestibulospinal reflex (from postural tests) and the developmental reflexes.

4.2.15.2 Tests for Posture/Vestibulospinal Reflex

This can be started by simple observation of the child. How is their posture? Newborns with poor tone may have a frog-leg posture. Children with balance difficulties will often hold on to their parent or to the walls or banister for support. A broad-based gait is a pointer of poor balance. Unusual gaits can be observed in cerebral palsy, neuropathy and hemiparesis. Keeping a few obstacles in the path of a walking child or engaging them to kick a football and observing how they manoeuvre these will prove useful. A child who is running around, rolling on the floor and climbing chairs is unlikely to have a significant balance problem! The principle of postural tests is to reduce the visual and proprioceptive inputs, thereby uncovering vestibular dysfunction (Valente 2011).

- Romberg's test: the child stands with feet together, and sway is noted with eyes both open and closed. A variation is the sharpened Romberg's test whereby this stability is evaluated in a heel-to-toe stance.
- Foam test: the child stands on foam with eyes open and closed and sway is noted.
- Unterberger's test: the child is asked to march on the spot with the eyes closed and the deviation is noted.
- Tandem gait: the child walks heel to toe and steadiness is noted.

The postural tests are limited by lack of specificity for vestibular dysfunction and paucity of normative data for children.

4.2.15.3 Tests for Eye Movements and VOR

The VOR in children is dependent on the attention and state of arousal of the child, unintended ocular fixation due to light leaks and difficulty with head stabilisation during testing. Examination of children is helped by using child-friendly visual targets (e.g. stickers, toys). Begin by looking for a squint and spontaneous nystagmus. The best way to look for vestibular nystagmus is by using Frenzel's or Video-Frenzel's glasses in the central, right and left gaze (angle of gaze should be <30°). Smooth pursuit is best checked with a toy and optokinetic nystagmus with a striped drum with child-friendly pictures.

Halmagyi's Head Thrust

The child's head is gently rotated by approximately 30° in the yaw plane (about the vertical body axis) while asking the child to focus on the examiner's nose. A rapid head thrust is incorporated ensuring maintenance of visual fixation. A 'catch-up' saccade indicates loss of function of the ipsilateral lateral semicircular canal.

Head-Shaking Nystagmus

The child's head is briskly rotated in the yaw plane with eyes closed for about 30s. The eyes are then opened and examined preferably using Frenzel's/Video-Frenzel's glasses. Vestibular asymmetry causes nystagmus beating away from the side of the lesion.

Vibration-Induced Nystagmus

This can be done with a vestibular vibrator applied to the mastoid process for approximately 10s. The test also elicits vestibular asymmetry. The nystagmus begins when the vibration is applied and beats opposite to the direction of the lesioned side.

Dynamic Visual Acuity

Children may be evaluated with modification of the Snellen eye chart using child-friendly characters. The child is asked to read this chart from a distance of 1.5 m with the head steady. A baseline visual acuity is obtained. The child's head is rotated in the yaw plane at approximately 1–2 Hz. A loss of three lines or more of visual acuity may indicate a VOR deficiency.

4.2.15.4 Tests for Neonatal Reflexes

In the article of O'Reilly et al. (2011), various approaches are presented.

Moro Reflex

This is elicited by holding the child supine and allowing its head to drop by approximately 30° in relation to the trunk. There is extension and abduction of the arms with fanning out of the fingers followed by adduction of the arms at the shoulder and crying. This reflex normally disappears by the age of 5–6 months. Its presence before this age is indicative of vestibular function.

Farmers Rotation Test

The baby is held at arm's length (facing the examiner) and rotated in one direction around the examiner. There is a deviation of the eyes and head in the direction of the rotation, in the presence of vestibular function. This response can be elicited up to the age of 6 weeks. At a later age, the nystagmus supersedes the eye deviation.

Parachute Reflex

The child is held face down horizontally and moved downward suddenly. This causes an extension and abduction of the lower limbs and outstretched hands. A backward and sideward parachute reflex can also be elicited. This can occur beyond the age of 5 months and is indicative of vestibular function.

Head Righting Reflexes

These develop by the age of 4–6 months. The child's trunk is held 30° from the vertical, and a normally responding infant will tilt its head so as to remain vertical. At about age 5 months, the child will also move the lower limbs away from the side to which they have been tilted.

4.2.15.5 Other Tests: Dix-Hallpike Positional Test

This involves rapidly taking the child from a seated to a lying back position with the head turned to one side (right or left). The eyes are observed for nystagmus. The child is then rapidly taken to the seated position and the eye observation is repeated. The presence of horizontal, rotatory, geotropic nystagmus with vertigo after a short latent period and fatigue on repeated testing occurs in benign paroxysmal positional vertigo (BPPV).

4.2.15.6 Vestibular Investigations

Adequate preparation for the tests is important. Vestibular sedatives are withheld for 24–48 h prior to testing, and it is important that the child eats only a light meal before the appointment.

Electronystagmography and Video-Oculography

These are techniques used for recording eye movements during rotational chair testing. They can also be used for recording eye movements for gaze, smooth pursuit, saccades and optokinetic nystagmus. It is important to understand the differences between child and adult traces, and normative data should be collected. Testing in a dark room, the need for placing electrodes or goggles and the rotational chair stimulus itself make these tests challenging in children. Furthermore, inattention and alertness will influence responses.

Video Head Impulse Test (vHIT)
could be used successfully to test dizzy children (Khater and Afifi 2016). This test provides vestibular ocular reflex analysis of high-frequency vestibular activity of the horizontal and vertical semicircular canals. It is based on Halmagyi's head thrust response. With the video head impulse test, eye movements can be recorded by a high-speed lightweight video camera and mini-gyroscopes fitted to eye glasses (MacDougall et al. 2009; Petrak et al. 2013).

Computerised Rotational Chair Testing
The response to impulsive and sinusoidal rotation indicates the presence of vestibular function. The limitation is that this test assesses the overall vestibular function rather than for individual ears. The advantage is that children may sit on their mother's lap and this test is better tolerated than the caloric test. Using this method, young infants can be examined for VOR. The gain, phase and time constant of the nystagmus is calculated. In the event that recording of the nystagmus is difficult, simple observation with an infra-red camera is useful in detecting per-rotatory and post-rotatory nystagmus. VOR gain increases linearly as a function of age from 3 to 9 years (Casselbrant et al. 2010).

Bithermal Caloric Testing
Warm and cool irrigation of water or air may be used. This test allows individual ear testing of vestibular function and, from the Jongkees formula, will give the canal paresis and directional preponderance. Studies of ice-cold caloric responses in infants indicate that nystagmus is observed by the age of 6 months in full-term infants (Eviatar and Eviatar 1979). Practically, children younger than 5 years of age may not tolerate this test well.

Computerised Dynamic Posturography
The test can be used in children as young as 3–6 years of age (Foudriat et al. 1993). The sensory organisation test (SOT) is the commonest subtest used. This test consists of six conditions of varying combinations of fixed and moving platforms and visual surroundings done with eyes open or closed. The child must try to maintain the best balance possible despite conflicting clues. Normative data should be obtained, although it has been shown that younger children perform worse than older ones (Valente 2007). Special adaptations should be made for testing children. Information may be gained regarding how well a patient integrates visual, vestibular and proprioceptive cues and whether there is an over-dependence on one modality.

Vestibular Evoked Myogenic Potentials Test (VEMPs)
Both cervical and ocular VEMPs (cVEMPs and oVEMPs) have been done in children to evaluate the integrity of the otolith system (Valente 2007; Wang et al. 2008; Lin et al. 2010). cVEMPs are commonly recorded from the sternocleidomastoid muscle and test the vestibulocollic reflex, whereas the oVEMPs assess the otolithic VOR. Rectification methods may be employed to correct for the difference in background muscle activity. Latency, threshold and asymmetry may be measured. VEMPs are well tolerated and can give information on individual ear otolith function. VEMPs have been demonstrated in neonates and children and the wave latencies may be shorter than in adults (Valente 2007).

Subjective Visual Vertical/Subjective Visual Horizontal (SVV/SVH) Test
This test involves setting a linear marker to the vertical or horizontal in a dark room, in the absence of visual clues. The patient is asked to adjust the marker to his/her subjective vertical/horizontal. The degree of deviation is recorded. This can be done in older children but head restraint may be required to avoid the effect of head tilt. The values may be abnormal in acute unilateral vestibular lesions.

4.2.16 Evaluation of Speech Communication in Hearing-Impaired Children

Antoinette Am Zehnhoff-Dinnesen
and Mona Hegazi

4.2.16.1 Introduction: Relation of Hearing, Language and Speech

According to Aslin and Smith (1988) and Carney (1996), basic sensory perception (sound detection) is followed by coding perceptual representations (phonetic discrimination) and cognitive/linguistic processing (word recognition). These levels are mirrored in speech production by primitive vocalisations, complex vocal utterances (babbling) and phonemic or syllabic speech patterns (Eisenberg et al. 2007). Hearing loss (HL) in early childhood impairs the development of speech recognition and speech production by hindering the generation of correct recognition categories, linguistic and motoric patterns. Recognition of word boundaries, of syllables, of prosodic elements of speech, of sound patterns in words is basically essential for language development in early infancy.

Results in speech recognition and production depend on the type and degree of hearing loss, onset of manifestation, age at detection and start of intervention, additional handicaps, kind and quality of hearing device supply, communication mode, support by parents and intensity of therapeutic training.

Typical findings in hearing-impaired children, dependent on the degree of hearing loss, may be:

- Prolonged phase of primitive vocalisations.
- Delay in onset of babbling and differences in babbling behaviour, less consonantal types.
- Delay in development of phonemic/syllabic speech patterns.
- Lagging behind in vowel and consonant production.
- More problems in recognising consonant than vowel contrasts.
- More problems in recognising consonant manner and rear place than consonant voicing and front place.
- Substitution particularly for fricatives and affricates.
- Mild to moderate hoarseness.
- Nasal resonance problems (Eisenberg et al. 2007).

Furthermore, school achievement and academic chances may be impaired by hearing loss-related disorders of speech and language development.

Evaluation of speech communication in hearing-impaired children will be presented in this section concerning:

- Communication mode (oral-aural, manual, combined, total).
- Nasality and voice function.
- Non-verbal communication.
- Receptive language/comprehension with/without lip reading, narrative and supralinguistic skills, expressive phonetic, phonological levels, semantic levels, working memory and word finding, morphological, syntactic levels, prosody, intelligibility, pragmatics.
- Auditory and visual perception.

For assessment of kinaesthetic and tactile perception see Sect. 11.10; oral motor examination protocol and assessment of speech sound development see Sects. 11.4 and 11.5; details of literacy (phonological awareness, reading, writing) see Volume 2, Part III.

In recent years, evaluation of speech and language development in hearing-impaired children has focused on testing oral language in children with cochlear implants in comparison with children with hearing aids and normal-hearing children. Often-used tests and exemplary results are presented.

The choice of test material may be motivated by the aim to evaluate signal processing strategies, the intention to identify perceptual processes or the purpose to detect individual promotive or hindering factors (Kirk et al. 2012). Only a selection of tests can be included in this article. For further reading, see e.g. the systematic review from da Silva et al. (2011) on Instruments to Assess the Oral Language of Children fitted with a Cochlear Implant, and the book on Clinical Management of Children with Cochlear Implants by Eisenberg (2016).

4.2.16.2 Evaluation of Communication Mode

In a first step, the communication mode used in the education of the child should be clarified. The most common types are:

Oral Communication

The use of residual hearing to develop oral communication is emphasised.

- Auditory-Verbal: This method maximises the use of residual hearing to develop spoken language and restricts the use of visual cues, speech reading (lip reading) and signs.
- Auditory-Oral: This method maximises the use of both residual hearing and speech reading (lip reading) to develop spoken language.

Manual Communication

This method refers to communication by using the hands without dependence on verbal communication:

- Sign Language: A visuospatial language that uses handshapes, movements and locations of the hands, facial expressions and other body movements; each sign in a sign language is like a word in a spoken language; sign language is a real language with its own grammar rules.
- Fingerspelling: Each letter in any language is represented by a sign and words are simply spelt letter-by-letter.
- Cued Speech: This method uses eight handshapes—none of which are derived from sign languages—to represent consonants and four hand placements around the face to represent vowels.

Simultaneous Communication 'Sim-Comm'

Sign language and spoken language are simultaneously used.

Total Communication

Any means of communication is utilised such as formal sign language, fingerspelling, natural gestures, speech, lip reading, listening with amplification, pictures and writing.

4.2.16.3 Evaluation of Nasality and Voice Function

Nasal Resonance Disorders in Hearing Loss

Abnormal resonance in children with hearing loss (HL children) may be explained by an uncoordinated velopharyngeal function (Kim et al. 2012) due to the absence of complete auditory feedback. By auditory perceptual evaluation, the type of nasality may be defined:

- Hypernasality, typical in children with sensorineural hearing loss.
- Cul-de-sac resonance (typical in children with sensorineural hearing loss, caused by muffled airflow near the lower pharynx and incomplete velopharyngeal closure).
- Hyponasality, typical in children with conductive hearing loss.
- Mixed nasality, e.g. sensorineural hearing loss and adenoids, for details see Volume 2, Part I Speech Disorders (Dysglossia/Nasality/Velopharyngeal Insufficiency).

Henningsson et al. (2008) developed, as a working group, a set of five parameters with hypernasality, hyponasality, audible nasal air emission or nasal turbulence, consonant production errors and voice disorder, also considering speech understandability and speech acceptability. They presented guidelines for scoring procedures in relation to these parameters.

The Nasometer (Kay Elemetrics Corp.) is considered the most reliable tool for objectively evaluating resonance disorders (Van Lierde et al. 2005). The Nasometer (Kummer 2008) (Kay Elemetrics Corp.) is a computer system that measures the proportion of acoustic energy produced in the oral and nasal cavities during speech and calculates the proportion of nasal and oral resonance as a nasalance score: nasal acoustic energy divided by the (sum of nasal and oral energy) × 100 = nasalance percentage.

The MacKay-Kummer SNAP Test-R in the revised version from 2005 comprises a syllable-repetition subtest (oral + /a:/, oral + /i:/, nasal + /a:/, nasal + /i:/), a prolonged sounds subtest (/a:/, /i:/, /s:/, /m:/), a picture-cued subtest (sentences) and a paragraph (reading) subtest (https://www.researchgate.net/publication/282586585_SNAP_TEST_II_Score_Sheet_32505).

By such a test in combination with Nasometer measurements, nasalance scores for oral (bilabial, alveolar, velar and sibilant) and nasal phonemes may be obtained (Nguyen et al. 2008).

Kim et al. (2012), in addition to nasalance tests by nasometer, used the 'vertical focus of resonance' (VFR), for evaluation of perceptual rating, which focuses on the resonance energy in the frontal, throat, pharyngeal and nasal locations. Their results showed inappropriate coordination of velopharyngeal function in HL subjects and that the air flow and the resonance energy were not released from the resonance cavity in this group.

Baudonck et al. (2015) studied nasalance and nasality in 36 children with cochlear implants (CI children), 25 children with hearing aids (HA children) and 26 normal-hearing children (NH children) at the age of 9 years. The objective assessment of nasalance values was performed with the Nasometer, perceptual evaluations of nasality by two experienced speech therapists on the basis of a nominal rating scale with consensus evaluation. Nasalance values were lower in CI and HA children for nasal stimuli and higher in oral stimuli than those of NH children. In addition, larger cul-de-sac resonance was found in CI and HA than in NH children. According to the perceptual evaluation, HA children were more hypernasal than NH children.

Naso-video-endoscopy may be used to exclude organic causes.

Voice Changes in Hearing Loss

Lack of auditory feedback in hearing-impaired children has effects on voice function with incoordination of intrinsic and extrinsic laryngeal muscles, and with disturbed contraction and relaxation of antagonistic muscles. Higher fundamental frequency, lack of loudness control and variable abnormal voice quality features have been reported in HL children, as well as incomplete mutational voice disorder or puberphonia. Voice has also been described as being monotonous because of the lack of prosodic information and acquisition of melodic patterns of language (Nickerson 1975). Nowadays, voice quality parameters found in children with profound hearing loss are more normalised than in former times, owing to the high technical standard of hearing aids and cochlear implants, and newborn hearing screening, early detection and intervention.

Garcia et al. (2010) found more altered voice quality in 62 children with profound HL supplied with cochlear implants than in such children wearing digital hearing aids, dependent on the degree of HL and the type of hearing prosthesis. The worst results were observed in children with analogue hearing aids. The children had to produce a sustained vowel /a:/ for 4–5 s. For evaluation of voice quality the authors focused on the analysis of F_0, jitter and shimmer. The control group comprised 54 NH children.

According to results in NH children, the authors defined a range of normal values for children 7–8 years old: F_0 253–270 Hz, jitter $\leq$1.250%, shimmer $\leq$0.400 dB.

The following quality values were achieved in children with profound hearing loss:

- Digital hearing aid users:
  F_0 265.50 Hz, jitter 1.009%, shimmer 0.486 dB.
- Cochlear implant users:
  F_0 287.93 Hz, jitter 1.344%, shimmer 0.526 dB.
- Analogue hearing aid users:
  F_0 323.80 Hz, jitter 1.999%, shimmer 0.687 dB.

Most important factors were degree of HL, type of prosthesis and hearing threshold reached with the prosthesis. The hearing age also has to be considered. Maturation of control mechanisms and adaptation of neuromuscular abilities to acquired hearing control by hearing devices have to be taken into account. The voice quality values were more normalised than found in the time before access to high technical standard hearing devices.

Campisi et al. (2006) described values of F_0, jitter and shimmer in 21 profoundly deaf children within the normal range and emphasised the importance of measuring Fundamental Frequency variation (vF0) and Peak Amplitude variation (vAM). According to their results, auditory deprivation causes reduced long-term control of frequency and amplitude during sustained phonation.

The phoniatrician/pedaudiologist has to be aware of possible functional effects by an insufficient hearing threshold reached with the prosthesis. In case of dysphonia, laryngoscopy with flexible optics may be necessary. Auditory perceptual analysis of the voice (throatiness, breathiness, hoarseness) and the average speaking pitch may be possible on the basis of spontaneous utterances. Depending on age, questionnaires, pitch range, standardised, phonetically balanced texts and acoustic analysis methods may be applied, the latter working with vocal expressions lasting a few seconds (Fuchs et al. 2007). For more details, see Sect. 5.16.

4.2.16.4 Evaluation of Non-verbal Communication

Preverbal Communication Skills

To study preverbal communication skills in HA or CI children, the Tait video analysis is a suitable method for e.g. vocal turn-taking, non-looking vocal turns, gestural turn-taking, gestural autonomy and vocal autonomy (Tait et al. 2010). Vocal and early verbal developments may be monitored by video and audio recordings during parent–child interaction sessions, also observing developmental landmarks. Transcription should be performed by at least two experienced listeners as a consensus transcription procedure. Frequency of vocalisation, age at consistent babbling, consonantal inventory (place, manner), vowel inventory (height, place), mean syllable structure level and patterns of syllable complexity in dependence on age are the parameters relating to vocal measures (Moeller et al. 2007a).

Sign Language Assessment

An assessment tool of signed language skills is necessary to determine children's level of signed language proficiency, to monitor children's progress, to develop teaching goals and to give information to the parents.

The Assessing British Sign Language Development: Receptive Skills Test (BSL RST) (Herman et al. 1999) was developed for children aged 3–11 years. The BSL RST comprises a vocabulary check by a picture-naming task of 24 items and a video-based receptive test with 40 test items. The test items check grammatical structures, including negation, number and distribution, verb morphology and noun–verb distinction (Enns and Herman 2011).

Sign language raters should look at the candidate's performance in the following components:

- Sign production (its use and clarity of signs).
- Vocabulary knowledge.
- Use (or lack of use) of grammatical features.
- Fluency of the language to convey ideas, thoughts and opinions during the interview.
- Level of comprehension or receptive skills to judge the ease of understanding of what was signed.
- Use of culturally appropriate sign conversational strategies such as eye contact, appropriate turn-taking in dialogue and interruptions.

According to Johnston (2004), the BSL RST is the first worldwide standardised test of any signed language, normed on a population and tested for reliability.

An overview of existing sign language tests is given on the webpage http://www.signlang-assessment.info/index.php/home-en.html. These tests concern:

- Development of a sign language (L1).
- Learning a foreign sign language (L2).
- Linguistic research, e.g. concerning morphology, syntax.

4.2.16.5 Evaluation of Receptive Language/Comprehension with/without Lip Reading, Narrative Skills, Supralinguistic Skills, Evaluation of Expressive Language with Phonetic, Phonological Levels, Semantic Levels, Working Memory and Word Finding, Morphological, Syntactic Levels, Prosody, Intelligibility and Pragmatics

The assessment of the developmental speech and language status of children is intensively explained in Sect. 11.3. The aim of this section is to present test instruments that are used for the assessment of children with hearing loss. In recent years, evaluation of speech communication in hearing-impaired children has focused on speech and language development of CI children in comparison with that of HA and NH children. A variety of test instruments is used for oral language assessment. Da Silva et al. (2011) performed a systematic literature survey on instruments assessing oral language in CI children and found 74 different tests, questionnaires and inventories used in different versions. We present the most-often used tests according to their results, and tests found in more current literature.

Evaluation of Receptive Language/Comprehension with/without Lip Reading, Narrative Skills, Supralinguistic Measures

While evaluating receptive language skills, testing should be done in the auditory-only mode and in the audiovisual mode. If necessary, signing cues have to be used (Archer and Crosby-Quinatoa 2009). Before evaluation:

- The child's amplification should be checked.
- The testing environment should be quiet and free of visual distractions.
- The examiner should sit next to the child's best hearing ear (Archer and Crosby-Quinatoa 2009).
- Inadequate lighting of the examiner's face should be avoided and the child should watch him or her.

Non-formal assessment of language comprehension entails evaluating the child's understanding of speech aspects such as following a direction, answering a question, participating in a conversation and paraphrasing what has been said.

According to Kyle et al. (2013), prelingual children already use visual speech processing, which is important for phoneme discrimination/phoneme boundaries, and speech-reading ability improves similarly with age in deaf and in NH children. The authors emphasise the impact of speech-reading skills on word reading ability and vice versa.

Testing of lip reading should be performed at different psycholinguistic levels:

- Word level (lexicon and knowledge of using phonetic/semantic features are needed).
- Phrase/sentence level (higher-order linguistic skills and good working memory are needed).

It has to be taken into account that speech-reading accuracy decreases with complexity and length of the psycholinguistic requirement.

One example of formal testing is the Test of Child Speechreading (ToCS) developed by Kyle et al. (2013) which is a valid and reliable assessment of speech-reading ability in school-aged children:

- For testing of words/sentences the child watches a silent video clip of the male or female speaker saying the target word/sentence and then clicks on the correct picture out an array of four.
- For testing the comprehension of short stories the child sees a silent video clip of the male or female speaker telling a short story and is asked two questions by the tester, the child answers the question by selecting the correct picture from an array of four.

According to the systematic review of da Silva et al. (2011), the most-often used tests in CI children for receptive language are the Peabody

Picture Vocabulary Test (PPVT) (see Dunn and Dunn 2007), the receptive parts of the Reynell Developmental Language Scales (RDLS) (see Edwards et al. 2011) and the Clinical Evaluation of Language Fundamentals (CELF) (for latest version, see Wiig et al. 2013). All these tests are available in different versions and translations.

A useful test to assess auditory comprehension is part of the fifth edition of the Preschool Language Scale (PLS-5) (Zimmerman et al. 2011) for children from birth to 7 years 11 months of age.

The Northwestern University Children's Perception of Speech Test (NU-CHIPS) (Elliott and Katz 1980), a closed-set picture-pointing task with four pictures per page, is designed for children with a vocabulary recognition age of at least two and a half years (Dobie and Van Hemel 2004).

The Common Phrases Test (six lists of ten sentences) measures the understanding of common phrases used in everyday situations. The material can be presented in the auditory-only (A), visual-only (V) and auditory + visual modality (AV) (Robbins et al. 1995). In 27 children with cochlear implants, the performance in the A condition was correlated with the ability to integrate visual speech information in the AV condition, which seems to be of predictive value in estimating the speech perception benefit with hearing devices (Kirk et al. 2012).

Kirk et al. (1995) found that CI children recognise acoustic-phonetic similarities among words and memorise words into similarity neighbourhoods in long-term memory. The Lexical Neighborhood Test (LNT) comprises two lists of 50 monosyllabic words, the Multisyllabic Lexical Neighborhood Test (MLNT) two lists of 24 two-to-three syllable words (audio-recorded in single-talker and multiple-talker conditions). In the MLNT, half of the words are easy because they are common in the language of young children and there are only few words that can be confused because of phonemic similarity. Half of the words are not easy and less common in early-acquired vocabulary and may be confused with more phonetically similar words.

On the basis of words used to develop the LNT and MLNT, five-to seven-word sentences were constructed including three key words. Twelve children with CIs, aged 5–14 years, showed better performance in the sentence than in the word task, and in sentences with lexically easy rather than lexically hard key words (20 test sentences, two lists, one with easy, one with hard key words) (Eisenberg et al. 2002).

For the Multimodal Lexical Sentence Test for Children (MLST-C), sentences by five male and five female talkers were audiovisually recorded to consider real-world listening. Twenty-one sentences were presented in the A, V and AV condition to 31 children in the age 4–12 years with HA or CI or both. Performance was poorer in the A than in the AV condition (perception of key words 81% and 91%, respectively), HA children correctly performed in 93%, CI children in 79% (Kirk et al. 2011).

Boons et al. (2013) studied *narrative skills* by the Bus Story subtest of the Renfrew Language Scales (Renfrew 1997) in 70 CI children (5–13.3 years) in comparison with NH children. CI children in general mentioned less-essential and subsidiary elements. The Comprehensive Assessment of Spoken Language (CASL) (Carrow-Woolfolk 1999) comprises amongst others *supralinguistic measures* to investigate if the child is able to comprehend complex language when meaning cannot directly be deduced from lexical or grammatical information.

Evaluation of Expressive Language with Phonetic, Phonological Levels, Semantic Levels, Working Memory and Word Finding, Morphological, Syntactic Levels, Prosody, Intelligibility and Pragmatics

According to da Silva et al. (2011), the most-often used instruments for expressive language in HL/CI children are the expressive parts of the Reynell Developmental Language Scales (RDLS) (see Edwards et al. 2011), The MacArthur Communicative Development Inventories to assess lexical development (words, gestures, sentences) (MCDI) (Fenson et al. 2007), the Meaningful Use of Speech Scale (MUSS) (Robbins and Osberger 1990) and the expressive part of the Clinical Evaluation of Language

Fundamentals (CELF) (for latest version, see Wiig et al. 2013). All these instruments are available in different versions and translations.

A useful test to assess expressive language in children from birth to 7 years 11 months is the corresponding part of the fifth edition of the Preschool Language Scale (PLS-5) (Zimmerman et al. 2011).

Evaluation of expressive language in hearing-impaired children should comprise phonetic, phonological, semantic, morphological, syntactic, prosodic and pragmatic levels:

Basic Phonetic Evaluation
This method was introduced by Ling (1976). The tester produces a target sound and asks the child to imitate it. According to this author, the following skills were assessed:

- Vocalising on demand.
- Producing sound patterns: loud or soft, high or low pitched, sustained or brief.
- Producing all diphthongs and vowels with control.
- Producing consonant with /a/, /u/ and /i/.
- Producing initial and final consonant blends.

Phonetic Transcription
Teoh and Chin (2007) performed phonetic transcriptions of 22 CI children to document the production of sounds with articulatory errors and distortions. The children labelled pictures, and the responses were recorded, digitised and edited. The transcription was performed with spectrographic support by two independent transcribers in phoneme-by-phoneme consensus.

Most common findings were:

- In place of articulation: inventories of coronal fricatives, nonstandard affricates, allophonic variants of /l/.
- In manner of articulation: substitution of dental stops for dental fricatives, spirantisation (i.e. the substitution of a fricative for a plosive), use of ejectives, glottalisation, flapping errors, partial nasality, gliding.
- In voicing: final obstruent devoicing, aspiration of voiced stops, unaspirated initial voiceless stops.
- In vowels: substitution of centralised vowels for /u/, errors of vowel length, use of nasal vowels for nasal consonants, lenition, monophthongisation, use of nonstandard diphthongs.

Archer and Crosby-Quinatoa (2009) use among others the Structured Photographic Articulation Test-Dudsberry II (by Dawson and Tattersall (2001), useful for ages 3–9 years) based on photographs of the golden retriever Dudsberry and the Arizona Articulation Proficiency Scale (Fudala 2001), a quick method for identifying misarticulations and most sensitive at preschool and early elementary school levels.If a child knows how to articulate a sound correctly, this does not imply that the usage is correct in his spoken language.

Phonological Assessment
This method investigates which phonetic elements (phonological contrasts) are used to achieve contrast of meaning in a specific language.

- Concerning vowels, any substitutions, neutralisation, diphthongisation and nasalisation of vowels are described.
- Concerning consonants, at least two presentations of all consonants of the language in initial, medial and final word positions are checked. Misarticulations of consonants are described in terms of voiced-voiceless errors, omission or distortion of initial and medial consonants, omission of consonants in blends, distortion of final consonants, substitution of one consonant for another, glottal replacement, final vowel additions and intrusive voicing between adjacent consonants. These non-developmental patterns should be differentiated from developmental processes such as final consonant deletion, reduplication, weak syllable deletion, cluster reduction, context sensitive voicing, depalatalisation, fronting (fricatives and velars), alveolarisation (stops and fricatives), labialisation (stops), stopping (fricatives and affricates), gliding (fricatives and liquids), deaffrication, epenthesis, and metathesis (Flipsen and Parker 2008).

To study early phonological development in children with and without hearing loss, Moeller et al. (2007b) analysed recorded samples of mother–child interactions from 21 NH children and 12 HL children during the age span of 16–24 months. They defined vocal play, babble, jargon (babbled sequences with the intonation contours of spoken phrases), unintelligible communicative utterances, and words or word attempts.

The Mean Syllable Structure Level in Words, Percentage of Vowels Correct, Percentage of Consonants Correct, Phonological Mean Length of Utterance, Proportion of Whole Word Proximity, Word Shape Match and Words with Final Consonants were items of their analysis. In addition, the authors used parents' reports of vocabulary development from 10 to 30 months of age and at 36 months of age, based on spontaneous productions in a picture-naming task, the Goldman–Fristoe Test of Articulation-2 (Goldman and Fristoe 2000).

At 24 months of age, the HL toddlers produced fewer and less-complex words and were less accurate in consonant and word production. Delayed or limited use of syllables with consonants, vowel errors and limited production of recognisable words were found as indicators of atypical development.

Evaluation of Semantics, Working Memory and Word Finding

Evaluating the meaning of words and utterances includes determining the number of single words uttered by the child, as well as evaluating complex use of vocabulary, including structures such as word categories, word relationships, synonyms, antonyms, figurative language, ambiguities and absurdities. In this respect, adjective, adverb, preposition, article and pronoun use is assessed. The response time in selecting vocabulary words is also considered (word-finding problems such as circumlocutions, repetitions, frequent pauses). Over-or under-generalisation and frequent use of empty words such as 'thing', 'that', or the routinised expression 'you know' are all noted.

Archer and Crosby-Quinatoa (2009) use e.g. the Expressive Vocabulary Test-second Edition (EVT-2) (by Williams 2007) in children with cochlear implants. The child has to perform more complex tasks than only to label the pictured object or action. It seems that nowadays, owing to newborn-hearing screening and modern hearing devices, children with profound HL are also able to acquire a normal vocabulary with time. Ramos et al. (2015) could not find a significant difference from testing semantics in 18 CI children (9 and 10 years old) in comparison with the normal standard of NH children.

Marchman and Fernald (2008) found in NH children relations between word-recognition speed and vocabulary at 25 months with expressive language, IQ and especially working memory at age 8.

May-Mederake (2012) saw good results in an active vocabulary test in 28 CI children with early implantation in the first 2 years of life, but compared with their normative peers a poorer phonological working memory for nonsense words. Scientific work has still to be done to clarify the relationships between early perception, word learning and later language skills (Schwartz et al. 2013). Testing working memory seems to be a necessary step. Storing and processing of information were studied by Nittrouer et al. (2013) in 48 NH and 50 CI children, 8 years old. In CI children, less accurate recall of serial order was observed than in NH children but the rate of recall did not differ. The authors concluded that only storage is impaired in CI children.

An example of a word finding test is the Word Finding Vocabulary Test, a part of the Renfrew Language Scales (Renfrew and Mitchell 2015).

Evaluation of Morphology and Syntax

Morphology assessment involves the evaluation of morphemes, the smallest units of language that have meaning.

A morpheme is a group of sounds that refers to a particular object, idea or action:

- Roots can stand alone (e.g. car, teach, tall).
- Affixes are bound, such as prefixes and suffixes, and when attached to root words change the meaning of the words (e.g. balls, baker, tallest, irresponsible).

Syntax assessment includes evaluating how the child uses the rules by which words are organised into phrases or sentences in their language. It refers to sentence structure.

This is typically assessed by referring to the mean length of utterance (MLU), the complexity of the sentence and word order in the sentence.

Boons et al. (2013) tested in 70 school-aged CI children (5–13.3 years) expressive morphological abilities by CELF Word Structure (CELF-WS) and expressive syntactic skills by CELF Formulating Sentences (CELF-FS), parts of the Dutch version CELF-4-NL (Kort et al. 2008). In comparison with the NH control group, the authors observed difficulties with morphological rules such as regular plurals, diminutives, irregular past participles, pronouns, comparative and superlative adjectives, demonstrative pronouns, articles and adjectives. Syntactical rules were more problematic for CI children with respect to nouns, verbs, adjectives, adverbs, conjunctions and prepositional expressions.

Testing of word ordering is part of the Test of Language Development: Intermediate (TOLD-I) (by Hammill and Newcomer 2001).

Evaluation of Prosody

Prosody is defined by supra-segmental features of speech: stress, intonation, tone and duration (Kent and Kim 2008). To acquire prosody is important for the HL child because it concerns transmission of meaning and intelligibility of its utterances.

Evaluation of prosody comprises:

- Fundamental frequency patterns.
  - Average pitch: normal, too high or too low.
  - Pitch contour: appropriate or inappropriate.
  - Intonation: monotone, excessive variability or insufficient variability.
- Stress (emphasised or prominent units) normal, excessive or reduced.
- Temporal factors.
  - Rate appropriate, slow (<2 syllables per second) or fast (>4 syllables per second).
  - Duration of consonants and vowels: normal, increased or decreased.
  - Pause (juncture): normal or prolonged.
- Phrasing: syllable/word repetitions or syllable/word revisions.

Chin et al. (2012) studied prosody production in 15 CI (6.00–10.33 years) and 10 NH children (4.00–14.08 years) with the Prosodic Utterance Production (PUP) task (Bergeson and Chin 2008). Adults rated the performance of declarative, interrogative, happy and sad sentences. The percentage of correct scores was lower for CI children and the lowest ratings concerned interrogative intonation.

Evaluation of Intelligibility

Speech intelligibility is either rated subjectively (poor, fair or good), quasi-objectively by rating scales, or by the ratio of intelligible words to the number of produced words (Ling 1976).

An example of a rating scale is the Speech Intelligibility Rating Test (SIR) (Cox and McDaniel 1989; Yoshinaga-Itano and Sedey 2000):

1. I always or almost always understand the child's speech with little or no effort.
2. I always or almost always understand the child's speech: however I need to listen carefully.
3. I typically understand about half of the child's speech.
4. I typically understand about 25% of the child's speech.
5. The child's speech is very hard to understand. I typically understand only occasional, isolated words or phrases.
6. I never or almost never understand the child's speech.

Chin et al. (2012) studied intelligibility in 15 CI (6.00–10.33 years) and 10 NH children (4.00–14.08 years) with the Beginner's Intelligibility Test (BIT; Osberger et al. 1994). This is a live-voice test of single sentences developed for CI children. The words are no longer than two syllables and are familiar to children. Adult listeners rated the performance in their study, the percentage of correct scores was higher for NH children than that of CI children, and better for children with longer hearing experience.

Evaluation of Pragmatics

Pragmatic rules are needed to create interaction and transfer meaning, and comprise e.g. turn-taking, continuing a topic, adjoining information or questioning.

In order to assess pragmatic skills, the clinician has to observe the child in spontaneous, unstructured conversation with a partner.

The following communication skills should be commented on (Prutting 1982; DuCharme 1983):

- Following conversation rules for a topic: turn-taking, introducing and maintaining a topic, revising a message to fit a change in topic, modifying a message to repair breakdown in communication, and terminating conversation appropriately.
- Using language for different purposes: greeting, requesting, informing, demanding, promising.
- Changing language according to the needs of a listener or situation: talking differently to a baby and to an adult, giving background information to an unfamiliar listener, speaking differently in a classroom and on a playground.
- Abstraction: using sarcasm, understanding/responding to sarcasm, using idioms appropriately, understanding/responding appropriately to idioms.
- Visual/gestural cues: using appropriate eye contact, facial and body postures appropriately, using appropriate proximity/distance and physical contact and responding appropriately.

In HL children, acquiring pragmatic ability is delayed. Less-skilled pragmatic abilities may be turn-taking, repair strategies and maintaining a conversation topic; they use too many instructions instead of questions and have difficulty in multi-talker conversations (Rinaldi et al. 2013). Rinaldi et al. (2013) used Prutting and Kirchner's (1987) pragmatic protocol in 11 CI children and 13 HA children in comparison with 13 NH children (7 years old). They assessed verbal (e.g. response to the partner, cohesion, choosing conversation topic), paralinguistic (e.g. intelligibility, prosody, voice intensity, fluency) and non-verbal aspects (e.g. eye gaze, facial expression, physical contact). The videotaped child–adult conversations were analysed by two judges. CI and HA children showed more inappropriate use of the different pragmatic abilities than NH children. Most problematic were contingency (continuing the same topic, adding information), response and adjacency (continuing the same topic, immediately after the utterance of the conversational partner). Delayed or a different acquisition of pragmatic abilities in comparison with NH children may be explained by fewer opportunities for observing and practising an appropriate model of communication, *delayed language acquisition and a* failure to hear important cues (Rinaldi et al. 2013).

4.2.16.6 Evaluation of Auditory Perception Skills

To assess auditory perception skills, the hierarchy presented by Erber in 1982 is still a useful tool:

- Awareness/detection: The child responds by demonstrating absence or presence of sound.
- Discrimination: The child has to respond to whether two or more stimuli are similar or different.
  - Supra-segmentals with differences in duration–intensity–pitch–stress.
  - Segmentals: initial sound vocabulary–words varying in number of syllables–words with the same consonants but varying vowels–words with the same vowel but varying consonants.
- Identification/recognition: The child responds by demonstrating recognition of what has been said by repeating or pointing to a picture or object as requested.
- Comprehension: The child demonstrates understanding of speech by:
  - Following a direction.
  - Answering a question.
  - Participating in a conversation.
  - Paraphrasing what has been said.
  - Answering questions about a story: open/closed set.

All these skills also to be tested in noisy environment.

Useful tools to measure auditory skills and progress over time may be the LittlEARS Auditory Questionnaire (May-Mederake et al. 2010) and the Evaluation of Auditory Responses to Speech (EARS) (Allum et al. 2000).

Among others the following tests are often used: the Early Speech Perception Test (Moog and Geers 1990), the Meaningful Use of Speech Scale (MUSS) (Robbins and Osberger 1990), the Meaningful Auditory Integration Scale (MAIS) (Robbins et al. 1991), the Test of Auditory Comprehension of Language (Carrow-Woolfolk 1985), the Ling 6 Sound Test (Ling 1989) and the Auditory Perception Test for the Hearing Impaired (Allen 2008).

For example, the BAS-II Digits Forward task (digit span) assesses auditory memory (GL Assessment 2011).

4.2.16.7 Evaluation of Visual Perception Skills

According to Berk (2000), the following parameters should be assessed for a basic visual perception evaluation: visual acuity, colour perception, focusing and tracking ability, depth perception, pattern recognition and object perception. For a full evaluation, the following should be assessed: visual coordination, visual discrimination, visual association, visual long-term memory, visual short-term memory, visual sequential memory, visual vocal expression, visual motoric expression, visual figure ground discrimination, visual spatial relationships and visual form perception. Examples of standardised tests are shown in Table 4.4.

Testing of visual memory may also be useful. The Leiter-R Memory Screen is standardised on a deaf sample (Roid and Miller 1997).

4.2.16.8 Evaluation of Phonological Awareness, Reading, Writing (Details See Volume 2, Part III)

Phonological Awareness

An important precursor of reading is the phonological awareness of syllables, rhymes and phonemes. In addition to the original test for phonological awareness by Bradley and Bryant (1983), a picture version has been developed by Harris and Beech (1998). The child is asked to point at two pictures out of three that share the same initial (e.g. boat, bow, rope), middle (hat, net, cat) or end sound (red, bed, pen).

To study phonological processing, Geers and Hayes (2011) used the following test instruments in 112 high school children with CI and found poorer phonological skills than in 46 NH peers:

- Woodcock Reading Mastery Test (WRMT) Revised (Woodcock 1987).
- Comprehensive Test of Phonological Processing (CTOPP) (Wagner et al. 1999).
- Children's Test of Nonword Repetition (CNRep) (Gathercole and Baddeley 1996).

Reading Assessment

In Part III of Volume 2, reading assessment is intensively presented. Examples of formal reading assessment in HL children are:

Table 4.4 Examples of standardised tests to evaluate visual perception skills

Name of the test	Skills	Age range
Motor-Free Visual Perception Test, Fourth Edition (MVPT-4) by Colarusso and Hammill (2015)	– Spatial relationship – Visual closure – Visual discrimination – Visual memory – Figure ground	4 through 80 years
Test of Visual Perceptual Skills, Fourth Edition (TVPS-4) by Martin (2017)	– Same as above plus: – Form Constancy – Visual sequential memory	5 through 21 years
Bender Visual-Motor Gestalt Test (Bender-Gestalt II) by Brannigan and Decker (2003)	– Visuospatial coordination – Visuomotor coordination	3 to 85+ years

- Test of Early Reading Ability: Deaf Hard of Hearing (TERA-D/HH) (Reid et al. 1991).
- Stanford Achievement Test for Hearing-Impaired Students (SAT-HI) (Gallaudet Research Institute 1983).

Geers and Hayes (2011) used the following tests in their study of 112 high school students with CI:

- Test of Reading Comprehension (TORC) (Brown et al. 1995).
- Peabody Individual Achievement Test (PIAT)-Revised (Dunn and Markwardt 1989).

Johnson and Goswani (2010) studied phonological awareness, vocabulary and reading in 21early and 22 late CI children, 16 HA children and 19 NH children (98–111 months old). They performed a rhyme test, an initial and final phoneme task, and for reading used the NARA-R test, the BAS-II single word reading subtest of the British Ability Scales and the Wordchains test (Miller Guron 1999), which measures visual word form familiarity. Phonological awareness, decoding, reading accuracy and reading comprehension were enhanced by early cochlear implantation.

Assessment of Writing

In Part 3 of Volume II, assessment of writing is intensively presented. Evaluation of writing involves areas such as writing traits (examples include ideas, organisation, word choice, sentence structure and mechanics), writing process (the child's engagement in planning, composing and revision) and kinds of writing (the child's ability to utilise a variety of forms, such as essay, stories and reports).

To perform an informal assessment, a representative writing sample (or samples) is (are) collected. An example of an analysis scale is the following 'Written words rating scale' (syntactic complexity evaluation from written text) (Levitt et al. 1987) (Table 4.5).

In CI children shorter, less-complex sentences containing more errors were observed (Spencer et al. 2003). Although many CI children may achieve age-appropriate skills in literacy, in 112 high school students with CI Geers and Hayes (2011) found poorer skills in phonological processing tasks, spelling, and written expression in comparison with 46 NH peers. The authors used a picture spelling test and the Expository Writing with NTID Scoring (Schley and Albertini 2005). The four scoring categories comprised organisation and content of the assay, language use (e.g. spelling, grammatical structures) and vocabulary use. Although a wide variability in literacy outcomes was reported, better literacy skills are expected in general in CI children implanted at younger ages (Sarant 2012).

Table 4.5 Written words rating scale (Levitt et al. 1987)

Rating	Category description
1	No useful output (no words related to test material)
2	Single words related to the test material (labelling only, incorrect word order)
3	Some evidence of syntactic structure (words in correct word order, or use of verbs. Repetitive, fixed word order is not counted)
4	Essentially complete structure, although errors may be present
5	Substantial output, essentially complete structure

With kind permission from American Speech-Language-Hearing Association ASHA

The Boehm Test of Basic Concepts (Boehm 1971) investigates basic concepts that are decisive for school performance. Children at risk for a learning difficulty can be identified from percentiles and performance ranges.

4.2.17 Occupational Therapy Examinations

Jill Massey

4.2.17.1 Occupational Therapy: Definition and Special Needs in Hearing-Impaired Children

Occupational therapy employs a client-centred approach focusing on enabling an individual to participate in a variety of occupations to enhance health and wellbeing. The term 'occupations' refers to everything people do in the course of their daily life (College of Occupational Therapists (COT) 2015).

Occupation within the context of children and young people includes aspects of self-care such as developing their independence in dressing, eating a meal and using the toilet; work or being productive within school, college and university or caring for others; and leisure socialising and playing with friends and participating in hobbies or sports (COT 2015).

Promoting engagement, developing independence and preparing children and young people for independence in future life are core occupational therapy values. Occupational therapists work with those whose occupations are affected by injury, illness or disability, by family situations, and during changes of circumstances.

The impact of a hearing impairment for children and young people on development of language is widely documented, but it can be wide ranging with a profound effect that is often overlooked. Children who are hearing-impaired engage in fewer interactions with hearing peers (Simeonsson et al. 2001; Stinson and Liu 1999). Without this interaction, they do not experience the same levels of social or academic group participation as their hearing peers, nor do they receive the social and academic benefits that such participation provides. Young people with hearing impairment have been observed to develop limited life skills (Akamatsu et al. 2005). It is assumed these students experience limited opportunities and miss the incidental learning prospects to develop independence in life skills compared with typically developing peers.

Children with a hearing impairment or deafness must rely on other sensory systems. Therefore, they have been identified to be at greater risk of delays in sensory processing, motor skills, balance and the ability to carry out complex motor sequences (Gheysen et al. 2007; Schlumberger et al. 2004; Russel and Nagaishi 2010). These delays or deficits can inhibit occupational performance and development in the areas of self-care productivity and leisure.

Occupational therapists should be an integral member of a collaborative multidisciplinary team working with a child or young person who has a hearing impairment, and use their unique occupational lens to evaluate and ameliorate participation and development of daily occupations, by utilising adaptive and compensatory approaches, alongside planning and implementing education for the child, young person, their family and other professionals working with the child.

4.2.17.2 Evaluation

Gathering Information and Interview

The occupational therapist's evaluation will include gathering information to form an occupational profile of the client. Initial referral information should include the student's type and degree of hearing loss, age of onset, cause of hearing loss, medical history comprising any additional disabilities and the student's level and preferred method of communication.

Through the use of a client-centred structured and semi-structured interview approach with the family, child and other key professionals such as the education team, the occupational therapist will then explore the child's daily life, routine occupations, needs and expectations, determine their strengths and how they are able to participate and identify any barriers or challenges that are influencing their successful participation.

In the case of interviewing a child with a hearing impairment, the occupational therapist will adapt their communication style to meet the needs of the student, depending on the student's preferred method of communication, age and literacy level. This may include use of simplified language, pictures and/or symbols; the most suitable method of communication should be discussed with the speech and language therapist and, where feasible, the specialist teacher of the deaf.

Observation

A fundamental part of the occupational therapist's evaluation will involve contextual observation of the child's participating in his daily occupations. Where possible this is best undertaken within the natural environment. Analysis of the child's occupational performance along with the information gathered enables the therapist to determine what supports or limits the child's ability to participate in home, community and school settings. Activity demands, client factors and contexts in which the child performs occupations form part of the therapist's comprehensive assessment.

Assessment Tools

Therapists also have a wide range of norm-referenced and criterion-referenced developmental assessment tools, which may typically be used in their practice, forming part of the comprehensive assessment. However, many rely on language for their standardised delivery; such tools need to be adapted or modified for their use with a child or young person with hearing impairment. Subsequently qualitative information can be taken and reported; standard scores should not be reported. Any reporting of information should include any amplification (if any) the children are using and details of how the assessment was modified taking into consideration their hearing impairment, e.g. their level of language and method of communication.

Goal Setting

Having identified areas of important occupations, the occupational therapist will work with the child, family and other key people to evaluate what helps or hinders their involvement in daily life roles and to set client-centred meaningful goals for occupational therapy provision. As well as directing intervention, the goals can be reviewed after intervention and used as an outcome measure to determine the effectiveness of therapy with the child or young person.

4.2.17.3 Intervention

Working collaboratively with the child or young person, their family and key professionals, the occupational therapist will develop possible solutions, such as exploring alternative ways of doing things, developing skills through adapted or simplified approaches, using task analysis or making changes to the environment to support participation.

Deaf children have been identified as being at increased risk (anywhere between 30 and 50% more likely) of mental health difficulties compared with their hearing peers. Access to high-quality, effective mental health services is a key standard of the Children's National Service Framework in the UK. Within the UK occupational therapists who focus on the mental health difficulties of a young person with hearing impairment play a central role within the specialist of National Deaf Child and Adolescent Mental Health Service (CAMHS) team of professionals. Communication can be challenging for deaf families; it is also recognised that, for a variety of reasons, the developmental pathways for deaf children differ from those of their hearing counterparts. The social-emotional mental health needs of the child or young person who is hearing-impaired need to be properly considered for intervention to be effective. A developmental occupational therapist will often work together with the National Deaf CAMHS team to promote effective outcomes (Beresford et al. 2008).

4.2.17.4 Conclusion

The occupational therapists' holistic approach to understanding the strengths of and barriers to a hearing-impaired student's participation in routines and activities in all aspects of their daily life can help to improve participation in all aspects of occupation through modifications or adaptations to the environment. It is critical for occupational therapists to form part of the multidisciplinary team supporting a child or young person with hearing impairment, in order to enable their maximum independence and engagement in meaningful occupation, social activities and opportunities for future life.

4.2.18 Evaluation of General Cognitive Developmental Stage

See Vol. 1, Part III Sect. 4.4.1.

4.2.19 Child Psychological Examinations Including Tests to Rule out Attention Deficit Disorders

See Vol. 1, Part I, Chap. 3, Sect. 3.5 and Part III, Chap. 11, Sects. 4.4.1 and 11.8.

4.2.20 Aetiological Assessment after the Diagnosis of a Permanent Hearing Loss[2]

Thomas Wiesner

4.2.20.1 Introduction

In the case of a child diagnosed with a hearing loss, the literature provides diverse lists of examinations that are recommended for its aetiological assessment (Gürtler in press). Yet most of these lists are quite general and do not specify, for example:

- The details that should be requested when ordering a certain examination.
- At what age the examination should be performed.
- Whether the examination must be repeated at certain intervals.
- Which kind of hearing loss requires which examinations.
- How the medical history and already existing test results affect the selection of additional examinations.

To ensure that the necessary examinations are performed at the right time, and that unnecessary examinations can be prevented, the following text gives guidelines to the questions: *Which tests, what are the goals and at which age?*

4.2.20.2 Proposal for a Stepwise Aetiological Assessment Process

The examinations necessary for an aetiological assessment should be proposed to the parents of all children with a permanent hearing loss at the beginning of the rehabilitation process:

- Aetiological assessments should be carried out in parallel with, and without delaying, the further multidisciplinary assessment of the hearing loss itself.
- The choice of tests has to depend on the prior clinical examination and the case history.
- The goals for this completive assessment after the diagnosis of the hearing loss are:
  - To supplement and specify the auditory diagnosis.
  - To initiate certain risk preventive actions (e.g. vaccination against *Haemophilus influenzae* and *Pneumococcus* in the case of a malformation of the internal ear, which increases the risk of meningitis as a complication of an ear infection).
  - To adjust and complete the information given to the parents in respect of the diagnosis, the therapeutic proposals and the follow-up.
- Any aetiological assessment needs informed consent of the parents.

Elements of the Aetiological Assessment

These include searching for a clue that may lead to a possible cause of the deafness:

- Looking for risk factors according to the list of the JCIH (Joint Committee on Infant Hearing 2007).
- Reconsidering the family history, including parents and relatives of three generations (a questionnaire with specific questions is helpful).
- All hearing-impaired children need a careful paediatric examination including a paediatric neurology evaluation and an ENT clinical examination, especially searching for signs such as:
  - A white wick, unpigmented cutaneous spots, different eye colours or blue crystal eyes in combination with a bilateral sensorineural hearing loss would point to the diagnosis of a Waardenburg syndrome.
  - Cervical fistulas and pits with ear deformities suggesting branchio-oto-renal (BOR) syndrome.
  - Cleft lip/palate, down-slanting eyes, coloboma, low-set small external ears and man-

[2]International Bureau for Audiophonology, Commission 12, adapted from the BIAP-Recommendation 12-7: Aetiological assessment after the diagnosis of a permanent hearing loss, April 2013, www.biap.org

dible and maxillary hypoplasia in association with a conductive type of hearing loss, which would possibly indicate Treacher Collins syndrome.
  - Palatal and lip clefts in association with choanal atresia, external ear deformity and facial paralysis, which might raise the suspicion of CHARGE association or similar syndromes.
  - Cleft palate, velopharyngeal dysfunction and congenital heart defects (often already detected by prenatal sonography) may suggest a microdeletion 22q11.2 syndrome (DiGeorge syndrome, velocardiofacial syndrome).
  - Microcephaly that might be seen in association with perinatal CMV (cytomegalovirus) or rubella infection or other events such as birth asphyxia or brain underdevelopment.
- For reducing the strain on the families, the recommended examinations should be combined as far as possible to keep the number of appointments low.
- The timetable (Table 4.6) and the list of recommended examinations are not strict rules to be followed automatically but a proposal that must be adapted to the special situation of every child and its family.

The order of the recommended examinations refers to a very efficient proposal of De Leenheer et al. (2011). This proposal heavily relies on an early genetic evaluation. As this may not be accepted by all patients, the concept was not fully endorsed by the BIAP, but the proposed flowchart can be found in the publication of De Leenheer et al. (2011).

Specifications for the Diagnostic Procedures Named in the Timetable 16.6 (See Numbering in Table 4.6)

1. The examination algorithm to assess a congenital CMV infection is presented in Fig. 4.36.
2. The chances and limits of genetic testing must be discussed with the parents, such as which diagnoses the genetic tests are looking for and whether and how the knowledge of a certain diagnosis is helpful in the management and treatment of the child. The parents must be informed of the potential likelihoods of heredity transmission, but also that the results of the genetic assessment might concern not only the deaf child but also other members of his family. The testing is only allowed with the parent's permission. The counselling of the parents should be done by a geneticist specialised in hearing disorders (or a hearing specialist specially trained in genetic counselling).

   For the genetic testing, it is necessary to have as far as possible the complete medical history, a clinical paediatric examination and the results of the above recommended aetiological assessment including the audiometric results of the family members.

   In case of an isolated cochlear SNHL, it is recommended first that a search for a mutation in connexin 26 and 30 genes be made, because it is the most frequent cause in this case.

   In case of a motor developmental delay and vestibular problems, it is recommended that Usher syndrome is sought, provided that there are no additional clinical signs, e.g. pointing to CHARGE or other syndromic conditions with a developmental delay, and vestibular and hearing problems.

   The decision on which kind of genetic test should be used will depend on whether a syndromic (Waardenburg, Pendred, Jervell, Alport, etc.) or an isolated non-syndromic cause of the hearing loss is being sought.

   In the case of a non-syndromic hearing loss, the selection of genetic tests will be influenced by the preceding diagnostic findings of:
   - Conductive or sensorineural.
   - Auditory neuropathy or auditory dyssynchrony spectrum (otoferlin).
   - Inner ear malformation or not.
   - Outer ear or middle ear malformation.
   - Genetic transmission mode shown by the family history (mitochondrial type? X-linked? dominant? recessive?)

Table 4.6 Timetable for recommended examinations in the aetiological assessment

Timetable									
Type of hearing loss		Sensorineural (SNHL)						Conductive	
Degree of hearing loss		Profound		Other degrees progressive		Other degrees stable			
	Examination	First test	Test repetition	First test	Test repetition	First test	Test repetition	First test	Test repetition
1.	CMV screening	A.s.a.p.		A.s.a.p.		A.s.a.p.		–	–
2.	Genetic	See remark in text							
3.	MRI	<12 m		A.s.a.p.	–	When possible without sedation		–	–
4.	CT scan	<12 m	–	–	–	–	–	When possible without sedation or before surgery	–
5.	Ophthalmological examination	6 m	Every year	6 m	Every year	6 m	Every year	6 m	Every year
6.	Searching for pre-and perinatal infections	<12 m A.s.a.p.	–	<12 m A.s.a.p.	–	<12 m A.s.a.p.	–	–	–
7.	Haematuria/ proteinuria screening + echo kidney	If malformation of external or middle ear	–	If malformation of external or middle ear	–	If malformation of external or middle ear	–	A.s.a.p.	–
8.	ECG	<6 m	Once at ~18 m	–	–	–	–	If CHARGE syndrome in CT	–
9.	ERG	>9 m	–	If clinical RP signs	–	–	–	–	–
10.	Vestibular tests	<6 m	If first abnormal and pre and post CI	A.s.a.p.	If motor delay	<12 m A.s.a.p.	If motor delay	If hypotonia or if CHARGE syndrome	If hypotonia or if CHARGE syndrome

The numbering in the timetable corresponds to the numbering of the more detailed explanations of recommended examinations in the text

Comment: In case of a mixed hearing loss, the CT scan should be done <12 m. If this CT scan shows an inner ear malformation, follow the recommendation for the 'SNHL—other degrees stable'

MRI magnetic resonance imaging; *CT* computed tomography; *ECG* electrocardiography; *ERG* electroretinography; *RP* retinitis pigmentosa; *CI* cochlear implant; *a.s.a.p.* 'as soon as possible'; *m* month of age

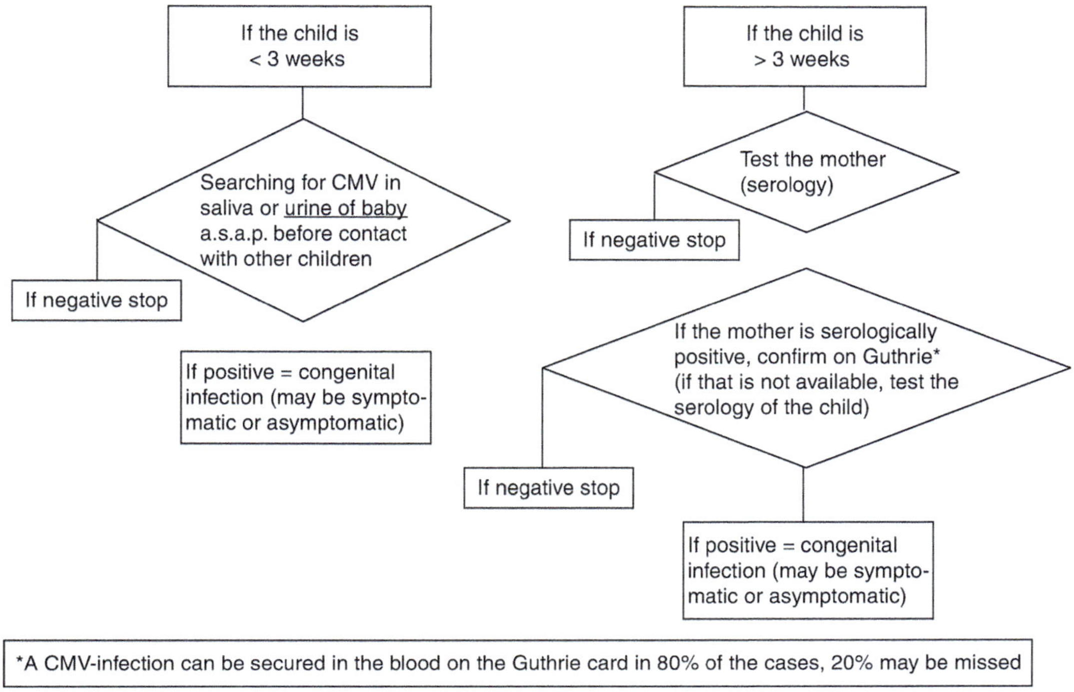

Fig. 4.36 Flowchart of an examination algorithm to assess a congenital CMV infection (Barbi et al. 2000; Boppana et al. 2011; Foulon et al. 2008, 2012; Soetens et al. 2008)

High-throughput next-generation sequencing (NGS) allows parallel screening of large panels of hearing-related genes with high accuracy, in a short time, at a cost lower than conventional Sanger sequencing (American College of Medical Genetics Expert Panel 2002). This can be achieved either by targeted capture of several dozens of genes or by direct sequencing of all exons present in the genome (so-called whole exome sequencing or WES). Targeted NGS screening would only detect genome variations in genes known to be involved in hearing loss. WES theoretically could uncover all DNA sequence variations, but laboratories that offer such WES may decide to filter the data and consider only pertinent genes (giving nevertheless the possibility of going back to the raw data to analyse further genes if necessary). Obviously, only targeted sequencing is convenient in a diagnostic setting. The strategy followed by the laboratory to which samples are sent must thus be clearly defined. At this point, the use of non-filtered WES data is limited to research. Parents must be informed before the examination whether the NGS screening will be in a diagnostic setting (i.e. focused on known hearing loss-causing genes) or whether the investigation is wider and may uncover unexpected negative findings, such as harmful mutations in genes predisposing to late-onset disorders. Genetic diagnosis and genetic counselling following the use of these new technologies require a close connection between clinicians and audiologists, clinical geneticists (or genetic counsellors) and molecular biologists, to avoid improper interpretation and for cross-validation between genotype and phenotype: even targeted NGS discloses a vast amount of DNA sequence variations whose significance may be unknown, or dubious. Genetic counselling based on NGS data may thus involve a number of ethical risks and questions that are not satisfactorily answered politically, juristically or by civil society.

3./4. Imaging should be performed by a specialist for paediatric radiology:

The decision whether to use a CT or MRI first will be influenced by whether one is searching for bony or soft tissue deficiencies (BAPA and BAAP 2008).

Temporal MRI scan and CT, general considerations:
- In case of a profound deafness.
- Before the end of the first year of life.
- For a CT a low radiation scanner should be used (e.g. cone beam scanner).
- A CT needs radiation but can be done so quickly that it can be performed during natural sleep (especially with very young children) or when under sedation.
- An MRI has no radiation but takes much longer and therefore normally needs general anaesthesia.
- Aim of temporal MRI: searching for a malformation of the:
- Vestibular aqueduct (dilation).
- Cochlear or vestibular fibrosis.
- Internal auditory canal.
- The auditory, vestibular and facial nerve.
- Central auditory pathways.
- Brain (lesions).
- Aim of CT: searching for a malformation of the:
- Ear (outer, middle and inner ear) and the vestibular organ.
- Internal auditory canal.
  Vestibular aqueduct (dilation).

5. **Aim** Searching for any impaired vision that might enhance the sensory deficit of the child and specifically for any signs of an 'oculo-auditory syndrome': coloboma, optic nerve abnormalities, oculomotor anomalies, refraction disorders, inflammation of the cornea or the retina, and cataract
   Exam Ophthalmological examination (incl. Ocular motricity study and funduscopy) done by a specialist experienced in examining young children. (The early funduscopy does not rule out an 'Usher syndrome type I', because the specific signs of a retinitis pigmentosa occur later in childhood!)
   For the indication of an electroretinogram, see Point 8.
6. As with some infections such as CMV, toxoplasmosis and rubella, neither the mother nor the child might show obvious clinical signs of the infection, so one should also search for the following prenatal and perinatal infections in cases of an isolated, idiopathic hearing loss:
   - CMV (see above)
   - Toxoplasmosis
     Determination of antibodies (IgM and IgG) against *Toxoplasma gondii* in the hearing-impaired newborn should be performed, except in cases where the mother was known to be immune before pregnancy.
   - Rubella
     If either maternal rubella immunisation by vaccination has not been performed or the maternal status is unknown, this diagnosis should be considered, and maternal and neonatal rubella-specific IgM and IgG should be determined.

As asymptomatic congenital infections of syphilis and herpes are very unlikely, routine serological screenings for these infections are not necessary in otherwise healthy hearing-impaired children.

4.2.20.3 Particular Situations Are an Indication for Complementary Testing

7. **Aim** Searching for a haematuria or proteinuria
   Exam Urine stick (a non-invasive procedure, but strong evidence to recommend this examination as a general screening is lacking; if any clinical signs of kidney malfunction occur, a thorough examination of the kidneys is necessary).
   Aim Searching for malformations of the kidney and urinary tract.
   Exam Kidney sonography, if there are even minor malformations of the ear or a history of urinary and renal symptoms.
8. **Aim** Searching for a prolongation of the QT interval in case of bilateral deafness (Jervell and Lange-Nielsen syndrome (BAPA and BAAP 2008)).
   Exam The ECG should be done by a paediatric cardiologist.
9. (see also Point 5)
   Aim Searching for 'Usher syndrome type I'. An abnormal ERG does not prove the Usher

diagnosis in all cases; therefore a genetic assessment is additionally necessary. The diagnosis of an Usher syndrome should be communicated to the parents only by a clinician with specific experience in the management of patients with Usher syndrome.
Exam An electroretinogram should be done in profoundly deaf children showing hypotonia or vestibular areflexia (not before the age of 9 months).

10. A vestibular examination should include otolithic functions and the semicircular canal functions.

4.2.21 Diagnostic Radiology

Sylva Bartel-Friedrich and Sabrina Kösling

4.2.21.1 Ear Malformations

Epidemiology

According to Weerda (2004), 50% of ENT malformations affect the ear. Congenital malformations (CMs) of the outer and middle ear occur mostly on the right side (58–61%), and the majority (ca. 70–90%) are unilateral. Inner ear CM may be found unilaterally or bilaterally. An incidence of 1:6000 to 1:6830 newborns has been reported for outer ear CM (Weerda 2004). Severe CM can be expected in 1:10000 to 1:20000 newborns (Ishimoto et al. 2005; Swartz and Harnsberger 1997; Weerda 2004). In terms of prevalence rates, the microtia is higher: ca. 2:10000 to 9:10000 births, depending on the data source (passive vs active surveillance systems) (EUROCAT 2013; Queißer-Luft and Spranger 2006; Schloss 1997).

CM can affect all three parts of the ear (outer ear (pinna and external auditory canal, EAC), middle ear, inner ear), not infrequently in combination. Inner ear CM frequencies of 11–47% in individuals with outer and middle ear CM have been reported (Kösling et al. 2009). CM of the middle ear can accompany CM of the outer ear at variable degrees and frequencies; according to Ishimoto, the ossicles are affected in 6–52% of cases, the round and oval window in 6–29%, the mastoid pneumatisation in 15–38%, the course of the facial nerve in 36–43% and the middle ear space in 0–15% (Ishimoto et al. 2005).

The most common form of CM is a combined deformity known as congenital aural atresia, involving severe CM of the pinna and the middle ear with the characteristic finding of an atretic EAC; there is accompanying CM of the inner ear in ca. 10% of cases, and the CMs are bilateral in 15–20% of patients. Nevertheless, the different embryogenesis of the outer/middle ear and inner ear results in CM of the outer or middle ear without inner ear CM and vice versa (Helms 1994). Overall, inner ear CM, middle ear CM and combined CM of all three parts of the ear are less frequent than congenital aural atresia.

Isolated middle ear CMs (often bilateral) without coexisting outer ear CM have been reported to occur in less than 10% of children with congenital conductive hearing loss (CHL) according to Lambert (2001).

The prevalence of inner ear CM in individuals with congenital deafness or sensorineural hearing loss (SNHL) varies from 2.3 to 28.4% depending on patient selection criteria. In groups of patients strictly selected for suspicion of CM, inner ear CMs were detected in 35% by means of CT and MRI, with MRI better at displaying the fine details (Kösling et al. 2003). In addition, as mentioned for CM of the outer and middle ear, the course of the facial nerve is found to be aberrant in ca. 15–32% of patients with cochleovestibular CM (Huang et al. 2012a).

CM can result from a developmental arrest, from irregular embryogenesis or from both, owing to spontaneous genetic mutations—this is the case for the majority of CM of the outer and middle ear—genetic transmission and exogenous factors (in about 10% of cases; e.g. teratogens such as retinoic acid, thalidomide and the immunosuppressant mycophenolate mofetil).

Congenital Malformations of the Outer and Middle Ear

Clinical Signs and Classification

CM of the outer ear can involve the orientation, position, size and relief pattern of the pinna; anotia may also occur. Anterior to the pinna, ear tags, ear sinus and ear pits may be found. The EAC can be atretic (aplastic) or hypoplastic. Middle ear CM can affect the configuration and size of the middle ear spaces and the number, size and configuration of the ossicles. There may be anomalies of the oval window and, rarely, of the round window. On the whole, it can be stated that there is normally a correlation between the degree of CM of the pinna and that of the middle ear with the corresponding CHL. Nevertheless, normal auricles with atresia of the EAC and albeit rarely microtia combined with normal EAC and normal tympanic cavity have been reported (Klaiber and Weerda 2002). Tables 4.7 and 4.8 list the most commonly used classifications for CM of the outer ear (Fig. 4.37).

Besides a wide range of findings within each grade of dysplasia, additional transitional forms have been noted, especially between grade II and grade III. Adapted from Weerda (2004) Thieme © 2004.

The classification of CM of the EAC according to Weerda (2004) includes three types, shown in Table 4.8.

The closely interrelated development of the EAC and the middle ear has led to the widely used classification of the combined CM termed congenital aural atresia according to Altmann (1955). Three degrees of severity are described, each based on its histopathological findings:

Table 4.8 Classification of EAC malformations according to Weerda (2004)

Type of CM	Signs of CM
EAC stenosis *type A*	Marked narrowing of the EAC along with an intact skin layer[a]
EAC stenosis *type B*	Partial development of the EAC with an atresia plate at the medial part[b]
Type C	Complete bony EAC atresia[c]

Adapted from Weerda (2004) Thieme © 2004

[a]Type A, compared with atresia, carries a much greater risk of cholesteatoma, beginning at a canal opening of 4 mm or less. In ears with a bony canal opening of 2 mm or less, the risk of cholesteatoma formation increases to 91% by the age of 12 years (Declau et al. 2008). Thus, surgery is recommended for canals of 2 mm or less

[b]Depending on concomitant middle ear malformations or conductive hearing loss, it may be advisable to implement hearing aid treatment

[c]Often it is advisable to implement hearing aid treatment in view of the frequently concomitant middle ear malformations with conductive hearing loss

First-degree CM:	*Stenosis of the EAC, normal or slightly hypoplastic tympanic cavity, deformed ossicles, well-aerated mastoid (*Fig. 4.38*)*
Second-degree CM:	*Blindly ending or absent EAC, narrow tympanic cavity, deformation and fixation of ossicles, decreased mastoid pneumatisation*
Third-degree CM:	*Absent EAC, absent mastoid pneumatisation (atresia plate), hypoplastic or rudimentary tympanic cavity, severely deformed ossicles (*Fig. 4.39*)*

Ossicular CMs include fusion of the malleus and incus, fixation in the epitympanic recess, bony ankylosis of the neck of the malleus to the atresia plate, hypoplasia of the manubrium of the malleus and absent malleus and incus.

According to Müller (1991), three degrees of severity of isolated middle ear CM can be differentiated:

Mild CM:	Normal configuration of the tympanic cavity, ossicular dysplasia
Moderate CM:	Hypoplasia of the tympanic cavity, dysplastic or aplastic ossicles
Severe CM:	Aplastic or cleft-like tympanic cavity

Stapes CMs frequently occur in isolated 'minor' (mild) middle ear deformities. The most common type of isolated ossicular chain CM is a combined deformity of the stapes superstructure and of the incus, especially of its long process and lenticular process. There are frequently incudostapedial joint fusions and aplasia or hypoplasia of the stapes superstructures, such as snapped-off stapes head; thickening, thinning and fusion of the stapedial crura; and masses of bony or fibrotic tissue between the crura. Stapes fixation can result from bony plates or from aplasia or dysplasia of the annular ligament. Moreover, stapes can be completely absent. On the basis of the frequent involvement of the stapes, Declau et al. (1999) proposed a modified classification.

Other changes viewed as malformations of the middle ear are cerebral spinal fluid (CSF)-middle ear fistulas (indirect translabyrinthine or direct paralabyrinthine CSF fistulas), congenital tumours

Table 4.7 Grades of dysplasia of the pinna with subgroups according to Weerda (2004)

Grade of dysplasia	Subgroups
I: First-degree CM	• Prominent ears • Macrotia • Cryptotia (pocket ear) • Coloboma (transverse cleft) • Scaphoid ear • Stahl ear • Satyr ear • Slight deformities (distinct Darwin tuberculum, absent crus of helix, deformities of tragus and antitragus) • Deformities of lobe (fixed lobe, hyperplasia or hypoplasia or aplasia or cleft of lobe) • Cup ear deformity type I • Cup ear deformity type IIa • Cup ear deformity type IIb
	Most structures of the normal pinna are recognisable. The reconstruction only occasionally requires the use of additional skin or cartilage
II: Microtia grade II, second-degree CM	• Cup ear deformity type III • Mini-ear ('concha-type microtia') – Hypoplasia of upper pinna – Hypoplasia of middle pinna – Hypoplasia (or aplasia) of lower pinna Often combined with dystopia and EAC stenosis, rarely with EAC atresia, ear drum CM possible
	Some structures of a normal auricle are recognisable. Partial reconstruction of the pinna requires the use of some additional skin and cartilage
III: Microtia grade III with anotia, third-degree CM	• Unilateral microtia grade III ('lobule-type microtia', Fig. 4.37) • Bilateral microtia grade III • Anotia often with dystopia and EAC atresia
	None of the normal structures of the pinna are recognisable. Total reconstruction requires the use of skin and large amounts of cartilage

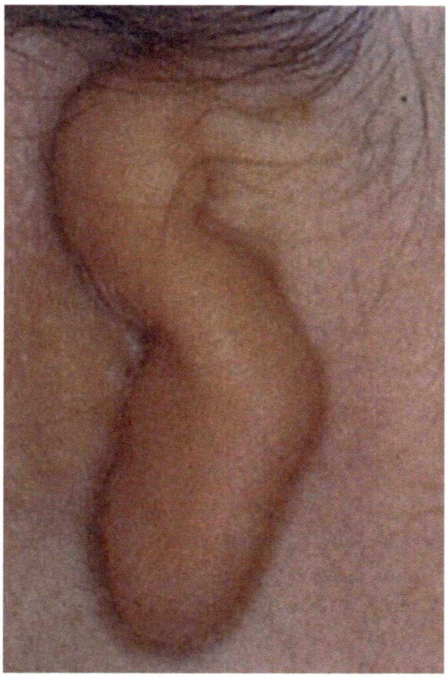

Fig. 4.37 Microtia grade III ('lobule-type microtia')

(epidermoid) and dermoids (see Sect. 4.2.23.2 of this section).

CM of the outer and middle ear may be found in syndromes (Table 4.9), most commonly Franceschetti (Treacher Collins) syndrome, Goldenhar syndrome and Klippel Feil syndrome (Fig. 4.40).

Table 4.9 also lists syndromes in which hearing loss is a frequent or major component, but where malformations are not commonly detected by imaging.

The diagnosis of CM of the outer and middle ear is based on clinical examination and imaging.

Clinical Examination

CMs of the outer and middle ear are diagnosed in early childhood in cases with deformities of the auricles or bilateral hearing impairment. If there is only unilateral hearing loss without external deformities, the diagnosis may be delayed. Thus,

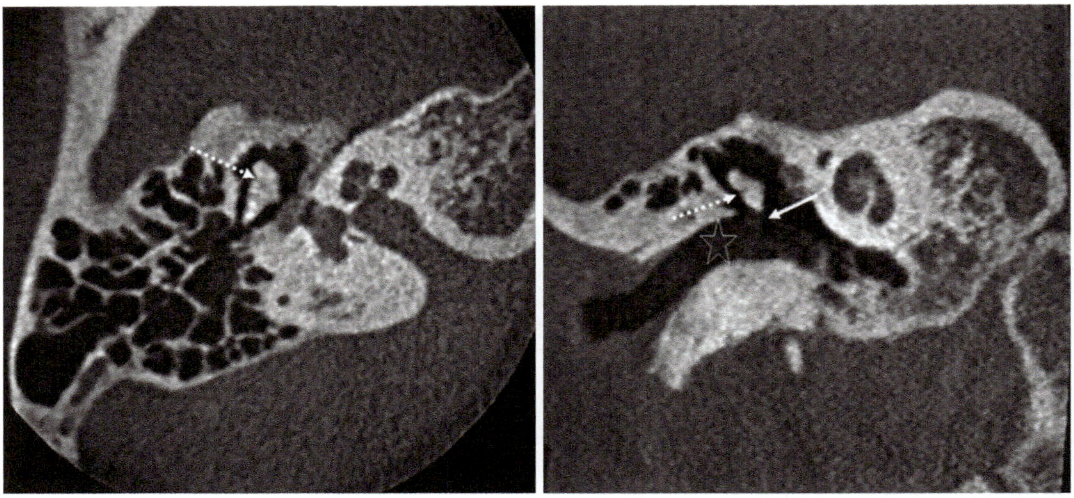

Fig. 4.38 CB-CT (A axial, B coronal) of a 13-year-old boy with unilateral auricular appendage, EAC stenosis and CHL of 45 dB. Narrowing of EAC (*star*), fused incudomalleolar joint (*dotted arrows*), absent malleolar manubrium (*arrow*), slightly smaller tympanic cavity than normal, normal pneumatisation and inner ear structures. Mild congenital aural atresia, grade I according to Altmann classification

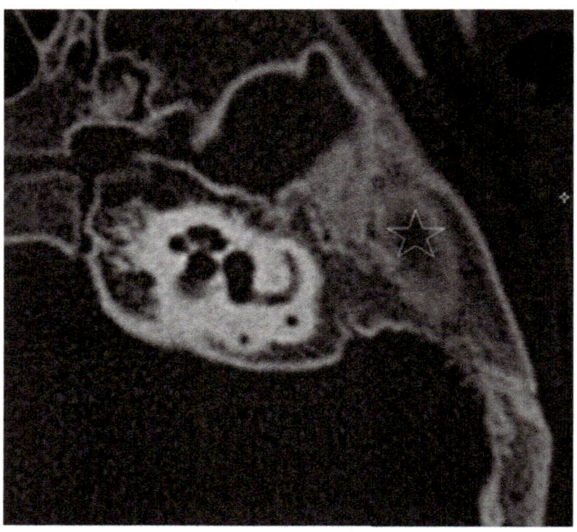

Fig. 4.39 Axial CT of a 6-year-old boy with unilateral microtia, atresia of EAC and severe CHL. Known Goldenhar syndrome. Absent tympanic cavity, broad atresia plate (*star*), normal inner ear. Severe congenital aural atresia, grade III according to Altmann classification

anamnesis plays an important role. The time of onset of the hearing problems should be established and other causes for hearing loss, e.g. infection, excluded. If CM is not suspected, CT is not frequently performed and the diagnosis is made during tympanotomy.

Newborns with CM of the outer ear must undergo detailed physical investigation of craniofacial structures for possible underlying syndromes. Each major branch of the facial nerve has to be carefully examined. Additional malformations should be excluded by an interdisciplinary team.

Auditory assessment is the most important functional investigation in patients with ear CM. Patients with CM of the outer and middle ear suffer from CHL of variable extent. Severe congenital aural atresia is often accompanied by a complete conductive sound blocking of about 60 dB. In cases of unilateral congenital aural atresia, early testing of the apparently normal contralateral ear is important in order to detect or exclude bilateral hearing loss.

The assessment includes reflex and behavioural audiometry, tympanometry (impedance measurement) and otoacoustic emissions (OAE), as well as auditory brainstem response testing in bone and air conduction. In older children, pure-tone and speech audiometry are added. Repeated audiometry may be necessary in young infants or in children who are otherwise difficult to test, or in patients with multiple malformations.

Imaging

Specific imaging of the temporal bone (not brain or skull imaging) has to be requested for patients

Table 4.9 Selected syndromes commonly associated with hearing loss and CM of the ear (Adapted from Beale and Madani 2008, Gorlin et al. 1990, Huang et al. 2012b)

Group of syndromes	Name of syndrome	Hearing loss			CM			
		CHL	SNHL	Mixed	Outer/middle ear	Inner ear	Facial nerve course	Not common on imaging
Otocraniofacial	Craniofacial microsomia, incl. Goldenhar	+	(+)	(+)	Pinna malformations, EAC atresia or stenosis, absent/abnormal ossicles, tegmen descent	IAC porus abnormally high	(+)	–
	Treacher Collins	+	(+)	(+)	Pinna malformations, EAC atresia, size-reduced attic/antrum, abnormal ossicles	Dysplastic lateral SCC	Altered	–
	BOR	+	+	+	EAC atresia or stenosis, abnormal ossicles	Hypoplasia of apical cochlear turn/ Mondini deformity, vestibular dysplasia, SCC hypoplasia, LVA, short/bulbous/funnel-shaped IAC, CND	Obtuse angle of anterior genu	–
	CHARGE	+	+	+	Pinna malformations, EAC atresia or stenosis, abnormal ossicles, absent windows	Mondini deformity, absent SCC, vestibular dysplasia, CND	Abnormal	–
	X-linked deafness (with stapes gusher)	+	+	+	–	Enlarged/bulbous IAC, widened cochlear aperture, absence/ deficiency of lamina cribrosa, cochlear hypoplasia, LVA	Widening of bony canal of labyrinthine segment	–
Cranio-synostoses	Crouzon	+	(+)		EAC atresia or stenosis, abnormal ossicles, petromastoid hypopneumatised, pyramid upward tilting	Large vestibule, dysplastic SCC	(+)	–
Otocervical	Klippel Feil and Wildervanck	+	+	+	Pinna malformations, EAC atresia or stenosis, abnormal ossicles	Mondini deformity, dysplastic SCC	(+)	–
	Pendred	–	+	–	–	Mondini deformity, modiolar deficiency, enlarged vestibule, LVA and sac	(+)	–

(continued)

Table 4.9 (continued)

Group of syndromes	Name of syndrome	Hearing loss			CM			
		CHL	SNHL	Mixed	Outer/middle ear	Inner ear	Facial nerve course	Not common on imaging
	Waardenburg	–	+	–	–	LVA, vestibule widening, decreased modiolus size, IAC hypoplasia, hypo–/aplasia of posterior SCC	(+)	–
Otoskeletal (bone dysplasias)	Osteogenesis imperfecta	+	+	+	Thin ossicles	Bone demineralisation within otic capsule	–	–
	Otodystrophies associated with sclerosis	–	–	+	(+)	Osteopetrosis with increased bone density	–	–
	Alport	–	+	–	–	–	–	+
	Jervell and Lange-Nielsen	–	+	–	–	–	–	+
	Norrie	–	+	–	–	–	–	+
	Stickler	–	+	–	–	–	–	+
	Usher	–	+	–	–	–	–	+

CM congenital malformation, *CHL* conductive hearing loss, *SNHL* sensorineural hearing loss, *BOR* branchio-oto-renal, *CHARGE* *c*oloboma, *h*eart, *a*tresia of the choanae, *r*etarded growth and development, *g*enital hypoplasia and *e*ar anomalies and/or deafness, *CND* cochlear nerve deficiency, *EAC* external auditory canal, *IAC* internal auditory canal, *LVA* *l*arge *v*estibular *a*queduct, *SCC* semicircular canal

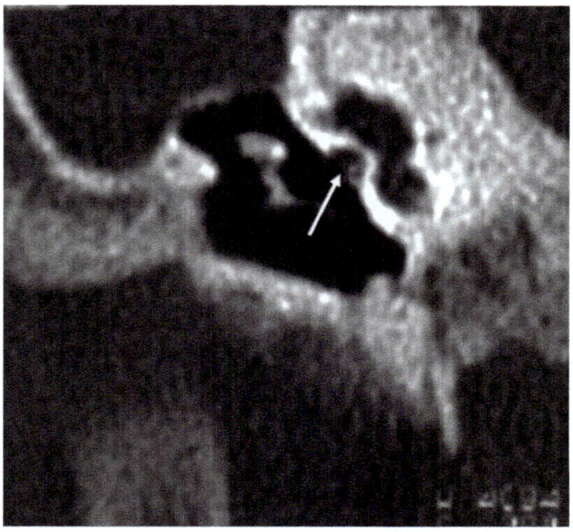

Fig. 4.40 Coronal CT of a 13-year-old boy with unilateral CHL of 40 dB. Known Klippel Feil syndrome. Moderate middle ear malformation and abnormal position of the facial nerve (arrow) in the oval window

with CM of the ear. CT or alternatively cone beam CT (CB-CT) is the method of choice in CM of the outer and middle ear. Conventional X-rays play no role in ear CM, and MRI delivers no diagnostic information. Diagnosis of CM requires optimal local resolution on CT. Primarily, this means low slice thickness (0.5–1 mm), use of a bone algorithm and a high zoom (small field of view). Radiation exposure can be lower than in tumour diagnostics, but cannot be as low as in low-dose CT of the paranasal sinuses because the increased image noise does not allow sufficient visualisation of small details, especially of the stapes. Nowadays a volume data set is acquired in only one plane from which images in any spatial orientation and of different character can be reconstructed.

CT and CB-CT have a high clarification rate in suspected CM of the outer and middle ear, including the detection of other causes of CHL. Only in a few cases can no cause be found. Even with modern techniques, it is difficult to diagnose isolated stapes fixation or visualise subtle detail of malformed ossicles. Nevertheless, CT or CB-CT is indicated in patients with suspected CM of the outer and middle ear and is absolutely necessary for presurgical planning.

The following structures and properties are analysed in detail:

Grade of temporal bone pneumatisation
Shape and width of EAC and tympanic cavity
Shape and localisation of ossicles, including interossicular joints
Presence and morphology of windows
Course of facial nerve and bony canal of internal carotid artery (ICA)
Tensor tympani muscle and Eustachian tube
Inner ear/internal auditory canal (IAC) (see sect. "Congenital Malformations of the Inner Ear")

High-grade CMs affect nearly all of these structures, while in low-and medium-grade CM, normal and malformed structures are coexistent.

The imaging correlates of malformed structures include:

EAC	Bony or fibrous atresia
Pneumatised cells	Reduced, absent
Tympanic cavity	Hypoplastic, split (then often opacified and filled with non-resorbed embryonic or fibrotic tissue), absent, extra-cavitation
Ossicles	Aplasia/hypoplasia of an ossicle or parts of it, dysplasia, conglomerations or clots, displacement, fixation of malleus or incus on the tympanic wall
Joints	Separation, fusion, fragility (incudostapedial joint may exist only as fibrous connection—This is not identifiable on CT)
Window	Narrowed, closed, absent

Additionally, the following variants (without functional deficit) can be demonstrated:

Facial nerve	Lateralisation/anterior displacement of the tympanic or mastoid segment, dehiscence of tympanic segment, duplications/rarely bifurcation of labyrinthine or mastoid segment, displacement in the oval window or through stapes crura
ICA	Aberrant, lateralisation in the middle ear with or without bony canal dehiscence
Bulbus v. jugularis	Elevation with or without diverticulum
Sigmoid sinus	Lateralisation, anterior displacement with or without diverticulum

Only variants of the facial nerve occur more often in patients with CM than in healthy individuals or patients with other diagnoses. Imaging has limitations in the detection of some subtle forms of stapes CM.

At some institutions presurgical rating is performed. The decision to operate depends primarily on the degree of middle ear development as reflected by the size of the tympanum and the status of the ossicles and of the windows. A commonly used CT-based scale (Table 4.10) has been developed by Siegert et al. (1996) and Siegert (2010).

Depending on the score and whether the malformation is bilateral or unilateral, these authors recommend surgical or conservative therapy (for more details see Sects. 18.4 and 18.5):

In bilateral malformations: Middle ear reconstruction of the better-hearing ear if the score is 15 or higher
In unilateral malformations: Middle ear reconstruction if the score is at least 20, following a frank discussion with the patient/parents
In patients with lower scores: Hearing aids only

Abnormal courses of arteries or of the facial nerve do not always preclude surgery, but they increase the risk of complications. Patients with a very atypical course of the facial nerve and those with severe middle ear malformations should not be considered for operative treatment. Thus, CT not only demonstrates suitability for surgery but also shows contraindications.

Table 4.10 CT score according to Siegert, Mayer and Weerda (Siegert 2010; Siegert et al. 1996; Weerda 2004)

Structures	Configuration	Points
EAC	Normal/fibrotic atresia/ bony atresia	2/1/0
Aeration of mastoid	Distinct/moderate/ absent	2/1/0
Size of tympanic cavity	Large/moderate/ eburnated	2/1/0
Aeration of tympanic cavity	Distinct/moderate/ absent	2/1/0
Facial nerve	Normal/slightly aberrant/strongly aberrant	4/2/0
Course of arteries and veins	Normal/slightly aberrant/strongly aberrant	2/1/0
Malleus and incus	Normal/dysplastic/ absent	2/1/0
Stapes	Normal/dysplastic/ absent	4/2/0
Oval window	Open/closed	4/0
Round window	Open/closed	4/0
Maximum score		28

With regard to further treatment strategies, the bony thickness of the calvaria can be measured and 3D reconstructions of the temporal bone made in patients scheduled for insertion of the well-established bone-anchored hearing aid (BAHA) or implantable hearing aids.

Congenital Malformations of the Inner Ear

Clinical Signs and Classification

Inner ear CMs cause hearing loss in ca. 20–30% of children with congenital SNHL. However, there is no clear correlation between severity of deformity seen on imaging and hearing loss. In some cases hearing loss develops after birth. This is particularly important in patients with large vestibular aqueduct syndrome (LVAS) or large endolymphatic duct and sac syndrome (LEDS). In these children, the onset of hearing loss may be delayed until adolescence or even longer (Bartel-Friedrich et al. 2008).

Aplasia, hypoplasia or dysplasia of the labyrinth and sensory patches in their entirety or in part has been described. Additionally, the vestibular aqueducts may be enlarged. The vestibuloacoustic ganglion cells are often reduced in number in inner ear CM. The IAC can also be affected by CM. Sennaroglu (2010) proposed a classification for cochleovestibular CM based on imaging and differentiated five main groups: malformations of the cochlea, of the vestibule, of the semicircular canals, of the IAC and of the vestibular or cochlear aqueduct. Cochlear CM (Table 4.11) has been divided into six categories of severity depending on the point of developmental arrest. In 2010, Sennaroglu (2010) updated their classification and provided more subgroups. For syndrome associations see Table 4.9.

The diagnosis of CM of the inner ear is based on clinical examination and imaging.

Clinical Examination

As also mentioned in Sect. 4.2.1.1, a newborn with hearing loss or deafness must undergo detailed physical examination of craniofacial structures for possible underlying syndromes. Additional CM should be excluded by an interdisciplinary team.

Table 4.11 Cochlear CM by time of developmental arrest according to Sennaroglu and Saatci (2002)

Cochlear malformations	Configuration
Michel deformity (arrest: Third week)	Complete absent of cochlear and vestibular structures, absent IAC, absent VA
Cochlear aplasia (arrest: Late third week)	Absent cochlea; normal, dilated or hypoplastic vestibule and SCC
Common cavity (arrest: Fourth week)	Cochlea and vestibule build a common space without internal architecture, IAC more enlarged than narrow, normal VA
Incomplete partition type I (cystic cochleovestibular malformation) (arrest: Fifth week)	Cystically enlarged cochlea without internal architecture, cystic dilated vestibule, enlarged IAC, normal VA
Cochlear hypoplasia (arrest: Sixth week)	Distinctly recognisable separation of cochlear and vestibular structures, small cochlea bud, absent or hypoplastic vestibule, narrow or normal IAC, normal VA
Incomplete partition type II (Mondini deformity) (arrest: Seventh week)	Cochlea with 1½ turns, cystically dilated middle and apical turn (cystic apex), nearly normal size of cochlea, slightly dilated vestibule, more enlarged IAC, enlarged VA

IAC internal auditory canal; *VA* vestibular aqueduct; *SCC* semicircular canal

Audiometry starts with the universal newborn hearing screening mostly by transient OAE (TOAE). Further investigations include tympanometry (impedance measurement), distortion product OAE (DPOAE) and early acoustically evoked potentials (auditory brainstem response, ABR). Older children are subjected to reflex and behavioural audiometric procedures, play techniques, pure-tone audiometry or speech reception threshold testing. The chosen test set depends on the age and development of the individual child. The objective measuring techniques (OAE and ABR in bone and air conduction) provide more reliable results. In the interests of accuracy, audiological testing should be repeated, particularly in young children and in patients with multiple malformations.

The testing of the labyrinthine vestibular organ has differential diagnostic value. The loss of the vestibular organ does not, however, exclude useful hearing.

Imaging

Nowadays MRI of the temporal bone should be preferred in suspected CM of the inner ear. CT or CB-CT may detect such CM in nearly the same proportion of cases, but MRI delivers more detail.

For morphological analysis of the labyrinthine structures in the IAC and cerebellopontine angle (CPA), thin-slice (<0.7 mm) 3D T2-weighted sequences are used. Native T1-weighted sequences have to be performed for the differentiation of pathologies with high T1 contrast (blood, fat). The contrast-enhanced T1-weighted sequence is most sensitive in the detection of inflammation or tumours as differential diagnoses. With the addition of diffusion-weighted imaging (DWI), the diagnosis of cholesteatomas/epidermoids is often possible. Temporal bone MRI is performed with thin slices and a high matrix. The investigation takes much longer than CT or CB-CT. In young children sedation or anaesthesia is necessary, which represents a major disadvantage.

For inner ear CM, the following structures are analysed:

Labyrinth	Fluid signal
Cochlea	Shape, number of turns, relation of scala vestibuli to scala tympani, modiolus
Vestibule	Shape
Semicircular canals (SCC)	Shape
Endolymphatic	Presence and width duct and sac
Internal auditory canal (IAC)	Width, presence of facial, cochlear, superior and inferior vestibular nerve

Vascular loops with contact to cranial nerves can be observed in the cerebellopontine angle (CPA) and IAC. These are mostly normal variants.

On CT or CB-CT, the modiolus and scala vestibuli/scala tympani are harder to recognise.

Cranial nerves in the IAC and CPA cannot be imaged. Rather than the endolymphatic duct itself, the canal through which it runs, the vestibular aqueduct, is visualised.

Compared with CM of the outer and middle ear, the clarification rate is lower in suspected inner ear CM. Only about 25% of cases have an imaging correlate. In other words, the imaging findings will be normal in the majority of patients.

The following changes are correlates of inner ear CM on MRI:

- Michel malformation: absent labyrinth and absent cochlear nerve.
- Mondini malformation: cochlea with normal basal but fused middle and apical turn, dilated vestibule and enlarged endolymphatic duct/sac (Fig. 4.41).
- Common cavity: fusion of cochlea and vestibule.
- LVAS = LEDS: large vestibular aqueduct (on CT: >1.5 mm)/large endolymphatic duct/sac (MRI) with or without other inner ear CM.
- X-linked deafness (final diagnosis by verification of defect gene): bulbous enlargement of IAC with defect of the bony margin to the cochlea, small cochlea without modiolus, enlarged labyrinthine facial nerve canal and enlarged canal of inferior vestibular nerve.
- Cochlear aplasia, hypoplasia of various grades (Giesemann et al. 2011) and incomplete partition (Sennaroglu 2010).
- Vestibule/SCC aplasia, hypoplasia, dilation, fusion of vestibule and SCC.
- IAC stenosis, hypoplasia or absence of nerves (Fig. 4.42).

In many, though not all, cases of inner ear CM and hearing loss appropriate for scheduling CI, hearing restoration can be successful (for further details see Sect. 18.6).

4.2.21.2 Paediatric Temporal Bone Tumours and Tumour-like Lesions

Tumours of the temporal bone are rare in childhood. Congenital temporal bone lesions include epidermoids (Fig. 4.43; congenital cholesteatoma: 2–4% of all cholesteatomas, white mass medial to an intact tympanic membrane with normal pars tensa and flaccida, ranging from intratympanic pearls to destruction of the temporal bone), lipomas and arachnoid cysts (Fig. 4.44). Mostly these lesions are incidental findings, rarely the cause of hearing loss. They can be demonstrated and diagnosed by imaging. Furthermore, paediatric brain tumours can involve the temporal bone and adjacent regions (cerebellopontine angle, brainstem, cerebellum, posterior cerebral fossa) and may be accompanied by SNHL (including central hearing loss) or CHL or both, depending on the location and spread of the tumour. Some examples are listed in Table 4.12.

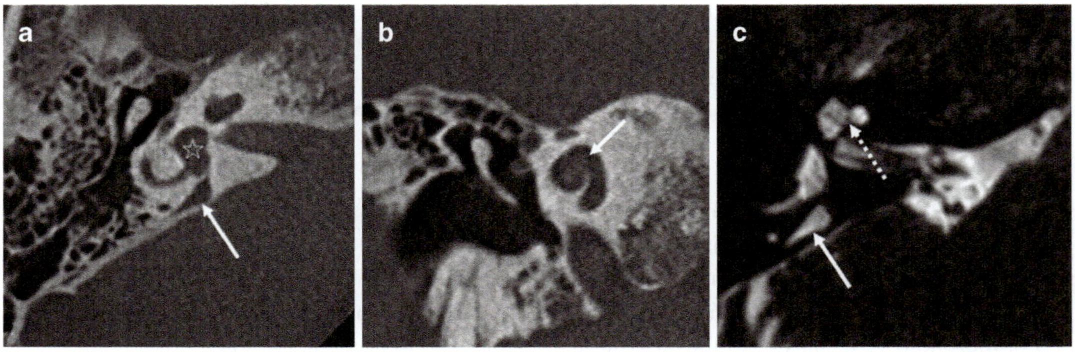

Fig. 4.41 CB-CT (**a** axial, **b** coronal) and axial T2-weighted MRI (**c**) of a 53-year-old woman, unilaterally nearly deaf. Mondini malformation: 1.5 cochlear turn (*arrow* in **b**), dilated vestibule (*star*), enlarged vestibular aqueduct (*arrow* in **a**) and endolymphatic duct (*arrow* in **c**). MRI additionally shows a hypoplastic modiolus (*dotted arrow* in **c**)

Fig. 4.42 T2-weighted MRI (**a** axial, **b**, **c** oblique sagittal reconstructions through the IAC) of a 5-year-old boy, nearly deaf on the right side. Absent cochlear nerve (*arrow*) and stenosis of right IAC

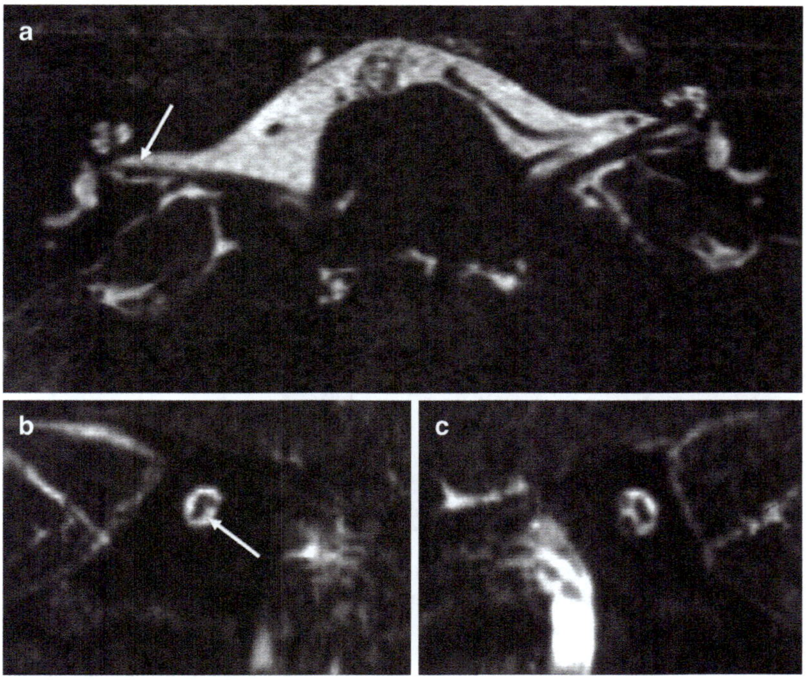

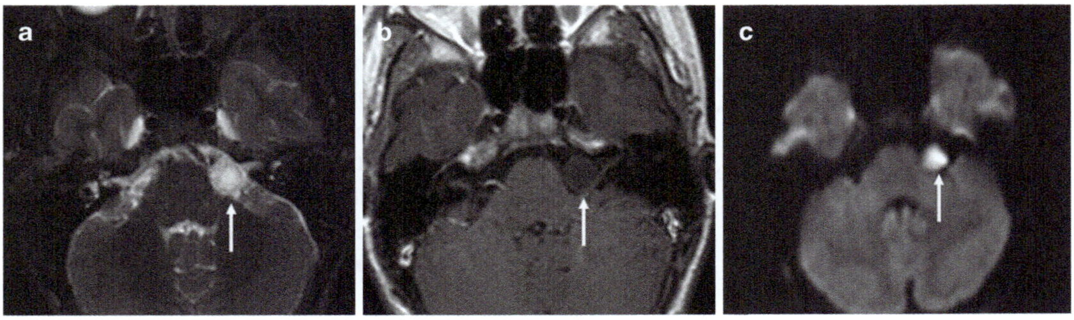

Fig. 4.43 Axial MRI (**a**) T2-weighted, (**b**) contrast-enhanced, (**c**) diffusion-weighted image showing an incidentally detected epidermoid in the left cerebellopontine angle (*arrows*) of right IAC

Examples of tumour-like lesions are cholesterol granuloma (rare in children, occurring anywhere from the middle ear to the petrous apex) and fibrous dysplasia.

Fibrous dysplasia is more frequent in the first two decades of life. It is a benign disease characterised by progressive replacement of normal bone elements with fibrous tissue, resulting in bone expansion. Temporal bone involvement, reported in ca. 20% of patients, can cause painless deformity and progressive CHL (occlusion of the Eustachian tube or of the EAC, or cholesteatoma formation secondary to obstruction) and sometimes SNHL (ca. 15% of patients, due to infection with ensuing cochlear destruction or to IAC stenosis and impingement of the eighth cranial nerve).

4.2.21.3 Imaging in Candidates for Cochlear Implantation

Before surgery can be planned, it has to be ascertained whether or not an electrode carrier can be implanted, whether complications are likely and whether electric signals will arrive at the central

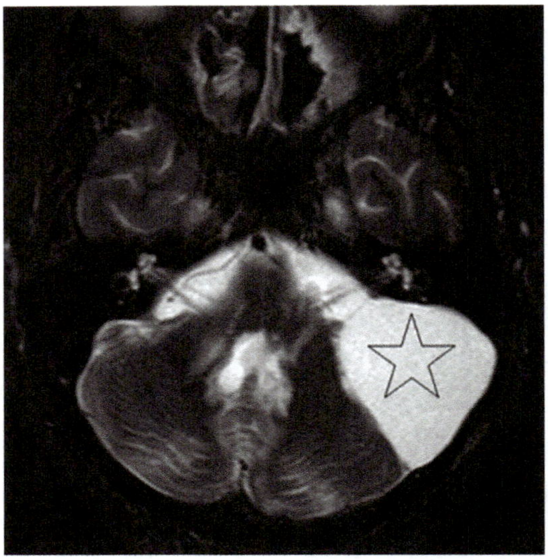

Fig. 4.44 Axial T2-weighted MRI showing an incidentally detected arachnoid cyst in the left cerebellopontine angle (*star*)

auditory cortex. To this end, imaging has to deliver the following information:

Configuration of the cochlea, detection/exclusion of fibrosis/ossification especially of the basal turn
Presence/absence of the cochlear nerve
Clarification of the individual anatomy including variants
Signs of gusher; inflammation

These points are best assessed by MRI and CT or CB-CT (Table 4.13).

According to Li et al. (2015), a stenosis of the internal auditory meatus or the cochlear nerve canal based on multi-slice spiral CT strongly hints at hypo-or aplasia of the cochlear nerve demanding an additional MRI. Differentiation between hypo-and aplasia is of prognostic value, as the degree of malformation correlates with the audiological outcome after cochlear implantation (Wu et al. 2015). Morlet et al. (2017) found in about half of cases with cochlear nerve deficiency vestibular anomalies and in about one-third cochlear abnormalities. The technical aspects and systematic reviewing are the same as described in Sect. 4.2.23.1.

Functional MRI (fMRI) has the potential to ascertain the integrity of the central auditory pathways, but is not yet widely used.

Some centres employ intraoperative imaging requiring special technical equipment (Aschendorff 2011), whereby surgically problematic cases can be monitored.

Immediately after operation the position of the electrode carrier is documented by imaging (Fig. 4.45). Different centres use different methods: X-rays in special projection, CT, CB-CT and digital subtraction angiography with 3D capability. Owing to its low radiation exposure and its insensitivity to metal artefacts, as well as its superior spatial resolution, CB-CT is most suitable for demonstrating the intra-cochlear localisation of the electrode carrier.

After the initial postoperative phase, CT or CB-CT may detect opacifications of the mastoidectomy cavity or ossifications of the labyrinth as signs of inflammation.

In the event that MRI is needed to clarify disease, the manufacturer must be consulted as to whether or not the individual CI can be investigated with the on-site MRI device. Devices with field strength greater than 1.5 T are currently not allowed. Recently, rotatable magnets within the CI were developed, which reduce the risk of dislocation, but continue to shadow the MRI image. Owing to the strong artefacts caused by the electrode carrier, the evaluation of the posterior fossa, including the temporal bone, is not possible after cochlear implantation.

4.2.22 Genetic Testing

Pavel Seeman, Simona Poisson-Markova, Eva Seemanova, Antoinette Am Zehnhoff-Dinnesen and Hanno J. Bolz

DFNB1, which is caused by mutations in the *GJB2* gene, is by far the most common type of hereditary hearing impairment. Mutations in *GJB2* are responsible for up to 50% of cases of early non-syndromic genetic hearing impairment with autosomal recessive (AR) inheritance (Snoeckx et al. 2005). Diagnostic *GJB2* testing is therefore offered in many laboratories worldwide. It should be the first test in patients with prelingual non-syndromic deafness. Certain *GJB2* mutations have different prevalences in

Table 4.12 Examples of paediatric central nervous system tumours assigned in part to the WHO histopathological categories

Tumours of neuroepithelial origin (56.4%[a])	Pilocytic astrocytoma (predominant in children 5–19 years of age) involving both the cerebellum and the brainstem; retrocochlear hearing loss can occur (Berg et al. 2005; Huang et al. 2012b; Mallur et al. 2008; Mirone et al. 2009)
Tumours of cranial and spinal nerves Tumours of the meninges	Meningiomas and nerve sheath tumours such as vestibular schwannoma within the temporal bone are rare in children. However, this entity diagnosed in a child, even if unilateral, should prompt confirmation or exclusion of a diagnosis of neurofibromatosis type 2 (NF-2). Hearing loss or tinnitus is described in ca. 20% of children, later diagnosed with this disease (Evans et al. 1999; Huang et al. 2012b; Neff and Welling 2005). In addition, NF-2 may be associated with multiple meningiomas and schwannomas of other cranial nerves
Lymphoma and haematopoietic neoplasms	Langerhans cell histiocytosis (also called histiocytosis X) can involve the temporal bone in ca. 20% of patients (De Foer et al. 2009; Fernández-Latorre et al. 2000; Robson et al. 1999). The disease results from clonal proliferation of Langerhans *cells*, abnormal cells deriving from *bone marrow*. Clinically, its manifestations range from isolated bone lesions to *multisystem disease*. In the multifocal unisystem subtype, fever, bone lesions and diffuse eruptions, usually on the scalp and in the ear canals, are characteristic. In cases with more extensive spread within the temporal bone, progressive otalgia, aural discharge, periauricular swellings and CHL can appear
Metastatic tumours	The most common metastatic neoplasms involving the temporal bone are leukaemia and neuroblastoma (Robson et al. 1999; Robson 2010). Depending on the site and size within the temporal bone, variable hearing loss can be present
Embryonal tumours (22.4%[a])	The 2006 Central Brain Tumor Registry of the United States (CBTRUS) reported that embryonal tumours, which encompass medulloblastomas, primitive neuroectodermal tumours and atypical teratoid/rhabdoid tumours (AT/RTs), are more prevalent among infants and children (0–4 years of age). Medulloblastoma is the second most frequent brain tumour in children after pilocytic astrocytoma and the most common malignant brain tumour in children (Gajjar et al. 2013). Originating from the cerebellar parenchyma and growing into the fourth ventricle and adjacent structures, medulloblastoma can lead to hearing loss combined with severe brain symptoms resulting from occlusion hydrocephalus
Mesenchymal tumours	Rhabdomyosarcoma (arising from immature mesenchymal cells that are committed to skeletal muscle lineage) is the most common primary malignancy of the temporal bone and is a highly aggressive lesion with a propensity for nervous system involvement and distant metastatic disease (De Foer et al. 2009; Robson et al. 1999). Clinical findings include a protruding tumour mass in the ear region, otorrhoea and bleeding from the outer ear canal, otalgia, hearing loss and facial weakness or palsy

[a]Frequencies according to Santi and Rushing (2013)

Table 4.13 Strengths of CT/CB-CT and MRI (Adapted from Huang et al. 2012a)

CT/CB-CT	MRI
Better for bone details (pneumatic cell system, location of jugular vein bulb, sigmoid sinus, internal carotid artery, ossicular chain, course of facial nerve in tympanic and mastoidal segment) Width of IAC Patency of bony cochlear nerve canal (if IAC is narrow) Fibrous versus osseous obstruction of cochlea Lower cost Less time Sparing with sedation or anaesthesia	Avoids radiation Superior soft tissue contrast High-resolution imaging of inner ear (fine details of cochlea) and brain Visualisation and fluid content of labyrinth Nerve courses in IAC and CPA

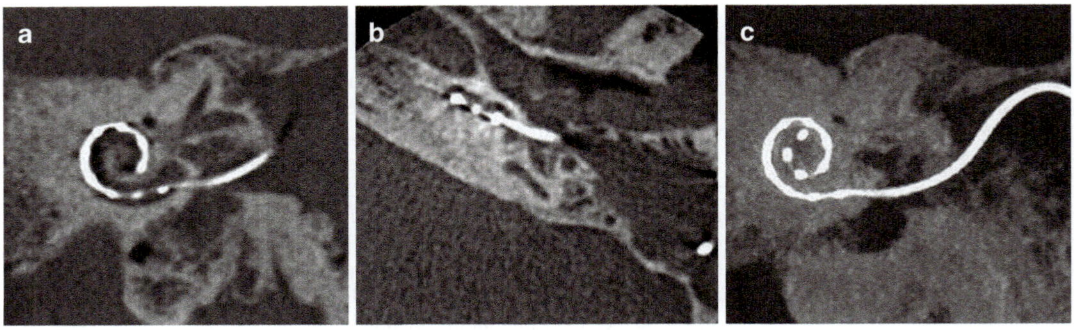

Fig. 4.45 CB-CT (an oblique coronal reconstruction, B axial, C maximum intensity projection) documenting correct position of an electrode carrier one day after implantation. At this time opacifications of the mastoidectomy cavity are normal postoperative changes

different populations. In Caucasian populations, initial diagnostic testing is therefore focused on the mutation c.35delG (Gasparini et al. 2000), in Asian populations on c.235delC (Yang et al. 2013), in Jewish populations on c.167delT (Morell et al. 1998; Sobe et al. 1999) and in Roma populations and in India on p.Trp24* (Minárik et al. 2003).

Attempts to correlate genotype and phenotype have shown a tendency of mutation c.35delG in *GJB2* to be more often related with severe to profound hearing loss (Beck et al. 2015).

Mutations in other known genes are less prevalent, and the probability of finding causal mutations in any other single gene in a patient previously excluded for DFNB1 is very low except of *STRC* gene (Marková et al. 2018). Testing mutations in the genes *STRC*, *SLC26A4*, *MYO15A* and *TMPRSS3* and in mitochondrial DNA is incidentally performed (Lechowicz et al. 2015), but recently developed genetic techniques, such as massively parallel sequencing (MPS), also called next-generation sequencing (NGS), allow testing of panels comprising all relevant genes (for non-syndromic deafness ~115) (Hereditary Hearing Loss 2019) in parallel for only a fraction of the cost of conventional sequencing. This new procedure improves the diagnostic yield for patients with already excluded mutations in the *GJB2* gene.

Even in cases with unilateral sensorineural hearing loss, genetic testing can be recommended according to the study of Gruber et al. (2016) showing *GJB2* mutations in 31.3% from affected children.

For further information, see Sect. 3.1 by Hanno J. Bolz.

Genetic testing has now begun to play a prominent role in diagnostics and genetic counselling, influencing the early management of disease and patients' subsequent quality of life. However, the importance of the physical examination when recommending genetic analyses should not be underestimated by clinicians.

4.2.23 Special Diagnostic Needs of Children with Multiple Handicaps: General Considerations

Mona Hegazi and Peter Matulat

4.2.23.1 Definition of Disability

The Convention on the Rights of Persons with Disabilities states to:

> provide those health services needed by persons with disabilities specifically because of their disabilities, including early identification and intervention as appropriate, and services designed to minimise and prevent further disabilities, including among children and older persons.—UN General Assembly (2007)

The primary nosological framework for the classification of diagnoses, disorders and health conditions is the International Classification of Diseases (ICD) (World Health Organization 1992). The International Classification of Functioning, Disability and Health (ICF)

(World Health Organization 2001) focuses on functioning and disability associated with health conditions. The children and youth version (ICF-CY) of the ICF was developed to take into account that:

> the manifestations of disability and health conditions in children and adolescents are different in nature, intensity and impact from those of adults.—World Health Organization (2007)

The ICF and ICF-CY provide a useful classification system with three levels: impairments, disabilities and handicaps. An impairment is primarily a problem of bodily function and structure (this part overlaps with the ICD). The term 'disabilities' includes impairments, activity limitations and participation restrictions. 'Handicap' refers to the result when an individual with an impairment or disability cannot fulfil a normal life role. 'Handicapped' is, however, not a medical term; it reflects the interaction between the individual's impairments and the social environment. The primary goal of these classifications is to allow the social participation of the handicapped child. Illum and Gradel (2015) found that a combination of the ICD and the ICF-CY could provide a helpful tool for the assessment of functioning in all children with different disabilities.

'Child with multi-handicaps' refers to a child who has more than one disabling health condition. The child typically has disabilities that are severe enough to require intensive support for handling the functions of daily living. In educational settings and according to the US Individuals with Disabilities Education Acts, the term 'multiple disabilities' refers to:

> concomitant (simultaneous) impairments (…), the combination of which causes such severe educational needs that they cannot be accommodated in special education programs solely for one of the impairments.—USC (2004)

4.2.23.2 Prevalence of Disabilities

A European Union-funded study found that 1.9% of families contain a child with a disability (Di Giulio et al. 2014). The lowest level was found in Lithuania (0.58%) and the highest in Poland (4.0%).

The prevalence of disabilities concomitant with hearing impairment can be estimated by two approaches:

- Recording how many people with hearing disorders show characteristics of other disabilities.
- Estimating the prevalence of hearing impairment among other disabilities.

Estimates of deaf or hard-of-hearing children with additional disabilities vary according to the approach used. Various reports and reviews (Holden-Pitt and Diaz 1998; Picard 2004; Gallaudet Research Institute 2013; Cupples et al. 2014; Wakil et al. 2014) have estimated that from up to 20 to 40% of deaf or hard-of-hearing children have accompanying disabilities.

The following disorders, which sometimes coexist in children with hearing impairments, can cause a wide range of different disabilities and handicaps:

- Intellectual disability.
- Disorders of psychological development:
  - Disorders of speech and language.
  - Disorders of scholastic skills.
  - Disorders of motor function.
  - Pervasive developmental disorders (e.g. autism spectrum disorders).
- Behavioural or emotional disorders:
  - Hyperkinetic disorders
  - Conduct disorders
  - Emotional disorders
  - Disorders of social functioning
  - Nonorganic enuresis/encopresis
- Visual disturbances and blindness
- Various syndromes and many other medical, physical or motor problems (e.g. CHARGE syndrome, *cytomegalovirus (CMV)* infection, meningitis, cerebral palsy, Goldenhar syndrome, Waardenburg syndrome, various trisomy disorders).

The more common disorders that coexist with hearing impairment are learning and intellectual disabilities (16%), developmental delay (6%), attention deficit disorders (5.4%) and impaired vision or blindness (5%) (Gallaudet Research Institute 2013).

In practice, doctors and therapists are also confronted with models of impairments, from other professions, that are not shared by mainstream medical theory. The theoretical model of sensory integration dysfunction, developed by occupational therapists to describe hyper-or hyposensitivity to stimuli, and applied kinesiology, often used by chiropractors, are two such examples.

According to Wiley et al. (2011), the proportion of additional disabilities experienced by people with hearing impairment is approximately similar across all degrees of hearing loss (mild, moderate, severe, etc.).

4.2.23.3 The Diagnostic Challenge

Additional disabilities are strong predictors of poorer auditory and speech-language outcomes (Cupples et al. 2014). The assessment of children with additional disabilities and different needs is challenging for doctors and therapists involved in medical and developmental diagnosis. The examiner must be aware of the child's individual needs and strengths, and the choice of diagnostic methods depends upon the communicative possibilities of the child. A person-centred multidisciplinary approach is recommended.

In practice, the assessment of hearing in children with hearing loss and additional impairments is challenging because of:

- The wide variety of individual limitations, competence and potential in different children with multiple handicaps (Marschark and Spencer 2003).
- The lack of clinical staff familiar with all communication styles that may be used.
- The lack of psychometric tests for hearing impairment appropriate for children with additional disabilities (Illinois Service Resource Center 2011).
- The presence of certain characteristics that influence the assessment. These include (Snell 2002):
  - Limited communication.
  - Difficulty in basic physical mobility.
  - Tendency to forget skills through disuse.
  - Trouble generalising skills from one situation to another.
  - Limited alertness.
- In general, the diagnostic procedure should answer the following questions:
  - What is the hearing condition and associated physical condition of the child?
  - Is the child able to perceive speech, vocalisations or environmental sounds?
  - Would the child benefit from hearing aids, amplification or noise reduction devices (such as an FM system) or cochlear implants?
  - What is the child's level of cognitive development?
  - In light of the above, what will the preferred mode of communication be?
  - Would this child benefit from talkers or other augmentative communication devices?

A full diagnostic profile for multi-handicapped children should include the assessment of the following areas (Center for Deaf and Hard of Hearing 2014):

- Audiological factors:
  - Age of onset and age of diagnosis.
  - Age at starting to use full-time amplification.
  - Auditory skills and use of residual hearing.
  - Effectiveness of hearing technology.
  - Aetiology of the hearing loss.
  - Type and degree of hearing loss.
- Behavioural factors:
  - Attitude and motivation level.
  - Psychosocial behaviour.
- Communication factors:
  - Augmentative communication devices; assistive technology.
  - Primary language.
  - Preferred mode of communication.
- Educational, social, developmental and medical factors:
  - Attendance consistency and stability.
  - Early education.
  - Family history including home language, cultural factors and hearing status of family members.

- Genetic history.
- Medical issues/concerns: risk factors.
- Visual status.

4.2.23.4 Evaluation of Cognitive, Social and Behavioural Functioning

In principle, an individual can be assessed with standard assessment batteries if he or she has normal auditory and visual modes of communication and can talk or respond adequately with at least one functional arm and hand (Johnson et al. 2001). If this is not possible, the use of developmental scales, which assess progress along a continuum rather than providing comparative performance data with peers, may be an appropriate alternative (Alvares and Sternberg 1994; Jones et al. 2007). With severe disabilities, it is important to conduct a functional skills assessment. This targets the skills needed in a given environment and activity and includes measures of social and adaptive functioning with a focus on basic life skills. It focuses on practical independent living skills. It also considers students' functioning in their environments and examines the process of learning and performance (Downing 2004).

Because speech and language therapists, clinical audiologists and teachers can provide important information regarding communication abilities, a multidisciplinary approach to psychological assessment is often best (Lutermann 2004).

In particular, visual or auditory disabilities combined with motor impairments or disabilities make accommodation and modification of the common testing conditions necessary. For these patients some hints for the adaptation of time/scheduling, test settings, administration/instructions, presentation format, response format and use of adaptive technology or computer-based testing can be found in the articles of Hill-Briggs et al. (2007) and Case (2005), which include:

- The adjustment of time limits and avoidance of speed tests.
- The substitution of tests that do not require motor responses.
- The management of test setting accommodation and accessibility.
- The use of adapted administration and responding, rather than self-administration.

Traxler (2000) points to the fact that deaf and hard-of-hearing children often have poor reading skills, which makes written instructions problematic and adaptations necessary. Children with a cochlear implant improve with respect to their readings skills (Vermeulen et al. 2007), but do not reach the level of normal-hearing children of the same age (Weisi et al. 2013).

However, one should always take into account that the adaptations above will often violate the assumptions of the test principle of 'standardisation' of the tests used.

Applied clinical and educational psychologists or neuropsychologists who work with children can use numerous psychological tests to evaluate intelligence (IQ), personality, adjustment, learning disabilities, memory difficulties, language skills, non-verbal skills, sensory and motor skills, executive functions and other neuropsychological skills.

Since not all tests are available in all languages, and country-specific norms are often lacking, recommendations of specific tests cannot be easily given.

To select a suitable test, the following questions should be answered:

- Can the test result produce information that helps answer one of the hypotheses concerning the child?
- Can the test items and the instructions be understood by the child in an appropriate style?
- Does the child have the communicative and motor skills required to respond to the test items?
- Are there national test norms for the age/sex/school grades of the child?

The starting point for a search could be special collections of psychological tests for deaf or hard-of-hearing children (Illinois Service Resource Center 2011) or test lists from members of the European Test Publisher Group (ETPG).

4.2.23.5 Visual Assessment

Visual impairment, as well as hearing impairment, has an impact on the child's cognitive, language, motor and social development.

The most common method of testing vision is to have the child verbally report what he or she sees. A satisfactory investigation is particularly challenging if the child has additional impairments. Visual function can be examined by functional and clinical vision assessments. Functional vision assessments focus on how children make use of their sight at school and play. In addition to careful observation of the child in their environment, electrophysiological techniques are used in order to assess the electrical activity of the visual pathway and occipital cortex of the brain. Children should also receive thorough eye examinations.

Two clinical visual acuity assessment techniques have gained wide acceptance for testing children with multiple handicaps (Mackie and McCulloch 1995), preferential looking (PL) and visual evoked potentials (VEPs):

- The preferential looking test (PL) is based on the fact that children prefer to fixate on patterned surfaces more than homogeneous ones and respond to visual stimuli by moving their eyes in the direction of the object of visual interest (Fantz 1965; Cohen and Cashon 2003).
- The visual evoked potential (VEP) is a bioelectrical signal generated in the visual cortex of the brain in response to visual stimulation.

4.2.23.6 Communicative Assessment

If a child with multiple disabilities communicates verbally, then standardised tests may be used for the evaluation of their communicative status (Guralnick 2000; Rowland 2005; Bagnato et al. 2007).

A functional communication assessment in preverbal children may consist of observing their behaviour in order to indicate different levels of particular communication skills that are suggested to be part of the language learning process (Johnson and Farroni 2007; Meltzoff and Brooks 2009; Van Hecke and Mundy 2007). The main steps are:

- Attending to and imitating faces and following a head turn:
  - Preferring to look at face-like stimuli.
  - Imitating basic facial expressions.
  - Following side-to-side head and eye movements.
- Dyadic interaction with persons and objects:
  - Looking at a caregiver during social interactions or at objects.
- Triadic interaction:
  - Sharing attention with an object with another person.
- Responding to joint attention:
  - Responding to caregiver's attempts to coordinate attention during play.
- Initiating joint attention:
  - Initiating interactions to coordinate attention with caregivers during play.

Augmentative and alternative communication (AAC) is used in children with severe speech-language impairments to compensate for spoken or written language (ISAAC—International Society for Augmentative and Alternative Communication 2016).

This includes:

- Facial expression and vocalisations.
- Gestures and sign languages.
- Communication books.
- Speech-generating devices (initiating or responding to communication by using hands, body parts, pointers, joysticks or switches and eye scanning devices).

The examination of the child's abilities and requirements for AAC should include their motor, visual, cognitive, language and communication strengths and weaknesses.

The evaluation should answer the following questions:

Receptive Language

- What types of communicative behaviour does this child understand (spoken words, manual signs, gestures, facial expressions, vocal intonation, picture symbols, object symbols, etc.)?

- What messages or communicative functions does this child appear to understand (directives, greetings, requests, etc.)?
- Is prompting and support needed for the child to respond to a communication?

Expressive Language

- How does the child make his or her needs and wishes known (body movements, gestures, facial expressions, vocalisations, words, sign language, picture symbols, object symbols, etc.)?
- Does the child's expressive behaviour appear to be intentional? Is it directed towards a goal? Does it appear that the child anticipates a response to the communication?
- How frequently does the child communicate?
- What specific messages or communicative functions does the child express (protests, requests, greetings, etc.)?
- Under what circumstances is the child most communicative (With whom? When? Where?)?
- Does the child need prompting or support to communicate clearly or consistently? What type of support?

4.2.24 Hearing Tests for Intellectually and Multiply Handicapped Children

Katrin Neumann

In paediatric audiology, the assessment of the hearing capacities of children with intellectual disabilities or multiple handicaps plays an important role and is particularly challenging. Intellectual disability has a prevalence of about 3% in Western countries. Persons with intellectual disability are at increased risk of hearing impairment. Permanent hearing impairment in persons with intellectual disability occurs in about one quarter of the cases (Hild et al. 2008; Neumann et al. 2008). This high prevalence is mainly related to genetic reasons, syndromes or chronic otitis media, such as in Down syndrome where hearing impairment has been reported in 28% (Van Schrojenstein Lantman-de Valk et al. 1994) to 73% of cases (Squires et al. 1986). Auditory synaptopathy/auditory neuropathy (AS/AN) also occurs. Earwax is another major problem, because its production and self-cleaning, as well as ear canal anatomy, often differ from that in non-disabled persons (Evenhuis 1995; Neumann et al. 2008). These hearing impairments often remain undetected or underestimated because of information deficits among the parents, persons in care and medical professionals and because the intellectually disabled themselves are often unable to recognise and indicate such problems, in particular children. About three-quarters of the bilateral hearing loss identified in persons with intellectual disabilities who underwent a hearing screening during the German National Special Olympic games (sports games for people with intellectual disabilities) were unknown at the time (Hild et al. 2008). Similar findings have been made regularly during national and international Special Olympics games (Hild et al. 2008; Neumann et al. 2006). A high prevalence of hearing loss and many of the described conditions hold true for a large part of multiply handicapped children, too.

Ear and hearing disorders in children with intellectual disabilities or multiple handicaps can be well rehabilitated if treated early and continuously. For instance, multiply handicapped children have been shown to benefit from cochlear implantation, despite the rehabilitation of perceptual and verbal expressive abilities progressing slower than for profoundly deaf children with no additional disabilities (Waltzman et al. 2000). After medical or surgical treatment of chronic otitis media, Shott et al. (2001) found normal hearing levels in 98% of children with Down syndrome and stated that aggressive, meticulous and compulsory diagnosis and treatment of chronic ear disease in these children provide significantly improved hearing levels. In particular, it is necessary to 'carry' children with chronic otitis media with effusion through their childhood until tube ventilation and middle ear conditions have stabilised. Most children need regular cleaning of their external ear canals and fitting or check-ups of their hearing aids or implants, examination for necessary ear surgery as well as speech and hearing rehabilitation, which in most cases takes more time than for typically developed children. These specific tasks belong to the profile of a paediatric audiologist: to ensure such regular examinations of the children and always to act from an integrated view with interdisciplinary case conferences and professional parent counselling, taking care that all necessary constituents of rehabilitation are in place.

If left untreated, hearing impairments of intellectually disabled or multiply handicapped children aggravate their social and communicative problems, in particular in the period of language development which is often delayed anyhow (Neumann et al. 2006). Additionally, central auditory and language processing problems that occur regularly in persons with intellectual disabilities or multiple handicaps have to be faced. It has been shown that central auditory difficulties at the brainstem level have to be expected in about three-quarters, and at the cortical level in nearly two thirds, of intellectually disabled adults, depending on the specific processing category (Neumann et al. 2008). Auditory discrimination thresholds for non-speech (frequency, tone duration and level) and speech stimuli (voiced/unvoiced consonants, place of articulation) are reported to be at the level of <4-to 6-year-old children (Neumann et al. 2014). Grammatical abilities for plural forming scored on average in the range of those of 4-year-old children (Neumann et al. 2014). Therefore, it is necessary to use a specifically adapted, simplified speech in the communication with persons with intellectual disabilities.

To face all these problems, both a newborn hearing screening and regular otological and audiological check-ups are necessary for intellectually and multiply handicapped children. In the Netherlands, for example, systematic hearing screenings and examinations for people with intellectual disability have been implemented (Evenhuis 1996). The International Association of Scientific Studies on Intellectual Disability (IASSID) has published an international consensus on the early identification of hearing and visual impairment in children and adults with intellectual disability (Evenhuis and Nagtzaam 1998). For the audiological assessment of hearing loss in children with intellectual disabilities or multiple handicaps, objective methods such as the measurement of otoacoustic emissions, stapedius reflexes and in particular AEP (auditory evoked potentials) are the methods of choice (Hoth et al. 2015). The estimation of the hearing threshold needs to be done with both wide-frequency and frequency-specific ABR (auditory brainstem response). During recent years, the improvement in ASSR (auditory steady-state response) and chirp-based AEP technologies, by an optimisation of the stimuli and signal statistics, has made them well-suited methods, also for frequency regions below 1 kHz, for diagnosing precisely the kind and degree of hearing loss and for fitting hearing instruments properly (Hoth et al. 2015).

In most cases ABR and ASSR recordings in intellectually and multiply disabled children have to be performed under general anaesthesia, taking into consideration all medical, physical and psychic conditions of the child and his family. A careful analysis of level-latency functions and level-amplitude functions of ABR enables the specification of the type of hearing loss, the extent of a sound conduction component and the presence of a recruitment in case of a sensorineural hearing loss. For the latter, the level-latency curve is steeper for lower sound levels and flows into the normative range for higher levels. For children with Down syndrome or craniofacial anomalies, a conductive or combined hearing loss is frequent, and it is often challenging to separate the single components of a hearing loss. A conductive component can be confirmed either by a bone-conduction ABR recording or by estimating the extent of a horizontal deviation of the wave JI latency from its normal range in an air-conduction ABR recording. It has to be considered that in case of paracentesis, which is performed frequently before an AEP measurement, remains of blood or secretion or inflammatory processes in the middle ear may lead to a non-permanent conductive component of a hearing loss.

A flatter than normal curve of the wave JV latency in the level-latency diagram may indicate a neural hearing disorder. Fig. 4.46 demonstrates an ABR finding of the right ear of a 2-year-old boy with a mitochondriopathy and a right-sided hearing loss with both a peripheral and a central

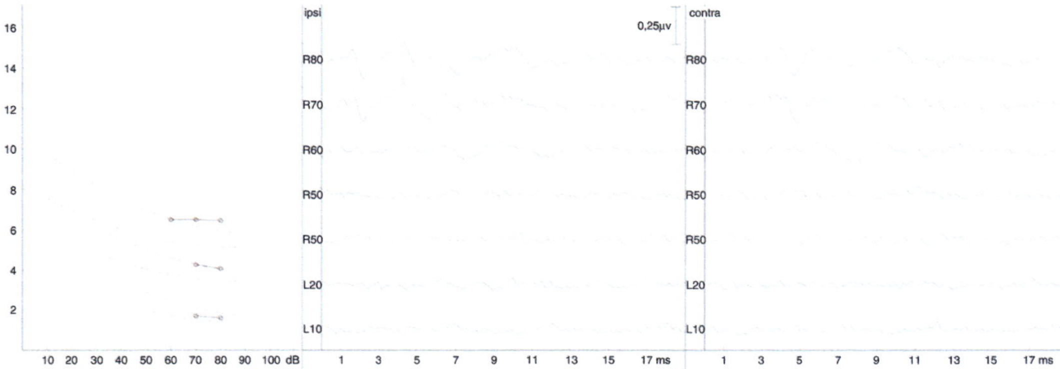

	JI	JII	JIII	JIV	JV	I-III	III-V	I-V	AI/V
R 80 A	1,60		4,05		6,45	2,45	2,40	4,85	
R 70 A	1,70		4,25		6,50	2,55	2,25	4,80	
R 60 A					6,50				
R 50 A									
R 50 A									
L 20 A									
L 10 A									

Fig. 4.46 ABR with click stimuli of the right ear indicating the peripheral and the central component of a right-sided hearing loss of a 2-year-old boy with a mitochondriopathy: stimulus-response threshold at 60 dB nHL with abnormal potential morphology, reduced amplitude of wave JV, immaturity-related elongated interpeak and absolute latencies and flat level-latency curves (Modified from Hoth et al. (2015)). Reprinted with permission from Springer Nature

component. In such cases the recording of middle and late-latency auditory evoked responses may indicate the central component and compensation of the hearing loss.

The safest method for the objective examination of the inner ear function is electrocochleography (ECochG), which demonstrates the sensorineural activity of pre-and postsynaptic processes during the transformation of acoustic stimuli in neural excitation. In intellectually disabled or multiply handicapped children, an ECochG is performed under general anaesthesia and mainly if there is a suspicion of a profound hearing loss or deafness or of an auditory synaptopathy/auditory neuropathy (AS/AN). The acoustic stimulation is performed via insertion phones and the recording by a needle electrode fixed on the promontory. The cochlear microphonics (CMs) and the summation potentials (SP) reflect the functioning of the outer and the inner hair cells and the compound action potentials (CAP) the functioning of the auditory nerve. For details see Hoth et al. (2015).

Pure-tone audiometry (PTA) has been shown to reveal reliable results for persons with intellectual disabilities, if performed properly. This includes suprathreshold training, short performance time and direct verbal or hand raising responses of the examined children if play audiometry is not understood satisfactorily. For younger or severely handicapped children, visual reinforcement audiometry or behavioural observational audiometry may reveal reliable results, too. Recently it has been shown that an adaptive self-assessment procedure such as the multiple-choice auditory graphic interactive check (MAGIC®) even assesses hearing thresholds with more sensitivity than a classical PTA (Neumann et al. n.d. in press). Results of speech audiometry are less reliable in most cases than those from PTA because it requires higher cognitive functions. Nevertheless, because it is needed for hearing aid or implant fitting and because a discrepancy between speech in quiet and in noise measurements indicates the neural or central component of the hearing difficulties, speech audiometry in quiet and noise shall be performed with tests adjusted to the cognitive capacities of a handicapped child.

Electrophysiological methods to assess central aspects of hearing difficulties of intellectually and multiply disabled children measure middle latency and late cortical evoked potentials. For example, the combination of normal PTA results, normal or near to normal ABR but disturbed perception of speech or music or environmental or animal sounds, a pathological reflex decay as well as degraded or lacking middle latency and late cortical evoked potentials indicates a central hearing loss (Hoth et al. 2015).

Procedures using speech or music or other complex stimuli have mainly been used for research purposes so far and may gain greater importance for the clinical routine assessment of auditory functions of children in the near future. Such methods include the measurement of cortical evoked responses in 32–64 up to 128 channels, event-related responses (ERP), ABR with complex sounds (cABR; Russo et al. 2010) and frequency-modulated auditory evoked responses (FMAER; Duffy et al. 2013), also called frequency following responses (FFR). These stimulation settings, which decode the quickly changing stream of segmented sounds such as speech or music, enable the hemisphere-specific analysis of the morphology and distribution of evoked potentials (brain mapping) on the cortical, subcortical and even brainstem level, or a dipole source analysis. They are particularly useful for neurologically motivated questions aimed at a precise localisation of a functional cerebral lesion or on the assessment of specific auditory processing capacities (Hall et al. 2011).

4.2.25 Management of Psychological Sequelae for Parents after Diagnosis

Peter Matulat and Mona Hegazi

> …and its [sic] not just a sentence, every word is important because you are hanging on to everything they say and you will remember every word that they say, it sticks in your mind. They need to really plan their sentences and their words because this is going to stay with you for the rest of your life.—Parent, Informing Families Focus Groups—Harnett (2007)

4.2.25.1 Parental Reactions and Coping

Parents of children who have been newly diagnosed with a hearing impairment usually have little or no experience with hard-of-hearing or deaf people. An appropriate emotional evaluation of an event depends greatly on previous experience, and most parents do not have a framework for making an appropriate evaluation. Perceived stress depends upon self-efficacy and the ability to master a situation by the individual's own competent action (Scholz et al. 2002). The initial emotions experienced after receiving a diagnosis of chronic illness—such as a hearing impairment—often include fear, shock, confusion, anger, frustration, depression, sadness, loneliness and blame (Kurtzer-White and Luterman 2003). In parents of newly diagnosed infants, these feelings may impede their natural interaction with the child (Horsch 2008; Spencer and Meadow-Orlans 1996; Koester and Lahti-Harper 2010).

The cognitive, emotional and behavioural strategies of parents' adaptation to the child's illness are called coping. Coping is process-orientated and has numerous interindividual variations. There are gender differences. Phase models are often used to describe the grieving process (Kricos 1993). Other authors focus more on the adaptation process (Ulrich and Bauer 2003).

Hintermair (2004) emphasised the importance of a sense of coherence (SOC)—in addition to experienced social support, the effects of the severity of the hearing loss and additional handicaps of the child—as a crucial personal resource in the coping process and as having a strong influence on the perceived quality of life. The Salutogenese model (Antonovsky and Sourani 1988) conceptualises the SOC as a combination of the subjective feelings of understandability, manageability and meaningfulness of the new situation.

4.2.25.2 Counselling and Intervention

Counselling and intervention are seen as the primary approach in helping to strengthen the resources of parents by promoting the ability for independent and self-determined action (empowerment). National principles and guidelines (Joint Committee on Infant Hearing 2013) and an international consensus statement (Moeller et al. 2013) on best practices for family-centred early intervention for children with hearing impairments have been created. Intervention programmes for parents and children have been developed (Holzinger et al. 2011; Reichmuth et al. 2013; Stredler-Brown and Abraham 2002). Early paedaudiologic care combined with family-centred educational intervention is predictive for a successful speech development of hearing-impaired children (Moeller 2000; Yanbay et al. 2014; Yoshinaga-Itano 2003; Meinzen-Derr et al. 2011; Fulcher et al. 2012).

Since a child with chronic illness will face new challenges in its childhood and adolescence (Compas et al. 2012; Laugen et al. 2016), the child's coping process must also be considered by doctors.

4.2.25.3 Informing Parents of the Diagnosis

The expectations of parents on the content and conditions of a medical diagnostic interview vary greatly between individuals. An evaluation of retrospective studies (Römer 2007) revealed that the following factors positively affect the experience for parents:

- The presence of a familiar person (e.g. a partner or close friend).
- Openness and directness of information sharing.
- Clarity of the information (including written information).
- Familiarity with the doctor.
- Awareness of support services.
- Opportunity to ask questions.

Very detailed descriptions of the necessary conditions for an appropriate setting can be found in the Irish national best practice guidelines for informing families of their child's disability (Harnett 2007). These hints are presented on the basis of the basic principles:

- Family-centred disclosure.
- Respect for child and family.
- Sensitive and empathetic communication.
- Appropriate and accurate information.
- Positive and realistic messages and hope.
- Team approach and planning.

These principles can certainly be applied to various diseases.

4.3 Basic Knowledge in Dentistry

Emmanuelle Noirrit-Esclassan, Maxime Rotenberg, and Ariane Hohoff

4.3.1 Introduction

Early diagnosis of skeletal, dental, occlusal, oral, facial and functional anomalies enables interceptive treatment to be started by the orthodontist, and coordination with possible orthophonic re-education; the latter is important, as speech pathologies and other functional disorders may have effects on orofacial morphology and vice versa.

Functional problems, skeletal discrepancies, malocclusions, agenesis of teeth, tooth anomalies and periodontal pathologies, which are frequently encountered in oro-facial-cranial syndromes with and without clefts, and also in non-syndromic orofacial clefts, need specific care. It is essential to give the patients and their families early warning of the importance of well-coordinated and precisely timed orthodontic, dental, periodontal, surgical, ENT, phoniatric, logopaedic and psychological treatment options, and the respective multidisciplinary therapeutic follow-up, in order to avoid further severe anatomical, functional, aesthetic, social and oral health-related quality of life consequences.

Oral health has considerable importance in a phoniatric assessment, and this is especially true for patients with oro-facial-cranial syndromes with and without orofacial clefting, and non-syndromic orofacial clefts, as all of them may present with velopharyngeal dysfunctions. According to Silva et al. (2018), daily performance of exercises related to phonetics provides the highest impact on oral health-related quality of life in non-syndromic cleft lip (CL) and cleft lip and palate (CLP) patients.

Results concerning a possible higher risk of dental decay in patients with clefts are contradictory (Howe et al. 2017; Worth et al. 2017; Abirami et al. 2022), but this special group has a higher risk of gingival inflammation (Veiga et al. 2017) and presents significantly higher rates of dental anomalies in the maxillary arch than unaffected controls in the deciduous, as well as in the permanent dentition (Howe et al. 2015).

More than 80% of patients with CL, CLP and cleft palate (CP) have malocclusions (Vettore and Sousa Campos 2011), compared with ≤48% of patients without (Ferro et al. 2016); thus, perfectly timed and well-coordinated orthodontic care in a multidisciplinary team is of special importance.

4.3.2 Dentofacial Dysmorphia in Orofacial Clefts

4.3.2.1 Objectives of Orthopaedic Treatment

- **At the skeletal level**

  Orofacial clefts are systematically associated with a growth anomaly, which has to be analysed in the three spatial dimensions. In *surgically treated* CLP, the maxilla is often transversally too small and sagittally too short owing to the scars in the soft tissues, which—over time—can restrict the growth of the bone, i.e. the 'functional matrix ... can have direct influence on the bone...' (Thilander 1995), a fact that was already described in the 'law of functional adaptation' by Roux (1881).

  In syndromic cases of the Occulo Auriculo Vertebral Spectrum (OAVS, e.g. Goldenhar syndrome (Vong and Funamura 2018), Treacher Collins syndrome, etc.), therapy is even more complex and combines orthopaedic treatment with orthognathic surgery (distraction, etc.) (Akram et al. 2015).

  - **In the transverse direction in Unilateral CLP** (UCLP), the muscular sleeves lead to an inward rotation of the small fragment (mostly leading to a unilateral crossbite) (Fig. 4.47).
  - **In Bilateral CLP** (BCLP), they lead to an inward rotation of both lateral fragments (mostly leading to a bilateral crossbite), while the premaxillary part is protruded. The aim of early correction is to obtain correct lateral occlusion, in order to prevent further—'crossbite caused'—maxillary growth restriction, and in the hope that the mandible will help to support maxillary growth and teeth will have enough space for eruption. Conservatively, true skeletal transversal widening of the median palatal suture (which, depending on the type of cleft, may or may not be present) can only occur when it is still open—it can already close at 15 years of age, but in some patients it might still be open until the age of 27 (Persson and Thilander 1977). After the midsagittal suture has closed, transversal expansion must either be surgically supported or the teeth must be tipped (see 'At the dental level, Occlusion') in order to compensate for a transversal malocclusion. The latter treatment, i.e. transversal dental tipping, is restricted to milder cases. After a correct transversal dimension in patients with palatal clefting has been reached, it should be retained life-long, as scar tissue could cause a relapse.
  - In the vertical direction, deep bite (Fig. 4.48) is mainly found in BCLP. Most

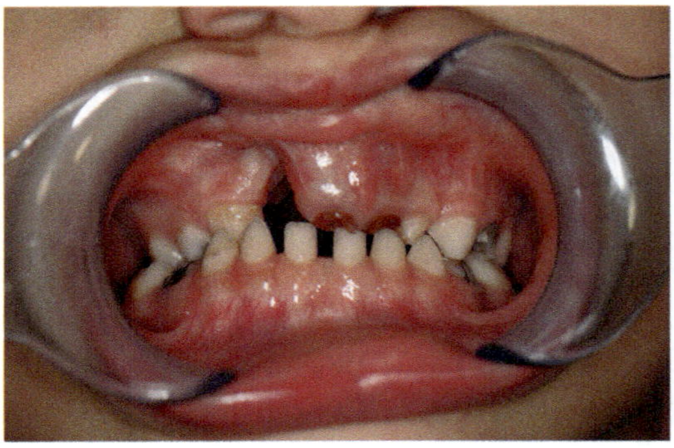

Fig. 4.47 Internal rotation of the small fragment in UCLP, lateral crossbite at the right side, agenesis of the right primary lateral incisor and severe tooth decay

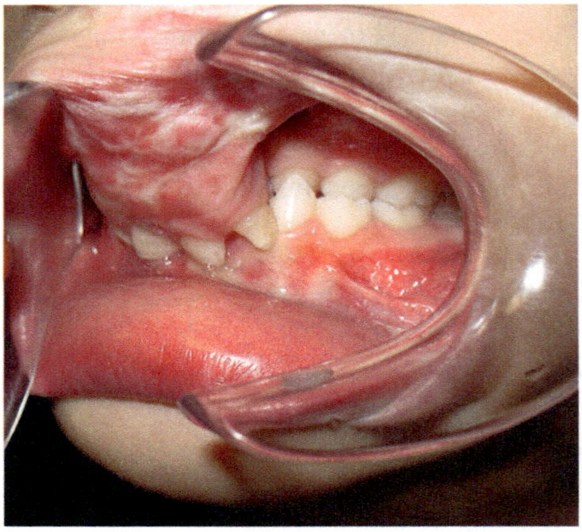

Fig. 4.48 Deep bite in BCLP

Table 4.14 Age at which teeth erupt, after Yeung and Chu (2014) (primary teeth) and the American Dental Association (permanent teeth) (2006)

Eruption	Primary teeth (mean age in months, rounded)	Permanent teeth (age in years)
Central incisors	7–11	6–8
Lateral incisors	10–15	7–9
Canines	18–21	9–12
First primary molar/ first premolar	15–18	10–12
Second temporary molar/second premolar	24–31	10–12
First permanent molar		6–7
Second permanent molar		11–13
Third permanent molar		17–21

of the time, this dysmorphia is primarily not corrected because it may be a good way to transmit the mandibular growth potential to the maxilla.

Correction of this specific problem in most instances starts when multi-braces are bonded to the teeth, usually after the second molars have erupted, i.e. at ages 11–13 (see Table 4.14).

 - **In the sagittal direction** anomaly of the sagittal axis may give rise to anterior crossbite (mandibular incisors anteriorly to maxillary incisors). What appears as mandibular prognathism is in fact maxillary retrognathism. If the patient is young enough, the orthodontist will stimulate sutural maxillary and midfacial growth with a combined intra-extra-oral device (protraction face mask) (Figs. 4.49a–c).

   Best results, i.e. more skeletal and less dentoalveolar corrections, are reached if this treatment has an early onset (5 years +). After the age of 9–10, prognosis for true skeletal correction worsens (Kim et al. 1999).

- **At the dental level**
  - **Occlusion** Dental occlusion is of major importance for oral functions. The desired occlusion can be imagined as a maxilla that covers the mandible just as a lid covers a box (Fig. 4.50).

    There is an approximately 2 mm vertical overlapping (so-called overbite) and 2 mm sagittal distance (so-called overjet) of the maxillary incisor edges on the mandibular incisor edges, a one tooth-to-two teeth occlusion in the sides, and the mesial cusp of the upper first molar occludes the mesio-and centro-buccal cusps of the lower first molar (Angle class I).

    Transversal skeletal widening of the median palatal suture (for conditions see 'At the skeletal level, in the transverse direction') or changing the bucco-lingual inclination of the teeth can sometimes compensate for a skeletal or dental transverse discrepancy (Schmid et al., 2022, 2023) (Figs. 4.51, 4.52a,b).

    If the distance between the teeth or jaws is too large, surgical intervention may be indicated, in which case the treatment course usually consists of orthodontic dento-alveolar decompensation (starting approximately at age 16.5); this will increase positional discrepancies in order to recover ideal occlusion after orthognathic surgery, which will be performed at age 18, i.e. approximately when growth has ceased. After surgery, orthodontic treatment will continue for a while in order to finish the occlusion.
  - **Superior labial support** In clefts, maxillary incisors are often positioned behind the mandibular incisors (anterior crossbite), because the lip scars exert considerable pressure ('push') on the teeth (surplus, palatal scars can exert considerable tension ('pull') on them). By giving these teeth a good position and the right labio-lingual inclination, correct occlusion, good labial support (which, among other factors, is essential for a physiological profile appearance), a harmonious smile and good conditions for speech/articulation might be obtained.
- **At the functional level.** Cheeks, lips, tongue and teeth are inseparably linked in their function. The orthodontist has to guide jaws, alveolar processes and teeth ('hardware') in order to create a frame favourable to good muscle function ('software'). Only if the hardware enables it, will functional re-education of the software by the orthophonist work, and vice versa, in the hope that both systems will stabilise each other.

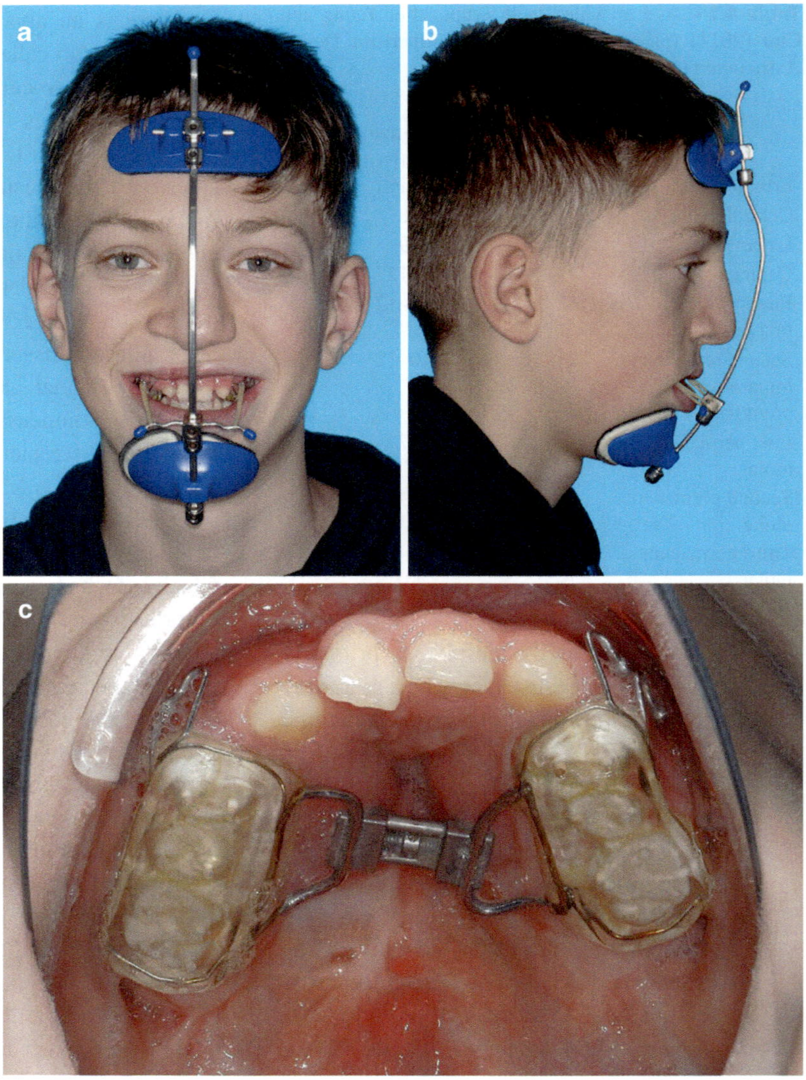

Figs. 4.49 (a–c) Depending on the area of transversal deficit, the screw for widening of the maxillary arch sometimes must be placed asymmetrically to the midline, as in this case. Figs. 4.49a–c with kind permission of the patient and his parents

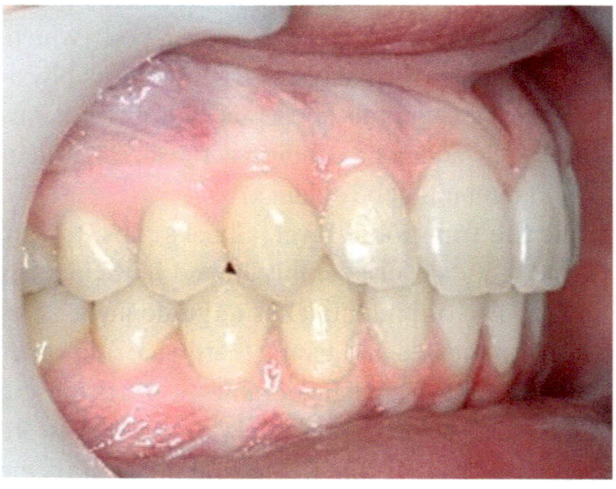

Fig. 4.50 Occlusion in angle class I

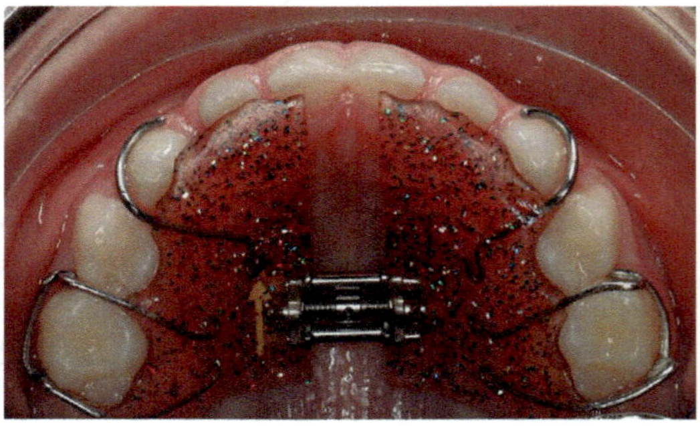

Fig. 4.51 Removable plate with expansion screw

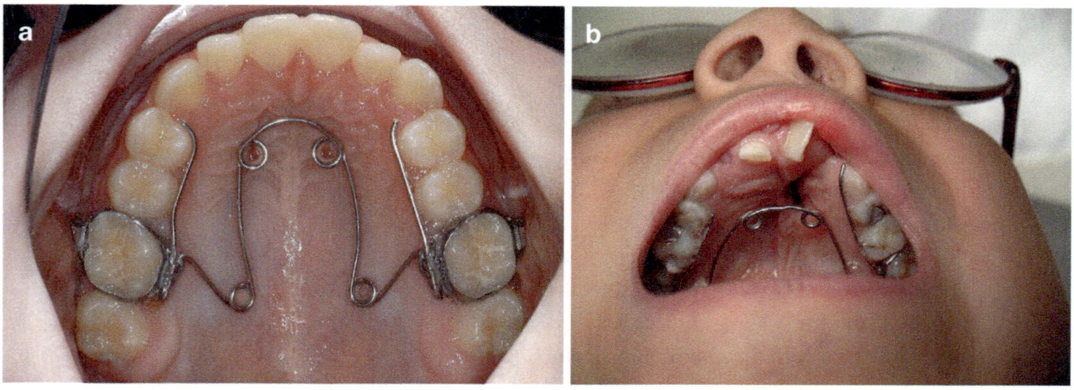

Figs. 4.52 (**a**) Expansion by quad helix . (**b**) The quad helix decompensates lateral crossbite

- **Creating space for the tongue:** Sufficient width, depth and length of the palate is essential for proper working of the tongue, and this can be conservatively obtained with the help of removable or fixed orthodontic appliances during the growth period, or surgically (often supported by orthodontics) after growth has ceased.
- **Controlling nasal ventilation:** By maxillary expansion, tongue position can be changed and nasal ventilation improved. Both reduce the risk of obstructive sleep apnoea syndrome (Iwasaki et al. 2013).

4.3.2.2 Therapy According to Age

- **In infants**

  Birth: (see Sect. 5.8) Infant orthopaedics with maxillary plates to guide the cleft segments has failed to prove its short-or long-term effectiveness in UCLP (Papadopoulos et al. 2012). In contrast, special palatal plates with a velopharyngeal extension have been proven to improve breathing significantly in various conditions (Robin sequence, craniosynostosis) (Müller-Hagedorn et al. 2017, 2018)

  - **In primary dentition**

    By around the third birthday, all primary teeth have erupted (Table 4.14). At approximately age 4–5, the child is usually cooperative enough to accept wearing an orthodontic appliance. Correction of the sagittal (Fig. 4.49) and transverse (Fig. 4.51) axis is the most urgent treatment issue and can be done with removable or fixed intra-extraoral appliances or their combinations.

  - **In mixed dentition**

    Fixed palatal expansion appliances such as the Quad Helix (Figs. 4.52) are anchored on the first permanent molars. The collateral effect of maxillary widening is an increase of the cleft width. This apparent worsening is usually necessary before the alveolar cleft osteoplasty, which, according to Theologie-Lygidakis et al. (2014):

    is usually performed at the age of 9–12 years, in the mixed dentition (so called secondary osteoplasty, in contrast to primary osteoplasty, which is performed in the primary dentition) when—from radiological observations—the root of the permanent upper cleft canine has gained approximately one half to two thirds of its final root length,

    might help to achieve a close-to-ideal alveolar morphology, to stabilise the maxillary arch, to eliminate an oronasal fistula, to create nasal and alar base support, as well as to reconstruct the hypoplastic pyriform aperture,

    might provide bony support for subsequent tooth eruption (mostly of the canine), might help to achieve orthodontic movement of teeth adjacent to the cleft side and for potential dental implant placement in cases of missing teeth,

    might help to improve speech, oral hygiene and periodontal health.

In cases of major growth deficiency, an extraoral force exerting anterior traction can be added (Fig. 4.49). This protraction face mask is worn at least 14 hours a day until correct overjet is achieved and can be combined with transversal widening of the maxilla or the dentition.

- **In permanent dentition**

  Once all permanent teeth (with the exception of the third molars and possibly retained teeth) have erupted, a multibracket technique can be used, after discussion with the maxillofacial surgeon. An interdisciplinary decision should be taken as to whether surgical orthognathic correction after growth has ceased is necessary (with decompensation and aligning of the teeth on their skeletal basis, implying a worsening of the occlusion until the date of surgery), or whether the result can be achieved by compensation movements of the dentition. Depending on the case, the treatment of dental agenesis can be done either by orthodontic space closure or by creating or preserving gaps for prosthodontic rehabilitation (Oosterkamp et al. 2010) or implants (Wermker et al. 2014). The latter should be placed only after growth has ceased.

4.3.3 Tooth Anomalies

The embryonic development of oral clefts and tooth buds is close in space, time and genes (Phan et al. 2016). Genetic and local developmental disturbances (interruption of the tooth bud by the cleft, inadequate blood supply etc.) can explain the more frequent anomalies of enamel structure, tooth number, size and eruption in these patients (Tannure et al. 2012). For diagnosis, the clinical examination has to be completed in most instances by panoramic X-rays—sometimes complemented with peri-apical radiographs—and in complex cases with cone beam computed tomography (CBCT) or computed tomography (CT).

4.3.3.1 Anomalies of Eruption

Neonatal teeth (Fig. 4.53) can be either prematurely erupted primary—most commonly—or supernumerary teeth (Rahul et al. 2018).

They occur more frequently in patients with UCLP and BCLP (Yilmaz et al. 2016) than in the general population (Wang et al. 2017). They can

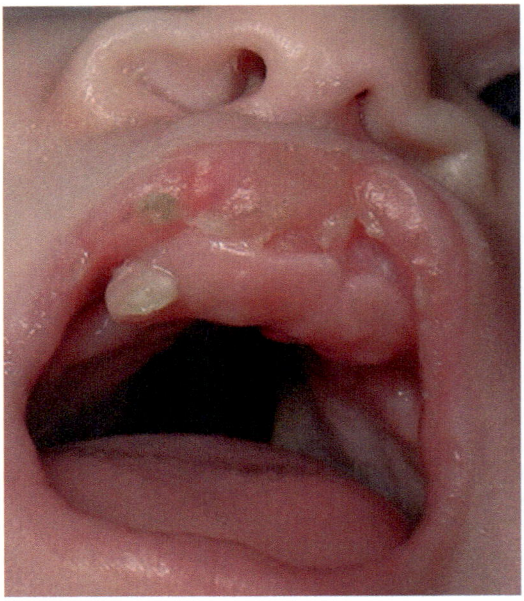

Fig. 4.53 Neonatal tooth in a bilateral cleft lip and palate

appear with hypoplastic enamel (Khandelwal et al. 2013) and incomplete roots (Malki et al. 2015). In the event they are mobile, they may be a risk for tongue ulceration and aspiration during breastfeeding (Rahul et al. 2018). In some instances, they can simply be extracted with a compress (N.B. in neonates, vitamin K substitution for this procedure might be necessary (Malki et al. 2015)). If there is an eruption delay of the teeth bordering the cleft, a differential diagnosis must be made with agenesis (Table 4.14).

4.3.3.2 Anomalies of Position

Ceft lip alveolus (CLA)/CLP is situated on the emergence zone of the lateral incisor. This tooth can erupt in an ectopic position (remote from its normal eruption site), e.g. on the edges of the cleft (Fig. 4.54a) or in the palate (Fig. 4.54b).

Teeth in the cleft area might also be crowded, rotated (Fig. 4.55) or impacted in the maxillary bone. Correction is usually achieved in the permanent dentition by orthodontic treatment with braces.

4.3.3.3 Anomalies of Number

Supernumerary teeth occur in about 20% of CLA or CLP (Fig. 4.56) in the primary (Suzuki et al. 2017) and permanent dentition (Tan et al. 2018; Sæle et al. 2017).

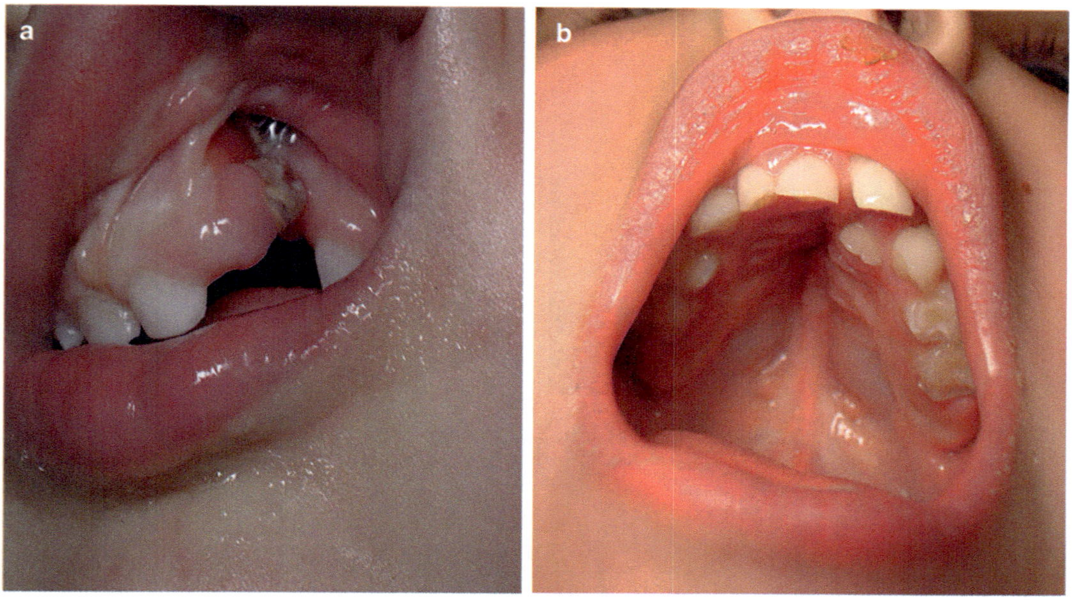

Fig. 4.54 (**a**) Eruption of a temporary lateral incisor with dysplastic enamel on the edge of the cleft. Secondary finding: the respective plaque accumulation. (**b**) Eruption of a deciduous lateral incisor in the palate

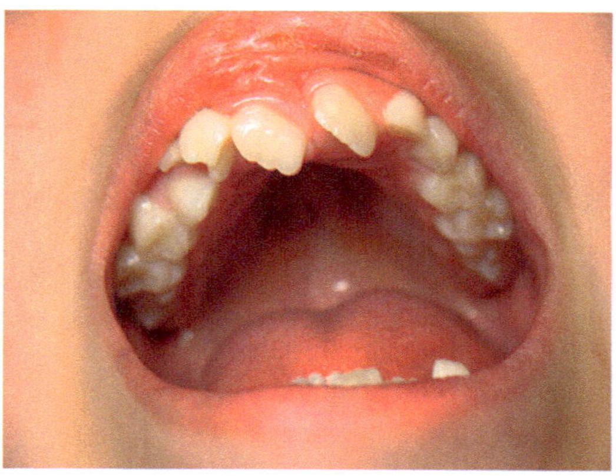

Fig. 4.55 Rotated permanent central incisors and lateral incisor with talon cup in a cleft lip

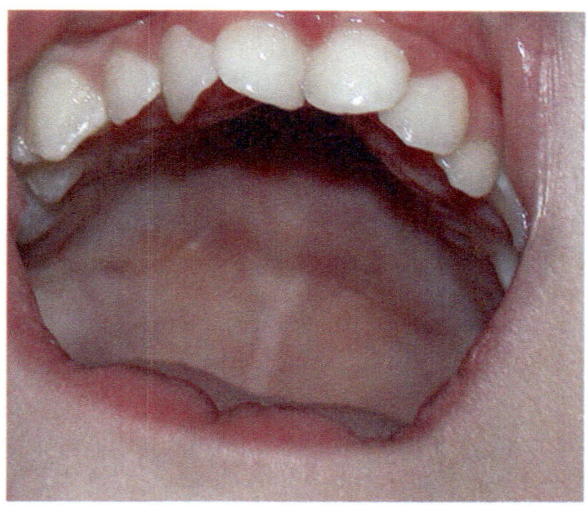

Fig. 4.56 Supernumerary lateral incisors in a bilateral cleft lip

They are mostly left in place in the primary dentition, but extracted from the permanent dentition. The maxillary lateral incisors are the most commonly missing teeth in the cleft area (Jamilian et al. 2016), with aesthetic, periodontal and restorative implications. The frequency of hypodontia increases with the severity of the cleft, and from the primary to the permanent dentition (Suzuki et al. 2017). Hypodontia may also be associated with syndromic clefts (e.g. Robin sequence, Van der Woude syndrome and EEC syndrome (ectrodactyly, ectodermal hypoplasia and clefting)). Maxillary growth is most severely deficient in patients with tooth agenesis and complete CLP (Antonarakis and Fisher 2015).

4.3.3.4 Shape Anomalies and Enamel Hypoplasia

Incisors may present a conoid shape associated with reduced size (microdontia), especially when

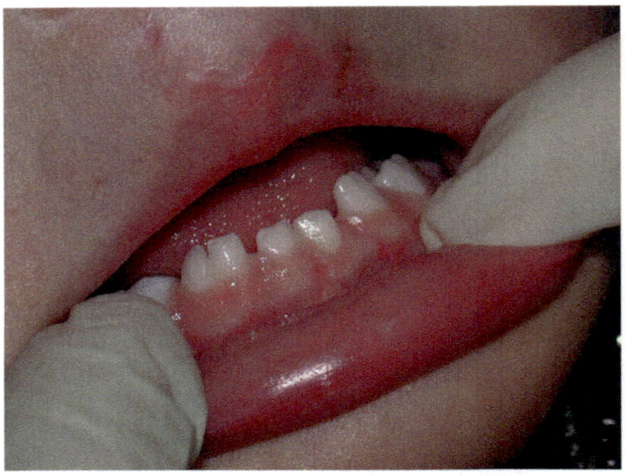

Fig. 4.57 Fusion of a lower lateral incisor with a canine

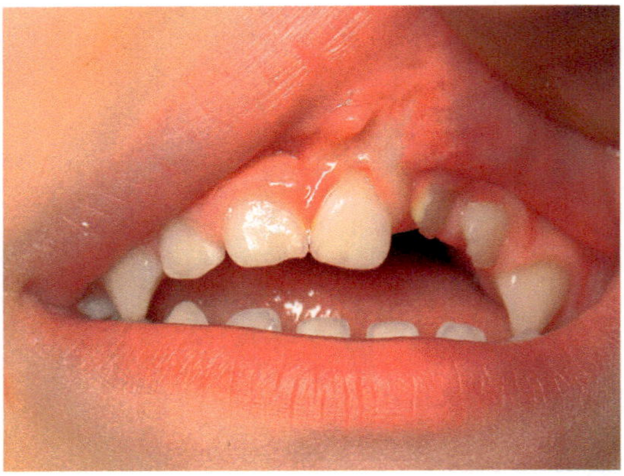

Fig. 4.59 Enamel hypoplasia of the mesial face (yellow patch) of the lateral incisor (near a supernumerary incisor)

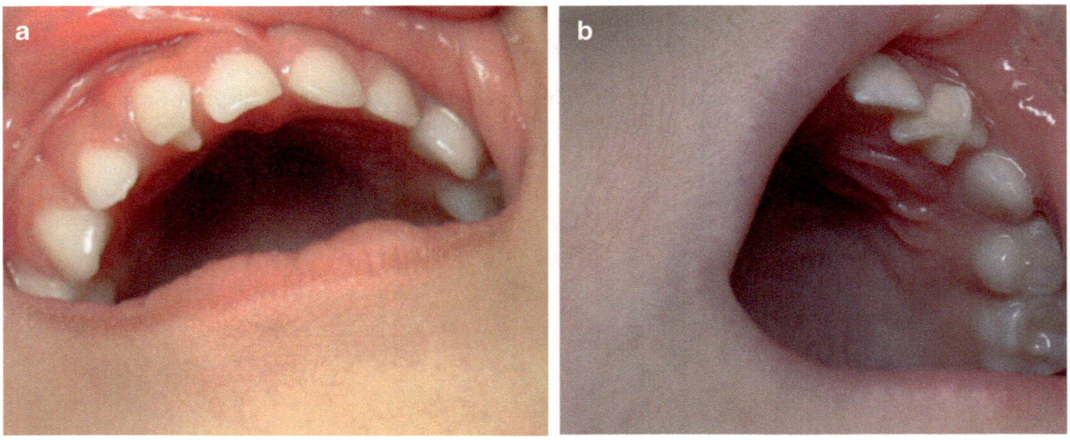

Figs. 4.58 (**a**) Supernumerary lateral incisor with talon cusp and (**b**) lateral incisor with talon cusp

there are two incisors, one on each of the cleft's edges. Some adjacent crowns may fuse (Fig. 4.57) (Fonseca-Souza et al. 2022).

Talon cusps in upper lateral incisors may also occur (Figs. 4.58a,b).

Enamel defects are more frequent in children with CL(P) in both the primary and permanent dentition, with anterior teeth most commonly affected (Sundell et al. 2016) (Fig. 4.59).

These defects increase the risk of development of dental cavities, which could have serious infectious consequences. Different restorative and aesthetic treatments can be proposed: in younger patients or less severe defects a bonded composite resin can be applied; in older patients with more severe defects, prosthetic rehabilitation can be performed (ceramic veneer, crowns…).

4.3.4 Caries Risk

According to a recent systematic review and meta-analysis (Worth et al. 2017), the prevalence of tooth decay might be higher in deciduous and permanent teeth of CLP patients, but the quality of the papers included in this publication was considered poor owing to incomplete descriptions of the participants. In contrast, a well-controlled study with a sufficient number of test subjects (Howe et al. 2017) did not show these differences for either dentition, but the authors speculate that this might be due to greater access to dental care preventing decay.

Preventive measures for tooth decay are to be found in Table 4.15 N. B. Different recommendations might exist between different countries and different professional societies; in the event of sys-

Table 4.15 Preventive measures for tooth decay

Birth till eruption of the first tooth	Eruption of the first tooth until <12 months		12 months ≤ 24 months	24 months ≤ 6 years	≥6 years
One tablet with fluoride and vitamin D daily	Tooth brushing up to 2 times daily		Tooth brushing 2 times daily	Tooth brushing 2–3 times daily	
	Either with or without toothpaste without fluoride and daily 1 tablet with fluoride and vitamin D	Or with toothpaste with fluoride[a] in the size of one grain of rice and daily 1 tablet with fluoride and vitamin D	With toothpaste with fluoride[a] in the size of one grain of rice Parents dose the toothpaste and brush their children's teeth	With toothpaste with fluoride[a] in the size of one pea Parents and day-care facility for children dose the toothpaste Child learns brushing, parents brush their children's teeth after the child has brushed	
Six dental visits for children up to 6 years[b]: 1st: 6th–9th month[b] 2nd: 10th–20th month[b] 3rd: 21st–33rd month[b] 3 further up to the age of 6[b]					One dental visit every 6 months[b]
					Hygiene aids (dental floss, interdental brushes) should be used in the interproximal spaces in addition[c] Fluoridated table salt should always be used in the home; by combining various preventive measures, it is possible to reduce caries considerably[c] In particular for patients with a high risk of caries, fluoride varnishes, gels or mouthwashes and participation in structured prevention programs should be recommended[c] For dental fissure sealing see below the table[d]

Table 4.15 (continued)

Birth till eruption of the first tooth	Eruption of the first tooth until <12 months	12 months ≤ 24 months	24 months ≤ 6 years	≥6 years
For measures in the event of radiotherapy see Harding (2017, 2018)				
Orthodontic control only in the event of clefts and syndromes[e]			Orthodontic control minimum once after all primary teeth have erupted[e]	Orthodontic control for all children and at adolescents at least once at the ages – 6–8[e] – 9–12[e] – 13–<18[e]

[a] Toothpaste with 1000 ppm fluoride
https://www.gesund-ins-leben.de/fileadmin/resources/files/PDFs/infografik_kariespravention.pdf
[b] https://www.bundesgesundheitsministerium.de/zahnvorsorgeuntersuchungen.html
[c] DGZMK (2016)
[d] https://register.awmf.org/assets/guidelines/083-002k_S3_Fissuren-Gruebchenversiegelung_2017-04-abgelaufen.pdf
[e] https://www.dgkfo-vorstand.de/fileadmin/redaktion/veroeffentlichungen/Stellungnahmen_Archiv/StellungZeitpunktKFOUnters.pdf

Indication for dental fissure sealing in permanent molars[d]:

- Fissures of patients with a higher caries risk (e.g. patients with caries in the primary dentition and patients who already have a cavitated permanent first molar)
- Caries-free but anatomically caries-susceptible fissure configurations
- Fissures with non-cavitated caries lesions
- Anatomically caries-susceptible fissure configurations in hypomineralized or hypoplastic teeth
- Fissures of patients with general diseases or bodily or mental special needs that can perform an effective daily oral hygiene only with restrictions
- Partly or totally lost fissure sealings should be renewed/repaired when the caries risk has not changed favourably

Indication for dental fissure sealing in deciduous molars or other permanent teeth than first molars can be considered in the event of an individual or tooth surface specific risk temic fluoride supply it is advisable not to swallow the tablets, but to suck them, as this builds up a fluoride depot in the gingiva, that is slowly released.

Additionally, parents should:

- Set a good example of oral hygiene and healthy food and drinks. Teeth must be in good condition and parents have to be careful not to transmit cariogenic bacteria to their children by testing food temperature with their childrens' spoon, as caries is a chronic bacterial disease.
- Focus on healthy, non-cariogenic food and drinks, and a tooth-friendly lifestyle for themselves and their children: neither should ever eat or drink (anything other than pure water) after brushing the teeth in the evening: secretion of saliva decreases during the night so it cannot play its protective role. With the exception of milk, which should be forbidden at bedtime, sweetened, caloric, acid drinks should be forbidden at any time.
- Prevent nibbling by their children: frequent food ingestion is much more cariogenic than the quantity of carbohydrates the food contains.
- Supervise tooth-brushing until their child is 10 years of age because first, the permanent teeth, which erupt around 6 years of age, have immature enamel sensitive to fluoride intake; second, tooth misalignment and the presence of scarring mucous flanges makes brushing much more difficult.

Practitioners must be aware that dental caries, especially in cardiac anomalies, may lead to endocarditis. The need for general anaesthesia for surgical procedures may present an opportunity for dental treatment to be carried out simultaneously, in young or uncooperative children.

In conclusion, a well-coordinated and precisely timed orthodontic, surgical, dental, periodontic, prosthodontic, ENT, phoniatric, speech therapist and psychological care is essential in patients with CL, CLA and CLP, to obtain the best skeletal, dental, occlusal, oral, functional, aesthetic, social and oral health-related quality of life results.

4.4 Basic Knowledge in Psychomotoric Development

4.4.1 Assessment of the Cognitive and General Developmental Status of Children

Christiane Kiese-Himmel

4.4.1.1 Introduction

Linguistic as well as cognitive abilities develop in mutual interdependence. Consequently, infants with delayed or disordered language development will achieve age-appropriate verbal intellectual functioning later than normal, and infants with delayed cognitive development, more specifically with cognitive deficits (e.g. limited capacity in phonological working memory, perceptual weaknesses), will learn language later.

There are also many genetic syndromes with behavioural phenotypes that affect language acquisition, given their association with learning disabilities or mental disability (significantly subaverage in intellectual functioning from IQ < 85), or a general developmental delay. Moreover, infants with foetal alcohol exposure often have impaired mental functioning and language learning problems. Children with other developmental disorders of speech and language associated with language-relevant comorbidities (synonym: nonspecific language impairment) often do not perform age-appropriately on measures of nonverbal intelligence. By definition, children with specific developmental disorders of speech and language (synonym: specific language impairment) display a significant discrepancy (two standard deviations or more below the average for their age) between receptive (or expressive) language abilities and age-level nonverbal intelligence and an average or higher psychometric intelligence. A valid and reliable assessment of a child's cognitive abilities and aptitude is the base for future clinical examinations and provides baseline data to monitor the effects of intervention.

4.4.1.2 Types of Diagnostic Assessment Approach

The *examiner* (usually a *qualified developmental* or *clinical psychologist*) has to be aware of the specific clinical question of the phoniatrician/pedaudiologist. This question determines the selection of the approach:

- Screening for developmental delay (before further assessment).
- Broad and in-depth assessment as well as the assessment tools such as:
- Clinical interview
- Parental report
- Behavioural checklist/questionnaire
- Observational assessment
- Normed and standardized test
- Test battery.

Normally, an intelligence test has to be administered to obtain an idea of a child's cognitive development status, which means his or her ability to solve problems by perception, verbal and nonverbal reasoning. There are many different types of test for measuring intelligence.

4.4.1.3 Pre-Assessment Information

A pre-, peri-or postnatal risk factor may limit (early) cognitive achievement of a child, and multiple risk factors may have cumulative effects on his or her development. Therefore, before testing a child, the examiner should obtain information on the history of the child (mainly history of maternal, pregnancy and perinatal conditions; (extremely) low birth weight; postnatal pathological conditions; physical developmental milestones; family history concerning hearing, language, academic difficulties; socio-economic status of the family) and results of physical examinations, additional existing diagnoses and medications, treatment histories or information from other professionals. Non-medical professionals (e.g. teachers) should only be contacted for information if parents/caregivers have given written permission.

4.4.1.4 General Principles for Psychometric Procedures in the Clinical Setting

An infant (till 1 year), a toddler (ages 1–3 years) or a preschooler (ages 3–5 years) has limited concentration, a short attention span, short interest levels and insufficient abilities to regulate its own behaviour compared with older children.

- The individual assessment should consequently take place in a neutral assessment context, be interesting for the child and be of a rather brief duration. It is recommended to take breaks or to perform several diagnostic sessions, if necessary.

Furthermore, the child's ability to interact and react adequately with an unknown person in an unfamiliar environment without the presence of a parent or another family member is relevant to the assessment situation.

- Since many children perform better in the presence of individuals to whom they have close relations, the examiner should provide or permit their presence (except in certain child-protection assessment situations in which a parent tends to interfere or to offer solutions to the child).
- The examiner should introduce himself or herself in the entry phase and describe the purpose of the meeting ('pre-diagnostic interaction').

The examiner has to bear in mind that tests have to be administered carefully in order to avoid diagnostic errors and to produce a reliable result that reflects the true level of cognitive functioning.

- The examiner must be informed about the methods of intellectual assessment and the theoretical underpinnings of the assessment tools, their characteristics, psychometric properties and limitations (e.g. handicaps accommodating assessment), be familiar with these and experienced with the tools. In general, the examiner should be experienced in working with children.

- Most importantly, aspects addressing the sensory integrity status and special needs such as motor disabilities of the child have to be taken into account. The latter are presumptions for a proper interpretation of the results in the context of all available information.
- Estimation of the general cognitive developmental stage should begin with demands or items that are within the child's capability. The examiner has to follow the instructions, examination and analysis procedures carefully, particularly the order in which the subtests have to be administered; to conduct the assessment tools accurately, in a fair and ethical manner; and to assure confidentiality. It is a breach of ethics for a psychologist to administer an intelligence test without the child's full understanding.
- Finally, the examiner should have the clinical skills required to interpret the assessment data appropriately, to synthesize them with all other available information into an overall picture and to communicate their relevance to other professionals (e.g. therapists) as well as family members in a sensitive way.

4.4.1.5 Aim of Psychometric Procedures

The main objective of psychometric procedures is the assessment of the general developmental status, more specifically the cognitive status (including the general intelligence level), in making classification and placement according to test scores, differential diagnosis or educational decisions and support needs. This is necessary to ascertain whether the child is at risk of cognitive developmental delay or exhibits:

- A major isolated development problem.
- A broad developmental delay up to a global retardation.
- Some cognitive weaknesses.
- A reduced verbal intelligence quotient (IQ).
- A learning disorder (IQ 70–84 according to ICD-10).
- A mental retardation (mild, IQ 50–69; moderate, IQ 35–49; severe, IQ 20–34; profound, IQ < 20).
- An intelligence score average or above normal ('high-ability' children).

The diagnosis involves testing and evaluation. Individual testing is much more reliable than testing in a group, but no single test can identify who is mentally handicapped. Multiple scores and several criteria must be combined in order to make this judgement—as for judging 'high-ability' children—given that genetic and contextual factors interact. In the light of brain plasticity during early childhood, cognitive disabilities may be modulated by environmental factors, such as the social or educational context, with consequences for the cortical development.

Amongst children with impaired cognitive functioning, other psychological problems often emerge. Subsequently, the child's pattern of strengths and weaknesses of cognitive competence has to be identified as a marker for his or her:

- Further developmental course.
- Therapy, training or another intervention success.
- Special education needs.
- Academic achievements and school performance.

4.4.1.6 Selected Examples of Assessment Tools

Infancy and childhood diagnostic assessments focus on special domains or on a broad range of development. The supposed cognitive developmental level at which the child functions and his or her history both influence his or her understanding of the tasks. Therefore, diagnostic instruments should be selected on the basis of the child's chronological age, medical and developmental history and their validity, reliability and user-friendliness (quick and easy to administer). Furthermore, the presence or absence of up-to-date standards or norms should be considered for the selection. Intelligence tests are the best available tools for revealing a child's cognitive functioning. The most popular assessment tools have been adopted from US, British or Dutch instruments.

Age Ranges

Infancy and Toddler Age

An infant or toddler with suspected language disability has to be assessed via a well-standardized, norm-referenced, valid and reliable *developmental scale*. It should be complemented by a description of the individual's functional difficulties and a *caregiver's evaluation of development and behaviour*, which has been shown to be as accurate as those administered by professionals in identifying children with developmental problems (Glascoe and Dworkin 1995).

Childhood

A child should first be assessed with a *nonverbal intelligence test* offering optimal psychometric properties in order to avoid problems in understanding and following instructions ('culture-fair assessment'). Most behavioural tests require a spoken response. Therefore, a verbal assessment may not be appropriate for children whose reduced speech intelligibility will invalidate the interpretation of responses. A language-free measure is also suitable for children with hearing loss, developmental disorder of speech and language, autism or test anxiety; for children from linguistically and culturally diverse backgrounds (e.g. migrant children); and for children who are difficult to test. Testing should be complemented by measures completed by parents (e.g. questionnaires).

Early Childhood Assessment Tools

Early childhood assessment tools are, for example, the single administered, norm-referenced *Bayley Scales of Infant and Toddler Development* (current version: *Bayley III*) from 1 to 42 months (Bayley 2006, 2014) or the *Griffiths Mental Development Scales Revised* from 2 to 8 years (Luiz et al. 2006). They measure, amongst other abilities, sensorimotor intelligence, receptive and expressive language and social-emotional behaviour, whereas intelligence tests focus more on cognitive abilities. That is, the skills evaluated by infant scales are not the same as those measured by psychometric intelligence tests. A useful adjunct to intelligence tests is measurement of cognitive processes underlying performance in intelligence tests, such as working memory capacity which is the base, amongst others, for an increase of other cerebral capacities, for example, the mental lexicon.

Example of Measures of Intelligence

Intelligence tests evaluate different components of mental functioning and assess cognitive development. A good example of *measures of intelligence* is the standardized and norm-referenced *Kaufman-Assessment Battery for Children* (*K-ABC*; Kaufman and Kaufman 1983) for children aged 2.5 through 12.5 years, which permits testing of hearing-or speech-language-impaired individuals or those with limited English proficiency. It comprises a multidimensional cognitive processing approach with items of little cultural content. A composite mental score results from the areas of 'sequential' versus 'simultaneous' information processing, investigated by several subtests. Furthermore, an achievement score and a nonverbal intelligence score can be calculated. In the meantime, a revision was published (*K-ABC-II*; Kaufman and Kaufman 2004) to make the test appropriate for a wider age (from 3 to 18 years) and for a wider range of abilities. The subtests are organized in three levels (ages 3; 4–6; 7–18 years). The *K-ABC-II* is—like the *K-ABC*—founded on Luria's neuropsychological model corresponding to learning abilities, sequential vs. simultaneous processing and planning ability and on the psychometric Cattell-Horn-Carroll approach of long-term and of short-term memory, visual processing, fluid reasoning and crystallized abilities (McGrew 2005). It yields a nonverbal composite and a mental processing fluid-crystallized index plus individual scale scores. Melchers and Melchers published the German version *K-ABC-II* (2015).

Latest Revisions of the Snijders-Oomen Nonverbal Intelligence Tests

Another example concerns the latest revisions (Tellegen and Laros 1993) of the popular *Snijders-Oomen Nonverbal Intelligence Tests: SON-R 2.5-7* comprising six subtests with separate total scores for the spatial performance and for the reasoning scale (Tellegen et al. 1998, 2009) and *SON-Revised 5.5-17* with seven subtests without a memory test, but with abstract reasoning and concrete reasoning tests, spatial tests and perceptual tests (Snijders et al. 1989). Both tests also provide a total intelligence score that indicates how an infant or a child performs in comparison with other children of the same age; and both tests are well suited for use with children of ethnic minorities (Tellegen and Laros 2005) as well as for mentally retarded, hearing-or speech-language-impaired and autistic children, because they do not need spoken language in administration. The *SON* tests are used in several countries, and test manuals are published in several languages. For example, a standardization of the SON-R 2.5-7 has been conducted in the Netherlands, Germany, the United Kingdom, Denmark, France, the Czech Republic, Portugal, Slovakia and Romania.

General Intelligence Functioning

The approach used in the family of the popular *Wechsler Intelligence Scale for Children* is based on the general intelligence functioning (highest 'g' loading), e.g. the *Wechsler Intelligence Scale for Children-IV* with an age range of 6 years to 16 years and 11 months (*WISC-IV*; Wechsler 2003), adapted for some European countries, e.g. Spain and the UK in 2004 and Germany in 2011. It comprises ten core subtests and five additional subtests that can be summed to provide four indices and one full scale IQ. Thus, it is a multi-trait/multi-method test. In the meantime, the fifth edition with 14 subtests has been published (*WISC-V Integrated*; Wechsler 2014); it is considered as a powerful upgrade for better understanding of a child's cognitive processes and for choosing of appropriate interventions.

The *Wechsler Preschool and Primary Scale of Intelligence* was originally developed by Wechsler in 1967 for preschoolers and young children (2 years 6 months to 7 years 7 months old). The test, now replaced by the *WPPSI-IV* (Wechsler 2012) with new processing speed subtests and reduced expressive language requirements, is available in many other European languages, e.g. Danish, Dutch, English (UK), Finnish, French, German, Icelandic, Italian, Lithuanian, Norwegian, Portuguese, Slovenian, Spanish and Swedish. Subtests exist for two age bands: 2 years 6 months to 3 years 11 months and 4 years 0 month to 7 years 7 months. For both, three levels of results are offered: full scale, primary index scale (verbal comprehension index; visual-spatial index; working memory index; fluid reasoning index; processing speed index) and ancillary index scale levels (vocabulary acquisition index; nonverbal index; general ability index; cognitive proficiency index).

Nonverbal Matrices

The nonverbal *Raven's Progressive Matrices* (measuring general intelligence) require the ability to recognize shapes/figures and their relationships, e.g. in childhood and for persons of limited intellectual ability. The brief intelligence measure *Coloured Progressive Matrices* (*CPM*), a 36-item test, has an age range from 5 to 11 years and the *Standard Progressive Matrices* (*SPM*) from 6 years to 16 years 0 month and from 17 years 0 month years of age upwards, a 60-item test used in measuring abstract reasoning and fluid intelligence. They are all unidimensional tests, but a useful nonverbal measure of overall cognitive functioning, and provide an overall intelligence score (Raven et al. 2004).

Alternative Testing Approaches

In addition, there are a number of alternative testing approaches and methods for estimating general cognitive developmental stage (e.g. neuropsychological-based assessment; learning tasks; informal play-based assessment) and more individually administered tests of intelligence that could not all be named and described in this brief overview.

4.4.1.7 Assessment Results

The assessment of both the child's cognitive processing abilities and of intelligence in an individually administered test indicates the intellectual level and profile as well as any delay or risk. This assessment information must be evaluated by the examiner in order to ensure that the results are valid and reliable and to determine a diagnosis (in combination with all clinical data) including both management and conclusions such as prognostic implications.

4.4.1.8 Forward Look

Frequently, re-evaluation ('follow-up') and consideration of environmental and biomedical variables are necessary:

- To identify whether a child has caught up his or her delay(s)
- To locate patterns of development (e.g. continuity; discontinuity; spurts; atypical)
- To monitor the further development processes in children at (high) risk (e.g. in case of preterm birth; very low-birth weight; persistent hearing impairment).

Nevertheless, high correlations between developmental infant assessment and the measurement of intelligence at later ages should not be expected, because intelligence is not a unitary construct. Comorbidity may be relevant for outcomes of cognitive development even when the nonverbal IQ is normal. Intelligence is also correlated with functional literacy and socio-economic status, and children who underachieve in educational systems may suffer a decline in their intelligence.

References

Abirami S, Panchanadikar NT, Muthu MS et al (2022) Dental caries experience among children and adolescents with cleft lip and/or palate: an umbrella review. Int J Clin Pediatr Dent 15(S-2):S261–S268

Akamatsu CT, Mayer C, Farrelly S (2005) An investigation of two-way text messaging use with deaf students at the secondary level. J Deaf Stud Deaf Educ 11(1):120–131

Akram A, McKnight MM, Bellardie H et al (2015) Craniofacial malformations and the orthodontist. Br Dent J 218(3):129–141

Alexiades G, Hoffmann RA (2008) Medical evaluation and medical management of hearing loss in children. In: Madell JR, Flexer C (eds) Pediatric audiology: diagnosis, technology, and management. Thieme, New York

Alfelasi M, Piron JP, Mathiolon C et al (2013) The transtympanic promontory stimulation test in patients with auditory deprivation: correlations with electrical dynamics of cochlear implant and speech perception. Eur Arch Otorrinolaringol 270(6):1809–1815

Allen SG (2008) Auditory perception test for the Hearing impaired-revised (APT/HI-R). Plural Publishing, San Diego, CA

Allen JB, Hall JL, Jeng PS (1990) Loudness growth in 1/2-octave bands (LGOB)—a procedure for the assessment of loudness. J Acoust Soc Am 88(2):745–753

Allum JHJ, Greisiger R, Straubhaar S et al (2000) Auditory perception and speech identification in children with cochlear implants tested with the EARS protocol. Br J Audiol 34(5):293–303

Altmann F (1955) Congenital aural atresia of the ear in men and animals. Ann Otol Rhinol Laryngol 64(3):824–858

Alvares R, Sternberg L (1994) Communication and language development. In: Sternberg L (ed) Individuals with profound disabilities. Pro-Ed, Austin, TX

American Academy of Audiology (2010) Guidelines for the diagnosis, treatment, and management of children and adults with central auditory processing disorder. http://audiology-web.s3.amazonaws.com/migrated/CAPD%20Guidelines%208-2010.pdf_539952af956c79.73897613.pdf. Accessed 29 Dec 2015

American College of Medical Genetics Expert Panel (2002) Genetic evaluation of congenital hearing loss. Genet Med 4(3):162–171

American Dental Association (2006) For the patient. Tooth eruption. The permanent teeth. J Am Dent Assoc 137(1):127. https://doi.org/10.14219/jada.archive.2006.0031

American Speech-Language-Hearing Association (1978) Guidelines for manual pure-tone threshold audiometry. ASHA 20(4):297–301

American Speech-Language-Hearing Association (1996) Central auditory processing: current status of research and implications for clinical practice. Am J Audiol 5(2):41–54

American Speech-Language-Hearing Association (2005a) (Central) Auditory processing disorders: the role of the audiologist. http://www.asha.org/policy/PS2005-00114.htm. Accessed 23 Sept 2013

American Speech-Language-Hearing Association (2005b) (Central) Auditory processing disorders (Technical Report). www.asha.org/policy. Accessed 12 July 2018

Amitay S, Ahissar M, Nelken I (2002) Auditory processing deficits in reading disabled adults. J Assoc Res

Otolaryngol 3(3):302–320. https://doi.org/10.1007/s101620010093
Antonarakis GS, Fisher DM (2015) Permanent tooth agenesis and maxillary hypoplasia in patients with unilateral cleft lip and palate. Plast Reconstr Surg 136(5):648e–656e
Antonovsky A, Sourani T (1988) Family sense of coherence and family adaptation. J Marriage Fam 50(1):79–92
Archer JC, Crosby-Quinatoa G (2009) Strategies for treating children with hearing impairment in the schools. http://www.asha.org/Events/convention/handouts/2009/1431_Archer_Jamy_Claire. Accessed 18 Mar 2017
Aschendorff A (2011) Imaging in cochlear implant patients. GMS Curr Top Otorhinolaryngol Head Neck Surg 10:Doc07
Aslin RN, Smith LB (1988) Perceptual development. Annu Rev Psychol 39:435–473
Australian Hearing (2013) CAPD service offered by Australian Hearing. http://www.hearing.com.au/capd-service-offered-australian-hearing/. Accessed 12 Mar 2015
Bagnato SJ, Wolfe PS, Rubina R (2007) How can we effectively assess for severe disabilities? In: Bagnato SJ (ed) Authentic assessment for early childhood intervention. Best practices. Guilford Press, New York, pp 178–204
Baguley D, McFerran D, Hall D (2013) Tinnitus. Lancet 9904:1600–1607
Barbi M, Binda S, Primache V et al (2000) Cytomegalovirus DNA detection in Guthrie cards: a powerful tool for diagnosing congenital infection. J Clin Virol 17(3):159–165
Barry JG, Moore DR (2014) Evaluation of Children's listening and processing skills (ECLiPS). MRC-T, London
Barry JG, Tomlin D, Moore DR et al (2015) Use of questionnaire-based measures in the assessment of listening difficulties in school-aged children. Ear Hear 36(6):e300–e313
Bartel-Friedrich S, Fuchs M, Amaya B et al (2008) Der erweiterte Ductus und Saccus endolymphaticus, Teil 2: Klinische Manifestationen. HNO 56(2):225–230
Baudonck N, Van Lierde K, D'haeseleer E et al (2015) Nasalance and nasality in children with cochlear implants and children with hearing aids. Int J Pediatr Otorhinolaryngol 79(4):541–545
Bayley N (2006) Bayley scales of infant and toddler development, 3rd edn (Bayley-III). Administration manual. Harcourt, San Antonio
Bayley N (2014) Bayley scales of infant and toddler development, 3rd edn (Bayley-III). Pearson Assessment, Frankfurt/Main (German version: Reuner G, Rosenkranz J (eds))
Beale TJ, Madani G (2008) Imaging of the deaf child. In: Graham JM, Scadding GK (eds) Bull PD Pediatric ENT. Springer, Heidelberg
Beck DL, Speidel DP, Petrak M (2007) Auditory steady-state response: a Beginner's guide. Hear Rev 14(12):34–37
Beck C, Pérez-Álvarez JC, Sigruener A et al (2015) Identification and genotype/phenotype correlation of mutations in a large German cohort with hearing loss. Eur Arch Otorrinolaringol 272(10):2765–2776
Benton C, Brough JE, Dodd MC (2004) Analysis of the middle ear. In: McCormick B (ed) Paediatric audiology 0–5 years, 3rd edn. Whurr Publishers, London
Beresford B, Greco V, Clarke S et al (2008) An evaluation of specialist mental health services for deaf children and young people. Social Policy Research Unit University of York, New York
Berg AL, Olson TJ, Feldstein NA (2005) Cerebellar pilocytic astrocytoma with auditory presentation: case study. J Child Neurol 20(11):914–915
Bergeson TR, Chin SB (2008) Prosodic utterance production. Indiana University School of Medicine, Manuscript
Berk LE (2000) Child development, 5th edn. Allyn and Bacon, Boston
Bischoff C, Klingelhöfer J, Conrad B (1989) Decay and recovery of the stapedial reflex by prolonged stimulation in the diagnosis of myasthenia gravis. J Neurol 236(6):343–348
Boehm AE (1971) Boehm test of basic concepts manual. Psychological Corporation, New York
Boons T, De Raeve L, Langereis M et al (2013) Expressive vocabulary, morphology, syntax and narrative skills in profoundly deaf children after early cochlear implantation. Res Dev Disabil 34(6):2008–2022
Boothroyd A, Cawkwell S (1970) Vibrotactile thresholds in pure tone audiometry. Acta Otolaryngol 69(6):381–387
Boppana SB, Ross SA, Shimamura M et al (2011) For the National Institute on Deafness and Other Communication Disorders CHIMES study. Saliva polymerase-chain-reaction. Assay for cytomegalovirus screening in newborns. N Engl J Med 364(22):2111–2118
Bradley L, Bryant PE (1983) Categorizing sounds and learning to read: a causal connection. Nature 301(5899):419–421
Brand T, Hohmann V (2002) An adaptive procedure for categorical loudness scaling. J Acoust Soc Am 112(4):1597–1604
Brannigan G, Decker S (2003) Bender visual-motor gestalt test, 2nd edn. (Bender-Gestalt II). http://www.wpspublish.com/store/p/2678/bender-visual-motor-gestalt-test-second-edition-bender-gestalt-ii. Accessed 27 Feb 2017
British Association of Paediatricians in Audiology (BAPA), British Association of Audiological Physicians (BAAP) (2008) Guidelines for the aetiological investigation of infants with congenital hearing loss identified through newborn hearing screening. http://www.baap.org.uk/Resources/Documents,GuidelinesClinicalStandards.aspx. Accessed Jan 2012
British Society of Audiology (2011a) Recommended procedure: pure-tone air-conduction and bone-conduction threshold audiometry with and without masking. British Society of Audiology, Berkshire

British Society of Audiology (2011b) Recommended procedure. Determination of uncomfortable loudness levels. British Society of Audiology, Berkshire

British Society of Audiology (2013) Recommended procedure: tympanometry. http://www.thebsa.org.uk/wp-content/uploads/2014/04/BSA_RP_Tymp_Final_21Aug13_Final.pdf. Accessed 5 Jan 2017

British Society of Audiology (2014) Tinnitus in children and teenagers. http://www.thebsa.org.uk/wp-content/uploads/2014/06/Paed-Tin-Guide-Pub-Consul-Compressed.pdf. Accessed 23 Feb 2017

British Society of Audiology APD SIG (2011a) Position statement: Auditory Processing Disorder (APD). www.thebsa.org.uk/images/stories/docs/BSA_APD_PositionPaper_31March11_FINAL.pdf. Accessed 28 June 2018

British Society of Audiology APD SIG (2011b) Practical guidance: an overview of current management of auditory processing disorder. www.thebsa.org.uk/images/stories/docs/BSA_APD_Management_1Aug11_FINAL_a_mended17Oct11.pdf. Accessed 28 June 2018

British Society of Audiology APD SIG (2018) Position Statement and Practice Guidance Auditory Processing Disorder (APD). http://www.thebsa.org.uk/wp-content/uploads/2018/02/Position-Statement-and-Practice-Guidance-APD-2018-1.pdf. Accessed 28 June 2018

Brown CJ (2003) Clinical uses of electrically evoked auditory nerve and brainstem responses. Curr Opin Otolaryngol Head Neck Surg 11(5):383–387

Brown VL, Hammill DD, Wiederholt JL (1995) Test of reading comprehension (TORC-3). ProEd Publishing, Austin, TX

Brunner M, Seibert A, Dierks A et al (1998) Heidelberger Lautdifferenzierungstest (HLAD). Westra Elektroakustik, Wertingen

Burns E, Arehart K, Campbell S (1992) Prevalence of spontaneous otoacoustic emissions in neonates. J Acoust Soc Am 91(3):1571–1575

Cacace AT, McFarland DJ (2013) Factors influencing tests of auditory processing: a perspective on current issues and relevant concerns. J Am Acad Audiol 24(7):572–589. https://doi.org/10.3766/jaaa.24.7.6

Campbell NG, Bamiou DE, Sirimanna T (2012) Current progress in auditory processing disorder. ENT Audiol News 21(2):86–90

Campbell NG, Grant P, Rosen S, Moore DR (2019) Auditory processing disorder in children. BATOD Foundation, London. http://www.meshguides.org/guides/node/1432

Campisi P, Low AJ, Papsin BC (2006) Multidimensional voice program analysis in profoundly deaf children: quantifying frequency and amplitude control. Percept Mot Skills 103(1):40–50

Canadian Interorganizational Steering Group for Speech-Language Pathology and Audiology (2012) Canadian guidelines on auditory processing disorder in children and adults: assessment and intervention. www.sac.oac.ca/sites/default/files/resources/Canadian-Guidelines-on-Auditory-Processing-Disorder-in-Children-and-Adults-English-2012.pdf. Accessed 28 June 2018

Carhart R, Jerger JJ (1959) Preferred method for clinical determination of pure-tone thresholds. J Speech Hear Disord 24:330–345

Carney AE (1996) Audition and the development of oral communication competency. In: Bess FH et al (eds) Amplification for children with auditory deficits. Bill Wilkerson Center, Nashville, pp 29–54

Carrow-Woolfolk E (1985) TACL-R: test for auditory comprehension of language, part 1. DLM Teaching Resources, Allen, TX

Carrow-Woolfolk E (1999) Comprehensive assessment of spoken language. American Guidance Service, Circle Pines, MN

Case JC (2005) Accommodations to improve instruction and assessment of students who are deaf or hard of hearing. Policy Report. Pearson Education, London

Casselbrant M, Mandel E, Sparto P et al (2010) Longitudinal posturography and rotational testing in children three to nine years of age: normative data. Otolaryngol Head Neck Surg 142(5):708–714

Center for Deaf and Hard of Hearing (2014) Guidelines for the assessment and educational evaluation of deaf and hard of hearing children in Indiana. http://www.state.in.us/isdh/files/Assessment_Guideline__finalized_January_2015.pdf. Accessed 13 Sept 2016

Chermak GD, Hall JW III, Musiek FE (1999) Differential diagnosis and management of central auditory processing disorder and attention deficit hyperactivity disorder. J Am Acad Audiol 10(6):289–303

Chermak GD, Tucker E, Seikel JA (2002) Behavioral characteristics of auditory processing disorder and attention-deficit hyperactivity disorder: predominantly inattentive type. J Am Acad Audiol 13(6):332–338

Chin SB, Bergeson TR, Phan J (2012) Speech intelligibility and prosody production in children with cochlear implants. J Commun Disord 45(5):355–366

Chou YF, Chen PR, Yu SH et al (2012) Using multi-stimulus auditory steady state response to predict hearing thresholds in high-risk infants. Eur Arch Otorrinolaringol 269(1):73–79

Cohen LB, Cashon CH (2003) Infant perception and cognition. Handbook of psychology. Dev Psychol 2:6389

Colarusso RP, Hammill DD (2015) Motor-Free Visual Perception Test-4 (MVPT-4). https://www.wpspublish.com/store/p/3303/motor-free-visual-perception-test-4-mvpt-4. Accessed 27 Feb 2017

Cole EB, Flexer C (2011) Children with hearing loss: developing listening and talking, birth to six. Plural Publishing, San Diego

College of Occupational Therapists (2015) Occupational therapy evidence fact sheet: occupational therapy with children and young people. https://www.cot.co.uk/sites/default/files/commissioning_ot/public/OT-with-

children-and-young-people-updated-April2015.pdf. Accessed 20 May 2015
Compas BE, Jaser SS, Dunn MJ et al (2012) Coping with chronic illness in childhood and adolescence. Annu Rev Clin Psychol 8:455–480
Coninx F (2005) Konstruktion und Normierung des Adaptiven Auditiven Sprach-Test (AAST). 100 Jahre Phoniatrie in Deutschland. 22. Jahrestagung der Deutschen Gesellschaft für Phoniatrie und Pädaudiologie, 24. Kongress der Union der Europäischen Phoniater. September 16th–18th, 2005, Berlin. http://www.egms.de/en/meetings/dgpp2005/05dgpp045.shtml#. Accessed 12 May 2018
Coninx F, Moore JM (1997) The multiply handicapped deaf child. In: McCracken W, Kemp L (eds) Audiology in education. Whurr Publishers, London, pp 107–135
Cox RM, McDaniel DM (1989) Development of the speech intelligibility rating [SIR] test for hearing aid comparisons. J Speech Hear Res 32(2):347–352
Cupples L, Ching TYC, Crowe K et al (2014) Outcomes of 3-year-old children with hearing loss and different types of additional disabilities. J Deaf Stud Deaf Educ 19(1):20–39
da Silva MP, Comerlatto AAJ, Bevilacqua MC et al (2011) Instruments to assess the oral language of children fitted with a cochlear implant: a systematic review. J Appl Oral Sci 19(6):549–553. https://doi.org/10.1590/S1678-77572011000600002
Dau T, Wegner O, Mellert V et al (2000) Auditory brainstem responses with optimized chirp signals compensating basilar-membrane dispersion. J Acoust Soc Am 107(3):1530–1540
Dawson JI, Tattersall PJ (2001) Structured photographic articulation test—DII. Janelle Publications, DeKalb, IL
De Foer B, Kenis C, Vercruysse JP et al (2009) Imaging of temporal bone tumors. Neuroimaging Clin N Am 19(3):339–366
De Leenheer EMR, Janssens S, Padalko E et al (2011) Etiological diagnosis in the hearing impaired newborn: proposal of a flow chart. Int J Pediatr Otorhinolaryngol 75(1):27–32. https://doi.org/10.1016/j.ijporl.21010.05.040
De Wit E, Neijenhuis K, Luinge MR (2017) Dutch position statement children with listening difficulties (translated version of the Dutch position statement Kinderen met Luisterproblemen). Federation of Dutch Audiological Centres, Utrecht
Declau F, Cremers C, Van de Heyning P (1999) Diagnosis and management strategies in congenital atresia of the external auditory canal. Br J Audiol 33(5):313–327. Review
Declau F, Van de Heyning P, Cremers C (2008) Diagnosis and management strategies in congenital middle and external ear anomalies. In: Graham JM et al (eds) Pediatric ENT. Springer, Berlin, Heidelberg
Delaroche M (2001) Audiométrie comportementale du très jeune enfant. De Boeck Université, Bruxelles
Delaroche M, Thiebaut R, Dauman R (2004) Behavioural audiometry: protocols for measuring hearing thresholds in babies aged 4-18 months. Int J Pediatr Otorhinolaryngol 68(10):1233–1243
Delaroche M, Thiebaut R, Dauman R (2005) Behavioural audiometric measurements obtained using the 'Delaroche protocol in babies aged 4-18 months suffering from bilateral sensorineural hearing loss. Int J Pediatr Otorhinolaryngol 70(6):993–1002
Delaroche M, Gavilan-Cellié I, Maurice-Tison S et al (2011) Is behavioral audiometry achievable in infants younger than 6 months of age? Int J Pediatr Otorhinolaryngol 75(12):1502–1509
DGZMK (Deutsche Gesellschaft für Zahn-, Mund-und Kieferhelkunde) (2016) DGZMK S2K Guideline Caries prevention in permanent teeth, status June 2016. https://www.awmf.org/fileadmin/user_upload/Leitlinien/083_D_Ges_fuer_Zahn-__Mund-_und_Kieferheilkunde/083-021le_S2k_Caries_prevention_2017-03.pdf. Accessed 5 Dec 2022
Di Giulio P, Philipov D, Jaschinski I (2014) Families with disabled children in different European countries. Families and Societies Working Paper Series (23). http://www.familiesandsocieties.eu/wp-content/uploads/2014/12/WP23GiulioEtAl.pdf. Accessed 13 Sept 2016
Dillon H, Cameron S, Glyde H et al (2012) An opinion on the assessment of people who may have an auditory processing disorder. J Am Acad Audiol 23(2):97–105. https://doi.org/10.3766/jaaa.23.2.4
Dobie RA, Van Hemel S (2004) Chapter 7: Hearing loss in children. In: Hearing loss: determining eligibility for social security benefits. National Academies Press, Washington, DC, pp 18–223. https://www.ncbi.nlm.nih.gov/books/NBK207837/. Accessed 12 Feb 2017
Dobie RA, Wilson MJ (1996) A comparison of t test, F test, and coherence methods of detecting steady-state auditory-evoked potentials, distortion-product otoacoustic emissions, or other sinusoids. J Acoust Soc Am 100(4 Pt 1):2236–2246
Downing JE (2004) Communication skills. In: Orelove FP et al (eds) Educating students with multiple disabilities: a collaborative approach. Paul H, Brooks, Baltimore
Dršata J, Havlík R et al (2015) Foniatrie—Sluch. Havlíčkův Brod, Tobiáš, p 136
DuCharme R (1983) The test of pragmatic skill. Pragmatic skills checklist from Communication Skill Builders. The Learning Clinic
Duffy FH, Eksioglu YZ, Rotenberg A et al (2013) The frequency modulated auditory evoked response (FMAER), a technical advance for study of childhood language disorders: cortical source localization and selected case studies. BMC Neurol 13:12
Dunn LM, Dunn DM (2007) Peabody picture vocabulary test, 4th edn. American Guidance Service, Circle Pines, MN

Dunn L, Markwardt FC (1989) Peabody individual achievement test-revised. American Guidance, Circle Pines, MN

Edwards S, Letts C, Sinka I (2011) The new reynell developmental language scales. GL Assessment, London

Eisenberg LS (2016) Clinical management of children with cochlear implants, 2nd edn. Plural Publishing, San Diego. http://pluralpublishing.com/publication_cmcci2e.htm. Accessed 28 Feb 2017

Eisenberg LS, Martinez AS, Holowecky SR et al (2002) Recognition of lexically controlled words and sentences by children with normal hearing and children with cochlear implants. Ear Hear 23(5):450–462

Eisenberg LS, Martinez AS, Boothroyd A (2007) Assessing auditory capabilities in young children. Int J Pediatr Otorhinolaryngol 71(9):1339–1350

Elberling C (1999) Loudness scaling revisited. J Am Acad Audiol 10(5):248–260

Elberling C, Don M, Cebulla M et al (2007) Auditory steady-state responses to chirp stimuli based on cochlear travelling wave. J Acoust Soc Am 122(5):2772–2785

Elliott LL, Katz DR (1980) Northwestern University children's perception of speech: (NU-CHIPS). Auditec of St Louis, St. Louis

Ellison J, Keefe D (2008) Audiometric predictions using SFOAE and middle-ear measurements. Ear Hear 26(5):487–503

Emanuel DC (2009) Acoustic reflex threshold (ART) patterns: an interpretation guide for students and supervisors. AudiologyOnline http://www.audiologyonline.com/articles/acoustic-reflex-threshold-art-patterns-875. Accessed 5 Jan 2017

Emanuel DC, Ficca KN, Korczak P (2011) Survey of the diagnosis and management of auditory processing disorder. Am J Audiol 20(1):48–60. https://doi.org/10.1044/1059-0889(2011/10-0019)

Enns C, Herman R (2011) Adapting the assessing British sign language development: receptive skills test into American sign language. J Deaf Stud Deaf Educ 16(3):362–374

Erber N (1982) Auditory training. Alexander Graham Bell Association, Washington, DC, pp 92–94

Erber NP, Alencewicz CM (1976) Audiologic evaluation of deaf children. J Speech Hear Disord 41(2):256–267

Esser G, Anderski CH, Birken A et al (1987) Auditive Wahrnehmungsstörungen und Fehlhörigkeit bei Kindern im Schulalter. Sprache-Stimme-Gehör 11:10–16

European Academy of Paediatric Dentistry (2009) Guidelines on the use of fluoride in children: an EAPD policy document. Eur Arch Paediatr Dent 10(3):129–135

European Surveillance of Congenital Anomalies (EUROCAT) (2013) Prevalence Tables. http://www.eurocat-network.eu/ACCESSPREVALENCEDATA/PrevalenceTables. Accessed 16 Apr 2013

Evans DG, Birch JM, Ramsden RT (1999) Paediatric presentation of type 2 neurofibromatosis. Arch Dis Child 81(6):496–499

Evenhuis HM (1995) Medical aspects of ageing in a population with intellectual disability: II hearing impairment. J Intellect Disabil Res 39(Pt 1):27–33

Evenhuis HM (1996) Dutch consensus in diagnosis and treatment of hearing impairment in children and adults with intellectual disability. J Intellect Disabil Res 40(Pt 5):451–456

Evenhuis HM, Nagtzaam LMD (1998) Early identification of hearing and visual impairment in children and adults with an intellectual disability. International Consensus Statement, IASSID, Edinburgh. http://iassid.org/pdf/sensory-imp-consensus. Accessed 16 Nov 2014

Eviatar L, Eviatar A (1979) The normal nystagmic response of infants to caloric and perrotatory stimulation. Laryngoscope 89(7 pt 1):1036–1045

Fabijańska A, Smurzyński J, Hatzopoulos S et al (2012) The relationship between distortion product otoacoustic emissions and extended high-frequency audiometry in tinnitus patients. Part 1: normally hearing patients with unilateral tinnitus. Med Sci Monit 18(12):CR765–CRC770

Fantz RL (1965) Visual perception from birth as shown by pattern selectivity. Ann N Y Acad Sci 118(21):793–814

Fenson L, Marchman VA, Thal DJ et al (2007) The MacArthur communicative development inventories: user's guide and technical manual, 2nd edn. Brookes, Baltimore

Ferguson MA, Hall RL, Riley A et al (2011) Communication, listening, cognitive and speech perception skills in children with auditory processing disorder (APD) or specific language impairment (SLI). J Speech Lang Hear Res 54(1):211–227. https://doi.org/10.1044/1092-4388(2010/09-0167

Ferm I, Lightfoot G, Stevens J (2013) Comparison of ABR response amplitude, test time, and estimation of hearing threshold using frequency specific chirp and tone pip stimuli in newborns. Int J Audiol 52(6):419–423

Fernández-Latorre F, Menor-Serrano F, Alonso-Charterina S et al (2000) Langerhans' cell histiocytosis of the temporal bone in pediatric patients: imaging and follow-up. AJR 174(1):217–321

Ferro R, Besostri A, Olivieri A et al (2016) Prevalence of occlusal traits and orthodontic treatment need in 14-year-old adolescents in Northeast Italy. Eur J Paediatr Dent 17(1):36–42

Fife T, Tusa R, Furman J et al (2000) Assessment: vestibular testing techniques in adults and children. Neurology 55(10):1431–1441

Flipsen PJ, Parker RG (2008) Phonological patterns in the conversational speech of children with cochlear implants. J Commun Disord 41(4):337–357

Fonseca-Souza G, de Oliveira LB, Wambier LM, Scariot R, Feltrin-Souza J (2022) Tooth abnormalities associated with non-syndromic cleft lip and palate: systematic review and meta-analysis. Clin Oral Investig

26(8):5089-5103. https://doi.org/10.1007/s00784-022-04540-8. Epub 2022 Jun 21. PMID: 35729285
Foudriat BA, DiFabio RP, Anderson JH (1993) Sensory organisation of balance responses in children 3-6 years of age: a normative study with diagnostic implications. Int J Pediatr Otorhinolaryngol 27(3):255–271
Foulon I, Naessens A, Foulon W et al (2008) A 10-year prospective study of sensorineural hearing loss in children with congenital cytomegalovirus infection. J Pediatr 153(1):84–88
Foulon I, Naessens A, Faron G et al (2012) Hearing thresholds in children with a congenital CMV infection: a prospective study. Int J Pediatr Otorhinolaryngol 76(5):712–717. https://doi.org/10.1016/j.ijporl.2012.02.026
Franks JR (2001) Hearing measurement. In: Goelzer B et al (eds) Occupational exposure to noise: evaluation, prevention and control. World Health Organization, Geneva, pp 183–232. http://www.who.int/occupational_health/publications/noise8.pdf. Accessed 9 Sept 2016
Fuchs M, Fröhlich M, Hentschel B et al (2007) Predicting mutational change in the speaking voice of boys. J Voice 21(2):169–178
Fudala JB (2001) Arizona articulation proficiency scale, 3rd Revision (Arizona-3). Western Psychological Services, Torrance, CA. http://li129-107.members.linode.com/downloads/compendium_instruments_publishers.pdf. Accessed 17 Mar 2017
Fulcher A, Purcell AA, Baker E et al (2012) Listen up: children with early identified hearing loss achieve age-appropriate speech/language outcomes by 3 years-of-age. Int J Pediatr Otorhinolaryngol 76(12):1785–1794
Gajjar A, Packer RJ, Foreman NK et al (2013) Children's oncology Group's 2013 blueprint for research: central nervous system tumors. Pediatr Blood Cancer 60(6):1022–1026. Review
Gallaudet Research Institute (1983) Norm tables: 1982 Stanford achievement test. In: Form E for use with hearingimpaired students, 7th edn. Gallaudet University, Washington, DC
Gallaudet Research Institute (2013) Regional and National Summary Report of data from the 2011–12 annual survey of deaf and hard of Hearing children and youth. Gallaudet University, GRI
Garcia JV, Rovira JM, González Sanvicens L (2010) The influence of the auditory prosthesis type on deaf children's voice quality. Int J Pediatr Otorhinolaryngol 74(8):843–848
Gasparini P, Rabionet R, Barbujani G et al (2000) High carrier frequency of the 35delG deafness mutation in European populations. Genetic analysis consortium of GJB2 35delG. Eur J Hum Genet 8(1):19–23
Gathercole SE, Baddeley A (1996) The children's test of non-word repetition. Psychological Corporation Europe, London
Geers A, Hayes H (2011) Reading, writing, and phonological processing skills of adolescents with 10 or more years of cochlear implant experience. Ear Hear 32(1):49S–59S
German Society of Phoniatrics and Pedaudiology (GSPP) (2014) Auditory processing and perception disorders: definition. Professional guidelines. German Society for Phoniatry and Pediatric Audiology
Germiller JA (2007) Hearing loss in children. In: Wetmore RF (ed) Pediatric otolaryngology: the requisites in pediatrics. Mosby Elsevier, Philadelphia
Gheysen F, Loots G, Van Waelvelde H (2007) Motor development of deaf children with and without cochlear implants. J Deaf Stud Deaf Educ 13(2):215–224
Gibbin KT (2007) Management of the deaf child. In: Graham JM et al (eds) Pediatric ENT. Springer, Berlin, Heidelberg
Giesemann AM, Goetz F, Neuburger J et al (2011) Appearance of hypoplastic cochlea in CT and MRI: a new subclassification. Neuroradiology 53(1):49–61
GL Assessment (2011) British ability scales, 3rd edn, The leading standardised battery for assessing children's current intellectual functioning. http://www.gl-assessment.co.uk/products/bas3. Accessed 10 Aug 2016
Glascoe FP, Dworkin PH (1995) The role of parents in the detection of developmental and behavioral problems. Pediatrics 95(6):829–836
Goldman R, Fristoe M (2000) Goldman-Fristoe-2 test of articulation. Pearson Assessments, Minneapolis, MN
Goodman S (2011) Comparison of high-frequency TEOAEs and DPOAEs for monitoring ototoxicity in pediatric cancer patients. Lecture presented at Illinois Speech-Language-Hearing Association. https://clas.uiowa.edu/sites/clas.uiowa.edu.comsci/files/groups/arl/pubs/goodman_isha_2011.pdf. Accessed 21 Jan 2017
Gorga MP, Johnson TA, Kaminski JR et al (2006) Using a combination of click-and tone burst-evoked auditory brain stem response measurements to estimate pure-tone thresholds. Ear Hear 27(1):60–74
Gorlin RJ, Cohen MM, Levin LS (1990) Syndromes of the head and neck, 3rd edn. Oxford University Press, Oxford
Govaerts PJ, Daemers K, Yperman M et al (2006) Auditory speech sounds evaluation (a(section)E): a new test to assess detection, discrimination and identification in hearing impairment. Cochlear Implants Int 7(2):92–106
Green DM (1976) An introduction to hearing. Lawrence Erdbaum Ass., New York
Gruber M, Brown C, Mahadevan M et al (2016) The yield of multigene testing in the management of pediatric unilateral sensorineural hearing loss. Otol Neurotol 37(8):1066–1070
Guralnick MJ (2000) In: Paul H (ed) Interdisciplinary clinical assessment of young children with developmental disabilities. Brookes Publishing, Baltimore
Gürtler N (in press) Studie: Prospektive multizentrische Studie zur Abklärung der Ätiologie der bilateralen kongenitalen Schwerhörigkeit. Nicolas Gürtler HNO-Klinik, Kantonsspital Aarau AG, Aarau

Hall JW (1999) Handbook of otoacoustic emissions. Singular Publishing Group, San Diego, p 643. ISBN: 1-56593-873-9

Hall JW, Bantwal AR, Ramkumar V et al (2011) Electrophysiological assessment of hearing with auditory middle latency and auditory late responses. In: Seewald R, Tharpe AM (eds) Comprehensive handbook of pediatric audiology. Plural Publishing, San Diego, CA, pp 449–482

Hammill DD, Newcomer PL (2001) Test of language development-intermediate, 3rd edn. http://cirrie.buffalo.edu/database/20818/. Accessed 4 June 2017

Harding J (2017) Dental care of cancer patients before, during and after treatment. https://www.nature.com/articles/bdjteam20178.pdf. Accessed 5 Dec 2022

Harding J (2018) Oral care in cancer: helping patients with tooth, gum and mouth problems. Br J Nurs 27(19):1106–1107

Harnett A (2007) Informing families of their child's disability. National best practice guidelines. In: Consultation and research report. The National Federation of voluntary bodies providing services to people with intellectual disability, Oranmore, Galway. ISBN: 978-0-9557833-0-2

Harris M, Beech JR (1998) Implicit phonological awareness and early reading development in prelingually deaf children. J Deaf Stud Deaf Educ 3(3):205–216

Haskins HL (1949) A phonetically balanced test of speech discrimination for children. Doctoral thesis, Northwestern University

Health and Safety Authority (2007) Guidelines on hearing checks and audiometry under the safety, health and welfare at work (general application) regulations 2007, control of noise at work. Health and Safety Authority http://www.hsa.ie/eng/Publications_and_Forms/Publications/Occupational_Health/audiometry.pdf. Accessed 9 Sept 2016

Heinz MG, Colburn HS, Carney LH (2001) Rate and timing cues associated with the cochlear amplifier: level discrimination based on monaural cross-frequency coincidence detection. J Acoust Soc Am 110(4):2065–2084

Helms J (1994) Mittelohrmissbildungen. In: Helms J (ed) Oto-Rhino-Laryngologie in Klinik und Praxis, vol 1. Thieme, Stuttgart, pp 545–563

Henningsson G, Kuehn DP, Sell D et al (2008) Universal parameters for reporting speech outcomes in individuals with cleft palate. Cleft Palate Craniofac J 45(1):1–17

Henry JA (2016) "Measurement" of tinnitus. Otol Neurotol 37(8):e276–e285

Henry JA, Meikle MB (2000) Psychoacoustic measures of tinnitus. J Am Acad Audiol 11(3):138–155

Henry JA, Stewart BJ, Abrams HB et al (2014) Tinnitus functional index—development and clinical application. Audiol Today 26(6):40–48

Henry JA, Griest S, Zaugg TL et al (2015) Tinnitus and hearing survey: a screening tool to differentiate bothersome tinnitus from hearing difficulties. Am J Audiol 24(1):66–77

Hereditary Hearing Loss (2019). http://hereditaryhearingloss.org. Accessed 20 June 2019

Herman R, Holmes S, Woll B (1999) Assessing British sign language development: receptive skills test. Forest Bookshop, Gloucestershire

Hild U, Hey C, Baumann U et al (2008) High prevalence of hearing disorders at the Special Olympics indicate need to screen persons with intellectual disability. J Intellect Disabil Res 52(Pt 6):520–528

Hill-Briggs F, Dial JG, Morere DA et al (2007) Neuropsychological assessment of persons with physical disability, visual impairment or blindness, and hearing impairment or deafness. Arch Clin Neuropsychol 22(3):389–404

Hind SE, Haines-Bazrafshan R, Benton CL et al (2011) Prevalence of clinical referrals having hearing thresholds within normal limits. Int J Audiol 50(10):708–716. https://doi.org/10.3109/14992027.2011.582049

Hintermair M (2004) Sense of coherence: a relevant resource in the coping process of mothers of hearing-impaired children? J Deaf Stud Deaf Educ 9(1):15–26

Holden-Pitt L, Diaz J (1998) Thirty five years of the annual survey of the deaf and hard of hearing children and youth: a glance over the decades. Am Ann Deaf 143(2):72–76

Holube I, Böld T, Gerdes T et al (2011) Internationales Sprachtestsignal (ISTS) als fluktuierender Maskierer im Satztest. 14. Jahrestagung der Deutschen Gesellschaft für Audiologie, March 9th–12th, 2011, Jena

Holzinger D, Fellinger J, Beitel C (2011) Early onset of family centred intervention predicts language outcomes in children with hearing loss. Int J Pediatr Otorhinolaryngol 75(2):256–260

Horsch U (2008) Dialog und Bildung in der Vorsprachlichkeit—Zur Situation hörgeschädigter Kinder in der Frühpädagogik. Sprache Stimme Gehör 32(1):18–25

Hoth S, Mühler R, Neumann K et al (2015) Objektive Audiometrie im Kindesalter. (Objective audiometry in children), 1st edn. Springer, Heidelberg

Howe BJ, Cooper ME, Vieira AR et al (2015) Spectrum of dental phenotypes in nonsyndromic orofacial clefting. J Dent Res 94(7):905–912

Howe BJ, Cooper ME, Wehby GL et al (2017) Dental decay phenotype in nonsyndromic orofacial clefting. J Dent Res 96(10):1106–1114

Huang BY, Zdanski C, Castillo M (2012a) Pediatric sensorineural hearing loss, part 1: practical aspects for neuroradiologists. AJNR Am J Neuroradiol 33(2):211–217. Review

Huang BY, Zdanski C, Castillo M (2012b) Pediatric sensorineural hearing loss, part 2: syndromic and acquired causes. AJNR Am J Neuroradiol 33(3):399–406. Review

Hugdahl K, Westerhausen R, Alho K et al (2009) Attention and cognitive control: unfolding the dichotic listening story. Scand J Psychol 50(1):11–22. https://doi.org/10.1111/j.1467-9450.2008.00676.x

Iliadou V, Ptok M, Grech H et al (2017) A European perspective on auditory processing disorder-current knowledge and future research focus. Front Neurol 8:622. https://doi.org/10.3389/fneur.2017.00622

Illinois Service Resource Center (2011) Guidelines for psychological testing of deaf and hard of hearing students. http://www.isrc.us/sites/default/files/pdf/psychguidelines2011.pdf. Accessed 13 Sept 2016

Illum ON, Gradel KO (2015) Assessing children with disabilities using WHO international classification of functioning, disability and health child and youth version activities and participation D codes. Child Neurol Open 28:1–9

ISAAC—International Society for Augmentative and Alternative Communication (2016). https://www.isaac-online.org/. Accessed 17 Mar 2016

Ishimoto S, Ito K, Yamasoba T et al (2005) Correlation between microtia and temporal bone malformation evaluated using grading system. Arch Otolaryngol Head Neck Surg 131(4):326–329

ISO 16832 (2006) Acoustics—loudness scaling by means of categories

ISO 60645-5 (2005) Electroacoustics—Audiometric equipment—Part 5: Instruments for the measurement of aural acoustic impedance/admittance

ISO 8253-1 (2010) Acoustics—Audiometric Test Methods—Part 1: Pure tone air and bone conduction audiometry

Iwasaki T, Saitoh I, Takemoto Y et al (2013) Tongue posture improvement and pharyngeal airway enlargement as secondary effects of rapid maxillary expansion: a cone-beam computed tomography study. Am J Orthod Dentofacial Orthop 143(2):235–245

Jamilian A, Lucchese A, Darnahal A et al (2016) Cleft sidedness and congenitally missing teeth in patients with cleft lip and palate patients. Prog Orthod 17:14. https://doi.org/10.1186/s40510-016-0127-z

Janse E, Newman RS (2013) Identifying nonwords: effects of lexical neighborhoods, phonotactic probability, and listener characteristics. Lang Speech 56(Pt 4):421–441

Jedrzejczak WW, Blinowska KJ, Kochanek K et al (2008) Synchronized spontaneous otoacoustic emissions analyzed in a time-frequency domain. J Acoust Soc Am 124:3720. https://doi.org/10.1121/1.2999556

Jerger J (1970) Clinical experience with impedance audiometry. Arch Otolaryngol 92(4):311–324

Jerger JF, Hayes D (1976) The cross-check principle in pediatric audiometry. Arch Otolaryngol 102(10):614–620

Jewett DL (1970) Volume conducted potentials in response to auditory stimuli as detected by averaging in the cat. Electroencephalogr Clin Neurophysiol 28(6):609–618

Jewett DL, Romano MN, Williston JS (1970) Human auditory evoked potentials: possible brain stem components detected on the scalp. Science 167(3924):1517–1518

John MS, Lins OG, Boucher BL et al (1998) Multiple auditory steady-state responses (MASTER): stimulus and recording parameters. Audiology 37(2):59–82

Johnson TA, Brown CJ (2005) Threshold prediction using the auditory steady-state response and the tone burst auditory brain stem response: a within-subject comparison. Ear Hear 26(6):559–576

Johnson MH, Farroni T (2007) The neurodevelopmental origins of eye gaze perception. In: Flom R et al (eds) Gaze-following: its development and significance. Lawrence Erlbaum Associates, Mahwah, NJ, pp 1–16

Johnson C, Goswani U (2010) Phonological awareness, vocabulary, and reading in deaf children with cochlear implants. J Speech Lang Hear Res 53(2):237–261

Johnson MR, Wilhelm C, Eisert D et al (2001) Assessment of students with motor impairments. In: Simeonsson RJ, Rosenthal SL (eds) Psychological and developmental assessment. Guilford Press, New York, pp 205–224

Johnston T (2004) The assessment and achievement of proficiency in a native sign language within a sign bilingual program: the pilot Auslan receptive skills test. Deafness Educ Int 6(2):57–81

Joint Committee on Infant Hearing (2007) Year 2007 position statement: principles and guidelines for early hearing detection and intervention. Appendix 1: risk indicators associated with permanent congenital, delayed-onset, or progressive Hearing Loss in childhood. Pediatrics 120:898–921. www.asha.org/policy. Accessed 11 June 2017. Reproduced with permission from Pediatrics

Joint Committee on Infant Hearing (2013) Supplement to the JCIH 2007 position statement: principles and guidelines for early intervention after confirmation that a child is deaf or hard of hearing. Pediatrics 131(4):1324–1349

Jones MW, Morgan E, Shelton JE (2007) Primary care of the student with cerebral palsy. J Pediatr Health Care 21(4):226–237

Jozefowicz-Korczynska M, Ciechomska EA, Pajor AM (2005) Electronystagmography outcome and neuropsychological findings in tinnitus patients. Int Tinnitus J 11(1):54–57

Kaufman AS, Kaufman NL (1983) Kaufman assessment battery for children. American Guidance Service, Circle Pines, MN

Kaufman AS, Kaufman NL (2004) Kaufman-assessment battery for children, 2nd edn (KABC-II). AGS Publications, Circle Pines, MN

Keith RW (2009) SCAN–3:C tests for auditory processing disorders for children. Pearson, London

Kemp D (1978) Stimulated acoustic emissions from within the human auditory system. J Acoust Soc Am 64(5):1386–1391

Kemp D (2002) Otoacoustic emissions, their origin in cochlear function, and use. Br Med Bull 63:223–241

Kent RD, Kim Y (2008) Acoustic analysis of speech. In: Ball MJ et al (eds) The handbook of clinical linguistics. Blackwell, Malden, MA, pp 360–380

Kentish RC, Crocker SR, McKenna L (2000) Children's experience of tinnitus: a preliminary survey of children presenting to psychology department. Br J Audiol 34(6):335–340

Khandelwal V, Nayak UA, Nayak PA et al (2013) Management of an infant having natal teeth. BMJ Case Rep 2013:bcr2013010049. https://doi.org/10.1136/bcr-2013-010049

Khater AM, Afifi PO (2016) Video head-impulse test (vHIT) in dizzy children with normal caloric responses. Int J Pediatr Otorhinolaryngol 87:172–177

Kim JH, Viana MA, Graber TM et al (1999) The effectiveness of protraction face mask therapy: a meta-analysis. Am J Orthod Dentofacial Orthop 115(6):675–685

Kim EY, Yoon MS, Kim NH et al (2012) Characteristics of nasal resonance and perceptual rating in prelingual hearing impaired adults. Clin Exp Otorhinolaryngol 5(1):1–9

Kirk KI, Pisoni DB, Osberger MJ (1995) Lexical effects on spoken word recognition by pediatric cochlear implant users. Ear Hear 16(5):470–481

Kirk KI, Eisenberg LS, French BF et al (2011) The multimodal lexical sentence test for children: performance of children with hearing loss. Paper presented at the 13th symposium on cochlear implants in children, Chicago, IL, 14–16 June 2011

Kirk KI, Prusick L, French B et al (2012) Assessing spoken word recognition in children who are deaf or hard of hearing: a translational approach. J Am Acad Audiol 23(6):464–475. https://doi.org/10.3766/jaaa.23.6.8

Klaiber S, Weerda H (2002) BAHA bei beidseitiger Ohrmuscheldysplasie und Atresia auris congenita. HNO 50(10):949–959

Koester LS, Lahti-Harper E (2010) Mother-infant hearing status and intuitive parenting behaviors during the first 18 months. Am Ann Deaf 155(1):5–18

Korczak P, Smart J, Delgado R et al (2012) Tutorial auditory steady-state responses. J Am Acad Audiol 23(3):146–170

Kort W, Schittekatte M, Compaan EL (2008) CELF-4-NL: clinical evaluation of language fundamentals-vierde-editie. Pearson Assessment and Information BV, Amsterdam

Kösling S, Jüttemann S, Amaya B et al (2003) Stellenwert der MRT bei Verdacht auf Innenohrmissbildung. Fortschr Röntgenstr 175(12):1639–1646

Kösling S, Omenzetter M, Bartel-Friedrich S (2009) Congenital malformations of the external and middle ear. Eur J Radiol 69(2):269–279. Review

Kricos P (1993) The counseling process: children and parents. In: McCarthy P, Alpiner J (eds) Rehabilitative audiology: children and adults, 2nd edn. Williams and Wilkins, Baltimore, MD, pp 211–237

Kuk FK, Tyler RS, Russell D et al (1990) The psychometric properties of a tinnitus handicap questionnaire. Ear Hear 11(6):434–445

Kummer AW (2008) Chapter 14. In: Cleft palate and craniofacial anomalies: effects on speech and resonance, 2nd edn. Thomson Delmar Learning, New York

Kunze S, Nickisch A, von Voss H et al (2016) Stapediusreflexe von Kindern mit und ohne auditive Verarbeitungs-und Wahrnehmungsstörungen. HNO 65(4):328–336. https://doi.org/10.1007/s00106-016-0271-2

Kurtzer-White E, Luterman D (2003) Families and children with hearing loss: grief and coping. Ment Retard Dev Disabil Res Rev 9(4):232–235

Kuwada S, Batra R, Maher VL (1986) Scalp potentials of normal and hearing-impaired subjects in response to sinusoidally amplitude-modulated tones. Hear Res 21(2):179–192

Kyle FE, Campbell R, Mohammed T et al (2013) Speechreading development in deaf and hearing children: introducing the test of child speechreading. J Speech Lang Hear Res 56(2):416–426

Lambert PR (2001) Congenital aural atresia. In: Bailey BJ (ed) Head and neck surgery—otolaryngology. Lippincott Williams & Wilkins, Philadelphia, pp 1745–1757

Laugen NJ, Jacobsen KH, Rieffe C et al (2016) Predictors of psychosocial outcomes in hard of hearing preschool children. J Deaf Stud Deaf Educ 21(3):259–267

Lechowicz U, Pollak A, Oldak M (2015) Novel trends in the molecular genetics of hearing loss. J Hear Sci 5(3):9–13

Lehnhardt E, Laszig R (eds) (2009) Praxis der Audiometrie. Thieme, Stuttgart, New York, p 140

Lesinski A, Littmann X, Battmer RD et al (1997) Comparison of preoperative electrostimulation data using an ear-canal electrode and a promontory needle electrode. Am J Otol 18(6 suppl):88–89

Levitt H, McGarr N, Geffner D (1987) Development of language and communication skills in hearing-impaired children: introduction. ASHA Monogr 26:1–8

Li Y, Yang J, Liu J et al (2015) Restudy of malformations of the internal auditory meatus, cochlear nerve canal and cochlear nerve. Eur Arch Otorrinolaringol 272(7):1587–1596

Lightfoot GR (1979) Air-borne radiation from bone conduction transducers. Br J Audiol 13(2):53–56

Lightfoot GR (2000) Audiometer calibration: interpreting and applying the standards. Br J Audiol 34(5):311–316

Lightfoot GR, Hughes JB (1993) Bone conduction errors at high frequencies: implications for clinical and medico-legal practice. J Laryngol Otol 107(4):305–308

Lightfoot G, Kennedy V (2006) Cortical electric response audiometry hearing threshold estimation: accuracy, speed, and the effects of stimulus presentation features. Ear Hear 27(5):443–456

Limberger A, Bohnert A, Lippert KL et al (2007) Verschiedene Sondentöne in der Tympanometrie. Paper presented at 78th annual meeting of the German Society of Oto-Rhino-Laryngology, Head and Neck Surgery, Munich, 16–20 May 2007. German Medical Science GMS Publishing House, Düsseldorf. http://www.egms.de/static/en/meetings/hnod2007/07hnod042.shtml. Accessed 30 Dec 2016

Lin K, Hsu Y, Young Y (2010) Brainstem lesion in benign paroxysmal vertigo children: evaluated by a combined ocular and cervical vestibular-evoked myogenic potential test. Int J Pediatr Otorhinolaryngol 74(5):523–527

Ling D (1976) Speech and the hearing-impaired child: theory and practice. Alexander Graham Bell Association for the Deaf, Washington, DC

Ling D (1989) Foundations of spoken language for the hearing-impaired child, vol 11. Alexander Graham Bell Association for the Deaf, Washington, DC, p 317

Lins OG, Picton TW (1995) Auditory steady-state responses to multiple simultaneous stimuli. Electroencephalogr Clin Neurophysiol 96(5):420–432

Luiz D, Barnard A, Knosen N et al (2006) Griffiths Mental Development Scales—extended revised: 2 to 8 years (GMDS-ER 2-8). Administration and Analysis Manual. http://www.hogrefe.co.uk/clinical-and-educational/child-development/gmds-er-2-8.html. Accessed 15 Nov 2016

Lutermann D (2004) Children with hearing loss and special needs. The Volta Review, Washington, DC

Luts H, Desloovere C, Wouters J (2006) Clinical application of dichotic multiple-stimulus auditory steady state responses in high-risk newborns and young children. Audiol Neurootol 11(1):24–37

MacDougall HG, Weber KP, McGarvie LA et al (2009) The video head impulse test: diagnostic accuracy in peripheral vestibulopathy. Neurology 73(14):1134–1141

Mackie RT, McCulloch DL (1995) Assessment of visual acuity in multiply handicapped children. Br J Ophthalmol 79(3):290–296

Madell JR, Flexer C (2008) Pediatric audiology: diagnosis, technology and management. Thieme, New York

Malki GA, Al-Badawi EA, Dahlan MA (2015) Natal teeth: a case report and reappraisal. Case Rep Dent 2015:147580. https://doi.org/10.1155/2015/147580

Mallur PS, Wisoff JH, Lalwani AK (2008) Steroid responsive fluctuating sensorineural hearing loss due to juvenile pilocytic astrocytoma involving the cerebellopontine angle. Int J Pediatr Otorhinolaryngol 72(4):529–534

Marchman VA, Fernald A (2008) Speed of word recognition and vocabulary knowledge in infancy predict cognitive and language outcomes in later childhood. Dev Sci 11(3):1–9

Margolis RH (1993) Detection of hearing impairment with the acoustic stapedius reflex. Ear Hear 14(1):3–10

Margolis RH (2015) The Vanishing Air-Bone Gap—Audiology's Dirty Little Secret. http://www.audiologyonline.com/articles/vanishing-air-bone-gap-audiology-901. Accessed 21 Oct 2016

Margolis RH, Wilson RH, Popelka GR et al (2015) Distribution characteristics of normal pure-tone thresholds. Int J Audiol 54(11):796–805

Marková SP, Brožková DŠ, Laššuthová P, Mészárosová A, Krůtová M, Neupauerová J, Rašková D, Trková M, Staněk D, Seeman P (2018) STRC gene mutations, mainly large deletions, are a very important cause of early-onset hereditary hearing loss in the czech population. Genet Test Mol Biomarkers 22(2):127–134. https://doi.org/10.1089/gtmb.2017.0155

Marschark M, Spencer PE (2003) Oxford handbook of deaf studies, language and education. Oxford University Press, New York

Martin N (2017) Test of visual perceptual skills–fourth edition (TVPS-4). Pro Ed, Austin

May-Mederake B (2012) Early intervention and assessment of speech and language development in young children with cochlear implants. Int J Ped Otorhinolaryngol 76(7):939–946

May-Mederake B, Kuehn H, Vogel A et al (2010) Evaluation of auditory development in infants and toddlers who received cochlear implants under the age of 24 months with the LittlEARS auditory questionnaire. Int J Ped Otorhinolaryngol 74(10):1149–1155

McGrew KS (2005) The Cattell-Horn-Carroll theory of cognitive abilities: past, present, and future. In: Flanagan DP, Harrison PL (eds) Contemporary intellectual assessment: theories, tests, and issues, 2nd edn. Guilford, New York, pp 136–181

Meikle MB, Vernon J, Johnson RM (1984) The perceived severity of tinnitus. Some observations concerning a large population of tinnitus clinic patients. Otolaryngol Head Neck Surg 92(6):689–696

Meinzen-Derr J, Wiley S, Choll ID (2011) Impact of early intervention on expressive and receptive language development among young children with permanent hearing loss. Am Ann Deaf 155(5):580–591

Meltzoff AN, Brooks R (2009) Social cognition and language: the role of gaze following in early word learning. In: Colombo J et al (eds) Infant pathways to language: methods, models, and research directions. Erlbaum, Mahwah, NJ, pp 169–194

Miller Guron L (1999) Wordchains: word reading test. NFER Nelson, Windsor

Miller CA, Wagstaff DA (2011) Behavioral profiles associated with auditory processing disorder and specific language impairment. J Commun Disord 44(6):745–763. https://doi.org/10.1016/j.jcomdis.2011.04.001

Minárik G, Ferák V, Feráková E et al (2003) High frequency of GJB2 mutation W24X among Slovak Romany (gypsy) patients with non-syndromic hearing loss (NSHL). Gen Physiol Biophys 22(4):549–556

Mirone G, Schiabello L, Chibbaro S et al (2009) Pediatric primary pilocytic astrocytoma of the cerebellopontine angle: a case report. Childs Nerv Syst 25(2):247–251

Moeller MP (2000) Early intervention and language development in children who are deaf and hard of hearing. Pediatrics 106(3):e43

Moeller MP, Hoover B, Putman C et al (2007a) Vocalizations of infants with hearing loss compared with infants with normal hearing: part I—phonetic development. Ear Hear 28(5):605–627

Moeller MP, Hoover B, Putman C et al (2007b) Vocalizations of infants with hearing loss compared with infants with normal hearing: part II—transition to words. Ear Hear 28(5):628–642

Moeller MP, Carr G, Seaver L et al (2013) Best practices in family-centered early intervention for children who

are deaf or hard of hearing: an international consensus statement. J Deaf Stud Deaf Educ 18(4):429–445
Moog JS, Geers AE (1990) Early speech perception test of profoundly hearing-impaired children. Central Institute for the Deaf, St. Louis, MO
Moore BCJ (2001) Dead regions in the cochlea: diagnosis, perceptual consequences, and implications for the fitting of hearing aids. Trends Amplif 5(1):1–34
Moore BCJ (2008) An introduction to the psychology of hearing, 5th edn. Academic Press, San Diego
Moore DR (2012) Listening difficulties in children: bottom-up and top-down contributions. J Commun Disord 45(6):411–418. https://doi.org/10.1016/j.jcomdis.2012.06.006
Moore DR, Hunter LL (2013) Auditory processing disorder (APD) in children: a marker of neurodevelopmental syndrome. Hear Balance Commun 11(3):160–167
Moore JM, Thompson G, Thompson M (1975) Auditory localization of infants as a function of reinforcement conditions. J Speech Hear Disord 40(1):29–34
Moore BCJ, Huss M, Vickers DA et al (2000) A test for the diagnosis of dead regions in the cochlea. Br J Audiol 34(4):205–224
Moore DR, Ferguson MA, Edmondson-Jones AM et al (2010) Nature of auditory processing disorder in children. Pediatrics 126(2):e382–e390. https://doi.org/10.1542/peds.2009-2826
Moore DR, Rosen S, Bamiou D-E et al (2013) Evolving concepts of developmental auditory processing disorder (APD): a British Society of Audiology APD special interest group 'white paper'. Int J Audiol 52(1):1499–2027
Morell RJ, Kim HJ, Hood LJ et al (1998) Mutations in the connexin 26 gene (GJB2) among Ashkenazi Jews with nonsyndromic recessive deafness. N Engl J Med 339(21):1500–1505
Morlet T, Pazuniak M, O'Reilly R et al (2017) Cochlear nerve deficiency and brain abnormalities in pediatric patients. Otol Neurotol 38(3):429–440
Mueller G, Killion M (1990) An easy method for calculating the articulation ındex. Hear J 43(9):14–17
Mühlenberg L, Schade G (2012) Frühe akustisch evozierte Potentiale: Low-chirp-BERA versus notched-noise-BERA. (a comparison of low-chirp-and notched-noise-evoked auditory brainstem response). Laryngo-Rhino-Otologie 91(8):500–504
Müller KHG (1991) Missbildungen des Schläfenbeins. In: Mödder U, Lenz M (eds) Klinische Radiologie, Gesichtschädel, Felsenbein, Speicheldrüsen, Pharynx, Larynx, Halsweichteile. Springer, Berlin, p 170
Müller-Hagedorn S, Buchenau W, Arand J et al (2017) Treatment of infants with syndromic Robin sequence with modified palatal plates: a minimally invasive treatment option. Head Face Med 13(1):4. https://doi.org/10.1186/s13005-017-0137-1
Müller-Hagedorn S, Wiechers C, Arand J et al (2018) Less invasive treatment of sleep-disordered breathing in children with syndromic craniosynostosis. Orphanet J Rare Dis 13(1):63. https://doi.org/10.1186/s13023-018-0808-4
Munro KJ, Agnew N (1999) A comparison of inter-aural attenuation with the Etymotic ER-3A insert earphone and the Telephonics TDH-39 supra-aural earphone. Br J Audiol 33(4):259–262
National Acoustics Laboratory (2015) NAL position statement on auditory processing disorder. www.capd.nal.gov.au/capd-position-statement.shtml. Accessed 28 June 2018
National Centre for Health Statistics (2003) National health and nutrition examination survey: audiometry procedures manual. http://www.cdc.gov/nchs/data/nhanes/nhanes_03_04/au.pdf. Accessed 1 Sept 2016
Neff BA, Welling DB (2005) Current concepts in the evaluation and treatment of neurofibromatosis type II. Otolaryngol Clin N Am 38(4):671–684
Neumann K, Dettmer G, Euler HA et al (2006) Auditory status of persons with intellectual disability at the German special Olympic games. Int J Audiol 45(2):83–90
Neumann K, Ludwig A, Montgomery J et al (2008) Special Olympics as research platform of hearing disorders in people with intellectual disabilities. In: Wegner M, Schulke HJ (eds) Kieler Schriften zur Sportwissenschaft—Behinderung, Bewegung, Befreiung: Gewinn von Lebensqualität und Selbständigkeit durch Wettbewerb und sportliches Training bei Menschen mit geistiger Behinderung. Christian-Albrechts-Universität zu Kiel, Kiel, pp 25–28
Neumann K, Waschkies L, Thomas JP et al (2014) Hearing and communication situation of persons with intellectual disability (ID). Paper presented at the Coalition for Global Hearing Health conference, Oxford, July 25–26, 2014, book of abstracts
Neumann K, Rosenberger D, Euler HA et al (n.d.) (in press) The adaptive MAGIC® test measures fast and reliably the pure tone hearing threshold of persons with intellectual disabilities. Manuscript in preparation
Newman CW, Jacobson GP, Spitzer JB (1996) Development of the tinnitus handicap inventory. Arch Otolaryngol Head Neck Surg 122(2):143–148
Nguyen LH, Allegro J, Low A et al (2008) Effect of cochlear implantation on nasality in children. Ear Nose Throat J 87(3):138–143
Nickerson RB (1975) Characteristics of the speech of deaf persons. Volta Rev 77(6):342–362
Nickisch A, Gross M, Schönweiler R et al (2015) Auditive Verarbeitungs-und Wahrnehmungsstörungen (AVWS): Zusammenfassung und aktualisierter Überblick. HNO 63:434–438
Nittrouer S, Caldwell-Tarr A, Lowenstein JH (2013) Working memory in children with cochlear implants: problems are in storage, not processing. Int J Pediatr Otorhinolaryngol 77(11):1886–1898
Northern JL, Downs MP (2001) Hearing in children. Lippincott Williams & Wilkins, Philadelphia
O'Reilly R, Grindle C, Zwicky E et al (2011) Development of the vestibular system and balance function: differential diagnosis in the pediatric population. Otolaryngol Clin N Am 44(2):251–271

Oosterkamp BCM, Dijkstra PU, Remmelink HJ et al (2010) Orthodontic space closure versus prosthetic replacement of missing upper lateral incisors in patients with bilateral cleft lip and palate. Cleft Palate Craniofac J 47(6):591–596
Osberger MJ, Robbins AM, Todd SL et al (1994) Speech intelligibility of children with cochlear implants. Volta Rev 96(5):169–180
Papadopoulos MA, Koumpridou EN, Vakalis ML et al (2012) Effectiveness of pre-surgical infant orthopedic treatment for cleft lip and palate patients: a systematic review and meta-analysis. Orthod Craniofac Res 15(4):207–236
Persson M, Thilander B (1977) Palatal suture closure in man from 15 to 35 years of age. Am J Orthod 72(1):42–52
Petrak MR, Bahner C, Beck DL (2013) Video head impulse testing (vHIT): VOR analysis of high frequency vestibular activity. The Hearing Review http://www.hearingreview.com/2013/08/video-head-impulse-testing-vhit-vor-analysis-of-high-frequency-vestibular-activity/. Accessed 20 Apr 2017
Phan MF, Conte KD, Khandelwal CW et al (2016) Tooth agenesis and orofacial clefting: genetic brothers in arms? Hum Genet 135(12):1299–1327
Piaget J, Inhelder B (1969) The psychology of the child. Basic Books, New York
Picard M (2004) Children with permanent hearing loss and associated disabilities: revisiting current epidemiological data and causes of deafness. Volta Rev 104(4):221236
Picton TW (2011) Human auditory evoked potentials. Plural Publishing, San Diego
Picton TW, Ouellette J, Hamel G et al (1979) Brainstem evoked potentials to tonepips in notched noise. J Otolaryngol 8(4):289–314
Picton TW, John MS, Dimitrijevic A et al (2003) Human auditory steady-state responses. Int J Audiol 42(4):177–219
Potsic WP, Lando T (2012) Introduction to pediatric otology. In: Wetmore RF et al (eds) Pediatric otolaryngology: principles and practice pathways. Thieme, New York
Pruszewicz A, Obrębowski A (2010) Clinical audiology Edd.IV. Med Univ Poznań, Poznań
Prutting C (1982) Observational protocol for pragmatic behaviors' (clinic manual). Developed for the University of California Speech and Hearing Clinic, Santa Barbara
Prutting C, Kirchner D (1987) A clinical appraisal of the pragmatic aspects of language. J Speech Hear Disord 52(2):105–119
Queißer-Luft A, Spranger J (2006) Fehlbildungen bei Neugeborenen. Dtsch Arztebl 103(38):A 2464–A 2471
Rahul M, Kapur A, Goyal A (2018) Management of prematurely erupted teeth in newborns. BMJ Case Rep 2018:bcr-2018-225288. https://doi.org/10.1136/bcr-2018-225288
Ramos JA, Kristensen SGB, Beck DL (2013) An overview of OAEs and normative data for DPOAEs. Hearing Review http://www.hearingreview.com/2013/10/an-overview-of-oaes-and-normative-data-for-dpoaes/. Accessed 2 Nov 2016
Ramos D, Jorge JX, Teixeira A et al (2015) The impact of cochlear implant in the oral language of children with congenital deafness. Acta Medica Port 28(4):442–447. Epub 2015 Aug 31
Rance G, Roper R, Symons L et al (2005) Hearing threshold estimation in infants using auditory steady-state responses. J Am Acad Audiol 16(5):291–300
Raven J, Raven JC, Court JH (2004) Manual for Raven's progressive matrices and vocabulary scales. Updated. Harcourt Assessment, San Antonio, TX
Reichmuth K, Embacher AJ, Matulat P et al (2013) Responsive parenting intervention after identification of hearing loss by universal newborn hearing screening: the concept of the muenster parental Programme. Int J Pediatr Otorhinolaryngol 77(12):2030–2039
Reid DK, Hammill D, Wiltshire S, Hresko W (1991) Test of early Reading ability deaf or hard of Hearing (TERA-D/HH) Hresko. Pro Ed, Austin
Renfrew C (1997) Bus story test (Renfrew language scales), 4th edn. Winslow Press, Bicester
Renfrew C, Mitchell P (2015) Word finding vocabulary test (the Renfrew language scales). Routledge, London
Rinaldi P, Baruffaldi F, Burdo S et al (2013) Linguistic and pragmatic skills in toddlers with cochlear implant. Int J Lang Commun Disord 48(6):715–725. https://doi.org/10.1111/1460-6984.12046. Epub 2013 Jul 29
Rizzi MD, Dunham BP (2014) Congenital malformations of the nose and nasopharynx. In: Elden LM, Zur KB (eds) Congenital malformations of the head and neck. Springer, New York
Robbins AM, Osberger MJ (1990) Meaningful use of speech scale (MUSS). Indiana University School of Medicine, Indianapolis
Robbins AM, Renshaw JJ, Berry SW (1991) Evaluating meaningful auditory integration in profoundly hearing-impaired children. Am J Otol 12(Suppl):144–150
Robbins AM, Renshaw JJ, Osberger MJ (1995) Common phrases test. Indiana University School of Medicine, Indianapolis
Robinette M, Glattke T (2007) Otoacoustic emissions: clinical applications. Thieme, New York
Robinette MS, Cevette MJ, Probst R (2007) Otoacoustic emissions and audiometric outcomes across cochlear and retrocochlear pathology. In: Robinette MS, Glattke TJ (eds) Otoacoustic emissions: clinical applications, 3rd edn. Thieme Publishing, New York, pp 236–237
Robson CD (2010) Imaging of head and neck neoplasms in children. Pediatr Radiol 40(4):499–509
Robson CD, Robertson RL, Barnes PD (1999) Imaging of pediatric temporal bone abnormalities. Neuroimaging Clin N Am 9(1):133–155
Roid GH, Miller LJ (1997) Leiter international performance scale-revised. Stoelting, Wood Dale, IL

Römer TA (2007) Retrospektives Erleben von Eltern zur Diagnosestellung einer chronischen Stoffwechselerkrankung bei ihrem Kind. Dissertation, Universität Hamburg

Ross HW (1979) Wepman test of auditory discrimination (WADT): what does it discriminate. J Sch Psychol 17(1):47–54

Roux WH (1881) Der Kampf der Theile im Organismus. (the struggle of the parts in the organism.). Wilhelm Engelmann, Leipzig

Rowland C (2005) But what CAN they do? Assessment of communication skills in children with severe and multiple disabilities. Perspect Augment altern commun 14(1):1–5

Ruben JR (2001) The pediatric otolaryngic assessment of the child with a suspected hearing loss. In: Gerber SE (ed) The handbook of pediatric audiology. Gallaudet University Press, Washington

Russel E, Nagaishi P (2010) Service for children with visual or hearing impairments. In: Case-Smith J (ed) Occupational therapy for children, 6th edn. Maryland Heights, Mosby/Elsevier, Amsterdam, pp 744–784

Russo NM, Hornickel J, Nicol T et al (2010) Biological changes in auditory function following training in children with autism spectrum disorders. Behav Brain Funct 6:60

Sæle P, Østhus E, Ådalen S et al (2017) Pattern of clefts and dental anomalies in six-year-old children: a retrospective observational study in western Norway. Acta Odontol Scand 75(2):100–105

Santi S, Rushing EJ (2013) Tumors of the pediatric central nervous system. In: Keating RF et al (eds) Neurosurgery, 2nd edn. Thieme Medical Publisher, New York

Sarant J (2012) Cochlear implants in children: a review. The University of Melbourne Australia. http://cdn.intechopen.com/pdfs-wm/33875.pdf. Accessed 11 Aug 2016

Scherg M (1991) Akustisch evozierte Potentiale. In: Baumgartner A et al (eds) Psychiatrie, Neurologie, Klinische Psychologie. Kohlhammer, Stuttgart

Schley S, Albertini J (2005) Assessing the writing of deaf college students: reevaluating a direct assessment of writing. J Deaf Stud Deaf Educ 10(1):96–104

Schloss MD (1997) Congenital anomalies of the external auditory canal and the middle ear. Surgical management. In: Tewfik TL, Der Kaloustian VM (eds) Congenital anomalies of the ear, nose, and throat. Oxford University Press, New York, pp 119–124

Schlumberger E, Narbona J, Manrique M (2004) Nonverbal development of children with deafness with and without cochlear implants. Dev Med Child Neurol 46(9):599–606

Schmid JQ, Gerberding E, Hohoff A et al (2022) Non-surgical transversal dentoalveolar compensation with completely customized lingual appliances versus surgically assisted rapid palatal expansion in adults-the amount of posterior crossbite correction. J Pers Med 12(11):1893. https://doi.org/10.3390/jpm12111893. PMID: 36422069; PMCID: PMC9694179

Schmid JQ, Gerberding E, Hohoff A et al (2023) Non-surgical transversal dentoalveolar compensation with completely customized lingual appliances versus surgically assisted rapid palatal expansion in adults-tipping or translation in posterior crossbite correction? J Pers Med 13(5):807. https://doi.org/10.3390/jpm13050807. PMID: 37240977; PMCID: PMC10222191

Schmidt CM, Knief A, Deuster D et al (2007) Melatonin is a useful alternative to sedation in children undergoing brainstem audiometry with an age dependent success rate—a field report of 250 investigation. Neuropediatrics 38(1):2–4

Schmidt CM, Huebner JR, Deuster D et al (2012) A positive wave at 8 ms (P8) and modified auditory brainstem responses measurement in auditory neuropathy spectrum disorder. Int J Pediatr Otorhinolaryngol 76(5):636–641

Schmuziger N, Probst R, Smurzynski J (2004) Test-retest reliability of pure-tone thresholds from 0.5 to 16 kHz using Sennheiser HDA 200 and Etymotic research ER-2 earphones. Ear Hear 25(2):127–132

Scholz U, Gutiérrez-Doña B, Sud S et al (2002) Is general self-efficacy a universal construct? Psychometric findings from 25 countries. Eur J Psychol Assess 18(3):242–251

Schwartz RG, Steinman S, Ying E et al (2013) Language processing in children with cochlear implants: a preliminary report on lexical access for production and comprehension. Clin Linguist Phon 27(4):264–277

Sennaroglu L (2010) Cochlear implantation in inner ear malformations—a review article. Cochlear Implants Int 11(1):34–41

Sennaroglu L, Saatci I (2002) A new classification for cochleovestibular malformations. Laryngoscope 112(12):2230–2241

Shahnaz N, Bork K, Polka L et al (2009) Energy reflectance and tympanometry in normal and otosclerotic ears. Ear Hear 30(2):219–233

Sharma M, Purdy SC, Kelly AS (2009) Comorbidity of auditory processing, language, and reading disorders. J Speech Lang Hear Res 52(3):706–722. https://doi.org/10.1044/1092-4388(2008/07-0226)

Sherlock LP, Formby C (2005) Estimates of loudness, loudness discomfort, and the auditory dynamic range: normative estimates, comparison of procedures, and test-retest reliability. J Am Acad Audiol 16(2):85–100

Shetye A, Kennedy V (2010) Tinnitus in children: an uncommon symptom? Arch Dis Child 95(8):645–648

Shinjo Y, Jin Y, Kaga K (2007) Assessment of vestibular function of infants and children with congenital and acquired deafness using ice-water caloric test, rotational chair test and vestibular-evoked myogenic potential recording. Acta Otolaryngol 127(7):736–747

Shoman NM, Samy RN, Choo DI (2014) Congenital malformations of the ear. In: Elden LM, Zur KB (eds) Congenital malformations of the head and neck. Springer, New York

Shott SR, Joseph A, Heithaus D (2001) Hearing loss in children with down syndrome. Int J Pediatr Otorhinolaryngol 61(3):199–205

Siegert R (2010) Combined reconstruction of congenital auricular atresia and severe microtia. Adv Otorhinolaryngol 68:95–107

Siegert R, Weerda H, Mayer T et al (1996) Hochauflösende Computertomographie fehlgebildeter Mittelohren. Laryngo-Rhino-Otologie 75(4):187–194

Silva MARD, Balderrama IF, Wobeto AP et al (2018) The impact of nonsyndromic cleft lip with or without cleft palate on oral health-related quality of life. J Appl Oral Sci 26:e20170145. https://doi.org/10.1590/1678-7757-2017-0145

Simeonsson RJ, Carlson D, Huntington GS et al (2001) Students with disabilities: a national survey of participation in school activities. Disabil Rehabil 23(2):49–63

Sismanis A (2011) Pulsatile tinnitus: contemporary assessment and management. Curr Opin Otolaryngol Head Neck Surg 19(5):348–357

Slis IH, Snik AFM (1997a) Anatomie van het gehoororgaan. In: Peters HFM (ed) Handboek stem- spraak-taalpathologie. Bohn, Stafeu and Van Loghum, Houten, pp 51–56

Slis IH, Snik AFM (1997b) Werking van het gehoororgaan. In: Peters HFM (ed) Handboek stem- spraak-taalpathologie. Bohn, Stafeu and Van Loghum, Houten, pp 298–306

Smits C, Goverts ST, Festen JM (2013) The digits-in-noise test: assessing auditory speech recognition abilities in noise. J Acoust Soc Am 133(3):1693–1706

Smoorenburg GF, Willeboer C, van Dijk JE (2002) Speech perception in nucleus CI24M cochlear implant users with processor settings based on electrically evoked compound action potential thresholds. Audiol Neurootol 7(6):335–347

Snell ME (2002) Severe and multiple disabilities, education of individuals with multiple disabilities—definition and types of severe and multiple disabilities. http://www.encyclopedia.com/doc/1G2-3403200553.html. Accessed 13 Sept 2016

Snijders JT, Tellegen PJ, Laros JA (1989) Snijders-Oomen Non-Verbal Intelligence Test: SON-R 5.5-17. Manual and research report. Wolters-Noordhoff, Groningen

Snoeckx RL, Huygen PL, Feldmann D et al (2005) GJB2 mutations and degree of hearing loss: a multicenter study. Am J Hum Genet 77(6):945–957

Sobe T, Erlich P, Berry A et al (1999) Letter to the editor. High frequency of the deafness-associated 167delT mutation in the connexin 26 (GJB2) gene in Israeli Ashkenazim. Am J Med Genet 86(5):499–500

Soetens O, Vauloup-Fellous C, Foulon I et al (2008) Evaluation of different cytomegalovirus (CMV) DNA PCR protocols for analysis of dried blood spots from consecutive cases of neonates with congenital CMV infections. J Clin Microbiol 46(3):943–946

Spearman C (1904) "General intelligence," objectively determined and measured. Am J Psychol 15(2):201–209

Spencer PE, Meadow-Orlans KP (1996) Play, language, and maternal responsiveness: a longitudinal study of deaf and hearing infants. Child Dev 67(6):3176–3191

Spencer LJ, Barker BA, Tomblin JB (2003) Exploring the language and literacy. Outcomes of pediatric cochlear implant users. Ear Hear 24(3):236–247

Squires N, Ollo C, Jordan R (1986) Auditory brain stem responses in the mentally retarded: audiometric correlates. Ear Hear 7(2):83–92

Stapells D (2002) Cortical event-related potentials to auditory stimuli. In: Katz J (ed) Handbook of clinical audiology. Lippincott Williams & Wilkins, Philadelphia

Stapells DR (2011) Frequency-specific threshold assessment in young infants using the transient ABR and the brainstem ASSR. In: Seewald RC, Trahpe AM (eds) Comprehensive handbook of pediatric audiology. Plural Publishing, San Diego, pp 409–448

Stapells D, Oates P (1997) Estimation of the pure-tone audiogram by the auditory brainstem response: a review. Audiol Neurootol 2(5):257–280

Stavroulaki P, Apostolopoulos N, Segas J et al (2001) Evoked otoacoustic emissions—an approach for monitoring cisplatin induced ototoxicity in children. Int J Pediatr Otorhinolaryngol 59(1):47–57

Stenfelt S, Goode R (2005) Bone-conduction sound, physiological and clinical aspects. Otol Neurotol 26(6):1245–1261

Steindl R, Kunz K, Schrott-Fischer A et al (2006) Effect of age and sex on maturation of sensory systems and balance control. Dev Med Child Neurol 48(6):477–482

Stinson MS, Liu Y (1999) Participation of deaf and hard-of-hearing students in classes with hearing students. J Deaf Stud Deaf Educ 4(3):191–202

Stredler-Brown A, Abraham H (2002) Colorado home intervention program (CHIP) manual. The Keystone Project. Colorado School for the Deaf and Blind, Colorado

Stuart A, Stenstromb R, Tompkins C et al (1991) Test-retest variability in audiometric threshold with supra-aural and insert earphones among children and adults. Audiology 30(2):82–90

Studebaker GA (1967) Intertest variability and the air-bone gap. J Speech Hear Disord 32(1):82–86

Stürzebecher E, Cebulla M, Elberling C et al (2006) New efficient stimuli for evoking frequency-specific auditory steady-state responses. J Am Acad Audiol 17(6):448–461

Sundell AL, Nilsson AK, Ullbro C et al (2016) Caries prevalence and enamel defects in 5-and 10-year-old children with cleft lip and/or palate: a case-control study. Acta Odontol Scand 74(2):90–95

Suzuki A, Nakano M, Yoshizaki K et al (2017) A longitudinal study of the presence of dental anomalies in the primary and permanent dentitions of cleft lip and/or palate patients. Cleft Palate Craniofac J 54(3):309–320

Swartz JD, Harnsberger HR (1997) Imaging of the temporal bone, 3rd edn. Thieme, New York

Tait M, Nikolopoulos TP, De Raeve L et al (2010) Bilateral versus unilateral cochlear implantation in young children. Int J Pediatr Otorhinolaryngol 74(2):206–211

Tan ELY, Kuek MC, Wong HC et al (2018) Secondary dentition characteristics in children with nonsyn-

dromic unilateral cleft lip and palate: a retrospective study. Cleft Palate Craniofac J 55(4):582–589
Tannure PN, Oliveira CA, Maia LC et al (2012) Prevalence of dental anomalies in nonsyndromic individuals with cleft lip and palate: a systematic review and meta-analysis. Cleft Palate Craniofac J 49(2):194–200
Tellegen P, Laros J (1993) The construction and validation of a nonverbal test of intelligence: the revision of the Snijders-Oomen test. Eur J Psychol Assess 9(2):147–157
Tellegen PJ, Winkel M, Wijnberg-Williams BJ et al (1998) Snijders-Oomen Non-Verbal Intelligence Test. SON-R 2.5-7. Manual and research report. Swets Test Publishers, Lisse
Tellegen PJ, Laros JA (2005) Fair assessment for children from cultural minorities: a description of the SON-R non-verbal intelligence tests. In: Kopcanová D (ed) Quality education for children from socially disadvantaged settings. Commission of UNESCO, Bratislava, pp 50–73
Tellegen PJ, Winkel M, Wijnberg-Williams BJ et al (2009) Snijders-Oomen Non-Verbal Intelligence Test. SON-R 2.5-7. Manual and research report. Hogrefe, Göttingen
Teoh AP, Chin SB (2007) Phonetic transcriptions of children with cochlear implants. Poster presented at the 11th international conference on cochlear implants in children. Charlotte, North Carolina, 11–14 June 2007
Theologie-Lygidakis N, Chatzidimitriou K, Tzerbos F et al (2014) Development of surgical techniques of secondary osteoplasty in cleft patients following 12 years experience. J Craniomaxillofac Surg 42(6):839–845
Thilander B (1995) Basic mechanisms in craniofacial growth. Acta Odontol Scand 53(3):144–151
Thomsen KA (1955) The Metz recruitment test and a comparison with the fowler method. Acta Otolaryngol 45(6):544–552
Tlumak AI, Rubinstein E, Durrant JD (2007) Meta-analysis of variables that affect accuracy of threshold estimation via measurement of the auditory steady-state response (ASSR). Int J Audiol 46(11):692–710
Tlumak AI, Durrant JD, Delgado RE et al (2012) Steady-state analysis of auditory evoked potentials over a wide range of stimulus repetition rates: profile in children vs. adults. Int J Audiol 51(6):480–490
Traxler CB (2000) The Stanford achievement test, 9th edition: national norming and performance standards for deaf and hard-of-hearing students. J Deaf Stud Deaf Educ 5(43):337–348
Ulrich ME, Bauer AM (2003) Levels of awareness: a closer look at communication between parents and professionals. Teach Except Child 35(6):20–24
UN General Assembly (2007) Convention on the rights of persons with disabilities. http://www.refworld.org/docid/45f973632.html. Accessed 13 Sept 2016
United States Congress (USC) (2004) Individuals with Disabilities Education Act, 20
Valente LM (2007) Maturational effects of the vestibular system: a study of rotary chair, computerized dynamic posturography, and vestibular evoked potentials with children. J Am Acad Audiol 18(6):461–481
Valente L (2011) Assessment techniques for vestibular evaluation in pediatric patients. Otolaryngol Clin N Am 44(2):273–290
Van Hecke V, Mundy P (2007) Neural systems and the development of gaze following and related joint attention skills. In: Flom R et al (eds) Gaze-following: its development and significance. Lawrence Erlbaum Associates, Mahwah, NJ, pp 17–51
Van Lierde KM, Vinck BM, Baudonck N et al (2005) Comparison of the overall intelligibility, articulation, resonance, and voice characteristics between children using cochlear implants and those using bilateral hearing aids: a pilot study. Int J Audiol 44(8):452–465
Van Maanen A, Stapells DR (2010) Multiple-ASSR thresholds in infants and young children with hearing loss. J Am Acad Audiol 21(8):535–545
Van Schrojenstein Lantman-de Valk HJM, Havemann MJ, Maaskant MA et al (1994) The need for assessment of sensory functioning in ageing people with mental handicap. J Intellect Disabil Res 38(Pt 3):289–298
Veiga KA, Porto AN, Matos FZ et al (2017) Caries experience and periodontal status in children and adolescents with cleft lip and palate. Pediatr Dent 39(2):139–144
Vermeulen AM, van Bon W, Schreuder R et al (2007) Reading comprehension of deaf children with cochlear implants. J Deaf Stud Deaf Educ 12(3):283302
Vettore MV, Sousa Campos AE (2011) Malocclusion characteristics of patients with cleft lip and/or palate. Eur J Orthod 33(3):311–317
Vong A, Funamura J (2018) Multidisciplinary management of oculo-auriculo-vertebral spectrum. Curr Opin Otolaryngol Head Neck Surg 26(4):234–241
Wagner R, Torgesen J, Rashotte C et al (1999) Comprehensive test of phonological processing. ProEd Publishing Co, Austin, TX
Wakil N, Fitzpatrick EM, Olds J et al (2014) Long-term outcome after cochlear implantation in children with additional developmental disabilities. Int J Audiol 53(9):587–594
Walger M, Mühler R, Hoth S (2014) In: Hoth S et al (eds) Objektive Audiometrie im Kindesalter. Springer, Berlin, pp 140–157
Waltzman SB, Scalchunes V, Cohen NL (2000) Performance of multiply handicapped children using cochlear implants. Am J Otol 21(3):329–335
Wang S, Yeh T, Chang C et al (2008) Consistent latencies of vestibular evoked myogenic potentials. Ear Hear 29(6):923–929
Wang CH, Lin YT, Lin YJ (2017) A survey of natal and neonatal teeth in newborn infants. J Formos Med Assoc 116(3):193–196

Watson CS, Kidd GR (2009) Associations between auditory abilities, reading, and other language skills in children and adults. In: Cacace AT, McFarland DJ (eds) Controversies in central auditory processing disorders. Plural Publishing, San Diego, pp 217–242

Wechsler D (2003) The Wechsler Intelligence Scale for children, 4th edn. The Psychological Corporation, San Antonio, TX

Wechsler D (2012) Wechsler Preschool and Primary Scale of Intelligence–IV (WPPSI-IV). The Psychological Corporation, San Antonio, TX (German version; Petermann F, Daseking M, 2018)

Wechsler D (2014) Wechsler Intelligence Scale for Children, 5th edn (WISC-V). Pearson, Bloomington, MN (German version: Petermann F, 2017)

Weerda H (2004) Chirurgie der Ohrmuschel. Verletzungen, Defekte und Anomalien. Thieme, Stuttgart, pp 105–226

Wegner O, Dau T (2002) Frequency specificity of chirp-evoked auditory brainstem responses. J Acoust Soc Am 111(3):1318–1329

Weisi F, Rezaei M, Rashedi V et al (2013) Comparison of reading skills between children with cochlear implants and children with typical hearing in Iran. Int J Pediatr Otorhinolaryngol 77(8):1317–1321

Wermker K, Jung S, Joos U et al (2014) Dental implants in cleft lip, alveolus, and palate patients: a systematic review. Int J Oral Maxillofac Implants 29(2):384–390

Wiig EH, Semel E, Secord WA (2013) Clinical evaluation of language fundamentals–fifth edition (CELF-5). Pearson, Ontario

Wilber LA (2002) Calibration: puretone, speech, and noise signals. In: Katz J (ed) Handbook of clinical audiology, 5th edn. Lippincott Williams & Wilkins, Philadelphia, pp 50–68

Wiley S, Arjmand E, Meinzen-Derr J et al (2011) Findings from multidisciplinary evaluation of children with permanent hearing loss. Int J Pediatr Otorhinolaryngol 75(8):1040–1044

Williams KT (2007) Expressive vocabulary test, 2nd edn. http://images.pearsonclinical.com/images/Products/EVT-II/evt2.pdf. Accessed 4 June 2017

Wilson WJ, Arnott W (2013) Using different criteria to diagnose (central) auditory processing disorder: how big a difference does it make? J Speech Lang Hear Res 56(1):63–70

Wilson PH, Henry J, Bowen M et al (1991) Tinnitus reaction questionnaire: psychometric properties of a measure of distress associated with tinnitus. J Speech Hear Res 34(1):197–201

Woodcock RW (1987) Woodcock reading mastery test. Teaching Resources. Revised edition. American Guidance Services, Circle Pines, Allen, TX

World Health Organization (1992) International statistical classification of diseases and related health problems, 10th revision (ICD-10). WHO, Geneva

World Health Organization (2001) International classification of functioning, disability and health (ICF). WHO, Geneva

World Health Organization (2007) International classification of functioning, disability and health—children and youth. WHO, Geneva

World Health Organization (2013) WHO methods and data sources for global burden of disease estimates 2000–2011. WHO, Geneva. http://www.who.int/healthinfo/statistics/GlobalDALYmethods_2000_2011.pdf. Accessed 4 Jan 2017

Worth V, Perry RT, Ireland T et al (2017) Are people with an orofacial cleft at a higher risk of dental caries? A systematic review and meta-analysis. Br Dent J 223(1):37–47

Wu CM, Lee LA, Chen CK et al (2015) Impact of cochlear nerve deficiency determined using 3-dimensional magnetic resonance imaging on hearing outcome in children with cochlear implants. Otol Neurotol 36(1):14–21

Yanbay E, Hickson L, Scarinci N et al (2014) Language outcomes for children with cochlear implants enrolled in different communication programs. Cochlear Implants Int 15(3):121–135

Yang T, Wei X, Chai Y et al (2013) Genetic etiology study of the non-syndromic deafness in Chinese Hans by targeted next-generation sequencing. Orphanet J Rare Dis 8:85

Yeung CY, Chu CH (2014) A review of the eruption of primary teeth. OA Dentistry 2(1):7

Yilmaz RB, Cakan DG, Mesgarzadeh N (2016) Prevalence and management of natal/neonatal teeth in cleft lip and palate patients. Eur J Dent 10(1):54–58

Yoshinaga-Itano C (2003) From screening to early identification and intervention: discovering predictors to successful outcomes for children with significant hearing loss. J Deaf Stud Deaf Educ 8(1):11–30

Yoshinaga-Itano C, Sedey A (2000) Early speech development in children who are deaf or hard of hearing: interrelationships with language and hearing. Volta Rev 100(5):181–211

Ziegler JC, Pech-Georgel C, George F et al (2005) Deficits in speech perception predict language learning impairment. Proc Natl Acad Sci USA 102(39):14110–14115. https://doi.org/10.1073/pnas.0504446102

Ziegler JC, Pech-Georgel C, George F et al (2009) Speech-perception-in-noise deficits in dyslexia. Dev Sci 12(5):732–745. https://doi.org/10.1111/j.1467-7687.2009.00817.x

Zigmond AS, Snaith RP (1983) The hospital anxiety and depression scale. Acta Psychiatr Scand 67(6):361–370

Zimmerman IL, Steiner VG, Pond E (2011) Preschool Language Scales–Fifth Edition (PLS-5). Pearson Assessments, San Antonio

Rehabilitation and Prognosis of Dysglossia, Resonance Disorders and Velopharyngeal Insufficiency

5

Antoinette am Zehnhoff-Dinnesen, Wolfgang Bigenzahn, Monika Brunner, Philippe H. Dejonckere, Ilter Denizoglu, Doris-Maria Denk-Linnert, Florent Destruhaut, Rémi Esclassan, Lynn Marty Grames, Alexander Hemprich, Jenö Hirschberg, Ariane Hohoff, Mehmet Akif Kilic, Seo Simon Ko, Karel Neubauer, Lenka Neubauerová, Emmanuelle Noirrit-Esclassan, Ute Pröschel, Karen J. Reichmuth, Saskia Rohrbach-Volland, Robert J. Shprintzen, and Thomas Stamm

Jenö Hirschberg was deceased at the time of publication.

Supplementary Information The online version contains supplementary material available at https://doi.org/10.1007/978-3-031-25175-7_5.

A. am Zehnhoff-Dinnesen (✉)
Department of Phoniatrics and Pedaudiology, University of Münster, University Hospital Münster, Münster, North-Rhine Westphalia, Germany
e-mail: am.zehnhoff@uni-muenster.de

W. Bigenzahn
Private Practice, Lazarettgasse 25/1. Stock A-1090 Vienna, Formerly Medical University of Vienna, Vienna, Austria
e-mail: wolfgang.bigenzahn@chello.at

M. Brunner
HNO Praxis am Neckar, Heidelberg, Germany
e-mail: info@monikabrunner.eu

P. H. Dejonckere
Federal Agency for Occupational Risks, Brussels, Belgium

I. Denizoglu
Vocology Center, Egesante Medical Center, Izmir, Turkey

Vocology Centre, Izmir, Turkiye

Speech Language Therapy, Tinaztepe University Faculty of Health Sciences, Izmir, Turkey

Main Art Division of Opera, Dokuz Eylül University State Conservatory Vocal Arts Department, Izmir, Turkey

D.-M. Denk-Linnert
Division of Phoniatrics and Speech Language Therapy, Department of Otorhinolaryngology, Vienna, Austria
e-mail: doris-maria.denk-linnert@meduni.wien.ac.at

F. Destruhaut
Faculté d'Odontologie de Toulouse, Unité fonctionnelle de Prothèse Maxillo-Faciale, Toulouse, France

A. am Zehnhoff-Dinnesen et al. (eds.), *Phoniatrics II*, European Manual of Medicine,
https://doi.org/10.1007/978-3-031-25175-7_5

5.1 Coordination and Monitoring of Rehabilitative Measures of Dysglossia, Resonance Disorders and Velopharyngeal Insufficiency[1]

Ute Pröschel, Seo Simon Ko, Antoinette am Zehnhoff-Dinnesen and Alexander Hemprich

5.1.1 Cooperation Within the Multidisciplinary Team

Optimal care for children with cleft lip and palate and their families requires a special multidisciplinary cleft team, e.g. in a cleft centre or coordinated in a network based on a defined care pathway. All team members should be experienced and qualified professionals from the medical, surgical, dental or allied health disciplines. They all should have a major commitment to the treatment of clefts. The inner circle of the cleft team should consist of a maxillofacial surgeon, an orthodontist, a speech and language therapist and phoniatrician, an ENT surgeon, a pedaudiologist and a psychologist. The extended team should include an obstetrician, a geneticist, a paediatric dentist, a restorative dentist, a prosthodontist, a paediatrician, maxillofacial and dental technicians. Additionally, it is of great help to involve nurses who are specially trained in the feeding of children with clefts and dietitians to ensure macronutrient intake (Frederick et al. 2022) Assistance of a social worker should be offered. The cleft team should keep in touch with a regional support group where possible.

[1]Equal first authorship of all four authors

R. Esclassan
School of Dental Medicine, Department of Oral Rehabilitation, Marseille, France
e-mail: remi.esclassan@univ-amu.fr

L. M. Grames
Cleft Palate and Craniofacial Institute, St. Louis Children's Hospital, St. Louis, MO, USA

A. Hemprich
Maxillofacial and Facial Plastic Surgery, University of Leipzig, Leipzig, Germany
e-mail: hemprich@medizin.uni-leipzig.de

J. Hirschberg
Division of Pediatric Otorhinolaryngology and Bronchology, Saint John's Hospital, Budapest, Hungary

A. Hohoff
Department of Orthodontics, Medical Faculty of the University of Münster, University Hospital of Münster, Münster, Germany
e-mail: hohoffa@uni-muenster.de

M. A. Kilic
Department of Otorhinolaryngology, University of Health Sciences, Istanbul, Turkiye

S. S. Ko

HNO Praxis Rotkreuz, Rotkreuz, Switzerland
e-mail: hnorotkreuz@hin.ch

K. Neubauer
Clinic of Phoniatrics of University Hospital Prague, Charles University Faculty of Medicine, Prague, Czech Republic
e-mail: Karel.Neubauer@lf1.cuni.cz

L. Neubauerová
Philosophical Faculty of the University of Hradec Králové, Institute of Social Work, Hradek Kralova, Czech Republic
e-mail: lenka.neubauerova@uhk.cz

E. Noirrit-Esclassan
School of Dental Medicine, Department of Oral Rehabilitation, Marseille, France
e-mail: emmanuelle.noirrit@univ-amu.fr

U. Pröschel
Institute for Phoniatrics and Pedaudiology, Vestische Children's and Adolescents' Clinic, Datteln, Germany
e-mail: u.proeschel@kinderklinik-datteln.de

K. J. Reichmuth
Clinic of Phoniatrics and Pedaudiology, University Hospital Muenster, Münster, Germany
e-mail: karen.reichmuth@ukmuenster.de

S. Rohrbach-Volland
Praxis für HNO, Phoniatrie & Pädaudiologie, Berlin, Germany
e-mail: saskia@everskin.ch

R. J. Shprintzen
The Virtual Center for Velo-Cardio-Facial Syndrome, Manlius, NY, USA
e-mail: robert.schprintzen@vcfscenter.org

T. Stamm
Department of Orthodontics, Medical Faculty of the University of Münster, University Hospital of Münster, Münster, Germany
e-mail: stammt@uni-muenster.de

The special needs of each individual child and its family have to be respected. The parents or persons in charge of the child with the cleft should get accurate information about the cleft, its type, possible additional anomalies, the functional consequences, feeding methods and the treatment protocol. The information addressing the functional consequences should include information about the hearing, the speech, the teeth and jaws, possible problems in midfacial growth and the overall appearance of adolescents and adults with clefts. The latter may be accompanied by pre- and post-operative photographs of other patients with similar clefts. As well as obtaining the overall information, the parents should have the possibility to address their inquiries to the specialist of the field involved. Questions about the hearing should be answered by the ENT specialist or the pedaudiologist, questions about speech and language development should be addressed to the speech therapist and the phoniatrician.

The possible causes for the cleft should be listed and genetic advice should be offered if necessary. The verbal information should be supported by other material such as an information booklet from the cleft team, or a brochure from the cleft parent group. The psychologist should provide support to the parents in the grieving process, with the possible feelings of guilt and how to handle the reactions from others.

The care pathways of different cleft teams often differ in the timing of the surgical procedures. The parents or persons in charge of the children should be introduced to the generally planned procedures and the timeframe for treatment. Before each surgical measure the parents should be informed about the planned procedures, the approximate duration of the operation, the anaesthesiological concept, the postoperative pain management, the expected postsurgical recovery process, the duration of the hospitalisation and the care required after surgery.

Nearly all patients with cleft palate suffer from serous middle ear infections before the closure of the cleft of the soft palate. Owing to the middle ear problems, newborn hearing screening will often be conspicuous and additional inner ear hearing loss cannot be excluded before the insertion of grommets. Therefore, an ENT and audiological assessment should be carried out before the first operation is done. If a serious otitis media is found, the anaesthesia of the cleft operation should be used for the insertion of the grommets, too. The parents need to be informed about the procedure and the required postoperative care in this regard.

If inner ear hearing loss cannot be ruled out before the insertion of grommets, owing to the middle ear infection, there should be a hearing test 4–6 weeks after the operation.

However, even after the cleft of the soft palate is closed, some children will continue to have middle ear affections regularly after the grommets have been extruded. Thus, a continuous ENT and audiological assessment is necessary at least every six months during early childhood. Depending on the individual number of middle ear problems up to school age, the intervals may than be prolonged.

Serous otitis media always causes a more or less severe conductive hearing loss. If this lasts for more than 3 or 6 months per year, speech development may be affected. Persisting serous otitis media may also result in chronic middle ear infections, especially cholesteatomas. Therefore, grommets should be inserted again in case of persisting middle ear infections.

Before every maxillofacial operation the middle ear, its function and hearing of the cleft patient should be assessed in order to combine the operation and the insertion of grommets, if necessary, to reduce the number of operations under anaesthesia necessary for the child. In some cases the insertion of grommets may not be possible or advisable. Then an existing conductive hearing loss has to be compensated by properly adjusted hearing aids.

While the child with the cleft is growing up, speech development should be monitored and speech therapy should be initiated if necessary. Special attention needs to be given to a possible nasality of the speech. In case the comprehension of the child's speech is still considerably reduced owing to nasality at a pre-school age, velopharyngeal function needs to be assessed and possible surgical measures have to be discussed with the parents. In certain cases an adenotomy or even a tonsillectomy may sometimes be necessary before a velopharyngoplasty. Parents need to be informed about the possible development of postoperative nasality if their child has to undergo adenotomy or tonsillectomy for medical reasons. This is a common risk after these operations. However, the risk factor is clearly increased in patients with clefts of the soft palate.

If in adolescents or in young adults the maxillofacial surgeon plans a maxillary advancement, the cleft patient and his parents need to be informed that nasality may occur after the operation. The incidence of nasality cannot be predicted by evaluating velopharyngeal function. In some cases even pre-operatively existing nasality disappears. Most likely this is due to the reorganisation of the motor patterns and the changes in kinaesthetic feedback.

Table 5.1 gives an overview of the timing of the different procedures, but individual needs of the patient have to be considered. For further details, see e.g. information on the website of the American Cleft Palate–Craniofacial Association (2021) and Mink van der Molen et al. (2021).

In case of need, other or additional surgery may be indicated: e.g. repair of submucous cleft palate, correction of non-cleft Velopharyngeal Dysfunction (VPD), postoperative VPI, tonsillectomy/adenoidectomy, secondary surgeries, such as fistula repair.

5.1.2 Challenges to the Phoniatrician

The multidisciplinary nature of rehabilitative measures in dysglossia, resonance disorders and velopharyngeal insufficiency requires interdisciplinary exchange of medical and therapeutic reports, round table meetings with case conferences, or videoconferences between the experts. In the interdisciplinary context, one of the tasks of the phoniatrician may be to monitor the path from an anatomically determined point of view to a functionally orientated approach. Dealing with the upper respiratory and digestive tracts, the phoniatrician knows how orofacial and pharyngolaryngeal functions secure life and communication, interaction and ensure socialisation of the individual (Stelzig 2019). He works in close cooperation with the speech therapist, the dentist/maxillofacial surgeon and ENT professional. The provision of information and advice to parents or carers is essential.

A thorough head and neck examination, including perceptual evaluation scales and velopharyngeal closure measurements, must be performed to detect organic abnormalities, craniofacial dysmorphisms (cleft palate) or any syndromic stigmata. The assessment has to clarify whether nasal emissions are present in all non-nasal consonants, with any nasality related to a short or poorly moving palate or an excessively deep pharynx; whether nasal obstruction is related to enlarged adenoids and whether articulation errors are related to severe dysglossia or

Table 5.1 Overview on the timing of therapeutic measures (based on Cleveland Clinic 2018; NHS 2019; Mink van der Molen et al. 2021; ASHA 2022)

Birth to 6 weeks: feeding support (oral feeding as soon as possible), advice to parents, audiological testing, paediatric assessment, assessment of comorbidities
Birth to 3 months: as possible preparation of cleft lip surgery lip taping; nasal-alveolar moulding (NAM) (so far no evidence for long term benefits yet); devices for the gentle alignment of maxillary segments
3–6 months: first surgery cleft lip; nasal tip elevation
Control of middle ear status, if necessary insertion of grommets, combined with cleft surgery, often with cleft palate closure
Hearing tests 4–6 weeks after insertion of grommets to exclude combined inner ear hearing loss, otoscopy and audiological monitoring every 3–6 months, if necessary repetition of insertion of grommets, hearing aid supply
6–12 months: cleft palate surgery
Monitoring speech and language development to clarify indication of speech therapy; diagnosis of velopharyngeal insufficiency after primary palate repair and 6 months of speech therapy without adequate achievement
Monitoring hearing function and middle ear status every 6 months in early childhood, later depending on individual need prolonged intervals; at least until age of 5–6 years
5 years: in case of need surgical correction of velopharyngeal insufficiency (VPI)
In educational settings in case of permanent hearing loss Personal FM (Frequency Modulated) System transmitting audio signals by wireless radio frequencies or Bluetooth System
6(8)–10(12) years: alveolar bone grafting in case of a residual cleft alveolus, orthodontic treatment; dental hygiene
7–8 years: possibly palatal expansion
From early teenage years on: jaw orthopaedics and further different orthodontic measures; when adult teeth have erupted, control of facial growth
16–18 years in females, 18–21 years in males: orthognathic surgery; mostly maxillary advancement, in difficult cases bimaxillary procedures
Offer of genetic counselling (best before first surgery), assistance of a social worker and psychological support

dental malocclusions that require physical management (Brigger et al. 2009).

Functional exercises should be tried as a basic step according to symptoms, and their progression complemented with prosthetic and surgical approaches; in severe cases communication aids as a form of Augmentative and Alternative Communication (AAC) have to be applied. The main objective in treating speech disorders is to achieve correct articulation, adequate velopharyngeal function and normal oral-nasal resonance, in order to reduce this peculiarity in everyday life and its consequences for the quality of life. As distinctive features in language and speech development emerge in the toddler and preschool-age child, it is important to distinguish between speech disorders that are developmental, obligatory (related to structural deviations) and compensatory (learned articulation errors) (Brigger et al. 2009). When children with dysglossia, cleft or non-cleft velopharyngeal problems display articulation errors and resonance abnormalities, the developmentally appropriate articulation issues are addressed first, after elimination of compensatory misarticulations. Later, therapy also has to regard possible phonological errors (ASHA 2022).

When judging the potential for rehabilitation and establishing an attainable therapeutic goal, the following questions have to be addressed:

- When should speech therapy begin?
- How long should speech therapy take?
- What form of therapy should be taken?
- What are the principles, contents and goals of the speech therapy?

An early start of oral motor function-orientated speech therapy is desirable. Regular monitoring of the progress of functional exercises is of decisive relevance. Follow-up intervals of three to six months may be recommended, including paedaudiological and phoniatric assessments such as re-evaluation of the orofacial and pharyngolaryngeal situation, oro- and naso-pharynx, jaw and temporomandibular joints, and the dental apparatus in terms of morphology and functionality. The primary objectives are speech (articulation, nasality), food intake (biting, chewing, coughing, swallowing) and respiration. The benefit and necessity of speech therapeutic measures are of equal value as non-conservative and such conservative treatments as physiotherapy or psychotherapy.

An accompanying intensive functional exercise therapy of sufficient duration is obligatory, which depends on the following prognostic factors:

5.1.2.1 Communicative Strategies

Within speech therapy, the patient should acquire communicative strategies adapted to his speech intelligibility, his personality and psychosocial surroundings that can have essential influence on the course of the therapy.

5.1.2.2 Patient Motivation

The patient needs thorough advice and information about the nature of his disease and the therapeutic principles to become sustainably motivated. Suitable corrective techniques have to be carved out. All therapeutic measures need close cooperation with his parents or carers.

It must be guaranteed that qualified therapists are accessible to the patient (Schröter-Morasch and Ziegler 2005).

Case Study 5.1

The following case study describes a family's journey in finding the right specialist for an assessment and then in ensuring the appropriate input to meet the identified needs of their daughter.

A family reported early concerns centred on their baby's tongue, which seemed large, and then on her failure to meet most developmental milestones within the first 12 months. The child failed to produce adequate words or put anything in her mouth. The patient saw a paediatrician who described her as 'developmentally delayed' and referred her to a number of specialists: neurology, ENT, geneticist; but none of them came up with anything conclusive. At the age of two and a half years the patient's tongue still tended to hang out of her mouth and dribble ran down her chin. Because of her tongue and additional swallowing problems, she was referred to a phoniatrician.

The phoniatrician ruled out problems associated with swallowing but suspected oromotor dysfunction with dyspractical components that affected the ability to make and coordinate the movement of the tongue and lips etc. The patient had trouble sticking out her tongue or moving it from side to side and was still drooling. She took extra time to form words while speaking and used mostly vowel sounds ('aah-aah' instead of 'mama'). Furthermore, she refused to eat food that needs to be chewed. She did not only have a large tongue, but also did not know how to use it properly. The phoniatrician recommended weekly speech and language therapy.

The specialist assessments and therapeutic interventions included a tactile-kinaesthetic approach to guide her articulators (jaw, tongue, lips) manually through a targeted word, phrase or sentence. The technique developed motor control and the development of proper oral muscular movements, while eliminating unnecessary muscle movements, such as jaw sliding and inadequate lip rounding.

She additionally underwent exercises, such as smiling, pursing, blowing bubbles and performing lip massage to target lip mobility for the production of speech sounds involving the lips, such as /p/, /b/ and /m/. The specialist therapy worked well, and by the time the patient could keep her tongue in her mouth, she no longer dribbled and could say increasingly more understandable words.

5.2 Therapy for Active/Compensatory Misarticulations in Children with Cleft Palate or Velopharyngeal Dysfunction: A Motor Learning Approach

Lynn Marty Grames

5.2.1 Introduction

Children born with clefts of the palate, with or without cleft lip, and children with congenital velopharyngeal dysfunction (as frequently seen in the 22q11.2 Deletion Syndrome) may begin to babble and progress through the earliest stages of speech sound development with the inability to close the velopharynx. Nasalisation of oral stops, or sometimes fricatives, is common and is usually corrected with surgical correction of the palatal cleft, which is designed to separate fully the nose from the mouth and reconstruct the velopharyngeal mechanism. As many as 40% of children born with cleft palate, with or without cleft lip, may never require any speech therapy (Yen et al. 2017).

It is believed that some children, in an attempt to replicate the stops and fricatives of their primary language in the absence of velopharyngeal closure, develop alternative motor patterns for sound production that become a part of their phonological system, and then persist after the palate has been reconstructed. These are referred to as active misarticulations in Europe, Asia, Australia and New Zealand, or compensatory misarticulations in North America. Active/Compensatory Misarticulations (A/CMs) can render a child's speech poorly intelligible and are often considered challenging to treat. The estimated prevalence of these articulations varies widely across studies, but because they primarily occur in individuals with cleft palate or congenital velopharyngeal dysfunction, they are not routinely seen in the caseloads of paediatric speech-language pathologists (SLPs).

A/CMs are misarticulations that can, and should, be treated. Correction will not only normalise the child's speech intelligibility, but in some cases is needed for the medical team to make a decision about whether or not secondary surgery for velopharyngeal dysfunction is required.

5.2.2 What Are Active/Compensatory Misarticulations (A/CMs)?

Trost (1981) compiled a seminal description of the most commonly occurring A/CMs. Other authors have expanded and refined the list and definitions over time. The A/CMs most often seen and described are as follows:

- **Glottal Stop**: The airstream is stopped at the glottis as a consonant. If the airstream is forcefully stopped, a glottal plosive may result. The glottal stop may be the most common of the A/CMs. It may replace voiced or voiceless stops but may also replace fricatives. Henningsson and Isberg (1986, 1991) demonstrated that the velopharynx does not close when glottal stops are articulated, even in the presence of a fully functional velopharynx.
- **Pharyngeal Stop**: The pharyngeal stop may be voiced or voiceless, and is produced with the base of the tongue moving in a posterior vector to stop the airstream against the posterior pharyngeal wall. In some anatomical conditions, the tongue base may push the epiglottis against the posterior pharyngeal wall to produce the stop consonant. Whether or not the epiglottis is involved, the perceptual result is indistinguishable to the common ear, and the treatment techniques do not differ. Pharyngeal stops usually replace oral stop consonants.
- **Pharyngeal Fricative**: Pharyngeal fricatives can be voiced or voiceless and are produced in a lingual gesture similar to that of the pharyngeal stop, except that the air stream is constricted, rather than stopped, at the posterior pharyngeal wall. Garcia et al. (2014) demonstrated that velopharyngeal closure is reduced when pharyngeal fricatives are produced, but Eshghi et al. (2018), using Nasal RAM cannulas for analysis, suggested that velopharyngeal closure can occur on pharyngeal fricatives.
- **Nasal Fricative**: This is a fricative produced by forcing air through the nose. Zajac (2015) produced a detailed description of these articulations. Zajac characterised two types of nasal fricative: anterior and posterior. The anterior nasal fricative is produced with an open velopharynx, with frication occurring at the nares. Nasal grimacing may occur as a result of the attempt to produce frication at the nares. The posterior nasal fricative is produced with the air stream constricted at the partly-closed velopharynx, resulting in the characteristic nasal turbulent sound. As nasal fricatives are nasal consonants, the velopharynx does not close when nasal fricatives are produced.
- **Mid-dorsum Palatal Stop**: The mid-dorsum palatal stop is an oral stop consonant that often replaces [t,d], but that has also been described as replacing [k,g]. As described, the dorsum of the tongue stops the airstream at mid-palate, with elevation similar to that of [j]. While some describe the mid-dorsum palatal stop as developing in response to a palatal fistula, certainly not all children who develop mid-dorsum palatal stops have fistulas. The mid-dorsum palatal stop has been described as sounding like a cross between a lingua-alveolar stop and a lingua-velar stop. Others have described it as a distorted lingua-alveolar stop, almost as if [t,d] could be laterally distorted.
- **Ingressive Fricatives**: These are fricatives produced with an airstream that is ingressive, rather than egressive: the speaker is inhaling, rather than exhaling when the fricative is produced. Articulator placement may be accurate, or it may be inaccurate, and the fricative may be oral or nasal. The key feature is the direction of the airflow with which the fricative is produced. Ingressive fricatives can have an adverse effect on the fluency of speech because of the rapid shifts in airflow needed to use ingressive fricatives in rapid running speech.

While A/CMs may have their origin in the child's structural disorder, they do not generally correct spontaneously when the structural disorder is corrected. The child continues to use the learned motor pattern in linguistically appropriate ways. Unfortunately, because some of the A/CMs (glottal stops, nasal fricatives, pharyngeal fricatives) are produced with the velopharynx open, the child who uses these misarticulations may be inappropriately diagnosed with velopharyngeal dysfunction. Inappropriate diagnosis can lead to unnecessary surgery or delayed articulation therapy, both undesirable outcomes. The use of glottal stops, nasal fricatives or pharyngeal fricatives in an instrumental assessment of any kind would invalidate the assessment of velopharyngeal function, in the same way that use of nasal consonants would not yield a valid assessment of velopharyngeal function.

It is worth noting that all of these A/CMs, with the possible exception of the ingressive fricatives, are posterior to target, meaning that they occur somewhere posterior to the desired place of articulation. For children with multiple A/CMs, the therapeutic course may involve starting at the front of the mouth, and working posteriorly, in order not to continue reinforcing posterior articulation. This would mean that the process of developing consonants may not follow typical developmental trajectories. For example, consonants such as [s, z,ʃ, ʒ] and affricates might be taught and habituated before [k,g].

Ruscello and Vallino (2014) referred to these A/CMs as errors of motor learning. The child has the linguistic representation for the consonant but is using the incorrect motor pattern. Consequently, a language-based approach to therapy for these consonants, which is conducted without actually teaching the child to produce the correct motor pattern, may fail.

5.2.3 A Brief Motor Learning Overview

Ruscello and Vallino (2014) provide a succinct description of the motor learning process for speech sound therapy. The objectives of motor learning, according to the authors, are to:

1. Teach a new motor pattern (skilled movement)
2. Refine the motor pattern for optimal spatial and temporal control within the oral cavity
3. Enable practice with increasing rate and complexity
4. Advance from conscious to subconscious control

Ultimately, we want the child to be able to call up the motor pattern for the target speech sound easily and automatically, without having to think about it.

The first stage is the *Verbal-Cognitive stage*, which includes the teaching required to distinguish the desirable motor pattern from the undesired motor pattern, and all the pedagogy that is needed to teach the consonant in isolation. This includes teaching the child the names for the parts of the mouth that may be used in the teaching or cueing process, the reason that a new sound needs to be taught, and the teaching of the consonant itself in isolation.

The second stage is the *Motor stage*. It is in this stage that the new motor skill is refined spatially and temporally with continued practice. The practice is largely imitative, and decontextualised, meaning that it is done without adding linguistic load. It is desirable for the target motor pattern to become easy, automatic and readily called upon before linguistic load is added. An important objective of the motor stage is for the child to develop mastery of the motor skill without reliance on feedback: the child must be able to self-monitor.

Block practice is often used early in the motor stage. In block practice, syllables, words or phrases that each contain one or more tokens of the target, are practised one after another. This is useful for building motor pattern. Later, random practice is a useful addition to enhance refinement and retention. In random practice, some of the syllables, words or phrases do not contain any tokens of the target. This allows the child to enhance and fine tune the motor skill by practising when *not* to use it, and to be able to self-identify when the target is needed, when it is not needed, and if the production was correct.

The final stage of motor learning is the *Autonomous Stage*. It is in this stage that the motor skill is transferred from imitative practice to self-generated speech. Word and phrase imitation may be advanced to picture-naming or single-word question response (both are word-retrieval tasks, and by definition of a higher level of cognitive-linguistic complexity). Description and completion activities may follow. In addition, increased sequencing complexity may also be introduced, such as clusters and front–back contrasts, skills that will be needed for successful transfer to spontaneous speech.

5.2.4 Choosing and Facilitating Targets

In order for motor learning to be effective, one must teach the target consonant as a new motor pattern. Modelling alone will not facilitate motor learning. Facilitation of the consonant in isolation can often be accomplished by identifying appropriately articulated consonants that are already in the child's inventory, and using those to shape desired targets. For example, [b] can be taught from [m] with the nose plugged, and [p] can be facilitated by whispering [b]. Likewise, [d,t] can be shaped from [n]; [s,z] can be taught be prolonging [t,d], or by retracting from interdental placement as one would use for [θ]; [g,k] can be taught from [ŋ]. Other consonants, such as [m,f,v,θ], are generally easy to teach via direct imitation with verbal instruction.

5.2.5 Application of Motor Learning Principles in Treatment of Active/Compensatory Misarticulations

Case Study 5.2

It may be useful to examine a case study to see what motor learning looks like in therapy for a child with A/CMs. Our patient Mack had a history of cleft palate with micrognathia (Pierre Robin sequence). The micrognathia was treated in the neonatal period, but owing to his history of airway difficulties, the one-stage cleft palate repair was delayed until he was nearly fifteen months of age. He had bilateral myringotomies with ventilation tubes (grommets) placed in his tympanic membranes at the same time as his cleft repair to treat chronic middle ear effusions.

Early intervention skills included language stimulation. At 21 months of age, he presented with an intact palate (no fistula). Hearing sensitivity was normal bilaterally. Receptive language skills were age-appropriate. He used multisyllabic utterances to request, negate and comment, but was unintelligible to most listeners. His consonant inventory at the time consisted of [m,h,ŋ] as well as anterior and posterior nasal fricatives. He had no oral consonants of any kind, so there was no way to determine if his velopharynx was functional for speech purposes.

The first targets chosen were [p,b], as they were anterior, oral, easily visible, and would give us the earliest glimpse into his velopharyngeal function. His inventory already included [m], which could be used to facilitate production of [p,b]. Therapy began at 22 months of age and was conducted 1:1 for 60 min/week, with 45 min spent in direct treatment, then the mother joined for the last 15 min to observe, to calibrate listening and to discuss the home practice activity for that week.

5.2.5.1 Early Therapy: The Verbal Cognitive Stage

The verbal cognitive stage began with introduction to the therapy room, therapy procedures, and to help Mack learn that therapy time was fun. Age-appropriate picture story books with [p,b]-loaded words were introduced and read during each session. The therapist introduced 'nose sounds' by producing nasal fricatives, and 'mouth sounds' by producing [p,b], and explaining that talking with mouth sounds was good, because people would know what you were saying. Words that the therapist was going to be using in therapy were reviewed, such as nose, mouth and lips. An important skill that was taught was imitation of the therapist's actions. Mack was rewarded by earning pieces of puzzles or parts of Mr. Potato Head by imitating the therapist: first, gross motor actions, then fine motor, then mouth movements. Once he understood that he could have fun and be rewarded for imitating the therapist, consonant teaching could begin in earnest. For Mack, all of this was accomplished in one session.

He needed one more skill before we could begin teaching the consonant. He needed to learn to plug his nose. Since he was using nasal fricatives, nose plugging provided an easy way to 'turn off' the undesired articulatory path (the nose) in favour of the target path: the oral cavity. The nose plugging technique illustrated in Fig. 5.1 is useful in therapy and can be preferable to commercial nose plugs or to the therapist plugging the child's nose. It allows the child control over the nose plugging, and allows the therapist to see what the child's mouth is doing. It also allows the therapist to ascertain that the nose is completely plugged.

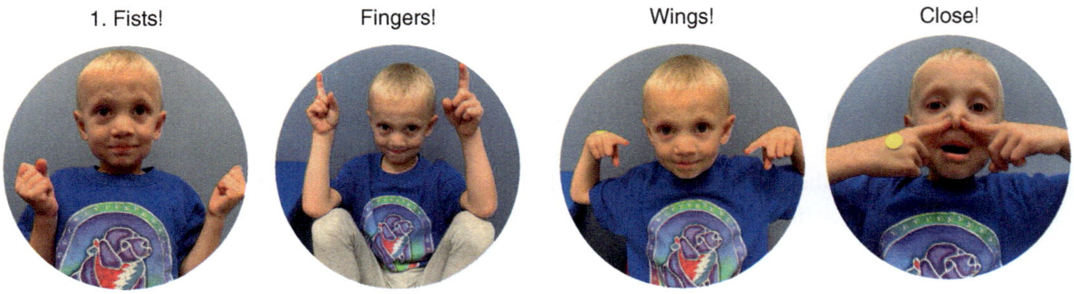

Fig. 5.1 The steps for teaching a child to plug their own nose. This technique, developed by Mary Blount Stahl at St. Louis Children's Hospital, is useful for giving the child control over nose plugging, and also allows the therapist to see the child's mouth, as well as their nose (©Marty Grames 2021. All photos used with parent permission)

As [b] is bilabial, the bilabial [m] was chosen as a facilitating context. First, Mack imitated [mamama] in slow, stretched repetitions. Then, [m] was continued, but the nose was plugged, to force an oral production. This established [bababaa], and much praise and excitement followed. Reading the age-appropriate picture story books with [p,b]-loaded words continued during each session. 100 consecutive correct productions are a useful way to solidify a simple motor pattern. Mack produced 10 tokens of the target, received a reward, and repeated until 100 accurate tokens were obtained. Whispering ensued to teach [pa], and this syllable was also practised until 100 correct productions were obtained. Home practice consisted of 'Give me 5!' with parent asking the child to produce five correct tokens at various times during the day. This allowed for short, but regular practice of the new skill.

5.2.5.2 The Motor Stage: Syllable Imitation

New vowels were introduced, so that [p,b] were practised in consonant-vowel (CV), vowel consonant (VC) and CVCV combinations. As his facility increased to more than 80% accuracy with syllable imitation, accurate imitated syllables were pushed immediately to word imitation: boo, boot, oob, tube, ooboo, booboo. However, syllable imitation did not stop until 100% accuracy was obtained. Ceasing work on skills that are foundational to speech production too soon can lead to carry-over problems later on. Home practice activities included syllable imitation, for example: ba, ab, baba, pa, ap, papa. Later in the day, parents would pick another vowel, and practice the same pattern. They were encouraged to do these very short practices four times per day.

5.2.5.3 Weaning from the Nose Plug

Once facility with syllable imitation was established, we attempted weaning from the nose plug. There are several ways one can attempt weaning. One method is to simply take the fingers off the nose, telling the child, 'see if you can make it just the same'. Another method is removing one finger first, so that only one side is plugged, practice that way for a while, and then remove the other finger. A third way is to gradually move the fingers up the nose to the bony aspect, at which point one can no longer close the nares. In Mack's case, we attempted the first method. He had developed a strong sense of the sound and feel of the targets [p,b], and was able to replicate them accurately, with good plosion, without the nose plugging. This was our first indication that Mack's velopharynx was capable of normal function. Had nasalisation occurred without the nose plug, we would have planned velopharyngeal imaging studies as soon as he was behaviourally ready and had accurate productions consistently for [p,b] at the phrase imitation level. But since he was capable of good plosion, we were able to continue therapy without nose plugging until it was time to teach a new oral consonant.

Word imitation followed syllable imitation, and words with the target in all positions were used, rather than focusing on a single position at once. No pictures are objects were used at this stage, so as not to advance linguistic complexity until the motor pattern was stable. However, some of the words that we imitated were words from the story books that we read each session. Home practice included words from a printed list, three times each (correctly), and parents were encouraged to practise a few words three times each four times per day.

As facility with word imitation increased, the words were pushed to phrases: ball, big ball, purple ball or baby, baby boy, baby girl. The last phrase is an example of the introduction of randomisation, adding words that do not contain the target, while the previous phrases are characteristic of block practice.

5.2.5.4 The Autonomous Stage

Once accuracy with phrase imitation was complete, we began to add linguistic load. Because we had a variety of picture story books with vocabulary that we had already practised in imitation, we had ready-made opportunities for picture naming (a word retrieval task), single word question response, simple sentence completion, and question response requiring more complex utterances, up to the child's level of linguistic sophistication. Figure 5.2 shows a diagram of the motor learning process for teaching a single consonant or an allophonic consonant pair from beginning to transfer to spontaneous speech.

For Mack, once [p,b] were established in spontaneous speech as best we could tell with our therapy tasks and parent report, we were ready to move to another allophonic pair of consonants. We taught [n], as it was not in his inventory, and once [n] was established in syllable imitation, we plugged the nose, and used the previously-described methods to teach [t,d], and used the motor learning approach to advance and transfer to spontaneous speech. Once [t,d] were established, we had an excellent foundation for facilitating [s,z]. After [s,z], we moved to [f,v], then to [ʃ,ʒ,t͡ʃ,d͡ʒ]. As mother was concerned that there could be psychosocial issues, we even addressed [l,ɾ,θ] at age five. Mack achieved fully normal speech by the time he began kindergarten, the first level of school. He did not require any secondary velopharyngeal management.

5.2.6 The Motor Learning Approach for an Older Child

The methods and pathway that are followed for a very young child, such as Mack, are essentially the same for an older child, but the activities and reinforcers are adapted to the child's age and interests. The motor stage is still imitative, in order to build a motor programme that the child can call up easily and automatically each time, so that when linguistic load is added, the child has the desired motor pattern ready to use.

If the child can read, word reading may be added at the same time that picture naming tasks are added in the autonomous stage. It is still advisable to use therapeutic activities that include picture naming alone, and word reading alone, so that both word retrieval and word attack skills can be addressed. As the child advances through the autonomous stage, reading activities

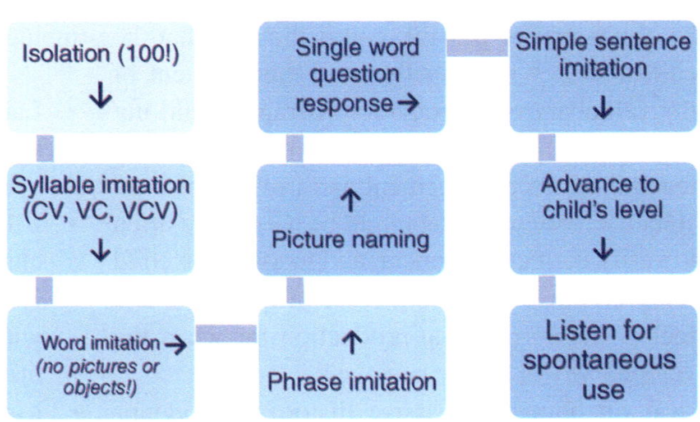

Fig. 5.2 The progression of the motor learning approach for a single consonant or allophonic pair in a young child. The shading of blocks reflects the three stages of motor learning (©Marty Grames 2021)

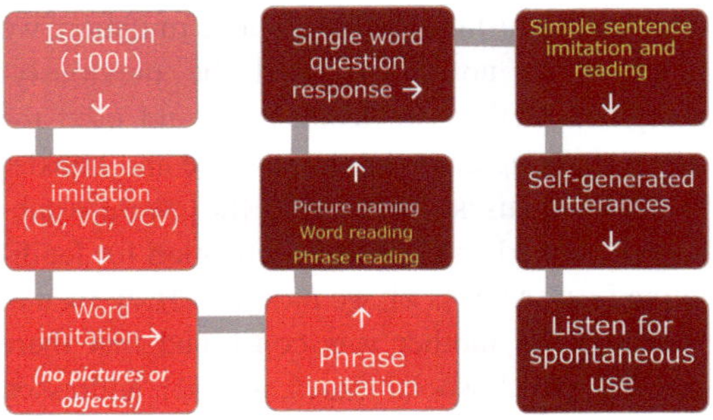

Fig. 5.3 The progression of the motor learning approach for a single consonant or allophonic pair in an older, literate child. The shading of blocks reflects the three stages of motor learning (©Marty Grames 2021)

can be used as well as more generative non-reading activities to promote transfer to spontaneous speech. Figure 5.3 shows a diagram of the motor learning process for a child who is able to read.

Additional information on motor learning approaches for children with cleft palate can be found in Hanley et al. (2023) as well as Kotlarek and Krueger (2023).

5.2.7 The Motor Learning Approach for the Child with Velopharyngeal Dysfunction

The methods and pathway that have been discussed above will still apply for the child who proves to have true velopharyngeal dysfunction. This may be discerned when the child weans from the nose plug, but despite best efforts reverts to nasalisation, or exhibits concomitant nasal emission with the accurate consonant production. In this case, we would consider the distortion to be obligatory, or passive, and is the sign that the child requires investigation and management of the velopharynx. Articulation therapy would not stop at this juncture. Therapy can continue to teach the correct placement and use for the consonants. Nose plugging might be used more often to verify correct placement, and to assist the child in developing an ongoing sense of the sound and feel of the correct oral production for when the velopharynx is finally managed.

If an obligatory/passive distortion is identified, there is no point in trying to force the child into making plosion. There have been instances of this occurring, in which the child developed a glottal stop co-production in order to approximate plosion. This resulted in a new, undesirable behaviour, which also had to be corrected with therapy. If obligatory/passive distortions occur, they should be accepted, as long as articulatory placement is correct, and a plan made for velopharyngeal assessment and management.

Speech therapy will correct articulation disorder, including those A/CMs that may sound like velopharyngeal dysfunction (glottal stops, nasal fricatives, pharyngeal fricatives). Speech therapy does not correct true velopharyngeal dysfunction.

5.2.8 Adaptive Articulations in Children with Craniofacial Differences

Children with oral structural differences, such as anterior crossbite, anterior open bite, significant anterior overjet or macroglossia, may produce consonants that *sound* accurate, but *appear* different if you are looking at the speaker's face. For example, some children with significant anterior crossbite may use an inverted labiodental production for [f,v] because this is an easier way to produce the accurate sound given the demands of rapid running speech. In the inverted labiodental production, the airstream is constricted with the lower incisors meeting the upper lip, instead of the usual upper incisors meeting the lower lip. It *sounds* exactly right but *looks* different. The key feature of adaptive articulations is that they sound completely normal if you are not looking at the speaker's face.

Other examples of adaptive articulations may include:

- Labio-dental productions for [p,b,m] in a child with lip incompetence or severe anterior overjet
- Bilabial fricative productions for [f,v] in a child with severe anterior crossbite
- Interdental placement for [t,d,s,z] in a child with severe anterior crossbite, open bite, or macroglossia
- Lingua-labial productions for [p,b,m] in a child with macroglossia

There is disagreement in the literature as to whether these articulations should be classified as compensatory for the oral structure (Golding-Kushner (2001) called them compensatory adaptations) or obligatory because of the oral structure (Peterson-Falzone et al. 2017 referred to them as adaptive oral misarticulations but classified them as obligatory). The classification may be important for research purposes, but likely makes little difference with regard to clinical functions. Are they truly misarticulations if they sound appropriate?

Three other questions occur with regard to adaptive articulations: first, should they be corrected if they occur naturally? The answer is likely not, as they are the child's best, and acoustically appropriate, articulatory adaptation to meet the demands of rapid running speech. Correcting to typical placement might not only be challenging but may result in a motor pattern that is unsustainable for rapid running speech. Second, will they require therapy for correction when the structure is corrected? The answer is usually not, as the child typically reorganises the motor pattern to adapt to the new structure once correction is made, without requiring further therapy. Third, are there instances when adaptive articulation should be taught? This may depend on specific situations, but the answer here could be yes.

For example, Jackson, aged 7, had bilateral complete cleft lip and palate and severe anterior crossbite. He used a nasal fricative as a substitution for [f,v], which required correction. He was capable of producing the traditional placement, but only with a slow rate, and with obvious facial strain. Consequently, a decision was made to teach a [f,v] as bilabial fricatives, a form of adaptive articulation. Jackson was able to eliminate the nasal fricative substitution, and to use the bilabial [f,v] in an acoustically, perceptually accurate way in rapid running speech without facial strain. In this instance, the decision to teach an adaptive articulation appeared to be the correct one.

Adaptive articulations are seldom discussed in training programmes or even at professional meetings. There may be value in discussing these more, as they may offer a useful tool for speech intelligibility in some individuals with a significant oral structural difference.

5.3 Physiotherapeutic Methods and Resistance Therapy in Velopharyngeal Dysfunction

Ilter Denizoglu and Mehmet Akif Kilic

5.3.1 Rationale of Physiotherapy for Velopharyngeal Dysfunction

Systems cannot be defined by a single component. Subsystems that generate a functional unit must be treated as a whole, because they interact during the defined function. The human velopharyngeal system is a complex structure that interacts with three vital functions: breathing, swallowing and speech. In this sense, a problem that exists in one of these functions inevitably affects others to varying degrees. They also use many of the same muscles but with differing patterns of activation. The physical modelling of these functions needs to be defined by muscle contraction patterns that create structural and functional features simultaneously. Each muscle contraction is a physical vector (Fig. 5.4), and two parameters define a vector: magnitude and direction. Various combinations of the vectors provide a certain pattern of motion. Physiotherapy aims to increase the efficiency (contraction and organisation) of the muscles that activate the system directly or indirectly.

The velopharyngeal port (VPP) is a three-dimensional functional structure that serves as a dynamic valve during speech and swallowing. Normal speech is dependent upon the functional and structural integrity of the velopharyngeal port. The oro-nasopharyngeal coupling function of the VPP during articulation of speech segments is a complex, dynamic, but mostly a voluntary process controlled by the motor cortex. It is a motor behaviour learned through speech and language development. On the other hand, similar movements for swallowing are primarily

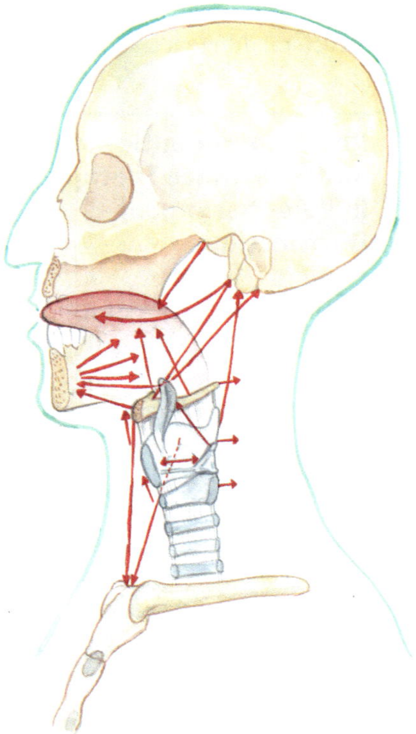

Fig. 5.4 The vector combination of muscles altering velar functions (From: Denizoglu (2020a), courtesy of Denizoglu) Denizoglu©2021

involuntary activities that originate from the brainstem (Shprintzen 2013).

Laryngeal and velopharyngeal valve mechanisms work in concordance during breathing, speech and swallowing (Flowers and Morris 1973). Speech, in this sense, seems to activate a chain reaction that increases the velopharyngeal activity. The muscles of the velar complex are intentionally considered in singing pedagogy. Many manoeuvres and exercises that are aimed at the velum are designed to reshape the vocal tract and control the vertical laryngeal position. The pre-yawn position is one of these examples for this relationship. Beyond their resonance function, the velar and pharyngeal muscles are active components of the dynamic laryngeal suspension system (Husler and Rodd-Marling 2007). This physiological fact, in addition to pedagogical and clinical experience, underlies the rationale for physiotherapy in velopharyngeal dysfunction (VPD) in certain patients.

The pharynx is a 12–14 cm muscular tube starting from the nasopharyngeal roof to the upper oesophageal sphincter, which resembles the trunk of an elephant. The muscles that contribute velopharyngeal port (VPP) closure and oral-pharyngeal phases of swallowing have a dominant role in articulation and formant tuning, and accordingly, laryngeal posturing. The VPP closure is the result of the velar and pharyngeal movements along antero-posterior, medial and vertical planes. The movement of those planes may differ between people (Skolnick et al. 1973).

The levator veli palatini muscle is the primary closing vector of the VPP by elevating the velum, but it does not mean that the VPP functions as a lid-valve; it operates as a sphincteric valve. In addition to the levator and tensor veli palatini muscles, others (stylopharyngeal, salpingopharyngeal, palatopharyngeal, superior constrictor pharyngeal) are related to velar movements vectorially and control this complex function. The anatomical borders of the velopharyngeal port can be defined anteriorly by the soft palate; laterally and posteriorly by the lateral and posterior pharyngeal walls. Especially during speech, the functional efficiency of this valve structure primarily depends on the velopharyngeal musculature, but the complex interactions and muscular connections make other muscular structures around the VPP (tongue, larynx, pharynx and jaw) influential on VPP function (Fig. 5.5).

VPD can be the result of anatomical/structural deficiencies (velopharyngeal insufficiency), neurological/neuromuscular causes (velopharyngeal incompetence) or behavioural maladaptations (velopharyngeal misuse). Velopharyngeal dysfunction may lead to resonation and articulation (primary and secondary) problems that impair the intelligibility of the speech. Management of the velopharyngeal dysfunction is dominantly surgical, but speech and voice therapy are inevitable after sufficient closure is obtained.

VPD has three dimensions: mechanical valve insufficiency (VPP closure), motor skill deficiency and behavioural disorder. In this sense, the management of VPD must be considered in different ways. The mechanical valve function is the primary issue. If there is a moderate or severe

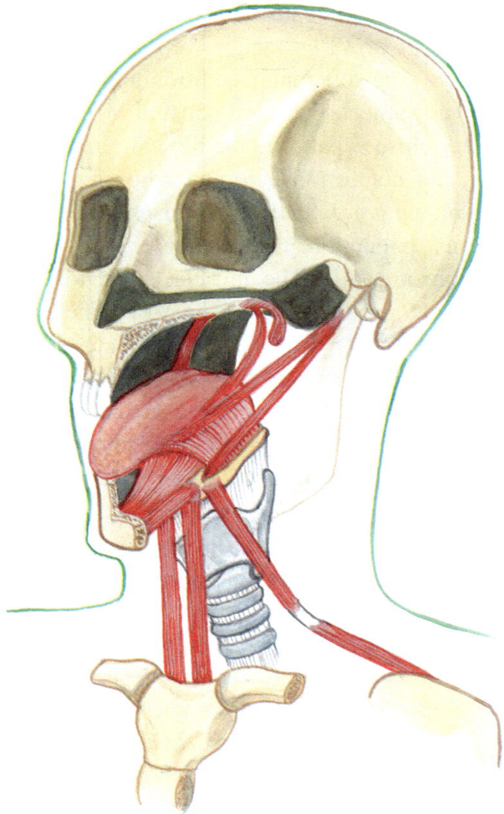

Fig. 5.5 Muscular relations between larynx, tongue and velum (From: Denizoglu (2020a), courtesy of Denizoglu) Denizoglu©2021

anatomical or neurological disorder that interferes with the valve function, attempts at speech correction will be unsatisfactory. In this case, surgical or prosthetic methods for providing velar closure may be considered in the first order. If the VPD is mild to moderate, and muscular rehabilitation seems to work, then physiotherapy procedures may be applied.

5.3.2 Physiotherapeutic Methods for VPD

Speech and other oral motor functions overlap to some degree in neural control, muscles deployed and movements performed (Kent 2015). Physical/behavioural therapy for hypernasality is a controversial approach historically. Physiotherapy for VPD may be indicated in postoperative cleft palate surgery, postoperative adenoidectomy (in some cases with predisposition to VPD), functional VPD and mild VPP insufficiencies due to neurological or anatomical problems. Muscular rehabilitation for VPD can be applied by various methods: muscular strength training (non-speech oral motor exercises, speech production exercises), stretching and range of motion (ROM) exercises, biofeedback and sensory stimulation.

Strength training may be used as a preparatory activity for the introduction of specific motor skill-learning programmes when muscle weakness is the dominant aetiology (Frontera and Lexell 2005). Strength training in VPD aims to provide a certain level of functional VPP performance before speech therapy. Resistance-assisted isotonic and isometric muscle exercises overload the VPP muscles above normal operating levels. Various non-speech oral motor exercises (NSOMT) and speech production-accompanied exercises have been proposed for muscular rehabilitation in VPD (Massengill et al. 1968; Ruscello 2008a, b; Kuehn et al. 2002; Clark 2005). NSOMTs have been defined by various authors to increase strength and improve muscle tone and ROM; modify tongue, lip and jaw resting postures; and improve muscular control and function through sensory stimulation (Ruscello 2008a, b). As the speech is not the only function of the VPP, NSOMTs may provide additional help for the VPP efficiency to some extent. Different approaches (Kuehn et al. 2002) have been applied for VPD since the 1940s, which began with non-speech exercises (blowing, sucking, swallowing). Velopharyngeal closure patterns and their underlying neuromotor control may differ for phonation, speech and non-speech activities (Moll 1965; Shprintzen et al. 1974). Moreover, inhibition of vegetative neural circuits might be necessary during phonation and speech (Netsell 1986). Despite being widely used, NSOMTs still lack enough literature support for their bringing clinical improvements. Phonation-assisted and/or speech-based interventions seem to be more efficient in communication disorders due to VPD (Ruscello and Vallino 2020).

Speech is a process incorporating coordinated movements of respiratory, laryngeal, velopharyngeal and oral articulatory gestures (Riski 2013). It is characterised by movements of low to moderate forces (relative to maximum forces measured during non-speech tasks) and high velocities, which makes it a suitable therapeutic tool for endurance and strength of the related muscles (Barlow and Burton 1990; Clark 2003). Speech-assisted exercises, thus, may increase contraction velocity in strength training. In order to strengthen the muscles related to velopharyngeal closure, a speech-production-assisted progressive resistance model was proposed by Kuehn (1991). In this therapeutic procedure continuous positive airway pressure (CPAP) is used as resistance source. CPAP provides increased nasal-pharyngeal air pressure that enables the upper airway to remain patent in patients with sleep apnoea by opposing the closure of the velopharyngeal valve during sleep (Kuna and Sant'Ambrogio 1991). The use of CPAP therapy has also been investigated in individuals diagnosed with hypernasality resulting from VPD. In response to the resistance provided by CPAP, it has been shown by EMG (Kuehn et al. 1993) that contraction of the levator veli palatini muscle is more forceful. Possible mechanism for the use of CPAP for VPD is the increased aerodynamic load in the velopharyngeal port to provide resistance training. Application of air pressure to the nasal surface of the velum provokes the velopharyngeal muscles to work against this load to create velopharyngeal closure during non-nasal speech productions. The muscles of VPP are thus strengthened through the principles of progressive resistance. Though with a limited number of patients, promising results exist in clinical studies for 'graded velopharyngeal resistance training' in VPD patients (Kuehn et al. 2002; Cahill et al. 2004; Kollara et al. 2014).

The stretching exercises are focused on ROM and may be applied by phonetic-based exercises and biofeedback (Shelton et al. 1966; Pamplona et al. 1999; Ysunza et al. 1997). Speech disorders in VPD patients, such as compensatory articulation disorder, may initially occur as a consequence of the VPD, producing a phonetic-based disorder. However, over time, these errors become incorporated into the patient's linguistic process, producing a phonologic disorder (Chapman 1993). Articulatory problems due to motor skill deficiency (verbal dyspraxia and dysarthria) in VPD benefit well from physiotherapy. The operant conditioning approach involves subjects who are capable of attaining normal closure patterns for blowing and whistling, but not for speech, and who are treated with blowing or whistling exercises with simultaneous phonation (Shprintzen et al. 1975; Shprintzen 1989). The muscles need to learn and develop how to close the VPP efficiently. Congenital VPD patients especially are able to learn the mother language with an articulatory deficit due to VPD. In addition to surgical correction and physiotherapy in moderate to severe VPD patients, a linguistic approach must be considered. A patent VPP that causes moderate to severe valve problems usually does not benefit from physical/behavioural therapy.

Biofeedback provides patients with ongoing physiological performance information that is typically not available to them, or has not reached a level of conscious introspection for VPP function (Ruscello 2008a, b). Visual feedback can be provided by instrumentation such as a nasalance meter (Kummer and Lee 1996) and video-pharyngoscopy (Ysunza et al. 1997). It seems to be an efficient assistance to speech therapy in improving motor skills, ROM, and to some extent, strength (Ysunza et al. 1997).

Sensory stimulation may be used to maintain the function of muscles as an auxiliary procedure. Two main forms may be applied: electrical and tactile stimulation. The electrical stimulation on the soft palate and pharyngeal walls may improve VPP function particularly when supported by home practice with tactile (touching the velum with Q-tips) stimulation and visual (mirror) feedback to incorporate the movements into speech (Yules and Chase 1969; Tash et al. 1971).

5.3.3 A Multidimensional Approach to VPD: DoctorVox Therapy

Phonation into tubes with one end immersed into water was introduced by Sovijarvi (Simberg and Laine 2007) to the paediatric group with hypernasality in order to improve the VPP. He used glass tubes and then started to use the procedure in voice problems. Sihvo (2017) proposed the use of silicone tubes in her 'LAX VOX tube exercise'. These exercises were modified and expanded by Denizoglu into the DoctorVox Voice Therapy Technique (DVT) (Denizoglu 2018).

The DVT programme (Denizoglu 2018, 2020a, b) is a four-level (preset, exploration, development, adaptation), three-dimensional (action plan, exercise, monitoring) schedule. In the first preset level, counselling, breath management and posture are studied. Primal sound is explored in the second level. The development level includes vocal exercises for an efficient and safe glottal closure pattern, to increase muscle strength and secure a pre-defined motor skill. In the last level (adaptation), the motor skill is transformed into a behaviour. Artificial elongation of the vocal tract and semi-occlusion are used as physical tools, and various devices have been developed for the DVT practice.

The DVT, as a physiotherapeutic approach to VPD, aims to strengthen the VPP muscles by applying oral-pharyngeal back pressure, stretching with phonatory exercises and speech production, and providing multilevel feedback during practice. Speech activities are obliged to be added to the exercises simultaneously. High back-pressure levels may be required gradually until VPP closure is obtained. In addition to a better VPP closure, therapeutic goals in the DVT programme for VPD patients include improved breath support, increased loudness, pitch variability, proper word stress and articulation.

DVT practice in VPD starts with counselling the patient and family. The process may take a long time. Patience and empathy are important, as even the child may not reveal the problem causing psychological stress. Forcing must be avoided, as parental pressure will not shorten the process; on the contrary, the patient may give up. Last but not least, 'play' is the motto of the whole practice in the paediatric population. Breath management must not be forced too much either, relaxation of the upper chest and shoulders during phonation is stressed in the preset level of DVT. Glottal and supraglottal hyperfunctional compensatory behaviour must be prevented. The possible physiological mechanism of the oral pressure-assisted speech exercises in DVT is the activation of the VPP muscles, not only the velar (the anterior wall) but also the posterior and lateral walls of the valve as a sphincteric function. The laryngeal and pharyngeal activity against back pressure is thought to support the muscles that affect VPP efficiency.

Phonation into the tube from the beginning may be tried with tube-only phonation or with a low back-pressure (1–2 cm H_2O) practice. The patient is given biofeedback by putting his or her index finger in front of the nose (to feel the nasal airflow) during phonation into the tube. At the beginning the nasal air leak may not be diminished with low back pressure. The back pressure is gradually increased by the DC-Valve (Fig. 5.6) until nasal leakage is diminished, if not stopped. Higher resistance levels (over 15–20 cm H_2O) though may vary with patient, and create a greater impact on nasal air leak during phonation into the device by experience. This is possibly because the larynx tends to rise and the VPP muscles contribute to this high resistance-assisted phonation. Bubbling is used as visual feedback for making the exercise more efficiently.

Basic DVT vocal exercises start with short vocalisations without giving much detail to the

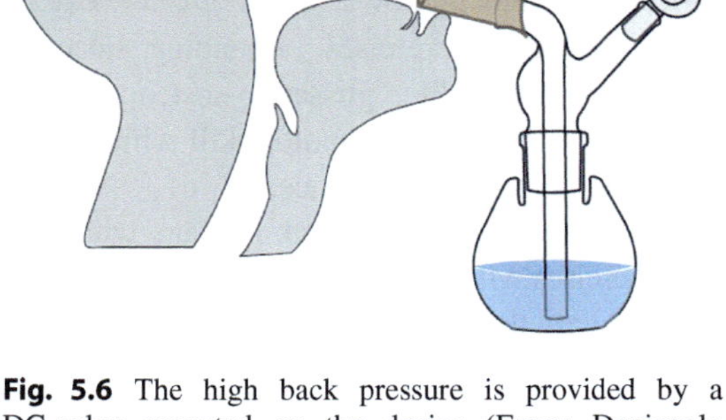

Fig. 5.6 The high back pressure is provided by a DC-valve mounted on the device (From: Denizoglu (2020a), courtesy of Denizoglu) Denizoglu©2021

patient, in order not to make the things complex. Later the duration of phonation against back pressure is elongated (the sostenuto exercise). The close-back vowels ([ɯ], [ʊ], [u]) may be preferred for the vocal tract shape that increases the VPP tension. Sostenuto (sustaining the same tone) may help to strengthen the muscles by isometric contraction. The sostenuto exercise may be executed in different pitches. Especially at high pitches, because the vertical larynx position tends to be elevated, the VPP function seems to be strengthened more efficiently owing to high levels of resistance. When completed to the point of fatigue, sostenuto may improve both strength and endurance.

Different muscle tonus states can be developed by a glissando (gliding between two tones) exercise. This tends to create an isotonic muscle contraction and stretching as a variation of strength training. Gliding between two pitches that succeeds without nasal emission includes not only glottal muscular contraction changes but also the whole vocal tract, including VPP and tongue muscles. Vocally untrained individuals especially tend to increase vertical larynx position and constrict the vocal tract at high pitches, which may not be a favourable behaviour in vocal pedagogy, but may be useful for VPD. The pitch range can gradually be extended beyond the ROM and a sostenuto can be added to the ascending glissando exercise. The most difficult pitch-based basic vocal exercise is staccato. In the staccato exercise, the patient is meant to phonate shortly into the tube abruptly and bubble the water, inhale from the nose and repeat this sequence quickly several times. This increased speed of contraction exercise seems to be particularly appropriate for strength training to improve VPP efficiency during speech because it targets movement velocity/power to a greater extent. Combined DVT exercises (ascending staccato-glissando, descending glissando-sostenuto, etc.) later aim to improve the motor skill while maintaining strength and endurance.

Phonating against high back pressure with various exercises will take approximately six weeks of practice until the velar muscles strengthen, depending on the individual. The high back-pressure phonation exercise should be practised 8–10 times a day, for 5 min each session at home. The follow-up is made by nasopharyngeal flexible endoscopy for efficient VPP closure in addition to nasometric and subjective assessments. When VPP closure in high back-pressure phonation is secured (nasal leakage has decreased or disappeared), the resistance is decreased to lower levels (3–5 cm H_2O). At this step, the oral mask is mounted (Fig. 5.7), and the linguistic load is started.

Ka ka ka syllables with non-nasal consonants ([ba ba ba], [da da da], [ta ta ta], etc.) are articulated into the oral mask while the nasal emission is being controlled. After securing the VLP closure in non-nasal consonants, the [m] and [n] phones are studied. Bubbling is used as visual feedback for the articulatory efforts but should be paused during nasal consonants. The phones before and after the nasal consonants during speech with the oral mask should create bubbles. This helps to control and master the VPP use for articulation and speech.

Simple phrases (counting, greeting, etc.) are started in the last step, and then oral mask reading is promoted. If the patient is non-literate, speaking into the oral mask may be practised in a playing condition, conversation, etc. Speaking with and without the oral mask can be practised and then compared by listening to recorded phrases

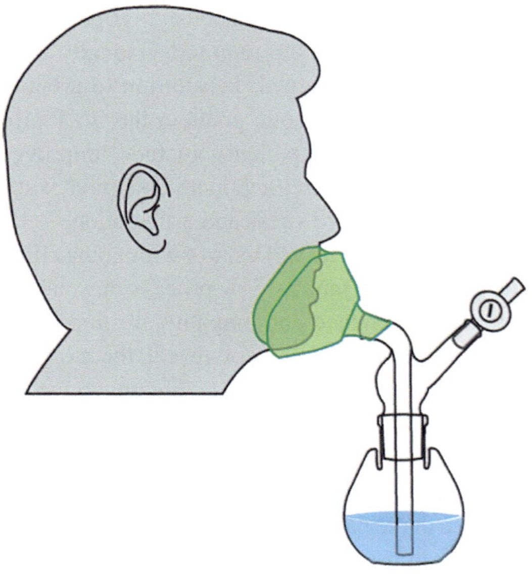

Fig. 5.7 Use of the oral mask at the DVT linguistic-load step (From: Denizoglu (2020a), courtesy of Denizoglu) Denizoglu©2021

together with the patient. In order to keep the muscle strength, the high-back-pressure exercises can be continued until the hypernasal speech is diminished or eliminated.

The efficiency of physiotherapy in VPD patients still has controversial areas to be clarified. Appropriate methods, patient selection, clinical efficiency mostly depend on experience. No single method is proven to be effective, the clinician needs to have a multidimensional approach. The DVT programme with assistance of oral-pharyngeal back pressure provides a multidimensional clinical approach for treatment of VPD, but also needs to be confirmed by multicentre-controlled clinical studies.

5.4 Orofacial Dysfunctions (Orofacial Myofunctional Disorders, OMD) with Special Focus on Paediatric Patients: Therapy

Doris-Maria Denk-Linnert
and Wolfgang Bigenzahn

5.4.1 Team Approach to Myofunctional Therapy

Myofunctional therapy (orofacial myofunctional treatment, OMT) is a crucial component of a multidisciplinary and multiprofessional team approach in OMD (Maspero et al. 2014). Besides otolaryngologists/phoniatricians and speech language pathologists, the following experts contribute to patient management: paediatricians, lactation consultants, orthodontists, oromaxillofacial surgeons, physical therapists, occupational therapists, certified orofacial myologists (US).

5.4.2 Precondition for Myofunctional Therapy

A precondition for myofunctional therapy is the elimination of ENT-specific problems before treatment can start; possible necessary ENT surgical procedures are:

- Adenoidectomy, tonsillotomy/tonsillectomy to ensure nasal breathing. Nasal breathing is crucial, because long-term mouth-breathing changes the natural resting position of the jaw, tongue and lips. This negatively influences growth patterns of the jaw and maxilla and often results in a significant malocclusion
- Tonsillotomy, frenulotomy (Zaghi et al. 2019) to enable a physiological tongue position and movement
- Paracentesis, ear grommet to ensure normal hearing in case of middle ear effusion

An individually tailored therapy must be established, taking into account the child's age, his or her physical and mental development (Fischer-Voosholz and Spenthof 2002; Godhard Blythe 2013; Hahn 1988). The classical concept of myofunctional therapy (MFT), according to Garliner (1974), is seen as a standard regimen in the fields of dental and oral medicine.

5.4.3 Treatment Goals of Myofunctional Therapy

These are to improve orofacial proprioception, tone and mobility in order to achieve (Homem et al. 2014):

- Physiological resting postures of the tongue, lips and jaw
- Nasal breathing and normalised respiration: mouth breathing is very common—up to 55% in the paediatric population (Abreu et al. 2008). This is due to the size of craniofacial structures in relation to the size of the tonsils or adenoids or both. One to 5% of the population suffers from obstructive sleep apnoea (Tan et al. 2015). Preterm infants are especially at risk
- Physiologically balanced muscle function of the tongue, lips, muscles of mastication and deglutition, as well as muscles of the face, head and neck
- Elimination of oral behaviour or habits that have a negative impact on growth of the face and dentition. The use of a pacifier is discussed controversially. The pros are, e.g. the

ability to soothe/comfort the child and a potentially decreased risk of sudden infant death syndrome. An increased incidence of acute otitis media, a possible negative influence on breast-feeding and on dental occlusion, is regarded as a con. The recommendations on how long a pacifier can be used vary and range from 6 months (recommendation of the American Academy of Pediatrics, with the aim of reducing the risk of ear infections) to a maximum of 24–36 months (Nelson 2012)
- Correction of abnormal chewing and swallowing patterns; initiation of physiological swallowing, resting postures of the tongue, lips, mandible, head and neck; correction of tongue thrust
- Elimination of parafunctional habits, bruxism or muscle clenching
- Correction of articulation disorders: traditional articulation therapy in patients with OMDs is often ineffective

5.4.4 Indications for Myofunctional Therapy

These comprise the *intended improvement of the functions* listed below (Billings et al. 2018):

- Nasal breathing after tonsillotomy/tonsillectomy/adenoidectomy and in sleep-disordered breathing and obstructive sleep apnoea (Diaféria et al. 2017; Guilleminault and Sullivan 2014; Camacho et al. 2015; Moeller 2018; Huang et al. 2019; Chuang et al. 2019), in adults (de Felício et al. 2018; Koka et al. 2021)
- Lingual mobility after frenectomy
- Stabilisation of occlusion during or after orthodontics or oromaxillofacial surgery (Homem et al. 2014). OMT in conjunction with orthodontic treatment helps to maintain closure of anterior open bites more than orthodontic treatment alone (Smithpeter and Covell 2010). Myofunctional treatment in deciduous and mixed dentition children is regarded to be promising, but the quality of the existing evidence is questionable (Koletsi et al. 2018). Positive effects of OMT on the clinical and electromyographic aspects of chewing in patients submitted to orthognathic surgery have been described (Prado et al. 2018)
- Infant chewing, feeding and swallowing
- Articulation: e.g. abnormal lingual dental articulatory placement (/t,d,l,n/), distorted production of /s, z/, nasal quality of vowels, distortion of velar sounds (/k,g/, 'ng')
- The elimination of dysfunctional oral habits is also an important part of myofunctional therapy
- Additional indications are symptoms of temporo-mandibular dysfunction and facial pain

5.4.5 Intervention Programmes for Myofunctional Therapy

Several intervention programmes are used, e.g.:

- **D Garliner's myofunctional therapy**
- The behaviourally orientated MFT aims at eliminating the aberrant orofacial functions. The therapy goals are as follows:
  - The recovery of normal muscle reflexes and muscular tone
  - The initiation of normal swallowing behaviour
  - The automation of the newly learnt swallowing pattern

The MFT therapy can be applied to children from the age of eight onwards and to adults who are undergoing an orthodontic treatment (Garliner 1974).

- **L Fischman's Viennese concept of therapy of orofacial dysfunctions**

  This therapy concept is based upon Garliner's MFT therapy, Bobath's Neuro-developmental Therapy (NDT, Bobath 1980) and the Neurofunctional Reorganisation (Padovan 1995). Children from the age of six onwards can be treated accordingly. The therapy comprises an intensive phase, a home-therapy phase as well as a final 'perfectioning phase'. Throughout the whole therapy patients should have regular follow-up with the treating ENT specialist/phoniatrician and dentist or orthodontist (Friedrich et al. 2013).

- **Regulation therapy by R Castillo-Morales**
  This therapy concept is beneficial for babies and children suffering from an oral motor disorder, a cerebral palsy, Down syndrome, Pierre–Robin sequence, Moebius syndrome or other cerebral lesions. Stimulation of areas in and around the mouth should begin as early as possible to facilitate neuromuscular reflex mechanisms and normal behavioural patterns, thus preventing a possible orofacial dysfunction (Castillo-Morales 1991).
- **'GRUMS-Heidelberg Group concept for myofunctional disorders'** (Lleras and Müller 1993)
- **Correcting dysfunctional habit patterns and oral hygiene**
  If sucking habits persist after the age of two years they may lead to morphological changes of the oral structures. Mostly anomalies of the teeth and jaw (malocclusion) occur. With regard to behavioural and psychological aspects, delicate emotional reminders to eliminate sucking habits are most effective (Conscious Habit Retraining). Further, an 'oral screen' (MVP—'Mundvorhofplatte', oral vestibular plate) can help minimise the sucking habits. The oral screen activates nose breathing and supports closure of the mouth.

With the appearance of the first teeth, parents should perform oral hygiene twice a day—in the morning and in the evening after the last food intake. An age-appropriate healthy diet is a vital factor to prevent tooth decay. Sugared drinks after oral hygiene must be avoided. A preventive intake of fluoride tablets should have already been started during pregnancy (endogenous prophylaxis) and continued during childhood (for primary teeth-exogenous prophylaxis).

In some cases, additional oral tools are used in addition to myofunctional therapy, such as straws, lip or bite blocks or appropriate food items.

5.4.6 Summary

Myofunctional, articulatory and ENT-specific problems occur at all ages, but are common in preschoolers and school-aged children. The differential diagnostics is a special phoniatric task within a multidisciplinary team. Only after history taking and a thorough phoniatric-logopaedic and myofunctional examination should an age-appropriate therapy programme be initiated.

However, in many cases, the surgical treatment of ENT-specific problems, such as adenoidectomy, tonsillotomy, tonsillectomy or frenulotomy (ankyloglossia!), is the precondition for a successful myofunctional therapy.

5.5 Biofeedback Nasopharyngoscopy for Cleft Palate Speech

Philippe H. Dejonckere

Unlike that of the lip, tongue and jaw muscles, the conscious sensorimotor control of the muscles of the velopharyngeal mechanism is—in most subjects—much less developed. Consequently, these muscles are less suited for verbally commanded exercise training in a context of speech rehabilitation. Further, auditory information is of little help in providing feedback on the adequacy of velopharyngeal closure. These have been the reasons for trying out other possibilities of biofeedback, such as the nasal mirror, the Sea-Scape, the Nasometer®, the HONC-instrumentation (Horii oral-nasal coupling score) and the nasopharyngeal endoscopy (Heller Murray et al. 2016).

In the 1970s and 1980s, technical developments of flexible transnasal endoscopes as well as imaging and recording material made possible (quasi-) unobtrusive 'live' visualisation of velopharyngeal morphology and dynamics, without impeding connected speech. Shelton (1975) showed that normal subjects were able to utilise videoendoscopic feedback to guide voluntary velopharyngeal movements. Siegel-Sadewitz and Shprintzen (1982) confirmed that a normal subject is able, after six sessions of twenty minutes visual feedback endoscopic training, to change velopharyngeal valving pattern at will during short samples of connected speech. This has led to its application in speech therapy.

Miyazaki et al. (1975) first mentioned the use of flexible fibreoptic nasopharyngoscopy as a tool for biofeedback in patients with repaired cleft of the palate, but no specific data were provided on the outcome. Shelton et al. (1978) applied the videoendoscopic feedback method to two adolescents with velopharyngeal closure deficit. The results indicated that the subjects more frequently approximated complete closure as the study progressed, but that improved performance was not established on an automatic level. Yamaoka et al. (1983) investigated 59 cleft palate patients with persistent velopharyngeal incompetence. The nasopharyngos copic biofeedback self-training was performed every two weeks for nearly one year. The results indicated that the patients who showed complete velopharyngeal closure during blowing or production of several speech samples were able to attain much improvement in all speech samples after one year of self-training. On the other hand, the patients who did not show complete velopharyngeal closure during all tasks failed to improve the velopharyngeal closing mechanism.

Witzel et al. (1989) reported positive results on three adult patients in promoting consistent closure of the velopharyngeal ports after pharyngeal flap surgery (a few nasopharyngoscopic feedback sessions of 30 min). They first identified the most appropriate starting point for biofeedback therapy, based on the sounds that produce the most extensive lateral wall motion or closure of the lateral ports. Then the patient was trained to move the velopharyngeal mechanism voluntarily without speech. The therapy continued moving from the sounds produced with the best closure of the lateral ports to those with the least amount of closure. Witzel et al. (1989) also reported successful elimination of a pharyngeal fricative in a 10-year-old child with repaired cleft lip and palate.

Ysunza et al. (1997) compared nine cleft palate patients receiving conventional speech therapy for correcting compensatory articulation, with eight patients receiving additional endoscopic feedback therapy. After 12 weeks, the authors found a clear, favourable effect on the negative movements of the lateral pharyngeal walls during speech in the biofeedback group, but not in the other. By using a multiple baseline design, Brunner et al. (2005) successfully tried the method in eleven patients (aged 7–30) with cleft palate and velopharyngeal dysfunction, who had all received conventional speech therapy without significant improvement. There were two biofeedback therapy sessions (20 min each) 6 weeks apart for each target speech sound (from 1 to 8 of them, depending on the patient). The authors noticed that it was more difficult to improve velopharyngeal closure for vowels than for consonants. However, even if the biofeedback training only concerned single sounds and syllables, velopharyngeal closure appeared to be improved as well as when the target sounds were produced within words and pre-structured sentences. According to the authors, 'patients gain new insights in articulatory and velopharyngeal valving processes, enabling traditional speech therapy to be continued on the basis of their extended knowledge and improved sensory control'.

Neumann and Romonath (2012) systematically reviewed the effectiveness of nasopharyngoscopic biofeedback in treatment of cleft palate speech. Their analysis of six studies reflects a quite low level of evidence and a broad heterogeneity concerning age range, intervention methods and outcome measurement. The authors concluded that this approach may be effective only in combination with traditional speech therapy in helping patients with cleft palate speech (particularly older children and adults) to optimise their velopharyngeal closure in articulation. There are no studies published measuring the effectiveness of nasopharyngoscopic feedback without additional treatments, such as secondary surgery or speech-language therapy.

5.6 Nasopharyngoscopic Biofeedback for Different Kinds of Velopharyngeal Insufficiency

Monika Brunner

Speech treatment of velopharyngeal dysfunction (VPD) in patients with cleft palate is challenging and time-consuming (Golding-Kushner 1995). In some patients, VPD persists, although the anatomical conditions of the repaired palate allow for adequate (or nearly adequate) velopharyngeal closure (VPC). In these patients, speech sounds remain hypernasal, and speech is hardly intelligible.

Non-speech exercises such as sucking and swallowing have not been found to transfer to speech (Kuehn et al. 2002) because VP closure patterns and their underlying neuromotor control differ between speech and non-speech activities (Hirschberg 1986). Conventional behavioural treatment of VPD has focused on improving the manner in which the VP muscles are used during speech and on shaping a different behavioural response. However, the latter is difficult because the patient does not have an idea or inner perception of the anatomical basis for the VPD. In particular, there are no proprioceptive sensations from the velopharyngeal sphincter. Conventional speech therapy does not provide any visually based facilitation of the motor response of the VP mechanism.

In seeking an alternative approach to treatment of VPD, I have considered the information provided by flexible nasopharyngoscopy to be an appropriate source of visually based treatment of VPD. The initial case studies of endoscopic biofeedback were reported by Yamaoka et al. (1983), Witzel et al. (1989), and Brunner et al. (1994). The method then was elaborated by Brunner et al. (1996, 1999, 2001, 2005) and tailored to different functional patterns of VPI (Brunner et al. 2007).

The different functional patterns we have found in our patients with VPD are the following:

- **VPD with motor coordination problems**
  Mis-timing of VP movements and voice onset/end
  Release of VP closure ahead of time
- **VPD with retracted articulatory placement**
  The back of the tongue and the epiglottis touch the posterior pharyngeal wall; the VP sphincter does not close
- **VPD with verbal dyspraxia**
  Motor speech planning disorder; regulation of muscle tonus is difficult
  Patients often achieve a good VP-closure in *voiced* stop sounds: /b/d/g/; however, no consistent closure in *voiceless* stop sounds: /p/t/k/. To compensate, these patients try to speak with an overly loud voice and forced muscle tension, which in consequence is not helpful for achieving complete VP closure
- **Phoneme-specific VPD**
  The sphincter is open only in specific sounds (often/s/without retracted articulation).

The therapeutic procedure of nasopharyngoscopic biofeedback is implemented as a standardised four-stage process (Brunner et al. 2001):

1. Introduction: learning the structures and function of VP closure
2. Experimentation: self-monitoring of articulation movements, guided by therapeutic instructions
3. Coupling: fusing visual perception and auditory perception with the aid of guided relaxation
4. Consolidation: transfer to spontaneous speech by means of a diary

One biofeedback session lasts an average of 20 min. We focus on the training of a target sound in isolation and during syllable production. We introduce the endoscope through the middle nasal meatus. At the posterior nasal choana, the endoscope provides a superior view of the VP mechanism with the soft palate, the lateral pharyngeal walls and the posterior pharyngeal wall. In patients with compensatory articulation, we advance the endoscope deeper into the pharynx to provide a view of the movement of the tongue and the epiglottis in speech.

The therapeutic stage of experimentation guided by instructions has to be differentiated according to the specific functional pattern of VPD:

1. **VPD with motor coordination problems**
Training the precision of timing under feedback control of the velopharyngeal sphincter
2. **VPD with retracted articulatory placement**
Using an endoscopic view of the tongue and epiglottis, we use a gradual transition from a correctly placed sound to the articulation of the

target sound. While gradually switching from a correct sound (e.g. /t/) into the target sound (e.g. /s/), the patients have to maintain the correct tongue placement of the first sound and slowly alter the other articulation features until the sound character of the target sound emerges. The image on the monitor provides the necessary feedback to capture the moment at which the tongue falls back into the incorrect position.

3. **VPD with verbal dyspraxia**
Provided with the view of the VP sphincter, patients learn to use adequate muscle tension while pronouncing the voiceless stop sounds.
4. **Phoneme-specific VPD**
These patients learn to control the direction of the airstream (nasal vs. oral) by using visual feedback of the VP closure.

Endoscopic biofeedback therapy for VPD yields quick and stable results because the motor learning process is directly reinforced (Ysunza et al. 1997; Brunner et al. 2005). Typically, improvement is achieved within a few sessions. Patients gain new insights into articulatory and VP valving processes, and they can then take this new knowledge and improved sensory control back to their traditional speech therapy. I see biofeedback therapy as an adjunct to, but not a substitute for conventional speech therapy (Neumann and Opitz 2013). This method should be used in cases when conventional speech therapy does not yield sufficient results (Neumann and Romonath 2011). In most cases two or three sessions (in phoneme-specific VPD even one session) might be sufficient to bring a new impulse and a new insight for continuing the normal speech therapy.

5.7 Augmentative and Alternative Communication

Karel Neubauer, Lenka Neubauerová, and Karen J. Reichmuth

The application of Augmentative and Alternative Communication (AAC) procedures to children and adults with speech communication disorders stemming from structural craniofacial malformations (manifestations of dysglossia, nasal disorders and velopharyngeal deficit) is a current concept of its use. AAC interventions are methods used to compensate for an individual's temporarily or permanently reduced communicative competence. Without supporting strategies such as AAC, reduced communicative competence may lead to reduced social participation, and therefore to a poorer quality of life.

The use of AAC in this target group of children and adults has three serious specific indicators:

- AAC procedures are used as an individual extension of clinical speech therapy procedures in cases where a specific complicating factor is present (illness, other somatic, psychogenic or social reasons) or where long-term persistent difficulties with incomprehensible speech. Even in these cases, it is mainly the use of augmentative procedures, not a complete alternative communication system that would replace speech communication (Škodová 2018; Young and Spinner 2020). This starting point applies especially to children with systemic craniofacial malformations. The typical early surgery for children with isolated cleft lip or palate or both, including velopharyngeal insufficiency, usually leads to sufficient and good speech intelligibility (Van Lierde et al. 2003; Ruda et al. 2012; Neubauerová and Neubauer 2018). This intervention includes paediatric surgical treatment and standard speech therapy, which aim to support feeding, speech motor skills and articulation, and reduce hypernasality.
- Children and adult persons with a speech disorder caused by isolated dysglossia or orofacial (muscular) dysfunction can understand language normally and can speak, but may have temporary or permanent difficulty being understood because of reduced intelligibility of their own speech. In some cases, the possibilities to express themselves successfully may be reduced as well. Because noticeably reduced speech intelligibility may lead to

reduced social participation, its severity and duration must guide the individual recommendation for AAC. The persons focused on in this category may correspond to the "supportive language group" outlined in target groups for AAC intervention—persons who temporarily use AAC in order to facilitate understanding of spoken language, as well as to express themselves, and persons who speak but have difficulty being understood (Von Tetzchner and Matrinsen 2000; Branson and Demchak 2009; Neubauerová and Neubauer 2018).

- The main indication for the use of AAC in the third target group of people is the presence of comorbidity and symptomatology of another serious communication disorder. So, AAC should be considered and recommended if craniofacial malformation or orofacial dysfunction is part of any broader or additional developmental speech and language delay, or if the child or their parents suffer from communication failure. In severe myofunctional disorders, such as myasthenia gravis and myotonic dystrophy, ASHA and WHO guidelines recommend AAC (ASHA 2005, 2015; WHO 2007). AAC comprises methods to compensate for temporary or permanent impairments, activity limitations and participation restrictions of individuals with severe disorders of speech-language production or comprehension (ASHA 2005). Recommending AAC to compensate for reduced communicative competence is also in line with the stated aim that any intervention or rehabilitation strategy is required to establish the best options for social participation and quality of life for the individual, determined by questionnaire, the aim of any intervention or rehabilitation (WHO 2007; Branson and Demchak 2009; Pless and Granlund 2012).

Orofacial myofunctional disorders and dysfunctions potentially predispose those with them to the use of AAC. Isolated speech disorders caused by peripheral myofunctional disorders do not usually lead to severely reduced speech intelligibility. AAC should be considered in children with Down's syndrome, in which the speech disorder is partly caused by macroglossia and orofacial dysfunction, and is a feature of a general developmental and language delay. In these children, early intervention including AAC is highly recommended and effective (Branson and Demchak 2009).

In the treatment of myasthenic disorders, there should be clear proof at the individual level of the potential benefit of indication AAC before its use. Myasthenia gravis can lead to severe speech disorders with changing and progredient severity (Engel 2012). Sjögreen et al. (2007) reported on a cohort of children and adolescents with myotonic dystrophy, in which moderately or severely reduced speech intelligibility was found in more than half, and some patients had no speech production capability. Following the guidelines of ASHA (2005) and ICF-CY (WHO 2007), short-term or permanent intervention with AAC can be given to these patients depending on the course of the disease. AAC is recommended for adults with speech disorders caused by progressive neuromuscular diseases. These individuals are less able to express complex communication needs successfully using their natural speech (Ball et al. 2012), leading to reduced social participation and therefore a reduced quality of life Given the positive effect of AAC on these individuals, AAC should be introduced early to children and individuals with a myasthenic disease. In such cases, AAC can supplement their natural speech and language repertoire and its development, and therefore enable more successful communication and participation.

If regular monitoring of speech intelligibility reveals noticeable reduction, intervention should include temporary or permanent AAC as well as advice on using AAC in daily communication at home as early as possible (Cress and Marvin 2003; Branson and Demchak 2009; Sevcik et al. 2008). The results of a meta-analysis by Walker and Snell (2013) found AAC intervention in children with disabilities to be equally effective across a broad spectrum of participants and interventions. AAC is more effective in younger children than in older children or adults. Good AAC intervention aiming in successful communication generally should include an individual multimodal combination of different communication forms

(Sevcik et al. 2008). The selection of the most appropriate form of AAC depends on the individual user's motor, visual, cognitive, language and communication strengths and weaknesses.

5.8 Overview of Oral Motor Devices in Functional Training of Oral Structures

Thomas Stamm and Ariane Hohoff

5.8.1 Background

Oral motor devices (OMD) are an unspecified group of aids that are used with the intention to improve skills necessary for proper oral motor function. Under the term "oral motor function", various functional processes are described in the scientific literature, from simple lip closure to complex processes such as swallowing, speech and breathing. In a narrower sense, *oral motor function* refers to the movement of oral soft and hard tissue (e.g. mucosa, muscles, jaws), including muscle tone and strength, coordination, speed and range of movement (Bean 2013). But for complex processes, such as salivation, more is needed; reflexes and morphological integrity of the oral and adjacent structures, as well as adequate spatial relationships to each other. It is therefore not surprising that different terminologies for similar and overlapping meanings of functional states exist: *oral motor/orofacial/orofacial sensorimotor; oral motor intervention/orofacial stimulation; oropharyngeal function; myofunctional; orofacial myofunctional; craniomandibular function.* In a broader sense, growth-directing concepts such as *functional orthopaedics, functional orthodontics* and *orofacial orthopaedics* are also meant.

The same diversity applies to therapeutic aids. A large number and variety of commercial materials are available under the name *oral motor devices/tools/objects/instruments/applicators; trainer; myobrace; guards.* The varied advertising is aimed not only at all medical professions dealing with the face, mouth, teeth and throat, but also at the consumer. Most manufacturers concentrate on the following areas: chewing, drinking, speech and other applications such as oral stimulation and tactile cues.

The understanding that an organism can adapt to changing conditions through functional stimuli has been known for a long time and probably goes back far beyond Darwin (1872): it has long been a key principle in the medical profession. However, it was the German anatomist Roux who understood the importance of the learning process (Fränkel and Fränkel 2001). According to Roux, the fundamental principle is

> … to learn new neuromuscular performance patterns and to provide security and ease in their performance by muscle exercises and training (Roux 1895)

Roux's hypothesis states that any improvement in (oral) function begins in the brain, namely with the individual will to perform a certain movement. In relation to the oral motor devices this means that a product should not only be a *passive* device but should also contain a learning component or should be instructed by a qualified practitioner.

A further factor which should be considered when measuring the success of these devices is the epigenetic potential of each individual to adapt to a certain condition. *Epigenetic* is meant here in the sense of physiology, the change of phenotypic characters due to external factors without modification of gene sequence (Ho and Burggren 2010). Put in simplified terms, a particular oral motor deficit is determined by internal (genetic) and external factors. The greater the genetic disturbance, the lower the epigenetic proportion that can be improved by exogenous factors, such as oral motor devices.

5.8.2 Effectiveness of Oral Motor Devices

The scientific literature on oral motor function focuses mainly on *feeding*, *speech*, *geriatrics*, *chewing* and *dysphagia*, while *dysphagia* overlaps almost 40% with *geriatric* disorders and almost 60% with *feeding* difficulties. *Chewing* also overlaps with *geriatrics* but only up to 12%.

5.8.2.1 Feeding Disorders and Dysphagia

The term oral motor intervention (OMI) is used for oral stimulation, oral support and non-nutritive sucking in feeding problems. A meta-analysis, which included 855 participants, evaluated the potential of OMI for improving oral feeding in preterm infants (Tian et al. 2015). It could be shown that OMI is associated with reduced transition time, shorter hospitals stays and increasing feeding efficiency. The OMIs comprised manual touching and soft tissue compression. The only used *device* was a pacifier of an unmentioned manufacturer. A distinction between manual and pacifier stimulation was not made, so that no statement could be made about the effectiveness of the pacifier in this work.

Patients with neurological impairments often suffer from dysphagia, a wide-ranging disorder that affects the oral preparation for swallowing. There is little evidence of the extent to which OMI has a positive effect on dysphagia. The last Cochrane review (Morgan et al. 2012) found only insufficient evidence from randomised controlled trials and only one intra-oral device could be identified from included articles: an oral screen (see Sect. 20.11, Fig. 25a, b).

Sjögreen et al. (2010) used this device to strengthen lip muscles and lip function. The authors found that the device led to higher muscle activity but could not automatically improve function. They point out that this kind of device can only be one part of the treatment and is not a substitute for speech therapy (Sjögreen et al. 2010).

Expiratory muscle strength training is one of many different procedures used in the treatment of Parkinson's disease (PD)-related dysphagia (López-Liria et al. 2020). The training can be supported by a device through which air flows for strengthening the expiratory muscles (for example, see Fig. 5.8).

Although a randomised trial revealed positive effects of this device on oropharyngeal function during swallowing (Troche et al. 2008), the device must be seen as only one component in the extensive rehabilitative therapy options for PD, which ultimately lead to an improvement in the degenerative function and quality of life (López-Liria et al. 2020).

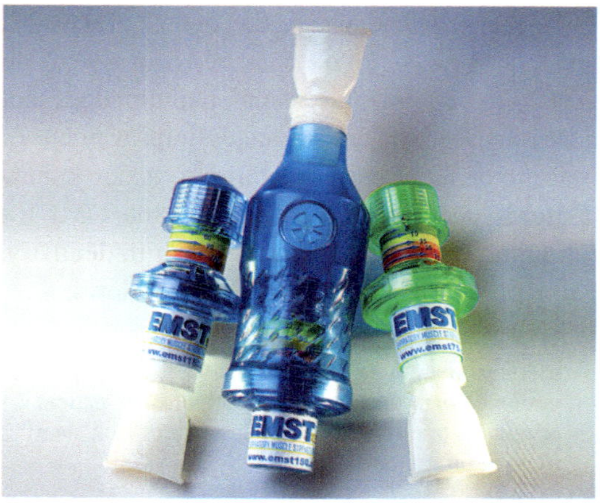

Fig. 5.8 Expiratory muscle strength trainer. Indications according to the manufacturer: enhancement of breathing, cough and swallow function (with kind permission of Aspire Respiratory Products, Cedar Point, North Carolina)

5.8.2.2 Geriatric Oral Care

With the increasing number of older people, the need for geriatric oral care is growing. Geriatric oral health includes not only prosthetic rehabilitation, but also the preservation of dental status, the maintenance of oral hygiene and the management of speech, chewing and swallowing difficulties due to drug-induced xerostomia or impaired physical or cognitive functions. An evaluation of 32 systematic reviews showed an association between poor oral hygiene and pneumonia as well as toothlessness and malnutrition (Ástvaldsdóttir et al. 2018). Oral rehabilitation is therefore mainly focused on the replacement of lost tooth structures. The latter, and the risk of serious disease that can occur in old age, could explain why OMI appears to play only a minor role in geriatric oral health. OMI is helpful in the transition from percutaneous endoscopic gastrostomy to oral feeding (Becker et al. 2011), but broad evidence of its application in geriatrics is not reflected in the literature (Ástvaldsdóttir et al. 2018).

In the broadest sense, the dental prosthesis, whether new or old, can be considered an OMD. Receiving an optimal denture does not necessarily guarantee automatic improvement of oral motor function. The ability to adapt to new dentures decreases with age, and the OMI for retraining mastication is not present in dentistry. Kumar et al. (2018) rightly state as follows:

> While anatomic restoration of general body parts is accompanied by a comprehensive training programme to motivate and rehabilitate the patient optimally, oral rehabilitation procedures lack such training programmes.

And to close the circle back to Roux they add:

> ... we propose that attention should also be directed towards the understanding of the brain and neuroplastic changes.

5.8.2.3 Speech Sound Disorders

Difficulties in producing speech sounds can have many causes, which range from benign vocalisation problems in the mixed dentition phase, to severe impairments due to structural or neurophysiological deficits. One treatment approach is non-speech oral motor treatment (NSOMT) whose introduction dates back to the beginning of the last century (Van Riper 1939). Speech sound is obviously the field where most OMDs were invented. Marshalla (2011) identified 86 different objects from NSOMT textbooks from 1939 to 1968. The general use of all listed objects was to manipulate the tongue, lips and jaw and also to touch the intra-oral soft tissues in order to achieve correct tongue position. They

> ... "were designed for children who present with different etiologies, degrees of impairment, and chronological age range." (Ruscello 2008b).

Several objects have identical functionality, whereby fingers, hands and teeth are also called objects (Marshalla 2011). The objects recommended in textbooks can be divided into the following categories: animal product, body part, cold object, eating utensil, food, glass object, heated object, liquid, metal object, musical instrument, paper object, plant-based object, rubber object, toy, wooden object, other specified and non-specified objects (Marshalla 2011).

Exemplarily some devices are mentioned in the following, which have survived and are nowadays available in modern design. Such objects as balls, horns, whistles, tactile, vibration and unknown pressure devices are involved in NSOMT (Strode and Chamberlain 1997). The functionality of these tools is based exclusively on statements from manufacturers, customers and other unscientific writings and activities. For example, horns should train inhalation, exhalation and mouth opening. Whistles should have a comparable effect, with different inherent difficulties to blowing. Tactile tools should help in diagnosing sensory-motor deficits and promoting awareness of the oral cavity. Vibration tools are used for stimulation of the different tissues of the oral cavity. The indications are very general and thus allow a wide range of applications.

Although these instruments have been used intensively by practitioners over many years, their effectiveness is disputed owing to the lack of sufficient evidence (Pillery 2008; Lee and Gibbon 2015). Counter arguments even come from speech-language pathologists themselves. Insufficient evidence and no demonstrable relationship between non-speech activity and speech are the main arguments against OMDs (Marshalla 2011). Clinical studies are limited and those available involve only a few patients. The most recent Cochrane review found no strong evidence regarding the treatment efficacy of non-speech oral motor treatment (Lee and Gibbon 2015). Another obstacle to scientific acceptance is the fact that NSOMT thrive in non-peer-reviewed sources such as continuing education events, marketed therapy tool websites, the popular press and instructional manuals with modernised vocabulary designed for practitioner and customers.

However, the constructive debate about the effectiveness of NSOMT continues, and the first methodologically sound studies on tools which have been used in speech training for more than 100 years (Marshalla 2011) are on their way.

5.8.2.4 Myofunctional Therapy and Removable Prefabricated Devices

Myofunctional therapy was introduced by Alfred P. Rogers at the annual meeting of the American Association of Orthodontists in 1918 (Rogers 1918). Rogers was a student of the influential orthodontist Edward Angle (see below) who suggested that restoration of the muscles would lead to normal orofacial function. It is theoretically difficult to separate myofunctional therapy from oral motor intervention, but because Rogers was an orthodontist, it is clear that myofunctional therapy is a special kind of orthodontic treatment. The purpose of myofunctional therapy is to enable orofacial function by using isotonic and isometric exercises that can be used in isolation or in combination with other forms of treatment. Without going into technical depth of the therapy, one can say that Rogers focused on a combination of body posture, muscle-bone interactions, psychology, exercises and the correction of habits and malfunction to produce a physiological occlusion. Rogers did not disparage the mechanical nature of the early orthodontic apparatus, but he stressed the physiological component as an aid in treatment and retention. With the decrease of the interest in Rogers' work over the years, both the orthodontic apparatus and myofunctional therapy have been developed to simplified, prefabricated *eruption control devices* (ECD) that are more or less supported by rudimentary exercise instructions.

In the mid-1970s, the American Speech-Language-Hearing Association (ASHA), the American Dental Association and the American Association of Orthodontics raised concerns regarding myofunctional therapy and demanded more clinical research (Shortland et al. 2021). The latest systematic review revealed that myofunctional therapy has been reported extensively in the scientific literature, but none of the multidisciplinary fields involved has been able to demonstrate clinical evidence (Shortland et al. 2021).

However, the prefabricated eruption guidance devices available today, whose effectiveness has been investigated, are Occlus-o-Guide® (Bergersen 1984), LM-Activator™ (Myrlund et al. 2014), Myobrace® (Čirgi et al. 2016) and Trainer System™ (Usumez et al. 2004). The latest systematic reviews showed low quality evidence that ECDs are less effective than orthodontic activators (Papageorgiou et al. 2019; Mohammed et al. 2020). Only one clinical trial showed that wearing an ECD is more effective than no treatment (Myrlund et al. 2014, 2015).

For the sake of completeness, it must be mentioned that with the increased attention on the treatment of obstructive sleep apnoea (OSA), prefabricated OSA devices have emerged from the ECDs and from mandibular advancement devices. The underlying principle here is not the oral motor intervention but only the advancement of the mandible.

5.8.2.5 Myofunctional Therapy and Removable Growth-Modifying Appliances

Appliances for modifying the direction of orofacial growth at an early stage are closely related to the terms *functional orthodontics, dentofacial orthopaedics and orofacial orthopaedics*. In the following, the term *appliances* is used because they are reserved for orthodontic specialists and custom-made individually for each patient after impression taking.

The theoretical concepts of removable growth-modifying appliances are similar to those of all the devices discussed here and can also be traced back to the beginning of the last century. Edward Angle, one of the more famous fathers of orthodontics, described the influence of *muscular pressure* as early as 1899 in his famous publication *Classification of Malocclusion*:

> … muscular pressure … is a far more important factor in relation to the study and correction of malocclusion than is generally recognized … powerful in maintaining inharmony in the sizes or relations of the arches and malocclusion of the teeth (Angle 1899)

Andresen and Häupl (1945) founded the concept of *functional orthodontic therapy/functional jaw orthopedics* and saw in their appliances the realisation of Wolff's law, which is that bone builds up and increases in strength when it is loaded by muscular pressure (Wolff 1899). It was Fränkel (1980), with his concept of *orofacial orthopaedics*, who introduced appliances requiring functional exercises for learning new ways of oral motor function and thus influencing growth direction in the orofacial region. The mentioned concepts are typical early treatments in the growing patient. The newest Cochrane review found evidence of low to moderate quality regarding early interventions' ability to reduce protrusion of upper front teeth (Batista et al. 2018) and the most recent meta-analysis proved the effectiveness of functional orthodontic appliances (Santamaría-Villegas et al. 2017).

5.8.2.6 Myofunctional Therapy and Removable Non-Growth-Modifying Appliances

Some removable appliances are used for oral motor interventions that are not intended to modify the direction of orofacial growth. The custom-made *oral screen* is one representative of these appliances, which was first described in 1913 by Harman Newell, who used this shield to treat mouth breathing (Newell 1913). Since then, the oral screen has been used as an individually custom-made shield (nowadays often prefabricated, see Sect. 20.11, Fig. 25a, b) for several indications.

Inconclusive evidence concerning the effectiveness was found for treatment of incompetent lips (Owman-Moll and Ingervall 1984; Thüer and Ingervall 1990) and tongue rest position (Knösel et al. 2011), whereas the oral screen improves lip force in patients with myotonic dystrophy type 1 (Sjögreen et al. 2010), improves lip force and swallowing capacity in stroke patients (Hägg and Anniko 2008; Wertsén and Stenberg 2020), relieves oesophageal dysphagia and reflux symptoms (Hägg et al. 2015) and improves oral function in Parkinson's disease (Baram et al. 2020). A possible explanation for the differing evidence of the above mentioned studies is provided by Hägg and Anniko (2008) who argue:

> "It is more plausible that treatment results are attributable to sensory motor stimulation and the plasticity of the central nervous system than to the training of the lip muscles per se."

The custom-made *palatal or stimulation plate* is a commonly used acrylic plate intended for early treatment of patients with oral sensorimotor disorders (Hohoff and Ehmer 1997, 1999; Hohoff et al. 1998). The principal aim is to stimulate adequate position of the tongue by stereognostic training and to achieve a reduction in drooling by developing sufficient lip tone and lip seal.

Various designs are available for the treatment of children with Down syndrome, and they are used in combination with the orofacial regulation therapy according to Castillo Morales (Hoyer and Limbrock 1990). For example, a bowl-shaped dorsal suction-knob should encourage the patient to take the tongue back and to close the mouth. Vertical ridges or small resin forms in the vestibular area facing the inner side of the upper lip are aimed at activating the perioral muscles. More used stereognostic bodies are moveable balls (Bäckman et al. 2003), acrylic bulbs (Bäckman et al. 2007) and moving pearls attached to a transverse wire.

The palatal plate has a positive effect on occlusion, oral motor function, facial expression and speech (Hohoff and Ehmer 1997, 1999; Korbmacher et al. 2004, 2006; Bäckman et al. 2007). The most recent systematic review proved the effectiveness of the plate (Javed et al. 2018). However, the majority of authors using the plate emphasise the importance of the accompanying physiotherapy, orofacial regulation therapy, according to Castillo Morales, as well as speech and language intervention.

5.8.3 Conclusion

Oral motor devices are, generally speaking, those that support a functional training of the oral structures, including the adjacent anatomy. All devices have emerged from similar treatment philosophies of different disciplines, which—and this is particularly striking—were all developed at the beginning of the last century. It is speculative to attribute these ideas of the founders to one point, but many of the explanations remind one of

> "use and disuse" (Darwin 1872)
>
> and
>
> "everything is interaction" (Humboldt 1803)

and refer to epoch-making works of Darwin, Humboldt and many scientific companions who shaped the dichotomous role of genetics and epigenetics.

Oral motor devices can be separated into two groups: (a) Custom-made, specially indicated, tailored to the individual patient, and (b) Prefabricated, non-customised, available for practitioners and consumers. The effectiveness of custom-made devices that have been reported in the literature is inconsistent. It appears that patients with degenerative functional impairment respond better to treatment, especially if a strict exercise regimen is involved. All authors emphasise that the device is only a part of the entire treatment.

A characteristic of the prefabricated devices is that they are accompanied by numerous advertising claims tailored to the consumer. Evidence about their effectiveness is lacking. When effects are present, they are more likely to be short term, in the context of an experienced practitioner, or compared with no treatment. The risk of worsening is always present when so-called 'do-it-yourself' treatments are performed.

5.9 Prostheses

Rémi Esclassan, Florent Destruhaut, Ariane Hohoff and Emmanuelle Noirrit-Esclassan

5.9.1 Introduction

Integrity of the palate and the velopharyngeal port is essential for guaranteeing physiological oral functions. The VP valve mechanism regulates nasal resonance during speech and is also involved in swallowing, blowing, sucking and whistling (Keyf et al. 2003). Cleft lip and palate (CLP), which is inevitably associated with velopharyngeal incompetence, may be treated by surgery, orthodontics, prosthodontics, speech therapy or a combined approach (Pinto et al. 2007). Starting at birth, the treatment of CLP requires combined action from a multidisciplinary team of which the prosthodontist is an important member (de Ladeira and Alonso 2012; Shaw et al. 2001).

5.9.2 Palatal Plates for Children with CLP

Around half of the cleft teams in Europe use presurgical infant orthopaedics (PSIO), which cover the palate without penetrating into the cleft (Shaw et al. 2001; Mossey et al. 2009). They were introduced by McNeil (1950) and later developed by Burston (1958) and Hotz et al. (1978) with the idea of guiding palatal growth, aligning maxillary arch segments, and separating nose and mouth, in order to improve feeding and establish a more physiological tongue position. These palatal plates are indicated in clefts involving the hard palate but not in purely labial, alveolar or velar clefts.

Different designs are used: passive or active (with springs or screws), removable or fixed (e.g. the Latham device with a pin fixation to the upper jaw, often used to retract the protruding premaxilla with intra-oral elastomeric chains with the idea of enabling less tension on the wounds after surgical reunion of the soft tissue parts (Allareddy et al. 2020), sometimes combined with extra-oral systems for nasoalveolar moulding (NAM) (Grayson and Cutting 2001) (Figs. 5.9, 5.10, and 5.11a, b)).

Active PSIO (NAM or Latham) are currently used by more than 40% of the cleft teams in the USA (Knösel et al. 2016). The fabrication of a PSIO, with a posterior extension closing parts of the velar cleft, requires an impression of the structure to be taken with a middle-fusing silicone-based material on a preformed acrylic tray (Figs. 5.12 and 5.13).

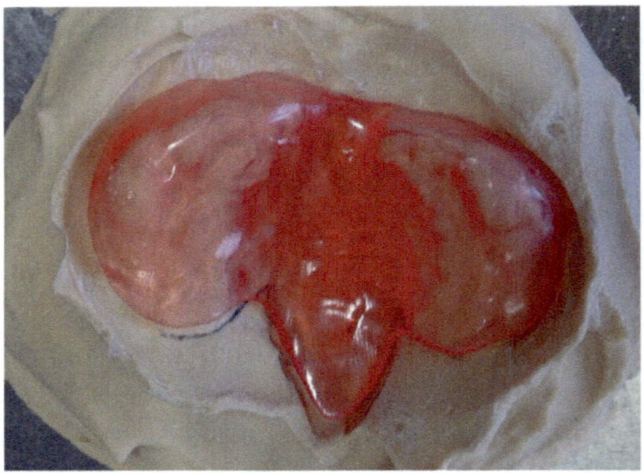

Fig. 5.9 Passive palatal plate (it sometimes has to be fixed with special adhesive)

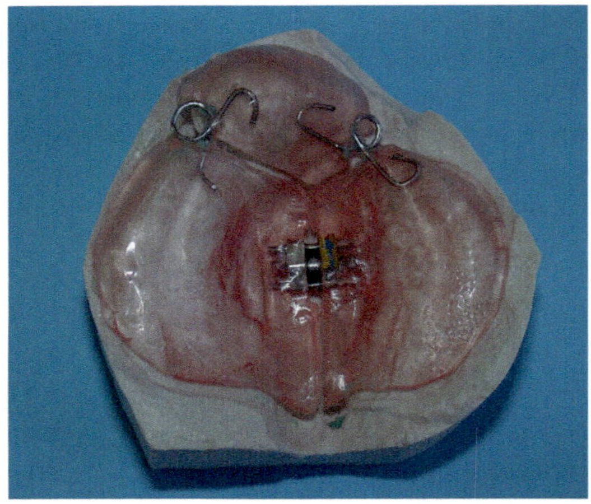

Fig. 5.10 Active palatal plate (it sometimes has to be fixed with special adhesive)

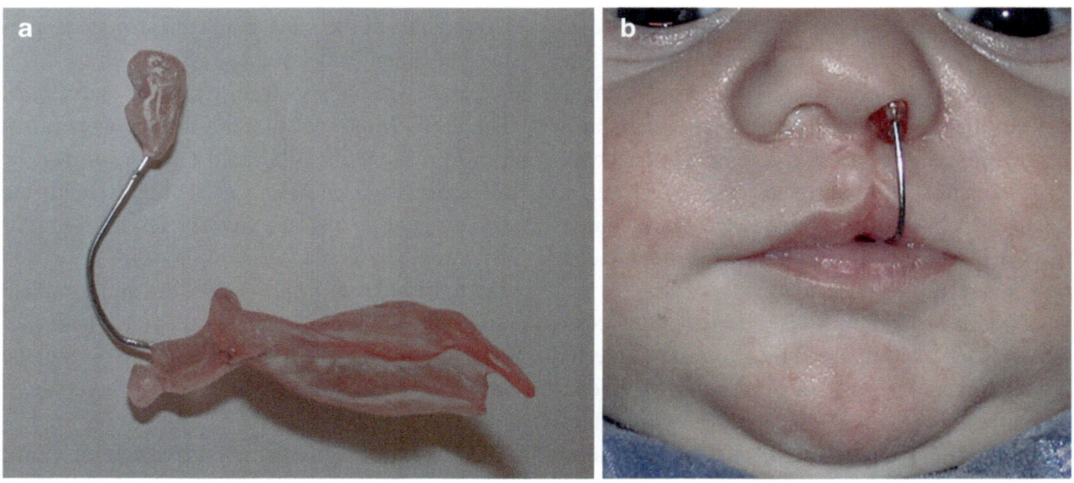

Fig. 5.11 (**a**) Nasoalveolar moulding appliance (NAM). (**b**) Infant with the NAM in place. This system can be retained by a system of elastics and tapes on cheeks

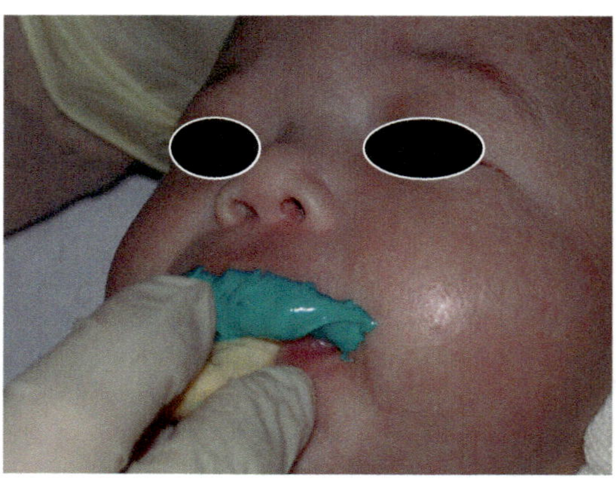

Fig. 5.12 Maxillary impression is taken with a resin tray and light body polyvinyl siloxane (silicone)

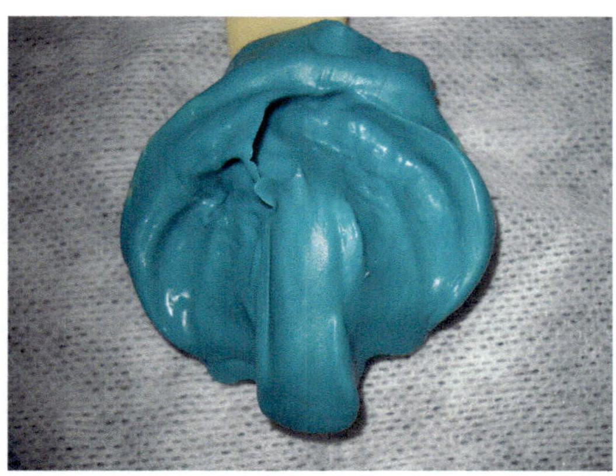

Fig. 5.13 Maxillary impression of a unilateral complete cleft lip and palate (not the same infant as in Fig. 5.12)

It is to be hoped that the procedure of analogue impressions will soon be replaced by intraoral scans (Fig. 5.14).

PSIO must be worn all day, except for cleaning, until veloplasty for two-step surgery or until palatoplasty for one-step surgery. As the child is growing, the appliance is usually renewed every two to three months, for a treatment duration depending on the therapeutic techniques and schedule (mostly from 6 to 13 months).

The effects of palatal plates are *very* controversial. Proponents of these appliances claim many benefits (Uzel and Alparslan 2011):

- Reduction of cleft width (Shetty et al. 2017) by stimulation of palatal shelf growth, which is thought to facilitate surgical closure
- Improvement in maxillary arch symmetry and stability (Shetty et al. 2017)
- Normalisation of lingual position and movements by preventing tongue intrusion into the cleft (Figs. 5.15a, b)
- Facilitation of feeding by providing a rigid opposite surface, allowing compression of the nipple (Goyal et al. 2014)
- Improvement in speech and language development at 2.5 years (Konst et al. 2004)
- Breathing and feeding improvement in Robin sequence thanks to a velar extension shifting the tongue forward-comparable to the effect of a laryngoscope (Buchenau et al. 2017) (Fig. 5.16a, b)
- Improvement of nasal symmetry, nasal tip projection, columella elongation and alveolar remodelling by pre-surgical nasoalveolar moulding (PNAM) by using an extra-oral extension to exert moulding pressure on the distorted nasal margin (Fig. 5.11a, b), associated with an early cheilorhinoplasty (Aihara et al. 2022; Likitkulthanaporn et al. 2024)

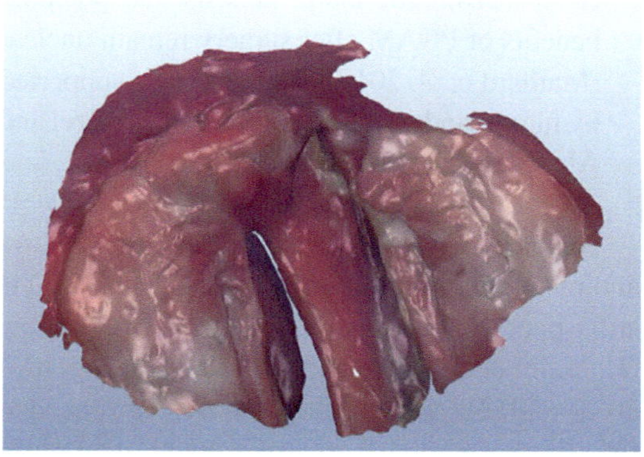

Fig. 5.14 Intra oral optical impression

Opponents of the use of the technique have reported that using a palatal plate:

- Is complex
- Implies more work and increased costs for the CLP team and the parents
- Depends on patients' and parents' cooperation (Masarei et al. 2007). Compliance is rarely taken into account although it might be proof of the quality of an orthosis and depend on the duration of the required wearing

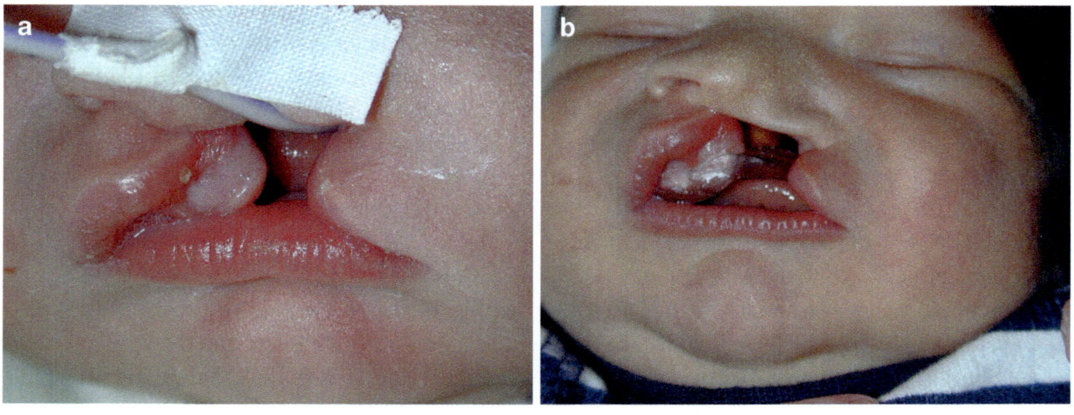

Fig. 5.15 (**a**) Infant with a unilateral cleft lip and palate. (**b**) Palatal plate prevents tongue intrusion into the cleft

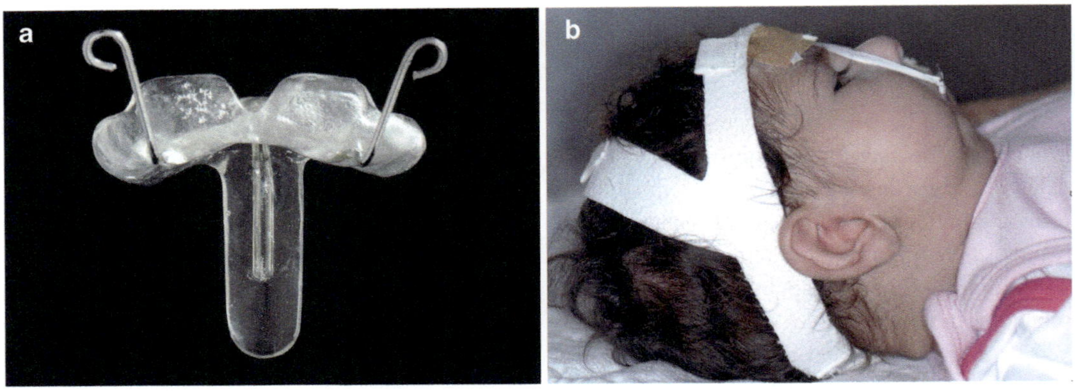

Fig. 5.16 (**a**) Tübingen pre-epiglottic baton plate/Tübingen palatal plate. The wire in the velar extension (middle of the picture) serves to prevent this part from fracturing. The right and left wires go from intra-orally to extra-orally (see panel (**b**)) for strip fixation on the face in order to prevent tipping of the appliance by the strong muscular forces of the tongue. (**b**) Tübingen pre-epiglottal baton plate—extra-oral view. In this infant, the appliance—in addition to the strip fixation on the face—had to be secured by some kind of "headgear", which was individually fabricated in the sewing department of the University Hospital of Münster

- Can be associated with bad fit of the plates, oral thrush and minor ulceration (Hosseini et al. 2017)
- Has no effect on mothers' satisfaction in motherhood (Prahl et al. 2008)
- Does not result in more effective feeding (Uzel and Alparslan 2011; Masarei et al. 2007; Prahl et al. 2005), deglutition (Knösel et al. 2016) or better general somatic growth (Prahl et al. 2005; Papadopoulos et al. 2012)
- Has no significant benefits for reducing oronasal fistula (Jodeh et al. 2019)
- Has no significant effect on the anterior and posterior arch width (Noverraz et al. 2015), on occlusion (Niranjane et al. 2014), on cephalometric angles indicating sagittal maxillary and mandibular skeletal growth pattern or on aesthetics of lip and nose (Ross and MacNamera 1994)
- Has no long-term effect on speech—early positive effects at age three (Konst et al. 2003a) fade away by the age of six (Konst et al. 2003b)
- Does not alter the need for subsequent revisionary surgery (Ross and MacNamera 1994)
- Sometimes needs additional taping (Cerón-Zapata et al. 2016), which could influence measurements. Effects of active plates are multifaceted and intertwined with the use of revision surgery and the price for getting better nasolabial results may be a worse dental arch and maxillo-mandibular relationship (Kornbluth et al. 2018). The claim persists that potential benefits of PNAM after surgery remain unclear (Maillard et al. 2017) and have to be supported by future randomised controlled trials (Uzel and Alparslan 2011; Hosseini et al. 2017)

According to the present systematic reviews and meta-analysis, scientific evidence on PSIO is still poor (Uzel and Alparslan 2011), low (Hosseini et al. 2017) and limited (Papadopoulos et al. 2012), and further studies are needed (Maillard et al. 2017). The aforementioned problems are in part due to low patient numbers, heterogeneity of surgeons´ skills and surgical primary and revisional procedures, taping (if performed), heterogeneity of plate design, timing and patients´/parents´ cooperation (Alqadi et al. 2023), which all make comparisons difficult. Therefore, in the future, PSIO should be evaluated as a part of a complete multidisciplinary protocol rather than as a treatment itself.

However, despite the lack of good evidence, PSIO is still widely used by many CLP teams; within those—according to local differences—the impressions are taken and the appliances are inserted and controlled either by specially trained orthodontists, paediatric dentists or prosthodontists.

5.9.3 Prosthetic Rehabilitation for Adults with CLP

According to Freitas et al. (2013), oral rehabilitation of adult patients with CLP is directly related to the severity of anatomical and functional alterations determined by the malformation and the age at treatment onset (Figs. 5.17a, b).

The ideal treatment is closure by bone graft and orthodontics, but when surgery is not possible or when the patient does not wish to undergo surgery, prosthetic rehabilitation can be necessary. Dentures may be fixed or removable, tooth or implant supported, and contribute directly and positively to the psychosocial aspects of the individual (Freitas et al. 2013). These treatments aim to re-establish aesthetics (e.g. by improvement of the profile at the upper lip), normal functioning (by preventing food and fluid leakage into and thus out of the nose) and VP closure (Pinto et al. 2007; Papadopoulos et al. 2012; Jodeh et al. 2019; Noverraz et al. 2015; Niranjane et al. 2014; Ross and MacNamera 1994), which contributes to better speech intelligibility.

According to Dhakshaini et al. (2015), three types of speech appliances can be used to assist speech production:

(a) A palatal obturator, serving for closing defects of the hard palate (most commonly fistulae) or velum (Fig. 5.18).
(b) A palatal lift prosthesis, which is used in cases of VP incompetence (also in children (Freitas et al. 2013)), elevates the velum at its natural bend and holds it in place against the pharyngeal wall. It is indicated if the velum is of sufficient length to achieve closure but doesn't move well enough to accomplish it. It has the disadvantage that it may potentially interfere with the production of nasal sounds and nasal breathing.
(c) A speech bulb obturator (also known as speech aid appliance) for VP insufficiency. The bulb courses upwards to fit behind the velum in the nasopharynx and fills the pharyngeal space. Breathing and sleeping can potentially be difficult with the bulb in place.

Classically, a palatal prosthesis for an adult individual with CLP is divided into three parts:

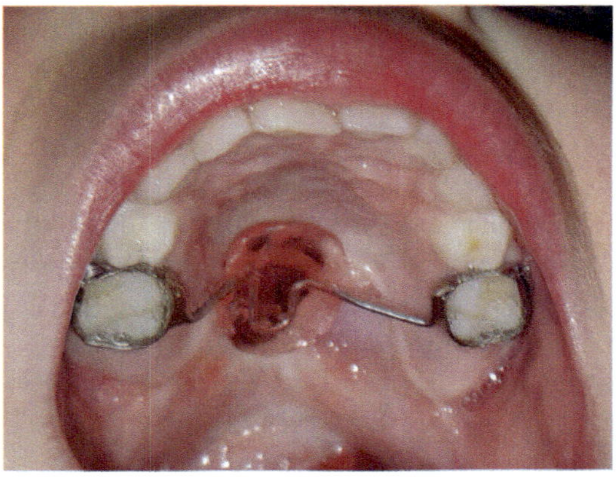

Fig. 5.18 Palatal fixed obturator in a child with fistulae, waiting for surgery

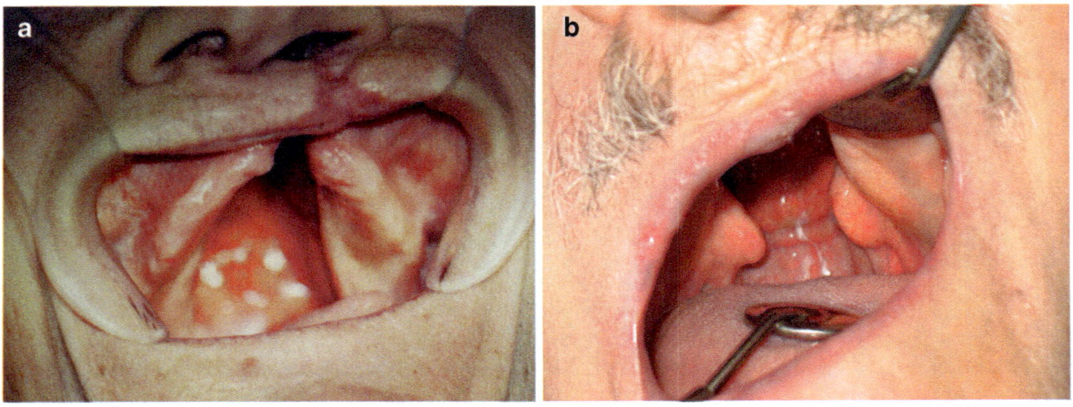

Fig. 5.17 (**a**, **b**) Adult patients with unrepaired cleft of the hard and soft palate

anterior, intermediate and posterior (Dhakshaini et al. 2015) (Fig. 5.19a, b).

The anterior portion corresponds to a conventional denture. It can be a removable partial denture, a complete denture, an over-denture or an acrylic plate (Freitas et al. 2013). This denture has the same function as other conventional dental prostheses: replacing missing teeth, restoring functions and providing acceptable aesthetics.

In patients with a deep nasopharynx, an intermediate portion is necessary to place and retain the posterior portion correctly. The latter is designed after the patient has used the prosthesis with the intermediate portion. To help to support the impression material and to avoid loosening, a brass wire of approximately 2 cm can be folded and polymerised to the end of the prosthesis. A small quantity of low-fusing impression material is placed on it and the device is inserted in the patient's mouth. The patient is allowed to wear this system for several minutes to become comfortable with its presence and is then asked by the speech pathologist to produce some phonemes, move the head and swallow (Fig. 5.20).

The enlargement of the prosthesis towards the pharynx must be progressive and very well tolerated to avoid discomfort and a gagging reflex (Pinto et al. 2007; Freitas et al. 2013); nasoendoscopy might be necessary (Hakan Tuna et al. 2009). When the nasal airway is completely occluded, the dentist must check that there is no area where the material is in overextension and that the patient tolerates the device correctly. Then the lift portion is replicated in acrylic resin, carefully finished and finally polished to ensure that there are no residual rough or sharp edges that may hurt the soft palate mucosa. Drinking liquid is the usual test to check the effectiveness

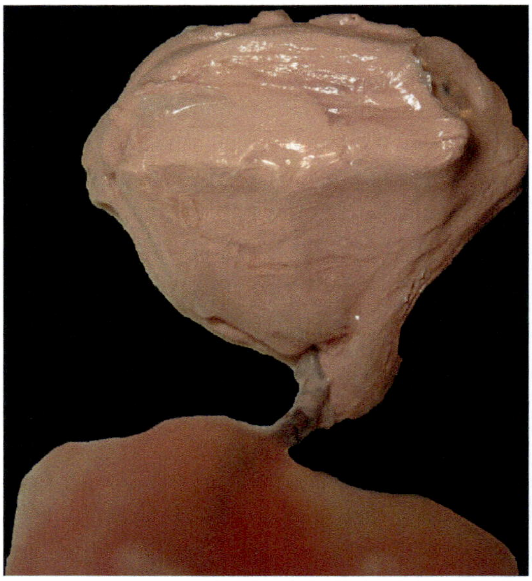

Fig. 5.20 Impression of the palatal defect with a zinc oxide eugenol impression material

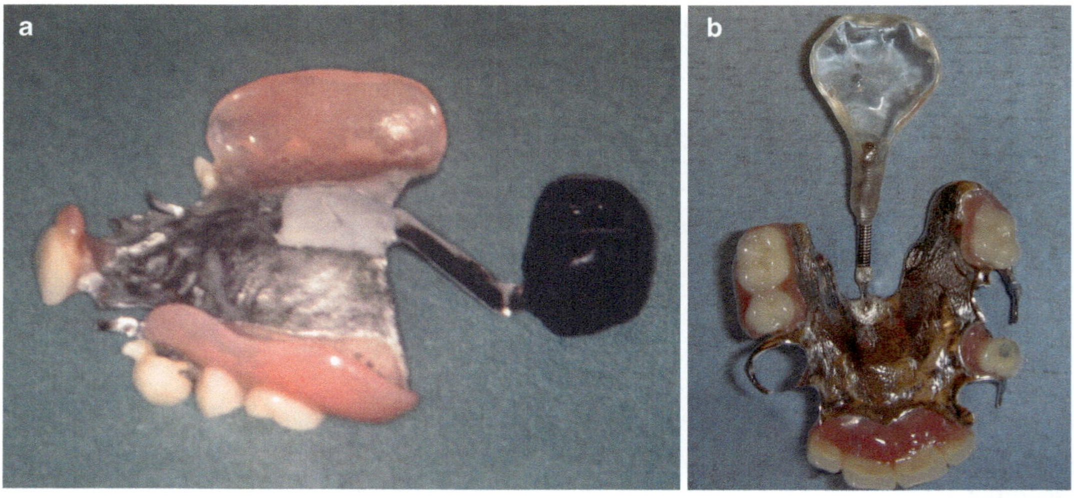

Fig. 5.19 (**a**, **b**) Palatal prostheses with a pharyngeal obturator. Note the three portions: anterior, intermediate and posterior

of the prosthetic closure. If the patient drinks in an upright position, liquid should not reflux into the nasal cavity (Hakan Tuna et al. 2009).

The defect's aetiology may determine the type of prosthesis that is indicated for the patient. In many cases, an interim prosthesis may be useful to get the patient accustomed to the feel of the prosthesis and the pressure exerted by the obturator (Raj et al. 2012) (Figs. 5.21 and 5.22).

Finally, in prosthodontic treatment of edentulous CLP patients with hard and soft palate defects, it is sometimes difficult to obtain a good result because of the weight of the prosthesis and the difficulty of establishing an atmospheric seal (Hakan Tuna et al. 2009), leading to loosening of the appliance from the palate. An effective speech-aid prosthesis must have a good retention and stability to improve the oral functions, which is often not achievable in the absence of teeth. In this case, and when it is medically and anatomically possible, osseo-integrated implants may be helpful to establish the support and mechanical retention needed to provide good prosthesis stability in such patients (Hakan Tuna et al. 2009; Abreu et al. 2007).

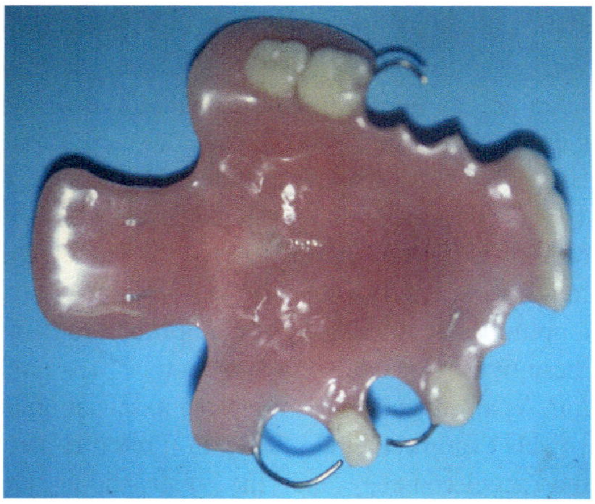

Fig. 5.21 Acrylic resin palatal lift prosthesis

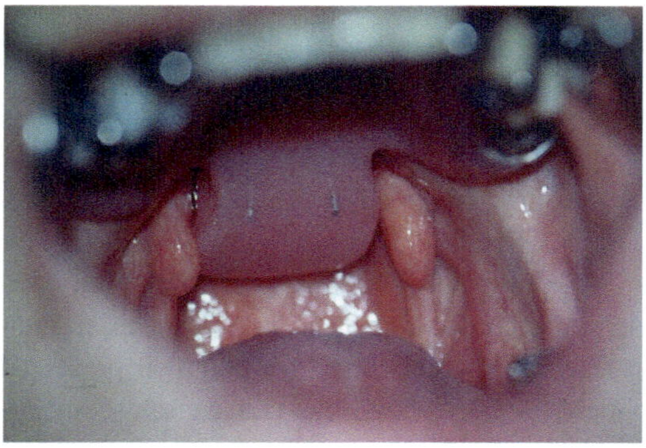

Fig. 5.22 Palatal lift prosthesis in place

The speech pathologist should work closely with the prosthodontist (Dhakshaini et al. 2015) to eliminate any compensatory articulation productions established before prosthetic management (Pinto et al. 2007; Freitas et al. 2013). Pinto et al. (2007) showed that a large majority of patients reported an improvement in their quality of speech and also felt comfortable with the help of the palatal prosthesis. Similarly, Nohara et al. (2010) reported a decrease in elevator muscle fatigue during speech in patients with a speech-aid prosthesis. A good prosthetic rehabilitation of CLP and VP dysfunction in children and adults in an interdisciplinary context helps to restore the oral functions and the aesthetics, and contributes directly and positively to the psychological state of the patient (Destruhaut et al. 2015).

The authors are most grateful to Pr. Philippe Pomar (PU-PH, Unité Fonctionnelle de Prothèse Maxillo-Faciale, Service d'Odontologie de Rangueil, Toulouse) and Dr. Jacques Dichamp (Stomatologue, Paris) for their precious advice and for some of the photographs included in this article. Many thanks also to Susan Becker for her help in the translation of this chapter.

5.10 Computerised Rehabilitation of Inappropriate Nasalisation

Antoinette am Zehnhoff-Dinnesen

5.10.1 Introduction

Principles of computerised rehabilitation (CR) aiming at developmental disorders of speech and language are presented in Sect. 13.6 in Volume 1. Special CR information related to stuttering is displayed in Sect. 10.5 in this volume. Technical aspects of CR are addressed in detail in Sect. 20.9 which concerns dysarthria/aphasia. Section 31.1 highlights telepractice options. Spectral speech analysis of hypernasality is presented as a diagnostic tool in Sect. 3.16, nasometry in Sect. 3.17 and nasopharyngoscopic biofeedback in the therapy Sects. 5.5 and 5.6.

In this section, an overview will be given of CR of inappropriate nasalisation by a disorder of the velopharyngeal valve. The velopharyngeal valve consists of the velum and the lateral and posterior pharyngeal walls. The space between these structures is called velopharyngeal port (VP port) or velopharyngeal sphincter (Fig. 5.23). Closure of the VP port should occur during swallowing, gagging, blowing, sucking and the production of non-nasal sounds (Shprintzen et al. 1974).

Velopharyngeal dysfunction (VPD) comprises velopharyngeal insufficiency (VPI) by structural deficits (e.g. in children with cleft palate), velopharyngeal incompetence (VPI) (e.g. by a neurological disease) and velopharyngeal mislearning (functional, e.g. owing to hearing impairment). VPD can cause pathological nasality and nasal air emission, hampering speech intelligibility and affecting listeners' attitude.

Nasality and its inappropriate alterations may be defined as:

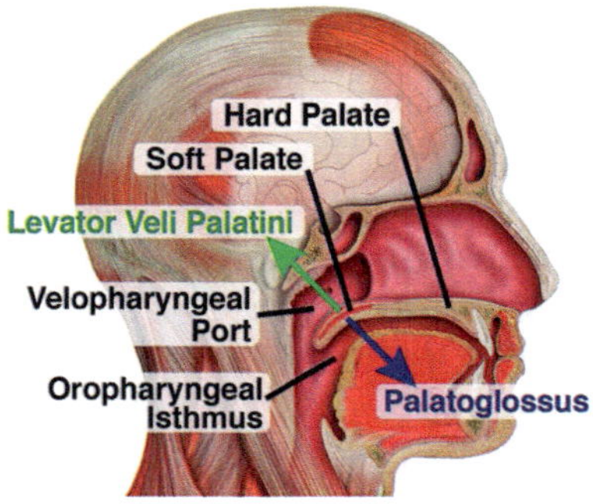

Fig. 5.23 Structures of the velopharyngeal valve and the velopharyngeal port. *M. palatoglossus* closes the oropharyngeal isthmus and acts as antagonist of the *M. levator veli palatini* (Reprinted from Anderson P, Fels S, Stavness I et al. (2019) Intravelar and Extravelar Portions of Soft Palate Muscles in Velic Constrictions: A Three-Dimensional Modeling Study. JSLHR (2019) 62(4):802–814 (adapted from image by Patrick J. Lynch, medical illustrator) (http://creativecommons.org/licenses/by/2.5))

Nasality is the percept of the nasalization of a voiced speech sound. When oral vowels are produced with an inappropriately open VP port, an excess of acoustic energy emanates from the nasal passages, which is perceived as hypernasality. In speech perceived as hyponasal, the VP port is closed to an inappropriate degree in sounds that are intended to be nasalized, resulting in reduction of the acoustic energy emitted through the nasal cavity (Heller Murray et al. 2016)

CR options offer therapeutic approaches and may be used as evaluation tools for monitoring therapy effects. In the following only a few examples can be presented.

5.10.2 Computerised Rehabilitation: Therapeutic Approaches

5.10.2.1 Accelerometry

In a case series of children with VPD, Cler et al. (2017) tested an interactive video game that provided real-time biofeedback on nasalisation by nasal accelerometry (recording vibrations of the nasal tissue during speech). The authors used the Horii Oral-Nasal Coupling Index (HONC; Horii 1980) in a filtered version. HONC is based on the ratio of nasal acceleration to acoustic output: the ratio of accelerometer and microphone-signal amplitudes is divided by the amplitude ratio of these two signals during production of the sound /m/. As an advantage in measuring nasalisation in vowels (Varghese et al. 2014), in filtered HONC the accelerometer and the microphone are bandpass-filtered. Figure 5.24 shows the headset with the microphone placed at a defined distance from the mouth and the Hot Spot accelerometer (K&K Sound, Coos Bay OR) fixed to the nasal skin with double-sided tape.

By using nasometry, aerodynamic measures and expert perceptual judgements, the extent of nasalisation was measured before and after therapy. Nasalisation decreased after training in four participants who used the system at home or at school, one participant discontinued his participation. The authors conclude that their presented video game offers an inexpensive and comfortable solution to supplement speech therapy. Further research is needed.

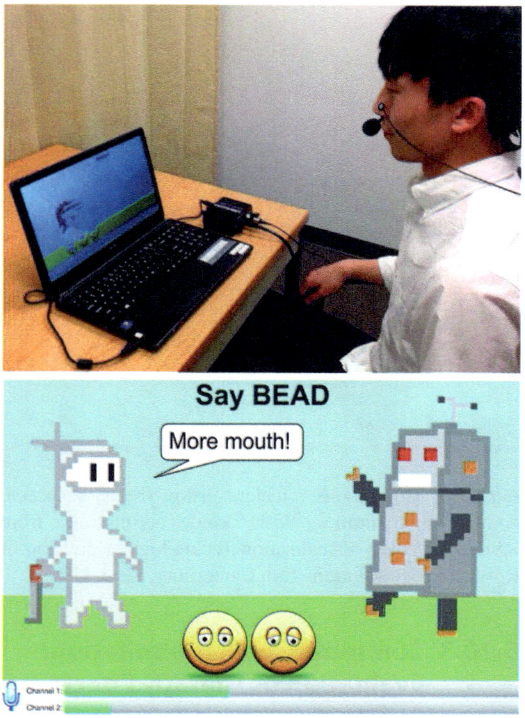

Fig. 5.24 Accelerometer, microphone and laptop in the upper part and a training example in the lower part: the robot wants the player/ninja to repeat the word 'bead' three times; after each repetition a smiley or frowny face indicates nasalisation quality; the latter corresponds to the next action of the ninja who is fighting the robot (Reprinted from Cler GJ, Mittelman T, Braden MN et al. (2017). Video Game Rehabilitation of Velopharyngeal Dysfunction: A Case Series. Journal of speech, language, and hearing research: JSLHR, 60(6S), 1800–1809, with permission from American Speech-Language-Hearing Association) (for the ebook permission will end after 5 years)

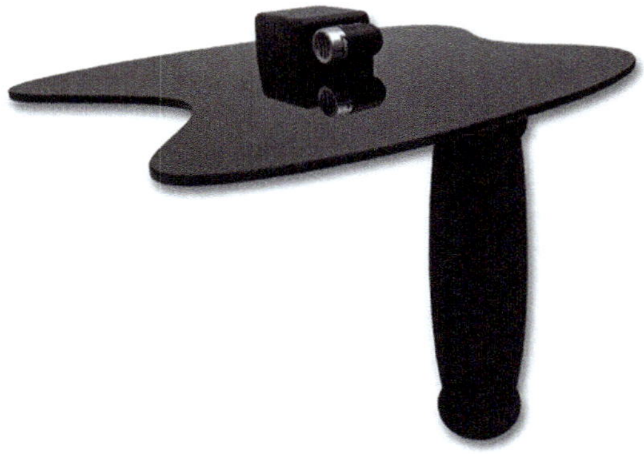

Fig. 5.25 Portable nasometry unit of icSpeech (https://icspeech.com/nasometry.html). With kind permission from icSpeech Speech Visualisation Technology, a division of Rose Medical Solutions Ltd, Canterbury, Kent, UK

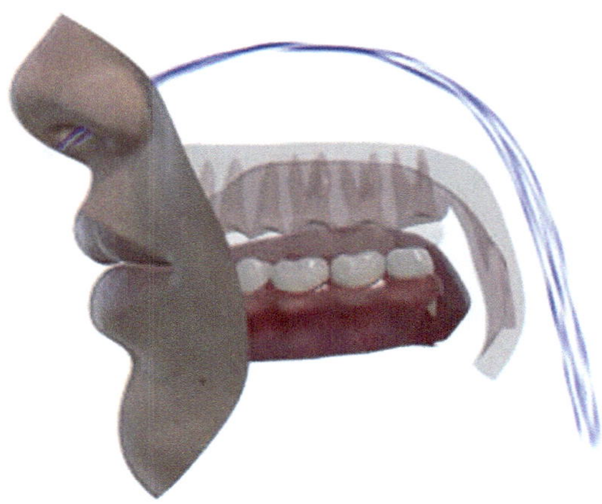

Fig. 5.26 Nasal airflow (lowered soft palate)

5.10.2.2 Nasometry

Nasalance (Bzoch 1989) is calculated in voiced sounds as a percentage of the nasal acoustic energy (sound pressure level SPL of sound emanating from the nose) in relation to the sum in SPL of nasal and oral acoustic energy (added from oral and nasal speech signals) (Fletcher et al. 1974). For visual feedback it can be presented in real-time.

The portable Nasometry Unit of icSpeech consists of highly directional nasal and oral microphones. The acoustic separator is placed above the upper lip (Fig. 5.25).

The NasalanceViewer 3D of icSpeech offers computer animation and 3D modelling techniques to illustrate the movements of articulators, the extent of velopharyngeal closure and nasal or oral airflow (Figs. 5.26, 5.27, 5.28, and 5.29).

An exemplary use of the software Nasalance Viewer can be found in Young et al. (2022). Further measurement systems of nasalance are explained in detail in Bressmann (2021).

5.10.2.3 Speech Analysis/Speech Recognition

Hsieh et al. (2015) developed and tested the user-friendly game Spokelt for children with cleft palate. Spokelt may be used on mobile devices. Sudro et al. (2021) used the cycle-consistent adversarial network (CycleGAN) method to

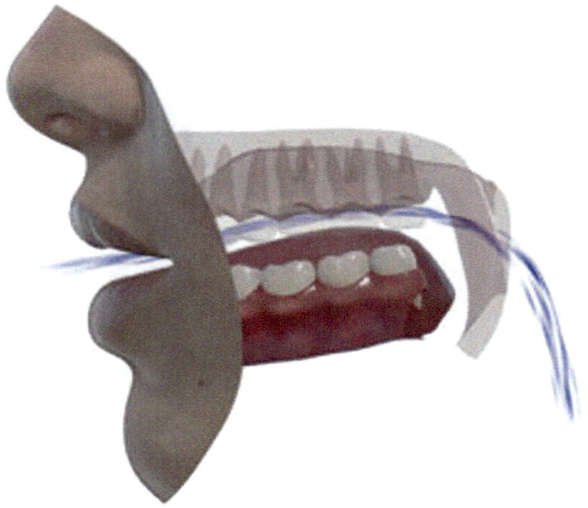

Fig. 5.27 Oral airflow (raised soft palate) (https://icspeech.com/nasometry.html). With kind permission from icSpeech Speech Visualisation Technology, a division of Rose Medical Solutions Ltd, Canterbury, Kent, UK

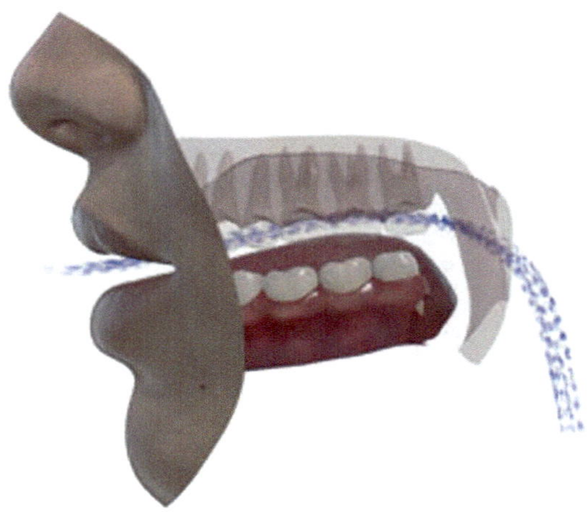

Fig. 5.28 Intermittent voiced airflow

enhance speech intelligibility of patients with cleft lip and palate (CLP). The system was trained in the Kannada language (India) by speech samples from 31 children with CLPs and 31 non-CLP controls. Objective measures and perceptual judgements confirmed speech intelligibility improvement. Future research is necessary.

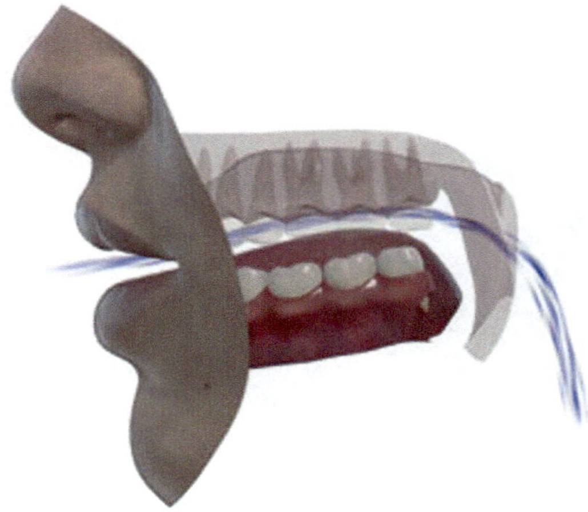

Fig. 5.29 Continuous voiceless airflow (https://icspeech.com/nasometry.html). With kind permission from icSpeech Speech Visualisation Technology, a division of Rose Medical Solutions Ltd, Canterbury, Kent, UK

5.10.3 Computerised Rehabilitation: Evaluation of Therapy Effects

5.10.3.1 Accelerometer

Heller Murray et al. (2016) used biofeedback in 48 adults with typical speech to change vowel nasalisation. They demonstrated the benefit of HONC for training control of nasalisation. Phonemic contexts (nasal or non-nasal) and the presence of augmentative visual feedback during training reliably predicted changes in nasalance scores from pre- to post-training.

5.10.3.2 Nasometry

Nasalance can be used for off-line analysis. For example, the NasalanceViewer 3D of icSpeech in real-time shows percentages of nasal speech, oral speech and nasalance during speech production. The Nasometer II (Model 6450) from PENTAX Medical provides objective measurements of nasalance and real-time processing for immediate biofeedback. Model 6500 also offers an intra-individual comparison of patient data during treatment and a comparison with norm data.

5.10.3.3 Speech Analysis/Speech Recognition

Seaward et al. (2018) presented an automated cleft speech evaluator (trained speech recognition engine) which achieved 85% agreement with SLP ratings interpreting resonance and articulatory cleft speech errors. Such an evaluation system allows outcome collaboration between cleft centres. Mathad et al. (2021) trained a deep neural network (DNN) to detect the presence of nasal acoustic cues with the aim to compute a speech analysis algorithm, the objective hypernasality measure (OHM). OHM results significantly correlated with the perceptual hypernasality ratings in the Americleft database and the New Mexico Cleft Palate Center database.

Zhang et al. (2020) used linear prediction methods to distinguish hypernasal from normal speech. Defining four grades from normal to severe hypernasal, the stabilised (SWLP) and the extended weighted linear prediction method (XLP) achieved classification accuracies from 83.9% to 97.5%. The study was based on Mandarin speech samples from 60 participants with cleft palate and 20 controls.

Young et al. (2022) developed a new system to detect hypernasality, based on broadband noise excitation at the nostrils (nRMD). In one participant, they could show a systematic difference between normal and hypernasal speech by the resulting transfer functions from the nRMD. In the frequency region 2–2.5 kHz, a peak present in normal speech decreased in centre frequency and amplitude in hypernasal speech. This promising result has to be validated by further research.

5.10.4 Conclusion

Facing pandemic situations or living in rural and under-served regions may be reasons for a more intensive application of CR in inappropriate nasalisation. Motivating games in the familial context may increase the compliance of patients and parents. The quality of speech analysis/speech recognition systems approximates perceptual judgements. CR therapy and evaluation tools may valuably assist SLP/logopaedic services.

5.11 General Principles of Drug Treatment (Sialorrhoea/Hypersalivation)

Saskia Rohrbach-Volland

5.11.1 Nomenclature and Pathogenesis

Hypersalivation describes an absolute or relative increase of saliva. The flow of saliva is called sialorrhoea. Hypersalivation and sialorrhoea can be used as synonyms. Drooling indicates the discharge of saliva from the mouth, and does not take into account the 'pooling' of saliva in the hypopharynx with the possibility of aspiration. An absolute overproduction is rather uncommon, whereas a relatively high amount of saliva is more often the case. Caused by decreased oromotor competence, defects in central nervous control or disturbed swallowing through neurological deficits, trauma or tumour (-resection), excess saliva can dampen lips, chin, hands, clothes and furniture, and enter the lower respiratory tract, causing infections such as bronchitis and pneumonia. Hypersalivation reduces social interaction and augments time and effort of the carers. If it is strongly developed, tracheotomy, as a protection of the lower airway, can often not be avoided and have a negative impact on the disease and on healthcare costs.

5.11.2 Diagnostics

Diagnostic procedures and therapeutic interventions have to be started soon after onset of hypersalivation and follow an interdisciplinary concept. Primarily, the focus should be on the examination of swallowing problems and orofacial myofunctional disorders: screenings and clinical assessments are followed by a differential examination of the orofacial functions, the larynx and a functional endoscopic evaluation of swallowing in adults and even in children (Reynolds et al. 2016). Videofluoroscopy can support the examination and provide important evidence of causes, therapy and development of the disorder (DeMatteo et al. 2005). New studies by real-time MRI show comparable results and will become of more clinical interest because of the absence of radiation burden (Olthoff et al. 2016).

5.11.3 Therapeutic Approaches

The improvement of the underlying disease, enhancement of oromotor function and eliminating malocclusions and dysphagia are the goals of the therapeutic approach. Surgical interventions such as myotomia of the oesophageal sphincter, and operations on the salivary glands or their ducts are reserved for rare and individual cases. If a modern 3D technique that protects the surrounding tissue is used, X-irradiation can reduce saliva. Because of its carcinogenic potential, it is applied only as the last resort in some diseases that cannot be influenced by other methods.

For acute hypersalivation, different drugs are available to reduce saliva flow. Atropine, transdermal scopolamine, ipratropium bromide and trihexyphenidyl (benzhexol) hydrochloride are used, but do have some limiting side effects through their anticholinergic impact (Bavikatte et al. 2012; De Simone et al. 2006; Hyson et al. 2002; Talmi et al. 1990; Lewis et al. 1994; Fairhurst and Cockerill 2011; Sockalingam et al. 2009; Mier et al. 2000). Different glycopyrrolates have been used, glycopyrronium bromide received clinical acceptance for on-label use with permission from the European Medicines Agency (EMA) in 2016 for application in children over 3 years of age.

Botulinum toxin plays a major role in the treatment of hypersalivation (Ellies et al. 2002a, b, 2004; Lim et al. 2006). Eight different serotypes are known (A–H), but only types A and B are used for clinical purposes. Botulinum toxins, produced by *clostridium botulinum*, an anaerobic bacterium, prevents the discharge of actylcholine from the presynaptic nerve terminal at the muscular or glandular synapses by changing the structural combination of different proteins (syntaxin, SNAP 25, synaptobrevin 2). Botulinum toxins are metalloproteases composed of a light chain (50 kDa, toxic subdomain) and a heavy chain (100 kDa, binding and transport domain), combined through two sulfide bridges. The anticholinergic effect is temporary and completely reversible: by 'sprouting' of transient nerve terminals, the therapeutic effect diminishes after a specific time before the original axon recovers and the sprouts disappear. This mechanism has different durations in neuromuscular versus autonomous synapses. The reason for this is yet to be determined.

Botulinum toxin A is available as onabotulinum toxin A (Botox®), incobotulinum toxin A (Xeomin®) and abobotulinum toxin A (Dysport®). In the USA, the use of incobotulinum toxin A for sialorrhoea was approved for use in adults in 2018, irrespective of the underlying disease. In Europe it was approved for adults in 2019 and in children in 2021 (Jost et al. 2021; Steffen and Rohrbach-Volland 2021). Such an approval has a tremendous influence on its use in the outpatient setting (for example liability and regress). A pivotal phase III placebo-controlled study of incobotulinum toxin A (incoBoNT/A) showed its superiority over placebo and confirmed IncoBoNT/A (up to 75 U, up to 4 cycles) as a well-tolerated treatment for sialorrhoea in children (Berweck et al. 2021). Botulinum toxin B is available as rimabotulinum toxin B (Myobloc™, Neurobloc®). The units of these four types (ona-, inco-, abo- and rima-botulinum) are not the same, equivalent units have to be respected. Even though rima-botulinum has the strongest anticholinergic effect on the autonomous nervous system (Ondo et al. 2004), it is used rather seldom because of the higher rate of the occurrence of antibodies against proteins of botulinum toxins (HA-HA1 and -HA3b subgroups).

Pre-requisites for botulinum injection include a differential anamnesis, an ENT-examination and an ultrasound of the salivary glands, in addition to specific examinations for the underlying disease. Other morphometric examinations such as a CT or MRI scan might be helpful in some cases. To assess hypersalivation clinically, different questionnaires exist and some use the cotton roll method to measure the amount of saliva and

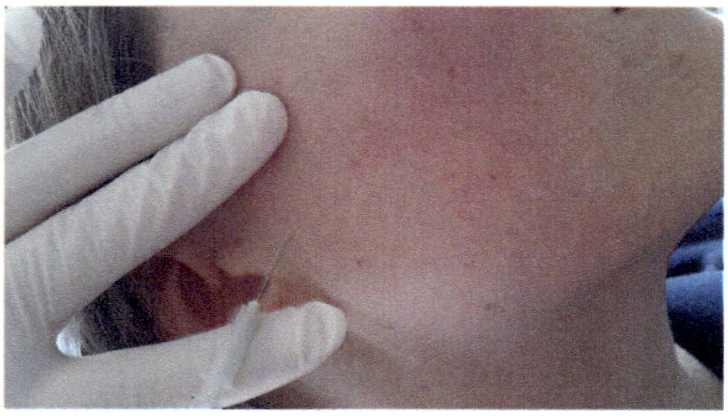

Fig. 5.30 Injection into the parotid gland

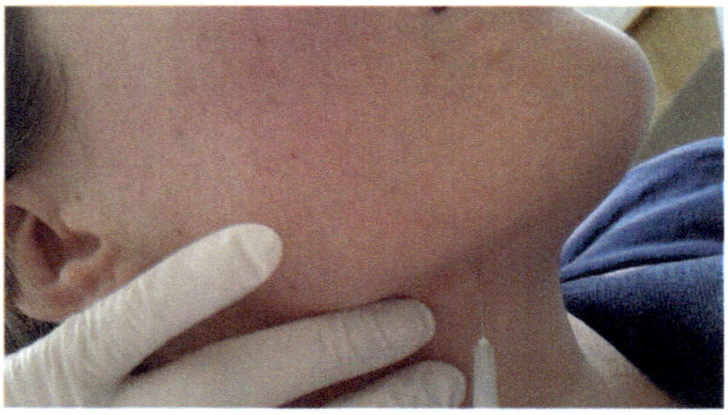

Fig. 5.31 Injection into the submandibular gland

its components quantitatively or qualitatively (Ellies et al. 2002b). This might also be useful to assess the therapeutic effect of treatment.

Botulinum toxin A is diluted in saline (for example 100 units onabotulinum toxin A in 4 ml sterile saline 0.9% (w/v) contains 2.5 units onabotulinum toxin A in 0.1 ml) and injected into the parotid and submandibular glands (Figs. 5.30 and 5.31) under ultrasound control to avoid the distribution into the muscles of the floor of the mouth, and thus prevent swallowing problems. The recommended dose is 100 units distributed on the parotid glands (30 units each) and submandibular glands (20 units each) with a re-injection interval of 16 weeks (Bäumer et al. 2018). The hazard of weakening the facial mimic muscles through injection into the pre-auricular facial nerve is negligible because the nerve itself does not have any cholinergic synapses. The therapeutic effect appears after approximately 3–7 days.

Side effects are rare and avoidable with a correct injection technique. Foreseeable side effects are infection, bleeding and local haematoma, as well as undesired weakening of musculature of the masseter muscle and muscles of the floor of the mouth, leading to dysphagia. In some cases, this occurs not because of incorrect injection but because of diffusion of the toxin into nearby muscles.

The injection of botulinum toxin in hypersalivation is effective, safe and has few side effects. Therefore, it has been recommended in current guidelines for the treatment of hypersalivation in different European countries (Bavikatte et al. 2012; Bäumer et al. 2018).

5.12 Principles of Craniofacial Surgery

Alexander Hemprich

5.12.1 Introduction

Craniofacial malformations were described by Herodotus, Hippocrates (fifth century BC) and later Galen (second century AD) in ancient Greece and Rome. In 1851, Virchow published nine forms of 'pathological skull shapes' which he described as a result of premature closure of the skull sutures naming this phenomenon 'craniosynostosis'. He also assumed a connection between a primary disturbance of skull structure with consecutive changes in the brain (Virchow 1851).

Today, the incidence of all forms of craniosynostoses is estimated at 1:2000 live births (Robin 1999).

The vast majority of them represent isolated (single suture) forms which can usually be treated well by a relevant operation in early childhood. On the other hand, there are more than 150 genetic syndromes including a craniosynostosis (Cohen 1995). The resulting deformities affect neurocranium (skull) and viscerocranium (face) alike. Owing to a rising intracranial pressure there is a risk not only for headaches/sleep disorders in infants but even more for the normal development of the child. In severe forms of craniofacial stenoses (M. Crouzon, M. Apert), the shallow orbits will result in an exorbitism, which may lead to an ophthalmopathy up to blindness.

Thus, it is necessary that an interdisciplinary surgical approach is undertaken by neurofacial and maxillofacial surgeons together at the age of 7–12 months to prevent the above named problems.

The differential diagnosis to a true craniosynostosis is a positional plagiocephaly where the sutures remain open but the skull undergoes a deformation by many external factors. In these cases, a conservative treatment may be sufficient if started within the first 6 months after birth.

5.12.2 Aetiology and Development of Neuro- and Viscero-cranium

The skull consists of a base formed out of a chondral matrix that influences the growth of the neuro- and viscero-cranium and a desmal bone matrix for the adjacent bones. The connection is formed by a membranous structure—the dura mater.

In the sixth embryonal week, the open chondral capsule is fully developed and can be seen as a primary growth centre, which means that the activity of the chondroblasts directs the further growth of the cartilaginous skull base (Joos 1995a). During further normal development, the base will lengthen, and the cranial vault will widen. Bony parts of the skull will adjust to the demand of the growing brain by apposition on the outside and resorption on the inside. The main place for bony growth happens on the edges. After the cessation of brain volume increase (end of the second decade), the sutures are closed by tight connective tissue (Enlow 1990) (Fig. 5.32).

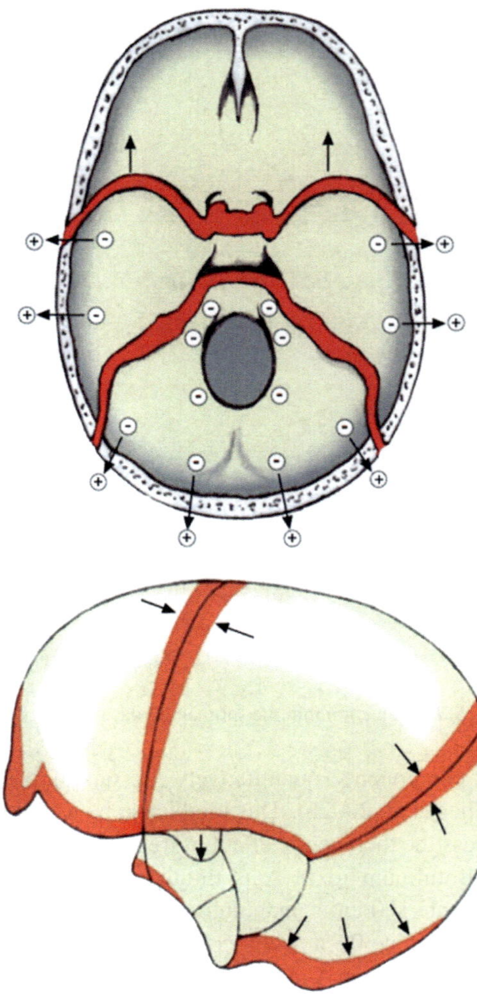

Fig. 5.32 Schematic illustration of skull base and calvarial growth ((after Enlow 1990) from Zöller JE et al. 2003, Kraniofaziale Chirurgie © 2002 Georg Thieme Verlag KG, Stuttgart, New York NY. With permission © Thieme Group)

In a normal child, brain volume triples in the first 12 months after birth and will reach 80% of the adult volume at the end of the second year (Fig. 5.33).

Thus, it is absolutely necessary that cranial sutures remain open until the brain has reached its full size.

Skull growth must be seen as a process that can be influenced by multiple internal (e.g. genetic defects, insufficient brain growth) and external factors such as metabolic disorders, foetal head constraint, irradiation (Cohen 1988). These may finally result in a *premature closure of a single or of several sutures*. Skull growth will then be obstructed perpendicular to the affected suture(s). Consequently, the growing brain seeks to gain room in the least obstructed direction so that skull growth has to continue uni- or bi-laterally opposite the affected region. Thus, the different deformities can easily be explained. In most cases, the growth disturbance of the neurocranium will also have an impact on facial growth (viscerocranium) to a different extent (see Sect. 15.3.5).

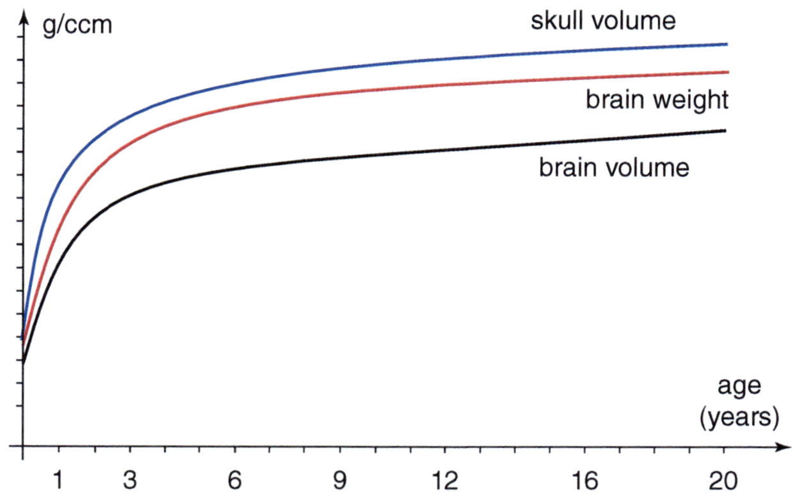

Fig. 5.33 Growth of brain and skull in the first 20 years ((after Boyd 1962) from Zöller JE et al. 2003, Kraniofaziale Chirurgie © 2002 Georg Thieme Verlag KG, Stuttgart, New York NY. With permission © Thieme Group)

Any *disturbance of the enchondral ossification of the skull base* at an early stage, however, will lead to severe craniofacial syndromes (Morbus Crouzon, Morbus Apert, Morbus Saethre-Chotzen, M. Pfeiffer) where a mutation of the FGFR2 gene (fibroblast growth factor receptor-2) on chromosome 10 is assumed to be the underlying cause. The prevalence of these syndromes is from 1:25,000 live births for M. Crouzon, 1:50,000 for M. Saethre-Chotzen and 1:100,000 for M. Apert and Pfeiffer (Ghali et al. 2019). The lack of a longitudinal development of the skull base leads to a grave dysmorphy of skull and face (brachycephalus).

5.12.3 Symptoms of Premature Skull Suture Closure

The symptoms of a premature closure of the skull sutures depend on time of onset, localisation and the affected numbers. The earlier the suture closure starts the more severe the growth obstruction will be. Thus, some mild forms of craniostenoses may not even need a surgical intervention whereas others will lead to a massive impairment of form and function. Depending on the main affected part there are different consequences for the neurocranium and the viscerocranium:

- Neurocranium
  - Chronically elevated intracranial pressure (headaches, sleeping problems, possible intelligence defects)
  - Decrease of cerebral blood perfusion (border zone infarction)
  - Cerebral atrophy with irreversible loss of brain functions
  - Obstruction of liquor circulation (possible hydrocephalus)
  - Damage to the optical nerve(s) (blindness)
  - Impairment of the psychosocial development
- Viscerocranium
  - Shallow orbits with exorbitism/protrusio bulbi, chronic keratitis, cornea erosions
  - Hypertelorism (with strabism)
  - Midfacial hypoplasia, obstructive sleep apnoea (chronic airway infections, severe development problems, right heart strain)
  - Dysgnathia (impaired maxillary-mandibular relation resulting in speech problems)

5.12.4 Diagnostics of Craniofacial Deformity

Usually, a craniofacial deformity can be diagnosed clinically early after birth. There are asymmetries of skull or face, which in mild cases, however, may be detected not before some weeks or even months have elapsed or the irregular development becomes obvious.

The examination of these children comprises a thorough clinical evaluation with a complete neurological and an ophthalmological status by a paediatrician, a maxillofacial and a neurosurgeon and an ENT colleague as well as an ophthalmologist and a geneticist. Quite often, a developmental deficit can be detected without extensive apparative measures.

If the fontanelles are no longer or just hardly present at the age of 4–6 months, an ultrasound scan will determine whether the sutures are still open. It has also proved effective to measure just the difference between the cranial diagonals with large calipers to find out whether the child has a positional plagiocephaly or a real single suture stenosis. In a positional plagiocephaly, the head is shaped like a parallelogram, whereas in a unilateral coronary synostosis the forehead is flat on the affected side with a bossing on the contralateral side (Ellenbogen et al. 2000) (see also Sect. 5.13.6)

Finally, 3D photogrammetrics are useful to take accurate records of the craniofacial development over several weeks/months. X-ray exposure should definitely be avoided in early infancy. Nowadays CT scans (cave: radiation!) in infants can almost be completely replaced by a 'Black Bone' MRI (magnetic resonance imaging) which is able to depict the bony structures of the skull so well that even 3-D models can be printed from these data (Eley et al. 2017). Thus, 'black' MRI may be seen as the standard method for imaging in these cases (Lethaus et al. 2021).

5.12.5 Classification of Craniosynostosis

Craniosynostoses can be classified according to three systems:

1. Skull shape
2. The affected skull sutures
3. Aetiology

5.12.5.1 Skull Shape

Virchow (1851) had already described nine forms of different skull shapes due to craniosynostosis. More recently Marchac and Renier (1982) summed up the possible malformations under therapeutic/surgical aspects to just five typical skull forms:

- Scaphocephalus, Trigonocephalus, Plagiocephalus: only one suture affected in most cases
- Oxycephalus, Brachycephalus: more severe forms due to the involvement of several sutures and the cranial base

This descriptive nomenclature has proven to be quite useful since the majority of diseases fit into this scheme, which in turn allows a certain standardised approach to surgery. Fine details and differences and the extent of the malformation cannot be described, however. Nevertheless, this classification has prevailed over those based on the affected sutures or on aetiology.

5.12.5.2 The Affected Skull Sutures

The exact knowledge of the affected sutures and their numbers give a more detailed knowledge of the whole region beyond the outer appearance. The extent and the severity of the malformation can be assessed satisfactorily and allow a precise operative planning. It may be necessary, though, to repeat imaging of the sutures (ultrasound, 'black' MRI but no CT scans!) several times in the first 5–9 months of the child since the process of a premature closure is often dynamic.

5.12.5.3 Aetiology

Craniosynostoses can be also be classified by the underlying aetiology:

(a) Primary craniosynostosis
In these cases, the bone building matrix has a developmental defect. Simple and isolated forms can be distinguished from more complex and syndromal types. So far, more than 150 syndromes are associated with craniosynostosis (Wang et al. 2016) with different incidence, genetics and variability. The best

known ones are M. Crouzon, M. Apert and M. Saethre-Chotzen

(b) Secondary craniosynostosis
This phenomenon is rather rare. When a child has a brain developmental disorder with a lack of brain expansion or even brain atrophy, there is no longer a stimulus from the dura to the surrounding bones for skull enlargement. Consequently, the sutures will be closed early resulting in a microcephalus. There are also secondary craniosynostoses induced by a hydrocephalus or a shunt (Wang et al. 2016) (Fig. 5.34).

(c) Metabolic craniosynostosis
These cases are also very rare. Some forms of hyperthyroidism or a hypophosphatasia can lead to craniosynostosis. In a recent study, maternal smoking and the intake of selective serotonin uptake inhibitors (psychotropic drugs) were identified as factors that may exacerbate incidence and severity of craniofacial abnormalities (Durham et al. 2019). The exact aetiopathogenesis is not known so far, but a multifactorial genesis with a genetic influence is the most probable cause.

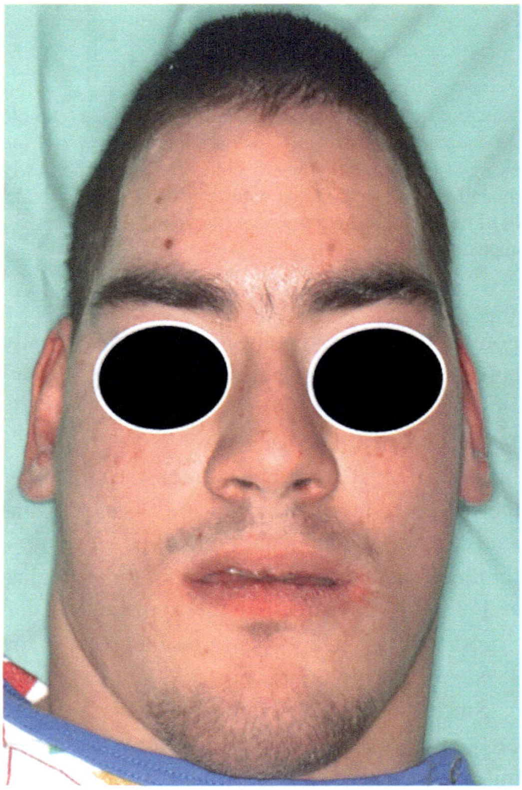

Fig. 5.34 Shunt-induced secondary craniosynostosis (courtesy of Prof. (em.) J. Bennek, Dept. of Pediatric Surgery, University Hospital of Leipzig, Germany)

5.12.6 The Most Typical Skull Deformities

5.12.6.1 Dolicho- or Scapho-cephalus

This is the most frequent deformity (about 50% of all cases) with a long and narrow head due to the premature closure of the sagittal suture. Forehead and especially the occiput show an increasing bossing. A bi-temporal deficit will also develop in the infratemporal region (Fig. 5.35a).

These children very often develop quite normally so that many parents are hesitant to have them operated. Arnaud et al. (1996), however, found significantly more normal patients in this group operated before than after the age of one year. The operation could not improve an already low mental level. Thus, the authors concluded that the indication for surgery at 8–10 months is not just a question of aesthetics.

Finally, it may be stated that the skull deformity worsens so that many patients are harassed by their peers at school. Thus, there is not an aesthetic but a psychosocial indication for a corrective operation.

Surgical therapy: In mild cases, an early (endoscopically assisted) strip craniectomy can be successful.

Since there is a tendency for a relapse, though, especially when the child is older than 1 year, the remodelling of the calvarial bones by a transverse widening and barrel stave remodelling may give better long-term results (Fig. 5.35b–d).

5.12.6.2 Plagiocephalus

This unilateral deformity makes up for about 25% of all craniosynostoses where the coronal suture is affected. There is a characteristic asymmetry with a flat forehead on the affected side and some bulging on the contralateral. Owing to shortening of the cranial base finally there will be a shift of the facial axis to the healthy side with a deformation of the nose. The orbital funnel

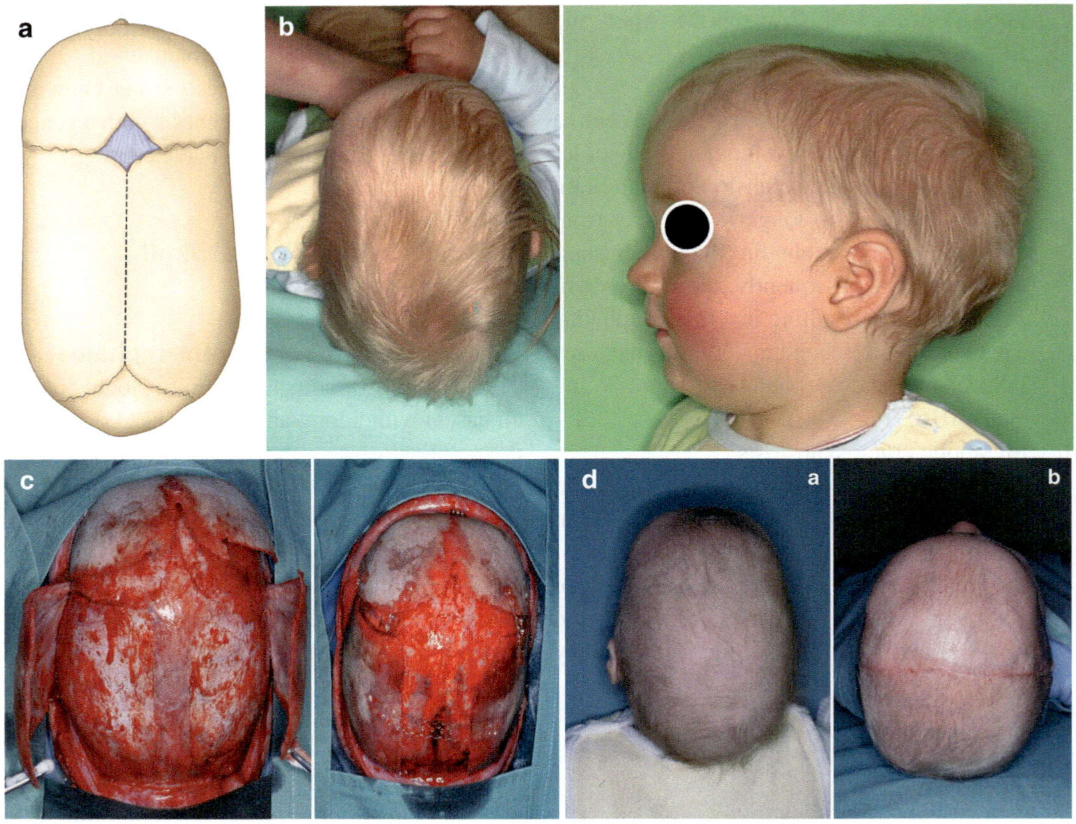

Fig. 5.35 (**a**) Schematic illustration of a scaphocephalus (after Recuero I I and Sanchez Aniceto G (2020) Craniosynostosis In: Ehrenfeld M, Futran N, Manson P, Prein J (ed.) Advanced craniomaxillofacial surgery. AO Foundation Thieme, Stuttgart, pages 464 and 465. Copyright by AO Foundation, Switzerland). (**b**) Typical scaphocephalus from above (l) and from the side (r); note the long and narrow skull. (**c**) Intraoperative view of the elevated frontal and temporal bones (left) and the newly modelled skull shape fixed with resorbable plates (right). (**d**) Pre- (left (a)) and 8 weeks post-operative (right (b)) appearance of the skull

appears flattened especially in the upper region. The lid axis will shift downward laterally. The occlusal plane will follow the affected side whereas the occlusion itself stays normal (Fig. 5.36a, b).

This craniosynostosis should also be operated upon by a cranioplasty depending on its extent to avoid severe facial deformities. The most important differential diagnosis to a unilateral coronal synostosis is a *positional plagiocephaly* due to a long lasting false positioning of the child's head in utero or later in early childhood. In these cases, the fontanellae are still wide open, and the head is mostly deformed like a parallelogram (Fig. 5.37a, b).

This is no indication for surgery but for conventional therapies such as consequent repositioning of the head, physiotherapy and finally helmet therapy (Jung and Yun 2020) (Fig. 5.38).

5.12.6.3 Trigonocephalus

In about 10% of all craniostenoses, the closure of the metopic suture (between the ossa frontalia) leads to the development of a midline crest in the forehead and a marked flattening of the frontolateral region also affecting the zygoma and the zygomatic arch. The eyes lie close together in the sense of a hypotelorism (Fig. 5.39a).

Since the onset of craniosynostosis is in the early intrauterine skull development, the deformity can usually be noticed very well just after birth. Normally this deformity is not accompanied by neurological disorders. Only in severe

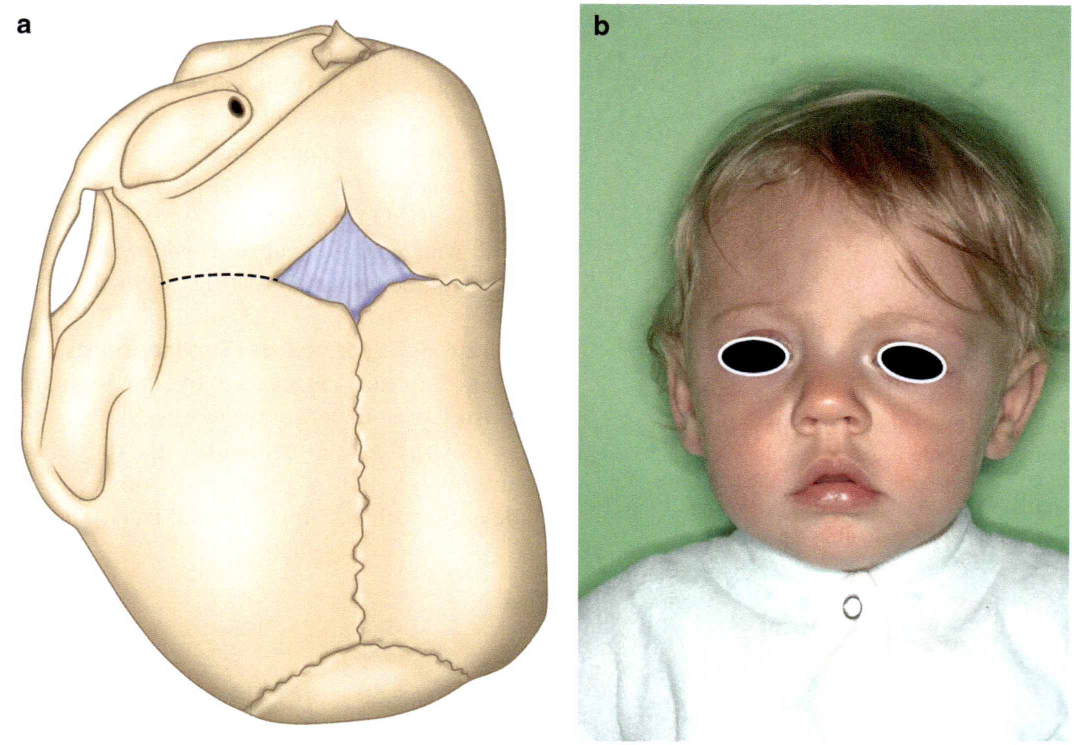

Fig. 5.36 (**a**) Schematic illustration of a plagiocephalus. Note the closed left coronal suture and the flat forehead and orbital rim on the left side with some bossing on the contralateral side (After Recuero I I and Sanchez Aniceto G (2020) Craniosynostosis In: Ehrenfeld M, Futran N, Manson P, Prein J (ed.) Advanced craniomaxillofacial surgery. AO Foundation Thieme Stuttgart, pages 464 and 465. Copyright by AO Foundation, Switzerland). (**b**) Clinical view of a child with a plagiocephalus; the lid axis of the left eye and the left supraorbital rim are shifted laterally downward

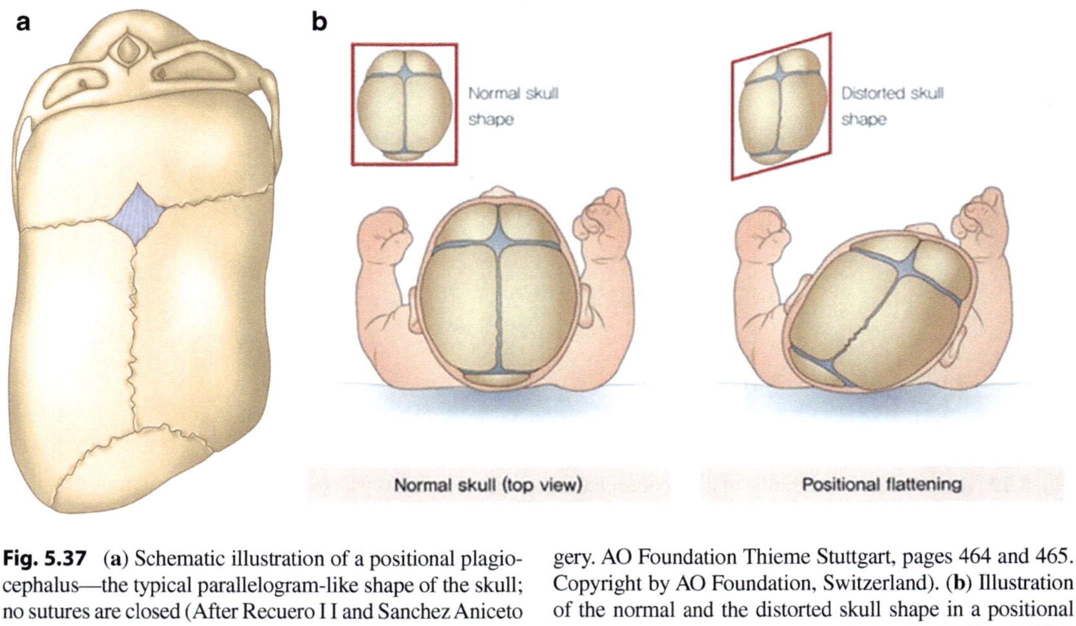

Fig. 5.37 (**a**) Schematic illustration of a positional plagiocephalus—the typical parallelogram-like shape of the skull; no sutures are closed (After Recuero I I and Sanchez Aniceto G (2020) Craniosynostosis. In: Ehrenfeld M, Futran N, Manson P, Prein J (ed.) Advanced craniomaxillofacial surgery. AO Foundation Thieme Stuttgart, pages 464 and 465. Copyright by AO Foundation, Switzerland). (**b**) Illustration of the normal and the distorted skull shape in a positional plagiocephaly (after Jung BK and Yun IS (2020). © 2020 The Korean Cleft Palate-Craniofacial Association)

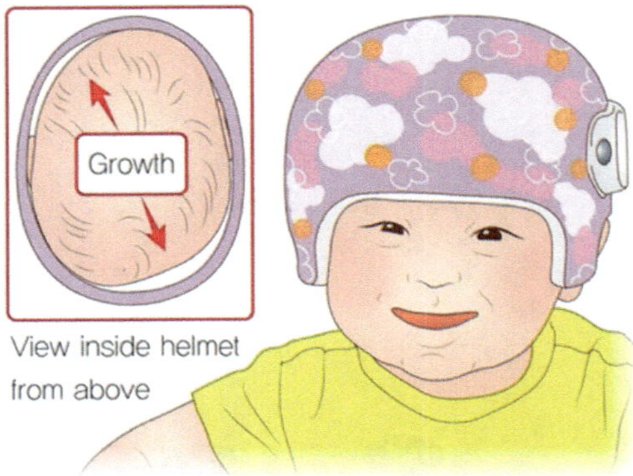

Fig. 5.38 Illustration of the principle of orthotic helmet therapy; pressure is exerted on the skull bulges and free room for development given on the other side (after Jung and Yun (2020). © 2020 The Korean Cleft Palate-Craniofacial Association)

forms is mental retardation possible, owing to the reduction of the space for the frontal lobes of the brain. There is a psychosocial indication for an operation, however, to help the child to achieve an inconspicuous appearance.

Treatment options: A classical fronto-orbital approach (FOA) is carried out (see also Fig. 5.45) with widening of the upper bandeau and remodelling of the frontal bones (Fig. 5.39b–d).

5.12.6.4 Oxycephalus (Turricephalus)

This deformity is caused by the premature closure of both coronary sutures. Skull growth is obstructed perpendicular to the closed sutures so that a high flat forehead will develop with flat upper orbital rims. Thus, an

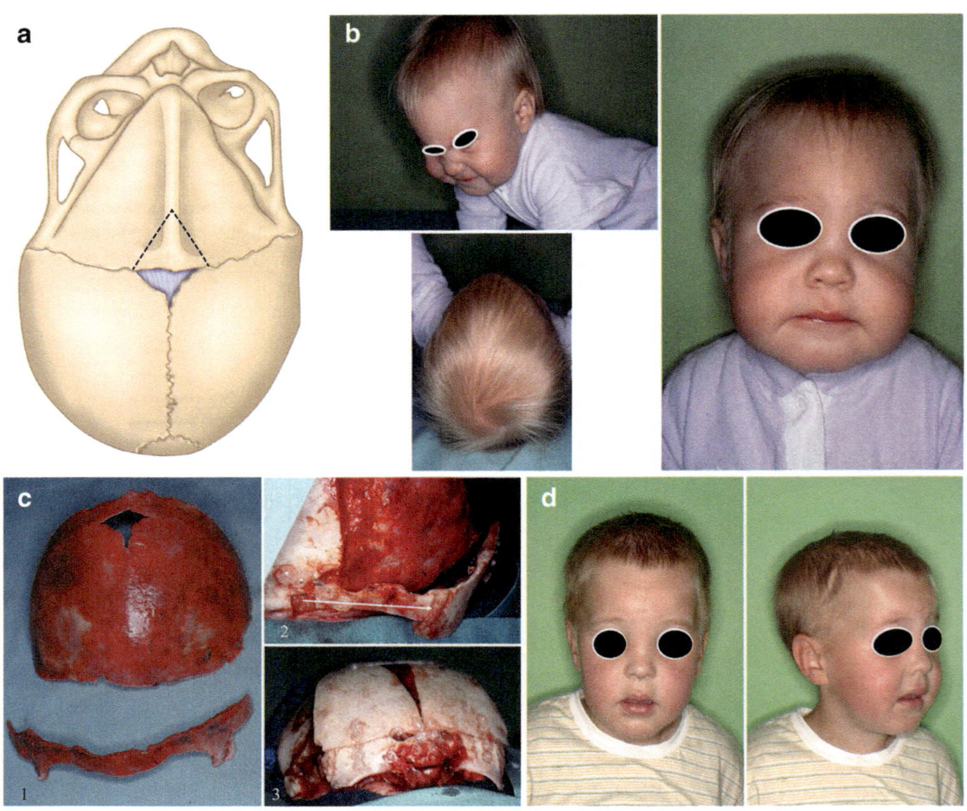

Fig. 5.39 (**a**) Schematic illustration of a trigonocephalus. Note the crest over the closed metopic suture and the resulting triangular shape of the forehead (After Recuero I I and Sanchez Aniceto G (2020) Craniosynostosis. In: Ehrenfeld M, Futran N, Manson P, Prein J (ed.) Advanced craniomaxillofacial surgery. AO Foundation Thieme Stuttgart, pages 464 and 465. Copyright by AO Foundation, Switzerland). (**b**) Clinical aspect of a typical trigonocephalus which can be clearly seen from above. (**c**) Intraoperative images with the elevated frontal bones and the upper bandeau (1), the marked forward movement of the upper bandeau which has been remodelled to abolish the midline triangle and give room for the frontal lobes (2); finally the fronto-orbital bones have been rearranged and fixed with resorbable plates (3). (**d**) The child 3 years after craniofacial surgery with a completely normal head

exophthalmos is a typical symptom although the infraorbital rim remains unaffected. If no other sutures are affected there is no direct growth disturbance of the viscerocranium (Fig. 5.40a–c).

In a great number of these patients, a higher ICP (intracranial pressure) develops so that there is a *strong indication for an early surgical correction!*

5.12.6.5 Brachycephalus

Here a premature closure of the coronary sutures is combined with that of the skull base sutures as well as the sagittal suture. This affects not only the growth of the neuro- but also the viscerocranium. The skull is short, wide and round. The orbital funnel is too short, so that these children have a marked exophthalmos.

Owing to the growth obstruction at the cranial base, a large compensatory bulging of the forehead and the temporal region will appear. If there is also a frontolateral bone constriction, there will be the clinical picture of a *Kleeblattschädel* (Clover leaf skull) (Fig. 5.41).

Regularly these children have a significantly increased ICP with the danger of mental retardation or visual disturbance. *Thus, there is an absolute indication for early surgery!*

5.12.6.6 Craniofacial Syndromes

In these cases, the premature closure of skull sutures can be combined with a great number of other deformities. The most common ones are:

M. Crouzon
M. Apert

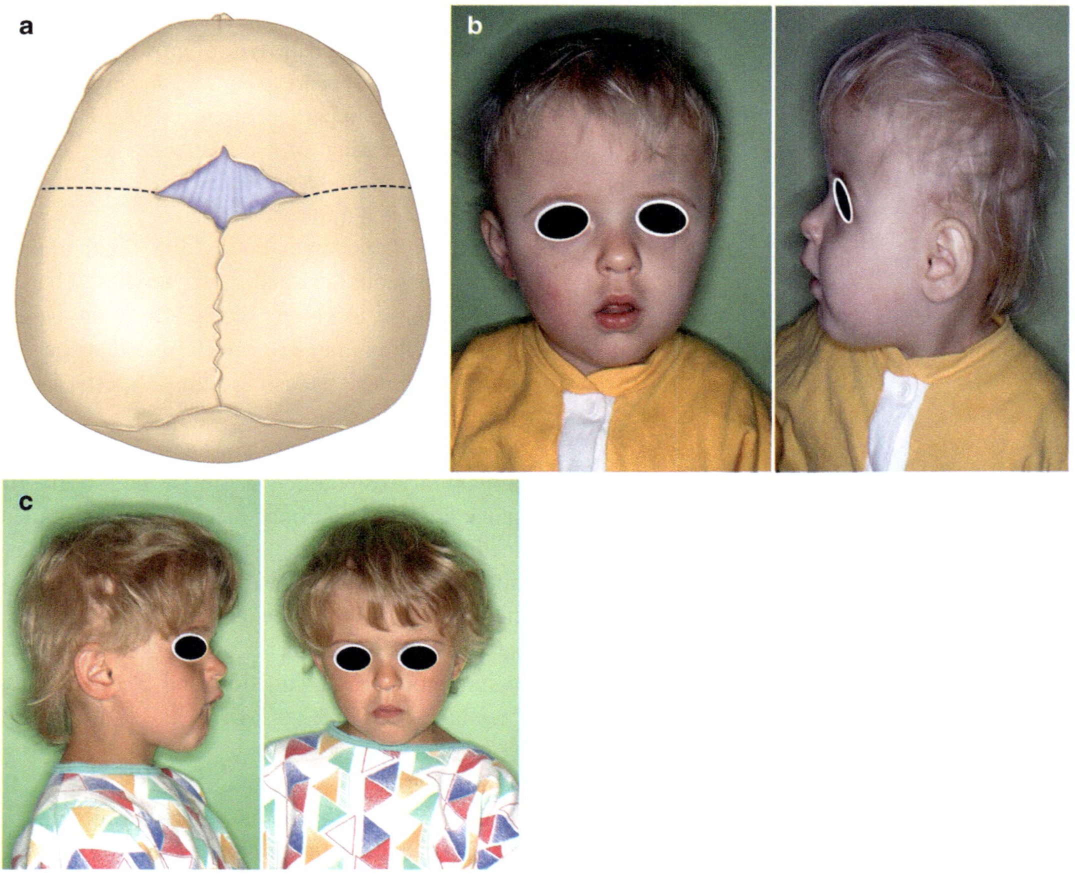

Fig. 5.40 (**a**) Schematic illustration of an oxy- (turricephalus). Note the closed coronal sutures and the short and wide skull (After Recuero I I and Sanchez Aniceto G (2020) Craniosynostosis. In: Ehrenfeld M, Futran N, Manson P, Prein J (ed.) Advanced craniomaxillofacial surgery. AO Foundation Thieme Stuttgart, pages 464 and 465. Copyright by AO Foundation, Switzerland). (**b**) One-year-old girl with the typical high flat forehead and flat upper orbital rim. (**c**) The same girl 3 years postoperatively with a normal physical and mental development

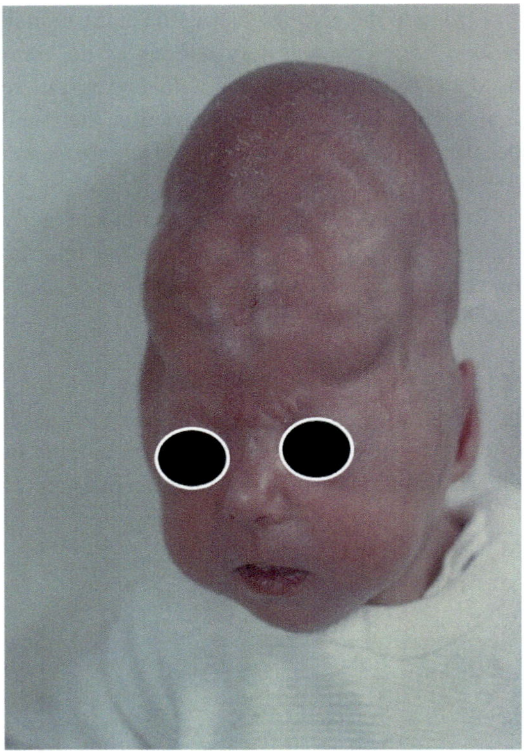

Fig. 5.41 Clinical case of a brachycephalus (a beginning frontolateral constriction—development of a Kleeblattschädel—can be seen) (courtesy of Prof. (em.) J. Bennek, Dept. of paediatric surgery, University Hospital of Leipzig, Germany)

M. Saethre-Chotzen
M. Pfeiffer
(for the aetiology see Sect. 15.13.2)

M. Crouzon (Craniofacial Dysostosis)

This is an autosomal dominant inherited syndrome first described by O. Crouzon (1912). The premature closure of the coronary, lambdoid and sagittal sutures, in combination with the also affected cranial base, leads to a brachycephalic skull with a severe midfacial hypoplasia and a marked exorbitism. This may often create ophthalmological problems due to an incomplete eyelid closure (cave: keratitis/corneal erosion, hypertelorism and strabism!).

The very short skull base will in consequence also result in a massive maxillary retrognathia with constriction of the posterior airway space. These children may consequently develop a severe form of an obstructive sleep apnoea syndrome (OSAS). Moreover calcified stylohyoid ligaments and fused vertebrae have been described. The mental development is not affected in most cases. Nevertheless an acute indication for an operation is given if the ICP rises.

Treatment options: At first, an FOA has to be carried out as early as necessary to relieve rising intracranial pressure, protect the eyes and foster a normal (cranial) growth pattern. Later, usually at the age of 7–9 years, a Le Fort III osteotomy has to follow in order to achieve normal maxillo-mandibular relations. In some cases, this may even have to be combined with a Le Fort I osteotomy to guarantee a good occlusion (Fig. 5.42a–d).

M. Apert (Acrocephalosyndactyly)

This syndrome is also autosomal dominant inherited. The majority of cases belong to new mutations, though. Since the coronary sutures are mostly affected, an oxycephalic type of growth is predominant. The face appears to be wide and hypoplastic. There are also hypertelorism, exophthalmos, strabism and hearing problems. Moreover, deeply positioned ears and a small upward bent beak-like nose are typical traits of M. Apert.

Finally, the characteristic, often bilateral dermal and osseous symmetric syndactylies of hands and feet have to be emphasised. In many cases, four fingers or toes are affected so that the so-called 'spoon hands' result (Apert 1906) (Fig. 5.43a).

Treatment options: In most cases, an FOA and bimaxillary osteotomy in the Le Fort I and III plane are required. Since there are more retained teeth and more maxillary deformations extensive—sometimes surgically assisted—orthodontic treatment is needed. In the end, a septorhinoplasty with rib grafts is necessary to assure good nasal function and a satisfactory facial appearance (Fig. 5.43b, c).

M. Pfeiffer

The Pfeiffer syndrome has a close resemblance to M. Apert. If the sagittal suture is also affected a more brachycephalic growth will result. In severe forms, there may also be cerebral, ventricular and ophthalmic problems. Another

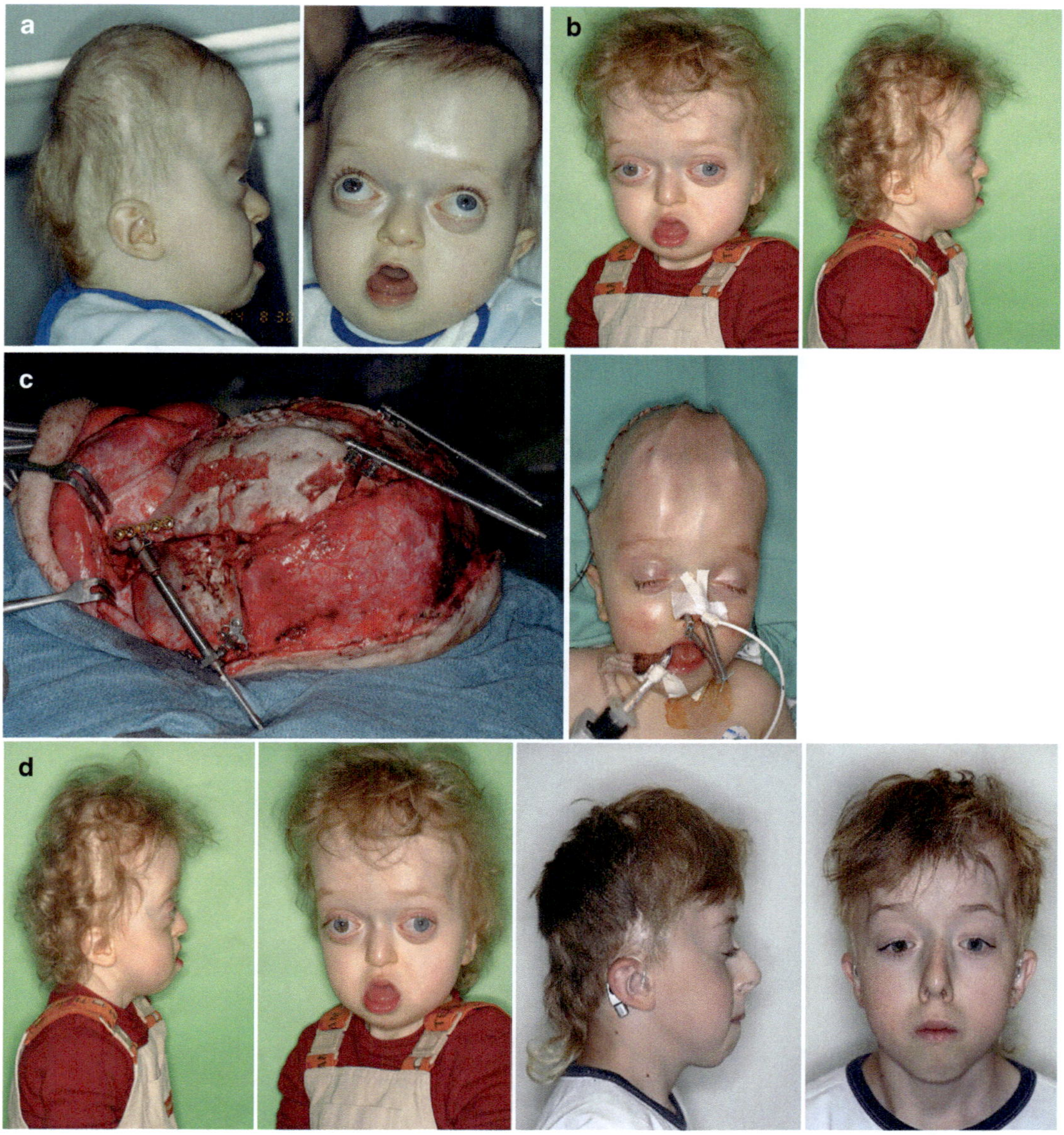

Fig. 5.42 (**a**) One-year-old boy with an M. Crouzon 3 months after an FOA; note the still existing exorbitism. (**b**) The same child at 34 months with a marked OSAS due to a severe midfacial hypoplasia and the resulting lack of tongue space. (**c**) Intraoperative view of the fronto-orbital and combined midfacial advancement for subcutaneous distractors; stabilisation with resorbable plates and two titanium plates at the abutment of the temporal distractors (left); the child at the end of the operation (3 mm distraction were initially performed). (**d**) The same boy at age 11 before (upper row) and 8 years after the above described operation (lower row) with an age-appropriate development. Photos with kind permission of the parents

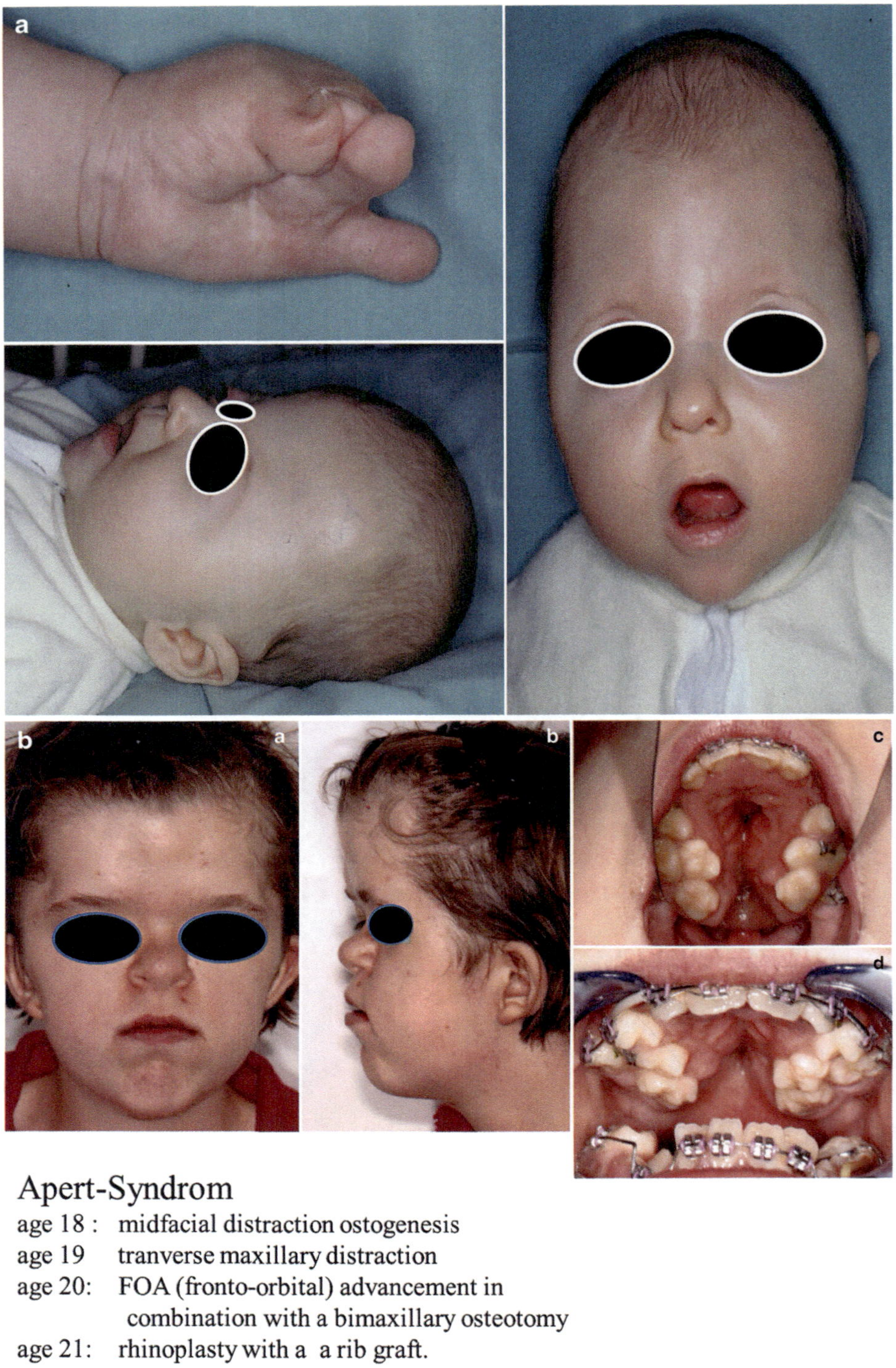

Fig. 5.43 (**a**) A newborn girl with an Apert syndrome; note the syndactyly of thumb and several fingers ('spoon hand'). (**b**) Another girl with an M. Apert at the age of 14 years; note the beak-like nasal malformation with the uplifted tip (a, b) and the Ω shaped maxillary arch (c, d). (**c**) The same patient (aged 22) four years after the end of the interdisciplinary treatment (maxillofacial and neurosurgeons and orthodontists) which finally included a septorhinoplasty one year ago; good physical and psychosocial development

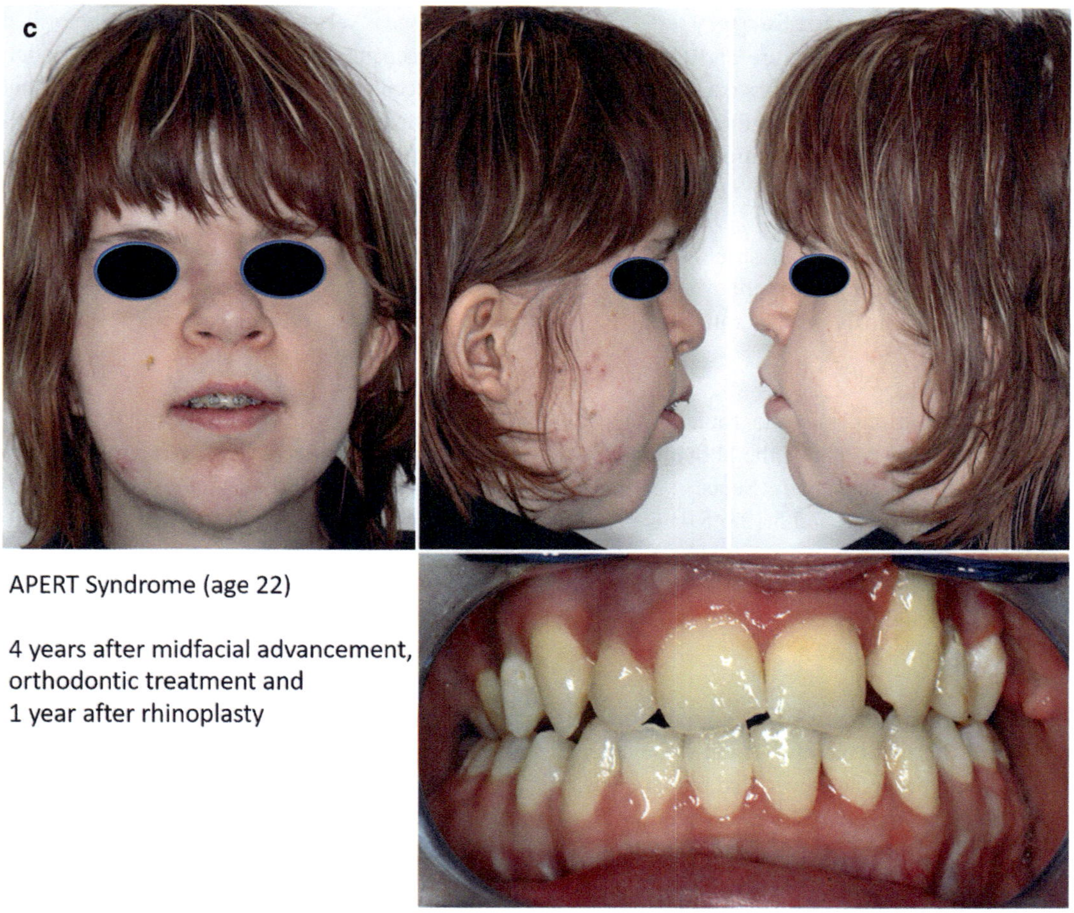

Fig. 5.43 (continued)

important difference includes the characteristic wide thumbs and big toes in various positions. Dermal syndactylies usually occur only between the second and third phalanges (Pfeiffer 1964).

M. Saethre-Chotzen

The Saethre–Chotzen syndrome is a special form of oxycephaly with an asymmetric skull deformity in combination with brachydactylies, klinodactylies, syndactylies and symphalangism (Saethre 1931; Chotzen 1932). There may also be an antimongoloid (oblique) lid axis, upward rotated nasal tip and nares and the characteristic deep hairline. Depending on the severity of this craniosynostosis it can be difficult to distinguish it from a M. Crouzon.

5.12.7 Surgical Correction of Craniosynostoses

Rising intracranial pressure (ICP) and mental impairment are linked. Even though the frequency of intracranial hypertension is higher the more sutures are involved in premature closure, monosutural craniosynostoses can be affected, too (Renier and Marchac 1988). The authors also found that mental deficiency in these patients is more frequent after the age of one year than before. Thus, surgical correction of craniosynostoses at an early age will stop further mental regression. An early operation will also contribute to the normalisation of facial development in non-syndromic cases.

5.12.7.1 Indication for Surgery

Depending on the very nature and the extent of sequelae of the craniosynostoses which can (rarely) be life threatening shortly after birth, there are absolute and relative indications for surgery.

- Absolute indication
  - Rising intracranial pressure
  - Psychomotoric retardation
  - Orbital stenosis with keratitis and bulbar luxation

These conditions may be found rather frequently in severe forms of the above mentioned craniofacial syndromes (Sects. 5.12.6.6.1, 5.12.6.6.2, 5.12.6.6.3, and 5.12.6.6.4)

- Relative indication
  - Scaphocephalus
  - Trigonocephalus

Some colleagues regard operations for these craniosynostoses as merely aesthetic. Geyer et al. (2005) could prove, however, that brain perfusion is restricted in these cases, too and will turn back to normal only after surgical correction of the malformation. A better mental outcome in scaphocephalies could be shown by Arnaud et al. (1996) in a group of children operated on before the age of one year.

5.12.7.2 Timing of the Operation

As early as 1927 Faber and Towne advocated an early prophylactic intervention in craniosynostoses to prevent blindness or least minimise craniofacial malformations during later growth. On the other hand, Müke (1972) still saw the indication for surgery only in the case of rising intracranial pressure. Finally, Joos stated in 1995 that a 'wait and see' strategy for the treatment of craniosynostosis is no longer justified since early operations (in most cases before the first birthday) will contribute significantly to normal craniofacial growth.

Cranio (facial) surgery at the age of 3–6 months would have the advantage of a thin bone which can be easily remodelled or removed. Re-ossification (initiated from the dura) of postoperative skull defects is almost guaranteed. On the other hand this juvenile bone is very weak so that the newly formed skull/midface may not be stable. The re-ossification potential decreases in the second half year of life but is still sufficient to close the bone gaps after craniotomy. After the third year of life, growth activity has diminished so much that postoperative re-ossification may not always be complete. Owing to all these facts the best time for cranio-orbital operations is the second half year of life unless rising intracranial pressure or severe eye problems need to be solved as emergency measures.

5.12.7.3 Development of Modern Craniofacial Operations

Beginning in the first half of the twentieth century, the so-called strip craniectomies were advocated where only the affected sutures were taken out (Faber and Towne 1943) (Fig. 5.44).

This resulted in many recurrences, though, due to the high re-ossification potential via the exposed dura. Finally, Tessier—the great French pioneer in craniofacial surgery—developed the fronto-orbital advancement in the 1960s. This meant uplifting of the complete frontal bone and releasing at least the upper bandeau (meaning the upper part of the orbit) (Tessier 1971a). Moreover, it is to his great merit to have combined intra- and extra-oral approaches together with the neurosurgeons in order to correct craniofacial syndromes in one step (Tessier 1971b). The use of bone transplants and wire osteosynthesis gave the advanced midface and calvaria a sufficient first stability but could not prevent some relapse.

Many more methods for cranioplasties were developed by different teams in the following years and described by Marchac and Renier (1982). Finally, Mühling (1986) introduced a standardised bilateral fronto-orbital advancement, including Tessier's idea of a tongue in groove technique for the safe advancement of the orbital bandeau by using miniplates for stabilisation of all parts (Fig. 5.45).

This omits the need for bone grafts in most of the cases and leads to predictable long-term results. In the last two decades, resorbable plates have increasingly replaced the titanium ones to avoid false plate migration and metal removal (Imola et al. 2001).

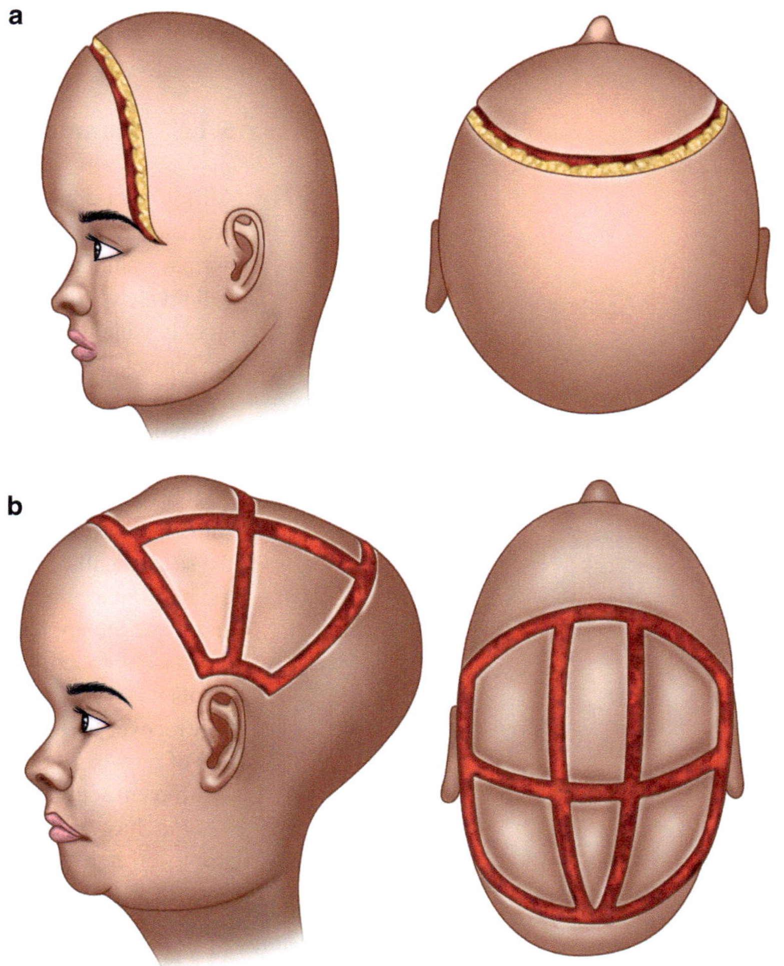

Fig. 5.44 Schematic illustration of strip craniectomies ((after Marchac and Renier 1982) from Zöller JE et al., Kraniofaziale Chirurgie © 2002 Georg Thieme Verlag KG, Stuttgart. New York. With permission © Thieme Group)

5.12.7.4 Complications

The most important problems related to craniofacial surgery are:

- Infections
- Bleeding
- Liquor fistulae
- Visual disturbances
- Brain damage

In 1979, Whitaker et al. issued a report on problems in a series of 793 craniofacial operations in 6 major craniofacial centres. They found an *overall complication rate of 16.5%* including:

- Postoperative bleeding 7.1%
- Infections 6.2%
- Liquor fistulae 2.2%
- Visual disturbance 0.12%
- Mortality rate 1.6%

These results could be significantly improved by hypotensive anaesthesia, a reduction in operation time, different surgical approaches, rigid fixation of all mobilised bones and extensive perioperative antibiotic therapy. In a similar more recent multicentre study with over 8000 patients, Bruce et al. (2018) found the markedly reduced *overall complication rate of only 8.6%* comprising:

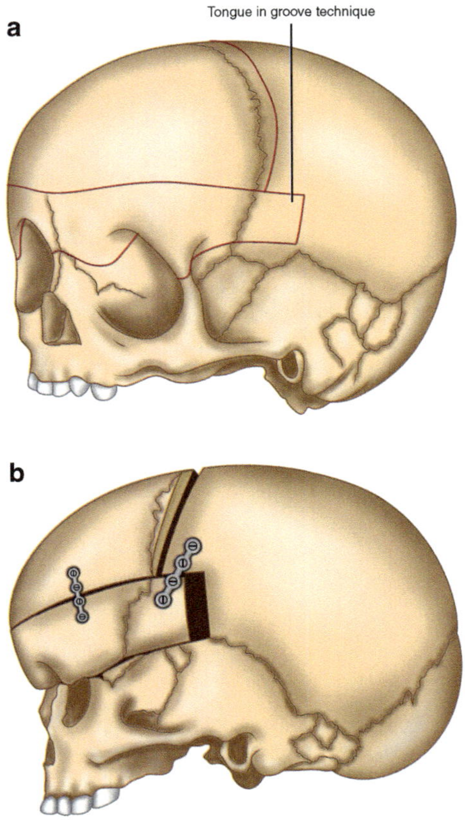

Fig. 5.45 (**a**) Standardised bilateral bone cuts for the fronto-orbital advancement by Mühling (1986), involving Tessier's tongue in groove technique (b) upper bandeau and frontal bone fixed in the new position by miniplates (after Mühling et al. 1994) from Zöller JE et al., Kraniofaziale Chirurgie © 2002 Georg Thieme Verlag KG, Stuttgart. New York. With permission © Thieme Group)

- Postoperative bleeding 3.3%
- Infections 0.3%
- Accidental puncture/laceration 1.2%
- Visual disturbance 0%
- Mortality rate 0%

Severe syndromic cases such as acrocephalosyndactyly presented with a higher complication rate of 22.9%, however. Finally, the authors advise performing craniofacial operations within the first year of life, since complication rates increased from 6.6% in the first 6 months over 10.3% from 7 to 11 months up to 13.9% from 12 to 36 months. These two studies clearly demonstrate the progress that has been achieved in craniofacial surgery. Some risks will always remain in such an operation, but they can definitely be outweighed by the benefit for these patients to lead a normal life.

5.12.8 Summary and Outlook

All forms of cranioplasties are done to release the prematurely closed skull sutures in order to allow a normal craniofacial development. Usually, the brain will fill the void after the surgical advancement very quickly without any problems. rCBF-brain-SPECT for a revelation of brain perfusion in infants with premature synostoses of cranial sutures could show a significant improvement of the perfusion after the widening of the scull (Geyer et al. 2005).

If no emergency exists (high intracerebral pressure), these operations should be performed within the second half of the first year of life. At this age, the best balance between too fast a re-ossification and no or incomplete re-ossification after craniotomy can be found. There is no need for bone transplants if rigid fixation is applied. The cranial bone will recover and form a complete scull. After the end of growth (2 years and older), there may be an insufficient scull remodelling.

One has to bear in mind, however, that a fronto-orbital advancement or cranioplasty may only lead to a small improvement of midfacial growth. In severe craniofacial anomalies, usually a Le Fort III osteotomy often in combination with a Le Fort I osteotomy has to follow at the age of 7–9 years to give the patient a normal facial appearance and a normal dental occlusion. In cases with a need of more than 10–15 mm forward movement of the midface distraction, osteogenesis may have to be applied.

5.13 Principles of Maxillofacial Cleft Surgery

Alexander Hemprich

5.13.1 Introduction

Clefts of lip, alveolus and palate belong to the more frequent congenital malformations with an incidence of about 1:500 births (ranging from 1:300 in Asia to 1:2000 in Africa).

The complete cleft is found in approximately 50%, the isolated cleft of the palate in about 30% and the cleft of lip and alveolus in about 10% of the cases, whereas rare forms of clefts make up the rest.

Such a cleft may eventually lead to problems in swallowing, hearing and speaking. Moreover facial growth and the development of the dental arches and dental occlusion will be affected.

Thus, a successful treatment concept can only be based on an interdisciplinary approach comprising maxillofacial surgeons or plastic surgeons with knowledge of facial and bone development, orthodontists, dentists, phoniatricians, paedaudiologists and speech language pathologists. The child also has to be taken care of by paediatricians, of course. In some cases, psychological counselling may be necessary for the parents and later for the small patients themselves.

In conclusion, it may be stated that the best long-term results will be achieved if patients with clefts are taken care of in a specialised cleft/craniofacial centre where regular interdisciplinary cleft clinics and panel discussions are offered. This principle had been established by Rosenthal as early as 1949 in Thallwitz close to Leipzig, Germany (Mühler 1995) and has become the standard in most cleft centres worldwide.

5.13.2 Presurgical Orthodontics

The use of presurgical infant orthopaedics (PSIO) with active palatal plates is still a question of debate. In a retrospective cohort study on 191 children in four cleft centres in North America, Kornbluth et al. (2018) concluded that active palatal plates or naso-alveolar moulding (NAM) may lead to a better aesthetic outcome but also to worse maxillary growth.

Only 16% of the children in centres using no active PSIO needed corrective orthognathic surgery later vs. 76% in centres applying active devices. The use of passive plates on the other hand, helps to prevent the alveolar segments from collapsing to the midline and has a beneficial effect in normalising the position of the tongue and its movements. This could be observed in an ultrasound study of 16 cleft children, in comparison with a similar group of non-cleft cases, by incorporating a passive palatal plate in the first 10 days post-partum (Hemprich and Dannhauer 2016). By adding a small median spur to the distal edge of the plate, a stimulation of the clefted palatal muscles could be noted which later facilitated the intravelar muscle plasty (Fig. 5.46). Such a plate should be worn permanently and adjusted about every 4–6 weeks until the closure of the hard palate at the age between 10–12 months.

5.13.3 Primary Surgical Procedures

It is agreed in most cleft centres that the lip–nose complex should be closed between four to six months of age, when the child has left the perinatal period and runs lower risks of complications, since heart, lungs and liver have matured and the child has itself produced blood. Some centres in France and Russia, however, advocate that the first procedure be done in the first weeks after birth in order to avoid psychological disorder for the parents (Bachy et al. 2002). The aesthetic long-term results were not better than in the group of children operated at 4–5 months of age, however, so that the question remains why a higher perioperative risk should be accepted for the infant, with only a small benefit on the side of the parents.

According to Delaire (1978), the main problem of cleft lip and alveolus is the disruption of the

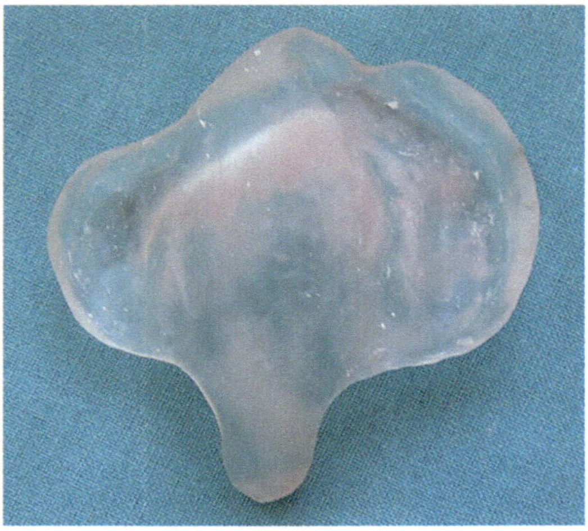

Fig. 5.46 Passive palatal plate for presurgical infant orthopaedics (courtesy of Prof. Karl-Heinz Dannhauer, Leipzig)

natural connection between the primary and the secondary facial growth centres. The nasal capsule including the nasal septum is part of the cartilaginous preformed skull base (primary autonomous growth centre) whereas the sutures between the cranial bones form the secondary growth centre. Thus, it is necessary to (re-)connect the upper part of the oral muscle ring (transverse part of the nasal muscle and the upper third of the orbicularis oris muscles) with the nasal septum. This will lead to a permanent gentle pull on the zygomatico-maxillary suture as long as there is the inherited (pre-programmed) forward–downward movement of the nasal capsule/nasal septum (Fig. 5.47).

Thereby, the formerly marked midfacial retrusions can be avoided. The meticulous reconstruction of the perioral and perinasal muscle rings, including a complete subperiostal uplift of the midfacial soft tissues, is the crucial point of lip/nose reconstruction done to foster normal midfacial development (Joos 1995b) (Fig. 5.48).

This is true for unilateral as well as bilateral clefts. The latter should always be closed in a single stage procedure, even over a protruding premaxilla leading to good lip–nose symmetry. There is no need for any surgical or orthodontical retruding of the premaxilla. The completed muscle ring will do this by itself in a couple of months (Fig. 5.49a–c).

Interestingly enough, the design of the skin incision, which had been highly valued in order to equalise the discrepancy in the length of the lip by straight line (Veau 1938), geometrical (Tennison 1952) and wave line (Pfeifer 1970) incisions or a rotation flap advancement (Millard 1958a), loses its importance when the lip stumps have been carefully dissected and reassembled in three anatomical layers (skin, muscle, mucosa) (Fig. 5.50a–e).

Muscle reconstruction will also contribute very much to a good result of the primary rhinoplasty, which is always part of the primary lip–nose closure. Utmost care has to be taken to create normal nasal ducts with a fully closed nasal floor to ensure good nasal breathing in the long run. To achieve this, the deviated cartilaginous nasal septum usually has to be mobilised from the premaxilla in its ventral third, and to be repositioned in the midline with one unresorbable suture.

Finally, the skin over the alar nasal cartilage on the cleft side is carefully elevated supraperi-

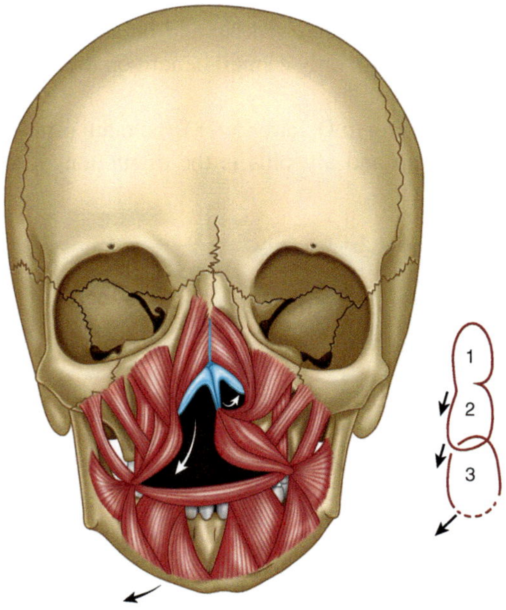

Fig. 5.47 Incomplete perioral and perinasal muscle rings; primary growth centre (blue), secondary growth centre (green) (courtesy of Professor Ulrich Joos, Münster, Germany)

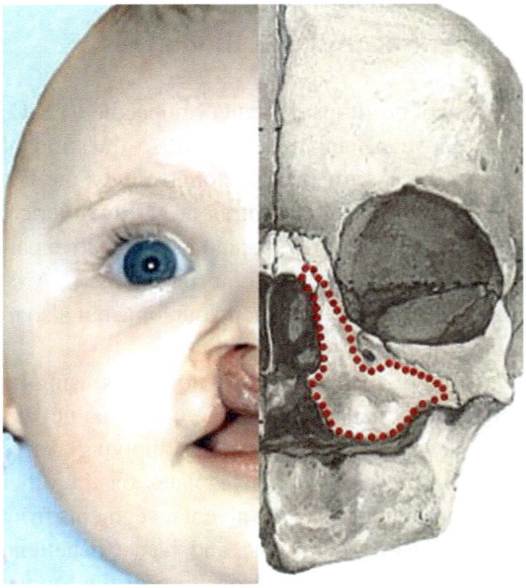

Fig. 5.48 Area of subperiostal elevation of the facial envelope (red dots)

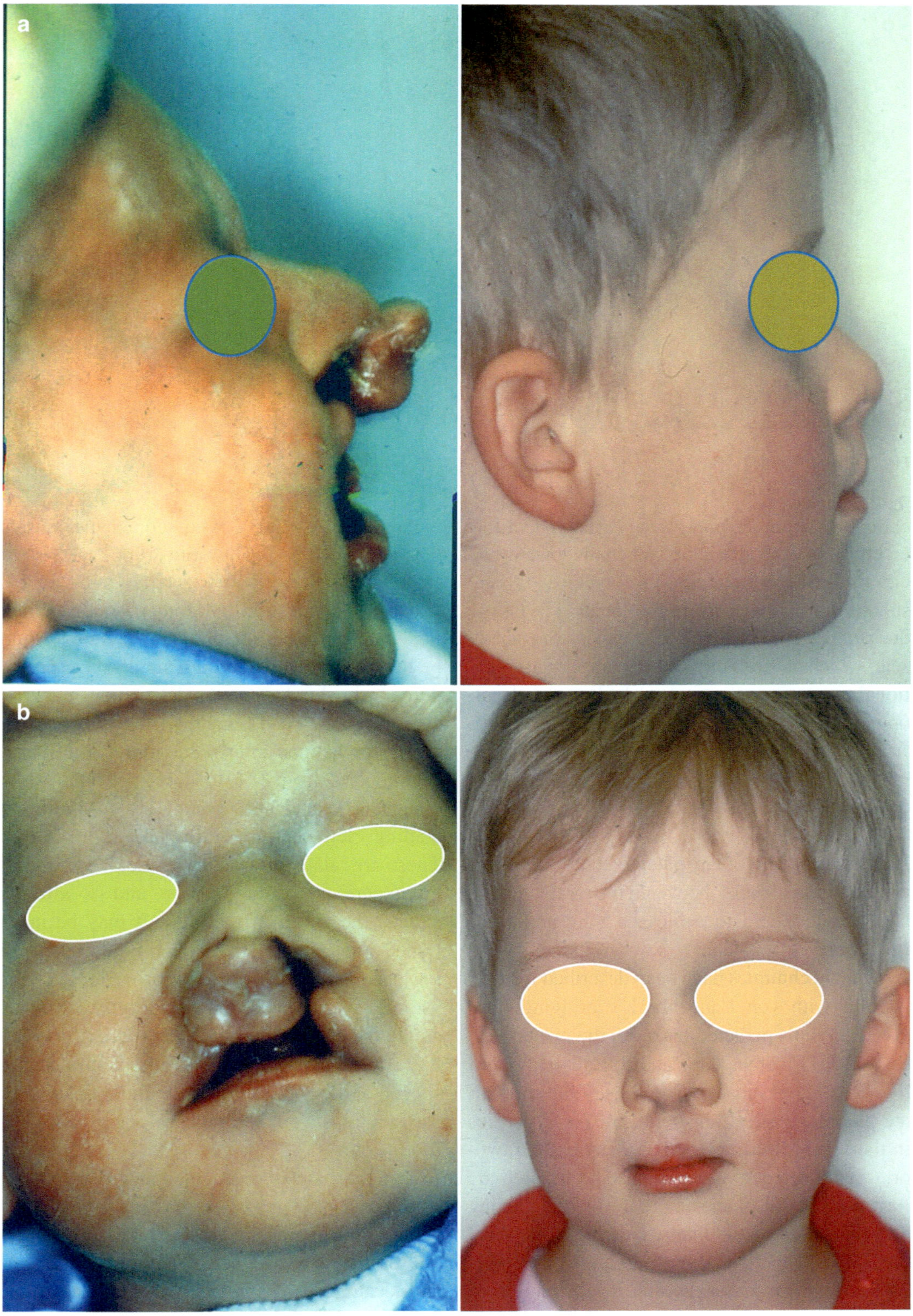

Fig. 5.49 (**a**) (upper 2 figures) (left) Markedly protruding premaxilla in a complete bilateral cleft (shortly after birth), (right) at the age of 5 years. (**b**) (middle 2 figures) Same child en face. (**c**) (lower 2 figures) Same child at the age of ten years (no secondary corrections performed!)

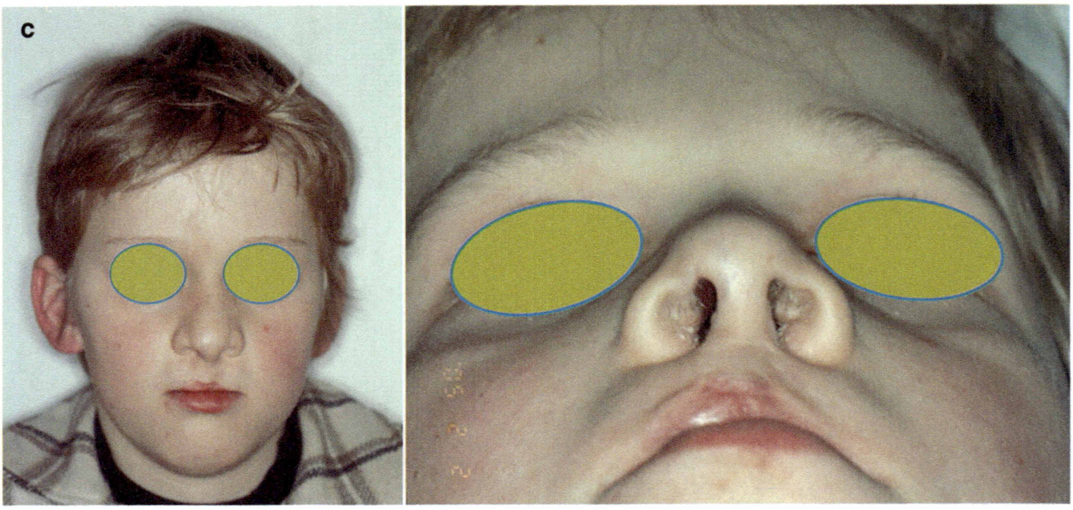

Fig. 5.49 (continued)

chondrally from the underlying cartilage to allow an uplifting of the nasal tip. When the lower muscle ring (m. orbicularis oris) is closed there should not be any pull on the labial skin before the suture. This will result in a very fine labial scar which is certainly a very important functional requirement for undisturbed speech development (Fig. 5.50e).

5.13.4 Palatoplasty

It must be the aim of any palatal reconstruction to ensure tight closure between the oral and the nasal cavities and to achieve a long and well-functioning soft palate.

Many techniques have been described for this, starting with von Langenbeck's bridging flaps (1862), Veau's pedicled flaps (on the palatal vessels) (1931), vomer flaps and different forms of the so-called pushback operations of the soft palate (Dorrance and Brainsfield 1946) or Z-plasties in the velum (Furlow 1986). In any case, a two- or three-layered closure should be assured by forming a nasal plane first, carefully realigning all velar muscles, and finally creating a good oral layer (Fig. 5.51a). No matter what technique is used, it is proven that the fine reconstruction of the complete intravelar muscle ring (Fig. 5.51b, c) will lead to good results, no matter which kind of flap had been used for the other layers.

Sommerlad (2003), who refined the muscle plasty initiated by Braithwaite (1966) and Kriens (1969), achieved 95–97% success rates for his palatoplasty, meaning that only a small amount of secondary speech-improving measures would be necessary. He also used a single-stage procedure closing hard and soft palate in one operation at the age of about 12 months.

As for fistulae after palatoplasty, the literature reports from 0% to 63%, overall (Losee et al. 2008) and still from 5.4% to 17.9% in leading cleft centres (Hardwicke et al. 2014). These are related to various surgical techniques, the experience of the surgeon, and (to a lesser extent) the width of the cleft. It may be mentioned that single-stage operations result in fewer fistulae than two-stage procedures or the use of a single layer vomer flap in the hard palate. In the end, a palatoplasty is successful when there remains no form of rhinophonia in the speech of the child, the ventilation of the middle ear functions well, and no nasal regurgitation of food occurs.

The mechanism of middle ear ventilation via Eustachian tube movement has been the subject of research for a long time. This is not only a question of a good reconstruction of the tensor and levator muscles in the velum, but also of a different relationship between the inner orifice of the tube and the velum itself in cleft palate patients. Thus, many children may need grom-

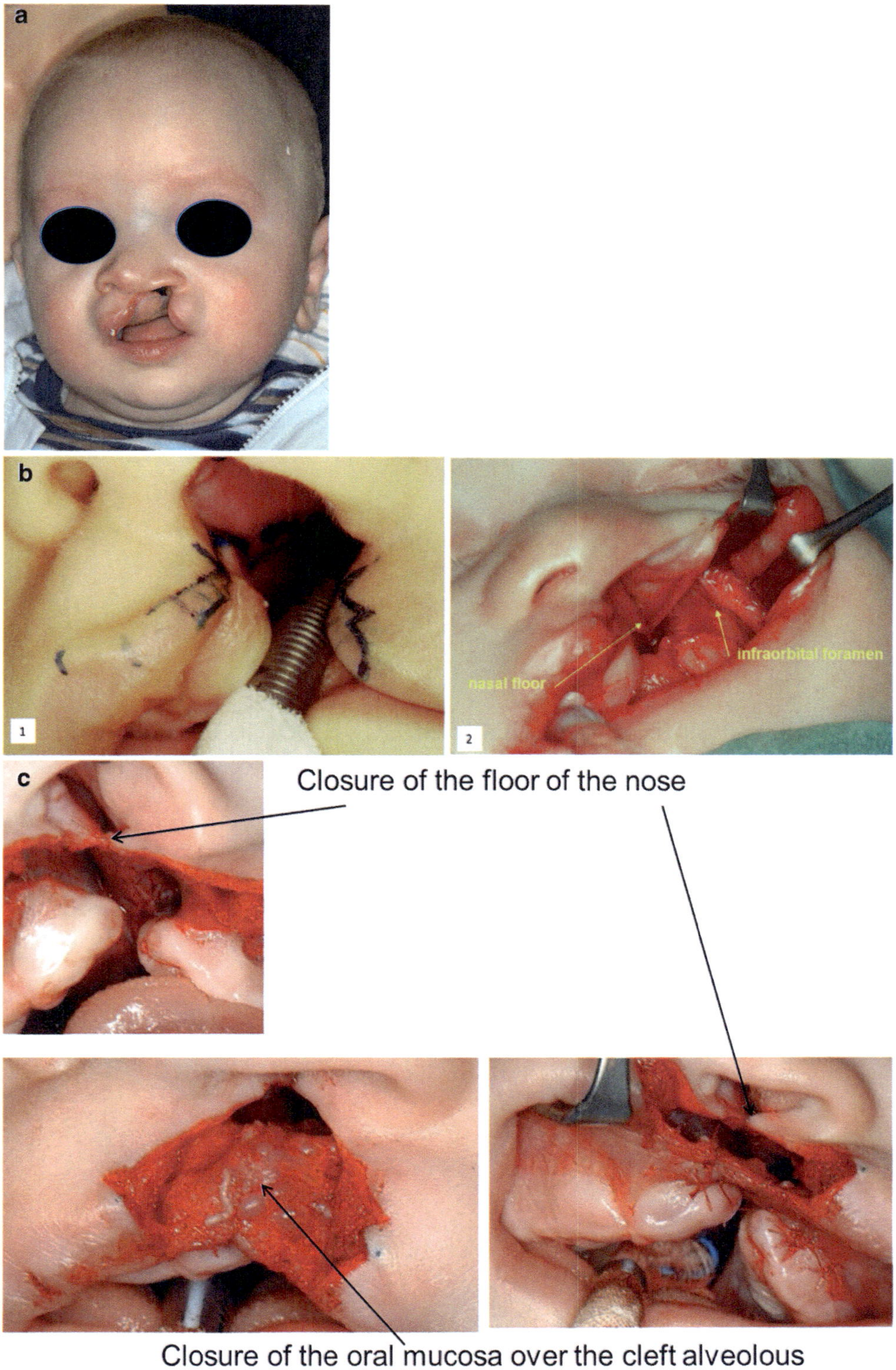

Fig. 5.50 (**a**) (top, left side) Unilateral complete cleft. (**b**) (top, middle) (1) Outline of the incision carefully omitting the columellar base. (2) After subperiosteal elevation of the midfacial soft tissues; suturing of the nasal floor started. (**c**) (top, right side) Closure of the nasal floor and the oral mucosa. (**d**) (bottom, left 4 figures) Closure of the perioral and perinasal muscle rings and the skin. (**e**) (bottom, right 2 figures) Child at the age of three years without any corrections

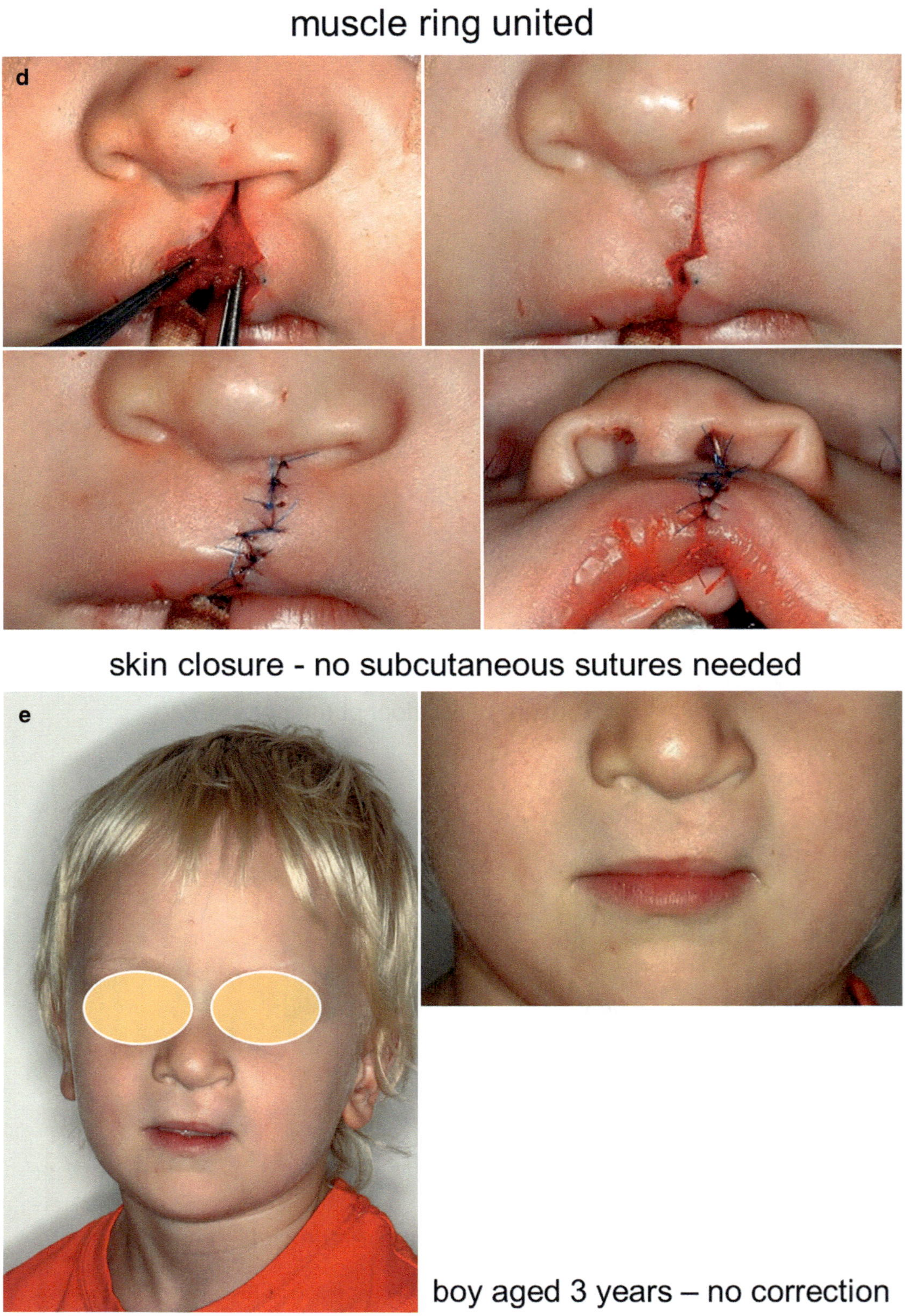

Fig. 5.50 (continued)

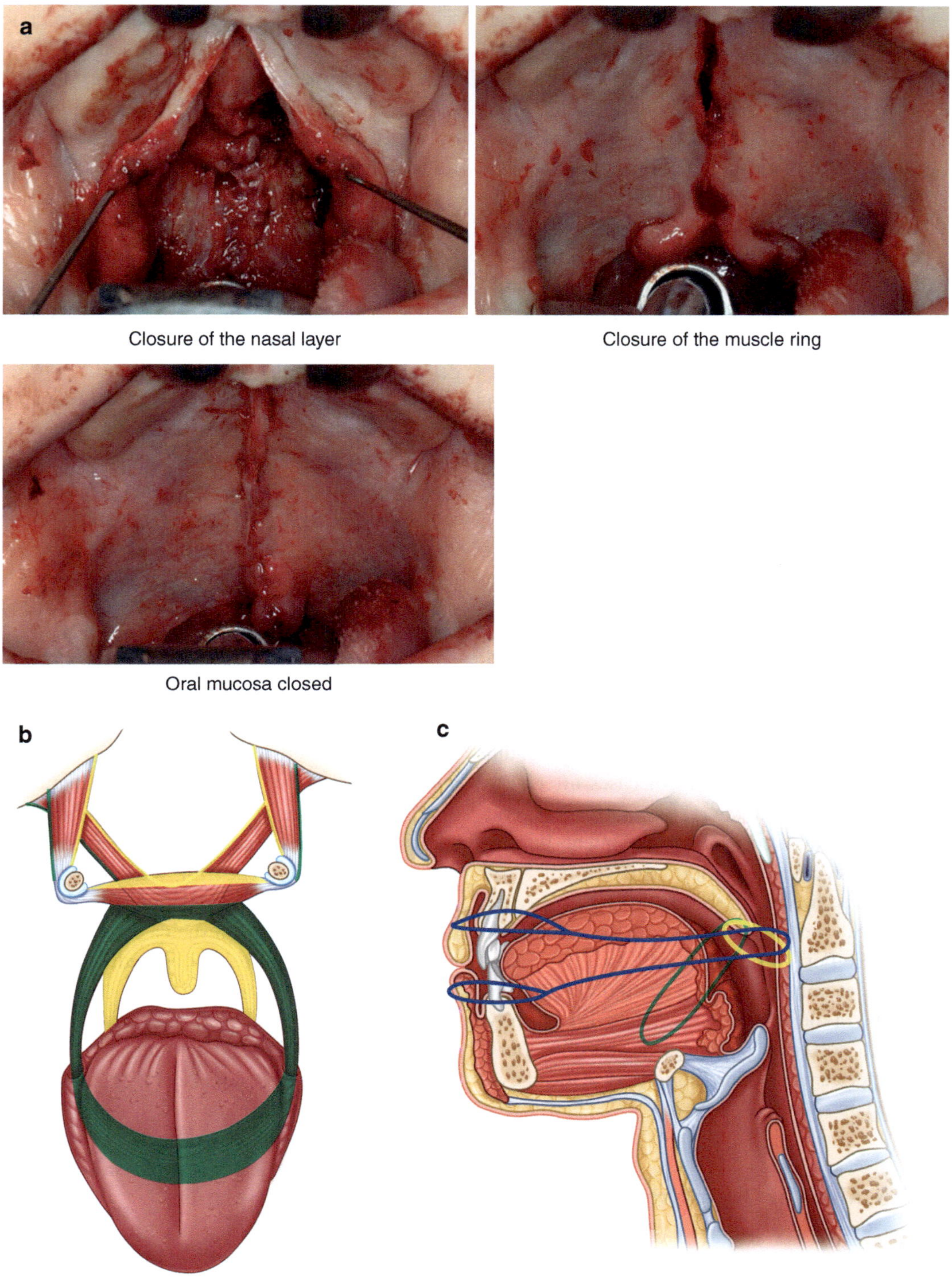

Fig. 5.51 (**a**) Closure of the velar cleft in three layers. (**b**) Schematic drawing of the anterior/upper (M. tensor and levator veli palatini) and posterior/lower (M. palatopharyngeus and M. palatoglossus) velar muscles; note the rectangular bend of the tensor muscle around the hamulus ossis pterygoidei (Modified from Voss and Herrlinger (1972) Taschenbuch der Anatomie II, Gustav Fischer, Stuttgart). (**c**) Lateral schematic view of M. palatopharyngeus (yellow), M. palatoglossus (green) and the labio-bucco-pharyngeal sphincter muscles

mets for some years to assure their middle ear function, even after a successful intravelar muscle plasty (Klockars and Rautio 2012).

The best timing for the palatoplasty is still debated. ENT surgeons and speech pathologists agree on an early closure (10–14 months of age) at the time of the onset of speech, whereas orthodontists are afraid of midfacial or at least dento-alveolar growth restriction due to scars with too early an intervention. They would like to postpone this procedure until the end of the first dentition (age 24–30 months).

In spite of many studies, no final conclusion can be made for the best timing of primary palatal surgery. The prospective randomised Scandcleft study (Lohmander et al. 2017), which evaluated four different approaches to palatal closure, did not find significant differences between the protocols, with the exception of the consonant formation in 5-year-olds. They performed better after an operation at the age of 12 months than with surgery at the age of 36 months. To date no problematic results in palatal growth have been found either, although long-term observations until the age of 18–20 years are pending.

In any case, no major growth inhibition could be observed in the majority of cases after very carefully performed interventions. Under good surveillance and consequent treatment by the orthodontist, a close to normal development of the dental arches and the midface can be expected in over 80% of all patients. In the remaining cases, a Le Fort I osteotomy will usually be adequate to establish regular mandibulo-maxillary relations. In the author's experience, it is usually harder to correct a pathological speech pattern than to perform orthognathic surgery at the age of 18–21 years.

5.13.5 Alveolar Ostoplasty

After the complete (soft tissue) closure of the uni- or bi-lateral cleft of lip, alveolus and palate, orthodontic follow up and treatment are a compulsory part of regular cleft clinics.

Usually, the lesser segment of the maxillary alveolus tends to turn inwards, especially when the second incisor is missing, which happens in up to 50% of all cases (Lourenço Ribeiro et al. 2003). Thus, the alignment of the upper maxillary arch has to be achieved by orthodontic measures followed by a cleft osteoplasty, usually with a bone graft from the hip (Boyne and Sands 1972) (Fig. 5.52).

This should happen when two thirds of the root of the cleft-sided canine have grown (age 8–11 years) so that the tooth can erupt through the grafted bone (Fig. 5.53a, b). This will not only lead to the formation of a normal alveolar socket for the canine but also stabilisation of the dental arch and support for the ala nasi.

The indication for the timing of this surgery has to be provided in close cooperation with the orthodontist. The morbidity of this operation is rather low, especially at a younger age when a trephine of 4–8 mm diameter is used to harvest the bone. There is only a 2–3 cm skin incision needed, which will usually leave a most inconspicuous scar. Low rates of surgical site infections (SSI) follow an intraoperative single-dose antibiotic regime (Naros et al., 2023). Children and adolescents may walk again on the day after surgery, using walking aids for some days in order to ease the load on the leg tissue.

In bilateral clefts, there is a tendency for both alveolar segments of the maxilla to move into the midline behind the premaxilla (even without any surgery), which necessitates early intervention to widen the dental arch with fixed orthodontic appliances bonded to the deciduous teeth (from the age of 2.5–5 years). In such a case, the alveolar osteoplasty has to follow immediately to stabilise the orthodontic results.

In adults, a tertiary cleft osteoplasty may be necessary for an implant to replace a missing tooth (mostly the lateral incisor) (Fig. 5.54a, b).

5.13.6 Secondary Corrections: General Principles

In spite of the surgeons' striving for perfection during all primary operations of clefts of lip, alveolus, and palate, it has to be expected that the results will not always live up to the expectations of the patient or the doctor or both. Moreover, complications may also be the reason for corrective surgery. It has

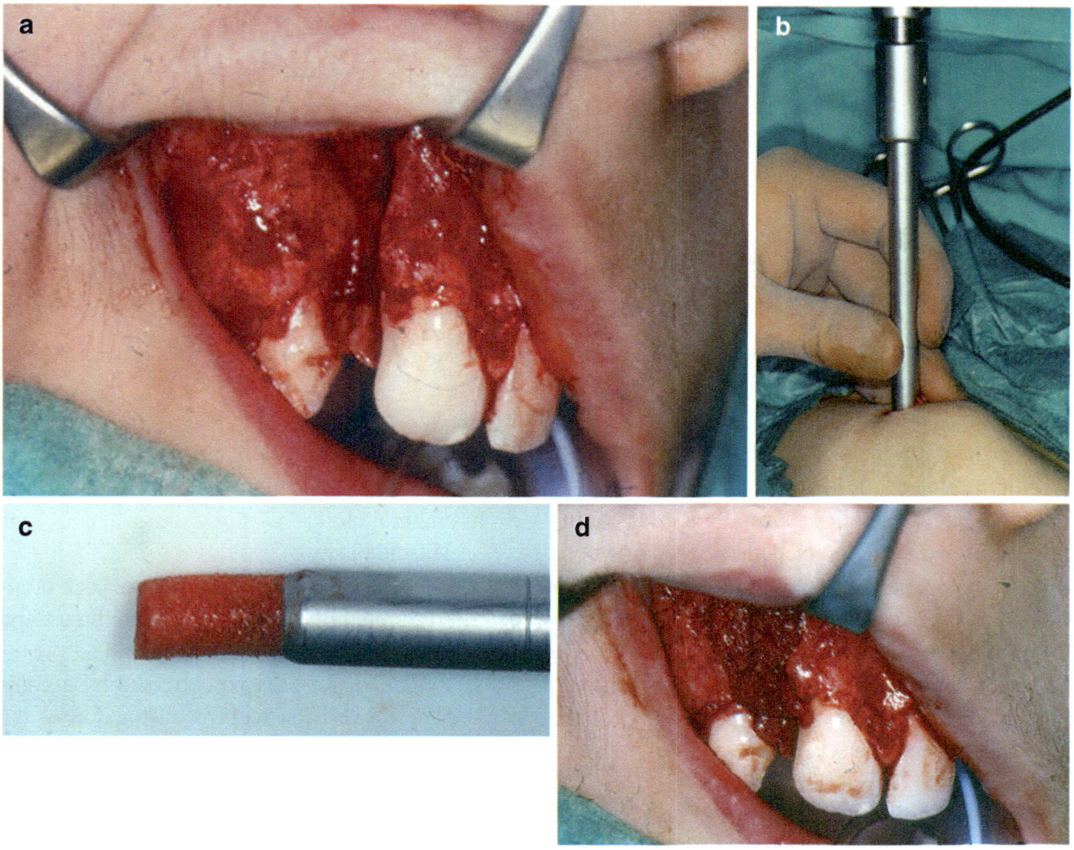

Fig. 5.52 Secondary osteoplasty: (**a**) exposed cleft alveolus, (**b**) bone harvesting from the iliac crest with a trephine, (**c**) cancellous bone cylinder, (**d**) bone graft stuffed into the alveolar cleft

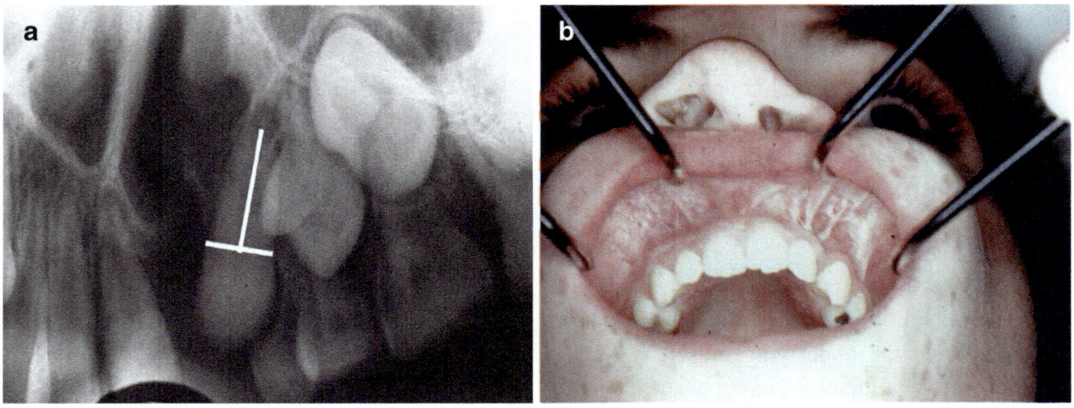

Fig. 5.53 (**a**) (left side) With two-thirds root growth. (**b**) (right side) Correctly erupted through the bone graft

proven to be extremely useful though, to wait for at least six months before another operation, because the wound-healing process has usually not been completed before this time.

In many primary lip closures, especially after Pfeiffer or Delaire, a shortening of the lip may be noted in the first 3–6 months postoperatively, before muscle function will achieve a normalisa-

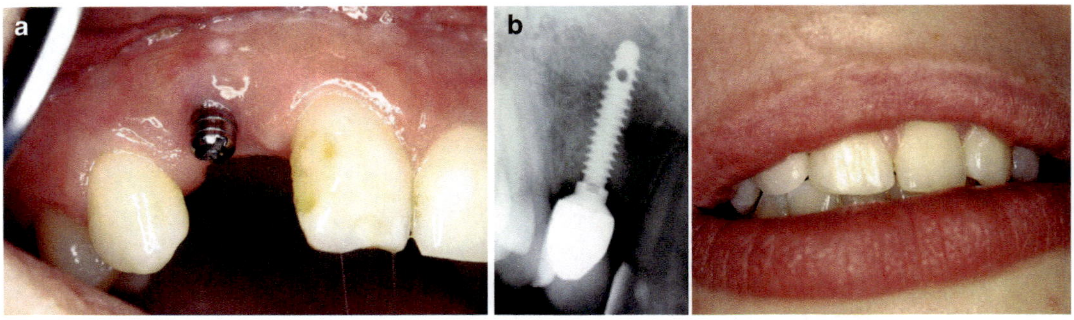

Fig. 5.54 (**a**) (left side) Dental implant inserted into the alveolar bone after tertiary osteoplasty. (**b**) (right side) Crown mounted on the implant in region 012

tion of the anatomical structures (lip symmetry) within the following 1–2 years (Fig. 5.55a–d).

This principle applies especially in cases of fistula repair in the palate. Such an area should not be touched before at least 6 months have elapsed after a fistula has been noted, and even though the parents may urge the surgeon to act earlier. Before a new operation is carried out, the wound should have healed completely with a completion of the scar formation; otherwise, there is a high risk of another wound dehiscence.

Finally, it must be stated that secondary corrections of clefts usually need a complete revision of all anatomical structures. The so-called 'small' scar excisions or 'little' skin flaps will rarely solve the complete underlying problem. Quite often it may be necessary to reopen the complete cleft and realign mucosa, muscles and skin in order to achieve good, long-lasting results.

5.13.7 Lip (Nose) Revisions

- In unilateral clefts
  - In cases of wound dehiscence, a wide and shortened scar can remain in the skin. Provided the underlying muscle has been correctly united, it may be sufficient to excise the scarred tissue with a wave line or rhomboid incision and to undermine the neighbouring area in order to gain length and achieve lip symmetry
  - If there is an irregular lip red/white border, a Z-plasty or a rhomboid excision may help. Care has to be taken, however, to keep an equal distance from the midline to the lateral philtrum edges on both sides
- In bilateral clefts
  - Muscle plasty

    If the perioral muscle ring has not been properly united, the philtrum appears broad and flat and the tip of the nose is pulled downwards. All this can be corrected by a complete lip revision with reconstruction of the orbicularis oris muscle and fixation of the transverse part of the nasal muscle at the nasal septum. This will not only lead to a normal appearance of the upper lip but also to a substantial improvement of the nose without dissection of the nasal cartilages (Fig. 5.56a, b) (Hemprich and Zieglowski 1996).
  - Columellar lengthening

    The columella may be very short after the closure of the lip white, resulting in a marked depression of the nasal tip, especially in wide bilateral clefts with a protruding premaxilla. At the age of about 4 years a forked flap can be prepared by using the scar tissue from both philtra of the lip to elevate substantially the tip of the nose. The shortened medial crura of the nasal cartilages can also be raised. This will usually result in a better patency of the nasal ducts. Finally the philtrum gains a normal width (Millard 1958b) (Fig. 5.57a–c). All this will give the child a normal appearance so that he or she will not be harassed during puberty. At the end of facial growth many patients though will still need a final rhinoplasty.

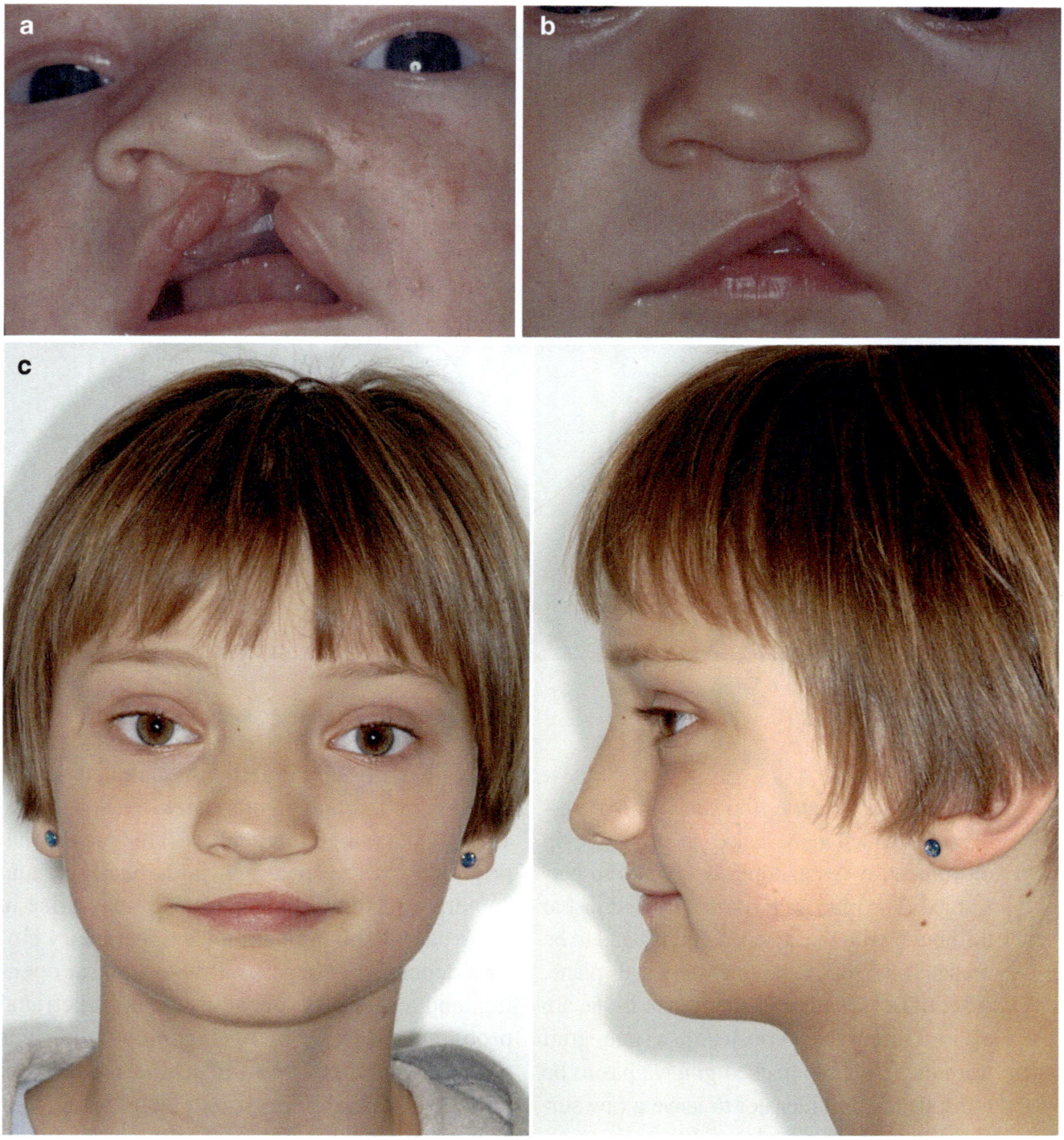

Fig. 5.55 (**a**) (top, left figure) Unilateral cleft lip with a very short medial stump (modified from Hemprich and Schiefke (2016) LKG: Spät/Korrekturbehandlungen. medupdate GmbH Wiesbaden with kind permission from medupdate GmbH). (**b**) (right figure) Significant shortening 5 weeks after lip closure (at age of 5 months) (modified from Hemprich and Schiefke (2016) LKG: Spät/Korrekturbehandlungen. medupdate GmbH Wiesbaden with kind permission from medupdate GmbH). (**c**) (2 figures) Good labial symmetry without any corrective procedure (age 6 years). (**d**) (below, 2 figures) Same patient at age 19 after 4 operations (lip/nose, palate, osteoplasty, (small) rhinoplasty

d

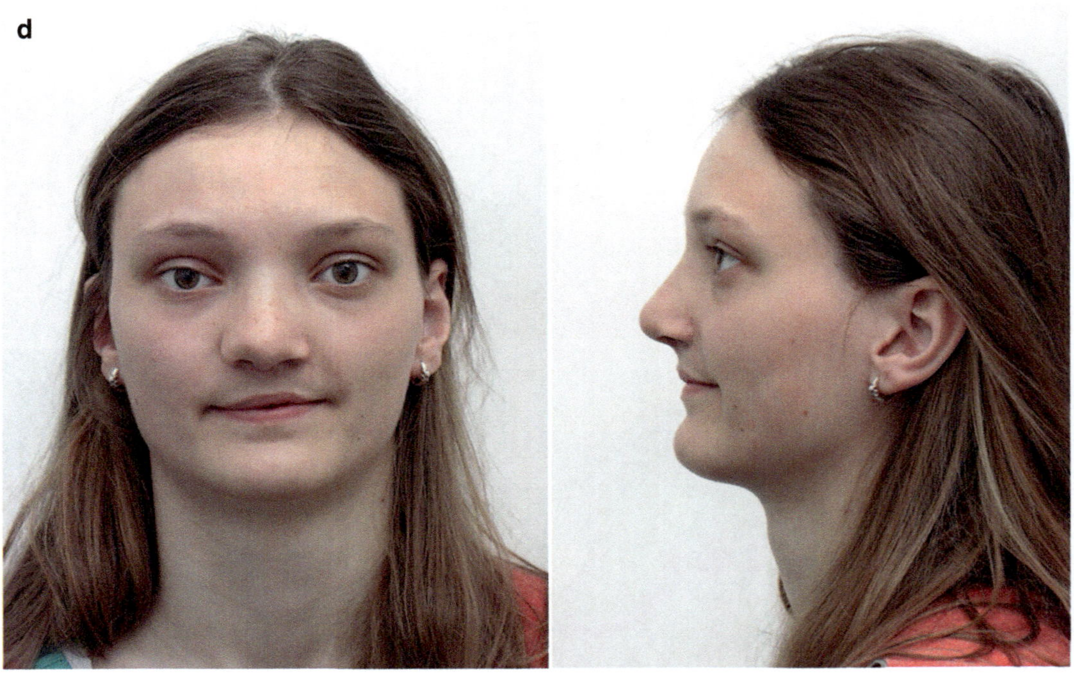

Fig. 5.55 (continued)

- Vestibuloplasty
  If there is too small or too short an oral vestibulum, which may cause an impaired lip movement, a vestibuloplasty should be performed. The mucosa has to be incised just at the border with the attached gingiva and to be prepared cranially on the periostal plane. After muscle fibres and connective tissue are excised from the periosteum, a free graft from the (palatal) attached gingiva has to be transplanted, in order not to leave a raw surface and to prevent a relapse. If speech development allows, this operation should be delayed until the eruption of the upper incisors, when at least a defined zone of attached gingiva has developed around the teeth.

5.13.8 Fistula Repair in the Palate

A pathological oro-nasal connection after failed wound healing or secondary wound dehiscence is called a fistula. The incidence in the literature ranges from 0% to 77.8%. Hardwicke et al. (2014) undertook a meta-analysis with 9294 patients included in 44 studies, and found fistula rates from 5.4% to 17.9% in leading cleft centres. This means that problems with speaking and hearing, and sometimes even with swallowing, may arise in these cases. The indication for a secondary closure depends on the size of the oro-nasal opening and especially on subsequent functional problems. In cases of open rhinophonia, it is possible temporarily to close the palatal gap with some dental impression material, to determine whether or not there will be a change in the patient's speech (nasality).

The main area for fistulae is the transition zone between hard and soft palate, followed by the area between the alveolus and the anterior part of the palate. If the size does not exceed 5 mm, a turn-over flap of the oral mucosa may be sufficient to create a nasal layer, and a (uni- or bi-lateral) von Langenbeck bridging flap for the oral closure. Utmost care has to be taken though, to prepare the flaps large enough so that they can be united over the fistula without tension.

In larger openings, different combinations of bridging or pedicled flaps, or both, may be neces-

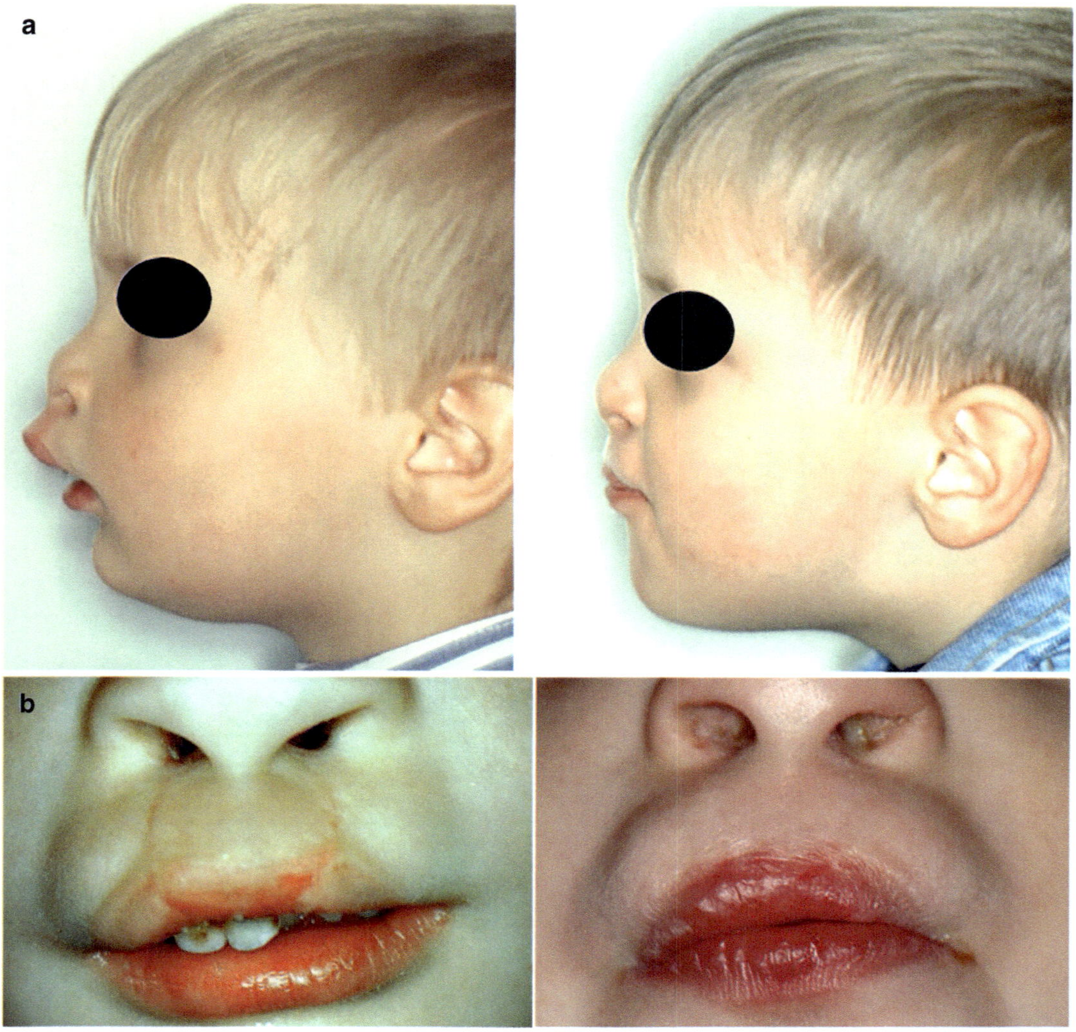

Fig. 5.56 (**a**) (left 2 figures) (left) Bilateral cleft lip after incomplete primary muscle plasty at age 3. Note the still protruding premaxilla. (right) Normal position of the premaxilla and better nasal growth two years after reconstruction of the perioral and perinasal muscle rings (modified from Hemprich and Schiefke (2016) LKG: Spät/Korrekturbehandlungen. medupdate GmbH Wiesbaden with kind permission from medupdate GmbH). (**b**) (right 2 figures) Same patient before (left) and 2 years after complete reoperation of the cleft lip/nose complex (right) (modified from Hemprich and Schiefke (2016) LKG: Spät/Korrekturbehandlungen. medupdate GmbH Wiesbaden with kind permission from medupdate GmbH). Note the better philtrum width and the better position of the nasal alae

sary. The relapse rate may rise to 30% if these rules are not strictly obeyed or a chronic infection is present at the palate and the maxillary teeth. The most difficult problem arises from a large recurrent fistula behind the premaxilla. This is the indication for a tongue flap (Mahajan et al. 2014) (Fig. 5.58a–c).

Sometimes, it may even be necessary to use a musculo-cutaneous flap from the antero-lateral thigh (ALT), which can be raised with the adjacent vessels and transplanted into the palate. The new blood supply will be provided by a microvascular connection to the buccal artery and vein (Bartella et al. 2021).

It must finally be noted that it is also possible to help a patient provisionally with a specially designed denture if a surgical correction is contraindicated for some reasons of general health.

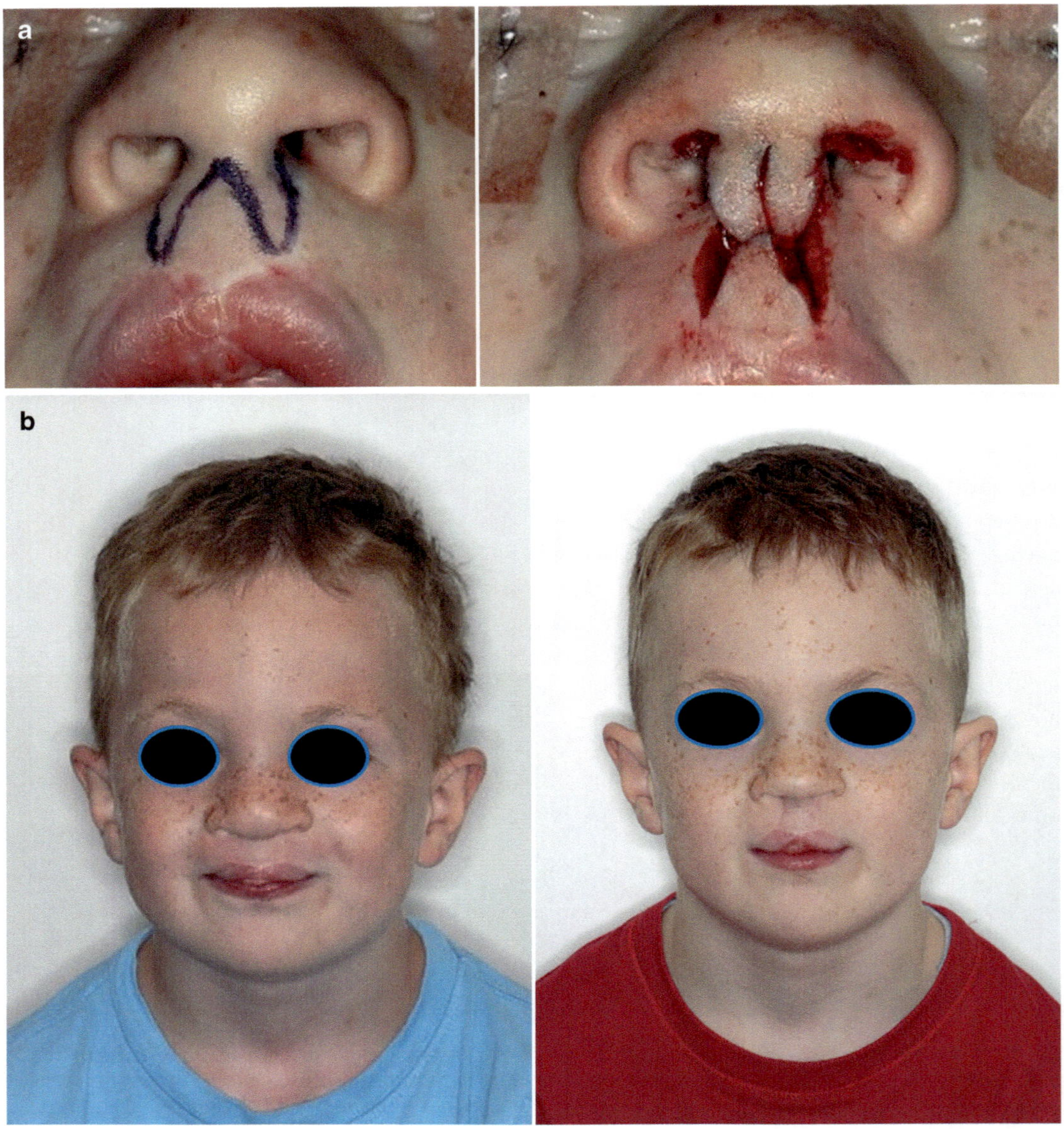

Fig. 5.57 (**a**) (top, left side) Forked flap for columellar lengthening. (**b**) (top, 2 right figures) 5-year-old patient with a bilateral cleft before (left) and one year after a columellar lengthening (right). Note the narrower philtral width. (**c**) (bottom, 2 figures) Lateral view of the same patient. Note the significant postoperative improvement of the columella and the nasal tip projection (right)

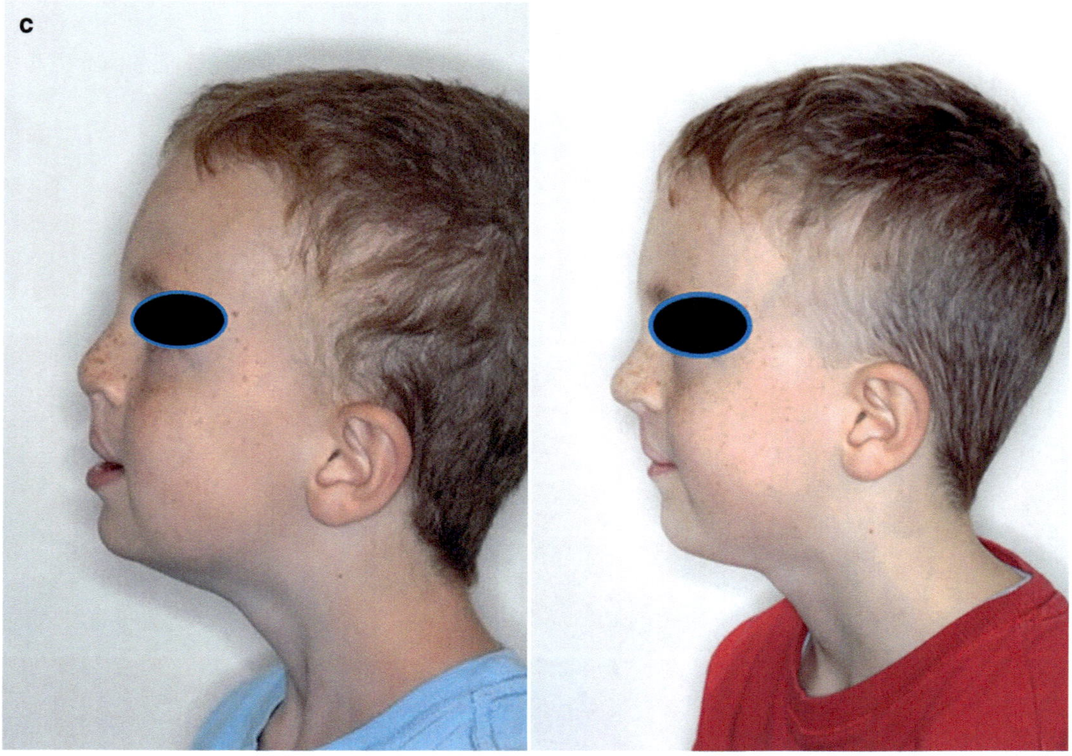

Fig. 5.57 (continued)

5.13.9 Speech-Improving Surgical Measures

See Sect. 5.14

5.13.10 Correction of the Cleft Nose Deformity

Even though primary rhinoplasty in cleft surgery has significantly contributed to the improvement of the results, more than 50% of patients are still not content with their facial aesthetics (Marcusson et al. 2002). They believe that a rhinoplasty is the most important operation for a better appearance (Meyer-Marcotty and Stellzig-Eisenhauer 2009). Basically, the cleft nose has the following characteristics:

- In *unilateral clefts*, there is a septal deviation, conchal hyperplasia and a cranial and lateral displacement of the ala nasi, leading to a drop of the tip of the nose on the cleft side.
- In *bilateral clefts*, there is a short columella due to the under-development of the medial crura of the alar cartilages, which will usually lead to a marked drop of the nasal tip with a pseudo hump in the supra-tip area and transversally open nares (Fig. 5.59).

5.13.11 Secondary Rhinoplasty

The aim of this procedure is the restoration of normal nasal anatomy (aesthetics) and function (breathing). In most cases, this must be combined in a lip–nose reconstruction, since facial (nasal) symmetry is based on tissues from lip and nose together. This includes the restoration of the perioral and perinasal muscle rings as well.

If there is still a substantial gap at the region of the cleft alveolus, a secondary osteoplasty should be performed beforehand in order to ensure a safe support of the alae nasi. In a number of cases, it may be sufficient to correct the

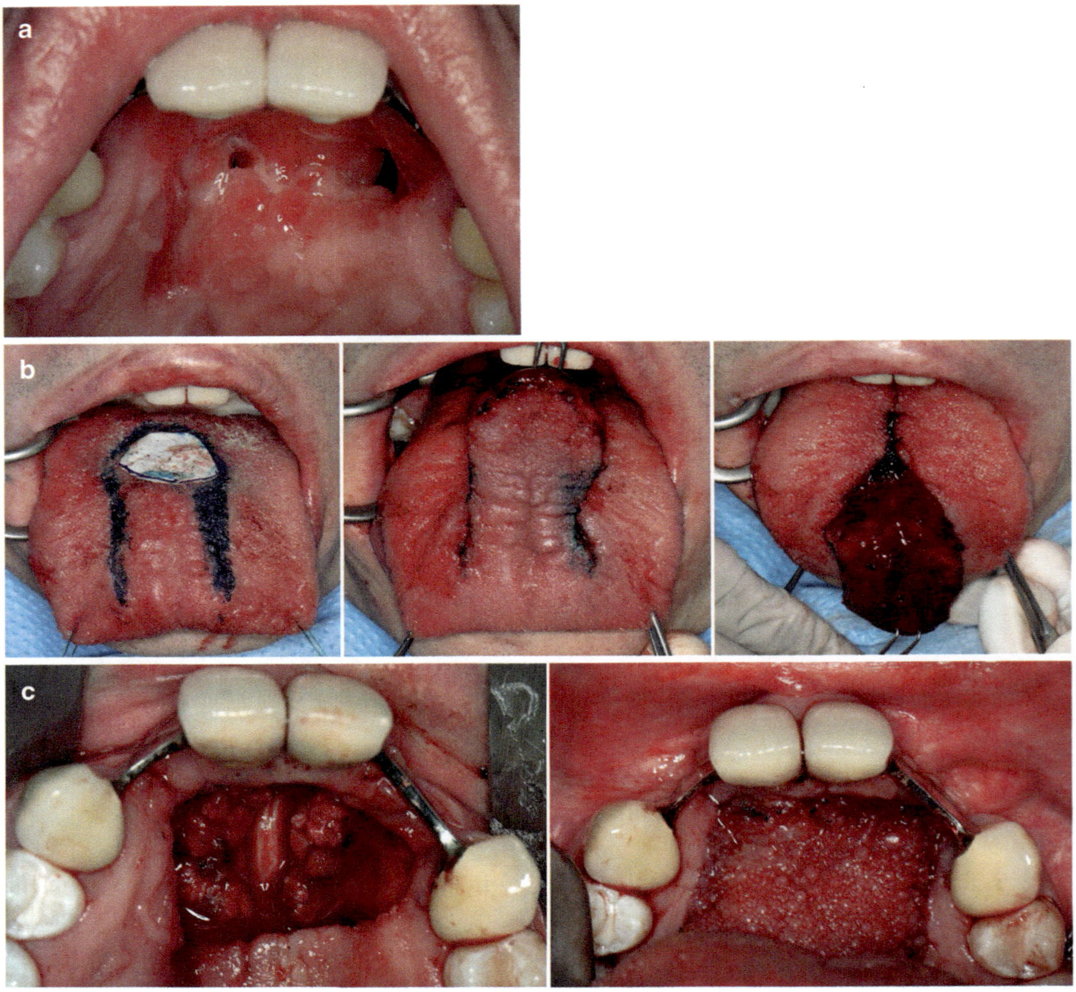

Fig. 5.58 (**a**) (top, left side) Remaining fistulae in the anterior palate after several attempts of closure. (**b**) (top, 3 figures) left: Outline of the tongue flap with an anterior pedicle, desired size of the flap marked by a template; middle: Flap raised; right: Partial closure of the tongue and raw surface of the flap. (**c**) (bottom, 2 figures) Nasal layer closed (left) and flap inserted as oral layer (right)

nasal septum and the alar cartilages. Very often the vomer (bony septum) has also to be straightened to achieve a normal passage for nasal breathing. Since the septo-vomerine transition zone is a main growth area though, a complete septorhinoplasty should not be performed before the end of facial growth, i.e. from the age of 14 years in girls and 16 years in boys.

The basis for this operation should be a facial analysis as described by Farkas et al. (1993). They could demonstrate that the naso-frontal and naso-labial angles are good tools to define the desired position of the nose. In most cases, the surgeon will choose an open approach to the inner nose. This enables him to make use of the (scarred) tissue in the upper lip which he can lift upwards to create a symmetric nasal tip. Moreover, he has to expose the nasal and septal cartilages, free them from their deviated position and suture them together to create a symmetric cartilaginous strut for the overlying skin. The septal deviation can be straightened by partially resecting the septal cartilage and the vomer, and moving the remaining parts to the midline.

In the end, there must be almost equal open nasal passages on each side to guarantee free

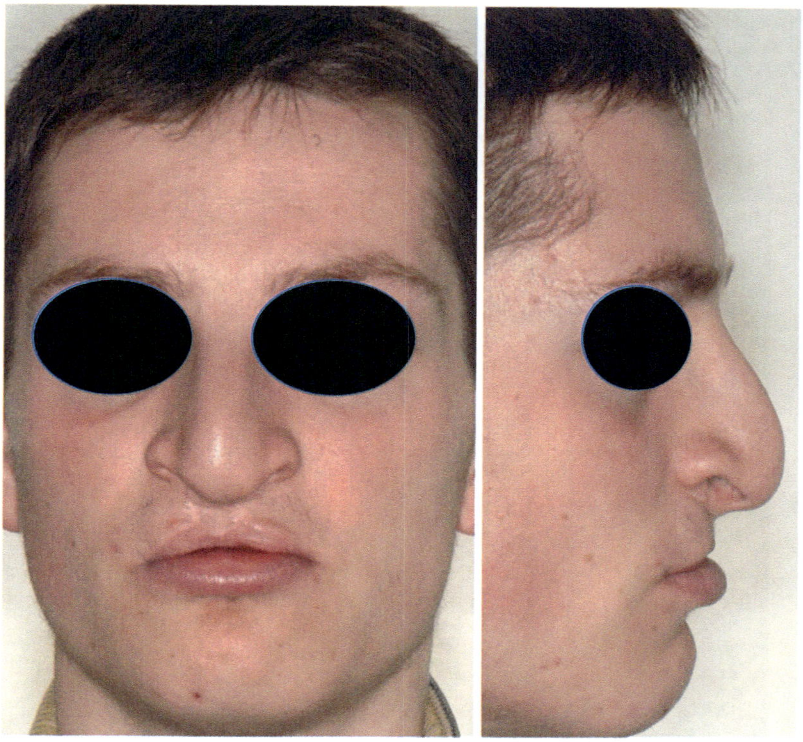

Fig. 5.59 Typical nasal deformity in a bilateral cleft: short columella, depressed nasal tip nasal hump, wide nares

nasal breathing. Before skin closure the perinasal muscles have to be fixed to the nasal septum, the anterior nasal spine and the perioral muscles, to form a complete ring. This will lead to functional support of nasal symmetry. Finally the nasal skin and the inner nasal mucosa have to be adapted by mattress sutures to avoid a haematoma and thereby an ugly inner scar formation with thick alae nasi (Fig. 5.60a, b).

It has proven to be helpful to let the patients wear nasal stents for several months postoperatively, in order to preserve the good result of (septo-)rhinoplasty. Long-term observations of more than four years have revealed 90% patient satisfaction, whereas only 69.2% of the medical experts saw a significant improvement of nasal appearance (Pitak-Arnnop et al. 2011).

5.13.12 Orthognathic Surgery

The incidence in cleft patients of a maxillary retrognathism, or even a midfacial retrusion, that needs a surgical correction ranges from 20% to 47.5% in the literature (Good et al. 2007). Here, the patient's face appears more concave, with deep nasolabial folds even in younger persons. The nasal cartilages lack support, so that the tip of the nose sinks down, which results in a low nasolabial angle (Fig. 5.61a). Finally, very often the occlusion shows an Angle Class III with a negative overjet of the front teeth (Fig. 5.61b). This can regularly have a negative influence on the patient's speech, too.

Many factors have been held responsible for this facial deformity, such as the method and timing of cleft palate closure, and the presence of early velopharyngeal flaps. Another important factor is the number of missing teeth in the maxilla. The indication for a Le Fort I osteotomy rises from 18.8% with a complete set of teeth to 86.4% with three or more missing teeth (Lai et al. 2015). In a long-term analysis of adult patients with and without an operated unilateral cleft palate, Liu and Chen (2018) demonstrated that intrinsic factors lead to a sagittal shortening of the posterior skull base, whereas the vertical growth of the maxilla is unimpaired. Finally, it may be stated

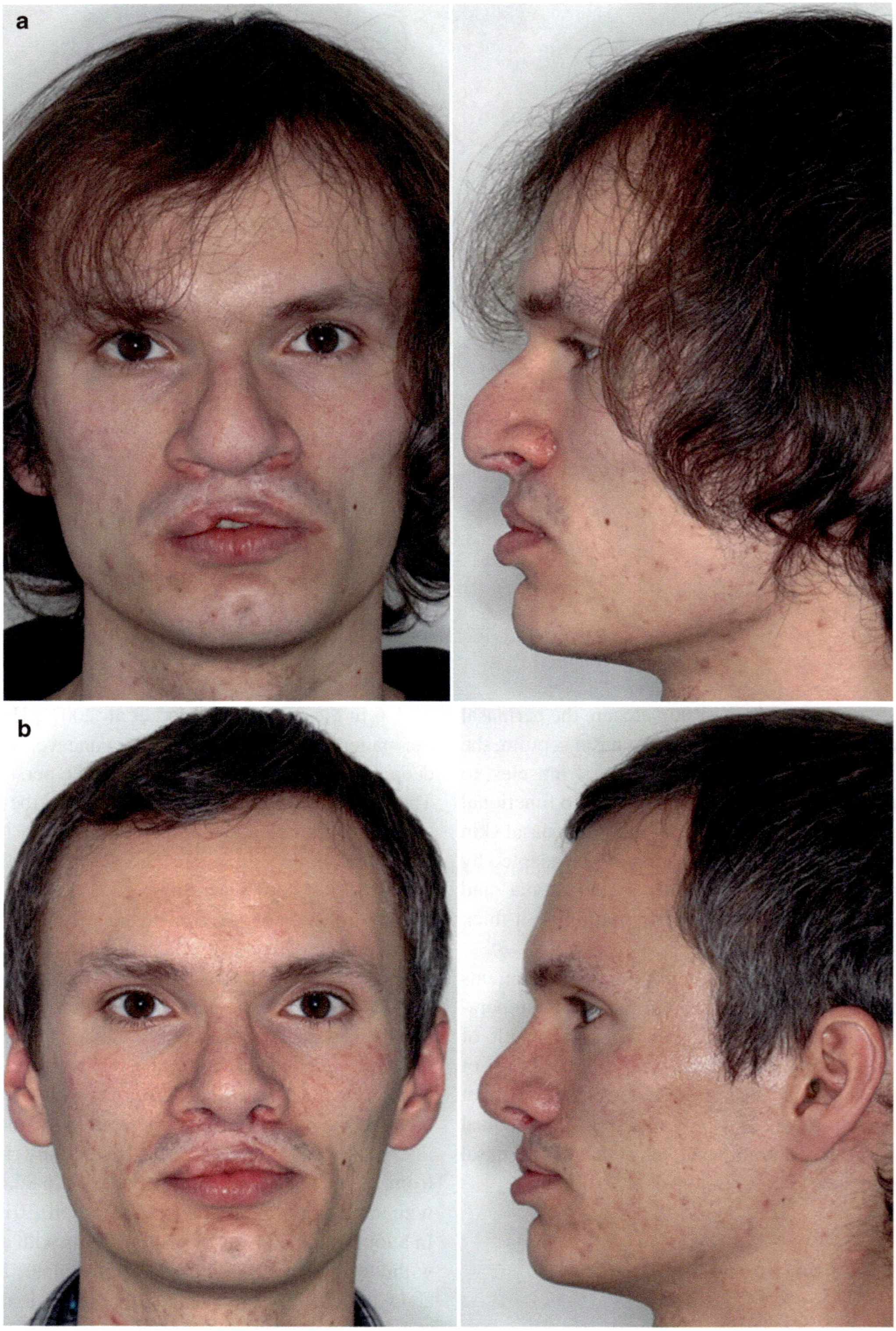

Fig. 5.60 (**a**) (left 2 figures) Cleft-related nasal deformity and whistle defect in the lip. (**b**) (right 2 figures) Same patient two years after a complete septorhinoplasty and lip revision

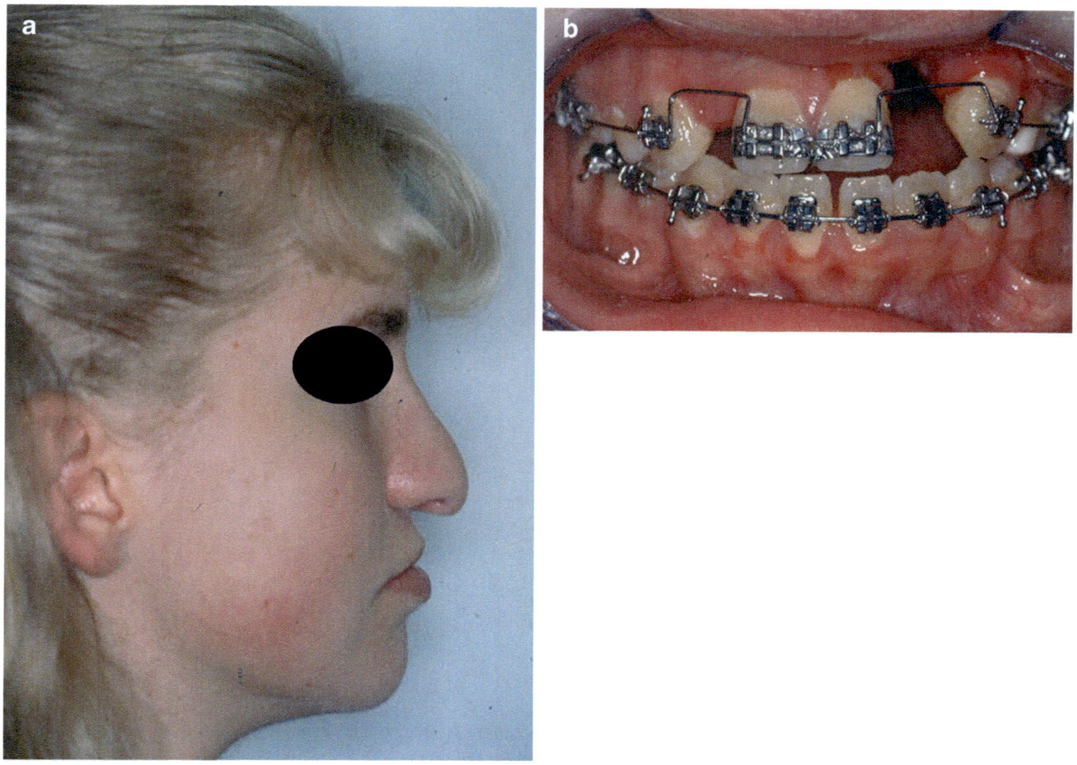

Fig. 5.61 (**a**) (left side) Typical cleft related maxillary retrognathism with low nasolabial angle and nasal tip depression. (**b**) (right side) Class III dental relationship

that skill and experience of the surgeon during the primary palatal closure have a great impact on the final results.

The decision for a maxillary advancement should always be based on the combined concepts of an orthodontist and a maxillofacial surgeon. Usually, there has to be an orthodontic treatment first, to align the teeth in maxilla and mandible into the postoperatively desired position before surgery. The final surgical protocol is based on a facial analysis in combination with a 2D or 3D imaging. In the majority of centres, the manufacturing of the surgical wafers for the intra-operative positioning of the jaws is still based on a mock operation of plaster casts individually mounted into an articulator. This will ensure that the surgeon can intraoperatively reach the planned position precisely. During the operation it must be ensured that the maxilla is mobilised so well that it can be moved forwards without any tension. The final fixation of the osteotomised bones is done by miniplate osteosynthesis. In adults, the long-term results are stable. A skeletal relapse of about 20% can be detected, which has no effect on the correctly achieved occlusion (Watts et al. 2015).

Owing to scars from the primary operations, resulting in a tight, soft tissue envelope over the midface, or to velopharyngeal flaps, there is a restriction of the forward movement of the maxilla by a conventional Le Fort I osteotomy to a maximum of 10 mm (Fig. 5.62a, b).

If larger movements prove to be necessary, a bimaxillary approach with simultaneous retropositioning of the mandible may be considered, if the facial profile allows this. Great caution has to be taken though, not to reduce the posterior airway space, which could result in an obstructive sleep apnoea. A good alternative to singular maxillary movements up to 30 mm is distraction osteogene-

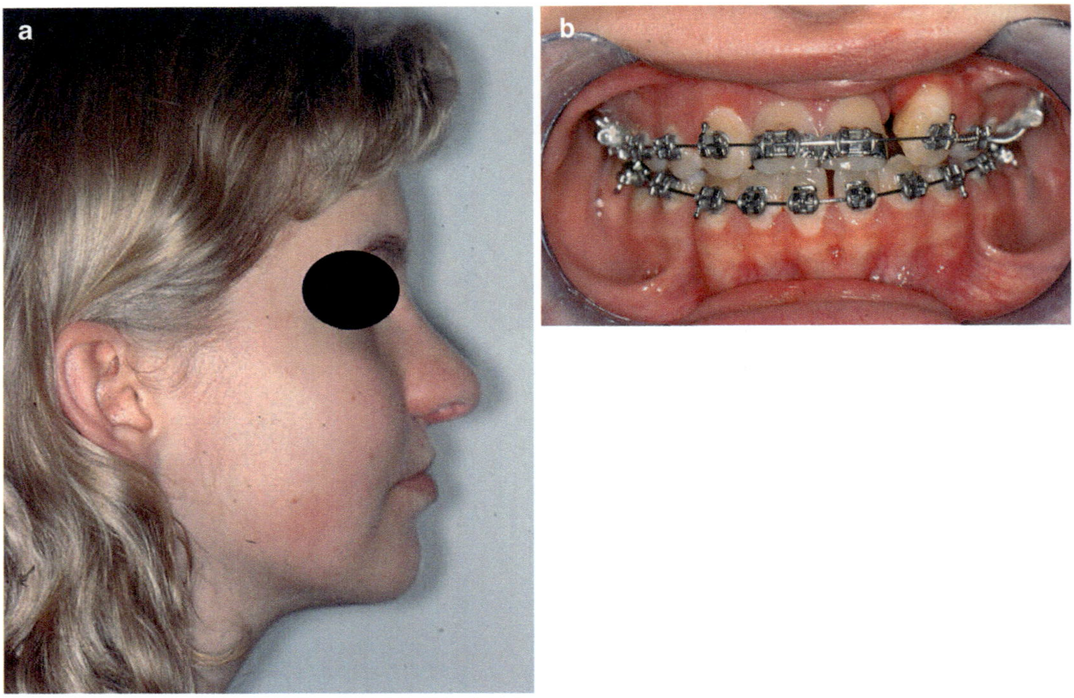

Fig. 5.62 (**a**) (left side) Same patient after maxillary advancement in the Le Fort I plane. Note the improvement of the nasolabial angle and nasal tip position without septorhinoplasty! (**b**) (right side) Normal overbite and overjet

sis (Hemprich and Hierl 2019) (Fig. 5.63a–c). An overcorrection of 15% should be planned, which will lead to stable long-term results.

It may be noted that a remarkable improvement of aesthetics, nasal breathing and mastication will always result from a forward movement of the maxilla. There is no deterioration in the velopharyngeal competence in any cases which had no speech problems before the treatment. In only 10% of the patients with a preoperative velopharyngeal incompetence, a velopharyngeal flap has been indicated.

More recently, the new philosophy of 'surgery first' has also been applied to cleft orthognathic cases. An extensive planning process is still performed by orthodontist and surgeon together, using 3D software and enabling the printing of the intraoperatively necessary wafers. The treatment itself starts with the operation. This leads to an immediate improvement of facial aesthetics and an overall reduction of treatment time. It can be demonstrated that tooth movements can be performed much faster in the more reactive (healing) bony tissue (Seo et al. 2019).

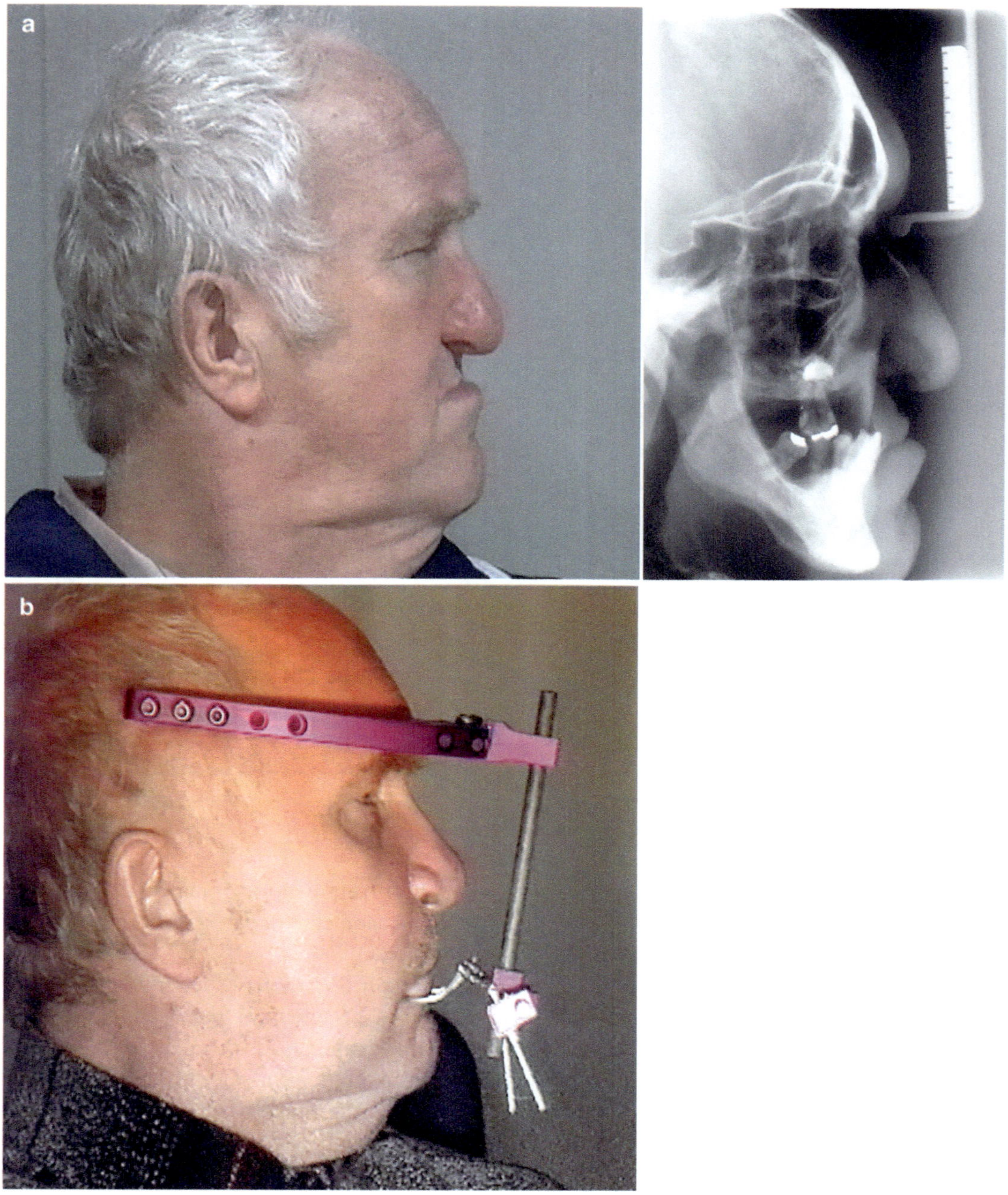

Fig. 5.63 (**a**) (left 2 figures) Marked maxillary retrusion in a bilateral almost edentulous cleft case (clinical aspect left), lateral side view X-ray (right). (**b**) (middle figure) External distraction device mounted. (**c**) (right 2 figures) Stable result of a 20 mm maxillary forward movement 2 years postoperatively. Note that the implants are inserted after successful midfacial distraction osteogenesis and tertiary osteoplasty

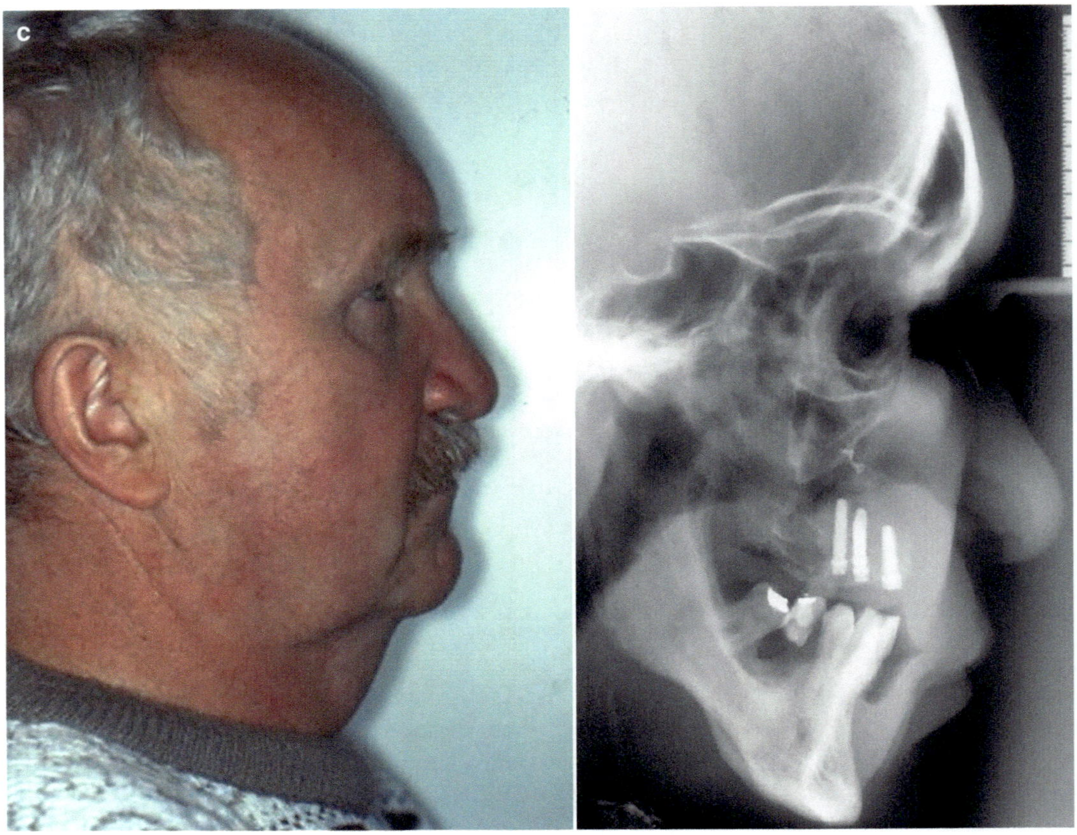

Fig. 5.63 (continued)

5.14 Speech-Improving Surgery

Jenő Hirschberg

5.14.1 Introduction

The soft palate is a very small part of the human body. Its importance, however, is far greater than its size. The velum together with the surrounding pharyngeal muscle, the so-called velopharyngeal (VP) sphincter, ensures the involvement and the smooth process of sucking, swallowing, speech, singing, blowing, whistling, yawning and breathing as well as middle ear ventilation—and thus—of hearing.

If for whatever reason the performance of the VP closure is insufficient, inadequate or disturbed, we speak of velopharyngeal insufficiency (VPI, velopharyngeal incompetence, palatal dysfunction). VPI may be organic or functional, congenital or acquired, and may be caused by structural anomalies or paresis (Hirschberg 1986) (Table 5.2).

In cases of VPI, one or several of the above functions are liable to be damaged. Judging the colourful symptoms of velopharyngeal insufficiency is a multidisciplinary task. The signs and symptoms of palatal dysfunction are primarily to be found in phonation and speech (Fritzell 1976); thus, the contribution of the phoniatrician in the diagnosis and therapy is considerable. However, as VPI is a borderline problem, the close co-operation with speech therapists (logopaedists), neurologists, otorhinolaryngologists, paediatricians, oral and maxillofacial or plastic surgeons is indispensable in early diagnosis and the choice of a suitable method of competent treatment.

The management types of VPI are as follows: speech therapy, surgery, prosthetic devices, others. Speech therapy is necessary and sufficient in about

Table 5.2 Classification of velopharyngeal insufficiency (Reproduced from Hirschberg (1986) Velopharyngeal Insufficiency. Folia Phoniatr Logop:221-276 with permission from Karger AG, Basel)

Form	**Subgroups**				**Most important causes**	
					congenital	*acquired*
Organic	*dynamic (paresis)*	*central*	supranuclear	neurogen	encephalopathy	tumor
			nuclear		nucleus aplasia (Moebius)	vascular alteration
						inflammation
		peripheric	peripheric neurogen		rudimentary paresis	degeneration
						polyneuritis (toxic, infectious)
			neuromyogen			compression
						trauma/tumor
			myoneurogen			poliomyelitis
						neural-muscular atrophy
			neuromuscular junction			myositis
			myogen	myogen		myasthenia gravis
						myopathies
	static-structural (anatomical changes)				cleft	
					submucous cleft	destruction (tumor, trauma)
					occult submucous cleft	
					shortening	cicatrisation (post-traumatic, post-surgical)
					deep nasopharynx (vertebral deformation)	
					anatomical disproportion	
Functional	*passive*				mental deficiency	mental deficiency
						hearing loss
					hearing loss	neurosis
						post-surgical pain
						habitual
	active					imitation
Combined forms					anatomical disproportion and dynamic disturbance	cicatrisation and functional VPI

80% of all VPI cases. If speech therapy fails, a surgical solution comes into consideration.

5.14.2 Surgical Indication

A pluridisciplinary attitude and individually determined therapy are important concomitants of the decision.

In general, surgery is recommended in those cases of organic VPI that imply a persistent condition (i.e. where a progressive process can be precluded), where no results can be expected on the basis of teachability tests or other examination data, or have been achieved by means of speech therapy of 4–6 months.

There are several circumstances that may influence the decision regarding surgery and surgical technique: age, mental level and hearing of the patient, the personal equation and attitude of the surrounding milieu to the surgery, the patient's anatomical status, measure of VPI, experience of the surgeon and the speech therapist. Before deciding upon surgery, consultation with the patient or the parents of the hypernasal child is indispensable, informing them about the expected results, the risks and about the not always easy postoperative days. It may happen that—on the basis of the examinations—it is obvious that speech therapy does not hold out much success (very short, cicatrised velum, serious hypernasality); in such a case surgery is nevertheless recommended at the very start. If the parents of the concerned child, however, are doubtful and or anguished, one should decide on a conservative treatment.

The purpose of the surgery is the cessation of hypernasality and nasal escape without forming a total obstruction of the velopharyngeal port. With surgical intervention the hyper-rinophony may be eliminated or decreased, and the anatomical basis of a postoperative speech therapy already auguring success may be created. The treatment of articulation disorders, after surgery, falls on the speech therapist.

The operative interventions performed on patients with VPI may be suitable not only to correct speech, but also at times swallowing: in cases of oropharyngeal dysphagia, the nasal regurgitation and aspiration of liquid and food may be impeded or decreased by the velopharyngeal surgery, but this is rare. Although velopharyngoplasties may occasionally affect swallowing and the extent of conductive hearing loss, undoubtedly the primary aim of these surgeries is the correction of voice, the timbre, the resonance; thus, these interventions may rightly be reckoned to belong to the domain of phonosurgery (Hirschberg 1990).

5.14.3 Age of Patient in Time of Surgery

The age of the patient at the time of surgery depends on many various factors. First of all on the patient's first visit with the physician or speech therapist because of his or her speech or swallowing complaints. It also depends on educational, traditional and geographical circumstances, but assuming favourable conditions, surgery at a young age is recommended. Most authors (Abyholm et al. 2005; Fukushiro and Trindade 2011; Isshiki et al. 1971) agree that better surgical results can be obtained in young children than in older ones or adults. In the opinion of Hirschberg (2012), the ideal age for velopharyngoplasty is around 4.5–5 years. The failure of speech therapy is revealed by this age and the child is sufficiently co-operative in the days following operation, which is not always easy. Moreover, if chosen, post-operative speech therapy can also be commenced before the age of schooling. The complication rate in young patients is also reduced (Bronsted et al. 1984; Isshiki et al. 1971), and the maxillofacial development is also more propitious if operation is performed before the age of 7 (Hirschberg and Rehák 1997).

5.14.4 The Person Who Performs the Surgery: Who Should Operate?

Established customs and different traditions in different countries determine the person who performs the operation for velopharyngeal insufficiency. According to an early survey (Hirschberg 1986), including data furnished by 42 experts from 30 countries, speech-correcting (velopharyngeal) operations are performed by plastic, oral and maxillofacial, and paediatric surgeons, otorhinolaryngology (ORL) specialists, as well as phoniatricians. As for competence, the Union of European Phoniatricians (UEP) took the view in 1982 that phonosurgery is an integrated part of phoniatrics. This standpoint can be accepted, provided that it is not a special branch of the medical profession that makes the decision on the selection of the surgeon. What is of importance, is that those who undertake the performance of these operations, should only be those, who are well versed in the question of velopharyngeal insufficiency; who have a thorough knowledge of the anatomy as well as the physiology of the VP area; who regularly perform such operations; and who can ensure, both before and after the operation, the participation—necessary for complex process of (re)habilitation—of all experts concerned. In other words, one can say that phoniatric preparedness for the performance of surgery for velopharyngeal insufficiency is by all means advisable.

5.14.5 Preoperative Diagnostics

The primary condition for a successful surgical therapy is a detailed investigation, the precise diagnosis before surgery. This investigation is indispensable and it should include each aspect of velopharyngeal insufficiency.

In observing the symptoms of VPI, our first task is to determine its cause. It should be realised—already at the first examination—that the speech disorder, the hypernasality, may be one or the only symptom of a disease or alteration affecting the entire constitution. Only if there is no such suspicion, or it can be precluded, i.e. there is not a pathological (neurological) process in the background, there is scope and basis for considering the surgical management.

As the signs and symptoms of VPI may be observable first of all in the field of voice and speech, the detailed analysis of these functions is of great significance. The correct perceptual, auditive evaluation of the speech is primary and indispensable in diagnosis: it constitutes the basis of any therapy. The parameters of all speech qualities (nasality, nasal escape, understandability, articulation, teachability) should be measured. The use of a five-point rating scale is proposed for the judgement and description of every speech attributes.

The secondary, additional and instrumental procedures serve for verification, validation or exclusion, and supplements the results and data gathering by routine examinations (see Chap. 3). According to the standpoint of the IALP (1999), the most essential and optimal instrumental procedures in cases of VPI are the following: nasopharyngoscopy, nasometry and—in cases of uncertain aetiology—neurological and electrophysiological examinations. Video(cine)fluoroscopy meanwhile is replaced by cine-MRI (Schenck et al. 2021).

5.14.6 Surgical Methods

Ever since Rosenthal (1924) and then Sanvanero-Rosselli (1955) renewed Passavant's (1879) and Schönborn's (1875) old surgical concept, many different kinds of surgical methods and techniques have been described, and the question of speech-improving operations has become one of the central subjects of the literature concerned with cleft palate and velopharyngeal insufficiency.

The most common and most frequently used techniques are as follows:

- Velopharyngoplasty (flap surgery)
- Sphincteroplasty
- Furlow plasty
- Augmentation

Formerly used but today rarely proposed methods:

- Push-back procedures
- Pharyngoplasties (creating a flap from the posterior pharyngeal wall without touching the palate; these techniques are nowadays counted as augmentation techniques)

5.14.6.1 Velopharyngoplasty

Posterior pharyngeal flap surgery, the so-called velopharyngoplasty, is the most commonly used operation to restore velopharyngeal competence. The essentials of this technique are to create a mucosa-covered fibromuscular flap from the posterior pharyngeal wall and suture it into the soft palate. Thus, a 'subtotal' obstruction is established between the mouth and nose in the midline, and two apertures are left beside the flap for the necessary nasal airflow. A sagittal and possibly circular velopharyngeal closure pattern seems to be ideal for this method. For more details, see Sect. 3.14.

The two more common versions of this technique are: the Schönborn-Rosenthal method with an inferiorly based pharyngeal flap (Fig. 5.64) and the superiorly based flap proposed by Sanvanero-Rosselli (Fig. 5.65).

The procedure is performed under general anaesthesia.

In the case of preparing an inferiorly based flap, a horizontal incision is first made in the nasopharynx as high as possible (at the site of the formerly removed adenoid), then at the two final points of the incision the cut will be continued vertically caudally. One should always account for the shrinkage of the prepared flap some months postoperatively: a flap cut too narrow will not guarantee any results. If surgery is indicated in case of velo-cardio-facial syndrome, careful inspection is necessary to detect aberrant carotid artery pulsations in the pharynx. Flap length is usually 2.5 cm. The tailor-made flap should be fixed into the layers of the velum. A well proven method of the fixation is to lay the pharyngeal flap on an apron flap formed and turned down from the soft palate. By the creation of the apron flap the velum elongates; thus, a longer receiving bed can be prepared to the flap (see Fig. 5.64).

In case of contemplating to dissect a *superiorly based flap*, a small vertical incision is made on a lateral side of the posterior pharyngeal wall. The prepared flap is then inserted into a pocket in the nasal side of the soft palate. The surgery may also be started below with an horizontal incision. Six to eight weeks before the velopharyngoplasty, adenoidectomy is routinely performed. After the operation careful observation is indispensable, watching for possible complications.

5.14.6.2 Sphincteroplasty (Sphincter Pharyngoplasty)

This is the second-most common surgical method for correcting hypernasality. The original concept of this procedure was described by Hynes (1950). It has since been modified and was widely promoted by Orticochea (1968, 1992). This technique involves the lysis of both palatopharyngeal muscles raised from the posterior tonsillar pillars. The prepared flaps are then rotated and transposed into a demucosalised recipient bed of the posterior pharyngeal wall or into a little inferiorly based flap

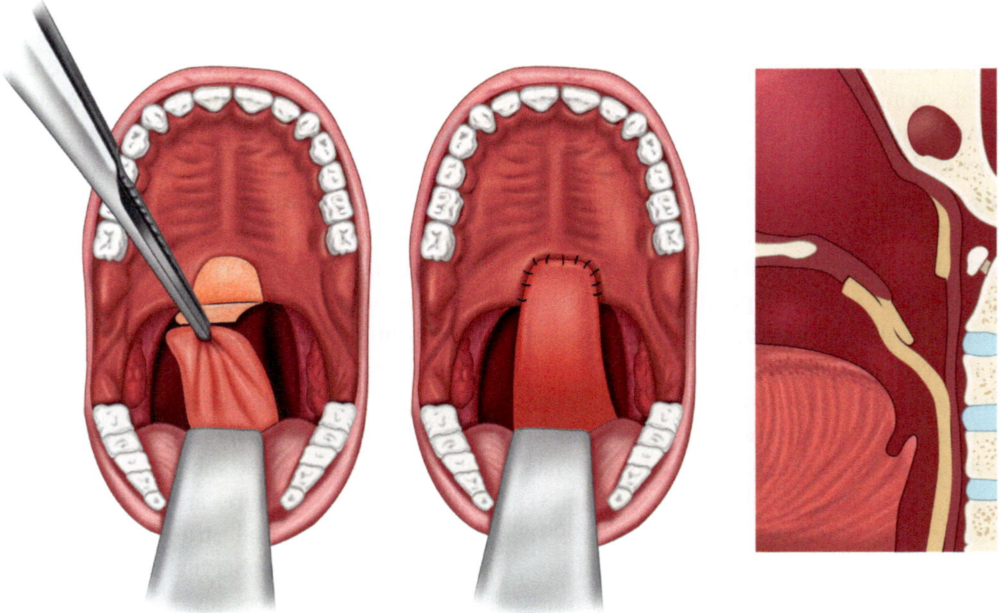

Fig. 5.64 Inferiorly based pharyngeal flap

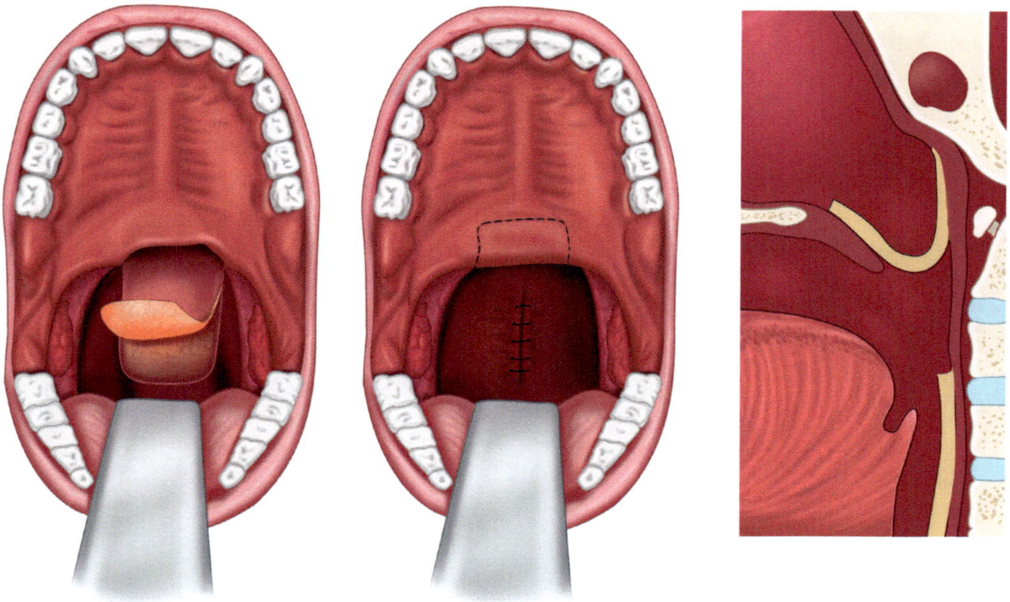

Fig. 5.65 Superiorly based pharyngeal flap

formed from the pharyngeal wall (Fig. 5.66). This technique preserves the motility of the soft palate and creates a 'dynamic' sphincter. Patients with good velar elevation, but poor lateral pharyngeal wall motion are good candidates for sphincter pharyngoplasty. The Orticochea methods can be used also secondarily, after failure of velopharyngoplasty.

5.14.6.3 Furlow Technique (Double-Opposing Z-plasty)

Furlow (1986) proposed his technique, the so-called intravelar palatoplasty, first for cleft palate repair. The essence of this surgery is that two opposite Z-plasty flaps are formed, one from the oral and the other from the nasal layer of both sides of the velum. One nasal layer is purely mucosal, and the opposite nasal layer is a mucosal-muscle flap. The oral flaps are similarly created. After adequate mobilisation, the nasal flaps are first transposed in a typical Z-plasty manner anteromedially and they are then sutured in the midline (Fig. 5.67). Closure of the oral side is performed similarly. It may be used, however, only in mild VPI cases, when the VP gap is no more than 5 mm.

5.14.6.4 Augmentation

Like Furlow plasty, the augmentation techniques may be recommended only for patients with small central velopharyngeal gap (3–4 mm). This intervention may be successful, primarily in cases with shortening of the soft palate, but can also be used secondarily, after failure of velopharyngoplasty. After the implantation, the pharyngeal wall bulges forward, and thus, the velopharyngeal port narrows (Fig. 5.68). A wide variety of materials have been implanted into the posterior pharyngeal wall, at the level of the first or second cervical vertebra, between the musculus constrictor pharyngis and the submucosa. At the beginning of the twentieth century, paraffin was used; later biological materials such as cartilage or fascia; afterwards plastics: teflon, silastic, proplast. Nowadays, autologous fat has been increasingly applied to augment the posterior pharynx (Leboulanger et al. 2011; Leuchter et al. 2012; Nicolas et al. 2011). This material has

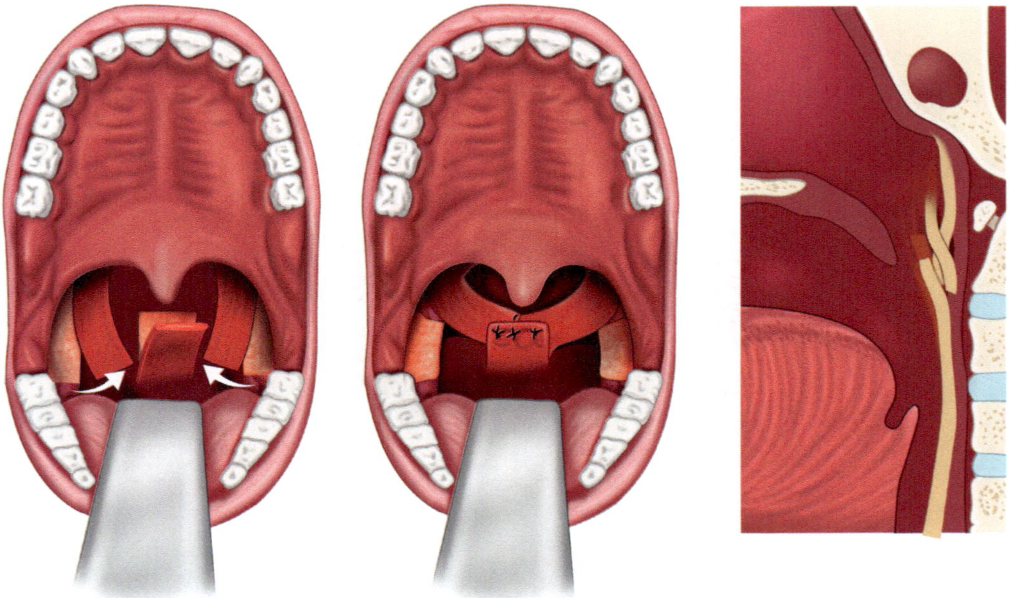

Fig. 5.66 Sphincteroplasty

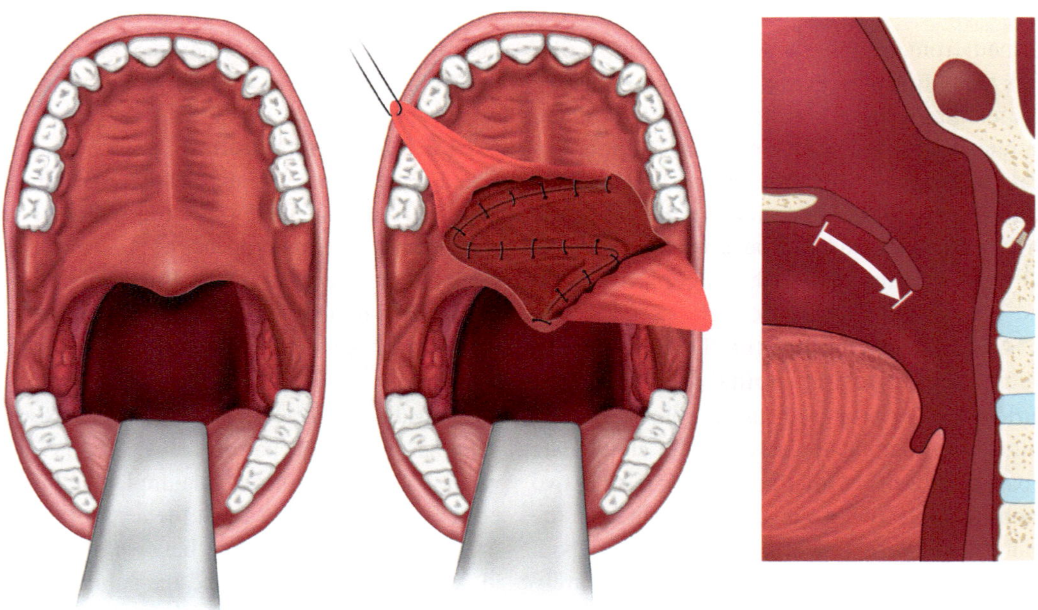

Fig. 5.67 Furlow technique

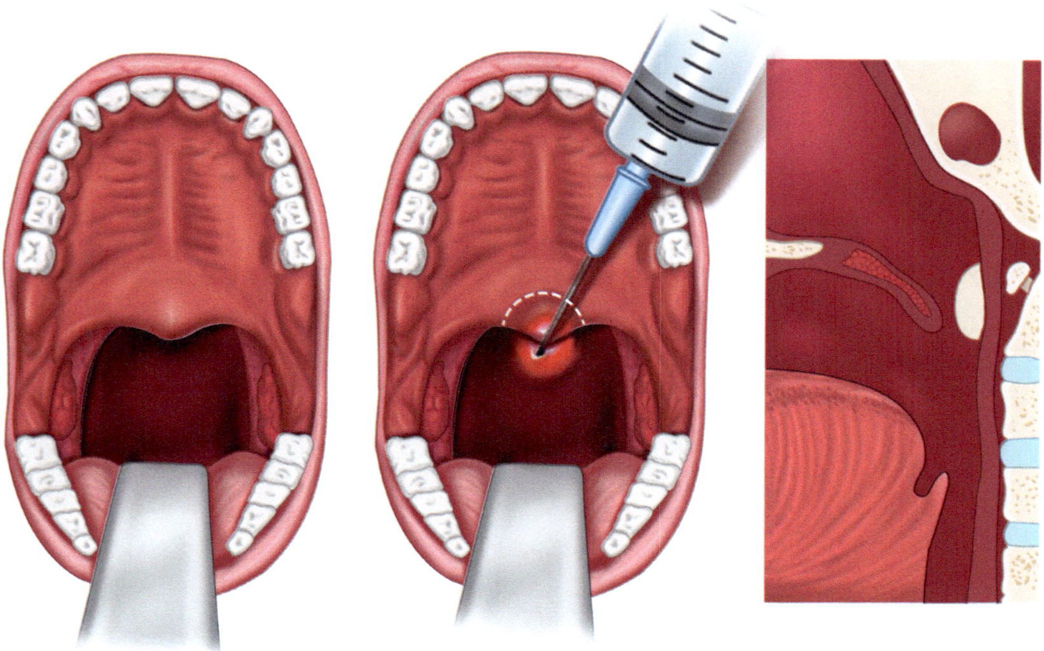

Fig. 5.68 Augmentation

numerous advantages: there is no foreign body reaction, immunisation, secondary migration or granulomas. Recent reports have described the use of calcium hydroxyapatite as injected material with auspicious results (Brigger et al. 2010).

5.14.6.5 Push-Back Procedures

The aim of these techniques is to lengthen the palate by means of mobilisation and caudal shifting of the soft tissues of the hard palate (Fig. 5.69). This technique is rarely successful and comes into question only in cases of moderate VPI. A disadvantage is a possible damaging consequence of this surgery: making free and irritation of the hard palate's significant area involves the risk of disorder in bone development.

5.14.7 Surgical Results

The anatomical results are excellent. It occurs rarely, in 1–2% of cases where the flaps do not adhere, the sutures are insufficient or the implanted material is resorbed or migrates. In a large Hungarian study, 21 pharyngeal flaps detached in 1104 surgeries for VPI (Hirschberg 2012). The functional results are also good. Independently of the various surgical techniques, speech improvement is—according to the literature—in the range of 62–98%, in general about 85–90% successful.

5.14.8 Factors Influencing the Surgical Results

- The age of the patient at the time of surgery (in younger children the results are better than in older ones or adults)
- Hearing and intelligence level of the patient (serious perceptive hearing impairment contraindicates the surgery; IQ should be over 50)
- Aetiology of VPI (in cases with structural anomalies, the results are better than in cases with paresis)
- A significant factor is the careful, detailed and instrumental preoperative diagnostics for judg-

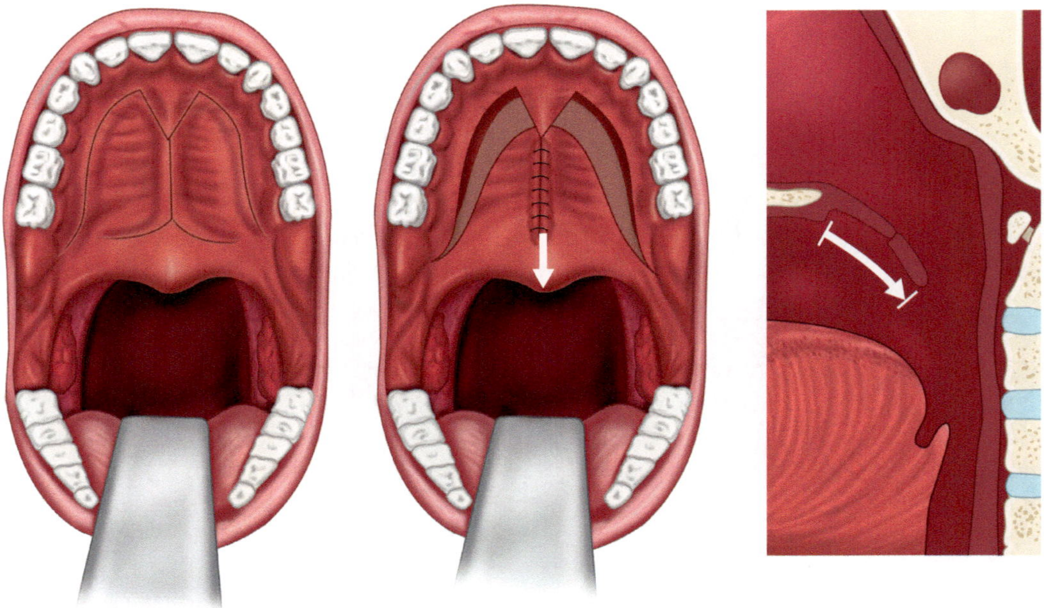

Fig. 5.69 Push-back procedure

ing the size and type of the velopharyngeal sphincter, important for choosing the adequate surgical method

- The postoperative anatomical status: the adequate width of the flap (in cases of velopharyngoplasty) and the motility of the lateral pharyngeal wall (Figs. 5.70a, b and 5.71a, b); each operative method has some advantages and disadvantages
- The experience of the operator and the routine of the speech therapist

Whereas by a superiorly based flap larger VP defects can be bridged and postoperative bleeding readily may be stopped, later corrections are easier in case of an inferiorly based flap which in addition offers less nasal obstruction (Hirschberg and Gross 2006). Wójcicki and Wójcicka (2011) compared the effectiveness of therapy in 84 patients with velopharyngeal insufficiency treated with different surgical methods: pharyngeal flap, sphincter pharyngoplasty, double Z-plasty and simultaneous Orticochea and Furlow operations. The evaluations of speech intelligibility, hypernasality and nasalance ratio were classified on a 1–5 point scale. Of the patients after pharyngeal flap, Orticochea, Furlow and Orticochea with Furlow operations, a good or very good outcome was achieved in 54%, 53%, 53% and 68%; and improvement in 25%, 27%, 38% and 23%.

5.14.9 Surgical Complications

Surgical complications are uncommon; one should, however, always take into account that it is not a vital or life-saving surgery but a speech-improving operation. Undesirable surgical consequences occur mostly after velopharyngoplasties. The two more serious complications of the velopharyngoplasty are postoperative bleeding and respiratory obstruction. Haemorrhage in the early postoperative period can cause aspiration which sometimes necessitates a tracheotomy. Among the late consequences with velopharyngoplasty, long lasting difficulty of nasal breathing and obstruc-

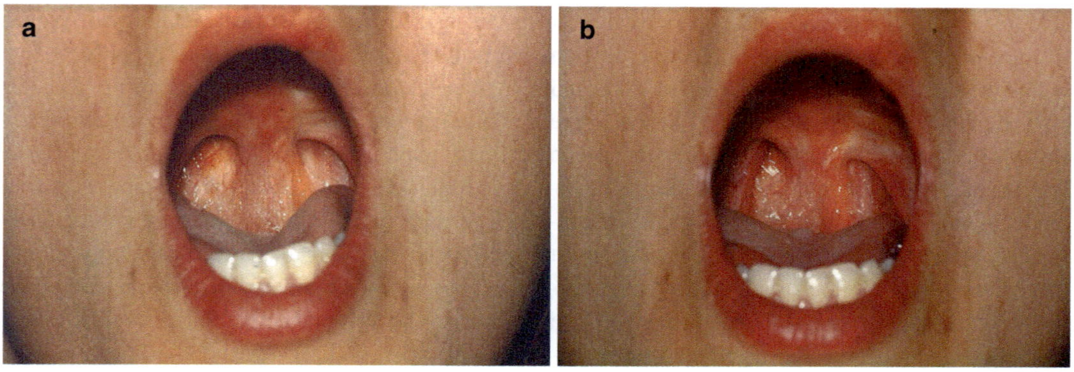

Fig. 5.70 (**a**) Inferiorly based pharyngeal flap in rest. (**b**) Pharyngeal flap during articulation

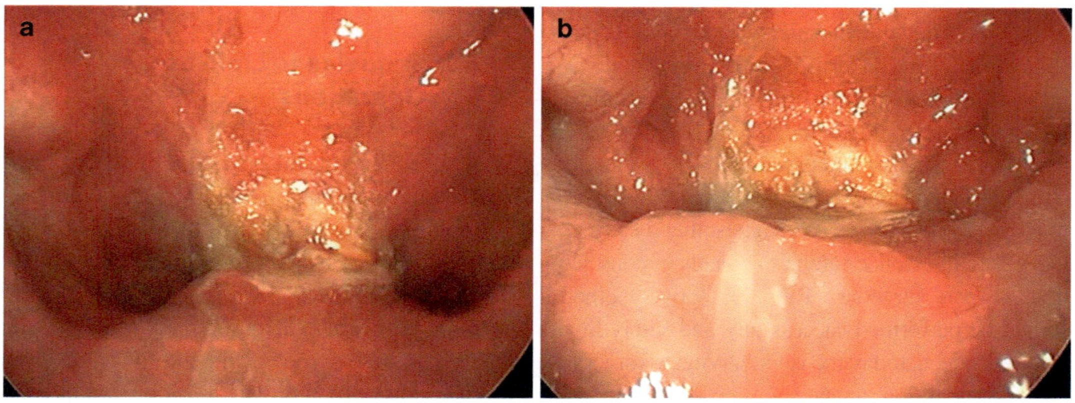

Fig. 5.71 (**a**, **b**) Nasopharyngoscopy with 30° rigid endoscope after velopharyngoplasty with superiorly based pharyngeal flap: appropriately sized flap with additional activity of the lateral pharyngeal walls and posterior pharyngeal wall resulting in a competent velopharyngeal sphincter, mucosa with tenacious mucus (**a**) in rest (**b**) articulating the stop consonant /p/ (with permission of Professor Siegmar Reinert, Department of Oral and Maxillofacial Surgery, Tübingen, Germany)

tive sleep apnoea (OSAS) may occur. It can happen, very rarely, that a total postoperative nasopharyngeal stenosis occurs after the velopharyngoplasty with chronic hyponasality. The remedies of these consequences vary: corticosteroid injections, dissolution of the cicatrices with a CO_2 laser or radio frequency radiation, constructing laterally based flaps or, a recently published technique, palatal eversion (Abdel-Fatah 2012). According to cephalometric measures (Hirschberg and Rehák 1997; Long and McNamara 1985), flap surgery also affects maxillofacial development; this effect is, however, not remarkable and it does not threaten the development of the harmonic configuration of the facial skull.

5.14.10 Summarising the Evaluation of Velopharyngeal Surgeries

The optimal time of the surgery is the age of 4½–5 years. At this age, if speech therapy fails, the child is already fairly co-operative in the difficult postoperative days and after surgery, and as still before schooling, enough time remains for the postoperative logopaedic management. Results of surgeries performed at an early age are significantly better than those in adults and at this age complications are fewer. The operation can be performed at a later age, but the results are not as good as at the age mentioned above. The surgery may be performed in multiply damaged individuals, too, but their IQ should be over 50. In the interest of choosing a suitable surgical method, the adequate operative type, it is imperative to perform a careful investigation before the surgery, for definition of the measure and type of the velopharyngeal closure. The aim of the surgery is to realise the most thorough speech improvement with the minimum of risk. A tailor-made plasty, considering the individual circumstances, assures optimal results. Nowadays, most surgeons prefer the velopharyngoplasty with superiorly based flap; for operative management of mild or moderate velopharyngeal insufficiency, sphincteroplasty, Furlow plasty or augmentation gains ground. In cases with sagittal type velopharyngeal closure, the pharyngeal flap surgery is generally recommended, while in patients with coronal or circular VP closure patterns, sphincteroplasty comes into question. Regarding the results, a significant factor is the experience of the surgeon. Hypernasality may be abolished or decreased in 85–90% of cases. Although the velopharyngeal surgery may have a few complications, one can suggest that these techniques are in essence safe in the hands of conscientious, expert surgeons. These operative methods should be performed successfully and safely in all centres. Indeed, today the velopharyngeal surgery is more of an art than science.

If surgery is contraindicated or the patient does not cooperate, application of prosthetic devices may come into consideration. Two types of them are known: the speech bulb and the palatal lift. The first, an obturator-like appliance, moderates the consequences of an anatomical defect or alteration of the palate; the aim of the palatal lift is the elevation of the velum. The two types of appliance may be combined.

5.15 Understanding Consequences of Various Surgical Procedures on Articulation

Alexander Hemprich and Ute Pröschel

5.15.1 Introduction

The functional outcome of surgical procedures depends on the extent of the cleft, the surgical procedures used and the individual (predisposition to scarring). The most critical anatomical regions regarding articulation are lip and soft palate.

A successful treatment of clefts of lip, alveolus and palate can only be achieved by an interdisciplinary team approach. The surgeon may play an important role in this context but can only contribute to give the child a good start by meticulously reconstructing the malformed anatomy. Early operations (before the end of the first year) have proven to be advantageous for the development of speech whereas later ones (24–30 months) are supposed to leave more room for an undisturbed midfacial growth (Lohmander et al. 2017).

5.15.2 Sequelae to Lip/Nose Operations

Even after a successful operation of the lip some tension and scars may remain and cause reduced lip mobility. This is especially true in bilateral clefts with a very much protruding premaxilla. In these cases the articulation of the labial phonemes is disturbed. Usually, the premaxilla will be pulled back by muscle force within the first 1–2 years after lip closure reducing lip tension substantially.

If the lip still appears to be fixed to the bone, however, a vestibuloplasty is indicated. The deeply attached mucosa of the upper lip will be incised on the border to the attached gingiva in the region between the two neighbouring teeth to the cleft. The complete supra-periostal upward preparation of the mucosa with removal of muscle and connective tissue fibres from the periosteum follows. Then the mucosa will be fixed to the periosteum about 10 mm cranially to the incision with fine resorbable sutures. Finally, it is necessary to cover the free periostal area with a free transplant of attached gingiva from the palate to prevent a substantial relapse (Fig. 5.72a–c). (For more details on lip/nose revisions, see Sect. 5.13)

5.15.3 Sequelae of Palatoplasty

The breakdown of a hard palate closure will leave fistulae (more details in Sect. 5.13). Depending on size and location they can influence speech by oronasal perflation from a small hiss to a snorkelling sound and finally to an

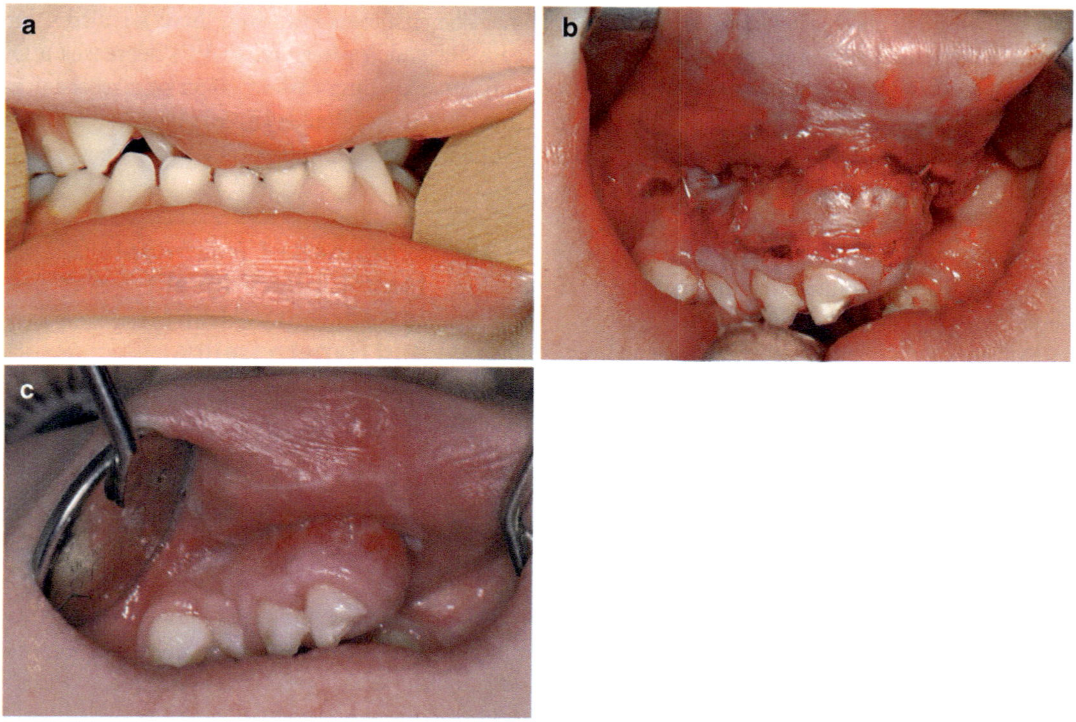

Fig. 5.72 (**a**) Left side: Fixed upper lip after bilateral lip closure. (**b**) Middle: At the end of a vestibuloplasty: mucosa shifted 10 mm cranially, periosteum covered by a split graft of attached gingiva from the palate. (**c**) Right side: Same patient 2 months later with a high vestibulum and a mobile upper lip

open rhinophonia. The patients may also notice nasal regurgitation of food. In all cases of a functional problem the fistulae have to be closed (more details in Sect. 5.13).

An insufficient reconstruction of the velum (especially mm. tensor veli palatini and levator veli palatini) and excessive scars in this region may result in hearing disorders, via malfunction of the Eustachian tube, and in conductive hearing loss and later a chronic serous otitis media and finally a cholesteatoma (Sect. 15.1, Chap. 15, Part IV, Vol. 1). The hearing handicap can result in indistinct articulation or—if not treated—in general delay of speech and language development.

Another severe problem after an insufficient velar closure is a velopharyngeal insufficiency (VPI). In light cases only a hypernasal sound may be noticed in the speech. In more severe ones the production of speech sounds is affected, too. Sometimes sounds cannot be articulated at all, are substituted by other sounds or articulated at false locations. The velopharyngeal insufficiency can be constant or inconstant, for example only prominent when the person is tired. Therapy of choice in VPI in the first 4–5 years is functional training.

Concerning sequelae on speech and language development and special diagnostics, see Chap. 9 and Sects. 11.3, 11.4, 11.5, Chap. 11, Vol. 1 and Sects. 3.9 and 3.10 in this volume.

5.15.4 Sequelae of a Velopharyngoplasty

In some patients with VPI, a functional therapy alone does not lead to comprehensible speech. In those cases speech improving surgery can be an option (see also Sect. 5.14). Before this operation, the removal of the adenoids should be considered. Otherwise, the nasopharynx will be very narrow, and the function of the Eustachian tube can be disturbed. This may result in the above-mentioned problems of conductive hearing loss and chronic middle ear affections (Sect. 15.1, Chapter 15, Vol. 1).

Following velopharyngoplasties, snoring might occur. Here, it is important to wait at least 6 months before any action is considered. The flap has a tendency to shrink substantially so that the result of this operation cannot be finally judged before this time. Shortly after surgery, the patients may take decongesting nose drops for some days/weeks and later take nasal showers with normal saline solution to eliminate the overshooting nasal mucus.

Rarely, an obstructive sleep apnoea syndrome (OSAS) may develop. If in severe cases, OSAS cannot be treated conservatively, and the release of the velopharyngeal flap from the base has to be taken into account. In the long-standing experience of the first author, a new velopharyngeal insufficiency rarely occurs, however, since a substantial (connective) tissue plus will remain at the flap's origin.

On the other hand, the underlying reason for an OSAS can also be a decreased tongue space due to a maxillary retrognathism which may be found in about 20% of the cleft patients (see also Sect. 5.13).

Finally, obesity is also one of the more important factors in developing an OSAS which should be treated before considering drastic surgical measures in the head and neck region.

5.15.5 Sequelae of Orthognathic Surgery

In more than 20% of the cleft patients, orthognathic surgery can be indicated to normalise their maxillo-mandibular relationship and thereby their facial profile. Since the problem lies in the retruded maxilla, the operation should be carried out by a maxillary advancement. In certain cases, a simultaneously performed moderate mandibular setback has proven to be useful. The singular mandibular setback should not be carried out any more, since this will definitely lead to a decrease of the posterior airway space (cave: OSAS!).

Maxillary advancement only results in the worsening of a *pre-existing or borderline VPI* in cases of extensive forward movements with midfacial distraction. No new cases of VPI occur in the other patients. However, there are also some cases in which preoperative VPI decreases after surgery. This might be an effect of a reorganisation of the velopharyngeal closure patterns (Hemprich and Hierl 2019) (see also Sect. 5.13).

5.16 Prognosis of Treatments for Velopharyngeal Insufficiency (VPI) and Hypernasality

Robert J. Shprintzen

5.16.1 Prognosis: Application and Meaning

Before discussing the commonly used term 'prognosis', one must ask the question, 'are we all thinking about the same thing when we are told that the prognosis is "good" or "excellent." Do all we clinicians or researchers define these parameters the same way?' In 1991, I published an article titled 'Fallibility of Clinical Research'. In it, I discussed the issue of definitions of success. In large part, the article was aimed at my disappointment as the Editor of the Cleft Palate-Craniofacial Journal that the reporting outcomes from surgical procedures for eliminating velopharyngeal insufficiency (VPI) were misleading and lacking scientific support. Besides the fact that very small sample sizes were typical in these studies (often 30 or fewer cases), statistics were applied incorrectly (Shprintzen 1991). It brought to mind the quotation from Mark Twain (the pen name of Samuel Langhorne Clemens):

> Most people use statistics like a drunk man uses a lamppost; more for support than illumination.

More importantly, outcomes were often judged by using ordinal rating scales (without equal intervals) with such small numbers of subjects that did not warrant analysis for 'significant' differences. Equally importantly, many of these studies used categorical classifications of improvement, such as 'no improvement, poor, some improvement, good improvement' without using terms such as 'normal resonance' or 'elimination of hypernasality'. Even the descriptions of preoperative speech were vague or misleading.

In my article, I was also critical of the frequent interchangeability of the terms 'speech' and 'hypernasality'. If an article reported that speech was improved, without explaining what that meant in terms of either nasal resonance or articulation, the validity of the study could not be claimed. In other words, the interpretation of the outcome depends on the choice of the postoperative evaluation. The proper way to assess the outcome is by using an imaging procedure, such as nasopharyngoscopy, to compare preoperative and postoperative presence or absence of VPI. If the postoperative imaging procedure shows no evidence of VPI, then the operation can be defined as a success. For scientific accuracy, the outcome must be measured to reflect the intent of the treatment. In the case of surgery for VPI, the goal is to eliminate VPI; either it is eliminated or it is not.

Although this might not seem relevant to prognosis, it is actually perfectly relevant. The word prognosis can be applied to the course of a disease, in order to predict the final outcome, including the course and extent of recovery. When applied to treatments, prognosis means a prediction of the likely outcome of a specific procedure (medical, surgical, behavioural, etc.). Prognoses help patients to understand their illness, the amount of time they will need to recover and whether or not they will suffer any long-term or permanent impairment. When a prognosis is provided in relation to surgery, medical management (including pharmaceutical treatment) or behavioural therapies, it helps a patient decide if they wish to move ahead with the treatment. The prognosis allows the patient to determine what risks are inherent in a particular treatment used to reach a certain goal. This is often referred to as the 'risk-to-benefit ratio'. Treating professionals often use their own experience and assessment of their outcomes to offer a prognosis. Others may cite medical literature, particularly if they have limited experience in performing a particular procedure. Sometimes a prognosis is offered purely on conjecture. In other words, there is no uniform method for offering a prognosis, which leads to an important question: how is the patient supposed to assess the accuracy of the prognosis?

5.16.2 Validity of Prognosis for VPI Treatments

Let me present a hypothetical situation to illustrate the difficulty of interpreting the value of a prognosis for treating velopharyngeal insufficiency. This situation is one that is commonplace and that probably most readers have experienced many times: a patient and his parents go to a surgeon for consideration of treatment of velopharyngeal insufficiency. The patient's speech is severely hypernasal and the family does not know very much about the techniques that can be applied to the problem.

The surgeon suggests the two operations that can be done, either a pharyngeal flap or a sphincter pharyngoplasty. The patient asks what the chance of success is for each procedure. The surgeon, who has done only a few pharyngeal flaps and a few sphincter pharyngoplasties, cites the literature; specifically outcomes from a recent report by Luo et al. (2020) who compared 30 cases who had a pharyngeal flap using the Hogan technique and 48 cases who had sphincter pharyngoplasties. In the study, there was no mention of whether the operations were done by one, two or more surgeons. There were two outcome measures: the presence or absence of VPI, and intelligibility of speech. For the pharyngeal flap method, VPI was eliminated in 25 out of 30 (83%) cases, as judged from listening, nasometry and fibreoptic nasopharyngoscopy. For the sphincter pharyngoplasty, VPI was eliminated in 29 out of 48 cases (60%). Inexplicably, the authors reported that seven cases of pharyngeal flap had mild hypernasal resonance, although only five were found to have VPI. How did two cases with velopharyngeal closure have hypernasal speech? The other outcome measure was based on accuracy of articulation and was better in the sphincter pharyngoplasty cases. This information was presented to the patient and his family who had no idea how to interpret that information.

Another patient with the same problem sees a different surgeon. This particular surgeon, a relatively recent graduate of a residency programme, does not cite the outcomes because only a few cases were done, and decided it was better to report literature on the procedure. Articles by Shprintzen et al. (1979), Chegar et al. (2007) and Ysunza et al. (2019) were cited, all of which reported a successful outcome of approximately 95%. With such a high success rate, the family is satisfied with the surgeon's information and decides to move forward, even though the surgeon had not yet done enough cases to calculate an actual percentage of his own success.

Still another patient with the same problem sees yet another surgeon, who had performed many surgical procedures for VPI. This surgeon has carefully tracked the cases over years and was confident of the outcomes of the procedure. Those outcomes were shared with the patient's family who trusted the information provided.

All three scenarios occur frequently, and in each case, the prognosis provided had different implications. In addition, the research reported for the first two cases had different designs, different criteria for success, and therefore, the true outcomes could not really be determined. Many articles in the literature make the major error of not determining success on the basis of what the operation was designed to do. In the case of the first scenario, the authors partially judge outcome from articulation. This is completely invalid because the surgery has only one purpose; to stop abnormal nasal resonance and nasal air escape during non-nasal speech. The surgery has nothing whatsoever to do with correcting articulation. Outcomes for VPI surgery can only be based on what the operation was designed to do—eliminate velopharyngeal insufficiency. Other studies include the mistake of using a rating scale to assess outcomes. It is common to see rank-ordered scales of 'no improvement, mild improvement, moderate improvement, major improvement', but leaving out a category of 'elimination of hypernasality'. Is it possible that even with major improvement, nasal resonance is still not normal?

The purpose of the paragraphs above is to demonstrate that prognoses are often subjective, and that this is especially true in the area of speech, resonance and voice outcomes. If the person offering the prognosis for a surgical procedure to resolve hypernasal speech says there is a 95% chance of 'improvement', does this mean the hypernasality is completely gone, or does it mean there is less hypernasality? If it is less hypernasality, is it still noticeable so that it would require treatment? Therefore, the prognosis should include the ability for the patient to ask the following questions and get answers to them:

1. Can you explain the operation and what it is supposed to do?
2. How does it do that?
3. How many of these operations have you done?
4. What percentage has been successful?
5. How do you define success?
6. How many cases have had complications, and what type of complications?
7. How many cases have had more surgery for the same problem?

The importance of these questions is to be able to determine what the prognosis represents. For disorders of velopharyngeal closure and hypernasal speech, the procedures applied to fix the problem are major operations with several significant risk factors, and the prognosis is important for calculation of the risk-to-benefit ratio.

It should be mentioned that the method for improving prognoses relative to treatment is highly dependent on clinicians' tracking outcomes diligently. Such tracking depends on using a standardised approach to valid and objective measures of 'success'. Outcome studies do not require publication unless the clinician wishes to share what is special about the results; they should be important to the individual clinician whose success in practice is dependent on successful treatments and realistic goals.

5.16.3 The Prognosis of Hypernasality Associated with Neurological Disorders

Hypernasality is a disorder that accompanies many diseases and clinical presentations. Most clinicians equate hypernasality with cleft palate.

Because clefting is a relatively common congenital anomaly and surgical reconstruction is focused on the palate early in life, it can be understood why the association with hypernasal speech and clefting is so strong. However, because palatoplasties result in the development of normal speech in most children with clefts, the frequency of secondary surgery for hypernasality is quite low in most locales. Hypernasality is more common in disorders that do not have clefting as a feature; these include neurological disorders, including cerebral palsy, myasthenia gravis, cerebrovascular malformations or injuries, brain and peripheral neoplasias, peripheral nerve damage, viral illnesses, trauma, and neurofibromatosis type 1 (Pollack and Shprintzen 1981).

The prognoses for correction of hypernasality are both variable and complex. In individuals with clefts that are non-syndromic, appropriate speech therapy is highly effective in correcting articulatory abnormalities, so that elimination of abnormal hypernasal resonance results in normal speech. However, hypernasality in most neurologically based hypernasality is accompanied by other neuromotor systems including dysarthria, voice abnormalities and apraxia. Resolution of hypernasality in such cases rarely leads to normal speech, and intelligibility remains poor. People with a neuromotor problem may close the velopharyngeal orifice intermittently but the closure is not often maintained. Hypernasality in neurologically based conditions are often caused by problems of timing of movements rather than lack of movement or anatomical anomalies. Such timing problems are often in synchrony with difficulty of movement of the oral articulators (lips, tongue, mandibles) and perceived as dysarthria. Correction of hypernasality alone, by creating a physical obstruction of the velopharyngeal office (either surgically or prosthetically), rarely results in good speech intelligibility. It has been observed both endoscopically and fluoroscopically that the velopharyngeal valve may close during the production of normally non-nasal pressure consonants, but open on the production of vowels. Therefore, during the utterance of the word 'prognosis', the valve will close on the production of the /p/, open during the /r/ and /o/, close on the /g/, open on the /n/ and the /o/, close on the /s/, open on the /i/, and close again on the /s/. In individuals with normal velopharyngeal function, the valve would be closed except for the production of the /n/.

For people with clefts who do not have neurological anomalies, the prognosis for normal speech is excellent when proper diagnostic and treatment techniques are applied (see Sect. 3.19), while the prognosis for normal speech for neurologically based disorders with or without clefts is poor. The severity of residual hypernasality and unintelligibility after surgery is dependent on the severity and permanence of the neurological or neuromotor problem. Because movements of the velopharyngeal valve are both variable and inconsistent in a neurologically based disorder, nasality is often perceived throughout the utterance even when velopharyngeal closure is achieved inconsistently. Therefore, the major emphasis in treatment should be to correct the articulation impairment and both the rate and rhythm of speech.

5.16.4 The Prognosis of Hypernasality Associated with Trauma and Neoplasia

Traumatic injury, neoplastic disease and cervical spine surgery are possible causes of incomplete velopharyngeal closure. Traumatic injury to the maxilla and palate can affect the structural relationship of the palate and velum to the surrounding pharynx; even if the velum is intact, an anterior defect in the hard palate will likely cause hypernasality even if velopharyngeal closure is achieved. If the brain is not impaired in the trauma, then surgical reconstruction or prosthetic restoration of the damaged anatomy will restore normal resonance, and in such cases the prognosis is excellent if such restorations are possible. Of course, articulation may be impaired by structural damage to the lips, tongue or dental arches, but the prognosis for resolution of those problems is also excellent if the neurophysiology of the brain and peripheral neurological pathways are functional.

Neoplasia often requires significant dissection of the surrounding tissues. Moreover, the use of radiation treatment, even when very targeted precisely, may have a negative effect on the texture of the mucosa and thin musculature of the palate and pharynx. However, if the brain is unaffected, reconstructive surgery or prosthetic management should have a positive prognosis, depending on the extent of the defect left by the removal of the neoplasia and surrounding tissues. It may even be that the defect left by ablative surgery requires a pharyngeal flap to make up for the tissue loss during reconstruction. Application of proper diagnostic procedures, in terms of knowing what the movement of the pharyngeal structures would be during attempts at phonation after management of the neoplasia, allows the surgeon to judge which method would be best in a postoperative reconstruction for closing the defect while also improving speech (see Sect. 3.19).

References

Abdel-Fatah G (2012) A new technique in treatment of nasopharyngeal stenosis. Int J Pediatr Otorhinolaryngol 76:879–882

Abreu A, Levy D, Rodriguez E et al (2007) Oral rehabilitation of a patient with complete unilateral cleft lip and palate using an implant-retained speech-aid prosthesis: clinical report. Cleft Palate-Craniofac J 44(6):673–677

Abreu RR, Rocha RL, Lamounier JA et al (2008) Prevalence of mouth breathing among children. J Pediatr 84(5):467–470

Abyholm F, D'Antonio L, Davidson Ward SL et al (2005) Pharyngeal flap and sphincteroplasty for velopharyngeal insufficiency have equal outcome at year postoperatively: results of randomized trial. Cleft Palate Craniofac J 42:501–511

Aihara Y, Yanagawa T, Sasaki M et al (2022) Nasal molding prevents relapse of nasal deformity after primary rhinoplasty in patients with unilateral complete cleft lip: An outcomes-based comparative study of palatal plate alone versus nasoalveolar molding. Clin Exp Dent Res 8(1):197–208

Allareddy V, Shusterman S, Ross E et al (2020) Dentofacial Orthopedics for the Cleft Patient: The Latham Approach. Oral Maxillofac Surg Clin N Am 32(2):187–196

Alqadi S, Qazali A, Altamimi R et al. (2023) Altamimi R, Abdouh I, Othman A, et al. Perception and Attitude of Parents of Children With Orofacial Clefts Regarding the Use of Presurgical Orthopedics and Feeding Obturators. Cureus 15(9):e46131

American Cleft Palate–Craniofacial Association (2021) Advancing patient care and research for individuals affected with cleft lip, cleft palate and other craniofacial anomalies. https://acpa-cpf.org/. Accessed 17 March 2022

Andresen V, Häupl K (1945) Functional orthodontics. In: The basics of the Norwegian system, 4th edn. Johann Ambrosius Barth, Leipzig

Angle EH (1899) Classification of malocclusion. Dental Cosmos 41:248–264

Apert E (1906) De l'acrocephalosyndactylie. Bull Mem Soc Med Hop Paris 23:1310–1330

Arnaud E, Renier D, Marchac D et al (1996) Mental prognosis in scaphocephaly. Arch Pediatr 3:16–21

ASHA (2005) Roles and responsibilities of speech-language pathologists with respect to augmentative and alternative communication: position statement. www.asha.org/policy. Accessed 31 August 2014

ASHA (2015) Speech-language pathology. Medical review. Guidelines American Speech-Language-Hearing Association. https://www.asha.org/siteassets/uploadedfiles/slp-medical-review-guidelines.pdf. Accessed 20 June 2021

ASHA (2022) Cleft lip and palate. https://www2.asha.org/PRPSpecificTopic.aspx?folderid=8589942918&section=Treatment. Accessed 19 March 2022

Ástvaldsdóttir Á, Boström A, Davidson T et al (2018) Oral health and dental care of older persons—a systematic map of systematic reviews. Gerodontology 35(4):290–304

Bachy B, Peron JM, Delcampe P et al (2002) Management of cleft lip and palate in university hospital of Rouen. Ann Chir Plast Esthet 47(2):150–154

Bäckman B, Grevér-Sjölander AC, Holm AK et al (2003) Children with down syndrome: oral development and morphology after use of palatal plates between 6 and 18 months of age. Int J Paediatr Dent 13(5):327–335

Bäckman B, Grevér-Sjölander AC, Bengtsson K et al (2007) Children with Down syndrome: oral development and morphology after use of palatal plates between 6 and 48 months of age. Int J Paediatr Dent 17(1):19–28

Ball L, Fager S, Fried-Oken (2012) Augmentative and alternative communication for people with progressive neuromuscular disease. Phys Med Rehabil Clin N Am 23(3):689–699

Baram S, Karlsborg M, Bakke M (2020) Improvement of oral function and hygiene in Parkinson's disease: a randomised controlled clinical trial. J Oral Rehabil 47(3):370–376

Barillas I, Dec W, Warren SM et al (2009) Nasoalveolar molding improves long-term nasal symmetry in complete unilateral cleft lip-cleft palate patients. Plast Reconstr Surg 123(3):1002–1006

Barlow SM, Burton MK (1990) Ramp-and-force control in the upper and lower lips: developing new neuromotor assessment applications in traumatically brain injured adults. J Speech Hear Res 33(4):660–675

Bartella AK, Halama D, Pausch NC et al (2021) Persistent fistula of the palate: cleft surgery meets microsurgery for the next rung of the ladder. Plast Reconstr Surg 147(1):178–179

Batista KB, Thiruvenkatachari B, Harrison JE et al (2018) Orthodontic treatment for prominent upper front teeth (Class II malocclusion) in children and adolescents. Cochrane Database Syst Rev 3(3):CD003452

Bäumer T, Beutner D, Degenkolb-Weyers S et al (2018) Update of the S2k guideline "Hypersalivation"; AWMF Registration Number 017-075; 2018. https://www.awmf.org/uploads/tx_szleitlinien/017-075m_S2k_Hypersalivation_2018-11.pdf. Accessed 11 January 2022

Bavikatte G, Sit PL, Hassoon A (2012) Management of drooling of saliva. BJMP 5(1):a507

Bean A (2013) Oral-motor skills BT - encyclopedia of autism spectrum disorders. Springer, New York, pp 2091–2092

Becker R, Nieczaj R, Egge K et al (2011) Functional dysphagia therapy and PEG treatment in a clinical geriatric setting. Dysphagia 26(2):108–116

Bergersen EO (1984) The eruption guidance myofunctional appliances: how it works, how to use it. Funct Orthod 1(3):28–29

Berweck S, Bonikowski M, Heakyung K et al (2021) Placebo-controlled clinical trial of incobotulinumtoxina for sialorrhea in children: SIPEXI. Neurology 97(14):e1425–e1436

Billings M, Gatto K, D'Onofrio L et al (2018) Orofacial myofunctional disorders. IAOM. http://iaom.com/wp--content/uploads/2018/10/OMD-Overview-IAOM.pdf. Accessed 9 January 2022

Bobath K (1980) A neurophysiological basis for the treatment of cerebral palsy. In: Clinics in developmental medicine Nr. 75 Spastics International Medical Publications. William Heinemann Medical Books Ltd, London

Boyd E (1962) Organ weights from birth to maturity: man, North American. Part I. Brain and lungs. In: Altmann PL, Dittmer DS (eds) Growth including reproduction and morphological development, 1st edn. Federation of American Societies for Experimental Biology, Washington, p 346

Boyne PJ, Sands NR (1972) Secondary bone grafting of residual alveolar and palatal clefts. J Oral Surg 30(2):87–92

Braithwaite F (1966) Some observations on cleft palate surgery. In: Schuchardt K (ed) Treatment of patients with cleft of lip, alveolus and palate. Thieme, Stuttgart

Branson D, Demchak M (2009) The use of augmentative and alternative communication methods with infants and toddlers with disabilities: a research review. Augment Altern Commun 25(4):274–286

Bressmann T (2021) Nasometry. In: Ball MJ (ed) Manual of clinical phonetics. Routledge, London

Brigger MT, Ashland JE, Hartnick CJ (2009) Diagnosis and treatment of velopharyngeal insufficiency. In: Hartnick CJ, Boseley ME (eds) Clinical management of children's voice disorders. Plural Publishing, San Diego, pp 225–244

Brigger MT, Ashiand JE, Hartnick CJ (2010) Injection pharyngoplasty with calcium hydroxylapatite for velopharyngeal insufficiency patient selection and technique. Arch Otolaryngol Head Neck Surg 136:666–670

Bronsted K, Liisberg WB, Orsted A et al (1984) Surgical and speech results following palatopharyngoplasty operations in Denmark 1959-1977. Cleft Palate J 21:170–179

Bruce WJ, Chang V, Joyce CJ et al (2018) Age at time of craniosynostosis repair predicts increased complication rate. Cleft Palate Craniofac J 55:649–654

Brunner M, Stellzig A, Decker W et al (1994) Video feedback therapy with the flexible nasopharyngoscope. Fortschr Kieferorthop 55(4):197–201

Brunner M, Stellzig A, Decker W et al (1996) New ways in speech therapy for cleft lip and palate. Sprache Stimme Gehör 20:116–122

Brunner M, Stellzig A, Decker W et al (1999) Biofeedback therapy of velopharyngeal insufficiency in cleft palate patients. In: Dejonckere P, Peters H (eds) Communication and its disorders: a science in progress. Nijmegen University Press, Nijmegen, pp 561–564

Brunner M, Stellzig A, Pröschel U et al (2001) Four-phase biofeedback for functional velopharyngeal insufficiency. In: Gross M, Kruse E (eds) Current phoniatric-paediatric aspects 2000/2001, vol 8. Median Verlag, Heidelberg, pp 146–150

Brunner M, Stellzig-Eisenhauer A, Pröschel U et al (2005) The effect of nasopharyngoscopic biofeedback in patients with cleft palate and velopharyngeal dysfunction. Cleft Palate Craniofac J 42(6):649–657

Brunner M, Dockter S, Pröschel U et al (2007) Forms of velopharyngeal dysfunction in cleft patients. HNO 55(11):851–857

Buchenau W, Wenzel S, Bacher M et al (2017) Functional treatment of airway obstruction and feeding problems in infants with Robin sequence. Arch Dis Child Fetal Neonatal Ed 102(2):F142–F146

Burston WR (1958) The early orthodontic treatment of cleft palate conditions. Trans Br Soc Study Orthod Dent Pract 9:41–56

Bzoch KR (1989) Communicative disorders related to cleft lip and palate. Pro-ED, Austin

Cahill LM, Turner AB, Stabler PA et al (2004) An evaluation of continuous positive airway pressure (CPAP) therapy in the treatment of hypernasality following traumatic brain injury: a report of 3 cases. J Head Trauma Rehabil 19(3):241–253

Camacho M, Certal V, Abdullatif J et al (2015) Myofunctional therapy to treat obstructive sleep apnea: a systematic review and meta-analysis. Sleep 38(5):669–675

Castillo-Morales R (1991) The orofacial regulation therapy. Pflaum Verlag, Munich

Cerón-Zapata AM, López-Palacio AM, Rodriguez-Ardila MJ et al (2016) 3D evaluation of maxillary arches

in unilateral cleft lip and palate patients treated with nasoalveolar moulding vs Hotz's plate. J Oral Rehabil 43(2):111–118
Chapman K (1993) Phonologic processes in children with cleft palate. Cleft Palate J 30(1):64–71
Chegar BE, Shprintzen RJ, Curtis MS et al (2007) Pharyngeal flap and obstructive apnea. Arch Facial Plast Surg 9(4):252–259
Chotzen F (1932) A peculiar familial developmental disorder (acrocephalosyndactyly, craniofacial dysostosis and hypertelorism). Monatsschr Kinderheilkd 55:97–122
Chuang LC, Hwang YJ, Lian YC et al (2019) Changes in craniofacial and airway morphology as well as quality of life after passive myofunctional therapy in children with obstructive sleep apnea: a comparative cohort study. Sleep Breath 23(4):1359–1369
Čirgi E, Kjellberg H, Hansen K (2016) Treatment of large overjet in Angle Class II: division 1 malocclusion with Andresen activators versus prefabricated functional appliances—a multicenter, randomized, controlled trial. Eur J Orthod 38(5):516–524
Clark HM (2003) Neuromuscular treatments for speech and swallowing: a tutorial. Am J Speech Lang Pathol 12(4):400–415
Clark HM (2005) Clinical decision making and oral motor treatments. The ASHA Leader, pp 8–9. https://doi.org/10.1044/leader.FTR3.10082005.8
Cler GJ, Mittelman T, Braden MN et al (2017) Video game rehabilitation of velopharyngeal dysfunction: a case series. J Speech Lang Hear Res 60(6S):1800–1809
Cleveland Clinic (2018) Cleft lip and palate. https://my.clevelandclinic.org/health/diseases/10947-cleft-lip-and-palate. Accessed 16 March 2022
Cohen MM (1988) Craniosynostosis update. Am J Med Genet Suppl 4:99–148
Cohen MM (1995) Craniosynostoses: phenotypic/molecular correlations. Am J Med Genet 56:334–339
Cress C, Marvin C (2003) Common questions about AAC services in early intervention. Augment Altern Commun 19(4):264–272
Crouzon O (1912) Dysostose cranio-faciale héréditaire (Hereditary craniofacial dysostosis). Bull Mem Soc Med Hop Paris 33:545–555
Darwin C (1872) The origin of species by means of natural selection, 6th edn. John Murray, London
de Felício CM, da Silva Dias FV, Trawitzki LVV (2018) Obstructive sleep apnea: focus on myofunctional therapy. Nat Sci Sleep 10:271–286
de Ladeira PRS, Alonso N (2012) Protocols in cleft lip and palate treatment: systematic review. Plast Surg Int 2012:562892. https://doi.org/10.1155/2012/562892
De Simone GG, Eisenchlas JH, Junin M et al (2006) Atropine drops for drooling: a randomized controlled trial. Palliat Med 20(7):665–671
Delaire J (1978) Theoretical principles and technique of functional closure of the lip and nasal aperture. J Maxillofac Surg 6:109–116
DeMatteo C, Matovich D, Hjartason A (2005) Comparison of clinical and videofluoroscopic evaluation of children with feeding and swallowing difficulties. Dev Med Child Neurol 47(3):249–257
Denizoglu I (2018) The DoctorVox voice therapy: simple and effective in voice therapy and vocal pedagogy. Vox Humana 14(3):36–41
Denizoglu I (2020a) Textbook of clinical vocology. Karaca Basim, Ankara
Denizoglu I (2020b) Voice therapy: a survey of methods and techniques. In: Zehnhoff-Dinnesen A, Wiskirska-Woznica B, Neumann K et al (eds) Phoniatrics I fundamentals- voice disorders-disorders of language and hearing development. Springer, Berlin, pp 456–457
Destruhaut F, Pomar P, Esclassan R et al (2015) Decision making for residual palatoalveolar cleft defects: a new classification. Int J Prosthodont 28(2):167–168
Dhakshaini MR, Pushpavathi M, Garhnayak M et al (2015) Prosthodontic management in conjunction with speech therapy in cleft lip and palate: a review and case report. J Int Oral Health 7(Suppl 2):106–111
Diaféria G, Santos-Silva R, Truksinas E et al (2017) Myofunctional therapy improves adherence to continuous positive airway pressure treatment. Sleep Breath 21(2):387–395
Dorrance GM, Brainsfield JW (1946) The push-back operation for repair of cleft palate. Plast Reconstr Surg 1:145–149
Durham E, Howie RN, Larson N (2019) Pharmacological exposures may precipitate raniosynostosis through targeted stem cell depletion. Stem Cell Res 40:101528. https://doi.org/10.1016/j.scr.2019.101528
Eley KA, Watt-Smith SR, Golding SJ (2017) "Black bone" MRI: a novel imaging technique for 3D printing. Dentomaxillofac Radiol 46:20160407. https://doi.org/10.1259/dmfr.20160407
Ellenbogen RG, Gruss JS, Cunningham ML (2000) Update on craniofacial surgery: the differential diagnosis of lambdoid synostosis/posterior plagiocephaly. Clin Neurosurg 47:303–318
Ellies M, Laskawi R, Rohrbach-Volland S et al (2002a) Botulinum toxin to reduce saliva flow: selected indications for ultrasound guided toxin application into salivary glands. Laryngoscope 112(1):82–86
Ellies M, Rohrbach-Volland S, Laskawi R et al (2002b) Successful management of drooling with botulinum toxin A in neurologically disabled children. Neuropediatrics 33(6):327–330
Ellies M, Gottstein U, Rohrbach-Volland S et al (2004) Reduction of salivary flow with botulinum toxin: extended report on 33 patients with drooling, salivary fistulas and sialadenitis. Laryngoscope 114(10):1856–1860
Engel AE (2012) Myasthenia gravis and myasthenic disorders. Oxford University Press, New York
Enlow DH (1990) The facial growth process. In: Enlow DH (ed) Handbook of facial growth, 3rd edn. Saunders, Philadelphia, pp 58–148
Eshghi M, Adatorwovor R, Crais E et al (2018) Lexical and grammatical development in 2-year-old children with and without repaired cleft palate. Poster at the

75th Meeting of the Cleft Palate and Craniofacial Association, Pittsburgh

Faber HK, Towne EB (1927) Early craniectomy as a preventive measure in oxycephaly and allied conditions with special reference to prevention of blindness. Am J Med Sci 173:701–711

Faber HK, Towne EB (1943) Early operations in premature cranial synostosis to prevention of blindness and other sequelae: 5 case reports with follow-up. J Pediatr 22:286–307

Fairhurst CB, Cockerill H (2011) Management of drooling in children. Arch Dis Child Educ Pract Ed 96(1):25–30

Farkas LG, Hajnis K, Posnick JC (1993) Anthropometric and anthroposcopic findings of the nasal and facial region in cleft patients before and after primary lip and palate repair. Cleft Palate Craniofac J 30(1):1545–1569

Fischer-Voosholz M, Spenthof U (2002) Orofacial muscular dysfunction. In: Clinic - diagnostics - holistic therapy. Springer, Berlin

Fletcher SG, Sooudi I, Frost SD (1974) Quantitative and graphic analysis of prosthetic treatment for "nasalance" in speech. J Prosth Dent 32(3):284–291

Flowers CR, Morris HL (1973) Oral-pharyngeal movements during swallowing and speech. Cleft Palate J 10:181–191

Fränkel R (1980) A functional approach to orofacial orthopaedics. Br J Orthod 7(1):41–51

Fränkel R, Fränkel C (2001) Clinical implication of Roux's concept in orofacial orthopedics. J Orofac Orthop 62(1):1–21

Frederick R, Hogan AC, Seabolt N, Stocks RMS (2022) An Ideal Multidisciplinary Cleft Lip and Cleft Palate Care Team. Oral Dis 28(5):1412–1417. https://doi.org/10.1111/odi.14213. Epub 2022 May 4. PMID: 35429208

Freitas JA, Almeida AL, Soares S et al (2013) Rehabilitative treatment of cleft lip and palate: experience of the hospital for rehabilitation of craniofacial anomalies/USP (HRAC/USP) - part 4: oral rehabilitation. J Appl Oral Sci 21(3):284–292

Friedrich G, Bigenzahn W, Zorowka P (2013) Phoniatrics and pediatric audiology. Introduction to the medical, psychological and linguistic basics of voice, language and hearing, 5th edn. Verlag Hans Huber, Bern

Fritzell B (1976) Palatal function. In: Hinchclifte R, Harrison D (eds) Scientific foundation of otolaryngology. W. Heinemann Medical Books Ltd, London, pp 484–493

Frontera WR, Lexell J (2005) Assessment of human muscle function. In: Lisa JA, Gans BM, Walsh NE (eds) Physical medicine and rehabilitation: principles and practice, 4th edn. Lippincott, Williams & Wilkins, Philadelphia, pp 139–154

Fukushiro AP, Trindade IEK (2011) Nasometric and aerodynamic outcome analysis of pharyngeal flap surgery for the management of velopharyngeal insufficiency. J Craniofac Surg 22(5):1647–1651

Furlow LT (1986) Cleft palate repair by double opposing Z-plasty. Plast Reconstr Surg 78(6):724–738

Garcia AF, Marino VC, Pegoraro-Krook MI et al (2014) Nasalance during use of pharyngeal and glottal place of production. Codas 26(5):395–401

Garliner D (1974) Myofunctional therapy in dental practice. Bartel Dental Co, Brooklyn

Geyer C, Foerster A, Hemprich A et al (2005) RCBF-brain SPECT for evaluation of brain perfusion in infants with premature synostoses of cranial sutures. Eur Surg 44(5):348

Ghali E, Tharanon W, Sinn D (2019) Craniofacial deformities: introduction and principles of management. In: Greenberg M, Schmelzeisen R (eds) Craniomaxillofacial reconstructive and corrective bone surgery, 2nd edn. Springer, New York

Godhard Blythe S (2013) Neuromotor school readiness, 1st edn. Verlag Hans Huber, Bern

Golding-Kushner KJ (1995) Treatment of articulation and resonance disorders associated with cleft palate and VPI. In: Sprintzen RJ, Bardach J (eds) Cleft palate speech management. A multidisciplinary approach. Mosby, St. Louis, pp 327–351

Golding-Kushner K (2001) Therapy techniques for cleft palate speech and related disorders. Singular, San Diego

Good PM, Mulliken JB, Padwa BL (2007) Frequency of Le Fort I osteotomy after repaired cleft lip and palate or cleft palate. Cleft Palate Craniofac J 44(4):396–401

Goyal M, Chopra R, Bansal K et al (2014) Role of obturators and other feeding interventions in patients with cleft lip and palate: a review. Eur Arch Paediatr Dent 15(1):1–9

Grayson BH, Cutting CB (2001) Presurgical nasoalveolar orthopedic molding in primary correction of the nose, lip, and alveolus of infants born with unilateral and bilateral clefts. Cleft Palate-Craniofac J 38(3):193–198

Guilleminault C, Sullivan SS (2014) Towards restoration of continuous nasal breathing as the ultimate treatment goal in pediatric obstructive sleep apnea. Enliven Pediatr Neonatal Biol 1(1):1–5

Hägg M, Anniko M (2008) Lip muscle training in stroke patients with dysphagia. Acta Otolaryngol 128(9):1027–1033

Hägg M, Tibbling L, Franzén T (2015) Esophageal dysphagia and reflux symptoms before and after oral IQoro(R) training. World J Gastroenterol 21(24):7558–7562

Hahn V (1988) Myofunctional therapy. A contribution to the interdisciplinary foundation from the point of view of the pedagogy of the speech impaired. Profil Verlag GmbH, Munich

Hakan Tuna S, Pekkan G, Buyukgural B (2009) Rehabilitation of an edentulous cleft lip and palate patient with a soft palate defect using a bar-retained, implant-supported speech-aid prosthesis: a clinical report. Cleft Palate-Craniofac J 46(1):97–102

Hanley L, Ballard KJ, Dickson A, Purcell A (2023) Speech Intervention for Children With Cleft Palate Using Principles of Motor Learning. Am J Speech Lang Pathol 32(1):169–189. https://doi.org/10.1044/2022_AJSLP-22-00007. Epub 2022 Dec 7. PMID: 36475751

Hardwicke JT, Landmini G, Richard BM (2014) Fistula incidence after primary cleft palate repair: a systematic review of the literature. Plast Reconstr Surg 134(4):618–627

Heller Murray ES, Mendoza JO, Gill SV et al (2016) Effects of biofeedback on control and generalization of nasalization in typical speakers. J Speech Lang Hear Res 59(5):1025–1034

Hemprich A, Dannhauer K-H (2016) Personal communication of unpublished data

Hemprich A, Hierl T (2019) Craniomaxillofacial distraction osteogenesis. In: Greenberg A, Schmelzeisen R (eds) Craniomaxillofacial reconstructive and corrective bone surgery, 2nd edn. Springer, New York, pp 787–844

Hemprich A, Schiefke F (2016) LKG: Spät/Korrekturbehandlungen (Cleft lip and palate: late/correction-treatments). Medupdate GmbH, Wiesbaden

Hemprich A, Zieglowski V (1996) First results of consequent muscular reconstruction in secondary cleft lip and nose repair. J Craniomaxillofac Surg 24(1):53

Henningsson GE, Isberg AM (1986) Velopharyngeal movement patterns in patients alternating between oral and glottal articulations: a cineradiographical study. Cleft Palate J 23(1):1–9

Henningsson GE, Isberg AM (1991) A cineradiographic study of velopharyngeal movements for deviant versus non-deviant articulation. Cleft Palate Craniofac J 28(1):115–118

Hirschberg J (1986) Velopharyngeal insufficiency. Folia Phoniatr 38(2-4):221–276

Hirschberg J (1990) Surgery of the velopharyngeal insufficiency – surgery of the velum. In: Milutinovicz Z (ed) Phonosurgery. Beograd, Naucna Knyiga, pp 53–72

Hirschberg J (2012) Result and complications of 1104 surgeries for velopharyngeal insufficiency. ISRN Otolaryngol 2012:181202. https://doi.org/10.5402/2012/181202

Hirschberg J, Gross M (2006) Velopharyngeal insufficiency with or without palate: diagnostics and therapy of hypernasality. Median-Verlag, Heidelberg

Hirschberg J, Rehák G (1997) Flap surgery: experience with 1030 operations and cephalometric investigation. Folia Phoniatr Logop 49:201–208

Ho DH, Burggren WW (2010) Epigenetics and transgenerational transfer: a physiological perspective. J Exp Biol 213(1):3–16

Hohoff A, Ehmer U (1997) Effects of the Castillo-Morales stimulating plate on speech development of children with Down's syndrome. A retrospective study. J Orofac Orthop 58(6):330–339

Hohoff A, Ehmer U (1999) Short-term and long-term results after early treatment with the Castillo Morales stimulating plate. A longitudinal study. J Orofac Orthop 60(1):2–12

Hohoff A, Seifert E, Ehmer U et al (1998) Articulation in children with Down's syndrome. A pilot study. J Orofac Orthop 59(4):220–228

Homem MA, Vieira-Andrade RG, Falci SG et al (2014) Effectiveness of orofacial myofunctional therapy in orthodontic patients: a systematic review. Dental Press J Orthod 19(4):94–99

Horii Y (1980) An accelerometric approach to nasality measurement: a preliminary report. Cleft Palate J 17(3):254–261

Hosseini HR, Kaklamanos EG, Athanasiou AE (2017) Treatment outcomes of pre-surgical infant orthopedics in patients with non-syndromic cleft lip and/or palate: a systematic review and meta-analysis of randomized controlled trials. PLoS One 12(7):e0181768

Hotz MM, Gnoinski WM, Nussbaumer H et al (1978) Early maxillary orthopedics in CLP cases: guidelines for surgery. Cleft Palate J 15(4):405–411

Hoyer H, Limbrock GJ (1990) Orofacial regulation therapy in children with Down syndrome, using the methods and appliances of Castillo-Morales. ASDC J Dent Child 57(6):442–444

Hsieh T-Y, Funamura JL, Roth C et al (2015) Developing a novel speech intervention iPAD game for children with cleft palate. JAMA Facial Plast Surg 17(4):309–311

Huang YS, Hsu SC, Guilleminault C et al (2019) Myofunctional therapy: role in pediatric OSA. Sleep Med Clin 14(1):135–142

Humboldt A (1803) Tagebücher der Amerikanischen Reise IX: Varia. Obs. Astron. de Mexico a Guanaxuato, Torullo, Tiluca, Veracruz, Cuba. Voy. De la Havana à Philadelphia. Geologie de Guanaxato, Volcans de Torullo et de Toluca. Voyage de Veracruz à la Havana et de la Havana à Philadelphia. Torulla, pp 95–196

Husler F, Rodd-Marling Y (2007) Singing: the physical nature of the vocal organ. Hutchinson Publishing Group, London

Hynes W (1950) Pharyngoplasty by muscle transplantation. Br J Plast Surg 3:128–135

Hyson HC, Johnson AM, Jog MS (2002) Sublingual atropine for sialorrhea secondary to parkinsonism: a pilot study. Mov Disord 17(6):1318–1320

IALP (1999) Cleft Palate Committee's proposal for treament and care of the individual with cleft lip/palate and/or velopharyngeal insufficiency. Folia Phoniatr Logop 51:138–139

Imola MJ, Hamlar DD, Shao W et al (2001) Resorbable plate fixation in pediatric craniofacial surgery: long-term outcome. Arch Facial Plast Surg 3:79–90

Isshiki N, Honjow I, Morimoto M (1971) Indication and the results of pharyngeal flap operation. Arch Klin Exp Ohr-Nas Kehlk-Heilk 200:158–168

Javed F, Akram Z, Barillas AP et al (2018) Outcome of orthodontic palatal plate therapy for orofacial dysfunction in children with Down syndrome: a systematic review. Orthod Craniofac Res 21(1):20–26

Jodeh DS, Buller M, Rottgers SA (2019) The impact of presurgical infant orthopedics on oronasal fistula rates following cleft repair: a meta-analysis. Cleft Palate-Craniofac J 56(5):576–585

Joos U (1995a) Die Behandlung kranio-fazialer Anomalien (The treatment of cranio-facial abnormalities). Dtsch Z Mund Kiefer Geschir 19:165–173

Joos U (1995b) Skeletal growth after muscular reconstruction for cleft lip, alveolus and palate. Br J Oral Maxillofac Surg 33(3):139–144

Jost WH, Steffen A, Berweck S (2021) A critical review of incobotulinumtoxinA in the treatment of chronic sialorrhea in pediatric patients. Expert Rev Neurother 21:1059–1068. https://doi.org/10.1080/14737175.2021.1979959

Jung BK, Yun IS (2020) Diagnosis and treatment of positional plagiocephaly. Arch Craniofac Surg 21:80–86

Kent RD (2015) Nonspeech oral movements and oral motor disorders: a narrative review. Am J Speech Lang Pathol 24:763–789

Keyf F, Sahin N, Aslan Y (2003) Alternative impression technique for a speech-aid prosthesis. Cleft Palate Craniofac J 40(6):566–568

Klockars T, Rautio J (2012) Early placement of ventilation tubes in cleft lip and palate patients: does palatal closure affect tube occlusion and short-term outcome? Int J Pediatr Otorhinolaryngol 76(10):1481–1484

Knösel M, Klein S, Bleckmann A et al (2011) Tongue position after deglutition in subjects with habitual open-mouth posture under different functional conditions. Orthod Craniofac Res 14(3):181–188

Knösel M, Fendel C, Jung K et al (2016) Presurgical orthopedics by drink plates does not significantly normalize deglutition in infants with cleft lip and palate. Angle Orthod 86(2):315–323

Koka V, De Vito A, Roisman G et al (2021) Orofacial Myofunctional Therapy in Obstructive Sleep Apnea Syndrome: A Pathophysiological Perspective. Medicina (Kaunas) 1;57(4):323

Koletsi D, Makou M, Pandis N (2018) Effect of orthodontic management and orofacial muscle training protocols on the correction of myofunctional and myoskeletal problems in developing dentition. A systematic review and meta-analysis. Orthod Craniofac Res 21(4):202–215

Kollara L, Schenck G, Perry J (2014) Continuous positive airway pressure (CPAP) therapy for the treatment of hypernasality: a single case study. Perspect Speech Sci Orofac Disord 24(2):48–58

Konst EM, Rietveld T, Peters HFM et al (2003a) Phonological development of toddlers with unilateral cleft lip and palate who were treated with and without infant orthopedics: a randomized clinical trial. Cleft Palate-Craniofac J 40(1):32–39

Konst EM, Rietveld T, Peters HFM et al (2003b) Language skills of young children with unilateral cleft lip and palate following infant orthopedics: a randomized clinical trial. Cleft Palate-Craniofac J 40(4):356–362

Konst EM, Prahl C, Weersink-Braks H et al (2004) Cost-effectiveness of infant orthopedic treatment regarding speech in patients with complete unilateral cleft lip and palate: a randomized three-center trial in the Netherlands (Dutchcleft). Cleft Palate Craniofac J 41(1):71–77

Korbmacher H, Limbrock J, Kahl-Nieke B (2004) Orofacial development in children with Down's syndrome 12 years after early intervention with a stimulating plate. J Orofac Orthop 65(1):60–73

Korbmacher HM, Limbrock JG, Kahl-Nieke B (2006) Long-term evaluation of orofacial function in children with Down syndrome after treatment with a stimulating plate according to Castillo Morales. J Clin Pediatr Dent 30(4):325–328

Kornbluth M, Campbell RE, Daskalogiannakis J et al (2018) Active presurgical infant orthopedics for unilateral cleft lip and palate: intercenter outcome comparison of Latham, modified McNeil, and nasoalveolar molding. Cleft Palate-Craniofac J 55(5):639–648

Kotlarek KJ, Krueger BI (2023) Treatment of Speech Sound Errors in Cleft Palate: A Tutorial for Speech-Language Pathology Assistants. Lang Speech Hear Serv Sch 17;54(1):171–188. https://doi.org/10.1044/2022_LSHSS-22-00071. Epub 2023 Jan 4. PMID: 36599098

Kriens OB (1969) An anatomical approach to veloplasty. Plast Reconstr Surg 43(1):29–41

Kuehn DP (1991) New therapy for treating hypernasal speech using continuous positive airway pressure (CPAP). Plast Reconstr Surg 88(6):959–966

Kuehn DP, Moon JB, Folkins JW (1993) Levator veli palatini muscle activity in relation to intranasal air pressure variation. Cleft Palate Craniofac J 30(4):361–368

Kuehn DP, Imrey BP, Tomes L et al (2002) Efficacy of continuous positive airway pressure for treatment of hypernasality. Cleft Palate Craniofac J 39(3):267–276

Kumar A, Kothari M, Grigoriadis A et al (2018) Bite or brain: implication of sensorimotor regulation and neuroplasticity in oral rehabilitation procedures. J Oral Rehabil 45(4):323–333

Kummer A, Lee L (1996) Evaluation and treatment of resonance disorders. Lang Speech Hear Serv Sch 27:271–281

Kuna ST, Sant'Ambrogio G (1991) Pathophysiology of upper airway closure during sleep. JAMA 266(10):1384–1389

Lai LH, Hui BK, Nguyen PD et al (2015) Lateral incisor agenesis predicts maxillary hypoplasia and Le Fort I advancement surgery in cleft patients. Plast Reconstr Surg 135(1):142e–148e

Leboulanger N, Blanchard M, Denoyelle F et al (2011) Autologous fat transfer in velopharyngeal insufficiency: indications and results of a 25 procedures series. Int J Pediatr Otorhinolaryngol 75:1404–1407

Lee ASY, Gibbon FE (2015) Non-speech oral motor treatment for children with developmental speech sound disorders. Cochrane Database Syst Rev 39(3):CD009383

Leuchter I, Schweizer V, Hohlfeld J et al (2012) Treatment of velopharyngeal insufficiency by autologous fat injection. Eur Arch Otorrinolaringol 267:977–983

Lethaus B, Grau E, Kloss-Brandstätter A et al (2021) Clinical Follow-Up in Orofacial Clefts-Why Multidisciplinary Care Is the Key. J Clin Med 10(4):842–851

Lewis DW, Fontana C, Mehallick LK et al (1994) Transdermal scopolamine for reduction of drooling in developmentally delayed children. Dev Med Child Neurol 36(6):484–486

Likitkulthanaporn A, Boonpratham S, Honglertnapakul Y et al (2024) Effects of nasoalveolar molding on nasolabial aesthetics in patients with cleft lip and palate during pre-adolescence: A systematic review and meta-analysis of retrospective studies. Orthod Craniofac Res 27(3):350–363

Lim M, Mace A, Nouraei SA et al (2006) Botulinum toxin in the management of sialorrhea: a systematic review. Clin Otolaryngol 31(4):267–272

Liou EJ, Subramanian M, Chen PK et al (2004) The progressive changes of nasal symmetry and growth after nasoalveolar molding: a three-year follow-up study. Plast Reconstr Surg 114(4):858–864

Liu X, Chen Z (2018) Effects of palate repair on cranial base and maxillary morphology in patients with unilateral complete cleft lip and palate. Cleft Palate Craniofac J 55(10):1367–1374

Lleras B, Müller L (1993) GRUMS (Heidelberg group concept for myofunctional disorders). Forum Logopädie 1:11–13

Lohmander A, Persson C, Willadsen E et al (2017) Scandcleft randomised trials of primary surgery for unilateral cleft lip and palate: 4. Speech outcomes in 5-year-olds - velopharyngeal competency and hypernasality. J Plast Surg Hand Surg 51(1):27–37

Long RE, McNamara JA (1985) Facial growth following pharyngeal flap surgery: skeletal assessment on serial lateral cephalometric radiographs. Am J Orthod 87:187–196

López-Liria R, Parra-Egeda J, Vega-Ramírez FA et al (2020) Treatment of dysphagia in Parkinson's disease: a systematic review. Int J Environ Res Public Health 17(11):4104. https://doi.org/10.3390/ijerph17114104

Losee JE, Smith DM, Afifi AM et al (2008) A successful algorithm for limiting postoperative fistulae following palatal procedures in the patient with orofacial clefting. Plast Reconstr Surg 122(2):544–554

Lourenço Ribeiro L, Teixeira Das Neves L, Costa B et al (2003) Dental anomalies of the permanent lateral incisors and prevalence of hypodontia outside the cleft area in complete unilateral cleft lip and palate. Cleft Palate Craniofac J 40(2):172–175

Luo X, Guo C, Yin H et al (2020) Comparison of Hogan pharyngeal flap and sphincter pharyngoplasty in postoperative velopharyngeal function. Br J Oral Maxillofac Surg 58(3):291–295

Mahajan RK, Chhajlani R, Ghildiyal HC (2014) Role of tongue flap in palatal fistula repair: a series of 41 cases. Indian J Plast Surg 47(2):210–215

Maillard S, Retrouvey JM, Ahmed MK et al (2017) Correlation between nasoalveolar molding and surgical, aesthetic, functional and socioeconomic outcomes following primary repair surgery: a systematic review. J Oral Maxillofac Res 8(3):e2. https://doi.org/10.5037/jomr.2017.8302

Marchac D, Renier D (1982) Craniofacial surgery for craniosynostosis, 1st edn. Little Brown, Boston

Marcusson A, Paulin G, Ostrup L (2002) Facial appearance in adults who had cleft lip and palate treated in childhood. Scand J Plast Reconstr Surg Hand Surg 36(1):16–23

Marshalla P (2011) Horns, whistles, bite blocks, and straws: a review of tools/objects used in articulation therapy by Van Riper and other traditional therapists. Int J Orofacial Myology 37:69–96

Masarei AG, Wade A, Mars M (2007) A randomized control trial investigating the effect of presurgical orthopedics on feeding in infants with cleft lip and/or palate. Cleft Palate-Craniofac J 44(2):182–193

Maspero C, Prevedello C, Giannini L et al (2014) Atypical swallowing: a review. Minerva Stomatol 63(6):217–227

Massengill R, Quinn GW, Picrell KL et al (1968) Therapeutic exercise and velopharyngeal gap. Cleft Palate J 5(1):44–47

Mathad VC, Scherer N, Chapman K et al. (2021) A Deep Learning Algorithm for Objective Assessment of Hypernasality in Children With Cleft Palate. IEEE Trans Biomed Eng 68(10):2986–2996. https://doi.org/10.1109/TBME.2021.3058424. Epub 2021 Sep 20. PMID: 33566756; PMCID: PMC9023650

McNeil CK (1950) Orthodontic procedures in the treatment of congenital cleft palate. Dent Rec 70(5):126–132

Meyer-Marcotty P, Stellzig-Eisenhauer A (2009) Dentofacial self-perception and social perception of adults with unilateral cleft lip and palate. J Orofac Orthop 70(3):224–236

Mier RJ, Bachrach SJ, Lakin RC et al (2000) Treatment of sialorrhea with glycopyrrolate: a double-blind, dose-ranging study. Arch Pediatr Adolesc Med 154(12):1214–1218

Millard DR (1958a) A radial rotation in single harelip. Am J Surg 95(2):318–322

Millard DR (1958b) Columella lengthening by a forked flap. Plast Reconstr Surg Transplant Bull 22(5):454–457

Mink van der Molen AB, van Breugel JMM, Janssen NG et al (2021) Clinical practice guidelines on the treatment of patients with cleft lip, alveolus, and palate: an executive summary. J Clin Med 10(21):4813. https://doi.org/10.3390/jcm10214813

Miyazaki T, Matsuya T, Yamaoka M (1975) Fiberscopic methods for assessment of velopharyngeal closure during various activities. Cleft Palate J 12:107–114

Moeller MR (2018) The emerging area of orofacial myofunctional therapy: efficacy of treatment in sleep disordered breathing bringing promise of a new field of medicine. Cranio 36(5):283–285

Mohammed H, Čirgi E, Rizk MZ et al (2020) Effectiveness of prefabricated myofunctional appliances in the treatment of Class II division 1 malocclusion: a systematic review. Eur J Orthod 42(2):125–134

Moll KL (1965) A cinefluorographic study of velopharyngeal function in normals during various activities. Cleft Palate J 2(2):112–122

Morgan AT, Dodrill P, Ward EC (2012) Interventions for oropharyngeal dysphagia in children with neurological impairment. Cochrane Database Syst Rev 10:CD009456

Mossey PA, Little J, Munger RG et al (2009) Cleft lip and palate. Lancet 374(9703):1773–17785

Mühler G (1995) The Wolfgang Rosenthal Clinic in Thallwitz—a historical review. Dtsch Z Mund Kiefer Ges Chir 19:191–194

Mühling J (1986) Zur operativen Behandlung der prämaturen Schädelnahtsynostosen (On the surgical treatment of premature skull suture synostoses). Med. Habilschrift. (Doctoral thesis) Univ. Würzburg

Mühling J, Sörensen N, Albert F et al (1994) Kraniofaziale Chirurgie im Kindesalter (Craniofacial surgery in childhood). Dtsch Ärztebl 91:1363–1366

Müke R (1972) New aspects of pathogenesis and therapy of craniosynostosis I. Acta Neurochir 26:191–250

Myrlund R, Dubland M, Keski-Nisula K et al (2014) One year treatment effects of the eruption guidance appliance in 7- to 8-year-old children: a randomized clinical trial. Eur J Orthod 37(2):128–134

Nelson AM (2012) A comprehensive review of evidence and current recommendations related to pacifier usage. J Pediatr Nurs 27(6):690–699

Netsell R (1986) A neurobiologic view of speech production and the dysarthrias. College-Hill, San Diego

Neubauerová L, Neubauer K (2018) Augmentative and alternative communication and clinical speech therapy practice. In: Neubauer K (ed) Compendium of clinical speech therapy. Portál, Prague, pp 697–713

Neumann S, Opitz M (2013) Effektivität sprachtherapeutischer Konzepte bei LKGS-Fehlbildung. MitSprache 45:5–26

Neumann S, Romonath R (2011) Effectiveness of nasopharyngoscopic biofeedback in clients with cleft palate speech – a systematic review. Logoped Phoniatr Vocol 37(3):1–12

Neumann S, Romonath R (2012) Effectiveness of nasopharyngoscopic biofeedback in clients with cleft palate speech: a systematic review. Logoped Phoniatr Vocol 37(3):95–106

Newell H (1913) Appliance for the prevention of mouth-breathing. Dent Cosmos 55:456–457

NHS (2019) Cleft lip and palate. https://www.nhs.uk/conditions/cleft-lip-and-palate/. Accessed 16 March 2022

Nicolas L, Marion B, Françoise D et al (2011) Autologous fat transfer in velopharyngeal insufficiency: indications and results of a 25 procedures series. Int J Pediatr Otorhinolaryngol 75:1404–1407

Niranjane PP, Kamble RH, Diagavane SP et al (2014) Current status of presurgical infant orthopaedic treatment for cleft lip and palate patients: a critical review. Indian J Plast Surg 47(3):293–302

Nohara K, Kotani Y, Sasao Y et al (2010) Effect of a speech aid prosthesis on reducing muscle fatigue. J Dent Res 89(5):478–481

Naros A, Naros CH, Awad D et al (2023) Antibiotic prophylaxis and surgical site infections in orthognathic surgery - a retrospective analysis. BMC Oral Health 23(1):688. https://doi.org/10.1186/s12903-023-03391-3. PMID: 37743500; PMCID: PMC10518949

Noverraz RLM, Disse MA, Ongkosuwito EM (2015) Transverse dental arch relationship at 9 and 12 years in children with unilateral cleft lip and palate treated with infant orthopedics: a randomized clinical trial (Dutchcleft). Clin Oral Investig 19(9):2255–2265

Olthoff A, Carstens PO, Zhang S et al (2016) Evaluation of dysphagia by novel real-time MRI. Neurology 87(20):2132–2138

Ondo WG, Hunter C, Moore W (2004) A double-blind placebo-controlled trial of botulinum toxin B for sialorrhea in Parkinson's disease. Neurology 62(1):37–40

Orticochea M (1968) Construction of a dynamic muscle sphincter in cleft palates. Plast Reconstr Surg 41:323–327

Orticochea M (1992) Method for the construction of sphincters in the human body: the birth of a new kind of medicine (editorial). Plast Reconstr Surg 90:469–473

Owman-Moll P, Ingervall B (1984) Effect of oral screen treatment on dentition, lip morphology, and function in children with incompetent lips. Am J Orthod 85(1):37–46

Padovan BA (1995) Neurofunctional reorganization in myo-osteo-dentofacial disorders: complementary roles of orthodontics, speech and myofunctional therapy. Int J Orofacial Myology 21:33–40

Pamplona M, Ysunza A, Espinosa J (1999) A comparative trial of two modalities of speech intervention for compensatory articulation in cleft palate children, phonologic approach versus articulatory approach. Int J Pediatr Otorhinolaryngol 49(1):21–26

Papadopoulos MA, Koumpridou EN, Vakalis ML et al (2012) Effectiveness of pre-surgical infant orthopedic treatment for cleft lip and palate patients: a systematic review and meta-analysis. Orthod Craniofac Res 15(4):207–236

Papageorgiou SN, Koletsi D, Eliades T (2019) What evidence exists for myofunctional therapy with prefabricated appliances? A systematic review with meta-analyses of randomised trials. J Orthod 46(4):297–310

Passavant G (1879) Über die Verbesserung der Sprache nach Uranoplastik. Arch Klin Chir 23:771

Peterson-Falzone SJ, Trost-Cardamone JE, Karnell MP et al (2017) The clinician's guide to treating cleft palate speech, 2nd edn. Mosby, St. Louis

Pfeifer G (1970) On a developmentally based procedure of closure of cleft lip. Dtsch Zahn Mund Kieferheilk 54:69–77

Pfeiffer RA (1964) Dominant hereditary acrocephalosyndactyly. Z Kinderheilkd 90:301–319

Pillery G (2008) Controversies surrounding nonspeech oral motor exercises for childhood speech disorders. Semin Speech Lang 29(4):253–256

Pinto JHN, da Silva Dalben G, Pegoraro-Krook MI (2007) Speech intelligibility of patients with cleft lip and palate after placement of speech prosthesis. Cleft Palate-Craniofac J 44(6):635–641

Pitak-Arnnop P, Hemprich A, Dhanuthai K et al (2011) Panel and patient perceptions of nasal aesthetics after secondary cleft rhinoplasty with versus without columellar grafting. J Craniomaxillofac Surg 39(5):319–325

Pless M, Granlund M (2012) Implementation of international classification of functioning, disability and health (ICF) and the ICF children and youth version (ICF-CY) within the context of augmentative and alternative communication. Augment Altern Commun 28(1):11–20

Pollack M, Shprintzen RJ (1981) Velopharyngeal insufficiency in neurofibromatosis. Int J Pediatr Otorhinolaryngol 3:257–262

Prado DGA, Berretin-Felix G, Migliorucci RR et al (2018) Effects of orofacial myofunctional therapy on masticatory function in individuals submitted to orthognathic surgery: a randomized trial. J Appl Oral Sci 26:e20170164. https://doi.org/10.1590/1678-7757-2017-0164

Prahl C, Kuijpers-Jagtman AM, Van't Hof MA et al (2005) Infant orthopedics in UCLP: effect on feeding, weight, and length: a randomized clinical trial (Dutchcleft). Cleft Palate-Craniofac J 42(2):171–177

Prahl C, Prahl-Andersen B, Van't Hof MA et al (2008) Presurgical orthopedics and satisfaction in motherhood: a randomized clinical trial (Dutchcleft). Cleft Palate-Craniofac J 45(3):284–288

Raj N, Raj V, Aeran H (2012) Interim palatal lift prosthesis as a constituent of multidisciplinary approach in the treatment of velopharyngeal incompetence. J Adv Prosthodont 4(4):243–247

Recuero II, Sanchez Aniceto G (2020) Craniosynostosis. In: Ehrenfeld M, Futran N, Manson P et al (eds) Advanced craniomaxillofacial surgery. AO Foundation Thieme, Stuttgart

Renier D, Marchac D (1988) Craniofacial surgery for craniosynostosis: functional and morphological results. Ann Acad Med Singap 17:415–426

Reynolds J, Carroll S, Sturdivant C (2016) Fiberoptic endoscopic evaluation of swallowing: a multidisciplinary alternative for assessment of infants with dysphagia in the neonatal intensive care unit. Adv Neonatal Care 16(1):37–43

Riski JE (2013) Speech, language, and velopharyngeal dysfunction: management throughout the life of an individual with cleft palate. In: Berkowitz S (ed) Cleft lip and palate diagnosis and management, 3rd edn. Springer, Berlin, pp 810–812

Robin NH (1999) Molecular genetic advances in understanding craniosynostosis. Plast Reconstr Surg 103(3):1060–1070

Rogers AP (1918) Muscle training and its relation to orthodontia. Int J Orthod 4(11):555–577

Rosenthal W (1924) Zur Frage der Gaumenplastik. Zentbl Chir 51:1621–1629

Ross RB, MacNamera MC (1994) Effect of presurgical infant orthopedics on facial esthetics in complete bilateral cleft lip and palate. Cleft Palate-Craniofac J 31(1):68–73

Roux W (1895) Developmental mechanics of organisms, 2nd edn. Engelmann, Leipzig

Ruda JM, Krakovitz P, Rose AS (2012) A review of the evaluation and management of velopharyngeal insufficiency in children. Otolaryngol Clin N Am 45(3):653–669

Ruscello D (2008a) An examination of nonspeech oral motor exercises for children with velopharyngeal inadequacy. Semin Speech Lang 29(4):294–303

Ruscello DM (2008b) Nonspeech oral motor treatment issues related to children with developmental speech sound disorders. Lang Speech Hear Serv Sch 39(3):380–391

Ruscello DM, Vallino LD (2020) The Use of Nonspeech Oral Motor Exercises in the Treatment of Children With Cleft Palate: A Re-Examination of Available Evidence. Am J Speech Lang Pathol 29(4):1811–1820. https://doi.org/10.1044/2020_AJSLP-20-00087. Epub 2020 Aug 5. PMID: 32755484

Ruscello D, Vallino L (2014) The application of motor learning concepts to the treatment of children with compensatory speech sound errors. Perspect Speech Sci Orofac Disord 24(2):39–47

Saethre H (1931) Pathogenese, erblichkeit und symptomatologie (a contribution to the tower skull problem (pathogenesis, heritability and symptomatology)). Dtsch Z Nervenheilk 117:533–555

Santamaría-Villegas A, Manrique-Hernandez R, Alvarez-Varela E et al (2017) Effect of removable functional appliances on mandibular length in patients with class II with retrognathism: systematic review and meta-analysis. BMC Oral Health 17(1):52. https://doi.org/10.1186/s12903-017-0339-8

Sanvanero-Rosselli G (1955) Verschluss von Gaumenspalten unter Verwendung von Pharynxlappen. In: Fortschritte der Kiefer- und Gesichtschirurgie, vol 1. Thieme, Stuttgart, p 65

Schenck GC, Perry JL, O'Gara MM et al (2021) Velopharyngeal muscle morphology in children with unrepaired submucous cleft palate: an imaging study. Cleft Palate Craniofac J 58:313–323

Schönborn G (1875) Über eine neue Methode der Staphylorraphie. Arck Klin Chir 19:527–531

Schröter-Morasch H, Ziegler W (2005) Rehabilitation of impaired speech function (dysarthria, dysglossia). GMS Curr Top Otorhinolaryngol Head Neck Surg 4:15

Seaward JR, Hallac RR, Vucovich M et al (2018) Improving the accuracy of automated cleft speech evaluation. J Craniomaxillofac Surg 46(12):2022–2026

Seo HJ, Denadai R, Pai Chien-Jung B et al (2019) Modern surgery-first approach concept in cleft-orthognathic surgery: a comparative cohort study with 3D quantitative analysis of surgical-occlusion setup. Clin Med 8(12):2116–2137

Sevcik R, Barton-Hulsey A, Romski M (2008) Early intervention, AAC, and transition to school for young children with significant spoken communication disorders and their families. Semin Speech Lang 29(2):92–100

Shaw WC, Semb G, Nelson P et al (2001) The Eurocleft project 1996–2000: overview. J Craniomaxillofac Surg 29(3):131–140

Shelton RL (1975) Panendoscopic feedback in the study of voluntary velopharyngeal movements. J Speech Hear Disord 40(2):232–244

Shelton RL, Arndt WB, Krueger AL et al (1966) Identification of persons with articulation errors from observation of nonspeech movements. Am J Phys Med 45(3):143–150

Shelton RL, Beaumont K, Trier WC et al (1978) Videoendoscopic feedback in training velopharyngeal closure. Cleft Palate J 15(1):6–12

Shetty V, Agrawal RK, Sailer HF (2017) Long-term effect of presurgical nasoalveolar molding on growth of maxillary arch in unilateral cleft lip and palate: randomized controlled trial. Int J Oral Maxillofac Surg 46(8):977–987

Shortland H-AL, Hewat S, Vertigan A et al (2021) Orofacial myofunctional therapy and myofunctional devices used in speech pathology treatment: a systematic quantitative review of the literature. Am J Speech Lang Pathol 30(1):301–317

Shprintzen RJ (1989) Research revisited. Cleft Palate J 26(2):148–149

Shprintzen RJ (1991) Fallibility of clinical research. Cleft Palate-Craniofac J 28(2):136–140

Shprintzen RJ (2013) The velopharyngeal mechanism. In: Berkowitz S (ed) Cleft lip and palate diagnosis and management, 3rd edn. Springer, Berlin, pp 741–758

Shprintzen RJ, Lencione RM, McCall GN et al (1974) A three dimensional cinefluoroscopic analysis of velopharyngeal closure during speech and nonspeech activities in normals. Cleft Palate J 11(4):412–428

Shprintzen RJ, McCall GN, Skolnick ML (1975) A new therapeutic technique for the treatment of velopharyngeal incompetence. J Speech Hear Disord 40(1):69–83

Shprintzen RJ, Lewin ML, Croft CB et al (1979) A comprehensive study of pharyngeal flap surgery: tailor-made flaps. Cleft Palate J 16(1):46–55

Siegel-Sadewitz VL, Shprintzen RJ (1982) Nasopharyngoscopy of the normal velopharyngeal sphincter: an experiment of biofeedback. Cleft Palate J 19(3):194–200

Sihvo M (2017) History of the LAX VOX tube exercise. Lambert Academic Publishing, Beau Bassin

Simberg S, Laine A (2007) The resonance tube method in voice therapy: description and practical implementations. Logoped Phoniatr Vocol 32(4):165–170

Sjögreen L, Engvall M, Ekström A et al (2007) Orofacial dysfunction in children and adolescents with myotonic dystrophy. Dev Med Child Neurol 49(1):18–22

Sjögreen L, Tulinius M, Kiliaridis S et al (2010) The effect of lip strengthening exercises in children and adolescents with myotonic dystrophy type 1. Int J Pediatr Otorhinolaryngol 74(10):1126–1134

Škodová E (2018) Speech communication disorders in anomalies of the orofacial system. In: Neubauer K (ed) Compendium of clinical speech therapy. Portál, Prague, pp 342–371

Skolnick ML, McCall GN, Barnes M (1973) The sphincteric mechanism of velopharyngeal closure. Cleft Palate J 10:286–305

Smithpeter J, Covell D (2010) Relapse of anterior open bites treated with orthodontic appliances with and without orofacial myofunctional therapy. Am J Orthod Dentofacial Orthop 137(5):605–614

Sockalingam S, Shammi C, Remington G (2009) Treatment of clozapine-induced hypersalivation with ipratropium bromide: a randomized, double-blind, placebo-controlled crossover study. J Clin Psychiatry 70(8):1114–1119

Sommerlad BC (2003) A technique for cleft palate repair. Plast Reconstr Surg 112(6):1542–1548

Steffen A, Rohrbach-Volland S (2021) Functional Hypersalivation in children and adults – therapy under consideration of recent guideline. Laryngorhinootologie 100:402–412. https://doi.org/10.1055/a-1355-7642

Stelzig G (2019) A phoniatric contribution to orofacial and pharyngolaryngeal functions. In: Codoni S, Spirgi-Gantert I, von Jackowski JA (eds) Function-orientated speech therapy. Springer, Berlin

Strode R, Chamberlain C (1997) Easy does it for articulation: an oral-motor approach. LinguiSystems, East Moline

Sudro PN, Kumar Das R, Sinha R et al (2021) Enhancing the intelligibility of cleft lip and palate speech using cycle-consistent adversarial networks. IEEE Spoken Language Technology Workshop (SLT), pp 720–727. https://doi.org/10.1109/SLT48900.2021.9383543

Talmi YP, Finkelstein Y, Zohar Y (1990) Reduction of salivary flow with transdermal scopolamine: a four-year experience. Otolaryngol Head Neck Surg 103(4):615–618

Tan HL, Kheirandish-Gozal L, Abel F et al (2015) Craniofacial syndromes and sleep-related breathing disorders. Sleep Med Rev 27:74–88

Tash EL, Shelton RL, Knox AW et al (1971) Training voluntary pharyngeal wall movements in children with normal and inadequate velopharyngeal closure. Cleft Palate J 8:277–290

Tennison CW (1952) The repair of the unilateral cleft lip by the stencil method. Plast Reconstr Surg 9(2):115–120

Tessier P (1971a) Chirurgie orbito-cranienne (Orbito-cranial surgery). Minerva Chir 26:878–904

Tessier P (1971b) The definite plastic surgical treatment of the severe facial deformities of craniofacial dysostosis. Crouzon's and Apert's diseases. Plast Reconstr Surg 48:419–442

Thüer U, Ingervall B (1990) Effect of muscle exercise with an oral screen on lip function. Eur J Orthod 12(2):198–208

Tian X, Yi LJ, Zhang L et al (2015) Oral motor intervention improved the oral feeding in preterm infants: evidence based on a meta-analysis with trial sequential analysis. Medicine 94(31):e1310. https://doi.org/10.1097/MD.0000000000001310

Troche MS, Sapienza CM, Rosenbek JC (2008) Effects of bolus consistency on timing and safety of swallow in patients with Parkinson's disease. Dysphagia 23(1):26–32

Trost JE (1981) Articulatory additions to the classical description of the speech of persons with cleft palate. Cleft Palate J 18(3):193–203

Usumez S, Uysal T, Sari Z et al (2004) The effects of early preorthodontic trainer treatment on Class II, division 1 patients. Angle Orthod 74(5):605–609

Uzel A, Alparslan ZN (2011) Long-term effects of presurgical infant orthopedics in patients with cleft lip and palate: a systematic review. Cleft Palate-Craniofac J 48(5):587–595

Van Lierde KM, De Bodt M, Baetens I et al (2003) Outcome of treatment regarding articulation, resonance and voice in Flemish adults with unilateral and bilateral cleft palate. Folia Phoniatr Logop 55(2):80–90

Van Riper C (1939) Speech correction: principles and methods. Prentice-Hall, Englewood Cliffs

Varghese LA, Mendoza JO, Braden MN et al (2014) Effects of spectral content on Horii Oral-Nasal coupling scores in children. J Acoust Soc Am 136:1295–1306

Veau V (1931) Division palatine. Masson, Paris

Veau V (1938) Bec-de-lièvre. Formes cliniques-chirurgie. Masson, Paris

Virchow R (1851) On cretinism, especially in Franconia, and on pathological skull forms. Verh Phys Med Ges Würzb 2:230–271

von Langenbeck B (1862) Uranoplasty by detachment of the mucous-periosteal palatal coating. Arch Klin Chir 2:205–287

Von Tetzchner S, Matrinsen H (2000) Introduction to augmentative and alternative communication. Whurr, London

Voss H, Herrlinger R (1972) Pocketbook of anatomy II. Gustav Fischer, Stuttgart

Walker V, Snell M (2013) Effects of augmentative and alternative communication on challenging behavior: a meta-analysis. Augment Altern Commun 29(2):117–131

Wang JC, Nagy L, Demke JC (2016) Syndromic craniosynostosis. Fac Plast Surg Clin N Am 24:531–543

Watts GD, Antonarakis GS, Forrest CR et al (2015) Is linear advancement related to relapse in unilateral cleft lip and palate orthognathic surgery? Cleft Palate Craniofac J 2(6):717–723

Wertsén M, Stenberg M (2020) Training lip force by oral screens. Part 3: outcome for patients with stroke and peripheral facial palsy. Clin Exp Dent Res 6(3):286–295

Whitaker LA, Munro IR, Salyer KE et al (1979) Combined report of problems and complications in 793 craniofacial operations. Plast Reconstr Surg 64:198–203

WHO (2007) Classification of functioning, disability, and health for children and youth (ICF-CY). http://apps.who.int/iris/bitstream/10665/43737/1/9789241547321_eng.pdf. Accessed 31 August 2014

Witzel AM, Tobe J, Salyer KE (1989) The use of videonasopharyngoscopy for biofeedback therapy in adults after pharyngeal flap surgery. Cleft Palate J 26(2):129–135

Wójcicki P, Wójcicka A (2011) Prospective evaluation of the outcome of velopharyngeal insufficiency therapy after pharyngeal flap, a sphincter pharyngoplasty, a double Z-plasty and simultaneous Orticochea and Furlow operations. J Plast Reconstr Aesthet Surg 64(4):459–461

Wolff J (1899) Die Lehre von der functionellen Knochengestalt (The doctrine of the functional bone shape). Virchows Arch Pathol Anat Physiol Klin Med 155(2):256–315

Yamaoka M, Matsuya T, Miyazaki T et al (1983) Visual training for velopharyngeal closure in cleft palate patients: a fiberscopic procedure (preliminary report). J Maxillofac Surg 11:191–193

Yen DW, Nguyen DC, Skolnick GB et al (2017) A comparison of the need for speech therapy after 2 palatal repair techniques. Ann Plast Surg 78(3):284–288

Young A, Spinner A (2020) Velopharyngeal insufficiency. In: StatPearls. StatPearls Publishing, Treasure Island

Young K, Sweeney T, Vos RR et al (2022) Evaluation of noise excitation as a method for detection of hypernasality. Applied acoustics. Acoustique appliqué. Angewandte Akustik 190:108639. https://doi.org/10.1016/j.apacoust.2022.108639

Ysunza A, Pamplona M, Femat T et al (1997) Videonasopharyngoscopy as an instrument for visual biofeedback during speech in cleft palate patients. Int J Pediatr Otorhinolayrngol 41(3):291–298

Ysunza PA, Chaiyasate K, Rontal M et al (2019) Comparison of three different surgical techniques for designing pharyngeal flaps according to findings of videonasopharyngoscopy and multiplanar videofluoroscopy. Int J Pediatr Otorhinolaryngol 120(2):123–129

Yules RB, Chase RA (1969) A training method for reduction of hypernasality in speech. Plast Reconstr Surg 43(2):180–185

Zaghi S, Valcu-Pinkerton S, Jabara M et al (2019) Lingual frenuloplasty with myofunctional therapy: exploring safety and efficacy in 348 cases. Laryngosc Investig Otolaryngol 4(5):489–496

Zajac DJ (2015) The nature of nasal fricatives: articulatory-perceptual characteristics and etiologic considerations. Perspect Speech Sci Orofac Disord 25:17–28

Zhang J, Yang S, Wang X et al (2020) Automatic hypernasality grade assessment in cleft palate speech based on the spectral envelope method. Biomed Tech 65(1):73–86

Zöller J, Kübler AC, Lorber WD et al (2003) Kraniofaziale chirurgie. Thieme, Stuttgart

Part II

Speech Fluency Disorders

Editors
Antoinette am Zehnhoff-Dinnesen,
Dobrinka Georgieva, Katrin Neumann,
Marie-Claude Monfrais-Pfauwadel

Lectors
Joseph Agius, Per Alm,
Susanne Cook, Sabine Van Eerdenbrugh,
Kurt Eggers, Dobrinka Georgieva,
Kenneth O. St. Louis, and J. Scott Yaruss

Basics of Speech Fluency Disorders 6

Ayoub Daliri, Harald A. Euler, Ahmed Geneid, Ludo Max, Katrin Neumann, Shelly Jo Kraft, Eva Seemanova, and John Van Borsel

6.1 Fluency Disorders: Definition and Classification

John Van Borsel

6.1.1 Fluency Disorder

Speaking is a rather complex human activity that involves a whole array of structures, muscles and brain regions. It takes some years to learn to speak but once speech has been acquired, it is a behaviour that largely happens automatically, smoothly, without any interruptions. When a speaker does interrupt the flow of speech, it is usually voluntarily. One may, for instance, pause for a second to think about the most appropriate word to use, or repeat a word or phrase to stress what just has been said. In some individuals, however, the flow of speech is interrupted beyond their control. They present what is generally called a fluency disorder. Various types of fluency disorder can be distinguished, the most common being stuttering and cluttering.

Eva Seemanova and Harald Euler were deceased at the time of publication.

Supplementary Information The online version contains supplementary material available at https://doi.org/10.1007/978-3-031-25175-7_6.

A. Daliri (✉)
Arizona State University, Tempe, AZ, USA
e-mail: Ayoub.Daliri@asu.edu

H. A. Euler · K. Neumann
Department of Phoniatrics and Pediatric Audiology, University Hospital Münster, University of Münster, Münster, Germany
e-mail: harald.euler@ukmuenster.de; Katrin.Neumann@uni-muenster.de

A. Geneid
Department of Phoniatrics and Otorhinolaryngology-Head and Neck Surgery, Helsinki University Central Hospital, Helsinki, Finland
e-mail: ahmed.geneid@hus.fi

L. Max
Department of Speech and Hearing Sciences, University of Washington, Seattle, WA, USA
e-mail: LudoMax@uw.edu

S. J. Kraft
Speech Language Pathology and Audiology, College of Liberal Arts and Sciences, Wayne State University, Detroit, MI, USA
e-mail: kraft@wayne.edu

E. Seemanova
Department of Child Neurology, 2nd Medical School of Charles University Prague, Prague, Czech Republic
e-mail: eva.seemanova@lfmotol.cuni.cz

J. Van Borsel
Faculty of Medicine and Health Sciences, Department of Rehabilitation, Ghent University, Ghent, Belgium
e-mail: john.vanborsel@ughent.be

A. am Zehnhoff-Dinnesen et al. (eds.), *Phoniatrics II*, European Manual of Medicine, https://doi.org/10.1007/978-3-031-25175-7_6

6.1.2 Stuttering

Stuttering, in British English also called stammering, is a fluency disorder that has been recognised for a long time but over the years has also been defined in divergent ways. One reason for the divergence is that the cause of stuttering is not clear. Especially in the past, definitions of stuttering were often based on assumptions about the aetiology and varied according to the causal theory adhered to. In recent times, it is more common to define stuttering by referring to its symptoms. The World Health Organization (WHO), for instance, defines stuttering as

> disorders in the rhythm of speech in which the individual knows precisely what he wishes to say but at the time is unable to say it because of an involuntary repetition, prolongation, or cessation of a sound (World Health Organization 1977, p. 202)

The first part of this definition makes it clear that stuttering is a speech disorder and not a language disorder. The problem is not with formulating ideas but with making words audible. The second part of the definition makes reference to three types of interruption that by many are believed to characterise stuttering, often called the primary symptoms of stuttering: repetitions, prolongations and blocks. They are speech interruptions that are exclusively seen in the speech of people who stutter and are sometimes called stuttering dysfluencies, less-typical dysfluencies or (referring to their occurrence) within-word dysfluencies. Interruptions that can also be found in the speech of speakers who do not stutter (for instance phrase repetitions and interjections such as 'eh, eh') are then called other dysfluencies, more-typical dysfluencies or between-word dysfluencies.

In addition to stuttering dysfluencies, people who stutter also tend to produce other dysfluencies more frequently than normal. It has further been suggested that in writing one reserves the spelling 'dysfluencies' (with 'y') to refer to the speech interruptions typical of stuttering and 'disfluencies' (with '*i*') to refer to speech interruptions in general, typical or not (Wingate 1984); this is not a rule, however.

Typical of people who stutter is that they may show all kinds of accompanying behaviour, often in an attempt to avoid or overcome their speech interruptions. This behaviour, called secondary symptoms, can be verbal or non-verbal. Some examples of verbal secondary symptoms are revisions (e.g. yesterday I went... visited my parents), incomplete sentences (e.g. And then I...) and substitutions of words (e.g. 'vehicle' for 'car'). Non-verbal secondary behaviour include pursing the lips, blinking the eyes or avoiding eye contact. In some definitions of stuttering, reference is made to the secondary symptoms. An example is the definition of the Special Interest Division on Fluency and Fluency Disorders of the American Speech-Language-Hearing Association (ASHA). Their guidelines state that

> Stuttering refers to speech events that contain monosyllabic whole-word repetitions, part-word repetitions, audible sound prolongations, or silent fixations or blockages. These may or may not be accompanied by accessory (secondary) behaviours (i.e., behaviours used to escape and/or avoid these speech events) (ASHA 1999, p. 6)

Apart from certain primary or secondary characteristics, the severity and impact of the occurring speech problem are sometimes also considered a defining characteristic of stuttering. Diagnostic criteria for stuttering according to the APA (2013), for instance, are:

1. Disturbance in the normal fluency and time patterning of speech (inappropriate for the individual's age) characterised by frequent occurrences of one or more of the following:
   (a) Sound and syllable repetitions
   (b) Sound prolongations
   (c) Interjections
   (d) Broken words (e.g. pauses within a word)
   (e) Audible or silent blocking (filled or unfilled pauses in speech)
   (f) Circumlocutions (word substitutions to avoid problematic words)
   (g) Words produced with an excess of physical tension
   (h) Monosyllabic whole-word repetitions (e.g. 'I-I-I I see him')

2. The disturbance in fluency interferes with academic or occupational achievement or with social communication
3. If a speech-motor or sensory deficit is present, the speech difficulties are in excess of those usually associated with these problems

6.1.3 Developmental and Acquired Stuttering

A striking detail in the definition of the World Health Organization (WHO) is that stuttering is described as 'disorders [plural] in the rhythm of speech', suggesting that more than one type of stuttering exists. One can indeed distinguish a number fluency disorders that could qualify as stuttering. One distinction that has been proposed is that between developmental and acquired stuttering. The majority of people who stutter started to do so in childhood, most often somewhere between the ages of 2 and 5 years. It is highly unlikely that a child starts to stutter for the first time after the age of 12 years (Johnson 1959; Yairi and Ambrose 2005). Stuttering is, therefore, often considered a developmental disorder. It should be noted, however, that most children start showing stuttering after having spoken fluently, or at least appropriately fluently, for their age. In this sense, stuttering is somewhat different from other developmental disorders such as dyslexia. Children with dyslexia do not lose a function that was already to some extent established.

While stuttering most often has its onset in childhood, speech disfluencies can nonetheless also occur for the first time later in life, beyond the typical childhood period. A number of conditions may be at the origin of the dysfluencies. The dysfluent speech may be the result of some brain damage (the most common condition), may be a side effect of the use of medication or may arise in a context of psychological or emotional trauma. Although the use of the label 'stuttering' in such cases has been contested in the past, it now seems an accepted practice also to refer to acquired dysfluencies as stuttering. One speaks then of acquired stuttering as opposed to developmental stuttering. Depending on the cause of the acquired dysfluency, more-specific labels are sometimes used. Thus, stuttering resulting from brain damage is usually called neurogenic stuttering; dysfluent speech as a side effect of medication is called drug-induced stuttering or less commonly pharmacogenic stuttering; dysfluent speech that is somehow associated with a psychological problem or an emotional trauma, formerly known as hysterical stuttering, is now commonly called psychogenic stuttering.

It should be admitted, however, that there is no consensus regarding the definitions and terminology referring to acquired stuttering. Over the years researchers and clinicians have used a whole array of terms, not all of which seem equally appropriate. Such labels as 'late-onset stuttering' and 'adult onset stuttering', for example, have sometimes been used as synonyms for acquired stuttering. However, children may also be the victim of brain damage and thus present with acquired stuttering. Drug-induced stuttering, for example, is sometimes classified under neurogenic stuttering, in spite of its very different cause and different possibilities with regard to diagnosis and therapy (unlike in stuttering due to brain damage, one can test if a drug causes dysfluencies by discontinuing the medication or changing its dose, and the latter actions may also be used therapeutically). In the case of neurogenic stuttering, one sometimes finds terms that refer to the nature or the localisation of the underlying brain damage such as 'stroke-associated stuttering' and 'cortical stuttering'. These labels may be quite correct to designate that in a given case the stuttering occurred in association with a stroke or resulted from a cortical lesion, respectively. They should not be used, however, as synonyms of neurogenic stuttering, as neurogenic stuttering can result from neurological conditions other than a stroke, and from lesions situated in parts of the brain other than the cortex. Moreover, these labels are misleading to the extent that they suggest the existence of distinct dysfluency patterns or symptom constellations associated with a particular aetiology or localisation of brain damage. Similarly, in cases of drug-induced stuttering it is not unusual to specify the drug that elicited the dysfluency. Thus, one speaks for instance of 'fluoxetine-induced stuttering' or 'theophylline-induced stuttering'. It is again important to note that these various labels do not necessarily refer to distinct types of dysfluency with a distinct symptomatology; on the contrary, the clinical picture in drug-induced stuttering appears to be quite heterogeneous. Different drugs may elicit stuttering with similar characteristics, and drugs belonging to the same pharmacological group, or even one drug, may evoke different symptoms in different patients. Other confusing terms are some older labels referring to other speech/language disorders such as 'dysphatic stuttering' and 'dysarthric, apraxic and dysnomic stuttering'. The problem with these labels is that, apart from again suggesting the existence of distinct subtypes of stuttering, they seem to broaden the label stuttering to include dysfluencies that are actually epiphenomena of another primary communication disorder, rather than genuine stuttering dysfluencies.

Some terminology recommendations with respect to the domain of acquired stuttering can be found in Table 6.1.

Table 6.1 Terminology of stuttering (for more details, see Van Borsel 2014)

Recommended terms
Acquired stuttering: most general term to refer to fluency problem that is not of developmental origin in an individual with no pre-existing stuttering
Psychogenic stuttering: subtype of acquired stuttering; dysfluency associated with a psychological problem or an emotional trauma. A psychopathological diagnosis need not be required
Neurogenic stuttering: subtype of acquired stuttering; dysfluency associated with acquired brain damage in an individual with no pre-existing stuttering; acceptable synonyms are neurologic(al) stuttering/stammering
SAAND, stuttering associated with acquired neurological disorders: subtype of acquired stuttering; most general term to refer to dysfluency associated with acquired brain damage; can also be used in individuals with pre-existing stuttering
Palilalia: subtype of neurogenic stuttering characterised by the repetition of words or phrases, often with increasing rapidity and decreasing voice volume, and mostly at the end of utterances. The number of repetitions may be impressive
Drug-induced stuttering: subtype of acquired stuttering; dysfluency associated with the use of medication; the drug can be specified (for instance fluoxetine-induced stuttering) with the understanding that the term does not denote a drug-specific pattern of dysfluency
Acceptable alternative terms
Acquired neurogenic stuttering: alternative term for neurogenic stuttering
Acquired psychogenic stuttering: alternative term for psychogenic stuttering
Uncommon terms, not recommended
Pharmacogenic stuttering: uncommon synonym for drug-induced stuttering
Neurologic stuttering: uncommon synonym for neurogenic stuttering
Neurological stammering: uncommon synonym for neurogenic stuttering
Misleading or confusing terms, to be avoided
Late-onset stuttering (but may be appropriate to refer to stuttering occurring for the first time beyond the typical childhood period and when the aetiology is as yet undetermined)
Adult-onset stuttering
Stroke-associated stuttering
Cortical stuttering
Idiopathic stuttering
Obsolete terms
Dysphasic/aphasic stuttering
Dysnomic stuttering
Dysarthric stuttering
Apraxic stuttering
Hysterical stuttering
Traumatic stuttering

6.1.4 Cluttering

This is a fluency disorder that on the one hand shows resemblances with stuttering, but on the other seems somehow different. Contrary to stuttering, cluttering is a disorder that for a long time hardly received any attention in the literature, to the extent that it has even been called 'the orphan' of speech language pathology. Even more than stuttering, cluttering is a disorder whose demarcation and definition are fraught with problems. According to Deso Weiss (1901–1971), one of the pioneers in the domain and the first to devote a whole book on cluttering, it is a speech disorder

> characterized by the clutterer's unawareness of his disorder, by a short attention span, by disturbances in perception, articulation and formulation of speech, and often by excessive speed of delivery. It is a disorder of the thought processes preparatory to speech and based on a hereditary disposition. Cluttering is a verbal manifestation of Central Language Imbalance, which affects all channels of communication (e.g. reading, writing, rhythm, and musicality) and behaviour in general (Weiss 1964, p. 1)

Clearly Weiss considers cluttering to be a multidimensional disorder and not only a speech disorder, as is stuttering. Others, however, define cluttering purely as a speech disorder. In Webster's Third International Dictionary, for instance, cluttering is described as

> a speech defect in which phonetic units are dropped, condensed, or otherwise distorted as a result of overly rapid agitated speech utterance (Merriam-Webster.com 2019)

Along with the lack of consensus on the nature of cluttering, one also finds in the literature a vast array of symptoms that have been considered typical of cluttering. Thus, a meta-analysis of 12 studies describing in total 29 participants diagnosed as 'clutterers' found that more than 50 different symptoms were mentioned as typical of cluttering (St. Louis 1996). Moreover, the type as well as the number of cluttering symptoms presented varied considerably from individual to individual.

A number of suggestions have been made in order to deal with the definitional problem associated with cluttering. One suggestion is that cluttering should be defined in terms of its 'lowest common denominator'. In this approach, one defines cluttering by referring only to its core features. As such, cluttering has been defined as

> a fluency disorder wherein segments of conversation in the speaker's native language typically are perceived as too fast overall, too irregular, or both. The segments of rapid and/or irregular speech rate must further be accompanied by one or more of the following: (a) Excessive "normal" disfluencies; (b) excessive collapsing or deletion of syllables; and/or (c) Abnormal pauses, syllable stress, or speech rhythm (St. Louis 2010)

Another suggestion is that of taking a spectrum approach (Ward 2012). In this view, cluttering-like symptoms can appear at a point on a spectrum between more normal and less normal examples, with at one end speech language output which would readily be regarded as 'cluttering', and at the other end behaviour that might be regarded as cluttering-like, but not for certain, warranting a diagnosis of cluttering.

Anyhow, the problem of defining and demarcating cluttering has had its impact on clinical practice. Up to now, there exists no proven valid and reliable instrument for diagnosing cluttering. Differentiating cluttering from stuttering especially remains a challenge.

6.1.5 Classification

Given the problems defining fluency disorders, it is not surprising that their classification too has been subject to discussion, with various attempts and revisions over the years. Table 6.2 shows how fluency disorders are coded and classified in the most recent version of International Classification of Diseases (ASHA 2019).

Table 6.2 Coding and classification of fluency disorders according to the International Classification of Diseases, Tenth Revision (World Health Organization 2016)

F80.8 Other developmental disorders of speech and language
F80.81 Childhood onset fluency disorder
Cluttering NOS
Stuttering NOS
Excludes1: Adult onset fluency disorder (F98.5)
Fluency disorder in conditions classified elsewhere (R47.82)
Fluency disorder (stuttering) following cerebrovascular disease (I69. withfinal numerals -23)
F98.5 Adult onset fluency disorder
Excludes1: Childhood onset fluency disorder (F80.81)
Dysphasia (R47.02)
Fluency disorder in conditions classified elsewhere (R47.82)
Fluency disorder (stuttering) following cerebrovascular disease (I69. with final numerals - 23)
Tic disorders (F95.)
R47.82 Fluency disorder in conditions classified elsewhere

(continued)

Table 6.2 (continued)

Stuttering in conditions classified elsewhere
Code first: Underlying disease or condition, such as: Parkinson's disease (G20)
Excludes1: Adult onset fluency disorder (F98.5)
Childhood onset fluency disorder (F80.81)
Fluency disorder (stuttering) following cerebrovascular disease (I69. with final numerals-23)
I69.023 Fluency disorder following non-traumatic subarachnoid haemorrhage
Stuttering following non-traumatic subarachnoid haemorrhage
I69.123 Fluency disorder following non-traumatic intracerebral haemorrhage
Stuttering following non-traumatic intracerebral haemorrhage
I69.223 Fluency disorder following other non-traumatic intracranial haemorrhage
I69.323 Fluency disorder following cerebral infarction
Stuttering following cerebral infarction
I69.823 Fluency disorder following other cerebrovascular disease
Stuttering following other cerebrovascular disease
I69.923 Fluency disorder following unspecified cerebrovascular disease
Stuttering following unspecified cerebrovascular disease

6.1.6 Conclusion

The normal flow of speech, as produced by most adult speakers, can be disrupted in various manners. Two main types of dysfluent speech are usually distinguished: stuttering and cluttering. Dysfluent speech may have various causes and manifest itself in various ways, however. Therefore, defining and classifying stuttering and cluttering is by no means a straightforward task.

6.2 Epidemiology of Stuttering: An Overview

Ahmed Geneid

6.2.1 Onset, Incidence, Prevalence and Genetic Background of Stuttering

Developmental stuttering is a speech disorder characterised by disruption in the forward movement of speech with disruptions including part-word or syllable word repetitions or sound prolongations or involuntary breaks in syllables or words.

Developmental stuttering is a speech disorder that nearly always starts in early childhood, at a mean age of 33 months (Yairi and Ambrose 2013), with 95% starting before the age of four years (Yairi and Ambrose 2005). Different studies estimated that 6–12% of children aged 2–4 will develop a stutter and that 15–25% of these speech impediments will persist to adulthood, resulting in approximately 1% prevalence in the adult population (Yairi and Ambrose 2013).

The life-span incidence of stuttering is approximately 5% (Guitar 2006). Recent studies point to a possibly higher incidence of 8–9% (Dworzynski et al. 2007; Felsenfeld et al. 2000; Reilly et al. 2009). The prevalence of stuttering has been documented to be around 0.7–1%, regardless of cultural background or social level. This has been documented through numerous investigations carried out since the beginning of last century (e.g. Okasha et al. 1974; Wallin 1916). Further studies also demonstrate a similar prevalence of little less than 1% (Craig et al. 2002; Van Borsel et al. 2006).

The disparity between the incidence and prevalence of stuttering has mainly been attributed to the natural recovery from it. Such natural recovery was known to be as high as 79% in a 16-year longitudinal study published in 1964 (Andrews and Harris 1964). Recent studies point to possibly similar, if not higher, recovery rates up to 85% (Dworzynski et al. 2007; Månsson 2000). Most of the studies on incidence and prevalence of stuttering have been in North America, Europe and Australia. The prevalence of stuttering is supposedly the same worldwide, and this has been confirmed with a few studies in Africa and Asia (Okasha et al. 1974). Accordingly, it can be presumed that the incidence of stuttering is also the same in different parts of the world.

Stuttering occurs more often in males than females in childhood, with more family history of stuttering among males (Ajdacic-Gross et al. 2010). Risk of incidence of stuttering rises to 5:1 in adolescents and adults (Yairi 1983). Such rise of incidence suggests that females may have a higher recovery rate during childhood (Seider et al. 1983). On the other hand, adult onset of stuttering is usually attributed to brain damage (De Nil et al. 2007; Preus 1981).

The genetic background of stuttering is no longer questionable. This has been confirmed by different studies (e.g. Wittke-Thompson et al. 2007; Lan et al. 2009; Kraft and Yairi 2012; Kang et al. 2010). For the current state and details, see Sect. 6.4. Neuroimaging research of the past two decades has provided important insight into the underlying mechanisms of stuttering in adults and young children (e.g. Chang et al. 2018). For details, see Sect. 8.6.

6.2.2 Race, Ethnicity, Culture and Socio-economic Status of Stutterers

Race, ethnicity, culture and socio-economic status do not seem to affect the above-mentioned prevalence rates. However, it may have an effect on the well-being of children who stutter, e.g. black and Hispanic children are less likely than White children who stutter to have many worries, to be unhappy or depressed, and less likely to have difficulties with emotions and concentration (Briley and Ellis 2020). Multilingualism among children imposes challenges on identifying and investigating stuttering among them, as it is likely that these children do have other challenges of going through more than one language when speaking; such challenges may produce more dysfluencies among this group (Byrd et al. 2020). Accordingly, monolingual stuttering guidelines may not be applicable among bilingual children (Eggers et al. 2019). Further studies are necessary to clarify if children with bilingual language development recover with a lower rate from early stuttering than monolingual children (Byrd et al. 2020). The parents' level of education seems to have an effect on the development of language among bilingual children (Richels et al. 2013). It is already known that at the age of 36 months, the parents' level of education and the total quality of child care, in addition to different parental words, are considered as significant predictors of child language (Pancsofar and Vernon-Feagans 2006). However, such findings still need to be supported by further studies.

6.3 Symptomatic Profile of Stuttering

Ahmed Geneid

6.3.1 Introduction

Stuttering is commonly defined as a disorder characterised by high frequency of involuntary interruptions of the forward flow of speech, regarded by the person who stutters (PWS) as 'stutters', which are often accompanied by a feeling of loss of control (Van Borsel and Tetnowski 2007; Guitar 2006; Curlee 1999). Usually, such instances are recognised by the stutterers themselves as well as the listener as stuttering.

In this regard, stuttering symptoms should be differentiated from symptoms of normal disfluency. Symptoms of normal disfluency include interjections, polysyllabic word and phrase repetitions. Excessive use of such normal disfluencies may call attention to the child's fluency abilities, but falls short of being stuttering (Conture 2001; Leclercq et al. 2017).

Symptoms of stuttering have been typically divided into external/overt and internal symptoms. Internal symptoms include, for example, emotional reactions and fear of talking. External symptoms are those related to speech and are often accompanied by facial or body movements. Such facial and body movements include nostril flaring, facial grimacing, rolling of the eyes, blinking, irregular breathing, etc.

6.3.2 Stuttering Disfluencies

Stromsta (1965) called intra-phonemic disruptions resulting in part sound or part syllable repetitions as the core behaviour of stuttering, with prolongations, tonic blocks and repetitions to be reactions or secondary features of stuttering. APA (2013) defines stuttering by its symptoms as a disturbance in the normal fluency and time patterning of speech (inappropriate for the individual's age), characterised by frequent occurrences of one or more of the following:

- Sound and syllable repetitions
- Sound prolongations
- Broken words (e.g. pauses within a word)
- Audible or silent blocking (filled or unfilled pauses in speech)
- Circumlocutions (word substitutions to avoid problematic words)
- Words produced with an excess of physical tension
- Monosyllabic whole-word repetitions

In addition, DSM-5 (APA 2013) defines three extra criteria:

- The disturbance causes anxiety about speaking or limitations of effective communication, social participation, or academic or occupational performance, individually or in any combination.
- The onset of symptoms is in the early developmental period. (Adults are diagnosed as adult-onset fluency disorder.)
- The disturbance is not attributable to a speech-motor or sensory deficit, disfluency associated with a neurological insult (e.g. stroke, tumour, trauma) or another medical condition, and is not better explained by another mental disorder.

For details, see Sect. 8.1.

6.3.3 Choral Effect of Stuttering

PWS usually do not show stuttering when reading in unison. Choral reading or unison speech, in which two or more people read or sing aloud the same material, is known to cause both immediate and dramatic reduction of stuttering (Andrews et al. 1983; Ingham 1984; Rami et al. 2005). These findings are a source of inspiration for some speech fluency treatments.

6.3.4 Speaking Rate

The speaking rate of stutterers is usually lower than those who do not stutter (Johnson 1961). However, such slow rates are not uniform and are correlated with the degree of severity, being much slower with severe stuttering (Andrade et al. 2003; Kelly 1994).

6.3.5 Concomitant Language and Phonological Disorders

Forty-four per cent of young children who stutter have concomitant phonological and language disorders. This percentage includes 32% with phonological disorders, 35% with language disorders and 33% with both phonological and language disorders (Arndt and Healey 2001). Studies investigating differences in speech and language skills in young children who do and do not stutter, however, have only found small group differences. Major developments in speech and language co-occur with the onset and early development of stuttering, which may explain the high comorbidity numbers.

6.3.6 Anxiety, Depression and Personality Dysfunction in Relation to Stuttering

Anxiety is a common characteristic of speakers who stutter. This has been repeatedly documented through a number of physiological measures, self-reported measures and scales (Travis et al. 1936; Ezrati-Vinacour and Levin 2004; Brutten 1963; Blumgart et al. 2010; Blood et al. 1994; St Clare et al. 2009).

Studies on depression among stutterers have given controversial results. Some reported high levels of depressive symptoms among stutterers (Tran et al. 2011), while others reported normal levels (Miller and Watson 1992; Bray et al. 2003).

Accordingly, it is not possible to draw a conclusion on depression and depressive symptoms among stutterers. It is worth mentioning that the number of studies on depression and stuttering is rather low, and few conclusions can be drawn from them. The same applies for personality dysfunction. Some studies have suggested that the experiences of stutterers during childhood result in serious personality dysfunction in comparison with the non-stuttering controls (Iverach et al. 2009a, 2010) and more specifically in mental health disorders (Iverach et al. 2009b) and anxiety disorders (Iverach et al. 2011). However, other studies have shown that personality disorders among the stutterers have rates that are similar to those in the general population (Manning and Beck 2013a, b). For details, see Sects. 8.3, 8.5, and 10.4.

6.4 Aetiology of Stuttering

Katrin Neumann, Harald A. Euler, Eva Seemanova and Shelly Jo Kraft

6.4.1 Aetiology of Persistent Developmental Stuttering

6.4.1.1 Contemporary Knowledge

The past decade of advancements in genetic and neuroimaging research has provided significant insights into the aetiology and pathophysiology of stuttering. From the contemporary state of knowledge, the aetiology of stuttering can no longer be described as unknown. Instead, persistent developmental stuttering can now be regarded as a central neurological disruption of motor-speech planning and production, characterised by childhood onset and a genetic architecture that is polygenic in nature. It has neuromorphological and neurofunctional correlates, likely caused by the genetic alterations and by compensatory processes, which are associated with stutter-typical disturbances of course, rhythm, motor, breathing, articulation and phonation of speech.

Research in the genetics of stuttering has proceeded from behavioural (quantitative) to biological genetics. Scientifically moving from a top-down approach (behavioural), to a bottom-up approach (biological), has enabled new genes to be identified. Despite this massive leap, there are still questions to be answered. For example, how many genes are involved in the complete profile for developing a stutter? And how are these genes passed down through families (Kraft and Yairi 2012)? Furthermore, as the function of genes is determined to a differing degree by the interaction between hereditary and environmental contributions, epigenetic factors undoubtedly play an important role for the multifactorial aspects of onset, severity, type, course and presentation.

6.4.1.2 Behavioural and Biological Genetics

By *behavioural-genetic* examinations, the genetic analysis of complex traits, the genetic component ('heritability') and the environmental component ('environmentality') of the variance of a phenotypical trait can be distinguished and quantified. *Biological genetics* aims to localise and identify genes that contribute to individually different expressions of a phenotypical feature.

6.4.1.3 Behavioural Genetics of Stuttering

Heritability of Stuttering

Developmental stuttering appears robustly in some families. While it may be easy to assume that this represents heritability, it can be far more complex. Most traits are complex in nature. For example, skin colour is regulated by more than 15 different genes, by behaviour, by the environment and by interactions of genes with the environment (epigenetics). Certainly we inherit genes for melanin production in the skin, but individuals may or may not spend time in the sun, may or may not wear sun-screen, and may or may not even live in a warm sunny climate. The interaction effects of what our skins has been exposed to across a life-span also contributes to the colour of our skin on any given day. Distinguishing the extent to which a particular trait is represented by what is genetically inherited from parents, versus learned from parents, versus caused by environmental contributions (or the interactions thereof), can be difficult. The classic approach to parsing apart heritability and environmentality is via twin, adoption and family pedigree studies. Heritability estimates the relative contribution of genetic and non-genetic differences to the total phenotypic variation in a population with respect to a trait or disease, and thus quantifies the fraction of phenotype variability that can be attributed to genetic variation. The phenotypic variability between individuals, with respect to a particular trait, is determined by the individual genome, population structure, the environment, chance and measurement error (Raj and van Oudenaarden 2008).

Heritability is not a natural constant, but is specific to a particular population within a particular environment. A phenotypic change can occur in a population of people without any genetic shifts to the architecture. For example, if environmental variation decreases for a phenotype, the broad effects on the trait gets reduced and results in less population variation. On the other hand, it may also increase if genetic variation increases, leading to more phenotypic variation among individuals. For example, the heritability of having ten fingers is relatively high at birth, as any deviation from ten fingers is mostly due to genetic factors, such as in polydactyly. As individuals age, however, fingers in the population get cumulatively lost in physical accidents. This increases the population variance through environmental impact and thus decreases the fraction of the phenotypic variance granted by genetic variation. As such, the adjective '*heritable*' must not be confused with the term '*hereditary*'. The fact that we have the nose in the middle of the face instead on the back of the head is hereditary, that is, constructed by genetic influence. The heritability of having the nose in the face, however, is nearly zero, because nearly no variation exists for that facial trait.

Heritability is difficult to measure, and epigenetic influence (i.e. the interaction effect of the environment with genes) may also depend on the nature of the genes involved. Genes may canalise a phenotype, making its expression independent from different environments. On the other hand, individuals with the same genotype may show different phenotypes because of phenotypic plasticity (the ability of an organism to change its phenotype in response to changes in the environment). On a molecular level, the transcriptional activity of some individual genes may change in association with environmental changes, while other genes do not react on the latter.

Behavioural genetic studies have confirmed a high heritability for developmental stuttering (Andrews et al. 1991; Fagnani et al. 2011; Felsenfeld et al. 2000; Howie 1981a, b; Ooki 2005). Although it has been observed that the tendency to stutter occurs more frequently among relatives, it was not before the 1930s that the incidence in families had been systematically studied (Bryngelson and Rutherford 1937) and that a genetic contribution to a higher incidence in certain families had been taken into consideration (Wepman 1939). Twin studies have enabled the study of genetic and environmental contributions to stuttering. Twin studies are powerful, because they consider a trait or disease with respect to different proportions of shared DNA (deoxyribonucleic acid) and shared environment. DNA is identical in monozygotic twins, as is their developmental environment in most cases. Both babies share a womb, upbringing, parenting and nutrition. Dizygotic twins are essential for comparing with monozygotic twins because, although they share only 50% of their DNA, they experience an almost identical environment such as womb, upbringing, parenting and nutrition. Typical siblings share 50% of their DNA (the same as dizygotic twins) but do not share exactly the same environment. Age differences between siblings contribute to environmental differences, as resources, living conditions, parenting and nutrition can shift significantly with time for any particular household.

When considering stuttering in twin studies, it has been observed that monozygotic twins are more frequently concordant (both affected) with respect to the probability of the occurrence of stuttering than reports of dizygotic twins. Respectively, 44.9% of identical twins both stutter compared to 12.0% of dizygotic twins as averaged over six studies weighted for sample size

(Andrews et al. 1991; Dworzynski et al. 2007; Felsenfeld et al. 2000; Godai et al. 1976; Howie 1981a). The heritability estimates for adults who stutter has been reported to be from 70% (Felsenfeld et al. 2000) to 84% (Fagnani et al. 2011; Ooki 2005; Rautakoski et al. 2012), suggesting that the larger part of the risk for developing a stutter (70–84%) is genetically inherited. For children who stutter, the heritability estimates have been reported somewhat lower, around 60% (Dworzynski et al. 2007). This could be due to sample sizes and the specific criteria utilised for diagnosis. Heritability has been shown to influence which children stutter into adulthood and which recover spontaneously without therapy (Ambrose et al. 1997; Dworzynski et al. 2007).

Heritability gives the percentage by which the occurrence of stuttering in a population is caused by genetic contributions. It does not allow for the implication of genetic influences for a single specific individual (e.g. 'Seventy per cent of *your* stuttering is genetically determined'). It is, however, feasible to make a prediction of the probability of stuttering in blood relatives of persons who stutter. Shared DNA alongside a shared environment provides a logical explanation for this phenomenon of expressing a shared trait. It is important to note, however, that there is not perfect concordance in developmental stuttering, even among those who share 100% of their DNA and their environment, as in monozygotic twins. We can conclude that the occurrence of stuttering in blood relatives predisposes for the manifestation of stuttering. In a non-selected population, the lifelong incidence of stuttering is about 5% for male subjects. By contrast, this incidence is 20% for fathers, brothers or sons of persons who stutter. Between female relatives the familial clustering is considerably lower (Kidd 1980). Relative risk estimates determined by pedigree studies provide only one component for the expression of complex conditions, diseases or disorders. While there is a strong genetic component demonstrated by heritability estimates, and a measurable environmental contribution, some of what is measured in phenotypic variability can only be attributed to random chance and unpredictable mutations during miosis and mitosis.

Environmentality of Stuttering

Considering the heritability estimates ranging from 70% to 84%, the remaining variance accounting for 15–30% is foremost attributed to environmental factors. The behavioural-genetic approach enables a distinction between (1) environmental influences, making siblings more similar to each other than to children from different families (shared environment) and (2) other environmental influences (non-shared environment). The behavioural-genetic findings largely agree that the aetiologically effective environmental influences on the occurrence of stuttering have to be attributed to the non-shared environment (Andrews et al. 1991; Fagnani et al. 2011; Felsenfeld et al. 2000; Ooki 2005). Therefore, it is unlikely that the speech and language environment of a child within the family contributes causally to the occurrence of stuttering. This insight contradicts older theories (e.g. diagnosogenic theory) (Johnson 1955), socialisation-theoretical assertions, and other popular assumptions. The parental style of education (e.g. high-performance requirements, high verbal demands) is not responsible for the occurrence of stuttering and even not a contributing factor. Some parents, however, reactively develop an unfavourable interactive behaviour (admonitions such as 'speak slowly', 'think before you speak', 'just take a deep breath and (then) remain (very) calm') with possible implications for the characteristics and severity of stuttering and its psychological sequelae for the child (e.g. insecurity, loss of communicative easiness).

The proportion of variance for non-shared (individual-specific) environments cannot be derived from behavioural-genetic findings. From a behavioural-genetic standpoint, the environment is not only restricted to the social environment. It includes all aspects and influences on development from the genome (including the intracellular environment), the physiological-anatomical and uterine environment during foetal development, as well as the social environment and stimulation after birth, not excluding the individual world of thought and experiences.

This complexity makes the behavioural-genetic, non-shared environment difficult to assess and makes a premature assignment to assumed aspects of the social environment assailable (Turkheimer and Waldron 2000). It is, therefore, possible that these environmental causes of stuttering are not (alone) grounded in the individual-specific social environment. Here, is where the non-shared environment of chance and randomisation also occurs. Individual development is a complex process, emanating from genes, which set in motion a network of interactions, with molecular, cellular, physiological, behavioural and social-environmental components that are additionally organised in various feedback loops, which also determine the impact of genes, e.g. their expression. Additionally, random physiological events can open individually different developmental paths (Molenaar et al. 1993). Monozygotic twins may differ in their fingerprints, handedness, hair whorls and laterality during folding their hands (right or left thumb above) despite identical genes. One monozygotic twin may develop stuttering and the other one may not, without individual-social experiences necessarily responsible for that difference.

The specific contribution of the non-shared environment to the occurrence of stuttering is difficult to specify on an individual-case basis. Retrospective attribution of causes to social or psychological events that preceded or paralleled the onset of stuttering (e.g. traumatic experiences) are typical attribution errors in which chance is mistakenly equated with causality.

6.4.1.4 Biological and Molecular Genetics of Stuttering

Principles of Molecular-Genetic Examinations of Disease

Genes are cohesive regions of DNA that carry information for the synthesis of RNA (ribonucleic acid) to be translated into protein. Within the protein-coding genes, the base sequence of nucleotides (subunits of the DNA) work together in triplets (called codons) to form specific amino acids that act as the building blocks of proteins that are then expressed throughout the entire body. The exact nature of each nucleotide results in the particular amino acid produced by that codon and thus encodes the information organisms need to survive and reproduce. Each genetic variation in the coding portions of the human genome has the potential to modify a trait or behaviour. DNA sequencing determines the primary structure of nucleotides by analysing fragments of each DNA molecule. It is used in medicine to identify, diagnose and treat certain conditions. A huge emphasis on molecular medicine including mRNA vaccines and gene therapies are being pioneered and implemented globally. Capturing the genetic architecture of a particular disease can pave the way for more informed diagnostic, preventive and treatment approaches.

Biological and molecular genetics give the most direct evidence for the aetiology of stuttering. Molecular-genetic examinations such as *linkage studies, analysis of candidate genes* and *genome-wide association studies (GWAS)* have contributed to our current biological knowledge about the genetic risk for stuttering. The two main methods employed are linkage and association studies. Both utilise *genetic markers*, which are clearly identifiable sequences of nucleotides in known genetic regions. These nucleotide sequences constitute observable variations among individuals and populations that are often linked to specific phenotypes. Because the properties and locations of the markers are known, they serve as reference points in linkage and association studies.

Linkage studies search for large chromosomal regions where candidate genes for a trait or disease are located in a family enriched for that phenotype. *Genetic linkage* is the tendency for genes that are located in close vicinity to each other on a chromosome to be inherited together during meiosis *(coinheritance)*. When DNA gets passed from one generation to the next in a single family, the co-transmission of the disorder is mapped. Alleles that are proximal to a marker will be coinherited, or linked. As the genetic inheritance of the condition is 'linked' to the corresponding genetic region that is passed from one generation to the next, this genetic approach is referred to as linkage. Linkage studies are very useful in the detection of rare variants. Sometimes these variants are singularly specific to the family being investigated and not representative of mutations at a population level.

However, they still serve to illuminate the neurobiological networks associated with the identified variants that help scientists select regions to explore further with population studies.

Association studies examine many common genetic variants in a case–control approach of unrelated individuals to see if any variant is frequently associated with a trait or disease in a group-wise comparison. Markers used in such studies are often identified by *polymorphisms* (variations in the DNA sequence). Different versions of the same gene are called alleles. When distinguishing between an allele (common genetic variant) and a mutation (rare genetic variant), geneticists look at the proportions of each polymorphism in the population. Genetic markers can be large—an entire extra 21st chromosome is a genetic marker for Down syndrome—or they may be as small as a single base-pair change, also known as a *single-nucleotide polymorphism* (*SNP*, pronounced 'snip'). An allele is one of several alternative forms of the same gene or same gene locus (generally a group of genes). Allelic differences may or may not be phenotypically observable. Almost all common SNPs have only two alleles. SNPs constitute about 90% of all genetic variants in the human genome, making them an ideal candidate for genetic analysis.

SNPs occur in both protein-coding and non-coding regions. In general, natural selection will fix the allele of the SNP to constitute the most favourable genetic adaptation (Barreiro et al. 2008). Since only 1–2% of the genome is protein-coding, most SNPs localise to non-coding DNA. As such, most polymorphisms are genetically and functionally meaningless to our current understanding of molecular genomics; however, they still prove to be useful in studies that localise these genetic variations affecting disease where disease alleles are present.

Linkage Studies, Candidate Gene Specification, Genome-Wide Association Studies, Biobank Discoveries, and Whole-Exome Sequencing in Stuttering

According to current theory, stuttering is regarded a complex polygenic condition encompassing various genes with different functional effects, acting in concert with gene–environment interactions and regulation. To what extent the latter contributes to the occurrence or persistence of stuttering has not yet been definitively explored. Linkage studies have localised more than a dozen different loci for stuttering on chromosomes 1, 2, 3, 5, 7, 9, 12, 13, 14, 15, 16, 18 and 21 (Kang et al. 2010; Kraft and Yairi 2012; Raza et al. 2013; Shugart et al. 2004; Suresh et al. 2006; Wittke-Thompson et al. 2007). Regions linked with stuttering and recovering from stuttering have been detected on chromosome 9. Linkage for persistent stuttering has been found on chromosome 15. Male-specific linkage has been found on chromosome 9, and female-specific linkage signal for stuttering on chromosome 21 (Suresh et al. 2006).

A substantial portion of the genetic architecture appears to be additive in nature, which may indicate a risk-threshold model. As such, the risk for persistent developmental stuttering would be normally distributed across a population, but would increase with more affected loci in any given individual. When a threshold is exceeded, typical motor-speech pathways are disrupted and phenotypical stuttering behaviour occurs as a result. According to this model, mechanisms regulated by gender must be protective in nature for females, or critical thresholds are lower for males to reflect the observed risk for persistent developmental stuttering as more than double for boys than for girls (Dworzynski et al. 2007).

Linkage analysis has several limitations. Very large DNA segments containing many genes are implicated when a statistically significant region is detected as a peak signal on a chromosome, making it difficult to determine which specific gene is driving the signal. Hence, additional investigations of these specific chromosomal regions to isolate candidate genes are necessary. Historically, family studies have provided only moderate evidence for linkage to stuttering (Kraft and Yairi 2012), and the overlap of findings from those studies are limited. Kraft and Yairi (2012) extensively reviewed linkage studies for overlapping signals and found only five chromosomes in association with stuttering that were reported in more than one study, and then not always in the same region of a chromosome. The outcome of a linkage analysis of 46 highly inbred Pakistani families with 144 stuttering and 55 non-stuttering participants (Riaz et al. 2005) may be confounded by the possibility that the detected linkages might reflect a single common mutation specific to these particular families of a founder nature (a single common ancestor), rather than chromosomal regions which may characterise stuttering in the overall population. Another weakness of linkage studies is the relatively low statistical power for complex disorders. Because there are many genes and a large number of chromosomal regions (often hundreds) shared by family members not associated with the disorder under study (Kraft and Yairi 2012), the correct transmission model must be incorporated into the linkage algorithm. Non-parametric linkage (without a specified inheritance model) can be performed, but it further reduces the power to detect causal variants. Early stages of genetic discovery are often without known transmission models, reducing the power of a linkage study. However, once linkage analysis has been performed and signals have been detected, the possible *candidate genes* under the peak require specification and *amplification* (i.e. the production of many identical copies of a DNA sequence of interest), the identification of polymorphisms or sequencing of neighbouring regions, genotyping of a control population, and the analysis of the functional relationship between alleles and the disease or trait of interest (Kraft and Yairi 2012).

Two studies have been performed with this approach. One of them compared a sample of Han Chinese who stuttered with a non-stuttering control group with respect to two genes known to be associated with ADHD (attention deficit hyperactivity disorder), a disorder that shows increased prevalence with stuttering (Lan et al. 2009). A mutation in DRD2 was identified in the stuttering group. DRD2 is a dopamine receptor gene that is very active in the reward centres of the brain. It has been identified as a reinforcement gene and theoretically fits well with models of dopamine excess, which has been found to occur in stuttering (Giraud et al. 2008). Validation of this gene for stuttering aetiology will require replication in larger cohorts.

In another linkage-based candidate gene analysis (Kang et al. 2010), researchers revisited regions on chromosome 12 reviewed earlier from the above-mentioned Pakistani families (Riaz et al. 2005). Several re-analyses in the Pakistani population and analyses in American-British people who stutter found mutations on the GNPTAB, GNPTG and NAGPA genes, which are involved in lysosomal function and transport (Kang and Drayna 2012). While mutations in NAGPA have not been associated with human disorders so far, mutations in GNPTAB and GNPTG cause mucolipidosis types II and III, i.e. rare lysosomal storage disorders, leading to pathology of bone, connective tissue, liver, spleen and brain. Biochemical studies of the mutant enzymes encoded by NAGPA have shown that the mutations found in stuttering reduce the overall cellular activity of this enzyme by about half, and that they result in deficits in intracellular processing that lead to a reduced cellular metabolite half-life. Although it is unknown so far how such deficits may lead to stuttering, these results stimulate new approaches to this pathology, including studies in mice carrying human stuttering mutations (Kang and Drayna 2012). Some criticisms oppose the generalisability of the named findings with these arguments: (a) chromosome 12 has not been confirmed as being associated with stuttering in any other linkage study (Shugart et al. 2004; Suresh et al. 2006; Wepman 1939) and in a GWAS (Kraft 2010); (b) the findings are based mainly on an extended Pakistani family which is highly inbred; (c) the conclusive association of lysosomal dysfunction with stuttering is not proven; (d) the GNPTAB mutation was only found in 4% of the sample of 316 unrelated stuttering subjects; (e) the NAGPA mutations were only found in 1% of the investigated persons who stutter (7 of 393). These numbers are too small for associating those genes causatively with stuttering. As of late, linkage studies have stalled and new technologies aimed at case–control GWAS designs have been gaining momentum.

Genetic association is the above-chance occurrence of two or more traits in a population, of which at least one trait is known to be genetic. It may occur between phenotypes, such as weight, between a phenotype and a genetic polymorphism, such as a SNP, or between two genetic polymorphisms. Association studies are based on the assumption that a heritable risk for a disease (or trait) is mostly referable to only a relatively small number of genetic variants, thus in *association* with the trait. Such studies test whether single-SNPs (of millions of them) or genotype frequencies differ between two groups of individuals, e.g. people who stutter and non-stuttering controls, on the basis of the condition that genotypes can be compared 'directly', i.e. with the sequences of the actual genomes. The fascinating aspect here is that such studies do not need a priori hypotheses for specific loci, genes or variants, making them applicable for such complex diseases as stuttering.

Association studies are expected to identify common variants (alleles) that are identifiable more in those affected than in unaffected subjects. Such alleles may directly affect disease risk or are in *linkage disequilibrium* with population statistics. This term is used in population genetics (the study of the distributions and changes of allele frequency in a population) for the non-random association of alleles at two or more loci, not necessarily on the same chromosome.

Association studies are more powerful than linkage studies for identifying genetic risk in complex disorders. *Genome-wide association studies (GWAS)* apply scanning markers across complete genomes (entire sets of DNA) of many unrelated individuals for detecting variations in association with a particular disease or trait. GWAS compare the DNA from large cohorts of people with the trait to cohorts of people without the trait by reading millions of genetic variants using SNP arrays (microscopic slides with open-ended probes targeted at specific sections of DNA with known sequencing). Current platforms can sample more than 5 million SNPs from a single participant. If one allele is more frequent in the patients, the SNP counts as 'associated' with the disease or trait. The associated SNPs mark a region of the human genome that potentially influences the risk of disease. GWAS are non-candidate-driven in contrast to gene-specific candidate-driven studies. These studies identify SNPs and other variants in DNA which are associated with a disease, but cannot specify cause on their own (Manolio 2010). GWAS enable the unique analysis of large population-based cohorts instead of small families, and sample across the whole human genome to detect variations that are only a single nucleotide in size. Association studies have been used to investigate other complex polygenic speech and language conditions such as autism, Tourette syndrome and developmental language disorders. GWAS appear to be most promising for gene discovery and replication in developmental stuttering (Kraft 2010). Ten candidate genes have been found with relevance to (a) neural development, (b) neural function and (c) behaviour (Kraft and Yairi 2012); however, a major necessity for the generalisability of such findings is replication. This requires collaborative genetic consortium projects with data sharing from multiple research sites using shared platforms, diagnostic criteria and methodology.

A global collaboration of investigators through the International Stuttering Project (ISP) collected nearly 1500 DNA samples from people who stutter and compared them to roughly 6800 matched controls of diverse ancestry (Polikowsky et al. 2021). The case–control design of a GWAS is powered to detect population-based variants among unrelated individuals. This study, published in 2021, identified SSUH2, a mutation found not only in people who stutter, but previously in studies of oral anatomy, dentition and tooth formation (Xiong et al. 2017). The pathophysiological mechanisms of SSUH2 for developmental stuttering are yet to be untangled; however, biological processes associated with SSUH2 that regulate the formation of oral anatomical structures, having an impact on extracellular organisation and migration, as well as nervous system development and morphogenesis, appear promising. Replication studies as well as imaging-genomics studies of SSUH2 are underway to elucidate the expression of this gene in the motor-speech pathway.

Historically, genetic investigations of stuttering have required the hand collection of DNA (saliva and blood) from participants. Recruitment efforts are time consuming and costly, as people are not hospitalised for stuttering, treatment approaches do not require pharmaceuticals or medical and surgical procedures, and individuals who stutter do not collectively amass with sufficient numbers at speech clinics to statistically power most studies. Under this premise, additional resources are required to make genetic discoveries for complex traits at a population level. The employment of electronic medical records, nationalised health-care systems and biological specimen repositories have become available to facilitate such genetic studies.

A recent study was able to map electronic health records to a biobank repository at Vanderbilt University (USA) for a genetic investigation of stuttering. Using a cohort of individuals data-mined for medical records with diagnostic codes for developmental stuttering or patient records with cohesive descriptions from the physician conclusive of developmental stuttering, a cluster of co-morbid conditions was identified (Pruett et al. 2021). These co-morbid conditions were highly correlated to those identified in many previous co-morbidity studies of stuttering, and include traits of speech and language development, tics, ADHD, social anxiety, allergies and inflammation (Arndt and Healey 2001; Blood et al. 2003; Donaher and Richels 2012), among others. A phenome-risk classifier (predictive risk for stuttering-model) was developed on the basis of the statistical significance of these conditions when compared with matched controls in the biobank who did not stutter. Population prevalence statistics suggest that more than 5% of a human database would represent individuals who stutter (life-time prevalence, i.e. having ever stuttered). Lack of medical treatment by physicians, as outlined above, results in a significant under-representation of patient files with a mention of developmental stuttering. To accommodate this invisible yet present patient group, the phenome-risk classifier was employed. This sophisticated algorithm was designed to predict who in the repository could be inferred to have a stutter (Shaw et al. 2021). Thus, a first-ever biobank GWAS was conducted. More than 9000 genotyped samples for those with the inferred stuttering phenotype were analyzed with nearly 100,000 controls. Two subsequent variants were identified as reaching genome-wide significance. The first, FAM49A, was located on chromosome 2 in European participants and ZMAT4 was identified on chromosome 8 in participants with African ancestry.

Both FAM49A and ZMAT4 are highly expressed in the brain. FAM49A is a signalling protein that has been previously associated with cleft palate. ZMAT4 is a zinc-finger protein that has been implicated in near-sighted vision and blood glucose-level regulation in African Americans. Looking at where these genes specifically express themselves in the brain is the next step to investigate their relationship to stuttering. Cortical regions of the motor cortex as well as robust expression patterns in the basal ganglia can be seen in the Allen Human Brian Atlas for both FAM49A and ZMAT4. Incidentally, both genes demonstrate a left-dominant expression pattern and are being studied further for direct pathogenic and neurogenic mechanisms driving speech production.

Environmental and behavioural factors such as stress, illness, diet, income, exercise, toxins, and pollution can significantly alter the way genes express themselves in the body. The dynamic of epigenetics is unique, as phenotypic changes can occur in the absence of a mutation in the DNA sequence. Behavioural and environmental contributions to the human experience have the ability to regulate genes via methylation, histone modification and RNA gene silencing. These three mechanisms of epigenetic regulation can turn off a gene entirely, prevent regions of the genome from being accessible for replication and thus expression, or block expression by binding non-coding RNA to portions of DNA.

How does this contribute to our perspective of stuttering? Stuttering is a complex polygenic condition, caused by the combined action of more than one gene. As polygenic disorders depend on the simultaneous presence of several genes, they are not inherited in monogenic Mendelian forms. *Whole-exome sequencing* is a procedure to selectively and efficiently sequence the protein coding regions of the genome (approximately 1.5% of DNA) as a more affordable but still effective alternative to whole-genome sequencing, as exon regions are thought to constitute about 85% of disease-causing mutations (Choi et al. 2009). Exome sequencing is particularly suited for discovering highly penetrant coding variants and possibly an unexplained proportion of disease heritability. Candidate genes for Mendelian disorders have been identified by exome sequencing a small number of unrelated affected individuals. This strategy may extend to diseases with more complex genetics and appears quite promising in the near future once larger sample sizes and appropriate weighting of non-synonymous variants according to their likely functional impact, such as stuttering, are undertaken. It has yet, however, to be applied.

Still, common genetic variants explain only a moderate fraction of heritable risk for common disease. Common variants are inherently non-deleterious, as they have a high prevalence in any given population and the individual expression has only a small effect on the organism. Larger more extreme effects on expression are not commonly found in populations, as social preference, selective mating and functional impact is substantial. Mutations of this nature are typically driven by rare variants displaying a large effect and are often family-, founder- or region-specific. When working to model polygenic risk for stuttering, we are looking for a large set of common variants, not a small set of rare variants. To power such studies sufficiently to detect population-wide common variants driving a complex polygenic condition such as stuttering, large-scale genome-wide association studies must be conducted.

6.4.1.5 Implications for the Future of Counselling, Therapy and Research

From the above findings regarding the genetic and environmentally associated underpinnings of persistent developmental stuttering, consequences can be derived for diagnosis, treatment and counselling of individuals who stutter and their families. Improved therapeutic outcomes and better long-term prognosis can be expected in the future (Yairi et al. 1996). We want to highlight that heritability does not preclude modifiability, as it is not a natural constant, and high heritability does not diminish the benefits of symptom-oriented therapeutic interventions, as it only indicates the proportion of variability attributable to genetic differences (Howie 1981a).

Understanding how genetic risk predominantly drives stuttering susceptibility alleviates parents from placing blame on environmental influences and has implications for the counselling of parents and their possible self-reproaches. Except for their hereditary dowry, parents do not make a causal contribution to the primary onset or occurrence of their child's stutter and are not responsible for its onset. In addition to the genetic influences on stuttering, the contribution of environmental factors has to be taken into consideration with more research because 'DNA is both inherited and genetically responsive' (Kang et al. 2010, p. 44). The gene–environment interaction has become an increasingly important research topic and may eventually become more accessible if we understand how to modify gene expression and mitigate the severity of symptoms. Perhaps preventive strategies or gene-induced recovery will become possible along the way (Ambrose et al. 1997). Corresponding biophysiological studies may soon follow the new genetic findings discussed in this section.

Gene therapies have made tremendous progress in the last decade. Clinical applications in cardiovascular disease, immunodeficiency diseases and neuropsychiatric disease such as Parkinson's disease, Alzheimer disease and some paediatric diseases are successfully being trialled and marketed (Gelfand and Kaplitt 2012). The complete aetiological architecture of stuttering has yet to be mapped, but definitive genetic variants contributing to risk and their organic-functional consequences have just recently been acknowledged. While the traits and types of behaviour of stuttering are still the focus of current stuttering therapies (which are inherently symptomatic and not causal), treatments are evolving as we gain more aetiological knowledge. Genetic research is tremendously important for all clinical aspects. Identifying, diagnosing and hopefully causally treating stuttering may be possible in the future by elucidating the contribution of certain genes to disrupt fluent speech production. It is also expected that treatment, in particular early treatment, might be more targeted than it has been in the past by modifying gene expression. Additionally, persistent stuttering after behavioural therapy should no longer be considered a treatment failure, as it may be more strongly attributed to a specific genetic predisposition (Yairi and Ambrose 2005). Genetic findings may also guide pharmaceutical approaches in a more targeted manner (Maguire et al. 2010), as it has for the treatment of Alzheimer's disease. It took only 10 years from the first identified causal genetic mutation in Alzheimer's disease to the first positive outcome of a gene therapy.

6.4.2 Aetiology of Syndrome-Associated Stuttering

In response to the fact that persistent developmental stuttering is associated with structural and functional cerebral changes, a German guideline on speech fluency disorders recently recommended that it (also) be referred to as 'originary neurogenic non-syndromic stuttering'. From this frequent form of stuttering, the rare syndrome-associated (persistent developmental) stuttering (referred to as 'originary neurogenic syndromic stuttering' in the German guideline) or the occurrence of stuttering-like symptoms, which is often associated with various genetic syndromes, should be distinguished (Neumann et al. 2016, 2017a, b). In particular, in Down syndrome, fragile X syndrome, Prader–Willi syndrome, Tourette syndrome, neurofibromatosis type I and Turner syndrome, stuttering is mentioned as a feature. However, a review of these syndromes demonstrates that affected individuals exhibit speech disfluencies, not all of which correspond to 'classic' stuttering. Some of these stuttering patterns are only characteristic of a certain syndrome or similar syndromes, as is the case with Prader-Willi syndrome or Tourette syndrome (Van Borsel and Tetnowski 2007). Many of the stutter-associated syndromes are characterised by varying degrees of intellectual disability, which likely contributes to a higher-than-average prevalence of stuttering compared with the typical population. This is not to claim that cognitive impairments are in any way causal to stuttering, but rather to suggest that their association with stuttering is more common because of limited cognitive abilities to mitigate or compensate for motor-speech disruptions in order to maintain or restore speech fluency. In syndromes with intellectual disability, speech disfluency patterns that are atypical of stuttering and sometimes clutter-like often occur and must be considered symptomatic for syndrome-associated cognitive and linguistic deficits such as word retrieval difficulties or lexical deficits (Coppens-Hofman et al. 2013).

6.4.3 Aetiology of Acquired Stuttering

If stuttering begins after the age of 12, an acquired neurogenic or psychogenic form of stuttering should be considered (Fig. 6.1) (Natke and Alpermann 2010; Neumann et al. 2016, 2017a, b). Psychogenic stuttering has recently often been referred to as functional acquired stuttering (Theys and De Nil 2022), a term that seems rather obfuscating. According to the ICD-11 nomenclature (WHO 2024), this type of stuttering belongs to category 6B60.5 (dissociative neurological symptom disorder, with speech disturbance) and should therefore be better referred to as dissociative stuttering. Neurogenic stuttering can occur at any time in life and is typically diagnosed with evidence of a temporal relation between the onset of stuttering symptoms and an acute or chronic brain injury. Compared with persistent developmental stuttering, acquired stuttering is rare and is usually distinguishable from the former by its aetiology, symptoms, age of manifestation and therapeutic influenceability.

6.4.3.1 Aetiology of Neurogenic Stuttering

Acquired neurogenic speech disfluencies are usually caused by acute or chronic injuries of the brain. As persistent developmental stuttering is also characterised by subtle structural and functional abnormalities of the brain, the former terminological distinction between developmental and

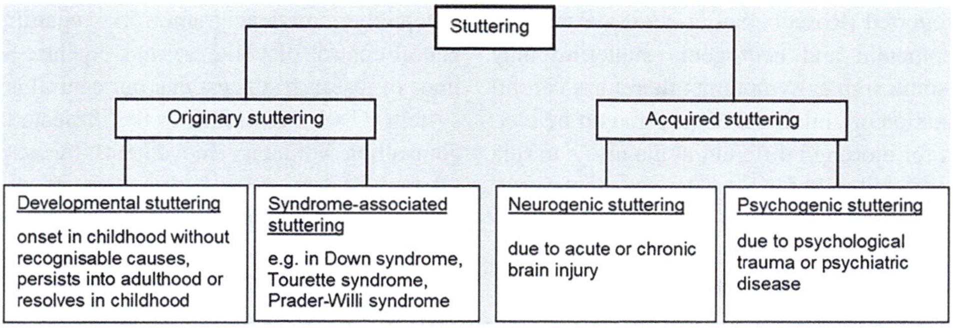

Fig. 6.1 Classification of stuttering according to its aetiology

neurogenic stuttering has limited applicability nowadays. A proposal to differentiate terminologically between originary neurogenic non-syndromic (persistent developmental) stuttering and syndromic stuttering as developmental forms of stuttering on the one hand and acquired neurogenic and psychogenic (or dissociative) stuttering on the other can be found, as mentioned above, in the German evidence-based guideline on speech fluency disorders (Neumann et al. 2017a, b). When diagnosing stuttering, attention should always be paid to symptoms of other neurological or neuropsychiatric disorders; if there are indications of acquired forms of stuttering, a comprehensive neuropsychological history and diagnosis is necessary.

Acute brain lesions such as strokes, intracerebral haemorrhage, asphyxia or head trauma may result in stuttering-like speech symptoms (Lundgren et al. 2010). Chronic or progressive neurological disorders such as Parkinson's disease also appear to be associated with a higher than average prevalence of stuttering (Maguire et al. 2012). In rare documented cases, neurogenic stuttering may be caused by drugs or medications (Van Borsel and Tetnowski 2007). Neurogenic stuttering may occur after diffuse, circumscribed, uni- or bi- lateral injuries in almost all regions of the brain (De Nil et al. 2007; Lundgren et al. 2010; Theys 2012; Theys et al. 2008, 2011, 2013). If caused by an acute brain damage, it is associated with a lesion in the left hemisphere in more than the half of cases. The temporal relationship between the acute lesion and the occurrence of stuttering symptoms is important for diagnosis. In most cases of neurogenic stuttering resulting from stroke or a trauma, onset of symptoms starts within one week after injury. Symptoms may, however, also occur weeks or even months later (Neumann et al. 2016, 2017a). Depending on the localisation, type and extent of brain lesions, the clinical picture of neurogenic stuttering is very heterogeneous, and individual trajectories and prognoses are inconsistent (Theys 2012; Theys et al. 2008). Stuttering symptoms may appear suddenly or gradually; a developmental stutter that may have existed before the injury may worsen, or already resolved symptoms may recur (De Nil et al. 2007). In cases of neurodegenerative brain injury, stuttering may develop slowly or suddenly. In many cases, neurogenic stuttering is associated with psychological symptoms and is accompanied by other communication pathologies such as aphasia or dysarthria. As in other forms of stuttering, severity may be exaggerated during episodes of increased cognitive or psychologic load.

Other neurogenic disorders of speech and language may worsen speech fluency and complicate the differential diagnosis of neurogenic stuttering. Disfluencies related to aphasia are clearly distinguishable from stuttering in most cases, because they accompany difficulties in word retrieval and in the expression of sounds, words and sentences. However, in cases of conduction aphasia (language disorders due to lesions of the arcuate fasciculus, which provides information transfer of perceived speech sequences from Wernicke's area to Broca's area, where speech production is planned), spasm-like repetition and self-correction attempts may occur, usually involving content words, and may be accompanied by stutter-like sound repetitions (Goodglass 1981).

Additionally, in cases of combined aphasia-apraxia patients, stutter-like symptoms have also been reported (Rosenbek et al. 1978). Persistent developmental and neurogenic stuttering may share some similar symptoms; therefore, careful examination of childhood history should be conducted for thorough differential diagnosis to rule out premorbid mild forms of developmental stuttering (De Nil et al. 2007; Jokel et al. 2007).

6.4.3.2 Aetiology of Psychogenic Stuttering

Though rare, psychogenic (or dissociative) stuttering almost always occurs suddenly and in association with psychological trauma or underlying psychiatric illness. It occurs in most cases after puberty, with no evidence of a chronic or acute neurological disorder (Mahr and Leith 1992). Unlike persistent developmental stuttering, the sex ratio ranges from 1:1 to 2.7:1 of females to males (Zückner and Ebel 2001). It is important to note that parents sometimes report that their child's stuttering began with psychological trauma (Yairi and Ambrose 1992). However, while an incisive psychological event could at best trigger a stuttering onset, a causal attribution of the development of clinical stuttering symptoms (typically between the ages of 2 and 6 years) to a psychogenic genesis of stuttering does not seem justified according to the generally accepted opinion of experts and researchers. Instead, such parental reports mostly reflect subjective causal attributions based on the coincidence in time of significant life events and do not allow for causal implications (Neumann et al. 2016, 2017a).

6.5 Speech and Non-speech Motor Characteristics of Stuttering

Ayoub Daliri and Ludo Max

6.5.1 Theoretical Framework: Feedforward and Feedback Control of Movements

Understanding the basic sensorimotor mechanisms underlying stuttering requires that we consider the relevant empirical findings in an accepted theoretical framework regarding the neural control of voluntary movements. Several lines of research suggest that our central nervous system (CNS) accomplishes the intricate task of controlling voluntary movements by acquiring internal models of the body's own effector systems and environment (i.e. internal representations of the motor-to-sensory transformations). These internal models can then be accessed to (a) determine the motor commands that will achieve a desired movement goal, (b) predict desired as well as undesired sensory consequences associated with the execution of those control signals and (c) optimise task-dependent feedback gains (Scott 2004; Shadmehr and Wise 2005; Shadmehr and Krakauer 2008).

Figure 6.2 schematically represents one possible conceptualisation of sensorimotor control. The model reflects a hybrid controller that resolves the dichotomy between feedforward and feedback theories of motor control. In the hybrid scheme, a control component (or control policy) generates a motor plan before movement onset, but it also sets the feedback gains that determine to what extent the planned motor commands will be modified on the basis of sensory information before and during the movement. Thus, the feedforward controller (upper three boxes in Fig. 6.2) determines and generates the motor commands that will achieve an intended movement goal. This is accomplished by accessing internal inverse models that are stored neural representations of which motor commands will result in the desired sensory consequences given the current properties of the system and environment (Shadmehr et al. 2010). The feedback controller (bottom two boxes in Fig. 6.2) adjusts movements not only on the basis of incoming sensory information but also by predicting the movements' sensory consequences with internal forward models and an efference copy of the motor commands (Shadmehr and Wise 2005). Internal forward models are stored neural representations of which sensory consequences will result from a set of motor commands given the current properties of the system and environment (Miall and Wolpert 1996). Using such sensory predictions, the CNS does not have to wait for sensory sig-

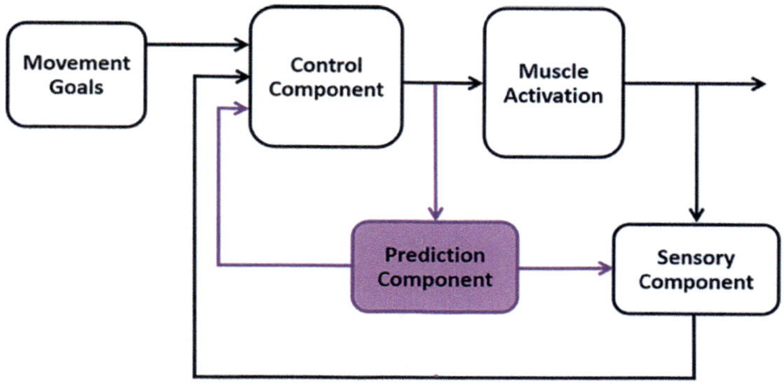

Fig. 6.2 Simplified representation of a contemporary model of sensorimotor control. Movements are pre-planned by a control component but also adjusted online by estimating the system's state from sensory predictions and actual sensory input

nals to indicate movement errors. Rather, it can correct motor commands in an anticipatory manner on the basis of the predicted outcome. In addition, sensory predictions influence the subsequent processing of real sensory inputs (e.g. differences in processing depending on whether the actual input matches the predicted input). At any given time, the best estimate of the system's state is obtained by combining the information that is available from predicted and actual sensory signals (Houde and Nagarajan 2011; Shadmehr et al. 2010).

Below, we summarise the results of selected studies on the involvement of sensorimotor deficiencies in stuttering. In each subsection, we describe which aspects of the described theoretical framework are more likely to be involved in completing the task.

6.5.2 Even the Fluent Speech of Individuals Who Stutter Is Subtly Different from That of Individuals Who Do Not Stutter

Acoustic and physiological methods have been used to investigate several characteristics of the perceptually fluent speech of stuttering speakers (i.e. speech that does not include noticeable moments of stuttering). The purpose of these studies was to examine speech that was not contaminated by stuttering itself (or by the speaker's reactions to the stuttering) and to determine whether subtle neuromotor differences between stuttering and non-stuttering speakers can be detected even in the absence of overt stuttering. In the context of the theoretical framework described above, these studies provide information about the combined use of both the feedforward pathway (i.e. planning and executing) and the feedback pathway (i.e. predicting, monitoring and correcting) as actual speech production involves both these components.

Acoustic studies analyse the speaker's sound output, for example the duration of various intervals in the speech signal. One example of a commonly used measure is the voice onset time (VOT), which is essential for distinguishing voiced and voiceless stop consonants (e.g. VOT is shorter in /b/ vs. longer in /p/). VOT is defined as the interval between the burst resulting from the release of an articulatory obstruction for a stop consonant and the onset of a periodic signal associated with vocal fold vibration for the subsequent vowel (Fig. 6.3). Thus, VOT reflects the elapsed time between an articulatory and a phonatory event in the production of a consonant–vowel syllable. Numerous researchers have found longer VOTs for stuttering speakers than for non-stuttering speakers, in particular for adult subjects (see Max 2004). In addition, stuttering speakers have also been reported to show more variable VOTs than non-stuttering speakers (Jancke 1994). It should be acknowledged, however, that there are also some studies that have failed to find such between-group differences (Borden et al. 1987; De Nil and Brutten 1991; Jancke 1994). This inconsistency appears to be due, in part, to factors such as sound and word characteristics (e.g. specific consonant, word length), subject characteristics (e.g. age, sex,

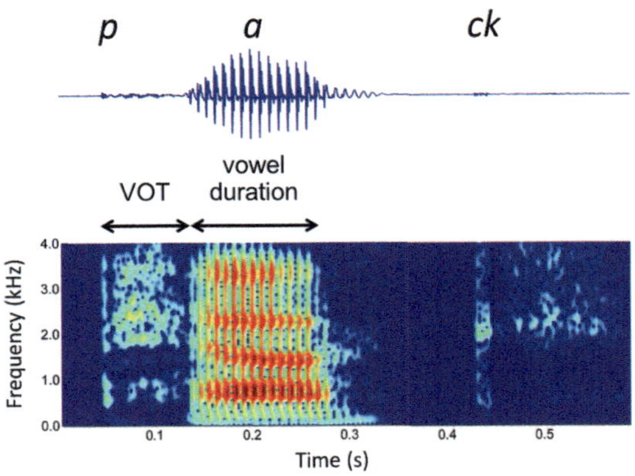

Fig. 6.3 Time domain representation (top) and time-frequency representation (bottom) of a production of the word 'pack'. Arrows indicate two measures commonly used in acoustic analyses of speech: voice onset time (VOT) and vowel duration. Frequency bands in red correspond to resonance frequencies of the vocal tract (formants)

speech rate, stuttering severity, prior treatment) and the number of completed trials (see below for more information on limited practice effects in stuttering speakers). Overall, however, VOT measurements are typically longer for stuttering speakers.

The above VOT data are described only as an example, and similar findings—i.e. generally longer durations and greater variability for adults who stutter, but with exceptions in some studies—have also been obtained for measurements of other acoustic intervals such as, among others, vowel duration (also illustrated in Fig. 6.3) and syllable or word duration (data reviewed in Bloodstein and Bernstein Ratner 2008). One consequence of these longer acoustic interval durations in stuttering speakers is that not only speech rate (i.e. syllables or words per minute, but often including pauses and disfluencies) but also articulation rate (i.e. the number of sounds produced per second, not including pauses or disfluencies) is slower in individuals who stutter than in individuals who do not (Bloodstein and Bernstein Ratner 2008).

Whereas the aforementioned studies have investigated stuttering individuals' temporal characteristics of speech production in the acoustic signal, several other studies have relied on direct kinematic measures of the involved articulatory movements. Tracking movements of the lips and jaw (and sometimes the tongue), these studies too have revealed that stuttering and non-stuttering speakers differ primarily in the duration of various movement intervals, with stuttering individuals showing longer durations between two articulatory events or between articulatory and phonatory events (e.g. Max et al. 2003; Zimmermann 1980).

Taken together, these acoustic and kinematic studies have made it clear that even the perceptually fluent speech of individuals who stutter differs, in subtle ways, from the speech of individuals who do not stutter. What remains unknown, especially in light of the fact that between-group differences have been found less consistently for stuttering vs. non-stuttering children, is whether the observed slowness in adults who stutter reflects a basic sensorimotor limitation or, alternatively, a preferred movement strategy that compensates for other, more fundamental deficits (Max 2004).

6.5.3 Reaction Times Are Longer in Individuals Who Stutter Than in Individuals Who Do Not Stutter

Another paradigm that has been widely used to examine the speech sensorimotor system of stuttering vs. non-stuttering individuals has focused on the ability to initiate movements under time pressure. In reaction time studies, subjects respond as fast as possible to a 'go' signal, either with a speech response or with a non-speech response such as a button press. In the context of our theoretical framework, this paradigm addresses the feedforward pathway, as movements are performed in a ballistic manner (with insufficient time for feedback corrections).

A large number of studies have investigated vocalisation-related reaction times of stuttering individuals by asking subjects to initiate a vowel, a syllable or a complete word as quickly as possible (Bloodstein and Bernstein Ratner 2008). With very few exceptions, these studies found that the reaction time of stuttering individuals is longer than that of non-stuttering individuals regardless of the linguistic or non-linguistic context of the motor response. Similar results have been reported from studies in which subjects responded with a non-speech act such as a button press or other finger movement (Max 2004).

Similar to the above studies on temporal aspects of perceptually fluent speech, reaction time studies with young children (below 7 years of age) have often found no between-group differences for stuttering vs. non-stuttering subjects (e.g. Anderson and Wagovich 2010; Arnold et al. 2005), whereas significant differences have been reported for older children (McKnight and Cullinan 1987). Thus, findings are again compatible with the possibility that the longer reaction times in stuttering individuals may reflect a learned strategy to compensate for underlying sensorimotor difficulties.

6.5.4 Motor Learning Is Limited in Individuals Who Stutter

When learning a new motor skill or refining a previously learned motor skill, the CNS builds or updates the internal models described above in our theoretical framework. That is, skilled motor performance is based on accurately determining the motor commands that will achieve a desired movement outcome (i.e. sensory state) and accurately predicting the desired as well as undesired sensory consequences of the planned motor commands (and compensating as necessary). Hence, stuttering individuals' ability to acquire and update these neural representations of the motor-to-sensory transformations involved in the control of voluntary movements can be investigated with various motor learning tasks.

From a review of reaction time studies, Smits-Bandstra (2010) concluded that stuttering and non-stuttering individuals differ in the extent of practice effects during sensorimotor experiments. Specifically, such practice effects may be more limited in stuttering individuals. This suggestion is interesting in light of the fact that one of the most studied aspects of stuttering is the adaptation effect—a gradual reduction in the frequency of stuttering over successive oral readings of the same material (Bloodstein and Bernstein Ratner 2008). Although several explanations have been proposed for this adaptation effect, the most compelling interpretation is that this fluency improvement is in fact due to motor learning (Max and Baldwin 2010; Max and Caruso 1998). For example, in a study by Max and Baldwin (2010), stuttering participants read a passage out loud five times during an initial session, five times during a retention session after 2 h, and five times during a second retention session after 24 h. The passages contained a mix of repeated sentences (occurring in each passage) and novel sentences (occurring in only one passage). Results showed a reduction in stuttering frequency for both the repeated and novel sentences, but with a greater decrease for the repeated sentences. Most importantly, after 24 h, the fluency improvement for novel sentences had been lost whereas the improvement for repeated sentences was partially retained. These results strongly suggest that motor practice does lead to improvements in speech fluency in individuals who stutter.

Comparing stuttering and non-stuttering speakers, De Nil and co-workers investigated motor learning by using sequence-learning tasks with speech (reading a sequence of syllables) or non-speech movements (tapping a sequence of finger movements) (Smits-Bandstra et al. 2006; Smits-Bandstra and De Nil 2013; Bauerly and De Nil 2011). The same studies also examined the effect of a concurrent secondary task on the rate of sequence learning. Results showed that stuttering individuals are slower in learning speech and non-speech sequences, as evident by smaller improvements in reaction time and movement duration. Stuttering individuals' performance was also more strongly affected by the secondary task. Moreover, during retention and transfer testing after 24 h, the stuttering group demonstrated slower and more variable performance than at the end of the initial practice session. In other words, the stuttering group did not maintain the level of skill acquired during the practice session. Namasivayam and Van Lieshout (2008) obtained similar results in a task in which subjects repeatedly produced bisyllabic non-words:

compared with a non-stuttering group, the group of stuttering speakers showed more limited changes in movement stability and coordination. In an arm movement study from our own lab, stuttering adults were less accurate in reaching to visual targets, and this deficit did not disappear with practice (Daliri et al. 2014).

More recently, a different type of learning has been investigated as a window into the central nervous system's updating of the internal models described above in our theoretical framework. Specifically, the input to a sensory feedback modality (for speech typically auditory feedback) is experimentally manipulated to alter the relationship between motor command inputs and sensory consequences. Hence, in order to produce accurate speech sounds, the system needs to update its internal representation of this relationship. In these paradigms, participants produce speech while hearing perturbed auditory feedback, and data analysis focuses on changes in the participants' speech output across the perturbed trials. One commonly used feedback perturbation involves a real-time shift in the frequency of one or more formants. As illustrated in Fig. 6.4, in studies with such formant shift perturbations, adults who stutter show very limited auditory-motor adaptation when compared with non-stuttering control participants (Daliri and Max 2018; Daliri et al. 2018). In one study that perturbed only the first formant, this between-group difference was observed only for adults and not for children (Daliri et al. 2018). However, in our ongoing work with a perturbation applied to all formants (identical to the shift used with adults in Fig. 6.4), the between-group difference is also present when comparing stuttering and non-stuttering children in the range 3–9 years of age (Kim et al. 2020).

Combined, these motor learning studies suggest that as a group, people who stutter learn speech and non-speech movements and movement sequences more slowly and less completely than those who do not stutter, and that their performance is more susceptible to interference by a secondary task. Additionally, stuttering individuals show reduced retention of any performance gains made during motor practice. Sensorimotor integration during learning appears to be limited in this population. On the other hand, individuals who stutter do show substantial benefits of motor learning in the form of reductions in speech dysfluency during repeated readings of the same material.

6.5.5 Sensorimotor Integration in Individuals Who Stutter Also Differs Outside of the Context of Motor Learning

In our theoretical framework, both predicted and actual sensory consequences are critical for correcting movements that will not achieve the

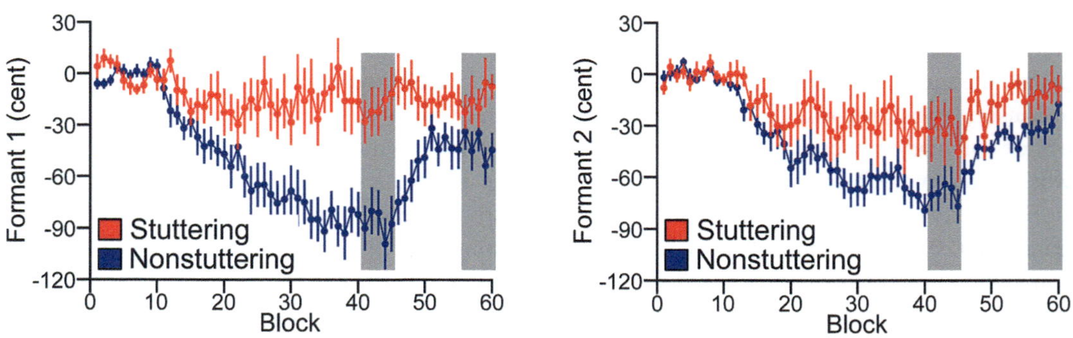

Fig. 6.4 Changes in acoustic speech output (Formant 1 on the left and Formant 2 on the right) when participants produced the monosyllabic words 'bed', 'bud' and 'baud' while hearing auditory feedback in which all formants were shifted 250 cents up in trial blocks 11–45 (one production of each word per block). Auditory-motor adaptation is substantially reduced in the stuttering group as compared with the non-stuttering group. Figure adapted from Daliri and Max (2018) with permission from Elsevier

desired outcome. In the previous subsection, we discussed the contribution of a mismatch between predicted and actual consequences to motor learning. If movement duration is sufficiently long, the detection of such a mismatch can also be used to correct movements online during execution. Stuttering adults' ability to implement online corrections—i.e. integrating predicted and actual sensory information to generate corrective motor commands that adjust ongoing movements—has also been investigated with sensory perturbation paradigms. In this case, sensory feedback is perturbed in random trials such that subjects cannot learn to adapt their movements in an anticipatory manner. Thus, quickly implemented corrections (compensation) occur within the individual trials that are perturbed, and the corrections are a reaction to incorrect sensory information rather than a result of sensorimotor learning. For example, Caruso et al. (1987) applied mechanical loads to the lower lip that perturbed its contribution to lip closure for the bilabial consonant in 'apa'. Results showed a significantly smaller compensatory response to the load perturbation in the stuttering group than in the non-stuttering group. More recently, two studies have demonstrated that stuttering subjects also show reduced compensatory responses to auditory perturbations such as pitch shifts (Loucks et al. 2012) and formant shifts (Cai et al. 2012). Hence, sensorimotor integration appears impaired in adults who stutter.

One intriguing possibility is that both the difficulty to update internal models appropriately during motor learning and the limited implementation of online corrections during ongoing movements relate to a common, more fundamental, problem with the use of sensory information for motor control. Stuttering individuals may be unable to use sensory prediction mechanisms to 'prime' task-relevant sensory systems. This, in turn, may affect the monitoring of afferent inputs for online feedback control, and result in feedback-based motor responses that are undesirable during self-generated voluntary movements (the latter is an idea that overlaps with suggestions by Zimmermann et al. 1981). Limited evidence consistent with this hypothesis had been available from work by McClean (1996) who demonstrated that, compared with fluent speakers, stuttering adults show less attenuation of mechanically-evoked lip muscle reflexes before the onset of speech (with lip muscle activity measured in speech trials vs. no speech trials). If participating sensory systems (auditory, somatosensory) are insufficiently modulated in terms of their response to self-generated afferent inputs, motor responses may be triggered that interfere with, and disrupt, ongoing movements. However, it remained unknown for a long time whether stuttering individuals' atypical sensorimotor responses at speech onset were in fact due to a lack of central modulation of sensory neural systems, and if so, whether a lack of such pre-speech sensory modulation occurs within the auditory system.

Over the last decade, we have studied these questions directly with electro-encephalography (EEG) and auditory-evoked potential analyses to quantify the modulation of cortical auditory activity elicited by probe tones delivered immediately before speaking vs. during carefully matched control conditions without speaking (Daliri and Max 2015a, b). By means of an experimental paradigm that we previously developed for work with typically fluent speakers (Max et al. 2008), we record long latency auditory evoked potentials (LLAEPs) in response to a pure tone stimulus presented during the delay phase of a delayed-response speaking task (subjects see a monosyllabic word on a computer monitor, silently read the word and prepare to produce it, but only produce it after a visual go signal is presented). These LLAEPs are compared with those in response to the same auditory stimulus presented during a silent reading task (subjects see a monosyllabic word on the computer monitor, silently read the word, and ignore the visual go signal) and, sometimes, an additional seeing task (subjects see non-linguistic symbols on the computer monitor and ignore the visual go signal). In an initial study with only fluent speakers, we found that—during speech movement planning—non-stuttering speakers showed a reduction in amplitude of the auditory N100 component in the LLAEP (Max et al.

2008). In later studies, however, we found that stuttering speakers did not show such auditory modulation: during speech movement planning, the stuttering speakers' auditory N100 amplitude did not differ from that observed during silent reading or seeing non-linguistic symbols (Daliri and Max 2015a, b, 2018; Max and Daliri 2019).

In our most recent pre-speech auditory modulation study, we added a condition in which the auditory feedback signal was experimentally delayed by 100 ms (a speaking condition that is fluency-enhancing for many individuals who stutter). Stuttering and non-stuttering adults were then compared for the amount of pre-speech auditory modulation in both the non-altered auditory feedback (NAF) condition and the delayed auditory feedback (DAF) condition. First, we confirmed that with NAF typically fluent speakers do show the modulation but stuttering speakers do not (Fig. 6.5a, b). Second, for the majority of non-stuttering participants, less modulation was observed in the DAF condition than in the NAF condition; however, most of the stuttering participants showed an increase, rather than decrease, in pre-speech auditory modulation in the DAF condition vs. the NAF condition (Fig. 6.5c). In fact, as a group the stuttering individuals showed a statistically significant modulation of the auditory N100 response only before speaking with DAF, and the between-group difference was no longer statistically significant in this condition.

It can therefore be speculated that (a) in individuals who stutter, an auditory-motor integration deficiency related to movement planning and sensory prediction may contribute to inefficient feedback monitoring when speaking with NAF, and (b) for at least some individuals who stutter, this deficiency is alleviated when speaking with DAF.

6.5.6 Conclusions

Overall, the studies included in this mini-review indicate that stuttering is associated with generalised sensorimotor deficits, in particular in the areas of sensorimotor integration and motor learning. The common finding of speech and non-speech movement slowness in individuals who stutter may reflect a preferred movement strategy that copes with the fundamental limitations in sensorimotor integration and learning. These results and interpretations are highly consistent with those from numerous neuroimaging studies suggesting abnormalities in the connectivity and functional interaction of premotor, motor and sensory brain regions in both children and adults who stutter (reviewed in Sect. 8.6).

6.5.6.1 Remark

This chapter is based on Max and Daliri (2018, 2019), both published open access under Creative Commons license CC BY 4.0.

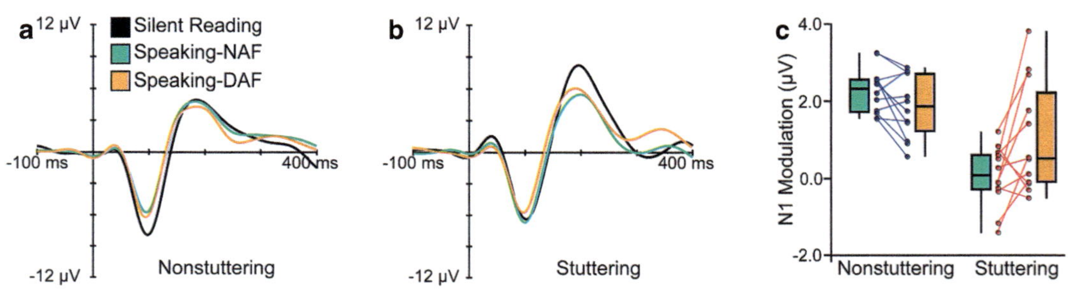

Fig. 6.5 Group average long latency auditory evoked potentials for non-stuttering (**a**) and stuttering (**b**) adults in a pre-speech auditory modulation paradigm. In non-stuttering speakers, the N100 response (i.e. negative peak ~100 ms after sound onset) to probe tones is modulated immediately before speaking with non-altered auditory feedback (NAF) or delayed auditory feedback (DAF) vs. silent reading. In stuttering speakers, this modulation is lacking when speaking with NAF. Most stuttering speakers show an increase in modulation with DAF (**c**), and the between-group difference is no longer statistically significant in this condition. Figure adapted from Daliri and Max (2018) with permission from Elsevier

References

Ajdacic-Gross V, Vetter S, Müller M et al (2010) Risk factors for stuttering: a secondary analysis of a large data base. Eur Arch Psychiatry Clin Neurosci 260:279–286

Ambrose NG, Cox NJ, Yairi E (1997) The genetic basis of persistence and recovery in stuttering. J Speech Lang Hear Res 40:567–580

Anderson JD, Wagovich SA (2010) Relationships among linguistic processing speed, phonological working memory, and attention in children who stutter. J Fluen Disord 35(3):216–234

Andrade CR, Cervone LM, Sassi FC (2003) Relationship between the stuttering severity index and speech rate. Sao Paulo Med J 121(2):81–84

Andrews G, Harris M (1964) The syndrome of stuttering. In: Clinics in developmental medicine, vol 17. William Heineman Medical Books Ltd., London

Andrews G, Craig A, Feyer A et al (1983) Stuttering: a review of research findings and theories circa 1982. J Speech Hear Disord 48(3):226–246

Andrews G, Morris-Yates A, Howie P et al (1991) Genetic factors in stuttering confirmed. Arch Gen Psychiatry 48:1034–1035

APA (2013) Childhood onset fluency disorder. In: Diagnostic and statistical manual of mental disorders, 5th edn. American Psychiatric Publishing, Arlington

Arndt J, Healey EC (2001) Concomitant disorders in school-age children who stutter. Lang Speech Hear Serv Sch 32(2):68–78

Arnold HS, Conture EG, Ohde RN (2005) Phonological neighborhood density in the picture naming of young children who stutter: preliminary study. J Fluen Disord 30(2):125–148

ASHA (1999) Terminology pertaining to fluency and fluency disorders: guidelines [guidelines]. Available via www.asha.org/policy. Accessed 18 September 2019

ASHA (2019) Available via https://www.asha.org/uploadedFiles/ICD-10-Codes-SLP.pdf. Accessed 18 September 2019

Barreiro LB, Laval G, Quach H et al (2008) Natural selection has driven population differentiation in modern humans. Nat Genet 40:340–345

Bauerly KR, De Nil LF (2011) Speech sequence skill learning in adults who stutter. J Fluen Disord 36(4):349–360

Blood GW, Blood IM, Bennett S et al (1994) Subjective anxiety measurements and cortisol responses in adults who stutter. J Speech Hear Res 37(4):760–768

Blood GW, Ridenour VJ, Qualls CD et al (2003) Co-occurring disorders in children who stutter. J Commun Disord 36:427–448

Bloodstein O, Bernstein Ratner N (2008) A handbook on stuttering. Delmar, Clifton Park

Blumgart E, Tran Y, Craig A (2010) Social anxiety disorder in adults who stutter. Depress Anxiety 27(7):687–692

Borden GJ, Kim DH, Spiegler K (1987) Acoustics of stop consonant vowel relationships during fluent and stuttered utterances. J Fluen Disord 12(3):175–184

Bray MA, Kehle TJ, Lawless KA et al (2003) The relationship of self-efficacy and depression to stuttering. Am J Speech Lang Pathol 12(4):425–431

Briley PM, Ellis C (2020) Behavioral, social, and emotional well-being in children who stutter: the influence of race-ethnicity. Logoped Phoniatr Vocol 46(4):171–179

Brutten EJ (1963) Palmar sweat investigation of disfluency and expectancy adaptation. J Speech Hear Res 6:40–48

Bryngelson B, Rutherford B (1937) A comparative study of laterality of stutterers and non-stutterers. J Speech Hear Disord 2:15–16

Byrd C, Werle D, Coalson G et al (2020) Use of monolingual English guidelines to assess stuttering in bilingual speakers: a systematic review. J Monolingual Billing Speech 2(1):1–23

Cai S, Beal DS, Ghosh SS et al (2012) Weak responses to auditory feedback perturbation during articulation in persons who stutter: evidence for abnormal auditory-motor transformation. PLoS One 7(7):e41830

Caruso AJ, Gracco VL, Abbs JH (1987) A speech motor control perspective on stuttering: preliminary observations. In: Peters HFM, Hulstijin W (eds) Speech motor dynamics in stuttering. Springer, New York, pp 245–258

Chang S-E, Garnett EO, Etchell A et al (2018) Functional and neuroanatomical bases of developmental stuttering: current insights. Neuroscientist 25(6):566–582

Choi M, Scholl UI, Ji W et al (2009) Genetic diagnosis by whole exome capture and massively parallel DNA sequencing. Proc Natl Acad Sci USA 106:19096–19101

Conture E (2001) Stuttering, its nature, diagnosis, and treatment. Allyn & Bacon, Boston

Coppens-Hofman MC, Terband HR, Maassen BA et al (2013) Dysfluencies in the speech of adults with intellectual disabilities and reported speech difficulties. J Commun Disord 46:484–494

Craig A, Hancock K, Tran Y et al (2002) Epidemiology of stuttering in the community across the entire life span. J Speech Lang Hear Res 45(6):1097–1105

Curlee RF (1999) Stuttering and related disorders of fluency, 2nd edn. Thieme Medical Publisher Inc., New York

Daliri A, Max L (2015a) Modulation of auditory processing during speech movement planning is limited in adults who stutter. Brain Lang 143:59–68

Daliri A, Max L (2015b) Electrophysiological evidence for a general auditory prediction deficit in adults who stutter. Brain Lang 150:37–44

Daliri A, Max L (2018) Stuttering adults' lack of pre-speech auditory modulation normalizes when speaking with delayed auditory feedback. Cortex 99:55–68

Daliri A, Prokopenko RA, Flanagan JR et al (2014) Control and prediction components of movement planning in stuttering vs. nonstuttering adults. J Speech Lang Hear Res 57(6):2131–2141

Daliri A, Wieland EA, Cai S et al (2018) Auditory-motor adaptation is reduced in adults who stutter but not in

children who stutter. Dev Sci 21(2):12521. https://doi.org/10.1111/desc.12521
De Nil LF, Brutten GJ (1991) Speech-associated attitudes of stuttering and nonstuttering children. J Speech Hear Res 34(1):60–66
De Nil LF, Jokel R, Rochon E (2007) Etiology, symptomatology, and treatment of neurogenic stuttering. In: Conture EG, Curlee RF (eds) Stuttering and related disorders of fluency, 3rd edn. Thieme, New York, pp 326–343
Donaher J, Richels C (2012) Traits of attention deficit/hyperactivity disorder in school-age children who stutter. J Fluen Disord 37:242–252
Dworzynski K, Remington A, Rijsdijk F et al (2007) Genetic etiology in cases of recovered and persistent stuttering in an unselected, longitudinal sample of young twins. Am J Speech Lang Pathol 16(2):161–178
Eggers K, Van Eerdenbrugh S, Byrd CT (2019) Speech disfluencies in bilingual Yiddish-Dutch speaking children. Clin Linguist Phon 34(6):576–592
Ezrati-Vinacour R, Levin I (2004) The relationship between anxiety and stuttering: a multidimensional approach. J Fluen Disord 29(2):135–148
Fagnani C, Fibiger S, Skytthe A et al (2011) Heritability and environmental effects for self-reported periods with stuttering: a twin study from Denmark. Logoped Phoniatr Vocol 36:114–120
Felsenfeld S, Kirk KM, Zhu G et al (2000) A study of the genetic and environmental etiology of stuttering in a selected twin sample. Behav Genet 30(5):359–366
Gelfand Y, Kaplitt MG (2012) Gene therapy for psychiatric disorders. World Neurosurg 80:S32
Giraud AL, Neumann K, Bachoud-Levi AC et al (2008) Severity of dysfluency correlates with basal ganglia activity in persistent developmental stuttering. Brain Lang 104:190–199
Godai U, Tatarelli R, Bonanni G (1976) Stuttering and tics in twins. Acta Genet Med Gemellol 25:369–375
Goodglass H (1981) The syndromes of aphasia: similarities and differences in neurolinguistic features. Top Lang Disord 1:1–14
Guitar B (2006) Stuttering: an integrated approach to its nature and treatment, 3rd edn. Lippincott Williams & Wilkins, Baltimore
Houde JF, Nagarajan SS (2011) Speech production as state feedback control. Front Hum Neurosci 5:82. https://doi.org/10.3389/fnhum.2011.00082
Howie PM (1981a) Concordance for stuttering in monozygotic and dizygotic twin pairs. J Speech Hear Res 24:317–321
Howie PM (1981b) Intrapair similarity in frequency of disfluency in monozygotic and dizygotic twin pairs containing stutterers. Behav Genet 11:227–238
Ingham RJ (1984) Stuttering and behavior therapy: current status and experimental foundations. College-Hill Press, San Diego
Iverach L, Jones M, O'Brian S et al (2009a) Screening for personality disorders among adults seeking speech treatment for stuttering. J Fluen Disord 34(3):173–186
Iverach L, Jones M, O'Brian S et al (2009b) The relationship between mental health disorders and treatment outcomes among adults who stutter. J Fluen Disord 34(1):29–43
Iverach L, O'Brian S, Jones M et al (2010) The five factor model of personality applied to adults who stutter. J Commun Disord 43(2):120–132
Iverach L, Menzies RG, O'Brian S et al (2011) Anxiety and stuttering: continuing to explore a complex relationship. Am J Speech Lang Pathol 20(3):221–232
Jancke L (1994) Variability and duration of voice onset time and phonation in stuttering and nonstuttering adults. J Fluen Disord 19(1):21–37
Johnson W (1955) A study of the onset and development of stuttering. In: Johnson W, Leutenegger RR (eds) Stuttering in children and adults. University of Minnesota Press, Minneapolis, pp 37–73
Johnson W (1959) The onset of stuttering: research findings and implications. University of Minnesota Press, Minneapolis
Johnson W (1961) Measurements of oral reading and speaking rate and disfluency of adult male and female stutterers and nonstutterers. J Speech Hear Disord 7(7):1–20
Jokel R, De Nil L, Sharpe K (2007) Speech disfluencies in adults with neurogenic stuttering associated with stroke and traumatic brain injury. J Med Speech Lang Pathol 15:243–261
Kang C, Drayna D (2012) A role for inherited metabolic deficits in persistent developmental stuttering. Mol Genet Metab 107:276–280
Kang C, Riazuddin S, Mundorff J et al (2010) Mutations in the lyosomal enzyme-targeting pathway and persisting stuttering. N Engl J Med 362:677–685
Kelly EM (1994) Speech rates and turn-taking behaviors of children who stutter and their fathers. J Speech Hear Res 37(6):1284–1294
Kidd KK (1980) Genetic modes of stuttering. J Fluen Disord 5:187–201
Kim KS, Daliri A, Flanagan JR et al (2020) Dissociated development of speech and limb sensorimotor learning in stuttering: speech auditory-motor learning is impaired in both children and adults who stutter. Neuroscience 451:1–21
Kraft SJ (2010) Genome-wide association study of persistent developmental stuttering. PhD thesis, University of Illinois at Urbana-Champaign, Urbana
Kraft SJ, Yairi E (2012) Genetic bases of stuttering: the state of the art, 2011. Folia Phoniatr Logop 64:34–47
Lan J, Song M, Pan C et al (2009) Association between dopaminergic genes (SLC6A3 and DRD2) and stuttering among Han Chinese. J Hum Genet 54(8):457–460
Leclercq AL, Suaire P, Moyse A (2017) Beyond stuttering: speech disfluencies in normally fluent French-speaking children at age 4. Clin Linguist Phon 32(2):166–179
Loucks T, Chon H, Han W (2012) Audiovocal integration in adults who stutter. Int J Lang Commun Disord 47(4):451–456

Lundgren K, Helm-Estabrooks N, Klein R (2010) Stuttering following acquired brain damage: a review of the literature. J Neurolinguistics 23:447–454
Maguire G, Franklin D, Vatakis NG et al (2010) Exploratory randomized clinical study of pagoclone in persistent developmental stuttering: the EXamining Pagoclone for peRsistent dEvelopmental Stuttering Study. J Clin Psychopharmacol 30:48–56
Maguire GA, Ngo J, Fonsworth PKIII et al (2012) Alleviation of developmental stuttering following deep brain stimulation of the ventral intermediate nucleus of the thalamus. Am J Psychiatry 169:759–760
Mahr G, Leith W (1992) Psychogenic stuttering of adult onset. J Speech Hear Res 35:283–286
Manning W, Beck JG (2013a) Personality dysfunction in adults who stutter: another look. J Fluen Disord 38(2):184–192
Manning W, Beck JG (2013b) The role of psychological processes in estimates of stuttering severity. J Fluen Disord 38(4):356–367
Manolio TA (2010) Genomewide association studies and assessment of the risk of disease. N Engl J Med 363:166–176
Månsson H (2000) Childhood stuttering: incidence and development. J Fluen Disord 25(1):47–57
Max L (2004) Stuttering and internal models for sensorimotor control: a theoretical perspective to generate testable hypotheses. In: Maassen B, Kent R, Peters HF et al (eds) Speech motor control in normal and disordered speech. Oxford University Press, Oxford, pp 357–388
Max L, Baldwin CJ (2010) The role of motor learning in stuttering adaptation: repeated versus novel utterances in a practice-retention paradigm. J Fluen Disord 35(1):33–43
Max L, Caruso AJ (1998) Adaptation of stuttering frequency during repeated readings: associated changes in acoustic parameters of perceptually fluent speech. J Speech Lang Hear Res 41(6):1265–1281
Max L, Daliri A (2018) A selective overview of sensory integration problems of speech and non-speech in individuals who stutter. Voice Speech Lang Pathol 23:81–97
Max L, Daliri A (2019) Limited pre-speech auditory modulation in individuals who stutter: data and hypotheses. J Speech Lang Hear Res 62(8S):3071–3084
Max L, Caruso AJ, Gracco VL (2003) Kinematic analyses of speech, orofacial nonspeech, and finger movements in stuttering and nonstuttering adults. J Speech Lang Hear Res 46(1):215–232
Max L, Daniels JC, Curet KM et al (2008) Modulation of auditory and somatosensory processing during the planning of speech movements. In: Proceedings of the 8th International Seminar on Speech Production, vol. 2, pp 41–44
McClean MD (1996) Lip-muscle reflexes during speech movement preparation in stutterers. J Fluen Disord 21(1):49–60
McKnight RC, Cullinan WL (1987) Subgroups of stuttering children - speech and voice reaction-times, segmental durations, and naming latencies. J Fluen Disord 12(3):217–233
Merriam-Webster.com (2019) Medical dictionary, "cluttering." https://www.merriam-webster.com/medical/cluttering. Accessed 18 September 2019
Miall RC, Wolpert DM (1996) Forward models for physiological motor control. Neural Netw 9(8):1265–1279
Miller S, Watson BC (1992) The relationship between communication attitude, anxiety, and depression in stutterers and nonstutterers. J Speech Hear Res 35(4):789–798
Molenaar PCM, Boomsma DI, Dolan CV (1993) A third source of developmental differences. Behav Genet 23:519–524
Namasivayam AK, van Lieshout P (2008) Investigating speech motor practice and learning in people who stutter. J Fluen Disord 33(1):32–51
Natke U, Alpermann A (2010) Stuttering. Insight, theories and methods of treatment, 3rd edn. Hans Huber, Bern
Neumann K, Euler HA, Bosshardt HG et al (2016) Pathogenesis, assessment and treatment of speech fluency disorders. Evidence- and consensus-based interdisciplinary S3 guideline. AWMF register number 049-013, version 1. 2016. http://www.awmf.org/leitlinien/detail/ll/049-013.html. Accessed 3 January 2022
Neumann K, Euler HA, Bosshardt HG et al (2017a) Stuttering and cluttering: pathogenesis, assessment, treatment. In: The guideline on speech fluency disorders. Peter Lang, Frankfurt am Main
Neumann K, Euler HA, Bosshardt HG et al (2017b) The pathogenesis, assessment and treatment of speech fluency disorders. Dtsch Arztebl Int 114:383–390
Okasha A, Bishry Z, Kamel M et al (1974) Psychosocial study of stammering in Egyptian children. Br J Psychiatry 124:531–533
Ooki S (2005) Genetic and environmental influences on stuttering and tics in Japanese twin children. Twin Res Hum Genet 8:69–75
Pancsofar N, Vernon-Feagans L (2006) Mother and father language input to young children: contributions to later language development. J Appl Dev Psychol 27(6):571–587
Polikowsky HG, Shaw DM, Petty LE et al (2021) Population-based genetic effects for developmental stuttering. HGG Adv 3:100073
Preus A (1981) Identifying subgroups of stutterers. University of Oslo, Oslo
Pruett DG, Shaw DM, Chen HH et al (2021) Identifying developmental stuttering and associated comorbidities in electronic health records and creating a phenome risk classifier. J Fluen Disord 68:105847. https://doi.org/10.1016/j.jfludis.2021.105847
Raj A, van Oudenaarden A (2008) Nature, nurture, or chance: stochastic gene expression and its consequences. Cell 135:216–226
Rami MK, Kalinowski J, Rastatter MP et al (2005) Choral reading with filtered speech: effect on stuttering. Percept Mot Skills 100(2):421–431

Rautakoski P, Hannus T, Simberg S et al (2012) Genetics and environmental effects on stuttering: a twin study from Finland. J Fluen Disord 37:202–210

Raza MH, Gertz EM, Mundorff J et al (2013) Linkage analysis of a large African family segregating stuttering suggests polygenic inheritance. Hum Genet 132:385–396

Reilly S, Onslow M, Packman A et al (2009) Predicting stuttering onset by the age of 3 years: a prospective, community cohort study. Pediatrics 123(1):270–277

Riaz N, Steinberg S, Ahmad J et al (2005) Genomewide significant linkage to stuttering on chromosome 12. Am J Hum Genet 76:647–651

Richels CG, Johnson KN, Walden TA et al (2013) Socioeconomic status, parental education, vocabulary and language skills of children who stutter. J Commun Disord 46(4):361–374

Rosenbek J, Messert B, Collins M et al (1978) Stuttering following brain damage. Brain Lang 6:82–96

Scott SH (2004) Optimal feedback control and the neural basis of volitional motor control. Nat Rev Neurosci 5(7):532–546

Seider RA, Gladstien KL, Kidd KK (1983) Recovery and persistence of stuttering among relatives of stutterers. J Speech Hear Disord 48:402–409

Shadmehr R, Krakauer JW (2008) A computational neuroanatomy for motor control. Exp Brain Res 185(3):359–381

Shadmehr R, Wise SP (2005) The computational neurobiology of reaching and pointing: a foundation for motor learning. MIT Press, Cambridge

Shadmehr R, Smith MA, Krakauer JW (2010) Error correction, sensory prediction, and adaptation in motor control. Annu Rev Neurosci 33:89–108

Shaw D, Polikowsky H, Pruett D et al (2021) Phenome risk classification enables phenotypic imputation and gene discovery in developmental stuttering. Am J Hum Genet 108:2271–2283

Shugart Y, Mundorff J, Kilshaw J et al (2004) Results of a genome-wide linkage-scan for stuttering. Am J Med Genet A 124A:133–135

Smits-Bandstra S (2010) Methodological considerations in the measurement of reaction time in persons who stutter. J Fluen Disord 35(1):19–32

Smits-Bandstra S, De Nil LF (2013) Early-stage chunking of finger tapping sequences by persons who stutter and fluent speakers. Clin Linguist Phon 27(1):72–84

Smits-Bandstra S, De Nil LF, Rochon E (2006) The transition to increased automaticity during finger sequence learning in adult males who stutter. J Fluen Disord 31(1):22–42

St Clare T, Menzies RG, Onslow M et al (2009) Unhelpful thoughts and beliefs linked to social anxiety in stuttering: development of a measure. Int J Lang Commun Disord 44(3):338–351

St. Louis KO (1996) A tabular summary of cluttering subjects in the special edition. J Fluen Disord 21(3-4):337–343

St. Louis KO (2010) What is cluttering? Defining cluttering in terms of its "Lowest common denominator". https://www.mnsu.edu/comdis/ica1/papers/stlouisc.html. Accessed 18 September 2019

Stromsta C (1965) A spectrographic study of dysfluencies labeled as stuttering by parents. Proceedings of the 13th Congress of the International Association of Logopedics and Phoniatrics, vol. 1, pp 317–319

Suresh R, Ambrose N, Roe C et al (2006) New complexities in the genetics of stuttering: significant sex-specific linkage signals. Am J Hum Genet 78:554–563

Theys C (2012) Unraveling the enigma of neurogenic stuttering: prevalence, behavioral characteristics and brain correlates. PhD thesis, Catholic University Leuven

Theys C, De Nil L (2022) Acquired stuttering: etiology, symptomatology, identification and treatment. In: Zebrowski P, Anderson J, Conture E (eds) Stuttering and related disorders of fluency. (4th ed) Thieme, New York NY, pp 260–276

Theys C, van Wieringen A, De Nil L (2008) A clinician survey of speech and non-speech characteristics of neurogenic stuttering. J Fluen Disord 33:1–23

Theys C, van Wieringen A, Sunaert S et al (2011) A one year prospective study of neurogenic stuttering following stroke: incidence and co-occurring disorders. J Commun Disord 44:678–687

Theys C, De Nil L, Thijs V et al (2013) A crucial role for the cortico-striato-cortical loop in the pathogenesis of stroke-related neurogenic stuttering. Hum Brain Mapp 34:2103–2112

Tran Y, Blumgart E, Craig A (2011) Subjective distress associated with chronic stuttering. J Fluen Disord 36(1):17–26

Travis LE, Tuttle WW, Cowan DW (1936) A study of heart rate during stuttering. J Speech Disord 1:21–26

Turkheimer E, Waldron MC (2000) The three laws of behavior genetics and what they mean. Curr Dir Psychol Sci 9:160–164

Van Borsel J (2014) Acquired stuttering: a note on terminology. J Neurolinguistics 27(1):41–49

Van Borsel J, Tetnowski JA (2007) Fluency disorders in genetic syndromes. J Fluen Disord 32(4):279–296

Van Borsel J, Moeyaert J, Mostaert C et al (2006) Prevalence of stuttering in regular and special school populations in Belgium based on teacher perceptions. Folia Phoniatr Logop 58(4):289–302

Wallin J (1916) A census of speech defects. Sch Soc 3:213

Ward D (2012) Cluttering: a spectrum perspective. https://www.mnsu.edu/comdis/ica1/papers/wardc.html. Accessed 18 September 2019

Weiss D (1964) Cluttering. Prentice-Hall, Englewood Cliffs

Wepman JM (1939) Familial incidence of stammering. J Hered 30:207

Wingate ME (1984) Fluency, disfluency, dysfluency, and stuttering. J Fluen Disord 9(2):163–168

Wittke-Thompson JK, Ambrose N, Yairi E et al (2007) Genetic studies of stuttering in a founder population. J Fluen Disord 32(1):33–50

World Health Organization (1977) Manual of the international statistical classification of diseases, injuries and causes of death, vol 1. World Health Organization, Geneva

World Health Organization (2016) International classification of diseases tenth revision. https://www.cdc.gov/nchs/icd/icd10cm.htm. Accessed 17 January 2022

World Health Organization (2024) International Classification of Diseases 11th revision (ICD-11), 2024-01 https://icd.who.int/browse/2024-01/mms/en. Accessed 19. 11. 2024

Xiong F, Ji Z, Liu Y et al (2017) Mutation in SSUH2 causes autosomal-dominant dentin dysplasia type I. Hum Mutat 38:95–104

Yairi E (1983) The onset of stuttering in two- and three-year-old children: a preliminary report. J Speech Hear Disord 48(2):171–177

Yairi E, Ambrose N (1992) Onset of stuttering in preschool children: selected factors. J Speech Hear Res 35:782–788

Yairi E, Ambrose NG (2005) Early childhood stuttering. In: For clinicians by clinicians. Pro-Ed, Austin

Yairi E, Ambrose NG (2013) Epidemiology of stuttering: 21st century advances. J Fluen Disord 38:66–87

Yairi E, Ambrose N, Cox N (1996) Genetics of stuttering: a critical review. J Speech Hear Res 39:771–784

Zimmermann G (1980) Articulatory dynamics of fluent utterances of stutterers and nonstutterers. J Speech Hear Res 23(1):95–107

Zimmermann GN, Smith A, Hanley JM (1981) Stuttering: in need of a unifying conceptual framework. J Speech Hear Res 24(1):25–31

Zückner H, Ebel H (2001) Erworbenes psychogenes Stottern bei Erwachsenen: Diagnostische und differentialdiagnostische Aspekte (Acquired psychogenic stuttering in adults: diagnostic and differential-diagnostic aspects). Sprache Stimme Gehör 25:110–117

7 Special Kinds of Speech Fluency Disorders

Dobrinka Georgieva,
Marie-Claude Monfrais-Pfauwadel,
and Nelly Suvi Tuuli Penttilä

7.1 Neurogenic Stuttering

Nelly Penttilä
and Marie-Claude Monfrais-Pfauwadel

7.1.1 Introduction

Stuttering is a speech disorder characterised by interruptions in speech fluency, manifesting commonly as repetitions (d-d-dog), prolongations (doooog) and blocks (d...og) (Guitar 2019). There are two clinical forms of stuttering: developmental stuttering and acquired stuttering (Junuzovic-Zunic et al. 2021). Developmental stuttering (DS) has its onset in childhood and may continue throughout one's lifetime (Boyle et al. 2018). Research suggests that developmental stuttering may stem from a complex interplay of genetic, neurophysiological, and environmental factors, rather than being solely a learned behavior or purely psychological phenomenon (Smith and Weber 2017). Contemporary perspectives increasingly recognize developmental stuttering as a unique speech pattern or a neurological trait, rather than merely a speech pathology, thus reducing stigma and promoting diverse communicative approaches (Boyle 2018). Acquired stuttering is not develo pmental but instead manifests in a formerly fluent speaker after a neurological or psychological episode. 'Neurogenic' stuttering (NS) belongs to the latter class (acquired stuttering). However, NS is often reported in the context of other speech, language or cognitive problems experienced by the patient, such as cluttering, verbal apraxia, dysarthria or aphasia (Krishnan and Tiwari 2011; Theys et al. 2011). Thus, differential diagnoses may be hard to achieve.

7.1.2 Aetiology and Origins of Neurogenic Stuttering

Both the incidence and prevalence of NS remain unknown, but the condition is generally considered a rare disorder (Cruz et al. 2018). Its origin can be traumatic (Jokel et al. 2007; Penttilä et al. 2019), vascular (Van Lieshout et al. 2007), degenerative (De Nil et al. 2009; Juste et al. 2018) or drug-

Supplementary Information The online version contains supplementary material available at https://doi.org/10.1007/978-3-031-25175-7_7.

D. Georgieva (✉)
Medical Faculty, Department of Neurology, Medical University of Plovdiv, Plovdiv, Bulgaria
e-mail: doby_logo@abv.bg

M.-C. Monfrais-Pfauwadel
Hopital Europeen Georges Pompidou, Paris, France

N. S. T. Penttilä
Faculty of Social Sciences, Tampere University, Tampere, Finland
e-mail: nelly.penttila@tuni.fi

A. am Zehnhoff-Dinnesen et al. (eds.), *Phoniatrics II*, European Manual of Medicine,
https://doi.org/10.1007/978-3-031-25175-7_7

induced (Krishnakanth et al. 2008; Van Borsel 2014). Stuttering may also be included in various and very different neurological conditions such as anorexia (Byrne et al. 1993), encephalitis (Chen and Peng 1993), epilepsy (Michel et al. 2004), PANDAS (Maguire et al. 2010) and Down syndrome (Bloodstein and Bernstein Ratner 2008).

NS has been associated with damage in all lobes of the cerebral hemispheres (Theys et al. 2013), as well as in the corpus callosum (Hamano et al. 2005), brainstem (Balasubramanian et al. 2003), cerebellum (Tani and Sakai 2011) and thalamus (Levine and MacDougall 2016). However, recent studies have reported a strong relationship between stuttering and basal ganglia circuits (Alm 2014; Chang et al. 2019; Levine and MacDougall 2016).

7.1.3 Clinical Characteristics and Associated Behaviour of Neurogenic Stuttering

It is sometimes difficult to differentiate the clinical characteristics of developmental stuttering (DS) from those of neurogenic stuttering (NS), as the cases vary (Lundgren et al. 2010; Van Borsel 2014). However, one can say that NS differs from DS in that people with DS produce more prolongations and blocks than people with NS (Jokel et al. 2007; De Nil et al. 2017; Guitar 2019). In addition, people with NS are more likely to stutter in tasks that are often found to be fluency-inducing, for example, reading. There is usually no anxiety or social phobia, as in DS, but in persisting cases, negative communication attitudes have also been reported in patients with NS. As found with DS, phenomena such as adaptation effects and instances of secondary behaviour have been reported in people with NS. In DS, stuttering frequencies vary in different tasks, and they also seem to vary in NS. The most frequent conditions inducing neurogenic stuttering are listed below.

7.1.3.1 Stroke

Recent reports suggest an incidence of stroke-related NS of 5.3% (Theys et al. 2011; De Nil et al. 2017). In a review by De Nil et al. (2017), data on co-morbid symptoms of 95 stroke patients were examined. NS as the only concomitant was reported in 28% of the cases, and the rest of the patients had either aphasia or dysarthria associated with NS. Aphasias influence both motor and language fluency of speech (Basso 2003). Most commonly, patients with aphasia suffer from language formulation difficulties (phonological approximations, impaired sentence processing, word-finding difficulties), which may sound like stuttering as they impinge on speech rhythm. However, NS after stroke is typically characterised as sound, syllable or single-word repetitions (De Nil et al. 2017). Blocks and prolongations are very rare. It must be recognised that many of these patients produce other disfluencies as part of their speech patterns, which differ from those typically labelled as stuttering. These other disfluencies may include phrase repetitions and revisions, sound groping, incomplete phrases, hesitations and interjections.

7.1.3.2 Closed Head Injury

Closed head injury is defined as an impairment in brain function due to an external physical force that damages brain tissue, with the primary pathology manifesting itself as, for example, a contusion, haemorrhage and diffuse axonal injury (Strasberg et al. 2016). Stuttering is typical after trauma in the pons, putamen, cerebellum, thalamus and basal ganglia (Theys et al. 2013). In addition, stuttering has been reported with specific types of pre-onset lesions, for example, a concussion with unconsciousness, and term birth with complications indicating hypoxia (Alm and Risberg 2007). Stuttering after a closed head injury is typically manifested as syllable, part word and word repetitions, as well as consonant prolongations (Jokel et al. 2007; Penttilä et al. 2019). Other disfluencies occur, but stuttering is the dominant disfluent characteristic. Only a mild task effect is noticed between different speech tasks (i.e. reading vs. conversation) (Jokel et al. 2007).

7.1.3.3 Side Effect of Medication

Stuttering can also be a side effect of medication (Shapiro 2011). Drug-induced stuttering has been reported, for example with theophylline (Movsessian 2005), antidepressants such as sertraline (Christensen et al. 1996) and fluoxetine (Guthrie and Grunhaus 1990), and with neuroleptic agents such as olanzapine (Bär et al. 2004) and clozapine (Begum 2005). It is important to note that the clinical picture in drug-induced stuttering appears to be quite heterogeneous (Van Borsel 2014). In addition, unique to drug-induced stuttering is that the causal factor can be removed, meaning that the possible reason for stuttering can be tested by discontinuing or replacing the drug or adapting the dose.

7.1.3.4 Epilepsy

NS as a manifestation of language-induced epilepsy has been described, for example the myoclonic kind is most likely to predispose to stutter-like disfluencies (Valenti et al. 2006). In addition, acquired aphasia with epilepsy, known as Landau–Kleffner syndrome, may generate this kind of fluency disorder (Tütüncüoğlu et al. 2002). Some antiepileptic drugs have been implicated in causing stuttering, including gabapentin, topiramate, phenytoin and lamotrigine (Valenti et al. 2006). Still, one must know that the relation between stuttering and medications for epilepsy is still very fragmentary, and there may be a difference in effect of different compounds.

7.1.3.5 Parkinson Disease

Parkinson disease (PD) is characterised by a progressive loss of dopaminergic neurons in the basal ganglia, leading to motor deficits of rigidity, bradykinesia and tremor, along with deficits in speech production affecting fluency (Goberman et al. 2010; Juste et al. 2018). The frequency and severity of disfluencies in individuals with PD have been reported to be greater than those in controls, and the majority of the disfluencies have been stuttering-like (repetitions, blocks, prolongations). Nevertheless, it is important to note that there are variations in speech symptoms among patients with PD. The most common stuttering-like disfluencies in speakers with PD are blocks and prolongations (61%) (Goberman et al. 2010); repetitions occur (39%). It has also been noted that the frequency of stuttering-like disfluencies varies in different speech tasks (higher disfluency frequency in monologue vs. reading).

7.1.3.6 Down Syndrome

Down syndrome is caused by a chromosomal defect, which leads to an intellectual disability impairing communication (Fawcett and Peralego 2009). It is estimated that the prevalence of stuttering in people with Down syndrome ranges from 10% to 45% (Kent and Vorperian 2013). Fluency disorder in people with Down syndrome is commonly manifested as repetitions, sound groping, long pauses and cluttering.

7.1.4 Assessment of Neurogenic Stuttering

First, detailed anamnestic information should be collected when assessing neurogenic stuttering. Key diagnostic questions include asking about the onset of stuttering, aetiology and stuttering symptoms (Theys et al. 2008). Individuals should be asked if there were any significant environmental factors, including starting medication, in the time period around the onset of stuttering. After clarifying the neurological background for stuttering, the possible coexisting speech disorders should be assessed. To assess aphasic symptoms, the Western Aphasia Battery (WAB; Kertesz 1982) or the Boston Diagnostic Aphasia Examination (BDAE; Goodglass and Kaplan 1972) can be used. As speech also may be non-fluent owing to dysarthria and apraxia of speech (Kent 2000), these motor speech disorders can be evaluated with the FDA (Frenchay Dysarthria Assessment-2; Enderby and Palmer 2008) and ABA-2 (Apraxia Battery for Adults-2; Dabul 2000), respectively.

There is no specific fluency assessment battery or standardised tests for neurogenic stuttering. However, fluency can be evaluated in several ways. First, a qualitative analysis of the pattern of symptoms should be reported. The clinician can analyse the speech patterns (repetitions, blocks, prolongations) in a spontaneous speech or reading task. As counting stuttered syllables can be difficult without experience, both the clinician and the patient can rate the severity of stuttering on a simple 0–9 scale adapted from Lidcombe Program (Onslow et al. 2017) (0 = no stuttering, 1 = extremely mild stuttering, to 9 = extremely severe stuttering). If objective measurement is required, a traditional severity scale for developmental stuttering called the Stuttering Severity Index-4 (SSI-4; Riley 2009) can be used. SSI-4 helps to examine the frequency of stuttering, the duration of stuttering moments and physical concomitants.

It is very important to remember that stuttering is a complicated communication disorder that can affect many aspects of a patient's life, e.g. relationships, career and quality of life (Yaruss 2007). Therefore, different self-assessment scales have been introduced, for example the WASSP (The Wright and Ayre Stuttering Self-Rating Profile; Wright and Ayre 2000). For a deeper self-assessment, the OASES (Overall Assessment of the Speaker's Experience of Stuttering; Yaruss and Quesal 2006), which is based on the ICF model (International Classification of Functioning, Disability and Health; WHO 2001), can be used. Finally, in cases where a communication disorder is suspected, speech and language pathologists should be consulted to ensure an accurate diagnosis and to start the treatment.

The assessment pattern for the clinician should involve:

1. Detailed case history
   (a) Aetiology
   (b) Onset of stuttering
   (c) History of developmental disorders
   (d) Medication
2. Assessing possible coexisting speech disorders
   (a) Aphasia
   (b) Dysarthria
   (c) Apraxia of speech
3. Assessing stuttering
   (a) Assessing features of stuttering (repetitions, blocks, prolongations)
   (b) Rating the severity on a 0–9 scale
   (c) Assessing other fluency patterns (speech rate, other disfluencies)
4. Patients' self-assessment of stuttering
   (a) Rating the severity on a 0–9 scale
   (b) WASSP (Wright and Ayre 2000)

7.1.5 Treatment

Neurogenic stuttering usually persists for a long time and responds poorly to treatment (Krishnan and Tiwari 2013; Cruz et al. 2018). Still, there are individual variations and cases where stuttering recovery has happened in some weeks or months. When planning treatment, the ICF can be used as the basis for both the diagnostic and the therapy process. The ICF focuses not only on the body functions—the stuttering moments—but also on the individual's activities and participation, as well as on factor that are personal (e.g. frustration, shame) and environmental (e.g. familial support, availability of adequate treatment) (Yaruss 2007).

Similar methods to those in developmental stuttering therapy (easy onset, rhythmical speech, slowing speech rate) can be used (Krishnan and Tiwari 2011; Van Borsel 2014). As NS rarely manifests as an isolated disorder, the rehabilitation of comorbid communication and cognitive disorders may be indicated, as alleviating their effects may also enhance fluency. In addition, if the person is expressing anxiety or concern about his fluency, therapy may include education about the disorder and counselling to change attitudes and perceptions. Finally, recent evidence suggests that there is no drug with proven efficacy in NS treatment despite several pharmacological trials (Cruz et al. 2018).

Acknowledgements We should like to express our great appreciation to Per Alm (PhD) for his valuable and constructive suggestions for writing this section.

7.2 Cluttering

Dobrinka Georgieva

7.2.1 Introduction

The aim of this section is to provide a comprehensive theoretical and practical approach to the definition, causes, assessment and treatment of cluttering. The complexity, diversity and variability of this fluency disorder are a challenge for the speech-language pathologist/phoniatrician.

7.2.2 Cluttering Awareness

Cluttering is a communication disorder that is known—but not well recognised—by the general public. Public attitudes towards cluttering have been documented in numerous countries (the USA (including Puerto Rico), Bulgaria, Turkey, Russia,

Norway, Poland, the UK, Malta and China) by using St. Louis's *Public Opinion Survey of Human Attributes–Cluttering* (*POSHA-CL*) (St Louis et al. 2010). The consistent finding is that adults from diverse cultures hold attitudes towards cluttering that are similar to their attitudes towards stuttering (as measured by a parallel stuttering instrument [*POSHA–S*]), but are somewhat less positive (e.g. St. Louis et al. 2011, 2014; Węsierska et al. 2014; Filatova et al. 2018). Even so, attitudes towards cluttering are unaffected by attitudes towards stuttering, indicating that the public appears to recognise these as two distinct fluency disorders. Adults also know fewer children or adults who clutter than those who stutter. The perspectives of fluency specialists and of clutterers themselves would be useful in identifying optimal standards against which any future efforts to change attitudes might be gauged (St. Louis et al. 2011, p. 103).

7.2.3 Terminology

Cluttering is an internationally accepted term with synonyms in several languages, including French (bredouillement), British English (stammering), German (Poltern), Italian (tartagliare), Spanish (tartajeo), Russian (спотыкание) and Bulgarian (запъване). In the late nineteenth century and first part of the twentieth century, scientists preferred terms such as Battarismuspolten, Paraphrasia, Glittering, Tumultossermonis, Balbutiement, Praeceps and Tachiphemia.

7.2.4 Definition of Cluttering

A proper definition should contain the basic characteristics and functions of what it proposes to identify. There is no agreed-upon definition of cluttering. According to Bakker (1996), the lack of a universally accepted definition of this multidimensional fluency disorder has impeded research, and has affected the development of successful clinical procedures. Traditionally, cluttering has been viewed as a fluency disorder thought to be congenital in nature. It is often identified as a syndrome owing to the myriad of symptoms reported to describe it (Tetnowski 2007). There are two main schools of thought regarding cluttering definition (Tetnowski 2007). The first considers cluttering to be primarily a speech disorder, and the second views it as a more complex language or cognitive disorder that manifests itself through the speech modality. It may include associated symptoms.

Below are a few popular definitions of cluttering. One of the leading authorities in this area, Weiss, suggests a descriptive classical definition or clinical symptoms definition.

The Weiss (1964) *clinical symptoms definition*

> Cluttering is a speech disorder characterized by the clutterer's unawareness of the disorder, by a short attention span, by disturbances in perception, articulation and formulation of speech and often by excessive speed of delivery. It is a disorder of the thought processes preparatory to speech and based on a hereditary disposition. Cluttering is a verbal manifestation of Central Language Imbalance, which affects all channels of communication (e.g. reading, writing, rhythm and musicality) and behavior in general—Weiss (1964) p. 1

St. Louis and Schulte (2011) share the European logopaedists and phoniatricians' position regarding a continuum from stuttering to cluttering with a spectrum of related conditions.

The Ward (2006) *spectrum definition*

> Cluttering is likely to contain one or more of the following elements: abnormally fast speech rate, or uncontrolled bursts of fast speech; reduced intelligibility due to over co-articulation and indistinct articulation; disturbances in language planning; greater and expected number of dysfluencies.—Ward (2006) p. 152

The World Health Organization (2007) *definition*

> A rapid rate of speech with breakdown in fluency, but no repetitions or hesitations, of a severity to give rise to diminished speech intelligibility. Speech is erratic and dysrhythmic, with rapid jerky spurts that usually involve faulty phrasing patterns.—WHO (2007) F98.6

The St. Louis et al. (2007a) *working definition*

> Cluttering is a fluency disorder, characterized by a rate that is perceived to be abnormally rapid, irregular, or both for the speaker (although measured syllable rates may not exceed normal limits). These rate abnormalities further are manifest in one or more of the following symptoms: (a) an excessive number of dysfluences, the majority of

> which are not typical of people who stutter; (b) the frequent placement of pauses and use of prosodic patterns that do not conform to syntactic and semantic constraints; and (c) inappropriate (usually excessive) degrees of coarticulation among sounds, especially in multisyllabic words.—St. Louis et al. (2007a) p. 299–300

The next description on cluttering is so called *lowest common denominator* (*LCD*) definition. It has gone through several revisions and incorporates multiple dimensions. According to Myers and Bakker (2014),

> the LCD is likely to be the most restrictive of definitions, especially in regard to the exclusion of the role of language encoding and pragmatics—Myers and Bakker (2014) p. 36

It is a very 'conservative perspective' including a limited number of core cluttering characteristics (Ward et al. 2015, p. 1).

The St. Louis and Schulte (2011) *refined working lowest common denominator* (*LCD*) *definition*

> Cluttering is a fluency disorder wherein segments of conversation* in the speaker's native language** typically are perceived as too fast overall***, too irregular****, or both. The segments of rapid and/or irregular speech rate must further be accompanied by one or more of the following: (a) excessive "normal dysfluencies" *****; (b) excessive collapsing****** or deletion of syllables; and/or (c) abnormal pauses, syllable stress, or speech rhythm.
>
> *Cluttering must occur in naturalistic conversation, but it need not occur even a majority of the time. Clear but isolated examples that exceed those observed in normal speakers are sufficient for a diagnosis
>
> **This may also apply to the speaker's mastered and habitual non-native language, especially in multilingual living environments
>
> ***This may be true even though syllable rates may not exceed those of normal speakers
>
> ****Synonyms for irregular rate include "jerky" or "spurty"
>
> ***** These dysfluences are often observed in smaller numbers in normal speakers and are typically not observed in stuttering
>
> ******Collapsing includes, but is not limited to, excessive shortening, "telescoping" or "overcoarticulating" various syllables especially in multisyllabic words—St. Louis and Schulte (2011) p. 241–242

According to St. Louis and Schulte (2011), in mathematics, the LCD is the smallest number that can be divided into the denominators of two or more fractions that are to be structured. Another way to consider an LCD definition is to determine the minimal number of necessary and sufficient conditions for a cluttering definition. In 2007, the First World Conference on Cluttering was held in Bulgaria, which resulted in the formation of the International Cluttering Association. This organisation has been trying to find consensus regarding the definition of cluttering (see http://associations.missouristate.edu/ica/).

7.2.5 Prevalence of Cluttering

There is a little empirical information regarding the prevalence of cluttering. St. Louis et al. (2007b) reviewed the following data:

- Becker and Grundman (1970) reported that 1.8% of 7-and 8-year-olds in a German School manifested cluttering.
- Freund (1952) reported that 22% of a group of stutterers also cluttered.
- Preus (1981) reported that 32% of 100 adolescent stutterers also cluttered.
- Pure cluttering appears to be rare (St. Louis and Myers 1997). Daly's (1996) data showed 5% of pure clutterers in the group of the fluency disorders, including 55% of pure stutterers (clients with such concomitant disabilities as reading difficulties or articulation disorders) and 40% representing the cluttering-stuttering group.

Although it is difficult to generalise, there are two scientific schools that have studied the relation between stuttering and cluttering. The first, represented by Freund, Preus and Weiss, holds that cluttering and stuttering are related disorders. Cluttering may lead to stuttering, or stuttering may have its roots in cluttering (Howell and Davis 2011, p. 69). Researchers who represent the second school of thought, such as Ward, Daly, Burnett-Stolnack, Myers and St. Louis, consider cluttering to be fundamentally different from stuttering (Howell and Davis 2011, p. 69).

7.2.6 Onset of Cluttering

This is possibly after 7–8 years of age, but it is not known for certain.

7.2.7 Causes of Cluttering: Pathogenesis

The aetiology of cluttering remains unclear, although much has been written about the multiple factors that influence its diverse range of symptoms and associated behaviour. The Czech phoniatrician Seeman (1970) gathered stuttering and cluttering in one nosological group. He was among the early researchers to postulate that cluttering results from a disturbance of the basal ganglia. One of the leading Belgian researchers, Lebrun (1996), wrote about a syndrome of acquired cluttering after brain damage (subcortical lesions) in adults.

The epidemiology of cluttering disorder is not well understood, although some studies have suggested a family predisposition (e.g. Ludlow et al. 1995).

> [It] is not possible to predict the heritability at this time, because no data that bear on this question have been published. If, however, this disorder is shown to have a high heritability …—Drayna (2011) p. 31

According to many researchers, heredity is an even better predictor of cluttering than stuttering, but there remains the need to prove the organic nature of cluttering (Daly 1996, p. 165).

As proposed by Alm (2011), a main mechanism of cluttering is a hyperactivation and dysregulation of the medial frontal cortex, which may be secondary to disinhibition of the basal ganglia circuits (for example as a result of a hyperactive dopamine system—p. 4). In Alm's (2007) dual premotor model of cluttering and stuttering, initiation of speech segments is cued by either of two parallel premotor systems, lateral and medial. Both fluency disorders are suggested as two opposite disturbances of the same function: insufficient versus premature release of speech motor segments by the medial premotor system. The dual premotor model emphasises that the motor functions of the basal ganglia are dependent on the complete circuit, the medial premotor system.

The dual premotor hypothesis of stuttering and cluttering postulates that:

- Stuttering and cluttering are disorders of the initiation of speech segments by *the medial premotor system.*
- The medial premotor system includes:
  - Circuit: cortical input ➔ basal ganglia ➔ thalamus ➔ frontal cortex (especially supplementary motor area—SMA).
  - Stuttering: insufficient initiation of speech segments.
  - *Cluttering:* premature initiation of speech segments.
  - Dysregulation may result in both disturbances in the same person (see Fig. 7.1).

There is evidence that the putamen is implicated in cluttering (Ward 2011, p. 41). Disruptions of this subcortical structure are associated with difficulties in the inhibition of inappropriate motor activity. It is suggested that cluttering disorder involves a breakdown in motor speech control that may be seen across a range of processing levels including planning, programming and execution. Somewhat more recently, Ward et al. (2015) examined 17 adults who clutter and 17 normally fluent control speakers. Their findings are related to theoretical predictions regarding the cluttering neural correlates. The evidence the authors obtained argue for an abnormal function in the basal ganglia and their cortical output target, the medial prefrontal cortex.

The causes of cluttering remain obscure and controversial (Sick 2014; Van Zaalen and Reichel 2015), and there is a continued tendency to view stuttering and cluttering as similar disorders.

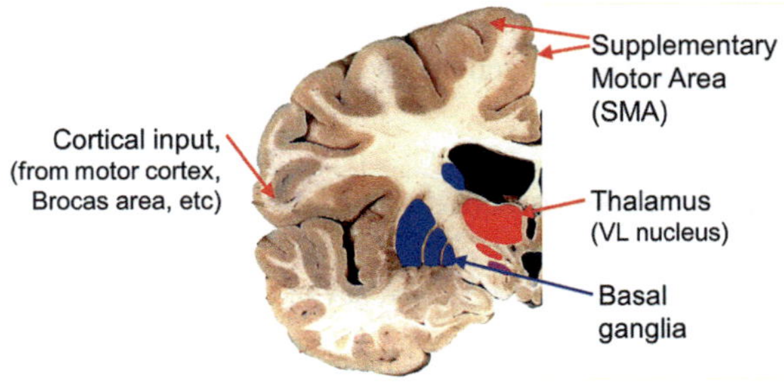

Fig. 7.1 Illustration of the dual premotor model from Alm 2007—with permission from Professor Per Alm, Lund University, Sweden

7.2.8 Characteristics of Cluttering

As a result of the cluttering definition controversies, it is very difficult to describe reliably its symptoms (Tetnowski 2007, p. 252). Daly (1996) believes that there are two types of cluttering symptoms: obligatory and facultative. He is of the opinion that there are four obligatory symptoms, six common facultative symptoms and other facultative symptoms (see Table 7.1).

Obligatory symptoms: there are four essential symptoms for the cluttering disorder diagnosis: (1) excessive number of whole-word or phrase repetitions; (2) poor thinking; (3) short attention span and poor concentration, and (4) lack of complete awareness of the problem.

Detailed discussion of the symptoms of cluttering can be found in Ward (2006) and Ward and Scott (2011). Analysing the speech errors in cluttering on the basis of Levelt's model of speech and language processing, Ward (2006) found that cluttering affects all levels of this processing: (1) conceptualisation, (2) formulation and (3) articulation, and postulated that all elements of speech could potentially be affected. According to Weiss,

> 'The majority of cluttering symptoms are facultative, i.e. often presented but not necessarily. Only a few are obligatory, i.e., symptoms which are always manifested and which clinch the diagnosis—Weiss (1964) p. 61–62

7.2.9 Assessment and Diagnosis of Cluttering

A framework that can accommodate the applications of all of these theoretical orientations is the World Health Organization's (WHO 2007) International Classification of Functioning, Disability and Health (ICF). This classification system is designed to accommodate theory as well as operational definitions and descriptions of illness and disabilities. It is intended to be context-inclusive and to be applicable to many cultures.

Cluttering is frequently misdiagnosed. According to Alm (2011), no single aspect is sufficient to determine the diagnosis; it is the cluster of symptoms and characteristics that constitute this syndrome.

Usually, children, adolescents and adults with disfluencies are referred to a speech therapist's office for stuttering or other fluency problems. The standard evaluation includes both informal and specific assessment.

Informal assessment focuses on (1) measurement of the person's automatic speech, (2) oral reading, (3) spontaneous speech, (4) auditory memory, (5) oral diadochokinetic skills and (6) written expression, and should begin after completion of the case history (Table 7.2).

The case history (questionnaire and interview) needs to include basic information regarding fluency problem, significant changes in the form of dysfluences after onset, delayed speech/language development, delayed motor development, a history of academic difficulties, a history of lack of awareness of the disorder, and a history of limited attention span. Questions about aggressiveness and impulsive personality are included as well. Since cluttering appears to have genetic roots, the case history particularly should include questions about family predispositions to fluency disorders, speech/language disorders and attention deficit/hyperactivity disorders. The specific assessment of cluttering is described in Table 7.3.

Table 7.1 Assessment findings and cluttering symptoms

Parameters	Symptoms	Features of cluttering (findings from literature)
Fluency	Obligatory	Excessive number of whole-word or phrase repetitions (Daly 1996; St. Louis and Myers 1997); Dysfluency in spontaneous speech, i.e. part word repetitions, word repetitions (Lees et al. 1996); Reduced prosody (both timing and pitch range) (Ward 2006)
Thinking	Obligatory	Poor organisation of thinking (speaking more quickly than the ability to formulate clear thoughts); lack of clarity of inner speech formulation (Daly 1996)
Attention span and concentration	Obligatory	Short attention span; inefficiency or inattentiveness to focus on details; poor auditory attention; poor concentration (Daly 1996). Distractibility/limited attention span; perceptual deficits (St. Louis and Myers 1997)
Awareness of the problem	Obligatory	Lack of complete awareness of own cluttering (Daly 1996). Impaired awareness of the problem (St. Louis and Myers 1997)
Language	Most Common Facultative	Language difficulties: word retrieval problems, word order difficulties, sentence simplification, use of fragmentary phrases. Many people who clutter have a poorly developed sense of language expression that affects grammar and syntax (Daly 1996); In spontaneous speech, limited range of grammatical structures and stereotypic use of coordinators; mean length of utterance is six words (Lees et al. 1996). Difficulties in word finding, planning of sentences and phrases, syntactic elements (Ward 2006). Reduced comprehension of vocabulary, lexical errors, syntactic errors, disorganised sentences (St. Louis and Myers 1997)
Tachylalia or excessive rate of speech	Most common facultative	Excessively rapid speech rate and impulsive speech patterns; festinating speech (more and more rapid); intraverbal acceleration (longer words contracted); avoidance of multisyllabic words; short responses to questions; arrhythmic speech (Daly 1996); high speech rate (Ward 2006). Speech rate in reading = 200 syl/min and speech rate in short fluent utterances = 240 syl/min; diadochokinetic rates are low (10 × /ptk/ in 12 s; norm = 5.7 s (Lees et al. 1996). Rapid articulatory rate, irregular rate (St. Louis and Myers 1997)
Auditory processing	Most Common facultative	Auditory imperceptiveness (Daly 1996)
Reading	Most common Facultative	Reading difficulties: the reading problem is the most prominent facultative symptom; skim sentences and paragraphs quickly, often missing syllables and entire words (Daly 1996). Reading comprehensive problems, oral reading difficulties (St. Louis and Myers 1997)

(continued)

Table 7.1 (continued)

Parameters	Symptoms	Features of cluttering (findings from literature)
Writing	Most common facultative	Writing difficulties: errors in cluttering people's writing abilities reflect their poor psychomotor coordination; clipping letters, omitting syllables, slurring substitutes, transposing words (Daly 1996). Writing problems (St. Louis and Myers 1997)
Speech and language development	Most common facultative	Delayed speech and language development (Daly 1996)
Rhythm	Facultative	Monotonous speech (Daly 1996)
Motor abilities	Facultative	Hyperactive, impulsive and restless (Daly 1996); reduced general motor coordination, reduced diadochokinetic rates, and hyperactivity (St. Louis and Myers 1997)
Physical size	Facultative	Many cluttering children are physically small for their age (Daly 1996)
Respiration	Facultative	Respiratory dysrhythmia; greater frequency of inhalations; tendencies to ignore punctuation and to talk in irregular spurts (Daly 1996)
Phonation	Facultative	Faulty breathing; various type of dysphonias possible; faulty patterns of phonation. Persons who clutter often begin sentences in a loud, explosive voice, and then dwindle to an unintelligible murmur (Daly 1996). Fo = 160 Hz on narrow band spectrography (norm = 98–165 Hz); maximum phonation time on /a/ = 12.28 s (norm = 25–35 s); difficulty on lowering and rising pitch on /a/; no pitch breaks apparent; vital capacity (max. of 3 trials) 1.2 litres (Lees et al. 1996). Abnormal timing and pitch range (Ward 2006); initial loud voice trails off to a murmur (Daly 1996; Bennett 2006); dysphonia (Daly 1996)
Articulation	Facultative	Articulation disturbances from mild dyslalia to congenital dyspraxia. Slurred articulatory productions, elision (omission of unstressed vowels or syllables), sound and word substitutions, vowel prolongations, interjections, skipping unstressed syllables, omitting small parts of speech (Daly 1996); poor articulation (Ward 2006); presence of developmental errors, vowel neutralisation, telescoping of syllables, cluster reduction, prosodic errors (St. Louis and Myers 1997)
Handwriting	Facultative	Tiny letter formation (Lees et al. 1996); handwriting problems (St. Louis and Myers 1997)
Personality	Facultative	Impulsive, hasty, impatient, forgetful, emotionally unstable, superficial, short-tempered, disorganised personality (Daly 1996)
Intelligibility	Facultative	Particularly difficult to understand on one word responses but also often unintelligible in connected speech (Lees et al. 1996)
Pragmatic skills	Facultative	Poor. Tend to speak before the listener is ready to attend (Lees et al. 1996)

(continued)

Table 7.1 (continued)

Parameters	Symptoms	Features of cluttering (findings from literature)
Intelligence	Facultative	Verbal IQ—91 (88–96 at 68% confidence level). Overall IQ score within average range. Visual IQ—77 (75–83 at 68% confidence level). Overall IQ score below average range (Lees et al. 1996). Deficit not due to reduced general intelligence (St. Louis and Myers 1997)

Table 7.2 Summary of the information required for a case history of a client with a cluttering disorder according to St. Louis and Myers 1997; St. Louis et al. 2007a

Obtain
Basic biographical information
Health, school and psychological history and data
Have the client describe
The cluttering disorder in his or her own words
Other people's reactions to the cluttering disorder
The effects of the cluttering disorder on his or her life
What he or she believes caused the cluttering disorder
The onset and development of the cluttering disorder

The theoretical and practical orientation of the speech-language pathologist/phoniatrician, as well as the purpose of assessment, will drive the selection of tools.

When a clinician suspects that the client may be cluttering (or possibly is exhibiting a combination of both stuttering and cluttering), it is recommended that specific instruments such as *Daly's Checklist for Possible Cluttering* (Daly 1996) *and Cluttering Treatment Planning Profile* (Daly 1996) be applied. Furthermore, it is suggested that the clinician complete the presented checklist by scoring each of the 33 items only after obtaining and reviewing all available information from the client's file (including medical, school and psychological reports). A score of 55 and above on the Daly's checklist strongly indicates a cluttering diagnosis.

When the clinician's diagnosis combines forms of cluttering–stuttering, it is good to consider that stuttering also affects the voice and voice characteristics: increasing pitch, prolongations with rising pitch, vocal tension, increased volume (loudness) in the moments of so-called struggle behaviour through a block. Pitch changes are atypical for cluttering and typical for stuttering (Daly 1996; Bennett 2006).

To assess pitch and intensity, speech therapists/phoniatricians can choose to assess these measures with instrumentation such as KayPentax's Computerized Speech Lab (CSL) and software such as the Real Time Pitch (RTP), Voice Range Profile (VRP) and Electroglottograph (EGG). The evaluation of pitch perturbations and amplitude perturbations can be extracted by using the MultiDimentional voice program (MDVP) of the CSL. The MDVP option provides quantitative assessment of voice quality, calculating over 20 parameters on a single sustained vocalisation.

7.2.10 Differential Diagnoses of Cluttering

Pure cluttering is rarely seen. Coexisting disorders that the clinician should assess include stuttering, articulation disorders, Attention Deficit/Hyperactivity Disorder (ADHD) and learning difficulties (St. Louis and Myers 1997).

7.2.10.1 Differential Diagnosis Between Cluttering and Stuttering

There exists a subgroup of clutterers who manifest stuttering behaviour, and stutterers who manifest cluttering behaviour; so-called combined forms. Usually clinicians have to differentiate cluttering from stuttering. Below related material is presented in Figs. 7.2 and 7.3.

7.2.10.2 Differential Diagnosis Between Cluttering and Other Concomitant Disorders

There is overlap between cluttering and motor disorders, central auditory processing disorders, autism spectrum disorder (Scaler Scott 2011), some neurological issues, as well as such congenital disorders as Down syndrome (Van Borsel 2011; Eggers and Van Eerdenbrugh 2018) and Fragile X syndrome (Hanson et al. 1986).

Table 7.3 Summary of the specific procedures used in the cluttering evaluation process

Obtain	Instruments for assessment
An audiocassette-or videotape-recorded sample of the client's speech (using standard reading passage)	
A description of the client's cluttering	
Evaluate	
Language: Receptive, expressive-verbal, expressive-written	The battery needs to include measurement of morphology (vocabulary and infections), syntax, and semantics Standardised and non-standardised measurements of expressive and receptive language
Speech: Fluency, rate, articulation, breathing, rhythm, reading, writing	Cluttering Severity Instrument by Bakker and Myers (2011) Stuttering severity instrument-4 (SSI-4) by Riley (2009); Andrews and Cutler (1974) S-24 Scale An articulation test
Pragmatics: Conversation, non-verbal and verbal communication	Pragmatic test Modified from Erickson (1969) scale of communication attitudes (S-24)
Motor: Motor control	Speech Motor Control—SPA test (Van Zaalen et al. 2009)
Cognition: Awareness, through organisation, memory, impulsivity	Predictive Cluttering Inventory (Daly and Cantrell 2006) Self-Awareness of Speech Index by St. Louis and Atkins (2005) An intelligence quotient (IQ) test if it is necessary Communication Attitude Test (CAT), Behaviour Assessment Battery (Brutten and Vanryckeghem 2006) Wright and Ayre Stuttering Self-rating Profile (WASSP), (Wright and Ayre 2000) Overall Assessment of the Speaker's Experience of Stuttering (OASES), (Yaruss and Quesal 2016)

Note: The instrument written in bold are specific for cluttering assessment; non-bold instrument could be used in the combined stuttering–cluttering disorders

7.2.11 Cluttering Treatment

Once the diagnosis of cluttering is determined, the speech-language pathologist/phoniatrician needs to decide whether treatment is indicated. Because of its specific nature, cluttering requires systematic interventions that need to be tailored to the special client's communication needs. Generally, these need to incorporate specific techniques tied to rate, language, pragmatics, and cognition.

Most popular in the speech therapy literature is Myers (1992) synergistic approach to cluttering treatment. This treatment outlines improvement in (1) fluency, (2) rate and rhythm, (3) articulation, (4) language functioning and (5) self-monitoring (Bennett Lanouette 2011).

Several constructs provide the framework for cluttering treatment: coexistence of speech/language functions, synergism, synchrony, coherence and cohesion. Synergism has to do with different parts of the communication system working together in a highly coordinated and well-timed way (St. Louis and Myers 1997, pp. 325–328). Specifically, the following principles and techniques are organised within the frame of prosody, fluency, articulation, language and pragmatic functions:

- **Principles and Techniques for Improvement of Prosody** (rate and rhythm) of speech—(1) systematic modulation of the speaking context starting from highly structured to short utterances; (2) coordination of respiratory, phonatory and articulation systems with linguistic junctures to provide appropriate stress patterns; (3) involvement of delayed acoustic feedback (DAF) to reduce speech rate and

Checklist for Possible Cluttering

Client ______________________ Date ____________ Age __________

Respond to each descriptive statement below. Your answer should reflect how well you believe the statement describes you.

	not at all	just a little	pretty much	very much
1. repeats syllables, words, or phrases	0	1	2	3
2. started talking late, onset of words and sentences delayed	0	1	2	3
3. fluency disruptions started early, no remissions, never very fluent	0	1	2	3
4. speech very disorganized, confused wording	0	1	2	3
5. silent gaps or hesitations common, interjections, many "filler" words	0	1	2	3
6. stops before saying initial vowel, no tension, no drawn-out vowels	0	1	2	3
7. rapid rate (speaks too fast), tachylalia, speaks in spurts	0	1	2	3
8. extrovert, high verbal output, compulsive talker	0	1	2	3
9. jerky breathing pattern, respiratory dysrhythmia	0	1	2	3
10. slurred articulation (omits sounds or unstressed syllables)	0	1	2	3
11. mispronunciation of /r/, /l/, and sibilants	0	1	2	3
12. speech better under pressure (during periods of heightened attention)	0	1	2	3
13. difficulty following directions, impatient/disinterested listener	0	1	2	3
14. distractible, attention span problems, poor concentration	0	1	2	3
15. storytelling difficulty (trouble sequencing events)	0	1	2	3
16. demonstrates word-finding difficulties resembling anomia	0	1	2	3
17. inappropriate reference by pronouns is common	0	1	2	3
18. improper language structure, poor grammar and syntax	0	1	2	3
19. clumsy and uncoordinated, motor activities accelerated or hasty	0	1	2	3
20. reading disorder is a prominent disability	0	1	2	3
21. disintegrated and fractionated writing; poor motor control	0	1	2	3
22. writing shows transposition of letters and words (omits letters and syllables)	0	1	2	3
23. left-right confusion, delayed hand preference	0	1	2	3
24. initial loud voice, trails off to a murmur, mumbles	0	1	2	3
25. seems to think faster than s/he can talk or write	0	1	2	3
26. above average in mathematical and abstract reasoning abilities	0	1	2	3
27. poor rhythm, timing, or musical ability (may dislike singing)	0	1	2	3
28. improper stress patterns of speech, poor melodic accenting of syllables	0	1	2	3
29. appears younger than age, small and/or immature	0	1	2	3
30. other family member with similar problem	0	1	2	3
31. untidy, careless, hasty, impulsive, or forgetful	0	1	2	3
32. impatient, superficial, and/or short-tempered	0	1	2	3
33. lack of self-awareness, unconcerned attitude over inappropriateness of many behaviors and responses	0	1	2	3
Total Score ________ Diagnosis ______________________				

Other relevant information determined by interviewer:

- identified in school as learning disabled ❑ yes ❑ no ❑ recommended for testing ❑ don't know
- currently receiving speech-language therapy ❑ yes ❑ no ❑ recommended for testing ❑ don't know
- comments ____

The Source for Stuttering & Cluttering

Fig. 7.2 Checklist for identification of cluttering—revised (Daly and Burnett 1999). . (Checklist for Possible Cluttering Note. Reprinted From Source for Stuttering and Cluttering (p. 178), by David A. Daly 1996, Austin, TX:PRO-ED. Copyright 1996 by PRO-ED, INC. Reprinted with permission)

Cluttering Treatment Planning Profile

Client ______________________ Date __________ Age ________

	undesirably different from normal -3	-2	-1	normal 0	+1	+2	desirably different from normal +3
A. Speech and Motor Coordination							
General							
(1) repeats syllables, words, phrases							
(5) silent gaps, hesitations, many "filler" words							
(6) stops before initial vowels							
(9) jerky breathing pattern, respiratory dysrhythmia							
(10) slurred articulation (omits sounds/unstressed syllables)							
(11) mispronunciation of /r/, /l/, and/or sibilants							
(19) clumsy and uncoordinated, hasty motor activities							
(21) poor motor control, disintegrated writing							
(27) poor rhythm, timing, or musical ability							
Suprasegmental Features							
(7) rapid rate (tachylalia), speaks in spurts							
(24) initial loud voice, trails off to murmur; mumbles							
(28) improper stress pattern							
B. Language and Cognition							
Auditory Comprehension							
(13) difficulty following directions, impatient listener							
Verbal Expression							
(16) word-finding difficulty, resembles anomia							
(17) inappropriate pronoun reference							
(18) poor grammar and syntax, improper language structure							
Written Expression							
(22) transposition/omission of letters and/or syllables							
Reading Comprehension							
(20) reading disorder is prominent disability							
Attention and Concentration							
(12) speech better under pressure for short periods							
(14) distractible, attention span problems							
Awareness							
(8) extrovert, high verbal output, compulsive talker							
(33) lack of self awareness, inappropriate behaviors							
Thought Organization							
(4) disorganized speech and language, confused wording							
(15) storytelling difficulty (trouble sequencing events)							
(25) thinks faster than can speak/write							
Reasoning/Problem Solving							
(26) above average math/abstract reasoning skills							
C. Behavioral — Pragmatic							
(31) untidy, careless, hasty, impulsive, or forgetful							
(32) impatient, superficial, short-tempered							
D. Developmental							
(2) started talking late, onset of sentences delayed							
(3) early fluency disruptions with no remissions, never very fluent							
(23) left-right confusion, delayed hand preference							
(29) immature, appears young for age							
(30) family member with same/similar problem							

The Source for Stuttering & Cluttering

Fig. 7.3 Inventory of characteristics that differentiate cluttering and stuttering disorders (Daly and Burnett 1999). (Cluttering Treatment Planning Profile Note. Reprinted From Source for Stuttering and Cluttering (p. 179), by David A. Daly 1996, Austin, TX:PRO-ED. Copyright 1996 by PRO-ED, INC. Reprinted with permission) enhance the intelligibility of speech—DAF set at 250 msec; (4) finger tapping technique application.

- **Principles and Techniques for Improvement of Articulation**—(1) misarticulation correction; (2) prolonged speech implementation through prolonged vowels within syllables and words; (3) continuing voicing modelling.
- **Principles and Techniques for Improvement of Language**—(1) reduction of word-finding problems; (2) specific therapy for semantics and syntax difficulties; (3) outlining the essential components of narratives; (4) written transcriptions of recorded speech implementation; (5) improvement of the pragmatic skills orientated to social competence development.
- **Principles and Techniques for Fluency Improvement**—(1) fluency and rate are strongly related with language function development; (2) 'linguistic fluency' or 'speech fluency' application; (3) application of easy voice onset technique and reduction in avoidance behaviour when the client presents stuttering components of dysfluency.
- **Principles and Techniques for Improvement Self-monitoring**—(1) awareness of cluttering through specific technique application: negative practice, using a list of 'danger signs' when speech gets 'into trouble'; (2) varying the rate of movement of other parts of the body; (3) listening examples of desired speech rates.
- **Principles and Techniques for Improvement the Client's Cognitive and Emotional Components associated with Speech**—(1) to cultivate positive attitude toward speech and communication; (2) to implement cognitive and attitudinal training (St. Louis and Myers 1997).

Because of cluttering's multidimensional nature, Myers (2011) described as an effective treatment construction of an A-frame to house therapy principles and approaches using a *cognitive-behavioural approach.* The foundation of this A-frame to house cluttering therapy is developing the client's meta-awareness (the cognitive component). The behavioural component includes: (1) the central role of rate control, and (2) the insulation of this A-frame to ensure success include the three Ms. of moderation, monitoring, modulation—to work on both the motoric and linguistic components of cluttering.

Ward (2011, p. 182) implements protocol, including possible areas of treatment during speech treatment phases: identification, monitoring and self-awareness, modification and maintenance.

7.2.12 Conclusion

This section has addressed an evidence-based practical approach to clinical cluttering assessment and intervention. It has included definitions of terms in current use and has also addressed some ways in which to proceed from measurement to logopaedic (speech-language therapy)/phoniatric management in order to improve fluency effectively and enhance the quality of life of people with cluttering.

References

Alm P (2007) The dual premotor model of cluttering and stuttering: a neurological framework. In: Bakker K, Raphael L, Myers F (eds) Proceedings of the first world conference on cluttering. Katarino, Bulgaria, pp 207–211

Alm P (2011) Cluttering: a neurological perspective. In: Ward D, Scaler Scott K (eds) Cluttering. A handbook of research, intervention and education. Psychology Press, Hove, New York, pp 3–29

Alm P (2014) Stuttering and the basal ganglia circuits: a critical review of possible relations. J Commun Disord 37(4):325–369

Alm P, Risberg J (2007) Stuttering in adults: the acoustic startle response, temperamental trials, and biological factors. J Commun Disord 40(1):1–41

Andrews G, Cutler J (1974) Stuttering therapy: the relation between changes in symptom level and attitudes. J Speech Hear Disord 39(3):312–319

Bakker K (1996) Cluttering: current scientific status and emerging research and clinical needs. J Fluen Disord 21(3–4):359–367

Bakker K, Myers FL (2011) Cluttering severity instrument [computer software and manual]. http://associations.missouristate.edu/ICA/Resources/Resources%20and%20Links%20pages/CSI%20software%20ALL/CSI_Software.htm. Accessed 27 Mar 2015

Balasubramanian V, Max L, Van Borsel J et al (2003) Acquired stuttering following right frontal and bilateral pontine lesion: a case study. Brain Cogn 53(2):185–189

Bär K, Häger F, Sauer H (2004) Olanzapine-and clozapine-induced stuttering. A case series. Pharmacopsychiatry 37(3):131–134

Basso A (2003) Aphasia and its therapy. Oxford University Press, Oxford

Becker KP, Grundman K (1970) Investigations on incidence and symptomatology of cluttering. Folia Phoniatr 22(4–5):261–271

Begum M (2005) Clozapine-induced stuttering, facial tics and myoclonic seizures: a case report. Aust N Z J Psychiatry 39(3):202

Bennett EM (2006) Working with people who stutter. A lifespan approach. Pearson Merrill Prentice Hall, Upper River, NJ

Bennett Lanouette E (2011) Intervention strategies for cluttering disorders. In: Ward D, Scaler Scott K (eds) Cluttering. A handbook of research, intervention and education. Psychology Press, Hove, New York NY, pp 175–197

Bloodstein O, Bernstein Ratner N (2008) A handbook on stuttering, 6th edn. Delmar, Clifton Park, NY

Boyle MP (2018) Enacted stigma and felt stigma experienced by adults who stutter. J Commun Disord 73:50–61. https://doi.org/10.1016/j.jcomdis.2018.03.004. Epub 2018 Mar 13. PMID: 29574262.

Boyle MP, Milewski KM, Beita-Ell C (2018) Disclosure of stuttering and quality of life in people who stutter. J Fluency Disord 58:1–10. https://doi.org/10.1016/j.jfludis.2018.10.003. Epub 2018 Oct 15. PMID: 30352701

Brutten G, Vanryckeghem M (2006) Behavior assessment battery for school-age children who stutter. Plural Publishing, San Diego CA

Byrne A, Byrne M, Zibin T (1993) Transient neurogenic stuttering. Int J Eat Disord 14(4):511–514

Chang SE, Garnett E, Etchell A et al (2019) Functional and neuroanatomical bases of developmental stuttering: current insights. J Neurosci 25(6):566–582

Chen WH, Peng MC (1993) Acquired stuttering in a patient with encephalitis. Kaohsiung J Med Sci 9(3):183–185

Christensen R, Byerly M, McElroy R (1996) A case of sertraline-induced stuttering. J Clin Psychopharmacol 16(1):92–93

Cruz C, Amorim H, Beca G et al (2018) Neurogenic stuttering: a review of the literature. Rev Neurol 66(2):59–64

Dabul B (2000) Apraxia battery for adults, 2nd edn. Pro-Ed, Austin, TX

Daly DA (1996) The source for stuttering and cluttering. LinguiSystems Inc., East Moline, IL, pp 157–197

Daly DA, Burnett M (1999) Cluttering: traditional views and new perspectives. In: Curlee RF (ed) Stuttering and related disorders of fluency, 2nd edn. Thieme Medical Publishers, New York, NY, pp 222–254

Daly DA, Cantrell RP (2006) Cluttering: characteristics labeled as diagnostically significant by 60 fluency experts. Paper presented at the Fifth IFA World congress of disorders of fluency, Dublin, July 25–28, 2006

De Nil L, Rochon E, Jokel R (2009) Adult-onset neurogenic stuttering. In: McNeil M (ed) Clinical management of sensorimotor speech disorders. Thieme, New York, NY, pp 235–248

De Nil L, Theys C, Jokel R (2017) Stroke-related acquired neurogenic stuttering. In: Coppens P, Patterson J (eds) Aphasia rehabilitation. Clinical Bartlett Learning, Burlington, MA, pp 173–202

Drayna D (2011) Possible genetic factors in cluttering. In: Ward D, Scaler Scott K (eds) Cluttering. A handbook of research, intervention and education. Psychology Press, Hove, New York NY, pp 29–33

Eggers K, Van Eerdenbrugh S (2018) Speech disfluencies in children with down syndrome. J Fluen Disord 71:72–84

Enderby P, Palmer R (2008) FDA-2: Frenchay dysarthria assessment-second edition Examiner's manual. Pro-ed, Austin, TX

Erickson RL (1969) Assessing communication attitudes among stutterers. J Speech Hear Res 12(4):711–724

Fawcett S, Peralego J (2009) Speech in individuals with down syndrome. Perspect Lang Learn Educ 16:109–116

Filatova YO, Song A, St. Louis KO (2018) Attitudes toward stuttering and cluttering by the Chinese public. In: Poster presented at the inaugural joint world congress of the international cluttering association (ICA), international fluency association (IFA) and international stuttering association (ISA). Hiroshima, Japan

Freund H (1952) Studies in the interrelationship between stuttering and cluttering. Folia Phoniatr 4:146–168

Goberman A, Blomgren M, Metzger E (2010) Characteristics of speech disfluency in Parkinson disease. J Neurolinguistics 23(5):470–478

Goodglass H, Kaplan E (1972) Boston diagnostic aphasia examination (BDAE). Lea and Febiger, Philadelphia PA

Guitar, B (2019) Stuttering : an integrated approach to its nature and treatment (Fifth edition). Wolters Kluwer, Alphen aan de Rijn

Guthrie S, Grunhaus L (1990) Fluoxetine-induced stuttering [letter]. J Clin Psychiatry 51:85

Hamano T, Hiraki S, Kawamura Y et al (2005) Acquired stuttering secondary to callosal infarction. Neurology 64(6):1092–1093

Hanson D, Jackson A, Hagerman R (1986) Speech disturbances (cluttering) in mildly impaired males with the Martin-bell/fragile X syndrome. Am J Med Genet 23(1–2):195–206

Howell P, Davis D (2011) The epidemiology of cluttering with stuttering. In: Ward D, Scaler Scott K (eds) Cluttering. A handbook of research, intervention and education. Psychology press, Hove, New York NY, pp 69–90

Jokel R, De Nil L, Sharpe K (2007) Speech disfluencies in adults with neurogenic stuttering associated with stroke and traumatic brain injury. J Med Speech Lang Pathol 15(3):243–261

Junuzovic-Zunic L, Sinanovic O, Majic B (2021) Neurogenic stuttering: etiology, symptomatology, and treatment. Med Arch 75(6):456–461. https://doi.org/10.5455/medarh.2021.75.456-461

Juste FS, Sassi FC, Costa JB et al (2018) Frequency of speech disruptions in Parkinson's disease and developmental stuttering: a comparison among speech tasks. PLoS One 13(6):e0199054

Kent RD (2000) Research on speech motor control and its disorders: a review and prospective. J Commun Disord 33(5):391–428

Kent RD, Vorperian H (2013) Speech impairment in down syndrome: a review. J Speech Lang Hear Res 56(1):178–210

Kertesz A (1982) The Western aphasia battery. Grune & Stratton, New York, NY

Krishnakanth M, Phutane V, Muralidharan K (2008) Clozapine-induced stuttering: a case series. Prim Care Companion J Clin Psychiatry 10(4):333–334

Krishnan G, Tiwari S (2011) Revisiting the acquired neurogenic stuttering in the light of developmental stuttering. J Neurolinguist 24(3):383–396

Krishnan G, Tiwari S (2013) Differential diagnosis in developmental and acquired neurogenic stuttering: do fluency-enhancing conditions dissociate the two? J Neurolinguist 26(2):252–257

Lebrun Y (1996) Cluttering after brain damage. J Fluen Disord 21(3–4):289–295

Lees RM, Boyle BE, Woolfson L (1996) Is cluttering a motor disorder? J Fluen Disord 21(3–4):282–287

Levine A, MacDougall K (2016) New-onset stutter after electrode insertion in the ventrocaudalis nucleus for face pain. World Neurosurg 90:703. https://doi.org/10.1016/j.wneu.2016.02.085

Ludlow C, Schultz G, Menedez L (1995) An investigation of a familial form of cluttering/stuttering. In: Proceedings of the First World Congress on Fluency Disorders, Munich, Germany, August 8-11, 2014, pp 655–658

Lundgren K, Helm-Estabrooks N, Klein R (2010) Stuttering following acquired brain damage: a review of the literature. J Neurolinguistics 23(5):447–454

Maguire G, Viele S, Agarwal S et al (2010) Stuttering onset associated with streptococcal infection: a case suggesting stuttering as PANDAS. Ann Clin Psychiatry 22(4):283–234

Michel V, Burbaud P, Taillard J et al (2004) Stuttering or reflex seizure? A case report. Epileptic Disord 6(3):181–185

Movsessian P (2005) Neuropharmacology of theophylline induced stuttering: the role of dopamine, adenosine and GABA. Med Hypotheses 64(2):290–297

Myers FL (1992) Cluttering: a synergistic framework. In: Myers FL, Louis KOS (eds) Cluttering: a clinical perspective. Far Communication, Leicester, pp 71–84

Myers FL (2011) Treatment of cluttering: a cognitive-behavioral approach centered on rate control. In: Ward D, Scaler Scott K (eds) Cluttering. A handbook of research, intervention and education. Psychology Press, Hove, New York, NY, pp 152–174

Myers FL, Bakker K (2014) Expert's saliency ratings of speech-language dimensions associated with cluttering. J Fluen Disord 42:35–42

Onslow M, Webber M, Harrison E et al (2017) The Lidcombe program treatment guide. https://www.uts.edu.au/sites/default/files/2018-10/Lidcombe%20Program%20Treatment%20Guide%20December%202017.pdf. Accessed 17 Jan 2022

Penttilä N, Korpijaakko-Huuhka AM, Kent R (2019) Disfluency clusters in speakers with and without neurogenic stuttering following traumatic brain injury. J Fluen Disord 59:33–51

Preus A (1981) Identifying subgroups of stutterers. Universitetsforlaget, Oslo

Riley G (2009) SSI-4: stuttering severity instrument examiners' manual, 4th edn. Pro-Ed, Austin, TX

Scaler Scott K (2011) Cluttering and autism spectrum disorders. In: Ward D, Scaler Scott K (eds) Cluttering. A handbook of research, intervention and education. Psychology Press, Hove, New York, NY, pp 115–133

Seeman M (1970) Relations between motorics of speech and general motor ability in clutterers. Folia Phoniatr 22(4):376–380

Shapiro D (2011) Stuttering intervention: a collaborative journey to fluency freedom, 2nd edn. Pro-Ed, Austin, TX

Sick U (2014) Poltern. Theoretische Grundlagen, Diagnostik, Therapie (cluttering. Theoretical basics, diagnostics, therapy). Thieme, Stuttgart, New York NY

Smith A, Weber C (2017) How stuttering develops: the multifactorial dynamic pathways theory. J Speech Lang Hear Res 60(9):2483–2505. https://doi.org/10.1044/2017_JSLHR-S-16-0343. PMID: 28837728; PMCID: PMC5831617

St Louis KO, Filatova Y, Coşkun M et al (2010) Identification of cluttering and stuttering by the public in four countries. Int J Speech Lang Pathol 12(6):508–519

St. Louis KO, Atkins CP (2005) Self-awareness of speech index (SASI). Authors, Morgantown, WV

St. Louis KO, Myers F (1997) Management of cluttering and related fluency disorders. In: Curlee RF, Siegal MG (eds) Nature and treatment of stuttering. New directions. Allyn and Bacon, Boston, MA, pp 313–332

St. Louis KO, Schulte K (2011) Defining cluttering: the lowest common denominator. In: Ward D, Scaler Scott K (eds) Cluttering. A handbook of research, intervention and education. Psychology Press, Hove, New York, NY, pp 233–254

St. Louis KO, Myers FL, Bakker K et al (2007a) Understanding and treating cluttering. In: Conture E,

Curlee R (eds) Stuttering and related disorders of fluency. Thieme, New York, NY, pp 297–325

St. Louis KO, Goranova E, Georgieva D et al (2007b) Public awareness of cluttering: USA, Bulgaria, Turkey, Russia. In: Bakker K, Raphael L, Myers F (eds) Proceedings of the first World Conference on Cluttering, Katarino, Bulgaria, pp 180–190

St. Louis KO, Filatova Y, Coşkun M et al (2011) Public attitudes toward cluttering and stuttering in four countries. In: Simon EL (ed) Psychology of stereotypes. Hauppauge, Nova Science Publishers, New York, NY, pp 81–113. https://www.novapublishers.com/catalog/product_info.php?products_id=23253

St. Louis KO, Sonsterud H, Carlo FJ et al (2014) Public attitudes toward—and identification of—cluttering and stuttering in Norway and Puerto Rico. J Fluen Disord 42:21–34

Strasberg S, Johnson E, Parry T (2016) "Stuttering" after minor head trauma. Am J Emerg Med 34(3):685. https://doi.org/10.1016/j.ajem.2015.07.056

Tani T, Sakai Y (2011) Analysis of five cases with neurogenic stuttering following brain injury in the basal ganglia. J Fluen Disord 36(1):1–16

Tetnowski JA (2007) Cluttering and concomitant disorders. In: Bakker K, Raphael L, Myers F (eds) Proceedings of the first world conference on cluttering. Katarino, Bulgaria, pp 252–260

Theys C, van Wieringen A, De Nil LF (2008) A clinician survey of speech and non-speech characteristics of neurogenic stuttering. J Fluen Disord 33(1):1–23

Theys C, van Wieringen A, Sunaert S et al (2011) A one year prospective study of neurogenic stuttering following stroke: incidence and co-occurring disorders. J Commun Disord 44(6):678–687

Theys C, De Nil L, Thijs V et al (2013) A crucial role for the cortico-striato-cortical loop in the pathogenesis of stroke-related neurogenic stuttering. Human Brain Mapp 34(9):2103–2112

Tütüncüoğlu S, Serdaroğlu G, Kadoğlu B (2002) Landau-Kleffner syndrome beginning with stuttering: case report. J Child Neurol 17(10):785–788

Valenti M, Rudolf G, Carré S et al (2006) Language-induced epilepsy, acquired stuttering, and idiopathic generalized epilepsy: phenotypic study of one family. Epilepsia 47(4):766–772

Van Borsel J (2011) Cluttering and down syndrome. In: Ward D, Scaler Scott K (eds) Cluttering. A handbook of research, intervention and education. Psychology Press, Hove, New York, NY, pp 90–99. https://www.who.int/publications/m/item/icd-10-updates-2007

Van Borsel J (2014) Acquired stuttering: a note on terminology. J Neurolinguist 27(1):41–49

Van Lieshout P, Bose A, Square P et al (2007) Speech motor control in fluent and dysfluent speech production of an individual with apraxia of speech and Broca'saphasia. Clin Linguistic Phon 21(3):159–188

Van Zaalen Y, Reichel I (2015) Cluttering. Current views on its nature, diagnosis, and treatment. iUniverse, Bloomington, IN

Van Zaalen Y, Wijnen F, Dejonckere P (2009) A test of speech motor control on word level productions: the SPA test. Int J Speech Lang Pathol 11:26–33

Ward D (2006) Stuttering and cluttering: frameworks for understanding and treatment. Psychology Press, Hove

Ward D (2011) Motor speech control and cluttering. In: Ward D, Scaler Scott K (eds) Cluttering. A handbook of research, intervention and education. Psychology Press, Hove, New York, NY, pp 34–44

Ward D, Scott KS (2011) Cluttering. A handbook of research, intervention and education. Psychology Press, Hove, New York, NY

Ward D, Connally EL, Pliatsikas C et al (2015) The neurological underpinnings of cluttering: some initial findings. J Fluen Disord 43:1–16

Weiss D (1964) Cluttering. Prentice-Hall, Englewood Cliffs, NJ

Węsierska K, St. Louis KO, Myszka A et al (2014) Comparison of attitudes towards cluttering among Polish SLTs and the general public in Poland using the POSHA-Cl. Poster presented at the 2nd World Conference on Cluttering, Eindhoven, The Netherlands, July 14–16, 2014

WHO (World Health Organization) (2001) International classification of impairments, disabilities, and handicaps: a manual of classification relating to the consequences of disease. World Health Organization, Geneva

WHO (World Health Organization) (2007) ICD—10. https://www.who.int/publications/m/item/icd-10-updates-2007

Wright L, Ayre A (2000) WASSP: Wright and Ayre stuttering self-rating profile. Speechmark, Bicester

Yaruss J (2007) Application of the ICF in fluency disorders. Semin Speech Lang 28(4):312–322

Yaruss JS, Quesal RQ (2006) Overall assessment of the Speaker's experience of stuttering (OASES): documenting multiple outcomes in stuttering treatment. J Fluen Disord 31(2):90–115

Yaruss JS, Quesal RW (2016) Overall assessment of the Speaker's experience of stuttering (OASES). McKinney, Texas: stuttering therapy resources. https://www.stutteringtherapyresources.com/pages/oases. Accessed 18 Jan 2022

8 Diagnosis and Differential Diagnosis of Speech Fluency Disorders

Charley Adams, Wolfgang Angerstein, Giovanna Baracca, Susanne Cook, Philippe H. Dejonckere, Matthias Echternach, Kurt Eggers, Ulrich Eysholdt, Franco Fussi, Ahmed Geneid, Tamás Hacki, Renate Haubrich, Katarzyna Karmelita-Katulska, Christiane Kiese-Himmel, Barbara Maciejewska, Nicole E. Neef, Katrin Neumann, Martin Sommer, František Šram, Jan G. Švec, Jitka Vydrová, and Bożena Wiskirska-Woźnica

František Šram was deceased at the time of publication.

Supplementary Information The online version contains supplementary material available at https://doi.org/10.1007/978-3-031-25175-7_8.

C. Adams (✉)
Communication Sciences and Disorders, University of South Carolina, Columbia, SC, USA
e-mail: charley@sc.edu

W. Angerstein
Phoniatrie und Pädaudiologie, Univ.-Klinikum Düsseldorf, Düsseldorf, Germany
e-mail: angerstein@med.uni-duesseldorf.de

G. Baracca
ENT Department, AO Niguarda Cà Granda, Milan, Italy

S. Cook
International Cluttering Association, Alexandria, VA, USA

P. H. Dejonckere
Federal Agency for Occupational Risks, Brussels, Belgium
e-mail: Philippe.deJonckere@kuleuven.be

M. Echternach
Division of Phoniatrics and Pediatric Audiology, Department of Otorhinolaryngology, Munich University Hospital (LMU), Campus Großhadern, Munich, Germany
e-mail: matthias.echternach@med.uni-muenchen.de

K. Eggers
Thomas More Campus Sint-Andries, Thomas More University College, Antwerpen, Belgium
e-mail: kurt.eggers@ugent.be

U. Eysholdt
Department of Medical Physics and Acoustics/Medical Physics and Cluster of Excellence Hearing4all, Carl von Ossietzky-Universität Oldenburg, Oldenburg, Germany
e-mail: ulrich.eysholdt@uni-oldenburg.de

F. Fussi
AudioPhoniatric Centre, Azienda USL Romagna, Ravenna, Italy

A. Geneid
Department of Otolaryngology and Phoniatrics – Head and Neck Surgery, Helsinki University Central Hospital, Helsinki, Finland
e-mail: Ahmed.Geneid@hus.fi

T. Hacki
Department of Otorhinolaryngology, Head and Neck Surgery, Semmelweis University Budapest, Budapest, Hungary

A. am Zehnhoff-Dinnesen et al. (eds.), *Phoniatrics II*, European Manual of Medicine,
https://doi.org/10.1007/978-3-031-25175-7_8

8.1 Stuttering Assessment

Kurt Eggers

8.1.1 Introduction

In clinical practice, parents of children of different age ranges, as well as adolescents and adults, present with questions and concerns about not speaking fluently. Primarily, parents of young children with speech disfluencies want to know from the doctor or the speech therapist whether the condition is stuttering or not. Parents, but also other caregivers and teachers, often ask themselves whether it is a normal phase in the speech development of the child. In the case of older children, adolescents or adults, one usually knows that it is stuttering, but one wants to know how severe it is, if it can improve or how to stop it. There is thus a clinical need to identify and evaluate the speech disfluencies in a more or less objective manner (Boey 2000).

The aim of this chapter is to provide doctors in training with a framework from which they can make a judgement as to whether the speech problem concerns normal or abnormal speech disfluencies. In the case of the latter, they will learn what exactly they need to look out for and evaluate more thoroughly. The most important thing, however, is an adequate and timely referral to a speech therapist specialised in diagnosing and treating fluency disorders, i.e. a fluency specialist.

Standardised tests are crucial tools in assessing children's communication skills (Gillam et al. 2009). Such tests allow speech therapists to determine whether there is a communication disorder, and if so whether it is mild, moderate or severe. Moreover, an accurate diagnosis contributes to the appropriate treatment of the disorder in question. At present there are many standardised instruments available that allow evaluation of children's speech and language skills. Gillam et al. (2009), however, state that only a limited number of standardised tools are available that allow fluency specialists to compare directly children's speech fluency with data from other children who stutter and children who do not. After all, according to Perkins (1980), speech therapists experience most difficulties in the differential diagnosis of the child who starts stuttering and the fluent-speaking child. Making a precise distinction between the two aforementioned groups at an early stage is therefore essential. Incorrectly diagnosing a child who stutters

R. Haubrich
Evangelisches Klinikum Niederrhein Duisburg-Nord, Zentrale Abteilung für Diagnostische und Interventionelle Radiologie, Duisburg, Germany

K. Karmelita-Katulska
Department of Neuroradiology, University of Medical Sciences in Poznan, Poznan, Poland

C. Kiese-Himmel
Phoniatrics/Pediatric Audiological Psychology, University Medical Center, Goettingen, Germany
e-mail: c.kiese@med.uni-goettingen.de

B. Maciejewska
Department and Clinic of Phoniatrics and Audiology, Poznan University of Medical Sciences, Poznan, Poland
e-mail: barbaramaciejewska@ump.edu.pl

N. E. Neef
Department of Diagnostic and Interventional Neuroradiology, Georg August University, University Medical Center Göttingen, Göttingen, Germany
e-mail: nicole.neef@med.uni-goettingen.de

K. Neumann
Department of Phoniatrics and Pediatric Audiology, University Hospital Münster, University of Münster, Münster, Germany
e-mail: katrin.neumann@uni-muenster.de

M. Sommer
Departments of Geriatrics and Neurology, University Medical Center Göttingen, Göttingen, Germany
e-mail: msommer@gwdg.de

F. Šram · J. Vydrová
Voice and Hearing Centre Prague, Prague 2, Czech Republic
e-mail: vydrova@medico.cz

J. G. Švec
Faculty of Science, Department of Biophysics, Palacky University, Olomouc, Czech Republic
e-mail: jan.svec@upol.cz

B. Wiskirska-Woźnica
Department of Phoniatrics and Audiology, Poznan University of Medical Sciences, Poznan, Poland

as a non-stutterer leads to the withdrawal of necessary clinical intervention. On the other hand, incorrectly diagnosing a child with normal disfluencies as a child who stutters might unnecessarily trigger the start of intervention.

In addition, the diagnosis of stuttering often follows a different course from the diagnosis of diseases in general medicine. Parents visiting their doctor with their child because of abdominal complaints, for example, expect the doctor to make a correct diagnosis on the basis of the symptoms, followed by a physical examination, thus excluding other conditions. In the case of stuttering, parents are generally aware of the problem and expect the fluency specialist to confirm or refute their suspicion. Upon confirmation of this, the specialist will then determine the nature of the stuttering and its severity on the basis of a thorough quantitative and qualitative analysis (Yairi and Seery 2015). Thus, most people seeking help already have a correct (self) diagnosis. Yairi and Ambrose (2005) describe how they have hardly ever disagreed with self-referred adults who diagnosed themselves as stuttering, or with parents who diagnosed their children's speech as stuttering. Moreover, both Curlee (1999) and Ambrose and Yairi (1999) report that their stuttering severity ratings are often close to those of the parents. Clinically, it is only seldom that there is a question of whether a child exhibits normal disfluencies or stuttering, and in these situations, a diagnosis in the more classical sense is required.

For a long time, several authors believed that the distinction between normal and abnormal disfluency was purely quantitative. However, there is sufficient evidence today that invalidates this vision and indicates that qualitative differences are also present (e.g. Yairi 1997, 2007; Yairi and Ambrose 2005). Indeed, Johnson et al. first supported this idea in 1959. Although there is no single type of speech disfluency that occurs only in children who stutter, a qualitative distinction can be made between normal and abnormal disfluencies, even in the initial stages of stuttering. Stuttering, in other words, is characterised by a complex pattern of specific speech disfluencies, their frequency, proportion and duration.

Although the overt speech disfluencies are the most characteristic symptom of stuttering, their diagnosis involves more than just determining whether there is stuttering. Therefore, the focus should not only be on the overt symptoms, but also on several covert aspects such as underlying cognition and emotions associated with stuttering, and the impact that stuttering has on the client's day-to-day functioning. According to the ICF model (e.g. Yaruss and Quesal 2004), the diagnostics of stuttering should consist of an assessment of the overt (core) symptoms and accompanying secondary behaviour (body function), the psycho-social load (person-related factors), communication and social behaviour (activity and participation) and environmental reactions.

Over the years, various objective instruments have been developed, based on the quantity and quality of the core symptoms and accompanying behaviour, allowing fluency specialists to determine if someone is stuttering, and how severe it is (Guitar 2013). Several questionnaires have also been developed (for parents, caregivers and clients themselves) giving insight into the cognitive and attitudinal components, as well as the consequences for everyday life. It is important for referring doctors to gain some basic knowledge of these instruments because recent research (Van Eerdenbrugh and Eggers 2020) has demonstrated a lack of knowledge in general practitioners and paediatricians of the criteria and instruments that can be used to diagnose and refer children who stutter.

8.1.2 Screening Procedure for Stuttering

Riley and Riley (1989) have developed a physician's screening procedure for detecting children who may stutter. While this brief 6-item questionnaire was not used much in the USA, it has been translated (with minor constructional differences) into several languages (Sandrieser and Schneider 2015; Stes and Boey 1997; Stotterfonds 2019) and is currently used frequently in such countries as Germany, Belgium and the

Netherlands. It is an easy-to-use questionnaire requiring information about the type and frequency of disfluencies, accompanying types of secondary behaviour, reactions of the child and others, and how long it has been since the abnormal disfluencies were first noticed. For each question, several answers are possible, some are categorised under 'normal behaviour' and others under 'borderline' or '(very) abnormal'. The questionnaire is jointly completed by the physician and the parents. From the total score different advice is given, ranging from further monitoring to referring the child to a fluency specialist. Similar instruments have been developed for specific languages, such as the Bochum-Aachener Stotterscreening (BASS; Neumann et al. 2015). The 'physician's checklist for referral' (see Fig. 8.1), developed by The Stuttering Foundation (2020), is based on the same principle.

The use of such screening instruments is not only an added value for doctors but also for other care providers and teachers who are concerned about the speech fluency of a child, and who want some more certainty about whether or not to refer them to a fluency specialist.

8.1.3 Assessment of Overt Symptoms

Stuttering is characterised by many overt symptoms, i.e. speech disfluencies and secondary, accompanying (motor) behaviour, and covert aspects such as the individual's affective and cognitive states, irrespective of the observably disfluent speech. The assessment of the overt stuttering symptoms involves listener judgement about the type and duration of the speech disfluencies and the associated behaviour.

PHYSICIAN'S CHECKLIST FOR REFERRAL

	The Child With NORMAL DISFLUENCIES Age of Onset: 1½ to 7 years of age	**The Child With MILD STUTTERING** Age of Onset: 1½ to 7 years of age	**The Child With SEVERE STUTTERING** Age of Onset: 1½ to 7 years of age
Speech behavior you may see or hear:	☐ Occasional (not more than once in every 10 sentences), brief, (typical ½ second or shorter) repetitions of sounds, syllables or short words, e.g., li-li-like this.	☐ Frequent (3% or more of speech), long (½ to 1 second) repetitions of sounds, syllables, or short words, e.g., li-li-li-like this. Occasional prolongations of sounds.	☐ Very frequent (10% or more of speech), and often very long (1 second or longer) repetitions of sounds, syllables or short words. Frequent sound prolongations and blockages.
Other behavior you may see or hear:	☐ Occasional pauses, hesitations in speech or fillers such as "uh," "er," or "um," changing of words or thoughts.	☐ Repetitions and prolongations begin to be associated with eyelid closing and blinking, looking to the side, and some physical tension in and around the lips.	☐ Similar to mild stutterers only more frequent and noticeable; some rise in pitch of voice during stuttering. Extra sounds or words used as "starters."
When problems most noticeable:	☐ Tends to come and go when child is: tired, excited, talking about complex/new topics, asking or answering questions or talking to unresponsive listeners.	☐ Tends to come and go in similar situations, but is more often present than absent.	☐ Tends to be present in most speaking situations; far more consistent and non-fluctuating.
Child reaction:	☐ None apparent	☐ Some show little concern, some will be frustrated and embarrassed.	☐ Most are embarrassed and some are also fearful of speaking.
Parent reaction:	☐ None to a great deal	☐ Most concerned, but concern may be minimal.	☐ All have some degree of concern.
Referral decision:	☐ Refer only if parents moderately to overly concerned.	☐ Refer if continues for 6 to 8 weeks or if parental concern justifies it.	☐ Refer as soon as possible.

Fig. 8.1 Physician's checklist for referral (The Stuttering Foundation 2020)

8.1.3.1 Normal Disfluencies Versus Stuttered Disfluencies

There are different types of speech disfluencies and through the years several speech disfluency classification systems have been developed. Conture (1997, 2001) differentiates between within-word and between-word disfluencies. Within-word disfluencies are produced significantly more frequently by people who stutter than by normally fluent speakers, and these types of speech disfluencies are also more prone to be considered by listeners as stuttered disfluencies. The most frequently used classification for disfluencies in published studies is that of Ambrose and Yairi (1999). They distinguish between 'stuttering-like disfluencies' (SLD) and normal disfluencies or 'other disfluencies' (OD). SLD are part-word repetitions (syllable or sound), single word repetitions, prolongations, blocks and broken words. OD are interjections, revisions of utterances, multisyllabic repetitions and phrase repetitions. Table 8.1 provides an overview of the different disfluency types, description and examples.

8.1.3.2 Frequency of Stuttered Disfluencies

Counting the speech disfluencies is a commonly used method for obtaining objective data on stuttering severity. This can be done by collecting a representative speech sample, counting the number of syllables or words that were stuttered, as well as the total number of words or syllables in the sample, and calculating the percentage of stuttered syllables or words. The way in which the speech sample is collected is important because one of the main characteristics of stuttering at a young age is its variability. A video-recording contributes to making analyses objective. The sample ideally consists of several minutes of spontaneous speech, at least 300 syllables, being representative of the stutterer's parents' experience outside the clinic. In younger children this can be collected by recording the interaction between the parent and the child, by playing, e.g. with a toy farm, or by asking the parents to bring a recording from home (quite often this is more valid). In older children and adults, this can be obtained by open questions. Closed questions, which can be answered with yes-no or short

Table 8.1 Categorisation, description and examples of the types of speech disfluencies, i.e. stuttering-like disfluencies (SLD) and other disfluencies (OD) (based on Ambrose and Yairi 1999; Eggers et al. 2019)

Disfluency type	Description	Example
SLD		
Monosyllabic word repetition	Repetition of a monosyllabic word	I II like it
Part-word repetition		
Sound repetition	Repetition of a sound within a word	She eats an aaa apple
Syllable repetition	Repetition of a syllable within a word	I ca ca cannot find it
Dysrhythmic phonation		
Prolongation	Prolongation of a sound resulting in an atypical duration of that sound	I want somemmmmilk
Block	Stopping airflow and sound during or before production of a sound	I like climbing ….trees
Broken word	Stopping airflow and sound in the middle of a vowel within a word	The door is o…pen
OD		
Multi-syllable word repetition	Repetition of a multisyllabic word	Yesterday yesterday I played …
Interjection	Filler words or non-linguistic sounds used within an utterance	When he um…um…
Phrase repetition	Repetition of a phrase within an utterance	I think I think it was yesterday
Revision	Correction of overt word choice errors, grammatical or phonological errors	Last week, last month we went …
Unfinished word (or sentence)	Abandoned or incomplete word	I have a do-

answers, should be avoided since they do not give a correct representation of the speech disfluencies. This is often combined with a reading sample of a standardised text. People who stutter sometimes avoid using specific words on which they often stutter in spontaneous speech, but when reading this is not possible. So, people who stutter and who also use a lot of avoidance strategies, will often stutter more when reading a text.

Conture (2001) states that while there are still no adequate norms for the frequency of speech disfluencies, from his experience people exhibiting three or more within-word disfluencies per 100 words show some degree of fluency problem. This is also in line with Ambrose and Yairi (e.g. 1999) who suggest a production of 3% SLD as a clinical threshold to diagnose 'stuttering'. For various languages, including English, Dutch, Spanish, German and French, this guideline of 3% does seem to be applicable (Ambrose and Yairi 1999; Boey et al. 2007; Carlo and Watson 2003; Eggers 2010; Leclercq et al. 2017; Natke et al. 2006; Pellowski and Conture 2002; Tumanova et al. 2014). Other guidelines are also being used, such as producing more than 10 disfluencies (of all types) per 100 words (e.g. Adams 1977; Guitar 2013) or the mean number of repetition units of 2 or higher (e.g. ye-ye-yesterday) per disfluency (e.g. Ambrose and Yairi 1999; Pellowski and Conture 2002). However, it is important to highlight, since bilingualism is gradually increasing, that most of these monolingual diagnostic guidelines for stuttering cannot be applied to a bilingual population, because bilingual children already produce a higher frequency of disfluencies (Byrd et al. 2020; Eggers et al. 2019; Saad Merouwe et al. 2024).

8.1.3.3 Secondary Accompanying (Motor) Behaviour

Besides the frequency of stuttered speech disfluencies, one must also qualify and quantify secondary accompanying speech and non-speech factors that affect and reflect speech fluency (Shapiro 2011). These types of secondary behaviour can be very diverse but include speech-related factors such as audible inhalations and exhalations linked to a stuttering moment; rises in pitch, reflecting additional laryngeal tension; sniffing and clicking sounds; visible oral and neck tension, such as jaw jerking, tongue protrusion and lip pressing. Non-speech factors include facial tension, eye movements, poor eye contact, head movements, movements of the extremities.

Children who do not stutter do not show these types of symptoms. While not all children who stutter develop these types of secondary behaviour, many do develop them, frequently within weeks or months after the onset of stuttering. This secondary behaviour can reflect the child's increasing awareness of stuttering and is often a coping mechanism to get out of or to prevent a stuttering moment. While the stuttered disfluencies (repetitions, prolongations, blocks) have a high degree of overlap between different children who stutter, the secondary behaviour is highly variable in each client, and therefore are quite often responsible for a very different clinical presentation of the client's symptomatology.

8.1.3.4 Overt Stuttering Severity

Several instruments have been developed to measure overt stuttering severity, such as the Stuttering Severity Instrument (SSI; Riley 2009) and the Test of Childhood Stuttering (TOCS; Gillam et al. 2009). The SSI is an established and widely used standardised test, which can be used with children and adults. It evaluates three components of stuttering, i.e. the frequency of stuttered disfluencies, the average duration of the stuttered disfluencies, and the physical concomitants or secondary behaviour.

For the frequency, a speech sample of at least 200 words is needed. Depending on the client's age, the client interprets a story from pictures or tells something spontaneously. In older clients this is combined with reading a standard text. Many fluency specialists collect more than one sample (e.g. in the home situation, by phone calls). The stuttered disfluencies are counted, and a syllable-based frequency is calculated and converted into a frequency task score. The duration is assessed by calculating the mean length of the three longer stuttering moments in the speech samples and converting it into a duration task score.

For the physical concomitants, the fluency specialist evaluates the secondary behaviour on a six-point scale, ranging from 0 (none) to 5 (severe and painful looking). The types of behaviour are placed in four categories, i.e. distracting sounds, facial grimaces, head movements and movements of the extremities. All the subscores are added to a physical concomitants task score. Finally, all the task scores are summed to provide a total score, which can be converted into a percentile and a severity equivalent, ranging from very mild, mild, moderate, severe, to very severe.

8.1.4 Assessment of Covert Symptoms

From the 1960s, the development of assessments focusing on the client's related cognitions, emotions and attitude towards the stuttering started to be developed (Ward 2006). This is crucial because overt symptoms may fluctuate over time depending on the situation and the period, resulting in an (overt) stuttering severity score that may inadequately reflect the severity and the impact of the disorder. Covert symptoms refer to feelings and thoughts, such as high levels of concern for listener reactions, fear of making a stutter, frustration when making a stutter, anxiety related to specific speaking situations, feelings of guilt and shame, but even depression (Eggers et al. 2022). These often result in an increase in the secondary accompanying behaviour such as struggling, avoidance or postponement. It is often assumed that this mainly occurs with older clients and that young children are not easily aware of their stuttering. Various studies (e.g. The KiddyCAT Vanryckeghem and Brutten 2007), however, have shown that children are already aware before the age of 3 that their speech is different from that of other children. Assessing these covert aspects can be done in an informal way during an interview (see for example Onslow et al. 2023), or in a more formal manner by using specially developed questionnaires probing the client's beliefs and feelings, such as Erickson's Scale of Communication Attitude (Erickson 1969) and the Wright and Ayre Stuttering Self-rating Profile (Wright and Ayre 2000).

In what follows, two widely used instruments that have been translated and validated in many languages will be discussed.

8.1.4.1 Behaviour Assessment Battery

The Behavior Assessment Battery (BAB; Vanryckeghem and Brutten 2001) is available for school-aged children (Brutten and Vanryckeghem 2007) and for adults (Vanryckeghem and Brutten 2018). Both versions contain different sets of self-reporting measures evaluating the affective, behavioural and cognitive dimensions of the experiences of people who stutter. Combined, they provide a broad overview of the covert symptomatology.

The Speech Situation Checklist-Emotional Reaction (*SSC-ER*), a 50-item questionnaire, investigates the extent to which a person experiences anxiety, fear or worry in particular speech situations. Clients are asked to respond to questions such as 'How do you feel when you talk to someone older than you?' The questionnaire includes different communication situations (e.g. talking in the classroom, making a phone call, talking to strangers, ordering in a restaurant). Clients have to indicate their emotional response by using a five-point Likert scale ranging from 1 (not afraid) to 5 (very much afraid).

The Speech Situation Checklist-Speech Disruption (*SSC-SD*) surveys the level of speech disruption in the same communicative settings as the SSC-ER. This time, the client rates the extent of their speech disruption on a scale from 1 (not at all disrupted) to 5 (very much disrupted).

The Behaviour Checklist (*BCL*) provides a way of indicating coping behaviour such as avoidance and escape (e.g. pausing before trying to say a feared word, avoiding eye contact) that the client typically uses before or during a moment of stuttering. Clients first evaluate whether they are using a certain coping behaviour, followed by the frequency with which they use it, ranging from 1 (very infrequently) to 5 (very frequently). The child version contains 50 items and the adult version 95 items.

The Communication Attitude Test (*CAT*), a 33-item questionnaire, provides insight into the way that clients think about their speech, and includes statements such as 'I don't worry about the way I talk' or 'Talking is easy for me', each of which has to be answered by true or false. For all these subtests, ratings are summed and compared with available age-appropriate norms.

8.1.4.2 Overall Assessment of the Speaker's Experience of Stuttering

Yaruss and Quesal (2016) developed the *Overall Assessment of the Speaker's Experience of Stuttering* (*OASES*) to obtain information about the totality of the stuttering experience as described by the ICF-model. The instrument assesses the overall impact of stuttering on school-age children, teenagers and adults. The questionnaire consists of 4 sections; each contains around 20 questions:

- Section 1 (general information) contains questions about the client's knowledge about stuttering and stuttering therapy, and the client's self-assessment of his speech.
- Section 2 (your reactions to stuttering) evaluates the client's affective, cognitive and behavioural reactions to stuttering.
- Section 3 (communication in daily situations) examines the difficulty of communicating in different age-related speaking situations, such as school, social activities and home.
- Section 4 (quality of life) contains questions providing information about the overall impact of stuttering on the client's life, such as interfering with communication, relationships and confidence (e.g. 'How much does stuttering stop you from saying what you want to say at school?', 'How much does stuttering interfere with your confidence in yourself?').

Every statement has to be answered on a five-point Likert scale, scores are summed for each section and divided by the number of items completed. All scores are combined into an overall impact score. Impact ratings range from mild, mild/moderate, moderate, moderate/severe, to severe.

8.1.5 Assessment of Children

Manning (2010) states that when evaluating the possibility of stuttering in young children, one needs to make two primary decisions: first, a judgement about the possible nature of the speech disfluencies, and second, whether they are within normal limits. In other words, normal disfluencies should be differentiated from abnormal, stuttered disfluencies; and if abnormal disfluencies are present, at what frequency (see 8.1.3 above). Moreover, both the child's awareness and reactions to the speech disfluencies, and the concern of parents, help inform the fluency specialist about whether a child is stuttering or not. Indicators of the child's awareness may be the presence of secondary accompanying behaviour, a change in the speaking behaviour (e.g. very outgoing, talkative at first but now much quieter, whispering) and reactions of the child to his own speaking difficulties (e.g. 'My mouth is stuck'). At this age, it is important to consider the concern of the parents but also to discover the nature of the family and the parent–child interaction.

Second, the fluency specialist needs to evaluate if the speech disfluencies are likely to be temporary or permanent; in other words, what the chances are of spontaneous recovery of the stuttering. Various studies have reported different recovery rates, with estimates ranging from 60% to 80%, with recent research pointing towards the higher recovery rates, especially in very young children (Yairi and Ambrose 2013). Given the uncertainty about the chronic nature of stuttering, the fluency specialist needs to make a well-balanced decision ranging from (in)formal monitoring of the speech disfluencies to the start of intervention. Factors that can guide this clinical decision-making process are predictors based on the work by Yairi and Ambrose (2005). Three subsets of criteria are distinguished: primary, secondary and other factors. The primary factors are family history (having no relatives who stutter gives a greater chance of recovery than having a family history of persistent stuttering), sex (stuttering is more likely to persist in boys than in girls), age at onset (stuttering beginning in older children is more likely to persist), development of the SLD (a downward trend in the number of SLD during the first year is a strong positive sign for eventual recovery), duration of the stuttering history (the longer the stuttering history beyond the first year, the higher the risk of persistence, especially in girls), length of the speech disfluencies (the continuing presence of several repetition units—e.g. ye-ye-ye-yes—and a more rapid rate of repetition are signs of higher risk), and the presence of prolongations and blocks (a decrease of these disfluencies is a sign for possible recovery). The secondary and other factors include such aspects as stuttering severity, concomitant disorders, awareness and affective reactions. Later studies have also revealed other influential factors such as temperamental constellation (Jones et al. 2020) and language profile (Leech et al. 2017).

In pre-school children, the gathering of information is primarily based on parent interview, parent–child interaction and child–clinician interaction; in school-age children, direct interviewing of the child about the stuttering is also appropriate, as is possibly a teacher interview.

8.1.6 Assessment of Adolescents and Adults

The primary decisions addressed in the assessment of children are of less importance in this age group: (complete) spontaneous recovery barely occurs at this age (Neumann et al. 2019) and the (self)diagnosis of stuttering has already been made. While the assessment can also involve interviews with parents, teachers and peers, as well as observation of the client interacting in different communicative situations, the perception of the clients about themselves and their circumstances are likely to be one of the more important aspects of the assessment procedure. In some adolescents, the assessment might be somewhat challenging because of denial of the problem or lack of motivation. Creating a secure environment of recognition enables the adolescent to feel understood (Shapiro 2011).

One of the easier techniques, yet potentially the most useful for obtaining the perspective of clients and their stuttering, is to have them respond to a number of questions designed to survey the range of their stuttering (Manning 2010): questions such as 'Why have you come to meet us today?' and 'What are your expectations?' Ask them to describe their stuttering, when it started, what they think causes the stuttering, if they have had previous treatments. Try also to get some insight into the impact of the stuttering by asking them how the stuttering is affecting their life, in what situations they experience the most disfluencies. Finally, their desire for change and motivation for starting fluency treatment, possibly impacted by previous (unsuccessful) treatment, should also be surveyed.

8.1.7 Summary

The goal of this section was to provide doctors with a framework for well-motivated clinical decision-making. The evaluation of the client's disfluent speech should be based on the type and frequency of the disfluencies, the presence of secondary accompanying behaviour and possible covert symptoms (see also Brundage et al., 2021). In case of stuttering, the client needs to be referred to a fluency specialist who, in consultation with the client or the parents, determines the need for starting direct or indirect treatment.

8.2 Psychomotor, Cognitive and Language Stages of Normal Children of Different Ages

8.2.1 Assessment of the Developmental Speech and Language Status of Children

Katrin Neumann

8.2.1.1 Normal Language Development: The Concept of Milestones and Border Stones

For the proper evaluation of the language status of a child, knowledge of the distinct age-appropriate developmental targets of the acquisition of a specific language is necessary. As for other domains of infant and child development, the concept of milestones and borderline stones is useful for characterizing important steps in the acquisition of the native language for each linguistic domain (Kliegman et al. 2011). As demonstrated in Table 8.2 for the example of German language acquisition, milestones indicate at which average age a child has reached domain-specific levels of competence. Border stones are distinct developmental targets that are reached by 90% of all normally developed children by a certain age (Michaelis 2004).

8.2.1.2 Diagnostics of Developmental Disorders of Speech and Language

For the diagnosis of developmental disorders of speech and language (DDSL), the separation of specific developmental disorders of speech and language (SDDSL) and DDSL with comorbidities has to be taken into consideration. Hence the first step of the diagnostic process is to seek comorbidities, because SDDSL is an exclusion diagnosis. Furthermore, DDSL have to be distinguished from socioculturally caused environmental language abnormalities, which do not need treatment but language input and training (see Sect. 9.8 in Volume 1).

Analysis of Spontaneous Speech

The analysis of spontaneous speech is an important tool in the diagnostics of developmental language deficits, and it complements language tests. It is based on the observation of the child during a guided game or a dialogue, mostly with adults (parents or examiner). It is important to create situations that stimulate the child to communicate.

Table 8.2 Time course of the normal German language acquisition (modified according to de Langen-Müller et al. 2012, with kind permission from Peter Lang GmbH, Internationaler Verlag der Wissenschaften)

Domain	Stage of development	Milestone (average age)	Borderline stone (age at 90th percentile)
Early language perception	Interest in human language ('eavesdropping')	Prenatally, first weeks of life	
	Perception of rhythmic and prosodic features of mother tongue	Prenatally, first weeks of life	
Development of vocalization	Crying	Birth	
	Cooing	Sixth to eighth week	
	Marginal babbling (testing of sound production)	Fourth month	
	Canonic babbling (syllables of consonants and vowels, e.g. *ba*)	Sixth month	Eighth to tenth month
	Reduplicated babbling (doubling of syllables, e.g. *baba*)	Eighth to tenth month	11th to 15th month
	Varying babbling (e.g. *bada*)	Eighth to tenth month	
Acquisition of the phonological system	Elementary sound inventory	12th month	
	Simple syllable structures (mostly open syllables)		
	Starting organization of the phonological system (use of sounds of the target language)	18th month	
	Starting to overcome phonological processes (systematic developmental changes of pronunciation of the target language)	2.5–4.5 year of life	
	Development of phonological awareness: detect syllables; 'clap' syllables; detect rhymes; detect initial sounds	About third year of life	
	Development of phonological awareness: detect and localize phonemes (smallest contrasting unit regarding meaning in the sound system), segmentation, analysis and synthesis of sounds into words	About fifth year of life	

(continued)

Table 8.2 (continued)

Domain	Stage of development	Milestone (average age)	Borderline stone (age at 90th percentile)
Acquisition of vocabulary	Starting to understand words	Ninth month	
	Understanding approximately 50 words	16th month	
	Pre-forms of naming (situation-dependent proto-words)	Tenth month	
	Purposeful usage of *mama* and *papa*	Tenth to 15th month	18th to 20th month
	Production of the first words (one-word utterances)	13th to 20th month at latest	18th to 20th month
	Production of at least 50 words	18th to 24th month at latest	24th month
	Vocabulary spurt	18th to 21th month	
	Stage 1: personal/social words (*yes*, *hello*), relational words (*there*, *on*), onomatopoeia, proper names, some nouns	12th to 18th month	
	Stage 2: noun growth, start of verb acquisition	19th to 30th month	
	Stage 3: verb growth, function words (*because)*, pronouns	30th to 36th month	
	Overextensions and underextensions (e.g. *dog*/*bow-wow* for naming all animals)	Second year of life	
	Acquisition of the hierarchical organization of the mental lexicon; understanding semantic relations	Third year of life till school age	
	Acquisition of word formation: compounding (composition, e.g. *front door*) + derivation (e.g. *heat → heater*; *sun → sunny*)	Second to fifth year of life	
Acquisition of grammar	Production of word combinations (two- or more-word utterances)	18th to 24th month at latest	25th to 26th month
	Increase of utterance length: at the age of 3 years, approximately 3 words per utterance on average	Third year of life	
	Production of simple syntactic structures	Third year of life	
	Decrease of omissions of obligatory constituents (e.g. subject)	Third year of life	
	Decrease of omissions of function words	Third to fourth year of life	
	Verbs in second position (*Lisa cake eat → Lisa eats cake* or *What eats Lisa?*)	30th to 36th month	
	Use of variable sentence types: declarative sentence, interrogative sentence, exclamatory sentence	30th to 36th month	
	Occurrence of subordinate clauses	36th month	
	Use of the definite article (*the*)	30th to 36th month	
	Correct subject-verb congruency (*I eat—she eats*)	Second to third year of life	
	Acquisition of the German case system, accusative at first, dative later	36th month to school entry age	
	Acquisition of the plural system	Second to sixth year of life	
	Acquisition of tempus markers	Third year of life	
	Temporary grammatical overextensions (*I runned away.*)	Third to fourth year of life	

(continued)

Table 8.2 (continued)

Domain	Stage of development	Milestone (average age)	Borderline stone (age at 90th percentile)
Development of conversational and narrative abilities	Eye contact with primary attachment figure	Third month	
	Early expression of communicative intentions via looking, gestures and vocalizations	First year of life	
	Triangular eye contact Establishing shared focus of attention	Ninth month	
	Adherence to turn-taking rules	Second year of life	
	Child relates to conversation partner in dialogue	18th month	
	Organization of topics in dialogue	Third year of life	
	Development of narrative competence; increasing coherence (content-related) and cohesion (formal connection of text elements) in narration	36th month to early school age	
	Understanding irony and metaphors	Sixth year of life	
Literary language acquisition	Logographic stage (recognition of frequent words)	Preschool age, early elementary school age	
	Alphabetic stage (linkage between sounds and letters)	Early elementary school age	
	Orthographic stage (learning of orthographic rules)	Elementary school age	

Speech and language-related behaviour and utterances of the child have to be documented. Video recordings may be helpful for language and interaction analyses and may also provide information on the parental communicative behaviour and style. From such informal observations, important information about phonetic-phonological, semantic-lexical, morphologic-syntactical and pragmatic-communicative abilities of a child can be gained. Furthermore, prosody, speech fluency and motivation to speak and to communicate as well as joyfulness of speaking may be analysed. For the evaluation of the spoken utterances, speech competence (the mastery of the speech-language systems) has to be distinguished from performance (the demonstration of the competence while communicating). Speech-language diagnostics aims to elicit as much as possible competence via performance within a short time (Neumann et al. 2009).

For a more thorough analysis of spontaneous speech, a detailed transcription, coding and analysis of language samples can be gained from audio or video recordings. Computer programs may be useful here, such as the Systematic Analysis of Language Transcripts (SALT) (Miller et al. 2011; SALT Software 2014) and the Computerized Language Analysis (CLAN) Program (MacWhinney 1995), which is a part of the Child Language Data Exchange System (CHILDES 2014), a database of speech audio files and text transcriptions in more than 20 languages serving as a central repository for first-language acquisition data (CHILDES 2014). Transcripts are necessary to calculate, for example, the mean length of utterances (MLU). This is a measure of linguistic productivity and language proficiency in children. It is the average number of morphemes per utterance contained in a sample of 100 utterances. The MLU is a benchmark of language acquisition, a good marker of DDSL, and may predict the further reading abilities of children (Bishop and Adams 1990; Rice et al. 2010). However, because the usefulness of MLU is questioned, it should not be used as the only diagnostic measure of language proficiency in children.

Examination of the Developmental Speech and Language Status with Informal and Nonstandardized Procedures

For a rough, informal evaluation of the phonetic-phonological, semantic-lexical and pragmatic competence of a child, simple test tools such as picture cards are suitable. Grammatical abilities might also be judged by using pictures that stimulate the production of specific grammatical structures, such as 'Brush your teeth!' to elicit the imperative or 'This is one apple, and these are two…?' for eliciting information on plural production (Neumann et al. 2011). The informal judgement of the types of language-related competence of a child requires the knowledge from professionals on the age-appropriate developmental targets (milestones) for each tested linguistic level (see Table 8.2).

Language Tests

The assessment of language skills should be performed with valid and normed tests, in order to get, as far as possible, examiner-independent, reproducible and reliable results. The use of only such tests enables the comparison of an individual test result with normal values, its interpretation and a differentiated evaluation of a child's language developmental status compared with the age norm. Comprehensive language tests that examine all or at least some linguistic levels have to be distinguished from tests that analyse only one type of competence, for example, vocabulary. The scores of single subtests of comprehensive tests ought not to be interpreted separately for different linguistic domains (grammar, vocabulary, etc.); otherwise such tests would reveal more children suspected of a DDSL than its prevalence (Neumann et al. 2011). In other words, if many subtests are performed, the probability is high by chance alone that at least one of them would indicate a deficit, which may lead to overdiagnosis. Therefore, a weighting system is required that evaluates test results according to the severity and prognosis of the specific deficiency.

Principles of the Interpretation of Test Values

Test results may be available as raw values or standardized values. Raw values are related to scores that result from an assignment prescription of a test. This could be, for example, the number of correct results in a language test or a sum score in a questionnaire test based on Likert scales ranging from 0 (does not fit at all) to 5 (fits perfectly). Raw values are useful (a) when related to reaching a cut-off value and as a base for (b) different categories (e.g. below average, average, above average) and (c) further transformations, e.g. in standardized values. Standardized values, on the other hand, are easier to interpret than raw values.

Example: A child has performed a speech perception test and has solved 6 of 10 items correctly. At first glance this suggests a quite good test result, which, however, may be oversimplified and wrong, because from the reference values it is clear that in the normative sample all children are able to solve five items correctly, and the majority of subjects even at least six items. A transformation of the raw value '6' into a standardized value, for example into the 10th percentile (to be interpreted roughly as: 90% of the subjects of the normative sample have solved more items) or a value that is even more related to the distribution of the normative values, such as the intelligence quotient, indicate a rather 'below average' result in this example (Petermann and Macha 2005).

A classical test construction is based on standard scales. For the tests applied during the assessment of DDSL/SDDSL, percentile scales, z scales, T scales, C scales and intelligence scales are used most frequently (Fig. 8.2). Standard scales enable the identification of the position of an examined child relative to a control sample. This requires an empirically gained reference frame from a sufficiently large, representative control sample. The named scales relate a test value to the average of the standard distribution and to the variance of the latter in order to answer the question: Is, or by how much is, the test score above or below the average?

The standardized values shown in Fig. 8.2 follow this sequence: (a) The average value of a distribution is identified. (b) A numerical value according to the chosen scale is attributed to the average. The percentile scale attributes the percentage of 50 to the average of the scale; the IQ scale, the IQ value 100; the z scale, the z value 0; the T scale, the T value 50; and the C scale, the value 5. (c) In order to interpret a test score, the spread of the distribution is of interest, in particular the distance between the average and the standard deviation (SD), because the test values on a specific scale are related to the SD. For example, the IQ scale subdivides the distance between the

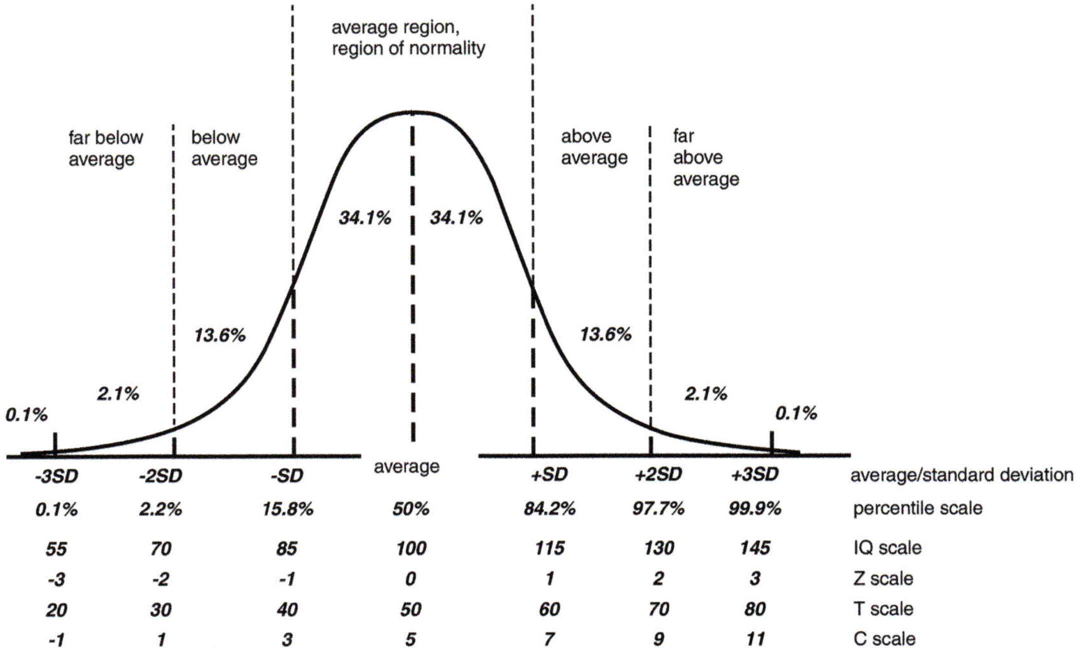

Fig. 8.2 Principles of generation of standard values and frequently used standard scales for the assessment of DDSL/SDDSL. Percentile, *z*-, *T*-, *C*- and intelligence (IQ) scales: selected standard values in a normal distribution (Gaussian curve) and convention of their interpretation. (Modified according to Petermann and Macha 2005 with kind permission from the authors)

average and one standard deviation into 15 scale units (an IQ value of 85 represents an intelligence that deviates 1 SD from the average downwards; an IQ of 70 indicates a deviation of 2 SD from the average downwards). The *T* scale attributes 10 points to the distance of the SD from the average. In this way each of the scales enables the quantification of direction and extent of a deviation from the average by a scale value.

The percentages given on the Gaussian bell curve of a normal distribution are useful for orientation. They indicate the proportion of subjects of a sample (e.g. the norming sample) which is in the respective performance range. Between −1 and +1 SD lie about 68.2% of all subjects, i.e. more than two thirds. Below −1 SD are located the worst 15.8% of the subjects of the normative sample related to the values of a specific test; below −2 SD, the worst 2.2%; and below −3 SD, the worst 0.1%.

Related to those reference values, the performance in a certain test can be interpreted. The region between −1 and +1 SD from the average is regarded as the average or normal region (~68.2% of all subjects), i.e. a *T* value of 43 or an IQ of 91 is 'average'. The deviation of a test value of more than one but not more than two SD from the average may be interpreted as 'below average' or 'above average' (13.6% of subjects are located on each side of the average distribution). The 'below average' region is often considered as a region of risk. Thus, a *T* value of 35 or the 12th percentile is 'below average' and an IQ value of 125 'above average'. Deviations of more than ±2 SD from the average may be named 'far below/above average' (2.2% on each side). A *T* value of 26 or the second percentile is thus 'far below average' and an IQ <70 as well (regarded an intellectual disability), and an IQ >130 is 'far above average' (intellectual giftedness) (Petermann and Macha 2005).

Diagnostic Criteria for Specific Developmental Disorders of Speech and Language

Four diagnostic criteria are defined for the diagnosis of an SDDSL (F80.1 and F80.2) according to the International Statistical Classification of

Diseases and Related Health Problems, the ICD-10 of the World Health Organization (2011), slightly modified by Dilling et al. (2008) and de Langen-Müller et al. (2012). They are based on the discrepancy between the language skills of a child and the age-related normative values and on the assumption of normality. According to this assumption, neurological, sensory, emotional, social or physical disorders, which could explain the language problems, are lacking. There is no reduced intelligence (IQ <85, as measured with a nonverbal intelligence test).

- Perceptive and expressive language skills, as assessed from standardized and normed tests, are 1.5–2 SD below the age-dependent normative values at one or more than one language/communicative level.
- The expressive and receptive language skills, as assessed by structured behavioural and linguistic analyses, are considerably below the average abilities of the age norm.
- The use and understanding of nonverbal communication are within the age norm.
- The assumption of normality is justified.

Additionally, the ICD-10 defines a double discrepancy criterion between cognitive and language competence: for an SDDSL diagnosis, language perception or language production of a child is below the level appropriate for his or her age. Additionally, the receptive/expressive language competence is 1–1.5 SD below the nonverbal IQ that is at least average (IQ ≥85) (see criteria 1 and 4). This criterion is, however, under debate.

A diagnostic algorithm as shown in Fig. 8.3 demonstrates the steps of an interdisciplinary diagnostics of a (S)DDSL and the subsequent interventions. If there is suspicion of an age-inappropriate language development, audiological assessment of the hearing of a child is inevitable. Thereafter, the language competence is assessed. A subsequent differential diagnostics does not follow a fixed scheme but depends on the specific symptoms (de Langen-Müller et al. 2012). If there is suspicion of an SDDSL, possible comorbidities have to be excluded.

Screening Tests for the Developmental Speech and Language Status

Parent questionnaires have been shown to be a useful screening for the language development status of young children (Dale 1991). Universal or regional screening tests at kindergarten or preschool ages, i.e. short and easy to perform and to analyze language tests, have been implemented in some European regions. They aim at the detection and support of children with language abnormalities by either language therapy or training, in order to ensure sufficient language competence at school entry. In most cases such screening can distinguish between children who have language abnormalities and those who do not. Only a few screening tests, such as the German Kindersprachscreening (KiSS.2), trichotomize between (a) normally developed children, (b) children who have sociogenically caused language abnormalities and who require language training and (c) those who are suspect for having a DDSL and need therapy (Neumann and Euler 2013).

In order to evaluate the validity of a screening, the proportion of children who fail it (REFER, screening-positive) and of those who pass it (PASS, screening-negative) have to be evaluated by comparing the results of the screening and those of reference language tests (gold standard) in a sufficient large, unselected sample of screened children. Furthermore, the proportion of false and correct positives (REFER rate) and false and correct negatives (PASS rate) have to be calculated (Table 8.3). From these values, sensitivity and specificity of the screening may be calculated, the most important validity criteria. Specificity measures the ability of language screening to detect children with normal language development correctly, and the sensitivity indicates the ability to identify children with language abnormalities correctly.

Sensitivity and specificity of screening are related to each other. This can be demonstrated by a receiver operating characteristic (ROC) curve, which shows the ability of screening to distinguish between two conditions such as PASS and REFER (Fig. 8.4).

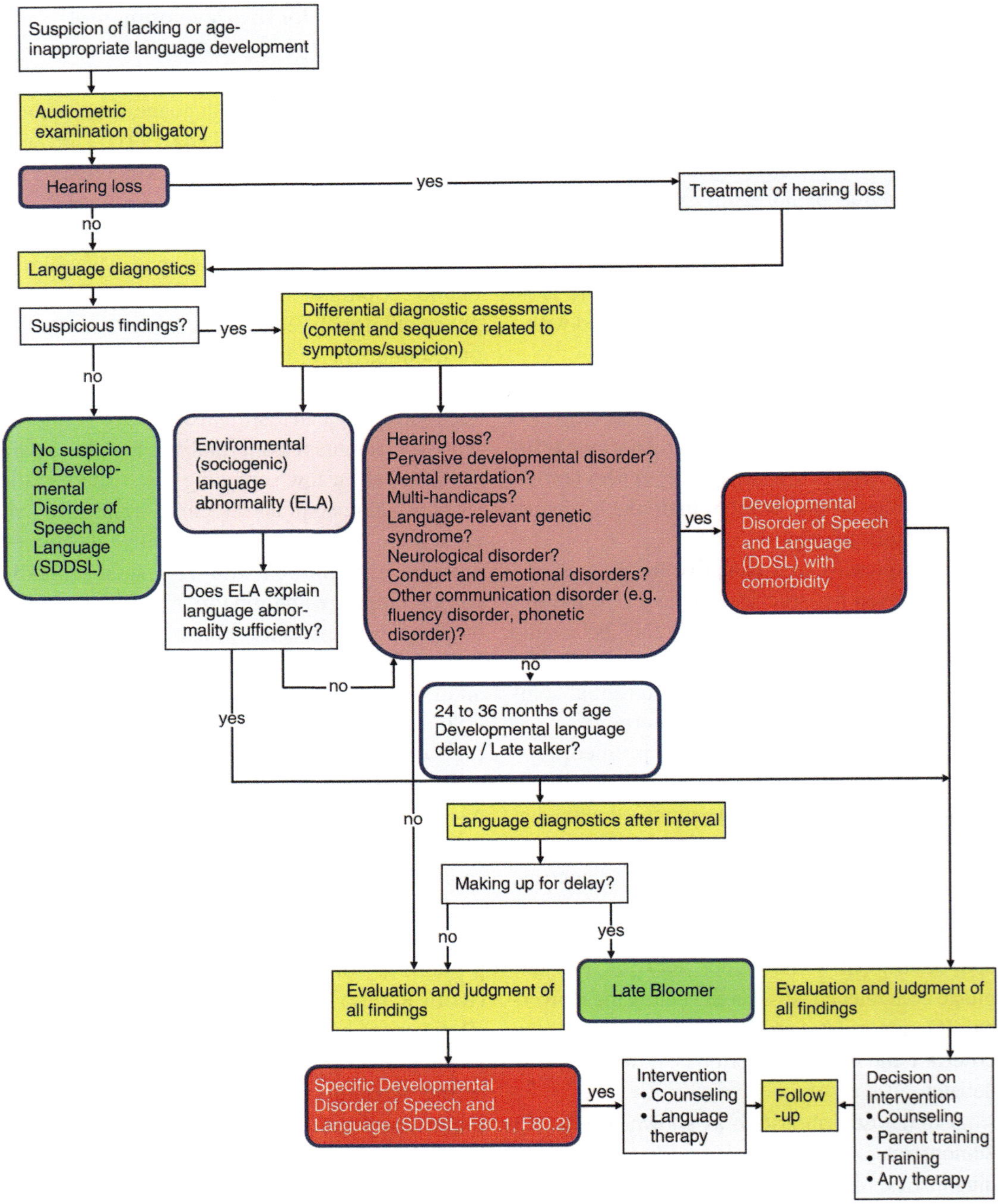

Fig. 8.3 Diagnostic algorithm for developmental disorders of speech and language. (Modified according to de Langen-Müller et al. 2012, with kind permission from Peter Lang GmbH, Internationaler Verlag der Wissenschaften)

For a PASS/REFER decision, a cut-off criterion has to be defined. Cut-off values may be derived from the prevalence of a disease. If the prevalence of SDDSL is given as 4–7% and that of DDSL with comorbidity estimates at least 3%, then diagnostic testing for DDSL should not reveal much more than 10% of children in a normal population who fail it, which is between −1 and −2 SD (see 'Diagnostic Criteria' in section "Language Tests"). For screening the borderlines

Table 8.3 Agreement between the results of language screening and diagnostic language assessment with language tests

		Diagnostic tests		
		DDSL (D+)	No DDSL (D−)	Total
Screening	REFER (S+)	**cp**	fp	cp + fp
	PASS (S−)	**fn**	rn	fn + cn
	Total	cp + fn	fp + rn	cp + fp + cn + fn

S+ screening-positive, *S−* screening-negative, *D+* diagnostics-positive, *D−* diagnostics-negative, *cp* correct positive, *cn* correct negative, *fp* false positive, *fn* false negative

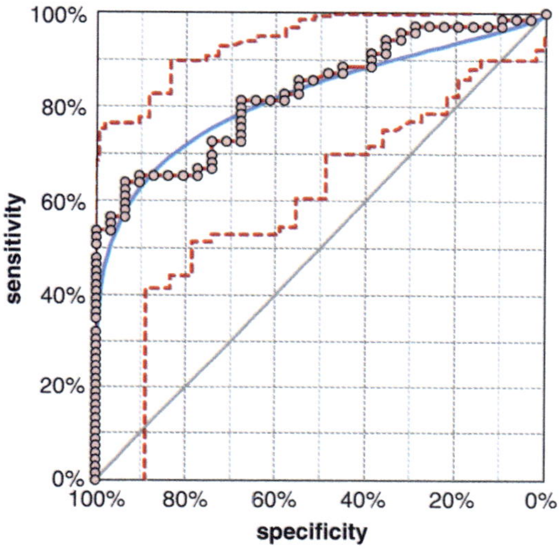

Fig. 8.4 Hypothetical ROC curve of a screening procedure. Because for ROC analyses the original proportions of false positives have been used, which are 1-specificity, the *x*-axis values descend from 100. The figure demonstrates an ROC curve (circles), a trend curve assuming a normal distribution of the data (blue curve), the upper and lower 95% confidence limits (dashed red lines) and the diagonal (grey line). The predictive power of a screening starts above the diagonal. The larger the AUC, the higher the validity of the screening. An increase in specificity in the decision algorithm of the screening results in a decrease of the sensitivity. An ideal curve would run rectangularly along the *y*-axis and the upper borderline of the diagram. (Image adapted from Keller 2014 with kind permission of Dr. Thomas Keller)

have to be extended, because a certain number of false positives (children who do not pass the test but have no DDSL) have to be accepted in order to minimize the number of false negatives (children who pass the test despite a DDSL). The cut-off value of a screening depends on a trade-off between the proportion of false negatives that is acceptable and that of false positives, which would increase the number of children who have to undergo follow-up diagnostics. It seems reasonable that screening should reveal about 15% of children who do not pass it in order to get the (at maximum) 10% of children who really have a DDSL from subsequent diagnostics.

The real language status of a child and the screening result for a given cut-off point can be compared in a contingency table (Table 8.3). In ROC curves the value pairs of specificity and sensitivity of a screening are drawn for all possible cut-off values. The area under the curve (AUC) indicates the validity of a screening. The more it approaches 1, the higher the validity.

Language screening programs are crucial because (a) children without language abnormalities are easier to detect than those with abnormalities (Law et al. 2000), (b) the language development for each specific linguistic competence has large variance and (c) there is often only poor evidence for a sufficient validity of a reference tests. Therefore, sensitivities and specificities of language screening that do not lie below 80% are assumed by convention to be acceptable (Petermann and Macha 2005; Plante and Vance 1994).

Examples of Language Screening, General and Specific Speech-Language Tests and Developmental Tests That Include Language Subtests

Tables 8.4, 8.5 and 8.6 show examples of valid and standardized language screening and general speech, language and developmental tests, which also include language subtests, for German- and English-speaking Europe.

8.2.2 Assessment of the Cognitive and General Developmental Status of Children

Christiane Kiese-Himmel

8.2.2.1 Introduction

Linguistic as well as cognitive abilities develop in mutual interdependence. Consequently, infants with delayed or disordered language development will achieve age-appropriate verbal intellectual functioning later than normal, and infants with delayed cognitive development, more specifically with cognitive deficits (e.g. limited capacity in phonological working memory, perceptual weaknesses), will learn language later.

There are also many genetic syndromes with behavioural phenotypes that affect language acquisition, given their association with learning disabilities or mental disability (significantly sub-average in intellectual functioning from IQ <85), or a general developmental delay. Moreover, infants with foetal alcohol exposure often have impaired mental functioning and language learning problems. Children with other developmental disorders of speech and language associated with language-relevant comorbidities (synonym: non-specific language impairment) often do not perform age-appropriately on measures of nonverbal intelligence. By definition, children with specific developmental disorders of speech and language (synonym: specific language impairment) display a significant discrepancy (two standard deviations or more below the average for their age) between receptive (or expressive) language abilities and age-level nonverbal intelligence and an average or higher psychometric intelligence. A valid and reliable assessment of a child's cognitive abilities and aptitude is the base for future clinical examinations and provides baseline data to monitor the effects of intervention.

8.2.2.2 Types of Diagnostic Assessment Approach

The *examiner* (usually a *qualified developmental* or *clinical psychologist*) has to be aware of the specific clinical question of the phoniatrician/pedaudiologist. This question determines the selection of the approach:

- Screening for developmental delay (before further assessment)
- Broad and in-depth assessment

as well as the assessment tools such as:

- Clinical interview
- Parental report
- Behavioural checklist/questionnaire
- Observational assessment
- Normed and standardized test
- Test battery.

Normally, an intelligence test has to be administered to obtain an idea of a child's cognitive development status, which means his or her ability to solve problems by perception, verbal and nonverbal reasoning. There are many different types of test for measuring intelligence.

8.2.2.3 Pre-assessment Information

A pre-, peri- or postnatal risk factor may limit (early) cognitive achievement of a child, and multiple risk factors may have cumulative effects on his or her development. Therefore, before testing a child, the examiner should obtain information on the history of the child (mainly history of maternal, pregnancy and perinatal conditions; (extremely) low birth weight; postnatal pathological conditions; physical developmental milestones; family history concerning hearing,

Table 8.4 Screenings, general developmental language tests and (The spelling *x;y* years in the table means *x* years and *y* months of age.) language-covering general developmental tests for German- and English-speaking Europe for the evaluation of a risk for a DDSL and other developmental disorders or delays

Method	Aim	Age-related test (year;month)					
		≤12 months	12–24 months	25–36 months	3–5 years	6–10 years	≥11 years
Screenings Parent questionnaires	Evaluation of a risk	ELFRA 1 (1;0) PLS-5 ST (0–7;11) MBCDI (0;8–3;1)	ELFRA 2 (2;0) ELAN (1; 4–2;2) FRAKIS (1;6–2;5) SBE-2-KT (1;9–2;0)[a,b] CDI (1;3–5;11) PLS-5 ST (0–7;11) LDS (1;6–2;11) MBCDI (0;8–3;1)	ELAN (1;4–2;2) SBE-3-KT (2;8–3;4) CDI (1;3–5;11) PLS-5 ST (0–7;11) LDS (1;6–2;11) MBCDI (0;8–3;1)	KiSS.2 (4;0–4;5)[b] SSV (3;0–5;0) LSV (4;0–6;5) BISC (preschool age) HASE (4;0–6;11) ETS 4–8 (4;0–8;11) CDI (1;3–5;11) PLS-5 ST (0;0–7;11) NSST S (3;0–7;11) LiSe-DaZ (3;0–6;11)[b]	ETS 4–8 (4;0–8;11) NSST S (3;0–7;11) LiSe-DaZ (3;0–6;11)[b]	
General developmental language tests and language-covering general developmental tests	Evaluation of a deviation from the age norm	PLS-5 (0;0–7;11) BISD III (0;1–3;6)	BISD III (0;1–3;6)	SETK-2 (2;0–2;11) PDSS (2;0–6;11) TELD, −2, −3 (2;0–7;11) NRDLS (2;0–7;5) WJ-III (2;0–90;0) BISD III (0;1–3;6) Vineland-II (0;0–90;0)	SETK 3–5 (3;0–5;11) PDSS (2;0–6;11) P-ITPA (4;0–11;0) BUEVA (4;0–5;11) HSET (3;0–9;0) TELD, −2, −3 (2;0–7;11) TOLD (4;0–17;11) NRDLS (2;0–7;5) CELF (5;0–21;0) CELF-P (3;0–6;11) WJ-III (2;0–90;0) BISD III (0;1–3;6) ITPA-3 (5;0–12;11) LiSe-DaZ (3;0–6;11)[b] TOLD-P:4 (4;0–8;11) Vineland-II (0;0–90;0) WRAT-4 (5;0–94;0)	PDSS (2;0–6;11) P-ITPA (4;0–11;0) BUEVA (4;0–5;11) SET 5–10 (5;0–10;11) HSET (3;0–9;0) TELD, −2, −3 (2;0–7;11) TOLD (4;0–17;11) NRDLS (2;0–7;5) CELF (5;0–21;0) CELF-P (3;0–6;11) WJ-III (2;0–90;0) ITPA-3 (5;0–12;11) LiSe-DaZ (3;0–6;11)[b] TOLD-P:4 (4;0–8;11) TOLD-I:4 (8;0–17;11) Vineland-II (0;0–90;0) WRAT-4 (5;0–94;0)	LTB-J (grade 9–10) TOLD (4;0–17;11) CELF (5;0–21;0) WJ-III (2;0–90;0) ITPA-3 (5;0–12;11) TOLD-I:4 (8;0–17;11) Vineland-II (0;0–90;0) WRAT-4 (5;0–94;0)

[a] Available in 34 languages
[b] Also suited for bi- and multilingual children

Table 8.5 Examples of specific language tests examining distinct linguistic skills for German- and English-speaking Europe

Diagnostic fields	Competence	Age-related test (year;month)					
		≤12 months	12–24 months	25–36 months	3–5 years	6–10 years	≥11 years
Basal or precursor functions							
	Verbal/phonological working memory				HASE (4;0–6;11) BISC (preschool age) Mottier (4;0–16;0) KiSS.2 (4;0–4;5) ETS 4–8 (4;0–8;11) AWMA (4;0–22;0) SSV (3;0–5;11)	HASE (4;0–6;11) BISC (preschool age) Mottier (4;0–16;0) AWMA (4;0–22;0) ETS 4–8 (4;0–8;11) MÜSC (first 5 school weeks)	AWMA (4;0–22;0) Mottier (4;0–16;0)
	Oral-motor skills			Check lists (e.g. Garliner; Giel & Tillmanns-Karus; Kittel)	Check lists (e.g. Garliner; Giel & Tillmanns-Karus; Kittel)	Check lists (e.g. Garliner; Giel & Tillmanns-Karus; Kittel)	
	Phonological awareness				TPB (4 to about 7 years) BISC (preschool age) ETS 4–8 (4;0–8;11	TPB (4 to about 7 years) MÜSC (first 5 school weeks) ETS 4–8 (4;0–8;11)	
Language competence							
Phonetics/ phonology	Articulation		PLAKKS-II (1;6–5;11)	PLAKKS-II (1;6–5;11) PDSS (2;0–6;11) GFTA-2 (2;0–21;11)	AVAK (children) PLAKKS-II (1;6–5;11) PDSS (2;0–6;11) KiSS.2 (4;0–4;5) TDA (3;0–8;0) GFTA-2 (2;0–21;11) PAT (3;0–8;11)	PDSS (2;0–6;11) TDA (3;0–8;0) GFTA-2 (2;0–21;11) PAT (3;0–8;11)	GFTA-2 (2;0–21;11)
	Phoneme discrimination			PDSS (2;0–6;11)	PDSS (2;0–6;11) KiSS.2 (4;0–4;5) Mottier (4;0–16;0)	PDSS (2;0–6;11) Mottier (4;0–16;0) BLDT (end of second grade)	

(continued)

Table 8.5 (continued)

Diagnostic fields	Competence	Age-related test (year;month)					
		≤12 months	12–24 months	25–36 months	3–5 years	6–10 years	≥11 years
Grammar	Morphology Perception			PDSS (2;0–6;11)	SETK 3–5 (3;0–5;11) PDSS (2;0–6;11) TROG-D (3;0–10;11) KiSS.2 (4;0–4;5) NSST (3; 0–7; 11 years) NRDLS (2; 0–7; 5) TTFC-2 (3;0–12;11) TOLD-P:4 (4;0–8;11)	PDSS (2;0–6;11) NSST (3;0–7;11) TROG-D (3;0–10;11) TTFC-2 (3;0–12;11) TOLD-I:4 (8;0–17;11) TOLD-P:4 (4;0–8;11)	TTFC-2 (3;0–12;11) TOLD-I:4 (8;0–17;11)
	Production		FRAKIS (1;6–2;5)	PDSS (2;0–6;11)	SETK 3–5 (3;0–5;11) ESGRAF-R (4–16 years) PDSS (2;0–6;11) KiSS.2 (4;0–4;5) NSST (3;0–7;11) TOLD-P:4 (4;0–8;11)	ESGRAF-R (4–16 years) PDSS (2;0–6;11) NSST (3;0–7;11) TOLD-I:4 (8;0–17;11) TOLD-P:4 (4;0–8;11)	ESGRAF-R (4;0–16;0) TOLD-I:4 (8;0–17;11)
	Syntax Perception			TSVK (2–8 years) PDSS (2;0–6;11) NRDLS (2;0–7;5)	TSVK (2;0–8;0) TROG-D (3;0–10;11) MSVK (5 year-end of first grade) SETK 3–5 (3;0–5;11) PDSS (2;0–6;11) KiSS.2 (4;0–4;5) NSST (3;0–7;11) NRDLS (2;0–7;5) TTFC-2 (3;0–12;11) TOLD-P:4 (4;0–8;11)	TSVK (2;0–8;0) TROG-D (3;0–10;11) MSVK (5 year-end of first grade) PDSS (2;0–6;11) NSST (3;0–7;11) NRDLS (2;0–7;5) TTFC-2 (3;0–12;11) TOLD-I:4 (8;0–17;11) TOLD-P:4 (4;0–8;11)	TTFC-2 (3;0–12;11) TOLD-I:4 (8;0–17;11)
	Production		ELFRA 2 (2;0) FRAKIS (1;6–2;5)	PDSS (2;0–6;11) NRDLS (2;0–7;5)	SETK 3–5 (3;0–5;11) PDSS (2;0–6;11) KiSS.2 (4;0–4;5) NSST (3;0–7;11) NRDLS (2;0–7;5) TOLD-P:4 (4;0–8;11)	PDSS (2;0–6;11) NSST (3;0–7;11) NRDLS (2;0–7;5) TOLD-I:4 (8;0–17;11) TOLD-P:4 (4;0–8;11)	TOLD-I:4 (8;0–17;11)

(continued)

Table 8.5 (continued)

Diagnostic fields	Competence	Age-related test (year;month) ≤12 months	12–24 months	25–36 months	3–5 years	6–10 years	≥11 years
Semantics and vocabulary	Semantics	ELFRA 1 (1;0)		PDSS (2;0–6;11) NRDLS (2;0–7;5) PPVT III (2;6–90;0)	Teddy-Test (3;0–8;6) MSVK (5 year-end of first grade) PDSS (2;0–6;11) KiSS.2 (4;0–4;5) NRDLS (2;0–7;5) PPVT III (2;6–90;0)	Teddy-Test (3;0–8;6) MSVK (5 year-end of first grade) NRDLS (2;0–7;5) PPVT III (2;6–90;0) TOLD-I:4 (8;0–17;11)	PPVT III (2;6–90;0) TOLD-I:4 (8;0–17;11)
	Vocabulary Perception (passive)	ELFRA 1 (1;0)		PDSS (2;0–6;11) PPVT III (2;6–90 years) NRDLS (2;0–7;5)	PDSS (2;0–6;11) KiSS.2 (4;0–4;5) TTFC-2 (3;0–12;11) CREFT-3 (5;0–89;11) PPVT III (2;6–90;0) NRDLS (2;0–7;5)	PDSS (2;0–6;11) CREFT-3 (5;0–89;11) TTFC-2 (3;0–12;11) TOLD-I:4 (8;0–17;11) NRDLS (2;0–7;5)	PPVT (14;0–60;0) CREFT-3 (5;0–89;11) TOLD-I:4 (8;0–17;11) TTFC-2 (3;0=12;11) PPVT III (2;6=90;0) PPVT German version (13;0–90;0)
	Production (active)	ELFRA 1 (1;0)	ELFRA 2 (2:0) ELAN (1;4–2;2) FRAKIS (1;6–2;5)	PDSS (2;0–6;11) NRDLS (2;0–7;5)	AWST-R (3;0–5;6) PDSS (2;0–6;11) KiSS.2 (4;0–4;5) CREFT-3 (5;0–89;11) NRDLS (2;0–7;5)	WWT 6–10 (6;0–10;0) PDSS (2;0–6;11) CREFT-3 (5;0–89;11) NRDLS (2;0–7;5) TOLD-I:4 (8;0–17;11)	CREFT-3 (5;0–89;11) TOLD-I:4 (8;0–17;11)
Pragmatics/ communication			Vineland-II (0;0–90;0) Das pragmatische Profil (0;0–10;0)	Vineland-II (0;0–90;0) Das pragmatische Profil (0;0–10;0)	MSVK (5 year-end of first grade) KiSS.2 (4;0–4;5) Vineland-II (0;0–90;0) Das pragmatische Profil (0;0–10;0)	MSVK (5 year-end of first grade) Vineland-II (0;0–90;0) Das pragmatische Profil (0;0–10;0)	Vineland-II (0;0–90;0)

Table 8.6 Register of examples of language screening tests, general and specific language tests and language-covering developmental tests for German- and English-speaking Europe

Test	Language	References
AVAK	German	Hacker D, Wilgermein H (2001) AVAK-Test mit CD-ROM Analyseverfahren zu Aussprachestörungen bei Kindern, 2nd. edn CD-ROM 2006) Reinhardt, München
AWMA	English	Alloway TP (2007) Automated working memory assessment (AWMA). Pearson, Oxford. Available via www.psychcorp.co.uk/product.aspx?n=1343&s=1492&cat=1356&skey=3909. Accessed 7 June 2014
AWST-R	German	Kiese-Himmel C (2005) Aktiver Wortschatztest für 3-bis 5-jährige Kinder – Revision. Beltz, Göttingen
BISC	German	Jansen H, Mannhaupt G, Marx H et al (2002) Bielefelder Screening zur Früherkennung von Lese-Rechtschreibschwierigkeiten. 2nd revised edn. Hogrefe, Göttingen
BISD III	English	Bayley N (2006) Bayley scales of infant and toddler development, 3rd edn. Harcourt Assessment Inc., San Antonio
BLDT	German	Niemeyer W (1976) Bremer Lautdiskriminationstest 2. Klasse BLDT, Herbig, Bremen
BUEVA	German	Esser G, Wyschkon A (2002) BUEVA – Basisdiagnostik umschriebener Entwicklungsstörungen im Vorschulalter. Hogrefe, Göttingen
CDI	English	Ireton H (1992) Child Development Inventory. Behavior Science Systems, Inc., Minneapolis Ireton H, Glascoe FP (1995) Assessing children's development using parents' reports: the Child Development Inventory. Clin Pediatr (Phila) 34(5):248–255
CELF	English	Semel E, Wiig E, Secord W (1995) Clinical evaluation of language fundamentals, 3rd edn. The psychological corporation, Harcourt Brace & Company, San Antonio
CELF-P	English	Wiig EH, Secord W, Semel E (1998) Clinical evaluation of language fundamentals – preschool (CELF-preschool). The psychological corporation, Harcourt Brace Jovanovich, San Antonio
CREFT-3	English	Wallace G, Hammill DD (1994) Comprehensive receptive and expressive vocabulary test, 3rd edn (CREFT-3). Pro-Ed, Austin
Das Pragmatische Profil	German	Dohmen A, Dewart H, Summers S (2009) Das Pragmatische Profil – Analyse kommunikativer Fähigkeiten von Kindern. Elsevier, München
ELAN	German	Bockmann AK, Kiese-Himmel C (2006) ELAN—Eltern Antworten. Beltz, Göttingen
ELFRA	German	Grimm H, Doil H (2006) ELFRA – Elternfragebögen für die Früherkennung von Risikokindern, 2nd revised edn. Hogrefe, Göttingen
EOWPVT-R	English	Gardner MF (2000) Expressive one-word picture vocabulary test – revised (EOWPVT). Academic Therapy, Novato
ESGRAF-R	German	Motsch HJ (2018) ESGRAF-R Testmanual: Evozierte Sprachdiagnose grammatischer Fähigkeiten, 2nd revised edn. Reinhardt, München
ETS 4-8	German	Angermaier M (2007) Entwicklungstest Sprache 4 bis 8 Jahre (ETS 4-8). Pearson Assessment, Frankfurt
FRAKIS	German	Szagun G, Stumper B, Schramm SA (2007) Fragebogen zur frühkindlichen Sprachentwicklung und FRAKIS-K (Kurzform). Pearson, Frankfurt
GFTA-2	English	Goldman R, Fristoe M (2000) Goldman-Fristoe Test of Articulation-2 (GFTA-2). American Guidance Service, Circle Pines
HASE	German	Schöler H, Brunner M (2008) HASE – Heidelberger Auditives Screening in der Einschulungsdiagnostik, 2nd revised edn. Westra, Wertingen
HSET	German	Grimm H, Schöler H (1991) Heidelberger Sprachentwicklungstest (HSET), 2nd revised edn. Hogrefe, Göttingen
ITPA-3	English	Hammill DD, Mather N, Roberts R (2001) Illinois test of psycholinguistic abilities, 3rd edn (ITPA-3). Pro-Ed, Austin

(continued)

Table 8.6 (continued)

Test	Language	References
KISS.2	German	Euler HA, Holler-Zittlau I, van Minnen S et al (2010) Psychometrische Gütekriterien eines Kurztests zur Erfassung des Sprachstandes vierjähriger Kinder. HNO 58(11):1116–1123 Neumann K, Holler-Zittlau I, Euler HA (2011) Kinder-Sprach-Screening "KiSS". Available via https://soziales.hessen.de/gesundheit/kinder-sprachscreening-kiss. Accessed 7 June 2014
LDS	English	Rescorla L (1989) The language development survey: a screening tool for delayed language in toddlers. J Speech Hear Disord 54:(4)587–599
LiSe-DaZ	German	Schulz P, Tracy R (2012) LiSe-DaZ. Linguistische Sprachstandserhebung – Deutsch als Zweitsprache. Hogrefe, Göttingen
LSV	German	Götte R (1976) Landauer Sprachentwicklungstest für Vorschulkinder LSV. Beltz, Weinheim
LTB-J	German	Barwitzki K, Hofbauer C, Huber M et al (2008) LTB-J - Leipziger Testbatterie zur Messung des formal-sprachlichen Entwicklungsstandes bei Jugendlichen. BBW, Leipzig
MBCDI	English	Fenson L, Marchman VA, Thal DJ et al (2007) MacArthur-Bates communicative development inventories: user's guide and technical manual, 2nd edn. Paul H. Brookes Publishing, Baltimore
Mottier	German	Kiese-Himmel C, Risse T (2009) Normen für den Mottier-Test bei 4- bis 6-jährigen Kindern. HNO 57(9):943–948 Risse T, Kiese-Himmel C (2009) Der Mottier-Test. Teststatistische Überprüfung an 4- bis 6-jährigen Kindern. HNO 57(5):523–528
MSVK	German	Elben CE, Lohaus A (2000) Marburger Sprachverständnistest für Kinder MSVK. Hogrefe, Göttingen
MÜSC	German	Mannhaupt G (2006) Das Münsteraner Screening zur Früherkennung von Lese- und Rechtschreibschwierigkeiten (MÜSC). Cornelsen, Berlin
NRDLS	English	Edwards S, Letts C, Sinka I (2011) The New Reynell Developmental Language Scales (NRDLS). GL Assessment, London
NSST	English	Lee, Lee LL (1969) Northwestern syntax screening test. Northwestern University Press, Evanston
NSST S	English	Ratusnik DL, Klee TM, Ratusnik CM (1980) Northwestern syntax screening test: a short form. J Speech Hear Disord 45(2):200–208
PDSS	German	Kauschke C, Siegmüller J (2009) Patholinguistische Diagnostik bei Sprachentwicklungsstörungen, 2nd edn. Elsevier, Heidelberg
PAT	English	Pendergast K, Dickey SE, Selmar JW et al (1984) Photo articulation test. Stoelting, Chicago
PPVT III	English	Dunn LM, Dunn LM (1997) Examiner's manual for the Peabody Picture Vocabulary Test-third edition (PPVT-III). American Guidance Service, Circle Pines
	German	Bulheller S, Dunn LM, Dunn LM et al (German edition) (2003) Peabody Picture Vocabulary Test: (PPVT); Manual. Swets Test Services, Frankfurt
P-ITPA	German	Ballaschk K, Hänsch S, Esser G (2010) P-ITPA. Potsdam-Illinois Test für Psycholinguistische Fähigkeiten. Hogrefe, Göttingen
PLAKSS-II	German	Fox A (2014) PLAKSS-II Psycholinguistische Analyse kindlicher Sprechstörungen-II, 1st edn. Pearson, Frankfurt
PLS-5	English	Zimmerman IL, Steiner VG, Pond RE (2011) PLS-5 Preschool Language Scales, 5th edn. Pearson, San Antonio
PLS-5 ST	English	Zimmerman, IL, Steiner VG, Pond RE (2011) Preschool Language Scale-5 Screening Test, 5th edn. (PLS-5 Screening Test). Pearson, San Antonio
Prüfbögen zur Mundmotorik	German	Garliner D (1989) Myofunktionelle Therapie in der Praxis - Gestörtes Schluckverhalten, gestörte Gesichtsmuskulatur und die Folgen - Diagnose, Planung und Durchführung der Behandlung. Hütig, Heidelberg Giel B, Tillmanns-Karus M (2004) Kölner Diagnostikbogen für Myofunktionelle Störungen. modernes lernen, Dortmund Kittel AM (2009) Myofunktionelle Therapie, 9th revised edn. Schulz-Kirchner, Idstein

(continued)

Table 8.6 (continued)

Test	Language	References
SBE-2-KT	German	Suchodoletz Wv, Sachse S (2009) Sprachbeurteilung durch Eltern, Kurztest für die U7 (SBE-2-KT). Available via http://www.kjp.med.uni-muenchen.de/download/SBE-2-KT.pdf. Accessed 7 June 2014
		Suchodoletz Wv, Sachse S (2009) Sprachbeurteilung durch Eltern, Kurztest für die U7 (SBE-2-KT), non-normalized translation in 33 languages. Available via https://www.kjp.med.uni-muenchen.de/download/SBE-2-KT.pdf. Accessed 13 April 2018
SBE-3-KT	German	Suchodoletz Wv, Kademann S, Tippelt S (2009) Sprachbeurteilung durch Eltern, Kurztest für die U7a (SBE-3-KT). Available via http://www.kjp.med.uni-muenchen.de/download/SBE-3-KT.pdf. Accessed 7 June 2014
SET 5-10	German	Petermann F, Metz D, Fröhlich LP (2010) SES 5-10. Sprachstandserhebungstest für Kinder im Alter zwischen 5 und 10 Jahren. Hogrefe, Göttingen
SETK-2	German	Grimm H, Aktas M, Frevert S (2000) Sprachentwicklungstest für zweijährige Kinder SETK-2. Hogrefe, Göttingen
	German	Grimm H, Aktas M, Frevert S (2010) Sprachentwicklungstest für drei- bis fünfjährige Kinder SETK 3-5, 2nd revised edn. Hogrefe, Göttingen
SSV	German	Grimm H, Aktas M, Kießig U (2003) Sprachscreening für das Vorschulalter SSV. Kurzform des SETK 3-5. Hogrefe, Göttingen
Teddy-Test	German	Friedrich G (1998) Teddy-Test. Hogrefe, Göttingen
TDA	English	Templin MC, Darley FL (1969) The Templin-Darley tests of articulation; a manual and discussion of articulation testing, 2nd edn. Bureau of Educational Research and Service, Division of Extension and University Services, University of Iowa, Iowa City
TELD, TELD-2, TELD-3	English	Hresko WP, Reid DK, Hammill DD (1981) Test of early language development. Pro-Ed, Austin, TX
TTFC-2	English	McGhee RL, Ehrler DJ, DiSimoni F (2007) Token test for children-second edition (TTFC-2). Pro-Ed, Austin, TX
TOLD-P:4	English	Newcomer PL, Hammill DD (2008) Test of Language Development-Primary, 4th edn (TOLD-P:4). Pro-Ed, Austin
TOLD-I:4	English	Hammill DD, Newcomer PL (2008) Test of Language Development-Intermediate, 4th edn (TOLD-I:4). Pro-Ed, Austin
TPB	German	Fricke S, Schäfer B (2011) Test phonologischer Bewusstheitsfähigkeiten, 2nd edn. Schulz-Kirchner, Idstein
TROG-D	German	Fox AV (2008) TROG-D - Test zur Überprüfung des Grammatik-Verständnisses, 3rd edn. Schulz-Kirchner, Idstein
TSVK	German	Siegmüller J, Kauschke C, van Minnen S et al (2010) Test des Satzverständnisses bei Kindern. Eine profilorientierte Diagnostik der Syntax. Elsevier, Heidelberg
Vineland-II	English	Sparrow SS, Balla DA Cicchetti DV (2005) Vineland Adaptive Behaviors Scales, 2nd edn (Vineland-II). American Guidance Service, Circle Pines
WJ-III	English	Woodcock RW, McGrew KS, Mather N (2001) Woodcock-Johnson-III Tests of achievement. Riverside Publishing, Itasca
WRAT-4	English	Wilkinson GS, Robertson GJ (2006) Wide Range Achievement Test - fourth edition (WRAT-4) professional manual. Psychological Assessment Resources, Lutz
WWT 6-10	German	Glück CW (2007) WWT 6-10. Wortschatz- und Wortfindungstest für 6- bis 10-Jährige. Urban & Schwarzenberg, München

language, academic difficulties; socio-economic status of the family) and results of physical examinations, additional existing diagnoses and medications, treatment histories or information from other professionals. Non-medical professionals (e.g. teachers) should only be contacted for information if parents/caregivers have given written permission.

8.2.2.4 General Principles for Psychometric Procedures in the Clinical Setting

An infant (till 1 year), a toddler (ages 1–3 years) or a preschooler (ages 3–5 years) has limited concentration, a short attention span, short interest levels and insufficient abilities to regulate its own behaviour compared with older children.

- The individual assessment should consequently take place in a neutral assessment context, be interesting for the child and be of a rather brief duration. It is recommended to take breaks or to perform several diagnostic sessions, if necessary.

Furthermore, the child's ability to interact and react adequately with an unknown person in an unfamiliar environment without the presence of a parent or another family member is relevant to the assessment situation.

- Since many children perform better in the presence of individuals to whom they have close relations, the examiner should provide or permit their presence (except in certain child-protection assessment situations in which a parent tends to interfere or to offer solutions to the child).
- The examiner should introduce himself or herself in the entry phase and describe the purpose of the meeting ('pre-diagnostic interaction').

The examiner has to bear in mind that tests have to be administered carefully in order to avoid diagnostic errors and to produce a reliable result that reflects the true level of cognitive functioning.

- The examiner must be informed about the methods of intellectual assessment and the theoretical underpinnings of the assessment tools, their characteristics, psychometric properties and limitations (e.g. handicaps accommodating assessment), be familiar with these and experienced with the tools. In general, the examiner should be experienced in working with children.
- Most importantly, aspects addressing the sensory integrity status and special needs such as motor disabilities of the child have to be taken into account. The latter are presumptions for a proper interpretation of the results in the context of all available information.
- Estimation of the general cognitive developmental stage should begin with demands or items that are within the child's capability. The examiner has to follow the instructions, examination and analysis procedures carefully, particularly the order in which the subtests have to be administered; to conduct the assessment tools accurately, in a fair and ethical manner; and to assure confidentiality. It is a breach of ethics for a psychologist to administer an intelligence test without the child's full understanding.
- Finally, the examiner should have the clinical skills required to interpret the assessment data appropriately, to synthesize them with all other available information into an overall picture and to communicate their relevance to other professionals (e.g. therapists) as well as family members in a sensitive way.

8.2.2.5 Aim of Psychometric Procedures

The main objective of psychometric procedures is the assessment of the general developmental status, more specifically the cognitive status (including the general intelligence level), in making classification and placement according to test scores, differential diagnosis or educational decisions and support needs. This is necessary to ascertain whether the child is at risk of cognitive developmental delay or exhibits:

- A major isolated development problem
- A broad developmental delay up to a global retardation
- Some cognitive weaknesses
- A reduced verbal intelligence quotient (IQ)
- A learning disorder (IQ 70–84 according to ICD-10)
- A mental retardation (mild, IQ 50–69; moderate, IQ 35–49; severe, IQ 20–34; profound, IQ <20)
- An intelligence score average or above normal ('high-ability' children).

The diagnosis involves testing and evaluation. Individual testing is much more reliable than testing in a group, but no single test can identify who is mentally handicapped. Multiple scores and several criteria must be combined in order to make this judgement—as for judging 'high-ability' children—given that genetic and contextual factors interact. In the light of brain plasticity during early childhood, cognitive disabilities may be modulated by environmental factors, such as the social or educational context, with consequences for the cortical development.

Amongst children with impaired cognitive functioning, other psychological problems often emerge. Subsequently, the child's pattern of strengths and weaknesses of cognitive competence has to be identified as a marker for his or her:

- Further developmental course
- Therapy, training or another intervention success
- Special education needs
- Academic achievements and school performance.

8.2.2.6 Selected Examples of Assessment Tools

Infancy and childhood diagnostic assessments focus on special domains or on a broad range of development. The supposed cognitive developmental level at which the child functions and his or her history both influence his or her understanding of the tasks. Therefore, diagnostic instruments should be selected on the basis of the child's chronological age, medical and developmental history and their validity, reliability and user-friendliness (quick and easy to administer). Furthermore, the presence or absence of up-to-date standards or norms should be considered for the selection. Intelligence tests are the best available tools for revealing a child's cognitive functioning. The most popular assessment tools have been adopted from US, British or Dutch instruments.

Age Ranges

Infancy and Toddler Age

An infant or toddler with suspected language disability has to be assessed via a well-standardized, norm-referenced, valid and reliable *developmental scale*. It should be complemented by a description of the individual's functional difficulties and a *caregiver's evaluation of development and behaviour*, which has been shown to be as accurate as those administered by professionals in identifying children with developmental problems (Glascoe and Dworkin 1995).

Childhood

A child should first be assessed with a *nonverbal intelligence test* offering optimal psychometric properties in order to avoid problems in understanding and following instructions ('culture-fair assessment'). Most behavioural tests require a spoken response. Therefore, a verbal assessment may not be appropriate for children whose reduced speech intelligibility will invalidate the interpretation of responses. A language-free measure is also suitable for children with hearing loss, developmental disorder of speech and language, autism or test anxiety; for children from linguistically and culturally diverse backgrounds (e.g. migrant children); and for children who are difficult to test. Testing should be complemented by measures completed by parents (e.g. questionnaires).

Early Childhood Assessment Tools

Early childhood assessment tools are, for example, the single administered, norm-referenced *Bayley Scales of Infant and Toddler Development* (current version: *Bayley III*) from 1 to 42 months (Bayley 2006, 2014) or the *Griffiths Mental Development Scales Revised* from 2 to 8 years (Luiz et al. 2006). They measure, amongst other abilities, sensorimotor intelligence, receptive and expressive language and social-emotional behaviour, whereas intelligence tests focus more on cognitive abilities. That is, the skills evaluated by infant scales are not the same as those measured by psychometric intelligence tests. A useful adjunct to intelligence tests is measurement of cognitive processes underlying performance in intelligence tests, such as working memory capacity which is the base, amongst others, for an increase of other cerebral capacities, for example, the mental lexicon.

Example of Measures of Intelligence

Intelligence tests evaluate different components of mental functioning and assess cognitive development. A good example of *measures of intelligence* is the standardized and norm-referenced *Kaufman-*

Assessment Battery for Children (*K-ABC*; Kaufman and Kaufman 1983) for children aged 2.5 through 12.5 years, which permits testing of hearing- or speech-language-impaired individuals or those with limited English proficiency. It comprises a multidimensional cognitive processing approach with items of little cultural content. A composite mental score results from the areas of 'sequential' versus 'simultaneous' information processing, investigated by several subtests. Furthermore, an achievement score and a nonverbal intelligence score can be calculated. In the meantime, a revision was published (*K-ABC-II*; Kaufman and Kaufman 2004) to make the test appropriate for a wider age (from 3 to 18 years) and for a wider range of abilities. The subtests are organized in three levels (ages 3; 4–6; 7–18 years). The *K-ABC-II* is—like the *K-ABC*—founded on Luria's neuropsychological model corresponding to learning abilities, sequential vs. simultaneous processing and planning ability and on the psychometric Cattell-Horn-Carroll approach of long-term and of short-term memory, visual processing, fluid reasoning and crystallized abilities (McGrew 2005). It yields a nonverbal composite and a mental processing fluid-crystallized index plus individual scale scores. Melchers and Melchers published the German version *K-ABC-II* (2015).

Latest Revisions of the Snijders-Oomen Nonverbal Intelligence Tests

Another example concerns the latest revisions (Tellegen and Laros 1993) of the popular *Snijders-Oomen Nonverbal Intelligence Tests: SON-R 2.5-7* comprising six subtests with separate total scores for the spatial performance and for the reasoning scale (Tellegen et al. 1998, 2009) and *SON-Revised 5.5-17* with seven subtests without a memory test, but with abstract reasoning and concrete reasoning tests, spatial tests and perceptual tests (Snijders et al. 1989). Both tests also provide a total intelligence score that indicates how an infant or a child performs in comparison with other children of the same age; and both tests are well suited for use with children of ethnic minorities (Tellegen and Laros 2005) as well as for mentally retarded, hearing- or speech-language-impaired and autistic children, because they do not need spoken language in administration. The *SON* tests are used in several countries, and test manuals are published in several languages. For example, a standardization of the SON-R 2.5-7 has been conducted in the Netherlands, Germany, the United Kingdom, Denmark, France, the Czech Republic, Portugal, Slovakia and Romania.

General Intelligence Functioning

The approach used in the family of the popular *Wechsler Intelligence Scale for Children* is based on the general intelligence functioning (highest 'g' loading), e.g. the *Wechsler Intelligence Scale for Children-IV* with an age range of 6 years to 16 years and 11 months (*WISC-IV*; Wechsler 2003), adapted for some European countries, e.g. Spain and the UK in 2004 and Germany in 2011. It comprises ten core subtests and five additional subtests that can be summed to provide four indices and one full scale IQ. Thus, it is a multi-trait/multi-method test. In the meantime, the fifth edition with 14 subtests has been published (*WISC-V Integrated*; Wechsler 2014); it is considered as a powerful upgrade for better understanding of a child's cognitive processes and for choosing of appropriate interventions.

The *Wechsler Preschool and Primary Scale of Intelligence* was originally developed by Wechsler in 1967 for preschoolers and young children (2 years 6 months to 7 years 7 months old). The test, now replaced by the *WPPSI-IV* (Wechsler 2012) with new processing speed subtests and reduced expressive language requirements, is available in many other European languages, e.g. Danish, Dutch, English (UK), Finnish, French, German, Icelandic, Italian, Lithuanian, Norwegian, Portuguese, Slovenian, Spanish and Swedish. Subtests exist for two age bands: 2 years 6 months to 3 years 11 months and 4 years 0 month to 7 years 7 months. For both, three levels of results are offered: full scale, primary index scale (verbal comprehension index; visual-spatial index; working memory index; fluid reasoning index; processing speed index) and ancillary index scale levels (vocabulary acquisition index; nonverbal index; general ability index; cognitive proficiency index).

Nonverbal Matrices

The nonverbal *Raven's Progressive Matrices* (measuring general intelligence) require the ability to recognize shapes/figures and their relationships, e.g. in childhood and for persons of limited intellectual ability. The brief intelligence measure *Coloured Progressive Matrices* (*CPM*), a 36-item test, has an age range from 5 to 11 years and the *Standard Progressive Matrices* (*SPM*) from 6 years to 16 years 0 month and from 17 years 0 month years of age upwards, a 60-item test used in measuring abstract reasoning and fluid intelligence. They are all unidimensional tests, but a useful nonverbal measure of overall cognitive functioning, and provide an overall intelligence score (Raven et al. 2004).

Alternative Testing Approaches

In addition, there are a number of alternative testing approaches and methods for estimating general cognitive developmental stage (e.g. neuropsychological-based assessment; learning tasks; informal play-based assessment) and more individually administered tests of intelligence that could not all be named and described in this brief overview.

8.2.2.7 Assessment Results

The assessment of both the child's cognitive processing abilities and of intelligence in an individually administered test indicates the intellectual level and profile as well as any delay or risk. This assessment information must be evaluated by the examiner in order to ensure that the results are valid and reliable and to determine a diagnosis (in combination with all clinical data) including both management and conclusions such as prognostic implications.

8.2.2.8 Forward Look

Frequently, re-evaluation ('follow-up') and consideration of environmental and biomedical variables are necessary:

- To identify whether a child has caught up his or her delay(s)
- To locate patterns of development (e.g. continuity; discontinuity; spurts; atypical)
- To monitor the further development processes in children at (high) risk (e.g. in case of preterm birth; very low-birth weight; persistent hearing impairment).

Nevertheless, high correlations between developmental infant assessment and the measurement of intelligence at later ages should not be expected, because intelligence is not a unitary construct. Comorbidity may be relevant for outcomes of cognitive development even when the nonverbal IQ is normal. Intelligence is also correlated with functional literacy and socio-economic status, and children who underachieve in educational systems may suffer a decline in their intelligence.

8.3 Diagnostic Interview of Parents/Partners/Other Relatives: Psychosocial Aspects

Susanne Cook and Charley Adams

8.3.1 Introduction

As part of the assessment of stuttering, it is important to interview family members and others familiar with the person who stutters. There is ample evidence that interviewing family members of children with other conditions, such as autism, Down Syndrome, ADHD, being deaf or hard of hearing is useful (e.g. Barkley and Edwards 2006; Prendergast et al. 2002; Sloper and Turner 1994). Barkley and Edwards (2006) state that a thorough evaluation 'requires integrating information from multiple sources', through multiple means. Along with semi-structured and structured interviews, they also list standardised behaviour rating scales as an important method of collecting information.

The World Health Organization's International Classification of Functioning (ICF) model provides a framework for assessing stuttering (Coleman and Yaruss 2014; Yaruss 2007; Yaruss and Quesal 2004, 2006). The part 'Activity and

Participation' of this model highlights the person's functional ability to communicate effectively in many situations. These include schools, the workplace, home, social situations etc. Some questionnaires are designed to assess behaviour in a variety of situations, as outlined by the ICF model. Two available questionnaires are the Overall Assessment of the Speaker's Experience of Stuttering (OASES, Yaruss and Quesal 2006) and the Wright and Ayre Stuttering Self-Rating Profile for adults (WASSP, Wright and Ayre 2000).

Interviewing parents, partners and other relatives about the communicative behaviour of the person who stutters may help to develop a clearer picture of that person, as suggested by a number of authors (e.g. Curlee 2007; Neumann et al. 2016; Ward 2006). One effective approach is the use of semi-structured and structured interviews, as outlined by Bosshardt (2008, 2010), Curlee (2007), Sandrieser and Schneider (2015) and Ward (2006). A small number of standardised questionnaires are available for the collection of information from different interviewees related to or associated with the person who stutters. The focus on interview partners changes with the age of the person who stutters. While for children, the major source of information will come from parents, and potentially from teachers, for adults this information might be collected from spouses or friends.

8.3.2 Diagnostic Interviews Related to Children Who Stutter

Limited questionnaires are available to assess directly the psychosocial impact of stuttering on the lives of children. For young children, there is for example the Communication Attitude Test for Preschool and Kindergarten children who stutter (KiddyCAT, Vanryckeghem and Brutten 2007; see Sect. 8.1) and the German questionnaire KES (Kinder Erleben ihr Stottern; Kids Experience their Stuttering, Walther 2009, 2015). For school-age children, there is the standardised Overall Assessment of the Speaker's Experience of Stuttering-School age (OASES-S, Yaruss and Quesal 2006, see Sect. 8.1). KiddyCAT assesses the attitude towards communication in children who stutter aged from 3 to 6 years with 12 yes/no questions; for example: 'Do words sometimes get stuck in your mouth?' or 'Do your parents like the way you talk?' A maximum of 12 points can be achieved, a higher number indicating a more negative attitude towards communication. KES assesses the experience of stuttering from the viewpoint of the child in the following areas: ability to communicate at home and preschool/school, reactions towards stuttering, quality of life. Sample questions include 'How easy is it for you to speak with other children?' or 'How often is it hard for you to speak?' Children indicate their answers on a three-point Likert scale with age-appropriate picture symbols. KES additionally provides an accompanying parent questionnaire, with matching questions from the viewpoint of the parent. This allows a comparison between the attitudes of the child and the perspectives of the parent. OASES-S measures the health-related quality of life of children who stutter aged 7–12 in the four areas of General Information, Your Reactions to Stuttering, Communication in Daily Situations, and Quality of Life. The questionnaire contains 60 questions on a five-point Likert scale. It provides an overall impact score as well as individual impact ratings for each part.

For young children, the person closest to the child (generally the parent or direct caregiver) is often the person who is able to give the most reliable input regarding the psychosocial impact the stuttering has on the child. In their study with preschool-age children, Tumanova and Backes (2019) collected information about children's attitudes towards speaking by using a direct questionnaire for the child. They used a parent report questionnaire to assess their child's tendency to experience negative emotions. Their findings showed that parents' beliefs were in line with how children experience their speech. Children who stutter showed a more negative communication attitude, and they were also rated by their parents as more fearful and prone to sadness compared with their non-stuttering peers. Similar findings were reported for Portuguese children who stutter, with parents generally providing comparable impact ratings. Differences emerged in families with a history of stuttering, where parents perceived the impact to be greater than the children did (Rocha, Yaruss & Rato 2020). Walther (2009), however, found a discrepancy between the rating of the parents and the responses of the children. In her study with preschool-age children who stutter, they rated their attitude towards and experience with stuttering as more negative than their parents. It should be noted that this study was conducted with children who were already diagnosed with stuttering. Guttormsen, Yaruss, and Bottegård Næss (2021) adapted the OASES-S to assess parents' perceptions of the impact of stuttering on their children aged 2 to 5 years. Parents in this study expressed confidence in their ratings and reported that stuttering had a negative impact on their children's lives. The authors suggested that if parents report an impact, it should be further validated by administering an age-appropriate test directly to the children.

Informal interviews can provide valuable insight in other ways. Parents/caregivers can indicate whether the child reacts emotionally or expresses concerns towards their disfluent speech, whether there is any suspected avoidance behaviour, or if speaking in different situations or with different communication partners seems to have an influence on the speech of the child (Curlee 2007; Sandrieser and Schneider 2015; Ward 2006). For example, the evaluator can ask 'Does the child often react emotionally or express concern about his or her disfluent speech?' (Curlee 2007 p. 8), 'How does the child deal with the disfluencies?', 'Are there any stigmatising reactions from the environment towards the child?' (Sandrieser and Schneider 2015). When inquiring about possible avoidance behaviour, the evaluator can for example ask, 'Is there any avoidance of words, situations or people?' (Ward 2006 p. 182), and further inquire if parents have noticed any changes in the child's personality since the onset of the disfluencies. It will also be helpful to determine if parents feel any guilt about their child's stuttering (e.g. Sandrieser and Schneider 2015; Ward 2006). These feelings can lead to conscious or subconscious reactions to the stuttering, which may in return contribute to more cognitive and emotional responses in the child (Pertijs et al. 2014). This can be addressed through parent counselling.

Formal questionnaires, such as the Observational Rating Scales available with the Test of Childhood Stuttering (TOCS, Gillam et al. 2009), provide valuable information about stuttering and related behaviour from parents, teachers and other individuals who are familiar with the child. The observational rating scale consists of two norm-referenced components: the TOCS Speech Fluency scale, and the TOCS Disfluency-Related Consequences scale. The Speech Fluency scale consists of nine questions related to overt observable behaviour, such as stuttering-like disfluencies, the length of a stuttering incidence or whether the child's fluency changes in different situations. The Disfluency-Related Consequences scale consists of nine questions focusing on reactions to stuttering, such as what the child does when disfluent, or how the child reacts to speech difficulties in general (Tumanova et al. 2018). These authors found that the TOCS Observational Rating Scales provided 'documentable, objective means to determine parental perception of and concern about their child's stuttering'.

Other important information can be obtained by interviewing teachers of children who stutter, either during a meeting or via a questionnaire (Ward 2006). This way a possible educational impact of the stuttering can be assessed, for example by asking if the child volunteers to read out loud, or raises his or her hand in class. Furthermore, questions should address social relationships of the child within the classroom, for example, how the child interacts during different class activities, with peers and teachers, or whether the child is teased or bullied and how this is being addressed (The Stuttering Foundation 2010; Ward 2006).

8.3.3 Diagnostic Interviews Related to Adolescents and Adults Who Stutter

Several standardised questionnaires are available for adolescents and adults who stutter, which serve to assess the impact of stuttering on their lives. Examples include the Overall Assessment of the Speaker's Experience of Stuttering for Teens, and for Adults (OASES-T and OASES-A, Yaruss and Quesal 2006), the German Fragebogen zum Sprechen (FzS, Cook 2013), and the Wright and Ayre Stuttering Self-Rating Profile (WASSP, Wright and Ayre 2000). OASES-T is an 80-item questionnaire for adolescents who stutter aged 13–17. OASES-A consists of 100 questions for people who stutter aged 18 and above. Both questionnaires include questions in the four domains of 'General Information, Reactions to Stuttering, Communication in Daily Situations, Quality of Life' on a 5-point Likert scale. Similar to OASES-S, these questionnaires provide an overall impact rating as well as impact ratings for each domain. FzS assesses the health-related quality of life for children and adolescents aged 8–17, and consists of 27 questions on a 6-point Likert scale. It addresses all four aspects of the ICF in the areas of general attitudes, feelings, different speaking situations and impact of stuttering, and results in an impact rating of stuttering on the person's life from no impact to very severe. WASSP is a self-rating profile for adults who stutter, and consists of 24 items on a 7-point Likert scale from none to very severe. Areas assessed are types of stuttering behaviour, thoughts about stuttering, feelings about stuttering, avoidance due to stuttering, disadvantages due to stuttering. The people who stutter rate the different aspects in each area, and results are displayed in a summary profile, which helps the therapist in the clinical decision making process.

Interviewing spouses or parents may provide further insight on the impact the fluency disorder has on the person who stutters (e.g. Ward 2006). Interviews with parents, spouses or partners are valuable in three domains. First, interviewers are likely to learn information that was not provided by the person who stutters, either by oversight or because it was withheld. Second, significant others provide a different perspective, which may or may not have been shared between them. Third, interviewers are likely to glean insight into the thoughts and beliefs about stuttering which are held by the interviewee. Each of these domains is important, as multiple perspectives have ramifications for therapy planning and potentially therapy success (Cook and Howell 2015). Ward (2006) states that input from parents of adolescents or teens who stutter, and spouses of adults who stutter, can help identify a potential mismatch between the perceptions of the person who stutters and that of their parent or partner. In a qualitative study with adolescents who stutter (mean age: 16.3), Landau (2011) found a significant discrepancy between perspectives of parents and the person who stutters on factors such as stuttering awareness, acceptance of stuttering and concerns about future prospects. Parents rated the stuttering of their children as more severe than their adolescent children did, and they expressed more concern for the future. These findings were partly confirmed by Cook and Howell (2015) in a quantitative study with adolescents who stutter (mean age: 14.1) and their parents. FzS (Cook 2013) was given to the participants, and a modified version to their parents before a therapeutic intervention. Children's and parents' answers showed a significant mismatch in the area of impact of stuttering on the child's life; parents rated the psychosocial impact of the stuttering on their child's life higher than the children did themselves. However, parents' and children's perspectives showed agreement in all other areas (information regarding the child's speech, emotions and different speaking situations). Svenning et al. (2021) examined how life partners of people who stutter perceive their loved ones' emotional reactions to speech situations, expectations of speech disruption, and communication attitudes, comparing these perceptions with the individuals' own ratings. They found that partners were generally in synch with the cognitive aspects of their partner's experience of stuttering.

8.3.4 Discussion

The aim of this section was to explore the importance of considering the viewpoints of parents, significant others or teachers of children and adolescents who stutter, when diagnosing their stuttering. This is especially important because formal questionnaires for measuring the psychosocial impact of stuttering on the person's life are not available for young children. Tumanova and Backes (2019) showed that parent input, gathered with structured questionnaires, was in line with children's experiences of their stuttering. Children whose parents expressed concerns regarding the speech fluency also showed a more negative attitude towards communication measured with the KiddyCAT (Groner et al. 2016). However, some studies with young children (Walther 2009) and adolescents (Cook and Howell 2015; Landau 2011) who stutter revealed that parents rated the stuttering of their children as more severe than their children. This might reflect the parents' concern for the child's future, or could suggest feelings of guilt, which could be important for therapy planning and parent education. It might be helpful to include parents in therapy sessions, and conduct awareness training related to stuttering and social-emotional aspects of the disorder. Sandrieser and Schneider (2015) suggest establishing parent groups in addition to direct intervention with the child. Topics for discussion in these parent groups could include general information about stuttering, the therapeutic approach, prospects and limitations about intervention, discussion of public and self-stigma surrounding stuttering, problem-solving strategies and resources for families. Through exchange with other parents who are or have been in the same position, concerns for the child's future can be addressed in an open and supportive environment. Collecting information from spouses/partners (significant others) or close friends of adults who stutter also can provide different viewpoints in speaking situations (Ward 2006), which can help with the therapy process. Beilby and colleagues explored the impact of stuttering on the quality of life of the individual's relationship with their significant other and found that both sides reported 'similar experiences in reactions to stuttering and perceived difficulties in communication' (Beilby et al. 2013, p. 14). The authors concluded that it would be beneficial for the success of therapy if the significant other would lend enhanced support during the clinical process.

8.3.5 Conclusion

For stuttering assessment, information collected in diagnostic interviews with parents, spouses or significant others can provide an in-depth picture of the individual's interaction with family members, friends, classmates, colleagues and others. Information can include behaviour during different life activities, such as within the family, in peer interactions, at school or work, and within the community. This input can be valuable for therapy planning and therapy success.

8.4 Evaluation of Voice Quality and Respiratory Function

Wolfgang Angerstein, Giovanna Baracca, Philippe Dejonckere, Matthias Echternach, Ulrich Eysholdt, Franco Fussi, Ahmed Geneid, Tamás Hacki, Katarzyna Karmelita-Katulska, Renate Haubrich, František Šram, Jan G. Švec, Jitka Vydrová, and Bożena Wiskirska-Woźnica

8.4.1 Methods of Non-instrumental Voice Examination and Voice Screening

Bożena Wiskirska-Woźnica

8.4.1.1 Introduction

The full non-instrumental assessment of the phonatory function of the larynx should include a medical history, adequately collected from the patient, as well as a physical examination (including respiration, hearing and velopharyngeal competence) and an auditory perceptual voice evaluation (Sataloff 2005a).

8.4.1.2 Diagnostic Interview

A medical history of voice disorders (Table 8.7) primarily consists of questions concerning the nature of the change in the timbre, the pitch, extent and loudness of voice, frequently reported hoarseness and its severity, any occurrence of episodes of voice loss and fatigability of voice. The history should be able to determine the onset and circumstances and effects of vocal problems, either sudden or prolonged, their appearance as an acute or chronic dysfunction, duration of the symptoms, any presence of a possible link to an excessive vocal effort, changes of voice quality during

Table 8.7 A medical history of voice disorders

Voice complaints	Timbre change Pitch Loudness Hoarseness Episodes of voice loss
Onset and nature of problems	Sudden/prolonged Acute/chronic Duration of symptoms Presence of fatigue voice Changes of voice quality during course of the day
Complaints accompanying phonation	Pharyngolaryngeal paraesthesia Dryness, irritation Sensation of having foreign body in the throat
Comorbidities	Respiratory tract infections Gastro-laryngeal reflux Neurological diseases, the use of medication Habits, e.g. smoking cigarettes Hormonal status (menstrual cycles, hormonal medications)
Occupational ailments	Onset and nature of voice complaints Daily loading of vocal organ Working conditions Number of working years

course of the day (e.g. in the morning voice problems in hypofunctional dysphonia, after voice load increasing voice problems in hyperfunctional dysphonia, alternating voice quality over the day in psychogenic dysphonia), infection or stress.

History taking should regard any complaints that may accompany phonation, such as pharyngolaryngeal paraesthesia, dryness, irritation or a sensation of having a foreign body in the pharynx and larynx. Moreover, questions in the medical interview should concern comorbidities, particularly respiratory tract infections, gastro-laryngeal reflux, neurological diseases, the use of medications, as well as any habits, especially cigarette smoking. In women, history taking should also involve the hormonal status: the regularity of menstrual cycles and the possible use of hormonal medications, including contraceptives or hormone replacement therapy. As far as professional voice users are concerned, it is necessary to establish the onset (after how many hours of using the voice) and the nature of voice complaints, the daily loading of the vocal organs, the working conditions and the number of years in the profession. In addition, information about systematic voice training during education and any former voice therapy may be useful (Aronson and Bless 2009).

8.4.1.3 Physical Examination Including Respiration and Velopharyngeal Competence

Any ENT examination should routinely pay special attention to the morphology of the vocal organ. Predominantly, palpation of the neck should be performed, with respect to the position of the larynx in relation to the other anatomical structures. The laryngeal skeleton and the surrounding structures should be palpated on respiration, phonation and swallowing. In particular, one should observe the formation of the thyroid cartilage and the laryngeal prominence, commonly known as the Adam's apple, more apparent in men. Furthermore, the *neck examination* includes observing any enlarged thyroid gland as well as the laryngeal vertical mobility (e.g. upwards on swallowing). The Bresgen grip is a frontal pressure on the thyroid cartilage notch. In cases of mutational falsetto, as a result of compression of the flexible thyroid cartilage, the voice drops immediately about an octave down into the chest register owing to relaxation of the overtensed vocal folds. It does not occur when the cartilage is calcified, e.g. due to age or hormonal disorders.

The physical examination assessing vocal functions of the *larynx* should include a routine examination of the larynx (see Sect. 8.4.1.3); voice emission technique including breathing; body posture; voice projection strategies; coordination between respiration, phonation and articulation; the indication of aerodynamic parameters (in particular, the maximum phonation time); and voice self-assessment (see Sect. 8.4.1.2). The examination of the larynx with an endoscope or a laryngeal mirror as indirect laryngoscopy should be performed at the very beginning. For phoniatric purposes, attention should be focused on the oropharynx - the valleculae epiglotticae and the shape of the epiglottis; on the hypopharynx - its shape, the size and symmetry of piriform sinuses and the glossoepiglottic and aryepiglottic folds; and on the larynx - the arytenoids cartilage region, vestibular folds, ventricles, colour, length, width and movement of the vocal folds, the shape of the glottis during phonation and the subglottal area, as well as the colour, moisture of the mucosa and the presence of any abnormal tissue.

In the process of voice assessment, it is essential to examine not only the larynx but the whole *vocal tract*: the oral and nasal cavities and naso-, oro- and hypopharynx. These cavities significantly contribute to the timbre and the proper resonance of the voice. The closure of the nasopharynx due to muscle obstruction of the soft palate on articulation of oral consonants prevents pathological nasality. The evaluation requires the estimation of the size of these cavities, the condition of the mucosa and any possible morphological changes. One should observe the following criteria:·the shape, symmetry and mobility of the tongue; the symmetry and mobility of the lips; the arrangement of the teeth and occlusion; the mobility of jaws and the mandible; the condition and the relationship of the hard and soft palate; the presence of abnormal movements as myoclonus; the symmetrical mobility of the soft palate and the uvula; the size and symmetry of the palatine tonsils, hypertrophy and signs of possible inflammation; the size of the adenoids; the condition of the nasal cavity and nasal turbinates; possible nasal obstruction; the presence of allergic symptoms including swelling and bruising of the turbinates; colour and moisture of the mucosa; and any pathological contents in the nasal cavities or in the nasopharynx.

The evaluation of conditions by means of the phonation technique should first assess the *activity of extrinsic and intrinsic laryngeal muscles.* One should assess whether the voice is produced freely without any hypercontraction of muscles. In case of vocal hyperfunctionality, there is an excessive, pathological muscle tension and distension of the veins of the neck. In the opposite condition, i.e. vocal hypofunction, phonation is carried out with a weakening of the laryngeal muscle activity (Sataloff 2005b).

8.4.1.4 Examination of Types of Respiration

Proper breathing technique is an essential condition for the normal voice, in particular for professional voice users. Significant also is the use of the appropriate manner of respiration (inhalation/exhalation). There are three patterns of breath support: upper thoracic/clavicular, abdominal/diaphragmatic and mixed thoracic/abdominal.

The upper thoracic/clavicular breathing involves the expansion of mainly the upper part of the chest. Ribs and abdomen are at relative rest. This type of breathing allows only partial filling of the lungs with air and the breath is defective. Breathing with a predominance of costal track called mixed thoracic/abdominal breathing consists of the ribs moving apart on the outside and slightly upwards, while the chest expands in the lateral dimension. The most appropriate and the most efficient, optimal manner for phonation is abdominal/diaphragmatic breathing. This type of breathing with a predominance of abdominal track occurs when the duration of the inspiration movement of the lower ribs is minimal and the diaphragm contracts and moves downwards. It increases the size of the chest forwards and backwards (Pruszewicz 1992). In singing, the deepest and most appropriate breath is characterised by high amplitude movements of the diaphragm, allowing a deep breath, and ample work of the muscles of the ribs guarantees the correct support breathing (appogio) (Fig. 8.5).

A properly produced voice should manifest the ability to use the whole resonator of the vocal tract. On clinical examination it is possible to evaluate the function of head resonators on phonation of memoranda combined with a vowel phonation [mmae], [mmo], and [mmi].

8.4.1.5 Examination of Velopharyngeal Competence

The assessment includes velopharyngeal competence. This plays an important role in the presence of a normal nasal resonance in the voice. Normally, only on emission of nasal vowels (e.g. /m/, /n/) is the function of the velopharyngeal

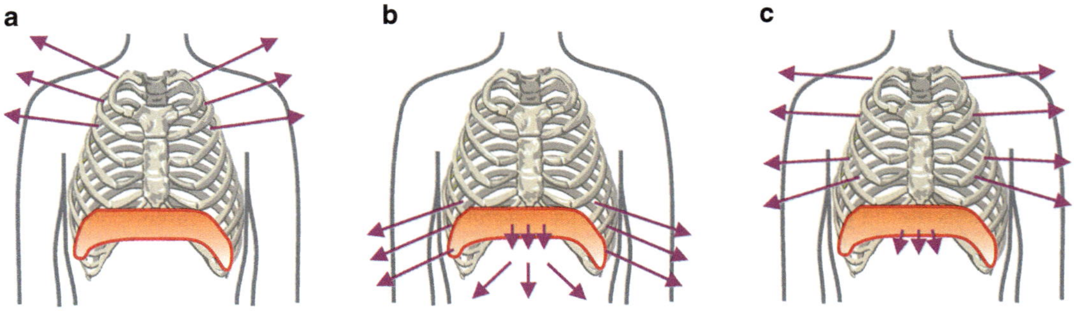

Fig. 8.5 Three patterns of breath support: (**a**) upper thoracic/clavicular, (**b**) abdominal/diaphragmatic and (**c**) mixed thoracic/abdominal

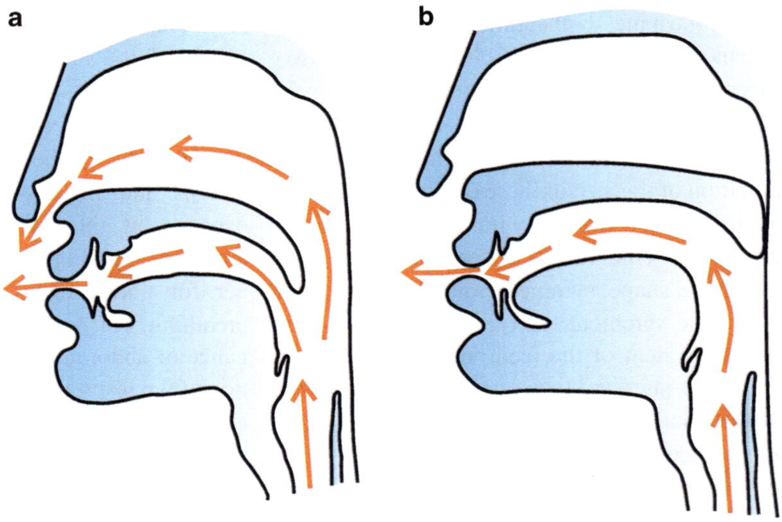

Fig. 8.6 The palatopharyngeal closure during production of (**a**) nasal and (**b**) oral sounds

sphincter physiologically incomplete, and the airstream enters the nose (Fig. 8.6).

On phonation of oral sounds, when the velopharyngeal valving is not properly controlled and the airflows into the nose, the vowels and nonnasal consonants have an improper hypernasal resonance (open nasality). In hyponasality, the velopharyngeal valving is also improperly controlled, which results in the absence of a nasal resonance on nasal consonants. The closed nasality (rhinophonia clausa—hyponasality) arises as a consequence of a difficult passage of air through the nose. Most frequently, this happens as a consequence of mucosal oedema or polyps in the nose as well as adenoid hypertrophy. The nasal sounds /m/ and /n/ sound like /b/ and /d/, and the voice becomes muted. If there is both velopharyngeal insufficiency and nasal obstruction, the nasality can be mixed.

The diagnosis of open nasality (rhinophonia aperta—hypernasality) is primarily based on the results of three tests:

- The Gutzmann test, which consists of pronouncing the vowel /a/ several times on compression and release of the wings of the nose, which normally does not change the sound. In case of the open nasality, the vowel sound on compression varies and is clearly darker.
- The Czermak mirror test involves placing an unheated mirror in front of the nostrils, and the patient is asked to pronounce the syllables composed of vowels and explosive consonants such as /pa-pa, ba-ba/. If open nasality occurs, the air is released through the nose in the form of a mist cloud visible on the mirror.
- In the Seeman test, one olive of the otoscope is placed in the patient's nostrils, and the second

one in the examiner's ear, while pronouncing vowels or consonants. If open nasality occurs, the murmur of the escaping through the nose can be heard (Pruszewicz 1992).

Otoscopy, performed as part of the ENT examination, may indicate possible changes in the middle ear, which as a possible cause of hearing loss may be the cause of abnormal phonation by means of its insufficient self-control. A pure tone *audiogram* should be performed in all cases of voice disorders owing to the feedback of hearing and voice.

8.4.1.6 Perceptual Evaluation of Voice Quality

The clinical evaluation of phonation (non-instrumental) should be started by identifying the timbre of spoken voice in the perceptual examination. *Voice quality* is a subjective concept from the auditory point of view. During the first contact with the patient, the assessment of voice disorders, as well as the evaluation of the efficacy of the treatment, is performed on the basis of the perceptual psychoacoustic evaluation of the voice (Bassich and Ludlow 1986). Hoarseness is the most common word that describes the quality of the voice characterised by noticeable noise components. It is a non-specific symptom caused mainly by irregularities of the normally almost periodic vibration of the vocal folds or lack of closure and most frequently accompanies organic diseases of the larynx (De Krom 1995). It can also be a symptom of innervation disorders of the larynx and occurs as a result of disturbed mechanisms of phonation in functional dysphonia. In addition, voice qualities are often described by the following words: harsh, breathy, rough, strained or squeezed.

It is important to mention that the same disease may lead to quite different manifestations in voice quality, and the same voice quality may have quite different causes of the underlying pathology (Kreiman et al. 1992, 1993). Thus, any deviant voice requires a complete physical examination (Bless and Baken 1992).

In order to standardise the terminology used to define dysphonia, a variety of *perceptual scales* have been developed to describe the quality of the voice (Dejonckere et al. 1993). Many phoneticians (Laver 1980), voice and speech physiologists and phoniatricians are convinced that it is necessary to create a universal scale for assessing perceptual voice. Currently, of many scales of subjective evaluation (de Bodt et al. 1996, 1997), e.g. the Stockholm Voice Evaluation Approach (Hammarberg 2000), Buffalo Voice Profile System (Wilson 1987), Laver's Vocal Profile Analysis Scheme (Laver et al. 1992), Consensus Auditory-Perceptual Evaluation of Voice (CAPE-V) (Karnell et al. 2007) and Newcastle Audio Ranking (NeAR) (Gould et al. 2012), the best known and the most widely used is the scale of the Japan Society of Logopaedics and Phoniatrics, the GRBAS scale (Hirano 1989).

The GRBAS scale describes the voice disorder with the use of five well-defined parameters: G, the grade of hoarseness; R, roughness, an audible impression of irregularities of the vibration of the vocal folds; B, breathiness, an audible impression of the air leakage through the insufficient glottal closure; A, an asthenic voice; and S, a strained voice. This scale has four degrees of intensity of disturbances, where '0' indicates a normal voice, '1' mild disturbance, '2' moderate disturbance, and '3' severe disturbance, with respect to all the parameters. Thus, a normal voice is described as follows: G0R0B0A0S0, which means a sonorous voice, without rough elements, produced with a soft attitude, and with a complete glottis closure, produced freely without any excessive muscle tension. Dejonckere et al. (2000) proposed to expand this scale with another parameter: I—instability of the voice (i.e. variability over time)—and then the scale will have the GIRBAS form. The shortened modification of the GRBAS scale excluding A and S owing to the proven low inter- and intra-rater reliability is the RBH scale (Wendler et al. 1986), where /R/ is roughness, /B/ breathiness and /H/ hoarseness. In research the perceptual evaluation should be performed by at least three independent examiners/judges, and then all the results should be averaged (Gerratt et al. 1993; Fang-Ling and Matteson 2014).

Additionally, it should be noted (Bough et al. 1996) that the features of an individual voice depend on the number of certain properties, and therefore apart from the personality and emotional state, one should take into consideration the current body temperature, the degree of rest and rehydration of the body and even the time elapsed from the last meal.

Moreover, the phoniatrician should estimate perceptually whether the *pitch* of the spoken voice is appropriate for the patient's age and gender and whether it is stable. The speech tasks for perceptual voice assessment is generally limited to a 5-s sustained phonation of the vowel sounds /ɑ/ and /i/, as well as a short reading of phonetically balanced texts, e.g. the Rainbow Passage for English language. The *mean speaking pitch* is different in male and female adults, and it changes with age. It is approximately 260 Hz (200–260 Hz, *g-c1*) and 130 Hz (100–130 Hz, *G-c*) in younger females and in males, respectively. The *vocal pitch range*, calculated as the difference between sung sounds at the lowest and highest pitch possible, should cover 1.5–2 octaves, and reaches, depending on the voice type, from d/c^1 to d^2/c^3 for females and D/c to d^1/c^2 for males. In running speech, an area of one octave is generally covered. Clinical observations are usually performed with respect to the patient's habitual pitch while speaking, in order to check whether it is too low or too high. Pitch is of striking importance for all kinds of professional speaking, especially for teachers, lecturers and public speakers. The physiological reference is the so-called indifference level, a pitch that is generated by a well-balanced action of all muscles involved with an optimal relation of muscular tension and vocal output. It is located at the transition area from the lower to the middle third of the pitch range.

This is the pitch that should be kept during speaking as the average or mean speaking pitch or at least to which it should be regularly brought back. Permanent upward deviation does not only mean an overloading of the speakers' voice apparatus but also that of the listener. As an effect of the so-called functional listening, listeners unconsciously mimic the speakers' muscular tension, get strained and tired and lose their attention.

For the purposes of complete voice evaluation, it is important to determine the *register of the voice*. The term 'register' means the type of voice, especially while singing, although the term may also refer to the mode of vibration (Niimi and Miyaji 2000). The laryngeal register reflects a specific mode of phonation. The physiological register (modal), called the chest tone, occurs because of the normal vibrations of the vocal folds and is a record of the fundamental frequencies that appear mainly while speaking. The term 'falsetto' (head tone) occurs at very high frequencies and is often slightly breathy with an incomplete glottal closure and vibration of the only free edges of the vocal fold, with the tension of the posterior part. A creaky voice, or glottal fry, occurs at very low frequencies by means of the vibration of the frontal parts of the vocal folds and a tight closure of the glottis (see also Sect. 4.5 in Volume 1).

A normal voice is produced with the appropriate *loudness*, not too loud and not too weak, and indicates the ability of the free and dynamic modulation of the volume.

The most important aerodynamic parameter of phonation is the measurement of the *maximum phonation time* (MPT) and the *s/z ratio* (Gelfer and Pazera 2006). MPT is the ability to pronounce the vowel /a/ freely at full exhaustion for as long as possible at a comfortable pitch and volume. According to Kent et al. (1987), for persons aged 17–41 years, on average it fluctuates between 15 s for women and 23 s for men and is reduced with age. Values depending on the age can range as low as 17.25–34.6 s for men and 12.10–26.5 s for women. The s/z ratio makes it possible to compare the ability to control airflow on phonation of the voiceless /s/ and voiced /z/, which is important for establishing the way in which the patient controls exhalation. In individuals with normal voices, the s/z ratio is near 1.0. Vital capacity (VC), measured parametrically by spirometry, is not a direct measurement of phonation but is used indirectly as a measure of lung function indicating the amount of air that can be used for phonation. Vital capacity is a combination of inspiratory reserve volume, expiratory reserve volume and tidal volume—this is total volume of air that can be inspired after total expiration (see Sect. 8.4.1.7). The average values of the normal vital capacity reach approximately 4800 mL for men and 3500 mL for women.

The *phonation quotient* (PQ) indicates the amount of air consumed on phonation and is obtained by division of the vital lung capacity by the maximum phonation time: PQ = VC/MPT. The normal values for this parameter vary from 145 to 269 mL/s for men and from 137 to 233 mL/s for women. Raes and Clement (1996) in their work presented the following results: for adult men at MPT 22.2 s and VC 4.800 mL, the PQ value was 269 mL/s; for women at MPT 18.4 s and VC 3.500 mL, the PQ was 233 mL/s.

The next issue to examine is *voice attacks*. There are three kinds of attack: the preferred soft mode—simultaneous, when the breath and the vibration occur at the same time; glottal, when vocal folds push against each other too strongly, making it difficult for them to vibrate; and breathy, when the breath occurs first and then the vocal folds begin to vibrate, but a gap in the incompletely closed glottis causes a portion of the air to be converted to the noise, rather than to the acoustic wave.

8.4.1.7 Articulation

Owing to the permanent interaction between vocal tract configuration and glottal function, proper articulation is also part of the specific technique of producing a normal voice. It should be characterised by a distinctive pronunciation of vowels and consonants, a moderate rate of speech and a mouth open wide with a suitable lowering of the mandible. What seems important is the ability of the correct movement of the lips, the palate (lifting and lowering) and the tongue.

8.4.1.8 Screening Methods

Screening is an investigation carried out in normal individuals to detect diseases in their early, subclinical stages. Screening of voice quality provides assessments to professional voice users, as well as candidates and students for occupations with special voice quality demands, or any lay person experiencing voice problems. Voice screening is also important for identification and early management of paediatric voice disorders, which can affect the child's education and psychosocial development. A screening method as a first step is usually based on a review of voice history to identify any potential problems or on questionnaire concerning vocal symptoms. It can be administered by health-care personnel in order to select persons for further examination by a phoniatrician and should include the assessment of voice quality and visualisation of vocal fold function. There are screening tests that can be used to measure different aspects of voice rapidly. They are generally based on questionnaire data and voice analysis, i.e. the assessment of the quality of voice, pitch, loudness, maximum phonation time, respiration and resonance. Questionnaires usually contain typical questions concerning voice complaints, duration of intensive voice and speech use, smoking, subjective voice function assessment (e.g. GRBAS scale) and voice self-assessment (e.g. VHI). Both questionnaire and voice analysis are non-invasive multi-parameter monitoring tools for early detection of potential voice disorders and therefore very useful in preventive health care in phoniatrics.

Methods of screening presented by scientists are based on a questionnaire and voice analysis that concern various groups of adults and children, e.g. the Voice Assessment Protocol for Children and Adults (VAP) (Haynes et al. 2006), Boone Voice Program for Children (Boone 1993; Boone et al. 2005), Quick Screen for Voice (Lee et al. 2004) and Screening Index for Voice Disorders (SIVD) (Ghirardi et al. 2013). There are also other voice screening tests based on only one parameter, e.g. the Glottal to Noise Excitation Ratio presented by Spanish scientists (Godino-Llorente et al. 2010). They confirmed that this acoustic parameter is a good choice for screening purposes in discriminating normal and pathological voices. Johnson et al. (2014) presented a voice screening over the telephone; it can differentiate spasmodic dysphonia from other voice disorders. Ohlsson et al. (2012) performed screening in teacher students using questionnaire Screen6 (Simberg et al. 2001) and the Swedish Voice Handicap Index. They found an association between the number of potential vocal risk factors and the number of voice symptoms.

There is no doubt that laryngoscopy is the most important information source for screening voice disorders. Awan et al. (2016) presented voice screening with the Cepstral Spectral Index of Dysphonia (CSID), which contains three reference standards: auditory perceptual estimation, Voice Handicap Index and laryngoscopic description. They suggested that this CSID method with acoustic voice analysis could be used as a potential screening tool for voice disorder identification. Pernambuco et al. (2016a, b) presented in Portuguese (there is not yet an English translation) a new tool for epidemiological screening voice in older adults: the Rastreamento de Alteracoes Vocais em Idosos (RAVI), i.e. Screening for Voice Disorders in Older Adults. This test consists of 16 questions related to sensations and perceptions associated with the voice. The authors emphasise that RAVI is the first voice-related self-reported questionnaire for identifying voice disorders in older adults. Several other countries, e.g. Scandinavian countries and Austria, have introduced many preventive programmes for professional voice users (Vilkman 2004; Schneider-Stickler et al. 2012).

Some of these screening procedures are useful practically and can be recommended, for example, the Quick Screen for Voice (Lee et al. 2004). It is a rapid and widely administered (by SPL) screening test for children that contains many aspects of voice, respiration and resonance; it has been validated in a large group of kindergarten and preschool children and is used as part of a comprehensive speech, language and hearing screening. The Screening Index for Voice Disorders (SIVD) has been proved to be an efficient tool for screening occupational voice disorders and can be used as an instrument of epidemiologic vigilance (Ghirardi et al. 2013). Voice screening procedures allow early detection of voice disorders in the subclinical stage and the administration of the treatment, rehabilitation and prevention; they can, if necessary, be used to dissuade people with voice dysfunction from the so-called voice professions.

8.4.2 Self-Administered Questionnaires for the Assessment of Voice Disorders in Normal and Professional Users

Franco Fussi and Giovanna Baracca

8.4.2.1 Introduction

Self-administered questionnaires are used to assess the impact of the health problems on the quality of life of the patients. The World Health Organization (1971) defines disability as:

> a restriction or lack of ability manifested in the performance of daily tasks

and handicap as

> a social, economic, or environmental disadvantage resulting from an impairment or disability.

Measuring the quality of life in case of a health problem, in addition to the physical examination, allows physicians to understand better the point of view of the patient related to his individual experience of a certain disease. An example of the different impacts produced by a voice problem follows: a vocal disability could increase when a patient is not able to speak at a certain pitch or loudness and a vocal handicap when a patient loses money because his voice becomes ineffective in communicating or performing. There is not necessarily a correlation between the results of the evaluation of dysphonia obtained by means of perceptive evaluation, video-laryngostroboscopy and acoustic/aerodynamic parameters and the severity of the subjective disturbance perceived by the patient in his daily life. Self-perceived impairment largely depends on how a person uses his voice. A professional speaker will be more strongly impaired by a breathy voice than a computer engineer; in the same way, a singer will face more serious consequences than a painter when his voice is hoarse. Self-assessment instruments, indeed, take into account the type of social activity, the environment where the voice is more utilised, the family habits, education, sex, gender, psychological traits and life style. The impact on the quality of life of a dysphonic problem is an important factor for clinicians not only to obtain a global evaluation but also to take the best therapeutic decision, in a field in which the prognosis is not with respect to life (quoad vitam) but with respect to health (quoad valetudinem). Moreover, questionnaires should be useful in providing a further element for measuring the outcomes of a voice treatment, be it surgical, pharmacological or rehabilitative.

8.4.2.2 List of Self-Assessment Questionnaires Utilised in Practice

In the literature, the administration of different types of questionnaire, all validated by means of statistical methodology, has demonstrated satisfactory psychometric qualities in terms of high internal consistency and test-retest reliability. Questionnaires are usually constituted by items individually scored on an ordinal scale from 0 to N, on the basis of how often each statement is experienced from the patient in daily life. The total score gives an indication of how the voice disorder creates annoyance in the life of the patient. The majority of questionnaires are also divided into subscales that score some specific aspects of the perception of the voice disturbance, such as the emotional, the physical or the social. The most well-known self-administration questionnaires include the Voice-Related Quality of Life (V-RQOL), the Voice Handicap Index (VHI), the Vocal Performance Questionnaire (VPQ), the Voice Activity and Participation Profile and the Voice Symptom Scale. There follows a brief description of each of these instruments.

The VPQ (Carding and Horsley 1992), developed in 1992, consists of 12 items concerning the physical and psychosocial impacts of a general voice disturbance on daily life. It has the advantage of being easily and briefly administered and demonstrates high internal consistency, but it does not investigate specific aspects of a voice problem. The VHI (Jacobson et al. 1997), validated in 1997, is the only self-assessment questionnaire that meets the criteria established by the Agency for Healthcare Research and Quality for determining disability in speech-language disorders. The VHI (Table 8.8), translated into and validated in more than 20 languages, is a 30-item questionnaire, each one scored from 0 (never) to 4 (always), differentiated into 3 subscales about specific domains of the impact of voice problems (emotional, functional and physical). The functional subscale investigates the consequences of a voice disturbance on daily activities (disability); the physical subscale is related to the perception of the dysphonia in terms of physical symptoms (impairment); the emotional subscale measures the effects on the emotional life of a voice problem (handicap). The maximum score of the VHI is 120; a score from 0 to 14 corresponds to no disturbance, from 15 to 28 to a slight disturbance, from 29 to 50 to a moderate disturbance and over 51 to a severe disturbance.

Jacobson et al. (1997) found that VHI has good psychometric properties and a correlation with patient judgment of the voice-disorder severity. Furthermore, VHI demonstrates a high correlation with the Dysphonia Severity Index (Wuyts et al. 2000), and it is a good index of the self-perception of the voice modification after vocal fold surgery. Available online since 2013 (Herbst et al. 2015), the DigitalVHI, a free open-source software application for obtaining Voice Handicap Index (VHI) and other questionnaire data, can be used when filling in the information. The software makes the VHI scores directly available for analysis in a digital form. Reduced versions of the VHI have also been validated, such as the VHI-10 (Rosen et al. 2004) and the VHI-9i (Nawka et al. 2009), comprised, respectively, of 10 and 9 items extracted from the original version, that can be comfortably utilised for their brevity and ease of administration. Another questionnaire that obtained similar results to those of the VHI-10 in terms of psychometric properties is the Voice-Related Quality of Life (V-RQOL) (Hogikyan and Sethuraman 1999), developed and validated in 1999, comprising ten items, divided into socio-emotional and functional-physical subscales. The Voice Symptom Scale (VoiSS) (Wilson et al. 2004) is a 30-item questionnaire developed in 2004 and able to assess communication problems, psychological impact, perception of voice characteristics and other respiratory symptoms. The Voice Activity and Participation Profile (VAPP) (Ma and Yiu 2001) is a 28-item questionnaire consisting of

Table 8.8 Voice Handicap Index (VHI)

		0	1	2	3	4
1	My voice makes it difficult for people to hear me					
2	I run out of air when I talk					
3	People have difficulty understanding me in a noisy room					
4	The sound of my voice varies throughout the day					
5	My family has difficulty hearing me when I call them throughout the house					
6	I use the phone less often than I would like					
7	I'm tense when talking with others because of my voice					
8	I tend to avoid groups of people because of my voice					
9	People seem irritated with my voice					
10	People ask, 'What's wrong with your voice?'					
11	I speak with friends, neighbours or relatives less often because of my voice					
12	People ask me to repeat myself when speaking face-to-face					
13	My voice sounds creaky and dry					

(continued)

Table 8.8 (continued)

		0	1	2	3	4
14	I feel as though I have to strain to produce voice					
15	I find other people do not understand my voice problem					
16	My voice difficulties restrict my personal and social life					
17	The clarity of my voice is unpredictable					
18	I try to change my voice to sound different					
19	I feel left out of conversations because of my voice					
20	I use a great deal of effort to speak					
21	My voice is worse in the evening					
22	My voice problem causes me to lose income					
23	My voice problem upsets me					
24	I am less outgoing because of my voice problem					
25	My voice makes me feel handicapped					
26	My voice 'gives out' on me in the middle of speaking					
27	I feel annoyed when people ask me to repeat					

(continued)

Table 8.8 (continued)

		0	1	2	3	4
28	I feel embarrassed when people ask me to repeat					
29	My voice makes me to feel incompetent					
30	I'm ashamed of my voice problem					

0 never; *1* almost never; *2* sometimes; *3* almost always; *4* always. Copyright with kind permission from the American Speech-Language-Hearing Association (ASHA)

five subscales focused on the self-perception of the severity of voice disturbances, impact on job activity and daily communication and impact on social relationships and emotional life. The answers are provided by the patient on a visual analogue scale (VAS).

The self-assessment instruments can play an important role in creating, in a brief time, an empathic relationship between dysphonic patients and clinicians, helping the latter to understand the real effect of a voice problem on daily living and functioning. In addition, it has to be taken into account that questionnaire answers are affected by several individual variables, such as family and community support, cultural background and so on. It is necessary to include the self-assessment evaluation in a multistep evaluation of voice, as recommended by ELS Guidelines (Dejonckere et al. 2001). Self-administered questionnaire results must be considered as an aspect of the multidimensional evaluation of a voice disorder, also including perceptual, videostroboscopic, acoustic and aerodynamic assessments. The utilities of the self-administration questionnaires must be considered in the diagnostic phase, when the idea of how the patient perceives the voice disorder can improve the clinician's choice on the best treatment. Moreover, by analysing the results, the clinician can help the patient to become aware of his problem and manage it. Comparison of the answers pre- and post-treatment, rehabilitative or surgical, indicates the level of satisfaction of the patient with the results of therapy.

8.4.2.3 Questionnaires for Special Kinds of Voice Disorders

Self-assessment protocols must be specific for special categories of patients with voice disorders. This is the reason that some special instruments have been created and validated for particular groups of dysphonic people. It has already been reported that self-evaluation questionnaires are influenced by several factors such as age, sex, specific disease patterns, occupation and others. Considering the age factor, it cannot be neglected that children's voice disorders must be evaluated with specific self-assessment instruments able to take into account the impact of dysphonia on daily paediatric life. The Pediatric Voice Handicap Index (pVHI) (Zur et al. 2007), comparable to adult VHI, is characterised by high internal consistency and high test-retest reliability. It is able to measure the impact of child's voice quality on overall communication, development, education, social and family life. It is composed of 21 items divided into three subscales, functional, physical and emotional, concerning how much the parents perceive the impact of their child's voice disturbance on his or her daily life. In this case, indeed, the questionnaire must be filled in by the child's parents. Ricci-Maccarini et al. (2013) validated a self-assessment questionnaire in Italian specific for children from 8 to 14 years of age, in which each child fills in the interview autonomously. It demonstrated good clinical validity and responsiveness to treatment in case of paediatric dysphonia. In 2012 Verduyckt et al. (2012) created and validated a new self-assessment questionnaire for paediatric use, capable of measuring in parallel the impact of children's voice disorders by themselves and their parents, the Pediatric Voice Symptom Questionnaire (PVSQ). It is valid, reliable and easy to administer in children from 6 years of age, when they are conscious of their vocal symptoms (Verduyckt et al. 2011). Another category of people usually affected by voice disorders in terms of low satisfaction with their voice parameters comprises transgenders, who often perceive their pitch too low and their voice disorder as a problematic factor in social life. In 2013 Dacakis et al. (2013) validated the Transgender Self-Evaluation Questionnaire able to provide a reliable self-report measure of vocal functioning in male-to-female transsexuals. It is structured as a self-administered interview composed of 30 items scored from 1 to 4 concerning voice problems in daily use experienced when living as a female. Another factor that must be taken in account is the awareness of the patient about his voice problem and his availability to modify his vocal strategies through a voice therapy. Some self-assessing instruments were created to be particularly useful in evaluating some variables important for the therapeutic choices. In particular, Epstein et al. (2009) created and validated the Voice Disability Coping Questionnaire (VDCQ), able to measure the coping processes in different patient groups. It is constituted by 4 coping subscales: 'social support', 'passive coping', 'avoidance' and 'information seeking' measured over 15 items. Coping in psychological medicine refers to the way in which people deal with the stress of illness. In case of voice disorders, this instrument helps people understand how to cope with voice problems. The questionnaire should be administered before voice therapy in order to address modification of coping and put it in relation to the outcomes.

8.4.2.4 Self-Administered Questionnaires for Professional Users

Singers constitute a specific population of professionals particularly at risk of voice problems. They are more likely to seek help and report problems related to their singing voice (Rosen and Murry 2000; Phyland et al. 1999). Singers represent 11.5% of all patients at voice consultations while constituting only 0.02% of the general population (Titze et al. 1997). Hoarseness frequently affects not only their speaking voice but also their singing voice and, consequently, their professional activity. This is partly due to the importance they give to their voice status, a critical social and occupational factor that can significantly affect their quality of life. The perception of a voice problem in singing is often related to specific symptoms, such as difficulty in the passaggio, vocal endurance and diminished range, aspects that are not assessed by the common self-assessment questionnaires. They are, indeed, more sensitive to vocal disabilities, which may have a higher impact on their quality of life than that of non-singers. Hence, to obtain a self-assessing instrument able to evaluate vocal disability in singers, in 2007, Cohen et al. (2007) created and validated a specific questionnaire, the Singing Voice Handicap Index (SVHI), aimed at measuring the physical, social, emotional and economic impacts of voice problems on the lives of the singers. The SVHI (Table 8.9) is a 36-item self-administered questionnaire that is used to assess difficulties related to voice health status typical of the singing professional, as demonstrated by its psychometric properties of reliability and validity. The items address symptoms frequently reported to phoniatricians and speech pathologists by singers. Each item must be individually scored on a 5-point Likert scale (ordinal scale) ranging from never (score of 0) to always (score of 4) (Likert 1932).

The SVHI has demonstrated higher sensitivity to clinical changes than the VHI in singers, proving the validity of the SVHI in measuring outcomes in the singing population. In fact, VHI may underestimate the level of handicap related to voice problems in performers, especially for certain pathologies able to produce severe consequences for the professional activity, for example, reflux or allergies. These disturbances affect the singing voice more severely than the speaking voice, so it is necessary to have a specific tool able to measure the impact of any kind of voice problem peculiar to the singing activity. It is important for a self-assessment instrument to recognise changes in singing voice health status after surgi-

Table 8.9 Singing Voice Handicap Index (SVHI) (Reprinted with kind permission of Prof. Seth Cohen, Durham, North Carolina, USA)

		0	1	2	3	4
1	It takes a lot of effort to sing					
2	My voice cracks and breaks					
3	I am frustrated by my singing					
4	People ask 'What is wrong with your voice?' when I sing					
5	My ability to sing varies day to day					
6	My voice 'gives out' on me while I am singing					
7	My singing voice upsets me					
8	My singing problems make me not want to sing/perform					
9	I am embarrassed by my singing					
10	I am unable to use my 'high voice'					
11	I get nervous before I sing because of my singing problems					
12	My speaking voice is not normal					
13	My throat is dry when I sing					
14	I've had to eliminate certain songs from my singing/performances					
15	I have no confidence in my singing voice					
16	My singing voice is never normal					
17	I have trouble making my voice do what I want it to					
18	I have to 'push it' to produce my voice when singing					
19	I have trouble controlling the breathiness in my voice					
20	I have trouble controlling the raspiness in my voice					
21	I have trouble singing loudly					
22	I have difficulty staying on pitch when I sing					
23	I feel anxious about my singing					
24	My singing sounds forced					
25	My speaking voice is hoarse after I sing					
26	My voice quality is inconsistent					
27	My singing voice makes it difficult for the audience to hear me					
28	My singing makes me feel handicapped					
29	My singing voice tires easily					
30	I feel pain, tickling or choking when I sing					
31	I am unsure of what will come out when I sing					
32	I feel something is missing in my life because of my inability to sing					
33	I am worried my singing problems will cause me to lose money					
34	I feel left out of the music scene because of my voice					
35	My singing makes me feel incompetent					
36	I have to cancel performances, singing engagements, rehearsals or practices because of my singing					

0 never; *1* almost never; *2* sometimes; *3* almost always; *4* always cal, pharmacological or rehabilitative treatments, and the SVHI demonstrates these properties in terms of clinical validity. The original English version of the SVHI has been translated into and validated in several languages, and it is utilised in different countries. Also developed and validated is an abbreviated version of the SVHI, the SVHI-10 (Cohen et al. 2009), composed of 10 items extracted from the 36 original, on the basis of the item-total correlation and better self-assessment of the voice disorders. SVHI-10 can be easily utilised to facilitate the assessment of the perceived handicap related to a singing voice problem, especially in the case of repeated administration or multidimensional assessment when the time for the evaluation is reduced.

Of course, singers constitute a peculiar population, but they are not so homogeneous: variables such as the singing styles performed, the amount of singing training and experience, the nature of singing demands and the performance environments can definitely affect the voice conditions of a singer and the perceived level of handicap. Voice disturbances, caused by vocal fold lesions, can in fact produce a different subjective disturbance depending on the number and duration of the performances, the amount of rehearsal needed and the characteristics of voice use during the performances. All these factors are influenced by the professional level and the singing style that a singer engages. Accordingly, singing style may be an important predictor of singing voice handicap requiring particular consideration. This evidence led Fussi (2005) and Moreti et al. (2012) to develop more specific self-assessment instruments, on the model of the SVHI, for the modern and classical singing voice. The two questionnaires, called the Classical Singing Voice Handicap Index (CSVHI) (Table 8.10) and the Modern Singing Voice Handicap Index (MSVHI) (Table 8.11), which are currently under validation on a large number of singers, are composed of 30 items grouped into 3 areas (impairment, disability, handicap). Each item is scored from 0 to 4 on the basis of how often it is experienced in the singing activity. The items are consistent with the peculiar use of the voice, depending on the singing style engaged. They investigate aspects of singing that can be perceived only in the case of a high level of self-confidence with their own voice. The two different instruments, for classical and modern singers, take into consideration the environments where singers perform; the theatre in the case of the classical style; open-spaces, restaurant or pubs in the case of modern style; the level of background noise that is minimum during the opera performance and could be very loud during parties; or other situations where modern singers often perform. Furthermore, the environments of classical concerts have similar acoustic characteristics, whereas modern music is performed in several different types of situations to which modern singers must adapt their voices each time. There are also some technical aspects in the use of voice that should be investigated differently for classical and modern singing: for the modern style, there is no definite vocal register as in classical, so the vocal texture is more adaptable to the repertoire. Singers in this case have the possibility of varying the timbre according to the songs, several times within the same performance, and to look for different vocal solutions. Classical style, conversely, needs homogeneous vocal emission and more rigour in the execution. It follows that performers can feel a different level of discomfort caused by a voice difficulty according to the singing style.

CSVHI and MSVHI are two specific instruments able to measure the level of handicap related to the singing voice differently for classical and modern styles and to evaluate peculiar aspects of the singing activity related to the singing style engaged.

In conclusion, the most utilised self-assessment questionnaires are the VHI for common dysphonic diseases, the PVHI for paediatric voice disorders and the SVHI for dysphonia in voice professional users.

Table 8.10 Classical Singing Voice Handicap Index (CSVHI)

		0	1	2	3	4
1	I have difficulties during the performance in the theatre with modification of my vocal efficiency					
2	My vocal warm up has to be prolonged					
3	I am forced to modify my vocal technique because my voice problem influences my usual technical control					
4	My singing problem forces me to modify or limit my repertoire					
5	My singing problem forces me to limit my usual study time					
6	I have difficulties during my performance with modification of my vocal efficiency					
7	I have to prolong the vocal rest between two performance					
8	I have to avoid changes in the vocal intensity during the pianissimo execution to mask my voice problem					
9	To mask my singing problem, I am forced to undergo continuous medical therapy					
10	My singing problem forces me to limit the use of my voice in my social life					
11	I feel more anxious than usual before performances					
12	People around me do not recognise my singing voice problem					
13	I am subjected to justified criticism from people around me					
14	I get nervous and less sociable because of my singing problems					
15	I get worried when someone asks me to repeat a vocalism or a sung phrase					
16	I feel that my career is in danger because of my singing difficulties					
17	My colleagues, managers and critics have noticed my singing difficulties					
18	I have to cancel performances and other professional commitments					
19	I avoid planning my next professional commitments					
20	I avoid speaking to people					
21	I have trouble managing my breathing					
22	I feel my sung emission breathy and weak					
23	I feel my sung emission is rough, with noise					
24	I have difficulties in controlling the intensity of the sound (vocal breaks)					
25	My vocal range is reduced					
26	I have difficulties in balancing vocal registers and resonance					

(continued)

Table 8.10 (continued)

		0	1	2	3	4
27	I feel I have to force to produce my voice					
28	The voice quality goes down during the performance					
29	My speaking voice is tired and worse after the performance					
30	The vocal efficiency is reduced at certain times of the day					

0 never; *1* almost never; *2* sometimes; *3* almost always; *4* always. Copyright with kind permission from OMEGA EDIZIONI s.a.s. di Giacomo Soncini & C., Torino, Italia

Table 8.11 Modern Singing Voice Handicap Index (MSVHI)

		0	1	2	3	4
1	I feel vocal fatigue from the beginning of the performance					
2	My speaking voice is hoarse and tired during a performance					
3	I am forced to modify my vocal technique because my voice problem influences my usual technical control					
4	My singing problem forces me to eliminate or limit certain songs from my repertoire, also with transposition of tonality					
5	My singing problem forces me to limit my usual study time					
6	I have difficulties during my performance with modification of my vocal efficiency					
7	I cannot stand more than two consecutive performances					
8	I have to ask the sound engineer for help to hide the alterations of my voice					
9	To mask my singing problem, I am forced to undergo continuous medical therapy					
10	My singing problem forces me to limit the use of my voice in my social life					
11	I feel more anxious than usual before performances					
12	People around me do not recognise my singing voice problem					
13	I am subjected to justified criticism from people around me					
14	I get nervous and less sociable because of my singing problems					
15	I get worried when someone asks me to repeat a vocalism or a sung phrase					
16	I feel that my career is in danger because of my singing difficulties					
17	My colleagues, managers and critics have noticed my singing difficulties					
18	I have to cancel performances and other professional commitments					
19	I avoid planning my next professional commitments					

(continued)

Table 8.11 (continued)

		0	1	2	3	4
20	I avoid speaking to people					
21	I have trouble managing my breathing					
22	My vocal performance changes throughout the day					
23	I feel that my voice is breathy and weak					
24	I feel that my voice is rough					
25	I have to strain to produce my voice					
26	My vocal efficiency varies in an unpredictable manner during the performance					
27	I try to modify my voice to make it better					
28	It takes a lot of effort to sing					
29	My voice is worse in the evening					
30	My voice tires easily during a performance					

0 never; *1* almost never; *2* sometimes; *3* almost always; *4* always. Copyright with kind permission from OMEGA EDIZIONI s.a.s. di Giacomo Soncini & C., Torino, Italia

8.4.3 Laryngoscopy, Stroboscopy, High-Speed Video and Phonovibrogram

Ulrich Eysholdt

8.4.3.1 Light Sources

Cold Light

Light projectors for medical endoscopy have been built since the 1930s. All techniques of light production have a common problem: the brighter the light, the higher the temperature of the equipment from unwanted heat generated. A heat-absorbing glass is built into endoscopy light projectors for the protection of the patient. Because of this, this equipment is not quite as hot, and the promotionally euphemistic name 'cold light source' is now applied. Clinically available cold light sources use light generated by excited halogen (F, Cl, Br) or inert (Xe, Kr) gas molecules and have a typical power consumption of 250–300 W. Halogen light is 'warm white' and is therefore more comfortable for the doctor during an examination. When working with a Xe or Kr source, the doctor must, however, first accustom himself and his perception to the blueish 'cold white' light.

LED

Currently, cold light source technology is being superseded by LED (light-emitting diode) light. Coloured LEDs (green, red, etc.) have been on the market for decades, but white light LEDs of sufficient luminance have only recently become available. LEDs are very suitable for clinical use: they need less power and generate much less heat than cold light technology, meaning that the tip of the endoscope does not become hot over time. Current LEDs (in 2015) do not have quite the same degree of brightness as conventional xenon cold light sources. LED light sources have another advantage for laryngoscopy: in contrast to cold light sources, LEDs do not fluctuate with the 50 Hz mains voltage. LEDs are therefore ideal light sources for high-speed video recording (HSV).

Stroboscopic Light

Stroboscopy is based on a special flashing light source which—in a medical application—is solely used for examination of the vibratory movement of the vocal folds. Laryngostroboscopy can be performed just as well by using a simple laryngoscopy mirror or any type of endoscope. Stroboscopy (from the Greek στρόβος *strobos*, meaning whirl or rotation, from the first mechanical stroboscopes that used rotating perforated discs to interrupt the light beam) is a method of visualising rapid movements that are impossible to be seen by the eyes alone because the chemical regeneration of rhodopsin in the retina of human eyes allows a maximum frequency of movement perception of only 20 Hz. However, stroboscopy is only appropriate for the visualisation of periodic movements, which are movements that repeat their spatial position. The moving object is illuminated by a rapid series of light flashes, the frequency of which is designated by the repetition rate of the movement. If the frequency of the light flashes is identical to that of the movement, then every light flash illuminates the object in the same phase, meaning that the object appears to the observer to be static ('stroboscopy in standstill'). If the frequency of light flashes is faster than the movement, the flash will illuminate the object earlier and reveal another phase of the periodic movement. The object will seem to move slowly ('stroboscopy in slow motion', an optical illusion). In laryngostroboscopy the apparent vibration of the vocal folds is lowered to 1 Hz. The visual representation is so convincing that the methodical constraints are often forgotten:

- **A** Stroboscopy only targets periodic (i.e. non-disturbed) vocal fold vibration during sustained phonation. The more irregular the vibration, the less effective the stroboscopy.
- **B** The virtual slow-motion movement of stroboscopy is a visual illusion only. A quantitative evaluation is technically possible but physically meaningless.

In technical terms, stroboscopy violates the Nyquist condition of Shannon's sampling theorem. Nonetheless, stroboscopy has been an important element of the diagnostic investigation of the voice since 1960.

8.4.3.2 The Endoscope

An endoscope is defined as an optical instrument that can be used to view a cavity from the inside through a narrow opening. The superposition principle of geometrical optics is utilised, which states that two crossing beams of light do not influence each other. Illumination and observation occur simultaneously in the same optical system. The size of an endoscope is given in 'mm diameter' (*D*) and sometimes in the older Charrière (Ch) unit of measurement, which corresponds to 'mm circumference' (conversion: $D = \mathrm{Ch}/\pi$, with $\pi = 3.14159 \ldots$ the circle constant). The length of the endoscope is unimportant for laryngeal endoscopy.

There are two main types of endoscope: rigid and flexible.

Rigid Endoscopy

Rigid endoscopes with a length of 3–50 cm are these days mainly used for examination of the upper respiratory tract. A typical rigid laryngoscope is a metal tube of 15–25 cm length that contains 'rod lenses' (glass cylinders with lens-shaped cavities that direct and focus light) as an imaging system. The light from the light source is directed laterally through a fibre-optic cable coupled to a semi-transparent beam splitter. At the tip of the endoscope, the light is reflected by a mirror and emitted. The reflection angle of this mirror defines the endoscope type (see Fig. 8.7). An angle of 70–90° is suitable for illuminating the larynx (90° is most common in Europe). Ninety degree or 70° laryngoscopes have today replaced the laryngoscopic mirror of the nineteenth century. The old term 'indirect' laryngoscopy is kept for this modern technique because the light is redirected at an angle. A 70° laryngoscope can be inserted a little deeper (and therefore be brought closer to the vocal folds), but a more subtle examination technique is required.

The image is observed through a magnifying eyepiece lens through which one can either directly look or to which a video camera can be attached. The eyepiece usually has fourfold magnification.

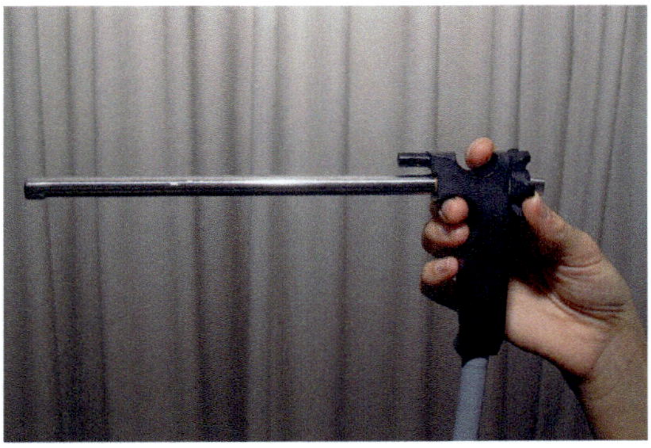

Fig. 8.7 Rigid endoscope 90°

Flexible Endoscopy

In contrast to the rigid endoscope, a flexible endoscope can be directed around a curve. Conventional flexible endoscopes have the same design as rigid endoscopes, except that they have a bundle of flexible fibre-optic cables instead of a rod lens. Flexible laryngoscopes are approximately 40 cm long, and the tip can be directed by control knobs near the eyepiece (see Fig. 8.8). In contrast to a bronchoscope, flexible laryngoscopes do not have a suction tube or working tube next to the light channel, and it is therefore possible to manufacture very narrow flexible laryngoscopes (max. 5 mm, in contrast with the 6–8 mm of a bronchoscope). However, a not insignificant loss of light occurs with fibre optics; the longer the endoscope, the greater the amount of light lost. This loss of light must be compensated for during observation, either by performing observations in a darkened room or by using electronic light amplification within the video chain.

COTT ('Chip-on-the-Tip')

Modern image sensors can be constructed so small that they can fit on the tip of a flexible laryngoscope. Image distortion must be corrected by an external computer, the camera processor. This 'chip-on-the-tip' technology produces very good images because it has almost no loss of light. It is, however, very expensive and is only used in combination with an HD standard high-quality video chain.

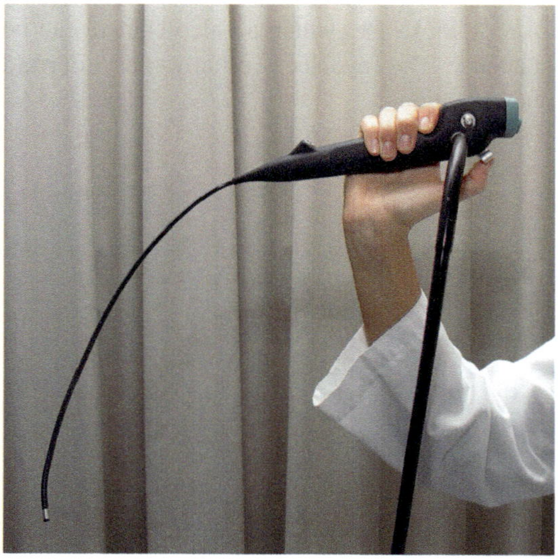

Fig. 8.8 Flexible endoscope

Transnasal Flexible Laryngoscopy

The flexible laryngoscope is inserted through the nose (inferior nasal meatus), and the tip is usually positioned in the oropharynx. The insertion phase must be uninterrupted and is often performed with mucosal anaesthesia to avoid patient discomfort. If the endoscope is inserted and positioned correctly, the patient is able to tolerate it well and can speak and swallow during the examination. This technique is used for 'fibre-optic endoscopic examination of swallowing' (FEES) (see Vol. 2, Chap. 6).

The endoscope can be inserted beyond the oropharynx if required to investigate specific issues. The tip is then positioned in the endolarynx or in the trachea but is less well tolerated here because the mucous membranes are more sensitive.

Rigid or Flexible?

Rigid and flexible endoscopic techniques are both types of indirect laryngoscopy. The technique used depends upon the country and local customs. Flexible laryngoscopy is prevalent in Japan, but 90° rigid laryngoscopy is more often found in Europe and the west coast of the USA, while 70° rigid techniques are more common on the east coast of the USA. In general, the luminance of the rigid endoscope is higher than that of the flexible endoscope, but this difference has less relevance these days because both techniques are typically combined with video recording, which essentially nullifies the difference. Analogue video techniques following S-VHS or U-matic high band have long since been replaced by digital recordings and data storage on computer. With digital video signals, weaknesses in the primary signal can easily be improved before storage (in jargon, 'Photoshopping'). Other differences between endoscopes exist and are measureable but play no role within clinical practice. 'Rigid or flexible'—previously a matter of faith—is now not a question of quality but a question of habit.

8.4.3.3 Indirect Laryngoscopy

The patient should be sat upright in a chair, with his bottom firmly against the backrest and his upper body bent slightly forwards (approximately 15°). With a 70° endoscope, the patient's head should be flexed dorsally, and the investigator should stand during the investigation. With a 90° endoscope, the patient's head is held normally and the investigator should sit down. With a flexible transnasal endoscope, the patient should be seated as comfortably as possible; the investigator should also be seated in a relaxed position and not just on ergonomic grounds: he must be able to use the footswitch of the stroboscope without losing balance. The magnifying laryngoscope is inserted through the oral cavity with the tongue outstretched, despite the fact that the uvular veli palatini must be pushed to the side with the tip of the endoscope. The investigator needs to be skilful in order to avoid gag and swallowing reflexes.

The patients should be asked to produce a vocal tone that they can hold over time, such as [hæ:]. Though this sound can hardly be produced with the endoscope in the throat, the intention alone makes the epiglottis rise, which permits a view into the larynx down to the glottis. When a patient is encouraged to produce this sound, the vocal folds, which are abducted for respiration, are then adducted. This transition of the larynx from respiratory to phonatory position can be visualised by laryngoscopy. A dynamic balance between the prephonatory tension of the vocal folds and the simultaneously raised subglottal pressure is generated within 80–150 ms, and the vocal folds begin to vibrate. This phase of prephonatory laryngeal alignment cannot be visualised by endoscopy, but once the vocal folds have established a steady oscillatory state (after 2–10 cycles of vibration), the voice level triggers the stroboscope, and the movement of the vocal folds can be observed in slow motion (Table 8.12).

Endoscopic imaging will continue to be improved by the advances in recording and analysis techniques afforded by video. The investigator should orientate himself on the monitor on which the 'moving image' is displayed. Despite the additional expenditure of time, it is common to record the video and assess it immediately after the actual investigation. It is important to concentrate on the management of the patient and the endoscope during the investigation itself in order to obtain good images.

Table 8.12 Transition from respiration to phonation

		Visible on laryngoscopy
Respiration	Vocal folds abducted, glottis open	Yes
Vocal insertion	Adductive movement of the vocal folds ('respiratory mobility')	Yes
	Prephonatory generation of • Vocal fold tension • Subglottal pressure	No
Phonation	Vocal fold adducted, glottis closed	Yes
	Vocal fold vibration ('phonatory mobility')	Only by using stroboscopic light or high-speed technology

The monitor must be orientated according to (a) the redirection of light in the laryngoscope and (b) the patient's ability to interpret it. 'Up' on the monitor is the dorsal direction, 'down' is ventral, and the 'right' side of the monitor is the patient's left and vice versa. This sounds trivial but in fact cannot be emphasised strongly enough: the most severe treatment errors within hospitals occur because of wrong-side procedures.

Figure 8.9 shows typical laryngoscopic images, (a) in respiration and (b) in phonation mode. The criteria for assessment of the images are adjusted according to Virchow's disease classification (malformation, degeneration, trauma, inflammation and tumour). A laryngoscopic finding should describe:

- The morphology of the endolarynx
  - Vocal fold configuration (free edges and surface)

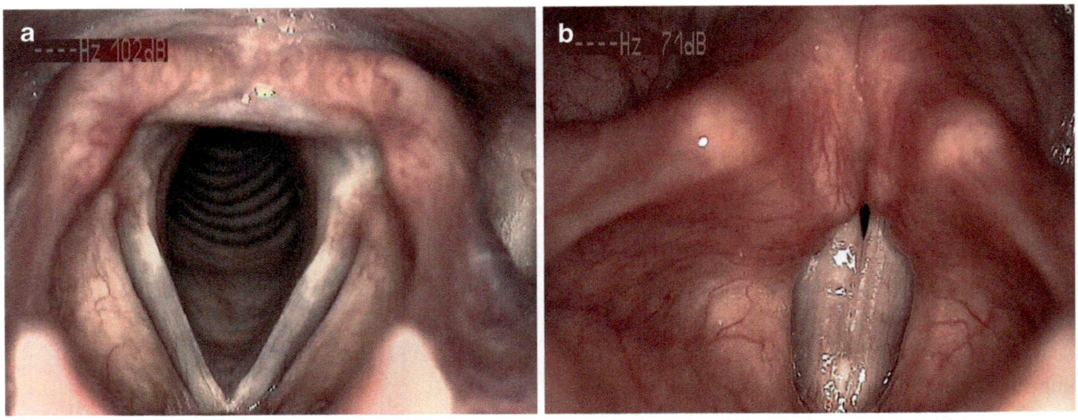

Fig. 8.9 Typical laryngoscopic images showing respiration in (**a**) and phonation in (**b**). (With kind permission from Prof. Tadeus Nawka, Berlin)

  - Inflammation
  - Trauma/haemorrhage
  - Neoplasia
  - Atrophy (degeneration)
  - Malformation
- Respiratory mobility
- Phonatory mobility

In order to orientate oneself rapidly, the triangular glottal opening, which is usually dark black, is bordered by the bright white vocal folds. The vocal folds, vestibular folds and arytenoids should be observed for the subsequent documentation of findings, and either the endoscope or the patient's head should be moved in order to look into the anterior commissure.

On phonation, the glottis closes and respiratory mobility is visible. Phonatory mobility (vibration of the vocal folds) cannot be visualised with a laryngoscope. This can be achieved by using stroboscopy (very widely used but methodically problematical; see section "Stroboscopic Light" A and B) and recording techniques in real-time resolution such as 1D videokymography (VKG) (see Sect. 8.4.1.5) or 2D high-speed video recording (HSV).

8.4.3.4 Visualisation of Vocal Fold Vibration

Vocal fold vibration, which has a frequency ≥100 Hz, is so fast it cannot be seen with the eyes. Video recording and technical devices to assist with observation are necessary in order to transform the speed of the vocal folds into a form that can be perceived. Such technology includes:

- Stroboscopy. Dispenses with detailed movement and reflects only a split-second recording of each vibratory cycle in which the vibrating vocal folds are illuminated by a flashing light source.
- High-speed video endoscopy (HSV). Records video with a high frame rate (≥4000 frames per second (fps), equating to 15–40 images per cycle. Videokymography (VKG) is a simplified, inexpensive variant but has associated limitations.

Both techniques are similar in that they involve connecting a video recorder to a laryngoscope. We tend to avoid the inconvenient word 'video(laryngo) stroboscopy' in clinical jargon and instead just use the terms stroboscopy or HSV endoscopy.

Stroboscopy

Stroboscopy has been widely used for decades (Schönhärl 1960; Hirano 1981); the recording apparatus has been substantially simplified and regularly adapted to current technology. Despite its underlying limitations, stroboscopy sometimes is thought of as a kind of secret weapon in voice diagnosis, even by many ENT physicians. However, stroboscopy is very well suited to the analysis of vocal fold vibration as long as the voice is no more than slightly disturbed.

The light source is a flashing light, which is set to the frequency of the patient's voice. The trigger signal is the fundamental frequency of the voice, which is continuously calculated by a microprocessor in the stroboscope. A very robust trigger signal for the stroboscope light source can be taken from EGG or from a contact microphone which the patient holds against the outside of his own larynx. Triggering by a microphone that is sensitive to airborne sound and is attached to the endoscope is simpler but gives a less robust signal: the airborne signal contains many harmonics, so it takes longer to identify the fundamental frequency (it may even be impossible within the appropriate time frame, by which time the stroboscope may have turned off).

Modern stroboscopic light sources can be triggered up to 600 Hz, at which frequency they can show an exact image for each vibratory cycle. Following the initial combination of all of the images from each vibratory cycle, a film of the moving image which appears to be slow motion can be shown on the monitor. Assessment criteria for video laryngoscopy are:

- Amplitude
- Mucosal wave
- Closure of the glottis
- Temporal and spatial symmetry of the vibration

All these parameters are highly dependent on pitch and loudness. Therefore, corresponding documentation is obligatory; otherwise the descriptions of any vibratory findings are definitely useless. The same is true for all methods used to assess vocal fold vibrations.

Consequently, a great deal of experience is required in order to evaluate and interpret results correctly. The complexity of voice function and its numerous mutual dependencies are difficult to interpret.

Amplitude denotes the distance of the vibrations of the vocal folds. Although the vocal folds vibrate in 3D rotatory movements, endoscopy only reveals a projection of the mediolateral component. This is interpreted as movement of the vocal muscle (musculus vocalis, thyroarytenoideus). The amplitude is smaller at higher frequencies (increased muscle tension resulting in lower vibratory mass) as well as at lower loudness. Amplitude is therefore best observed at a comfortable pitch and loudness for the patient (i.e. in the middle of his vocal range). It is categorised by using a four-step Likert scale: (1) enlarged, (2) normal, (3) small and (4) missing on both sides.

The phenomenon of the *mucosal wave* was first discovered by the use of stroboscopy. Mucosal waves are waves of the epithelium covering the vocal folds, which run laterally during the vibration of the medial edge of the vocal folds. They occur at the cranial and caudal surfaces of the vocal folds but are only observable at the cranial surfaces. Mucosal waves can only occur when the viscoelasticity of the lamina propria and Reinke's space is not impaired, when the epithelia of the vocal folds can be extended laterally within their own limits along the base. Mucosal waves are evaluated according to the following categories on stroboscopy:

1. Present
2. Restricted
3. Abolished
4. Extended/enhanced

where (1) corresponds to the normal condition and (2) and (3) indicate disruptions in viscoelasticity, which could have various causes (inflammation or tumour, or simply dysfunctional). Case (4) is essentially only found in Reinke's oedema, a specific type of chronic laryngitis featuring the pathological enlargement of Reinke's space and the build-up of gelatinous mucous.

The question of *glottal closure* (whether or not the glottis is closed completely) can only be answered by using stroboscopic or other visualisation techniques. As well as the binary decision:

- Glottis closed during phonation
- Glottis *not* closed during phonation

It is also important to describe the type of incomplete closure of the glottis. The following categories are distinguished:

- Ventral gap
- Dorsal gap
- Continuous chink-shaped gap
- Spindle-shaped gap
- Hour glass glottis
- Irregular gap

In principle, an incomplete glottal closure is considered to be pathological in most cases. One exception is the triangular dorsal gap in young women (the 'glottal chink'), which can also be observed during pubescent voice change in males (the 'mutation triangle').

The most complex stroboscopic evaluation category is *temporal and spatial vibration symmetry*. Human perception is very robust in the categories of shape, colour, size and texture but not very reliable for time-dependent processes. There are only two possible categories for evaluating the symmetry of vocal fold vibration with stroboscopy:

- Symmetrical
- (Clearly) asymmetrical

A European consensus paper proposed the use of quantitative values for stroboscopy, rather than the above categories. However, given the methodical restrictions and highly subjective nature of stroboscopy, this proposal is not sensible and suggests a level of accuracy that does not actually exist.

High-Speed Video (HSV)

High-speed video technology is well-established in sports coverage, where it is called slow-motion video. For laryngoscopy, it is not yet clinically established while being under evaluation. A high-quality HSV camera operating at 4000 fps (in comparison with the normal 25 fps) is required. This technology was first developed through military mass production and since then has become less expensive so that it can be used within medicine. To increase their recording rate, HSV cameras usually work in black-and-white mode. Indeed, HSV cameras exist that produce colour images with high temporal and spatial resolution. Using 4000 fps recording equipment, the camera takes 40 images during a single 100 Hz vibratory cycle and 16 images during a 250 Hz cycle. If the high-speed film is then played back at 25 fps, there is a time-stretch ratio of 1:160 which, in contrast to stroboscopy, is a true slow motion. HSV laryngoscopy is therefore always indicated in cases where the voice is so severely dysfunctional that stroboscopy cannot be reliably triggered.

An HSV camera can, in principle, be attached to any type of endoscope. However, at such a high recording rate, the video shutter is only open for approximately 10 μs, meaning that the intensity of the light is significantly reduced. To improve the luminance, HSV recordings are mostly created with 90° or 70° rigid laryngoscopes.

8.4.3.5 Data Compression: Phonovibrogram (PVG)

A 2-s video recording at a 1:160 time-stretch ratio takes 320 s (5 min 20 s) to watch: a clinically unacceptable duration. The only way to avoid this is by compressing the data, either by reducing the video image to a single line at the time of recording (videokymography, VKG) or by image processing after recording.

The phonovibrogram (PVG) is at present the only clinically evaluated data compression technique for HSV recordings. It uses post-recording image processing, in which the movement-relevant information is extracted from the whole HS video sequence and combined in a single image. The PVG is designed to visualise motion asymmetries between left and right vocal folds.

PVG Computation

The following calculation steps are performed for every individual image (step 0) of the HSV recording:

- Step 1: The glottis is segmented.
- Step 2: Anterior and posterior commissures are defined.
- Step 3: A connecting line is drawn from the anterior to the posterior commissure, called the main glottal axis. The main glottal axis is not a morphological structure; it simply indicates the line of symmetry.
- Step 4: Left and right vocal fold are distinguished, here indicated by colour.

- Step 5: The distance between the left or right vocal fold edge and the main glottal axis is now measured along the length of the axis, with the glottal opening either to the left or right. After this measurement, the remaining components of the image are completely removed.
- Step 6: Only the following image components are kept:
  - The left free edge of the vocal fold
  - The right free edge of the vocal fold
  - The anterior commissure
  - The posterior commissure
  - The main glottal axis
- Step 7: The image is then split up along the main glottal axis. The right vocal fold remains in position, and the left vocal fold (shown on the right side of the image) is rotated 180° around the posterior commissure. The length of the vocal folds (the main glottal axis) therefore appears to be doubled, as if the anterior commissure appears twice (as A_L at the top and A_R at the bottom).
- Step 8: In order to visualise them, the distance measurements from (Step 5), which define the glottal opening, are coded into red pixels. The wider the glottal opening, the brighter red of the corresponding pixel. The result is a column of red pixels of different brightness that is twice as long as the main glottal axis for each single video frame, showing the glottal opening left/right and ranging from the 'left' anterior commissure, over the posterior commissure, to the 'right' anterior commissure. By this procedure, each image of an HSV sequence is reduced to a column of coloured pixels, each of which represents the current glottal opening separated for left and right.
- Step 9: Steps 1–8 are applied to each single frame of the HSV sequence and produce as many pixel columns as there are video frames. Placed side by side, the columns form a 2D image showing the glottal opening over time, the phonovibrogram (PVG).

The ordinate is twice the main glottal axis, and the abscissa is time. The left side of the glottis is shown above the posterior commissure (point P), and the right side is shown below it. The parallel line that meets the abscissa at point P is the axis in relation to which the symmetry must be evaluated (Eysholdt and Lohscheller 2008).

Figures 8.10, 8.11, 8.12, 8.13, 8.14, 8.15, 8.16, 8.17, and 8.18 show PVG computation steps.

Evaluation of the PVG

A normal PVG of a clinical examination is shown in Fig. 8.19. Although it can be evaluated perceptually, a machine is usually used. The first step is to separate the oscillation cycles (Fig. 8.20). The regularity of the oscillation period is calculated; it corresponds to the acoustical jitter (Fig. 8.21). Within each cycle, the following measures are quantified and averaged over 40–200 cycles:

- Amplitude
- Right-left symmetry (Fig. 8.22)
- Glottal closure (Fig. 8.23)

Apart from mucosal waves, PVGs are evaluated from the same criteria as in stroboscopy.

Many more details of the movement can be quantitatively extracted from this technique.

Advantages of PVG visualisation include:

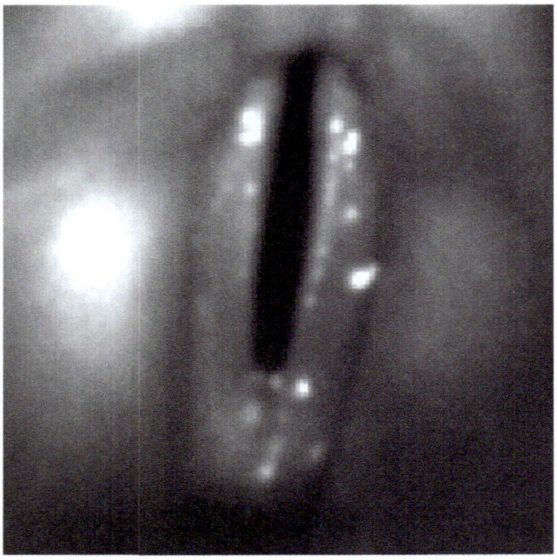

Fig. 8.10 PVG computation Step 0, the basis: Single image extracted out of a HS video sequence

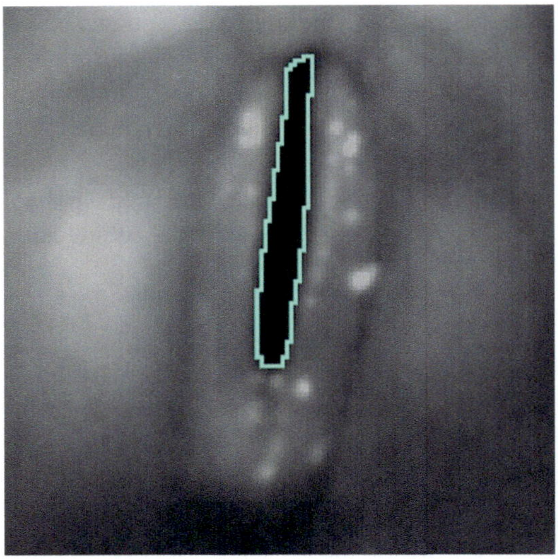

Fig. 8.11 PVG computation Steps 1 and 2: Segmentation of the glottis, i.e. detection of the vocal fold edges and anterior/posterior commissure

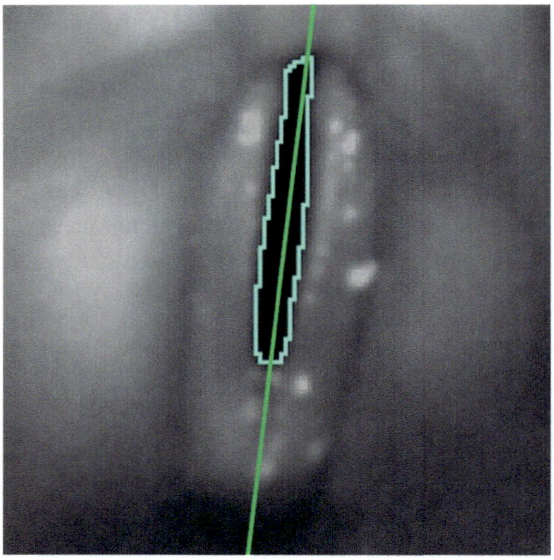

Fig. 8.12 PVG computation Step 3: Computation of the glottal midline (main axis)

- The possibility of evaluating the movement of left and right vocal folds independently.
- The speed and acceleration of each vocal fold can be measured at each position.
- The type of glottal opening and closure can be quantified.
- The symmetry of the movement can be quantified.

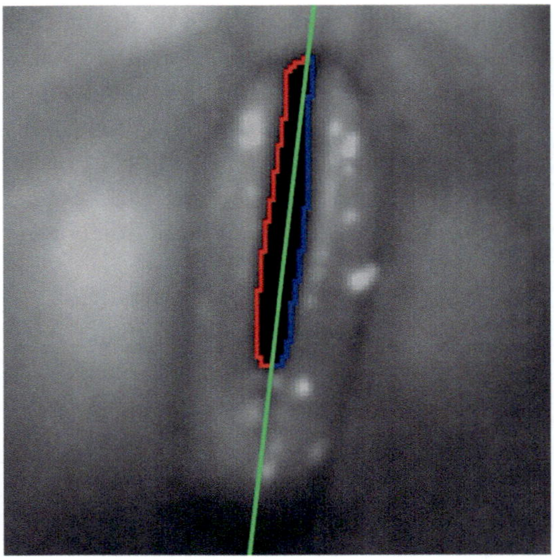

Fig. 8.13 PVG computation Step 4: Distinguishing between left and right vocal folds

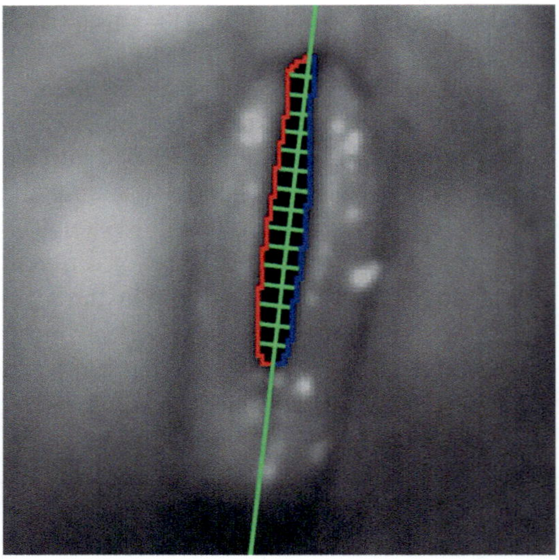

Fig. 8.14 PVG computation Step 5: Distance measurement between left/right vocal fold and glottal midline. After this, all image parts are suppressed except for the coloured structures

- The determination of irregular vibration modes (anterior-posterior).

These advantages of PVG over stroboscopy are not yet clinically used (Unger et al. 2016).

PVG is, at present, the only quantitative method of assessing vocal fold vibration. Because the

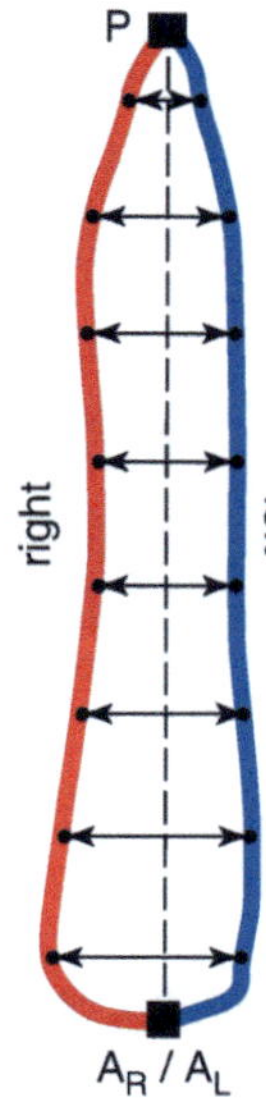

Fig. 8.15 PVG computation Step 6: Data-compressed laryngoscopic image after fading-off the non-moving parts. Components of the size-reduced image are: (1) Right vocal fold edge (red). (2) Left vocal fold edge (blue). (3) Anterior commissure A_L/A_R. (4) Posterior commissure P. (5) Glottal main axis (dashed), which is a reference line only

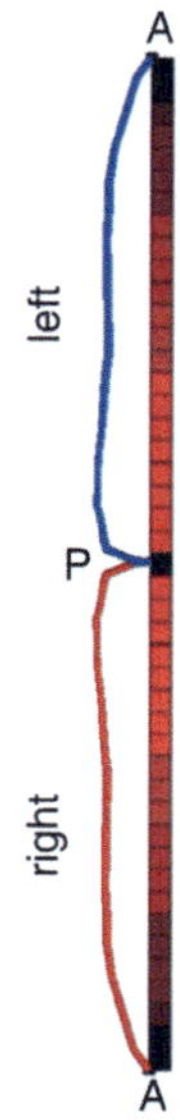

Fig. 8.17 PVG computation Step 8: the arrows from Step 7, which denote the side-dependent glottal widths, are replaced by red pixels. The wider the opening, the longer the arrow, the brighter the red pixel. All pixels together form a red vector containing the complete information about the glottal opening at the time T the image was taken

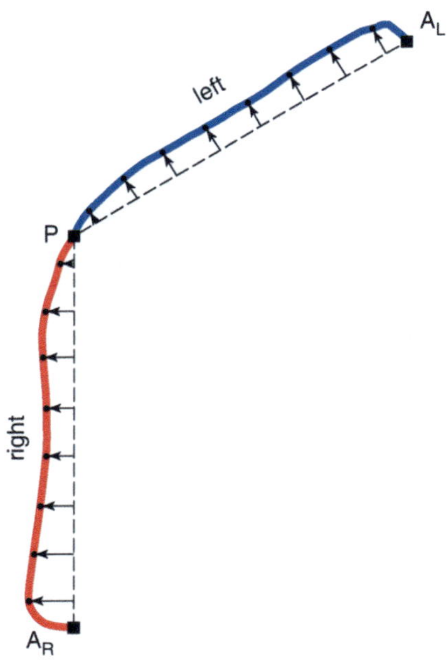

Fig. 8.16 PVG computation Step 7: the image is virtually split up along the dashed midline. The left vocal fold (blue) is rotated from the bottom up by 180° around P. Thus, the glottal length seems to be doubled, and the anterior commissure seems to appear twice (as A_L and A_R). The purpose of this visualisation procedure is to emphasise asymmetry between left and right

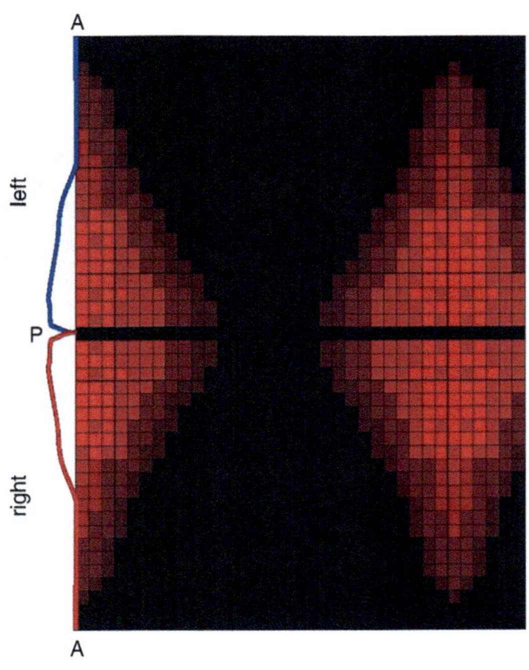

Fig. 8.18 PVG computation Step 9: Steps 1–8 are applied to each single image of the HS sequence. The resulting coloured columns are ordered side by side and form the PVG. This figure represents synthetic data, just for clarification of the image processing procedure

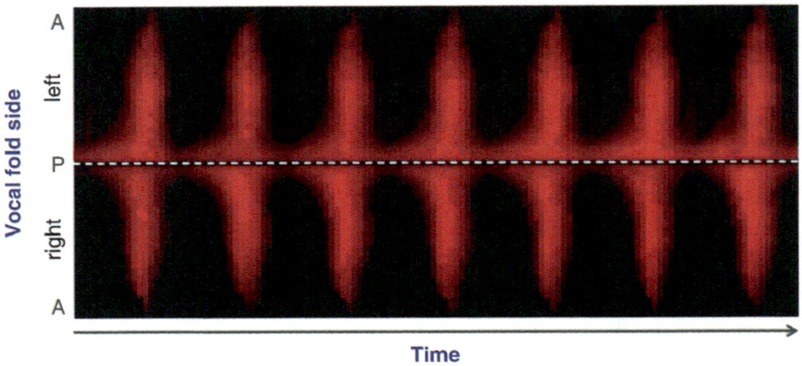

Fig. 8.19 Real PVG of a healthy patient

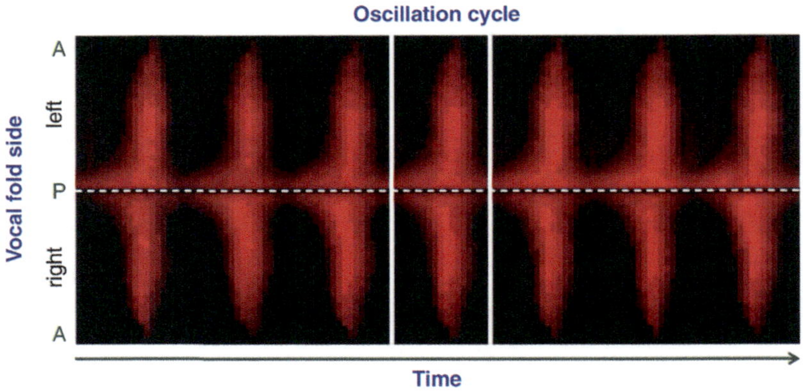

Fig. 8.20 PVG evaluation: identification of vibration cycles

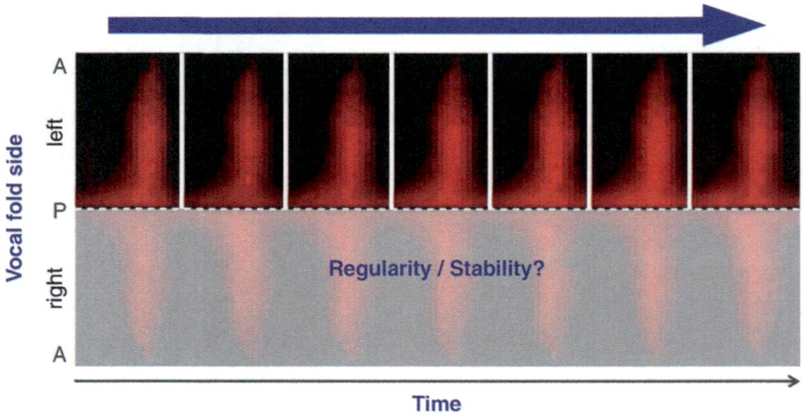

Fig. 8.21 PVG evaluation of regularity

technology is not very widespread, few people have clinical experience with PVG. The line between normal and abnormal/pathological patterns on PVG is still somewhat unclear, and it is not possible to predict the PVG pattern from the psychoacoustic impression from current models. Clinical observation so far indicates that a normal PVG is very variable and that many different PVG

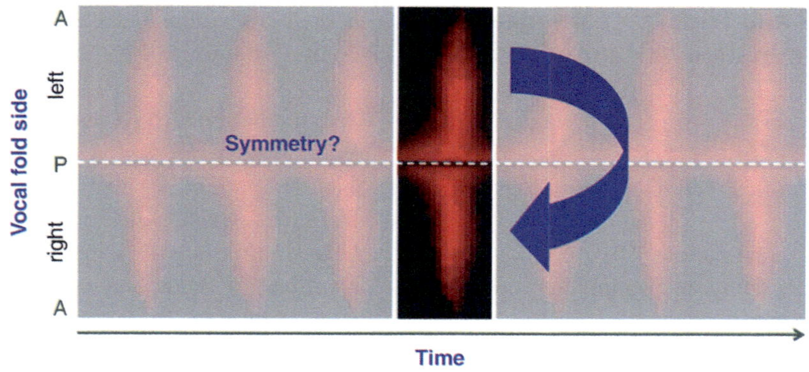

Fig. 8.22 PVG evaluation of symmetry

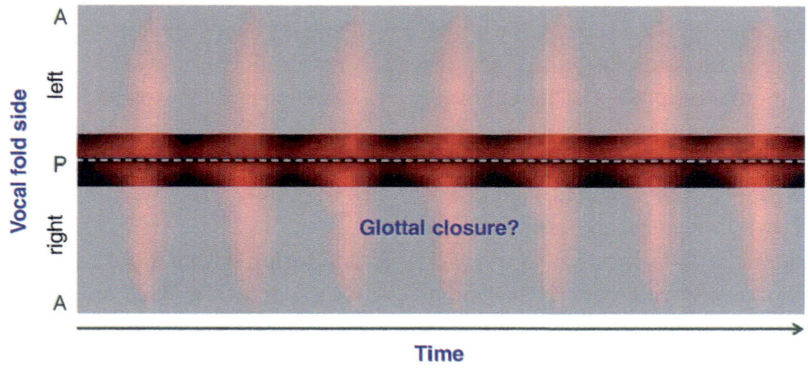

Fig. 8.23 PVG evaluation of glottal closure

patterns could result from a healthy voice. Clearly defined criteria for pathology only exist for organic voice disorders (e.g. polyps, Reinke's oedema, uni- and bilateral paresis, carcinoma, etc.), but HSV techniques are not necessary in such cases.

Asymmetrical modes of vibration are only visualisable by using PVG. These lateral differences can appear when phonatory contact at the midline between the vocal folds is too weak (right-left asymmetry, N cycles on one side over M on the other, N $\neq$ M, usually with $N = M + 1$). Anterior-posterior asymmetry (in which right and left vocal folds vibrate evenly but dorsal and ventral vocal folds have different frequencies) appears much less often. Whereas right-left asymmetry can result from various disorders, such as post-operative condition, paresis in recovery and others, anterior-posterior asymmetry belongs under the general term functional dysphonia. However, the reverse does not hold: functional dysphonia is only occasionally anterior-posterior asymmetry (Eysholdt 2014).

PVG cannot show any morphological criteria of the endolarynx. Redness resulting from inflammation, change in shape due to swelling or a tumour and change in mucosal texture: none of these can be seen on PVG. This is a consequence of the great degree of data compression and reduction, which focus only on moving areas of the vocal folds. PVG exclusively shows movement.

8.4.4 Tips and Tricks for Laryngeal Examination: A Handy Guide

Ahmed Geneid

The contents of this section comprise four parts:

- Before the examination
- Carrying out the basic examination
- Having a better view
- Other tricks

8.4.4.1 Talking with the Patient Before the Examination

In psychology, priming is an effect in which exposure to a certain stimulus influences the response to another stimulus. The exposure stimulus can be perceptual or semantic. In other words, if you start talking to the patient about the gag reflex, repeat the word and explain it too much, then you may end up getting a more frightened patient with a more sensitive gag reflex than his norm. If you start talking about how easy it is to examine the larynx and give the necessary information, then you may expect more cooperation from the patient.

Shaky hands searching for the instruments give the impression of a less experienced clinician. The reason may be that you just had too much coffee in the morning or that the examination room changed and it is your first time in the new room. However, the patient is not aware of your reasons and is just interpreting unconsciously the perceptual impression received from you.

Give the needed information, and if, for one reason or another, you have much time before the examination, then feel free to talk about voice and how stroboscopy works and shape the discussion to the cultural and educational background of the patient.

8.4.4.2 Carrying Out the Basic Examination

Positioning of the Patient

Laryngeal examination can be rendered quite simple for both the phoniatrician and the patient when the patient is positioned the right way. Adhere to the following steps and watch the video of positioning the patient:

- Ask the patients to sit with hips to the back as far as possible, with a straight back. Then ask the patient to lean the back forward from the waist with the head extended. Usually this is called the 'sniffing the air' position. In Scandinavia, where I work, I would hint that the patient take the position of a ski jumper.
- Be sure that patient's shoulders are down and relaxed. The more the patient raises them, the less space you will have inside the throat.
- Patient's hands are best resting on knees. Legs uncrossed.
- Remember that a patient's retraction of the head will limit your vision of the vocal folds. Reposition the patient's head to have a better view.

Examination with a Rigid Laryngoscope

After the patient is positioned, I usually opt for what I call a 'dry training', in which I ask the patient to protrude his tongue; I support it gently and ask the patient to have a sustained /ee:/ (as in 'see'). This dry training is done first without the laryngoscope. The idea is to teach the right position to the patient and ease fears about the examination. After this dry training, I start with positioning the rigid laryngoscope. My aim is not to touch the structures from the base of the tongue and backwards. If the patient has a quite sensitive gag reflex, then I would introduce the rigid laryngoscope while the patient is phonating, and then I ask the patient to breathe while the endoscope is there. The sound /ee:/ (as in 'see') is best taught to before the examination. During the examination, it is common that the patient is not able to produce it, so instruct him to think about it while phonating; this will get you the area of vision needed. Spray anaesthesia should be used if the gag reflex hinders the examination. Especially for stroboscopy, it can prevent the muscular hypertension that may influence the vibratory pattern, but on the other hand, the tactile-kinaesthetic feedback may be influenced too.

Examination with a Flexible Endoscope

Many patients tolerate the flexible endoscope better than the rigid. However, some cannot stand the idea of something going through their nose. Positioning of the patient is important here as well but without the need for a full 'sniffing the air' position.

I usually tend to use anaesthesia coupled with decongestant on a cotton probe rather than spraying Xylocaine, which causes more irritation. Choose the nostril side that is better anatomically and apply the anaesthesia and decongestant in the middle meatus of the nasal cavity if you would also like to assess the velopharyngeal port, otherwise you may find it enough to go through the lower meatus. Lidocaine jelly can also be used, taking care to apply it a few millimetres to the back from the scope lens to avoid disturbing the visualisation.

Hold the fibrescope in line with the nostril with your hands holding it below the level of the nose.

In functional endoscopic evaluation of swallowing, I prefer to carry it out without anaesthesia and also through the middle meatus. A decongestant can be applied. The idea is to avoid the anaesthetic leaking to the larynx and distorting the results of the examination. Another option is to apply a small amount of anaesthesia with a cotton probe to the front part of middle meatus.

- Using the middle meatus enables the examination of the velum much better than if you have the fibrescope on the floor of the nasal cavity.

Positioning of Observers

- In many cases there are people other than you and the patient in the examination room. They can be a nurse, spouse of the patient, students or other observers visiting your clinic. It is best if they are standing either behind the patient or in his blind spot. The patient may get quite distracted or even frightened by the reactions on the faces of the observers.

8.4.4.3 Having a Better View

Examining the Piriform Fossa

This can be done easily by blowing out the cheeks with the mouth closed. It is easier to perform with flexible nasofibrescopy. It also works well with the rigid laryngoscope and the patient rounding his lips around the laryngoscope and blowing his cheeks out.

Examining the Vocal Folds Closely Above and Below

Getting the endoscope quite close to the upper side of vocal folds during intermittent phonation can initiate the gag reflex, especially on touching the epiglottis or aryepiglottic folds. One way to avoid this is to move the endoscope down to the vocal fold level while the patient sustains phonation.

For certain patients, especially those with possible changes on the lower side of the vocal folds, you may want to get a closer look of the lower side of the vocal folds. Usually, it is quite tricky trying to get the scope down through the glottis without touching the vocal folds and starting a marked coughing episode. A nice trick for that deals with our innate reflex associated with inspiration, in other words the forced opening of the glottis during inspiration. Such forced opening is usually lengthened in duration with inspiration through only one nostril. Accordingly, with the flexible scope in one nostril, ask the patient to breathe in through the other while the mouth is closed. Apply a little pressure to close the nostril housing the flexible fibrescope. The result should be a long inspiration from the other nostril with sufficient opening of the glottis. This will give you the time to dip the tip of your fibrescope just below the vocal fold. Examine one vocal fold lower side at a time.

Visual Examination of the Valleculae and the Base of the Tongue

Visualising the valleculae and the base of the tongue with the rigid laryngoscope can be troublesome for a junior phoniatrician or laryngologist. It may give the feeling that the tongue base papillae and lingual tonsillar tissues are hypertrophied when they are not. palpation and the use of a laryngeal mirror should be performed when in doubt. It may add a few minutes to the examination time but will save unneeded consultations.

During flexible laryngoscopy, it is easy to get a better visualisation of this region by asking the patient to protrude the tongue.

Examining the Vertical Position of the Vocal Folds When Suspecting Superior Laryngeal Nerve Injury

A suspicion of superior laryngeal injury entails the need to examine the position of the vocal folds if they happen to be at different heights. Sometimes this can be easily detected if the difference is marked with one vocal fold hanging above the other. However, in many situations the difference in position may be quite small, and the monocular vision offered by the laryngoscope does not help in seeing it. In order to gain a binocular vision, you need to use both of your eyes. This can be done by using an otolaryngologic microscope and a laryngeal mirror. Focal distance should be changed to 35 cm from 20 cm, which is usually used for the ear.

8.4.4.4 Other Tricks

Stroboscope Is Not Available or Not Working

Stroboscopy or high-speed stroboscopy should always be used when carrying out laryngoscopic examination. However, if for one reason or another you do not have such possibility, then the vocal fold edge can be inspected while the vocal folds are abducted during respiration. This will enable you to assess with a sharp image the edge lesions that are usually blurred in phonation.

No Laryngoscope Available

Needless to say, you should really consider the administrative reason that left you, a phoniatrician, without your main tool. However, saving the day is possible. A nasal endoscope of 70° can be used for laryngeal examination; just remember to turn it upside down. The picture you get will be quite small in comparison with that from a laryngoscope. A laryngeal mirror combined with a microscope is also a good option and will enhance your experience in using such a demanding technique.

Working with Diplophonia and Triggering Problems

Stroboscopy is based on getting a stable audio signal from the patient. Irregularity of the signal will fail to trigger a regular series of light flashes, resulting in an inability to see to the vocal fold vibrations.

In cases of diplophonia, one good way of getting over this problem is to focus on one vocal fold at a time and search for the right frequency at which stroboscopy will work. This can be helped by asking the patient to phonate /ee:/ (as in 'see') at different frequencies following your examples. If this does not work, then one more trick that I use quite rarely is to have the stroboscope microphone attached to my neck rather than the patient's. By searching for the right frequency, you will get a better visualisation of the patient's vocal folds during vibration. You may end up seeing only one or two sustained phases of the vibration showing up a standstill pictures.

If the voice is relatively unstable, as it can be in cases of non-organic dysphonia, then ask the patient to phonate with closed lips. The result is elongation of the vocal tract by addition of the nasal cavities resulting in a more stabilised phonation.

Rigid Laryngoscopy and Fibrescopy for Children

Rigid laryngoscopy can work very well for children. The youngest I had was 3 years old. Refrain from using anaesthesia. Rigid laryngoscopy for children can be easier and more easily administered than nasofibrescopy, which requires more cooperation from the child.

Fibrescopy requires more preparation than rigid endoscopy. Use adrenaline or other constricting agents on a cotton bud to ensure more space for the fibrescope. I usually refrain from using Xylocaine spray owing to its irritating effect. The paediatric fibrescope has quite a small diameter that significantly limits the size of the obtained picture. However, it is better tolerated by small children. Requiring a paediatric fibrescope to drop from the middle to the lower meatus suggests that using an adult fibrescope is a better option. Adult fibrescopes can be used with children older than 5 years. Giving a lollipop to children is an excellent idea during fibrescopic examination. Its function in the examination is to make sure that the child is happily breathing through the nose resulting in opening of the velopharyngeal valve. Accordingly, the way will be open for the fibrescope from the nasal cavity downwards.

Acknowledgements Ideas mentioned in this article are the summation of what I have learned from colleagues or personally developed. The list of these colleagues is quite long. However, I am indebted to Nasser Kotby from Egypt, Per-Åke Lindestad from Sweden and Erkki Vilkman, Mari Markkanen-Leppänen, Teemu Kinnari and Maaria Ansaranta from Finland.

8.4.5 Videokymography

František Šram, Jan G. Švec, and Jitka Vydrová

8.4.5.1 Introduction: Videokymography (VKG) and Kymographic Techniques

The technique of videokymography (VKG) was developed as a low-cost, clinician-friendly version of laryngoscopic high-speed video (HSV) systems (Švec and Schutte 1996). It allows correct display of the patterns of vocal fold vibrations that cannot be properly visualised by stroboscopy (such as irregularities and instabilities, including severe hoarseness and register transitions). In contrast to the full HSV system, videokymography does not record the full images of the larynx but records only images from a single selected line at a high rate (currently 7200 line images per second). This reduces the amount of recorded data and makes the technique faster and less demanding on the recording and storage equipment than the full HSV. The VKG examination line can be placed at any location of the vocal folds. When captured, the line images are placed sequentially to form a new 'kymographic' image ('videokymogram', or in short 'kymogram') that displays the behaviour of the vocal folds at the specific selected location in real time.

The current generation videokymography (Qiu and Schutte 2006) utilises a special video camera (i.e. videokymographic camera) providing the kymographic images in real time, simultaneously and side by side with the standard laryngoscopic images of the vocal folds (Fig. 8.24). The immediate availability of the images makes the VKG method suitable for use in busy clinical practice, and it also distinguishes VKG from other HSV systems that can visualise or process the images only after the recording has taken place.

Apart from videokymography, which is based on a special video camera (hardware), the principle of kymographic imaging has also been applied to obtaining kymographic images from full high-speed videolaryngoscopic (*digital kymography*, DKG (Wittenberg et al. 2000)) and strobovideoscopic recordings (*strobo-videokymography*, SVKG (Isogai 1994, Sung et al. 1999)). In contrast to VKG, which displays the kymographic images immediately during the examination, the two latter methods employ special software to construct the kymograms from previously obtained high-speed laryngoscopic or videostroboscopic recordings. The advantages and disadvantages of these three kymographic methods are discussed by Švec and Schutte (2012).

In contrast to classical laryngoscopy, which aims at observing and evaluating the *structural appearance* of the vocal folds and of the laryngeal structures, kymography aims at observing and evaluating the *vibratory function* of the vocal folds and of the surrounding tissues. In this sense, the method aims at diagnosing the vibrational, rather than the structural, problems of the laryngeal tissues. Since voice is produced through vibration of laryngeal tissues, it provides a more detailed insight into the mechanism of voice disorders. *The method is especially useful for discovering vibrational problems in functional dysphonias where the vocal folds do not show any obvious structural abnormality, but the voice is impaired in some way.* The vibrational disorder problems reveal pathophysiological alterations of the vocal folds and surrounding tissues that are difficult to discover otherwise.

8.4.5.2 VKG Equipment and Examination Procedure

The basic equipment for videokymographic examination consists of (1) *a special videokymographic camera*, (2) *a laryngoscope*, (3) *a continuous light source of high intensity* (300 W xenon light is preferable), (4) *a standard video-*

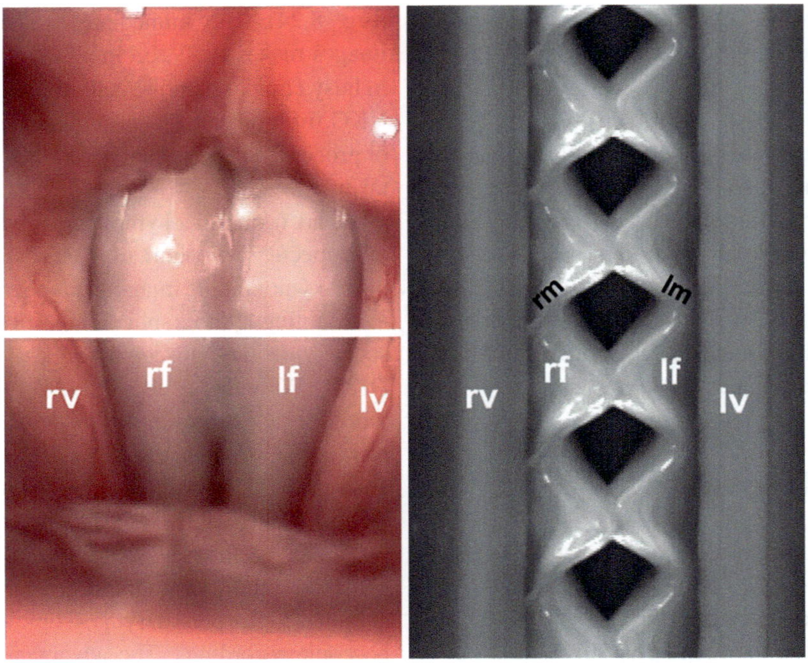

Fig. 8.24 The standard laryngoscopic (left) and VKG (right) images, which are delivered simultaneously by the second-generation VKG camera. The VKG image shows the normal behaviour of the vocal folds in time (40 ms duration, time running from top to bottom) at the location marked by the line in the standard image. The examined subject was a 43-year-old male without voice problems. Symbols used: *rf/lf* right/left vocal fold; *rv/lv* right/left ventricular fold; *rm/lm* right/left laterally travelling mucosal wave

capturing system (computer or a video recorder), (5) *a video monitor* and (6) *a microphone* for capturing the voice signal (Fig. 8.25).

Generally, the examination procedure in videokymography is similar to the video-laryngostroboscopic procedure. The difference is that the clinician should make sure that during the examination procedure, the measurement line for VKG images is placed at the desirable location on the vocal folds, perpendicular to the glottal axis. Useful tips and tricks on the VKG examination procedure can be found in the publication of Švec and Šram (2011).

8.4.5.3 Normal VKG Findings

Sustained phonations at a comfortable pitch and loudness (measures to be documented for later comparisons) should ideally present the following properties, which are well visible in the videokymographic images of the vocal folds (recall Fig. 8.24):

- Both vocal folds are vibrating.
- Ventricular folds are not vibrating.
- Vibrational amplitudes of both vocal folds are approximately similar.
- Vibrational frequencies of both vocal folds are approximately the same.
- The vibrations are regular.
- The vibrations are free of aberrations.
- The vocal folds touch each other during vibration at the place of maximum vibration amplitude.
- The closed phase takes from ca. 5 to 65% of period duration at the place of maximum vibration amplitude.
- The shape of lateral peaks (i.e. the turn from opening to closing) is sharp.
- Mucosal waves propagate laterally on the upper vocal fold surface.
- No large left-right phase asymmetry is present.

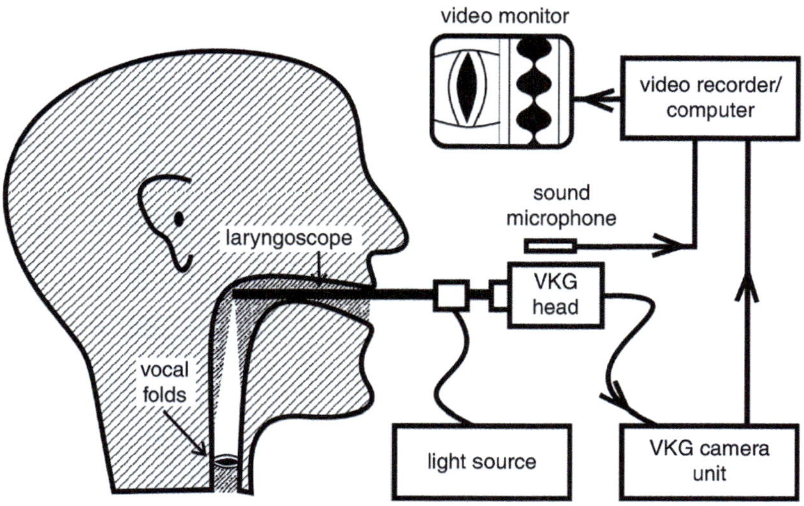

Fig. 8.25 The equipment setup for videokymography

The vocal fold vibrations vary when changing fundamental frequency (Fig. 8.26), loudness (Fig. 8.27) as well as vocal register (Fig. 8.28), so care should be taken to take these factors into account.

8.4.5.4 VKG Features in Voice Disorders

Alternations of vibratory features seen in VKG allow different types of vibrational disorders of the larynx to be distinguished (Fig. 8.29). The features and their possible causes are described in detail by Švec et al. (2007, 2009). Some of these are:

- *Completely Absent Vibration of the Vocal Fold* (Fig. 8.29a, rf)—a very serious finding, which can result from a tumour, scar or excessive vocal fold stiffness.
- *Partly Absent Vibration of the Vocal Fold*—can be observed, e.g. when the body of the vocal fold is stiff or in case of a dislocated vocal fold implant.
- *Absence of Glottal Closure* (Fig. 8.29b)—when observed at the place of maximum vibration amplitude at comfortable pitch and loudness, this indicates serious problems with vocal fold adduction. It is typical of voices with strong breathiness. It is a physiological finding in high-pitched or in intentionally breathy voices.
- *Large Cycle-to-Cycle Variability* (Fig. 8.29b, c)—is typical of largely irregular voices and can result, e.g. from left-right vocal fold asymmetry, from anterior-posterior vocal fold asymmetry or from excessively low vocal fold tension.
- *Large Left-Right Amplitude Differences*—indicate large structural differences between the left and right vocal folds. These can result from unilateral laryngeal pathological conditions, such as from, e.g. unilateral vocal fold paralysis.
- *Left-Right Frequency Differences* (Fig. 8.29b)—are mainly observed in subjects with different tension of the left and right vocal folds and lack of glottal closure. They occur most often because of unilateral vocal fold paralysis. The finding usually relates to biphonia or diplophonia.
- *Large Left-Right Phase Differences* (Fig. 8.29d)—are a sign of left-right asymmetry in tension or mass of the vocal folds. This finding can often be observed, e.g. in subjects with unilateral vocal fold paralysis with good glottal closure (i.e. after medialisation surgery) but may also be found in singers complaining of voice problems. Perceptually the voice may sound rather normal, but the asymmetry may limit the usable frequency range.

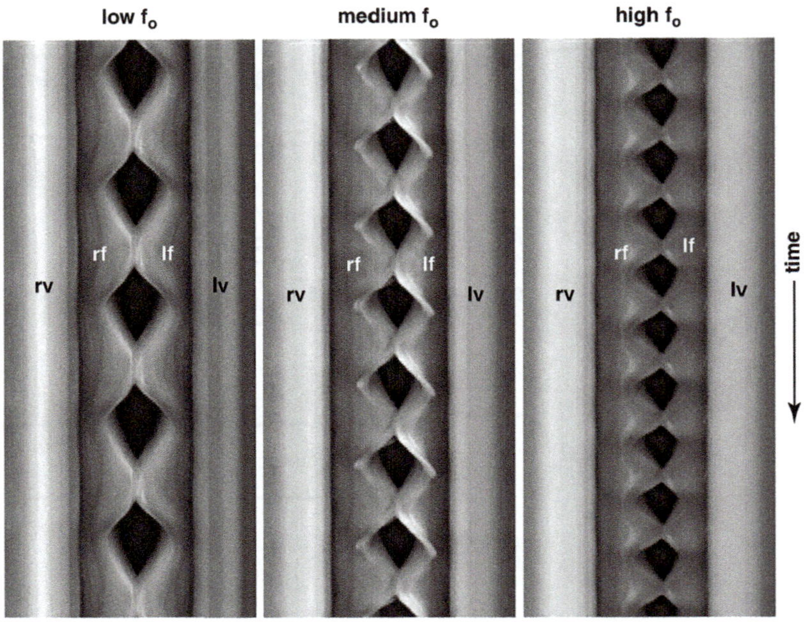

Fig. 8.26 The changes in vocal fold vibration due to increasing fundamental frequency (f_0) in a healthy male subject. Notice the increasing number of periods within the image (from left to right c. 5, 7¼ and 10 cycles, corresponding to the fundamental frequencies of c. 125, 181 and 250 Hz) and the decreasing amplitudes of vibration. The kymograms were obtained at the line perpendicular to glottal axis, in the middle of the membranous glottis. Total time displayed: 40 ms. For abbreviations see legend to Fig. 8.24

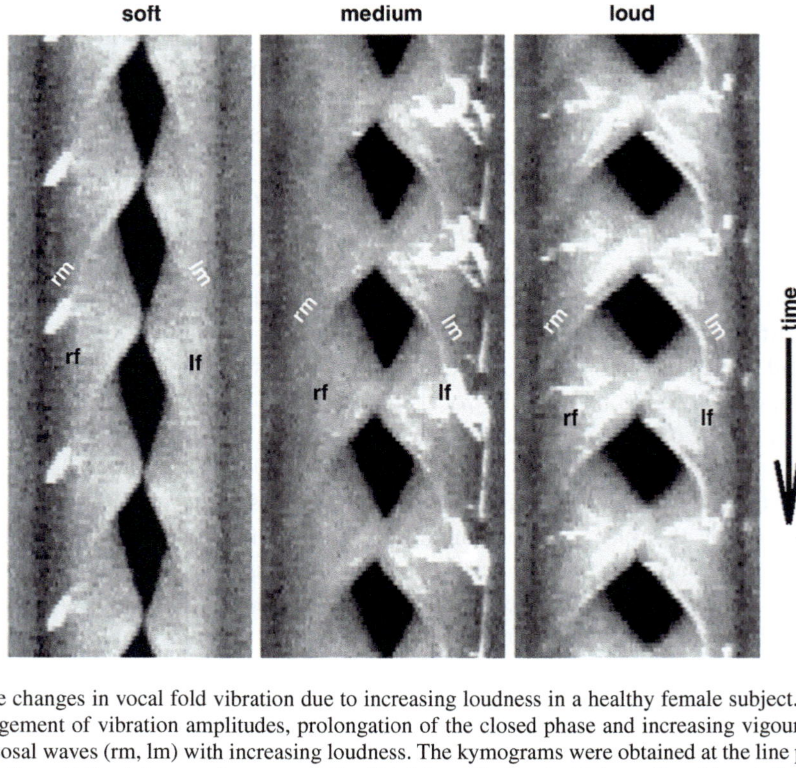

Fig. 8.27 The changes in vocal fold vibration due to increasing loudness in a healthy female subject. Notice particularly the enlargement of vibration amplitudes, prolongation of the closed phase and increasing vigour of the laterally travelling mucosal waves (rm, lm) with increasing loudness. The kymograms were obtained at the line perpendicular to glottal axis, in the middle of the membranous glottis. Total time displayed: 18.4 ms. For abbreviations see legend to Fig. 8.24

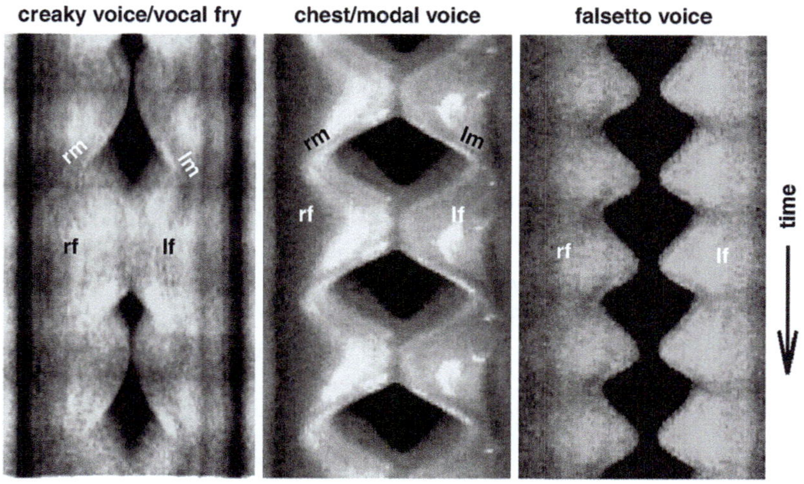

Fig. 8.28 The vocal fold vibration in different voice registers in a healthy male subject. Creaky voice/vocal fry register shows repetition of two different openings and smaller vibration amplitudes than in the typical pattern of the chest/modal register. The falsetto voice reveals no glottal closure, less sharp lateral peaks and reduced mucosal waves. In all the cases, the vibrations are left-right symmetric. The kymograms were obtained at the line perpendicular to glottal axis, in the middle of the membranous glottis. Total time displayed: 18.4 ms. For abbreviations see legend to Fig. 8.24

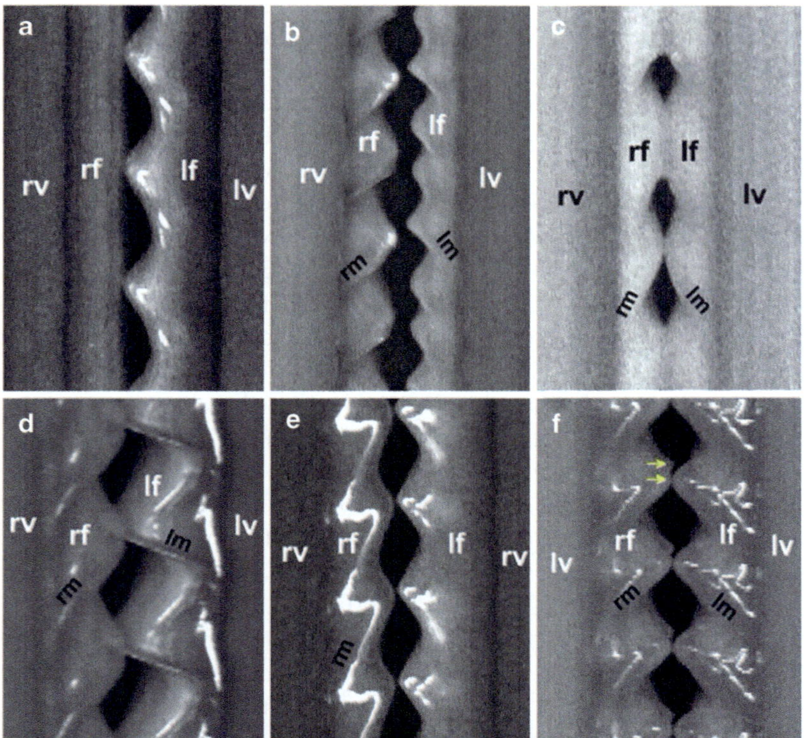

Fig. 8.29 Different types of vibration disorder of the vocal folds revealed in VKG images. Total time displayed in the VKG images: 18.4 ms (from top to bottom). (**a–f**) See the text. For abbreviations see legend to Fig. 8.24

- *Axis Shift During Closure* (Fig. 8.29d)—indicates left-right asymmetry in vocal fold tension or difference in level of the vocal folds.
- *Decreased Sharpness of Lateral Peaks* (Fig. 8.29a lf, Fig. 8.29e, rf)—indicates reduced vertical phase differences of the vocal folds, which may result from an excessively stiff mucosa on its medial surface.
- *Absent or Reduced Mucosal Waves on the Upper Vocal Fold Surface* (Fig. 8.29a, lf, Fig. 8.29e, lf)—indicate that the mucosa is excessively stiff on the upper vocal fold surface.
- *Sharpened Medial Peaks* (Fig. 8.29e, lf)—indicate a thinned edge of the vocal fold. It is observable when glottal closure is absent.
- *Ripple (Aberration)*—this is frequently observed anteriorly to a localised lesion on the vocal fold (nodule, polyp, cyst) when the lesion interferes with the vibrations.
- *Double Medial Peak (Aberration)* (Fig. 8.29f, rf-double arrow)—most often indicates the presence of a sulcus or furrow on the medial vocal fold surface.
- *Lack of Smoothness of Medial Peaks (Aberration)*—indicates defective medial vocal fold shape.
- *Large Vibration of Surrounding Tissues (e.g. Ventricular Folds or Aryepiglottic Folds)*—may be found in larynges exhibiting hyperfunction or compensating for glottal insufficiency. Sometimes it can be used voluntarily for special voice effects, e.g. in rock singing (Borch et al. 2004; Lindestad et al. 2001).

Co-vibration of Fluids—is a sign of too much fluid or mucus interfering with the vocal fold vibrations and causing slight irregularities of voice. This may be a result of laryngeal inflammation.

8.4.5.5 Clinical Examples

Case Study 8.1

A 63-year-old male suffering from dysphonia that arose after a cold and lasted for 4 months. He was a smoker (20 cigarettes daily).

VKG examination: Complete absence of vibration of the left vocal fold was revealed (Fig. 8.30, arrow).

Diagnosis: This raised a suspicion of tumorous infiltration of the left vocal fold. Laryngoscopy and histological exam revealed squamous cell carcinoma.

Therapy: Left-sided cordectomy.

Result: The patient comes for regular check-ups; currently he is in the fourth year without problems.

Case Study 8.2

A 52-year-old female, professional singer, member of the choir of the Prague Philharmonic Orchestra. Her original diagnosis was breast carcinoma for which she underwent complex therapy 2 years ago—breast ablation, radiotherapy and chemotherapy. Since then she had been on hormonal antioestrogenic medication (Arimidex). After the end of the therapy, she returned to the professional career of a choir singer. During the last 6 months, she experienced voice problems interfering seriously with her career—reduction of voice range, voice instabilities and hoarseness.

VKG examination (Fig. 8.31): Laryngoscopic view revealed slight structural unevenness of the posterior third of the right vocal fold. VKG view showed four abnormal vibrational characteristics revealing an impairment of vocal fold functioning: (1) large left-right phase asymmetry indicating different tensions of the two vocal folds; (2) axis shift during glottal closure, again indicating different tensions of the two vocal folds; (3) reduced sharpness of the right lateral peak indicating increased stiffness of the right vocal fold mucosa on the medial surface; and (4) reduced laterally travelling mucosal waves on the right vocal fold indicating increased stiffness of the mucosa of the right upper vocal fold surface.

Diagnosis: Chronic laryngitis with serious stiffening and potential scarification on the right vocal fold mucosa, most likely due to laryngopharyngeal reflux. Reflux episodes penetrating upper oesophageal sphincter were verified by using combined multichannel intraluminal impedance and pH monitoring (MIi-pH).

Therapy: PPI medications, reduced voice usage, work inability.

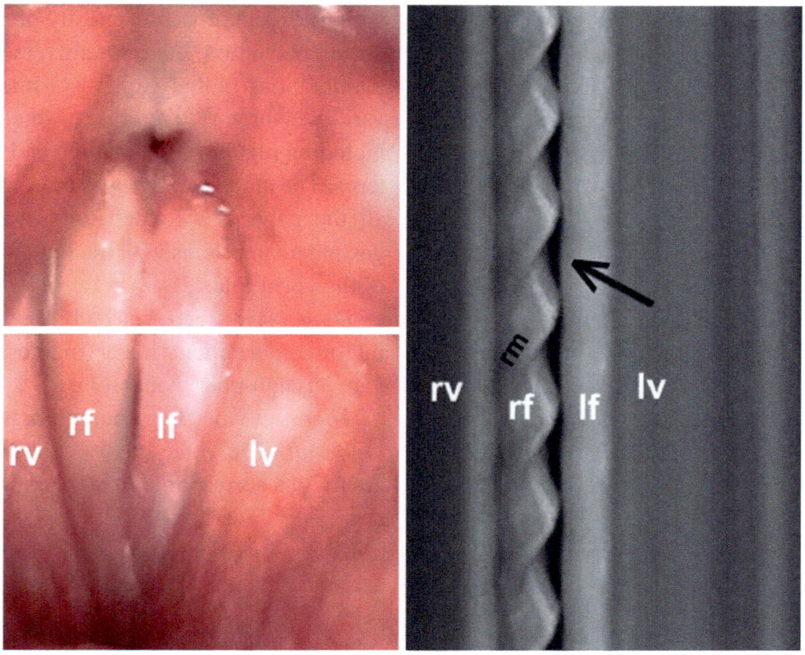

Fig. 8.30 VKG examination images of a subject with left vocal fold carcinoma. The left vocal fold shows complete absence of vibrations (arrow), while the right vocal fold shows normal vibratory behaviour. Total time displayed in the VKG image: 40 ms (from top to bottom). For abbreviations see legend to Fig. 8.24

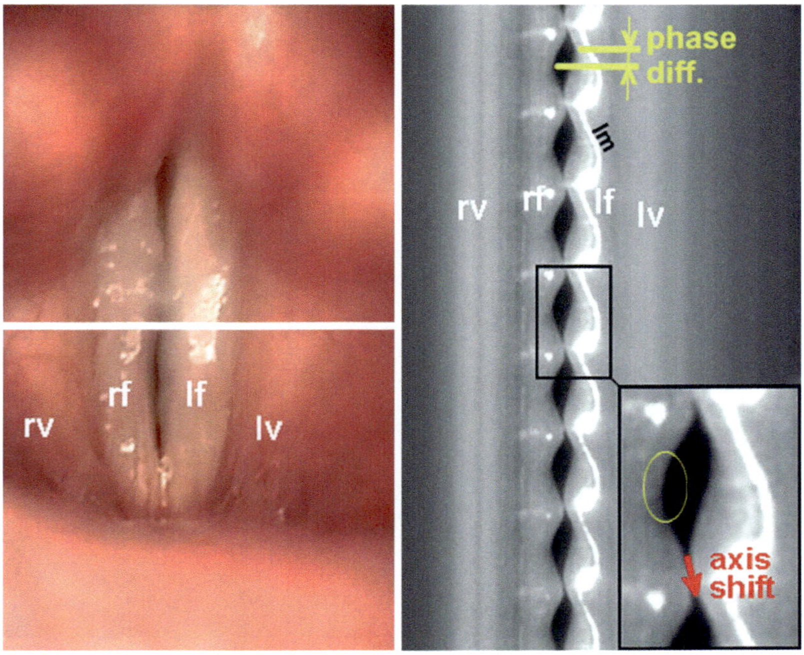

Fig. 8.31 VKG examination images of a female professional singer with decreased mucosal pliability of the right vocal fold. Notice (1) the left-right phase differences of the lateral peaks, (2) axis shift during glottal closure, (3) the markedly more rounded lateral peak on the right vocal fold (yellow ellipse) than on the left one and (4) hardly any presence of laterally travelling mucosal waves on the right vocal fold, whereas these are clearly present on the left one (lm). Total time displayed in the VKG image: 40 ms (from top to bottom). For abbreviations see legend to Fig. 8.24

Result: Presently the patient requests a disability pension. It is probable that the voice problems are partly related to stress from the primary carcinoma diagnosis. There is also a likely relationship to the Arimidex antioestrogen therapy, which is, however, unavoidable in the case of breast carcinoma.

Case Study 8.3

A 72-year-old male, retired accountant. The voice was husky, produced with an incorrect technique, usually pressed with breathiness, exhibiting poorly controlled changes in pitch and loudness.

VKG examination (Fig. 8.32): Laryngoscopic images showed rather normal-looking vocal folds with the vocal processes mostly pressed together during phonation. Intermittently, there was linear membranous glottal gap. VKG images revealed various vibratory patterns of the vocal folds, including regular, subharmonic and irregular patterns. The mucosal wave was present. Noticeably, all the patterns were left-right symmetric suggesting no problems with the left-right imbalance of the vocal folds.

Diagnosis: Aged voice, bilateral paresis m. interni, intermittent linear membranous glottal gap, laryngo-pharyngeal reflux.

Therapy: Voice hygiene, reflux treatment.

Result: The voice quality and the vibrational alterations correspond to the age of the patient.

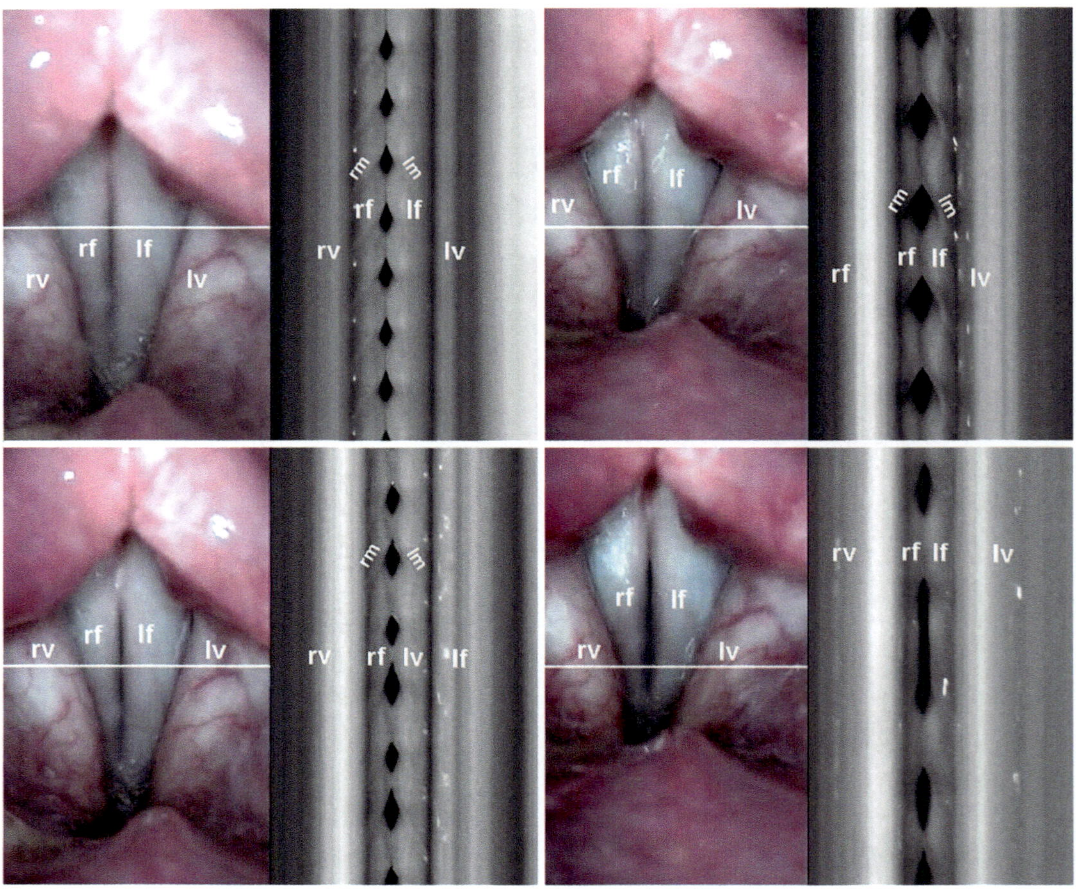

Fig. 8.32 Four VKG examination images of a male subject with an aged voice. Notice the variability of the vibration pattern of the vocal folds. Top: regular voice at higher (right) and lower (left) pitch. Bottom: dicrotic vocal fold vibration showing repetition of two glottal openings of different shapes at higher vocal fold tension (left) and irregular vocal fold vibration at lower vocal fold tension (right). Total time displayed in the VKG image: 40 ms (from top to bottom). For abbreviations see legend to Fig. 8.24

8.4.5.6 Summary

Videokymography is an optical laryngoscopic examination method that is mainly aimed at diagnosing vibration disorders of the vocal folds. These are the basic cause of voice disorders. A special videokymographic camera is used to capture the standard laryngoscopic video images simultaneously with the high-speed kymographic images showing the vibratory pattern of the vocal folds at a selected location. This also allows diagnosis of small alterations of the vocal fold vibrations. These alterations could result from inflammatory as well as from tumorous infiltration of the vocal fold tissues. Furthermore, it allows diagnosis of vocal fold mucosa impairments, small scars, submucosal blood vessel dilations and vocal fold oedema of allergic or hormonal origins. Visual clinical evaluation of the videokymographic pattern requires knowledge of the normal vocal fold vibratory pattern and of the correlation between the pattern alterations and the pathophysiology of the vocal fold tissue disorders. The method is very useful for early diagnosis of vocal fold cancer. It allows recognition of tissue pathology at the stages when the laryngoscopic or laryngostroboscopic images still look normal.

8.4.6 Stroboscopic and Kymographic Examinations of Lip Vibrations in Brass Musicians

Renate Haubrich and Wolfgang Angerstein

8.4.6.1 Introduction

Lip vibrations in brass musicians can be investigated and video-documented by stroboscopy and kymography. These non-invasive imaging techniques are relevant within the practice of musicians medicine for assessing the occupational (in) capacity of professional brass musicians. Helmholtz (1875) stated:

> Only two kinds of membranous tongues have to be considered as musical instruments: the human lips in brass instruments, and the human larynx in singing.

Sounds can be produced by vibration of the mucosal or muscular layers of the vocal folds. This is also true for the lips: the anatomical requirement for sound generation is the multilayered construction of both tone generators. In the larynx, the mucous membrane is connected to the vocal ligament and vocal muscle via a thin layer of connective tissue (Reinke's space). This multilayered construction of the vocal folds is also referred to as the 'body-cover model' (Hirano 1974; Story and Titze 1995). A similar multilayered construction also exists in the lips (internally to externally: the mucosa, submucosa with glands, orbicularis oris muscle, subcutis and epidermis) (Tillmann 1997; Paulsen 2010; Welsch 2006).

Phoniatricians have used imaging methods to examine high-frequency vibrations of the vocal folds for many decades (stroboscopy, Schönhärl 1960; Luchsinger 1949; Oertel 1878, 1895; Böhme and Gross 2001; kymography, Böhme and Gross 2001; Šram et al. 1998; Gall et al. 1971; Gross 1985). Therefore it is obviously justified to employ stroboscopy and kymography when lip vibrations of brass musicians are examined. Martin (1942) developed a method by which lip vibrations of a French horn player could be investigated stroboscopically. Damsté (1966) compared the vibrations of a singer's vocal folds to the vibrations of the lips of a trombonist. Kymographic studies of a trombonist's lip vibrations were described by Šram and Švec (2000).

8.4.6.2 Occupation-Specific Diseases

> *Embouchure* is the word that wind instrumentalists use to describe the way the mouth is held during performance. It is derived from the French *bouche*, meaning mouth. The definition of embouchure normally refers to the lips and facial muscles, but the teeth and jaw are integral to its function and the embouchure could not function without them.
> Campos (2005)

When this complex interaction of various muscle groups gets out of control, embouchure problems result: the physician Flesch (1925) reported on a trumpeter with

> convulsions in the orbicularis oris. The patient could not blow a tone.

Similar difficulties of the lower lip were described by the neurologist Singer (1926):

> The lower lip of a trumpeter slid off the mouthpiece 'as if paralysed'. Tones of a certain pitch could not be blown anymore (…). But there was no pain involved, only the feeling of a heavy 'chunk' in the mouth (cheek), the outblown airjet seemed to flee between the upper lip and the mouthpiece.

These painless disease patterns are nowadays called 'embouchure dystonia'. In early stages, the disease manifests as a:

> subtle deficiency of sound production, mainly in a certain register, a certain style or a clearly defined dynamic range.
> Altenmüller and Jabusch (2008)

Later the disease expands to the whole ambitus and all dynamic ranges of the instrument. Then, control over the embouchure, articulation and breathing cannot be ensured for any kind of playing technique. Quite likely the sound will break off, and side tones will appear. Air leaks can occur besides the mouthpiece; brass players may have spasms or tremor of the involved musculature (Altenmüller and Jabusch 2008). Furthermore, tremor of the lips, involuntary closure of the lips ('liplock') and locking of the jaw can be experienced in embouchure dystonia (Frucht et al. 2001; Frucht 2009). The Meige syndrome in brass players is a combination of embouchure dystonia with blepharospasm (Frucht et al. 2001; Frucht 2009).

Even a rupture of the orbicularis oris muscle is possible when the lips are tensed excessively (especially when playing very high pitches) (Arcier and Vernay 1994; Papsin et al. 1996; Donnet et al. 1996; Planas 1982, 1988; Maneiro 2014). A prominent patient who suffered from rupture of the lip musculature was Louis Armstrong. 'Satchmo's syndrome' (Planas 1982) is characterised by fatigability of the lip musculature and the inability to produce high pitches, often accompanied by pain (Papsin et al. 1996; Donnet et al. 1996; Maneiro 2014; Liu and Hayden 2002). An injury of the orbicularis oris muscle can force the brass musician to stop playing temporarily or may result in a permanent occupational incapacity, with serious economic consequences (Maneiro 2014). In the literature an operative reconstruction of the orbicularis oris muscle is highly recommended (Papsin et al. 1996; Planas 1982, 1988; Sullivan 1989).

Functional diseases (embouchure dystonia (Altenmüller and Jabusch 2006a)) as well as organic lesions of the lips (soft tissue wounds (Bumiller 1936), pressure-induced neuropathy (Zeller 1985; Loock and Lorenz 1981; Schuppert and Altenmüller 2000) and Satchmo's syndrome (Arcier and Vernay 1994; Planas 1982, 1988; Maneiro 2014)) can lead to an incapacity for work in brass players. Landeck (1974) reported that in the vast majority of brass players with chronic lesions of the lip, an early retirement or an occupational retraining is inevitable.

Thirteen per cent of German orchestra musicians have to give up their profession for health reasons (Böckelmann and Schneyer 2009), about 1% of professional musicians suffer from occupation-specific dystonia (musicians dystonia) (Altenmüller and Jabusch 2006b; Rozanski et al. 2015). Damage of the lip nerves due to pressure exerted by the mouthpiece is recognised as a pathogenetic agent for an occupational disease in brass players (BK-Nr. 2106, Ärztl. Sachverständigenrat beim Bundesministerium für Arbeit u. Sozialordnung (BMA) 2002). Thus, musicians dystonia as an 'occupation-specific and occupational disease' should be included in the schedule of occupational diseases (Rozanski et al. 2015). Assessment of the embouchure function in brass players is therefore relevant for entitlements from institutions for statutory accident insurance and prevention.

8.4.6.3 Methodology

Brass musicians lips are observed while playing by using a rigid endoscope inserted into a bore hole of the mouthpiece.

The optimal position for the bore hole can be determined separately for each individual mouthpiece. This is done by positioning the 70° endoscope above the cup of the mouthpiece so that the outer rim of the mouthpiece is completely visible through the endoscope. The distance between endoscope tip and outer rim is measured and mirrored on a horizontal axis along the outer rim. This measurement defines the optimal position for the bore hole. The bore hole is drilled at a 70°

angle into the cup of the mouthpiece, and a thread is tapped into it.

A guiding sleeve with a knurled screw is subsequently screwed into the hole (cf. Fig. 8.33, lower image). The 70° endoscope (cf. Fig. 8.33, upper image) is inserted into the guiding sleeve and fixed with a coupler.

Fine adjustments may be done by turning the knurled screw of the guiding sleeve slightly upwards or downwards, depending on the configuration of the mouthpiece (semi-spherical or conical cups). Lighting is provided by a fibre optic cable, screwed onto the endoscope. The mouthpiece is connected to the instrument, and a stroboscopy or kymography camera is clipped onto the endoscope (cf. Fig. 8.34).

An airborne-sound microphone mounted on a stand approximately 1 m from the bell of the instrument triggers the stroboscope. Alternatively, a contact microphone can be placed on one cheek, near the corner of the mouth.

For the observation of lip vibrations, this standardised device with fixed coupling between endoscope and camera on the one hand and mouthpiece with instrument on the other hand is suitable. Thus, motion artefacts (e.g. generated when using freehand endoscopy) are avoided. In contrast to the depiction of the vibrating lips via fenestrated mouthpieces, this technique allows the instrument to be played without loss of air. Near-real playing conditions are created by using the musician's own instrument with a modified commercial quality mouthpiece.

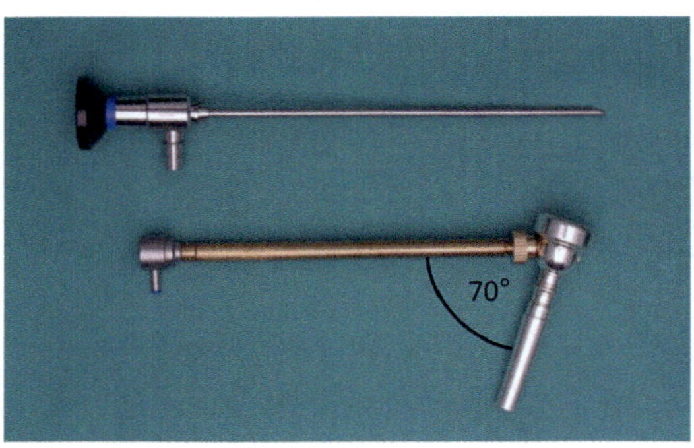

Fig. 8.33 Trumpet mouthpiece with fixed guiding sleeve and a separate 70° endoscope (© Mauersberger 2016)

8.4.6.4 Examination

Before the examination, the musicians should be asked to play 'dry' (i.e. without moistening the lips with saliva), and the mouthpiece should be slightly warmed (e.g. through submerging it in warm water) in order to reduce misting of the optics from the player's breath.

Examination of lip vibrations begins after an individual warm-up period. The exercises that are to be played should be passages consisting of various dynamics (pianissimo to fortissimo), articulations (staccato and legato) and pitches. They should cover the entire technical spectrum of the instrument in order to imitate the player's 'natural strain' (such as in a concert or opera) as closely as possible.

8.4.6.5 Evaluation

Stroboscopy

Vibration Phases

Opening, closing, open and closed phases of the lip vibration cycle can be distinguished by stroboscopy, analogously to those of the vocal folds (Böhme and Gross 2001; Nawka 2012).

During the opening phase (see Fig. 8.35; 45–180°), the distance between the lips increases. In the closing phase (see Fig. 8.35; 180–315°), the upper and lower lips come closer to each other. The complete time period during which the lips are open (see Fig. 8.35; 45–315°) is known

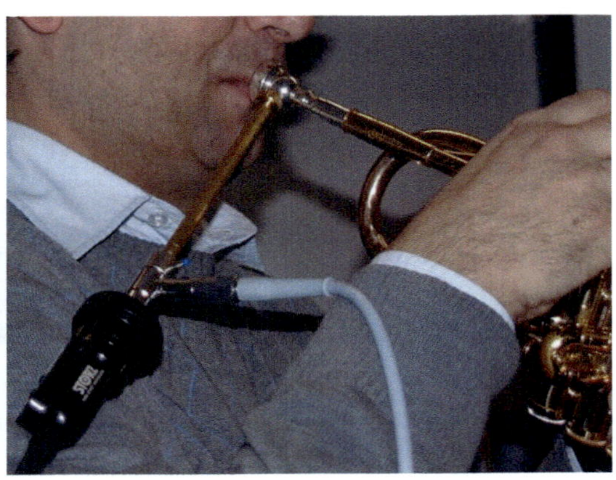

Fig. 8.34 Trumpeter's examination by a mouthpiece with lateral bore hole, guiding sleeve, attached endoscope and camera (© Mauersberger 2016)

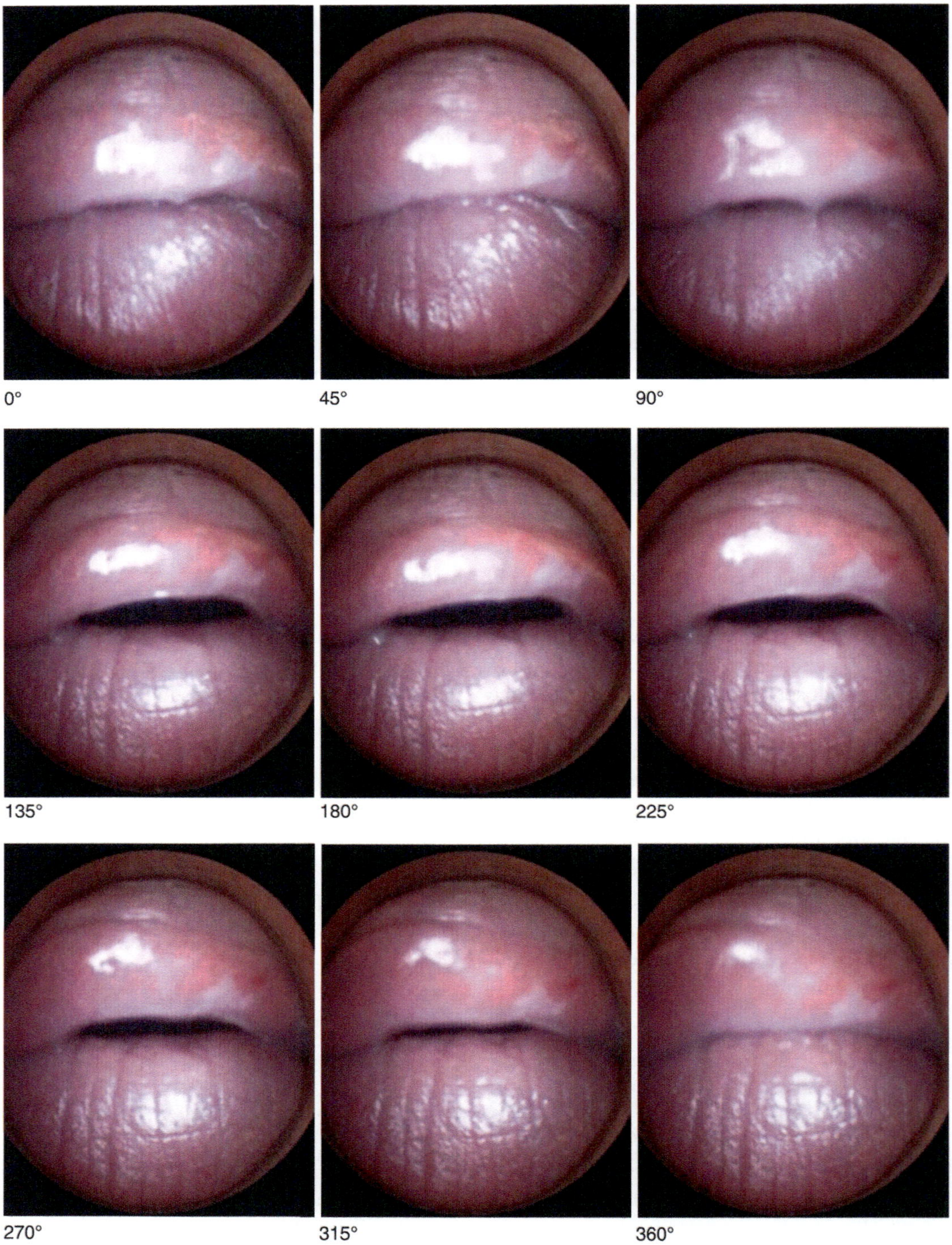

Fig. 8.35 Stroboscopic vibration cycle of a trumpeter's lips (266 Hz, C4, mezzo forte) (© Mauersberger 2016)

as the open phase. The open phase is therefore the sum of the opening and closing phases. In the closed phase (see Fig. 8.35; 0° und 360°), the oral fissure is completely shut.

Embouchure Types

Various embouchure types of brass players were described by Leno (1971, 1974, 1995, 2009) through stroboscopic visualisation and were more precisely distinguished by Reinhardt (1973): by mouthpiece position and direction of exhaled airstream, upstream or downstream types can be classified (Leno 1971, 1974, 1995, 2009). The downstream type (see Fig. 8.36) is characterised by a prominent upper lip, which directs the airstream downwards into the mouthpiece. The mouthpiece is positioned high (Leno 1971, 1974, 1995, 2009; Wilken 2009). The upstream type (see Fig. 8.37) is characterised by a prominent lower lip, which directs the airstream upwards into the mouthpiece. The mouthpiece is positioned low. This embouchure type is much less common than the downstream type (Leno 1971, 1974, 1995, 2009; Wilken 2009).

The embouchure type depends on the individual anatomy (including positioning of the teeth, distance between oral fissure and columella base and lip morphology) and cannot be trained (Wilken 2009). Upstream and downstream types are possible with both high embouchure (mouthpiece closer to the nose) and low embouchure (mouthpiece closer to the chin) (Wilken 2009).

Functional Analyses

As for the vocal folds, the vibrating lips of a brass player should be initially assessed for the sufficiency of lip closure and phase synchronicity (comparison of upper and lower lip vibrations). In addition, mucosal waves can often be observed on the vibrating lips, analogously to the displacement of the marginal edge of the vocal folds (see Fig. 8.38).

Seidner and Eysholdt (2005) identify the displacements of the marginal edge of the vocal folds as

> movements of the superficial mucosa sliding on a gliding layer [...] over the muscle.

Similar

> movements of the superficial mucosa [...] over the muscle

also exist on the lips.

Functional mucosal distensions are occasionally seen, which presumably arise through the

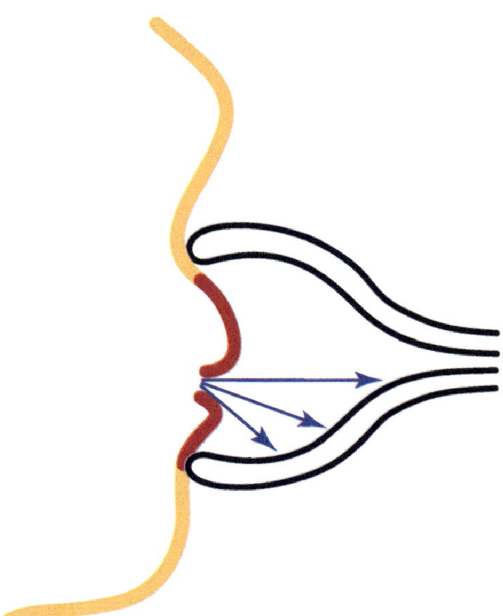

Fig. 8.36 Downstream type (© Mauersberger 2016)

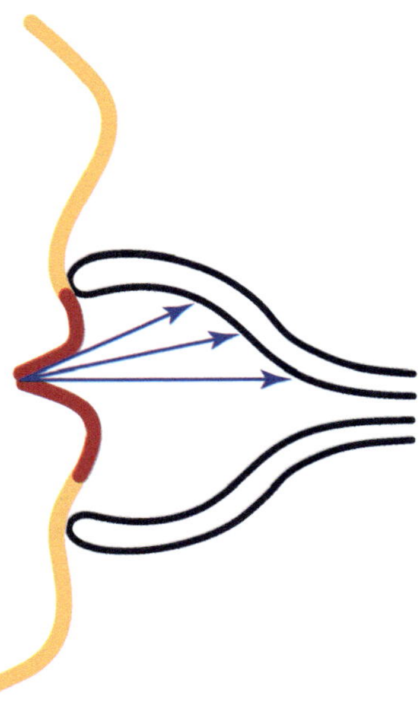

Fig. 8.37 Upstream type (© Mauersberger 2016)

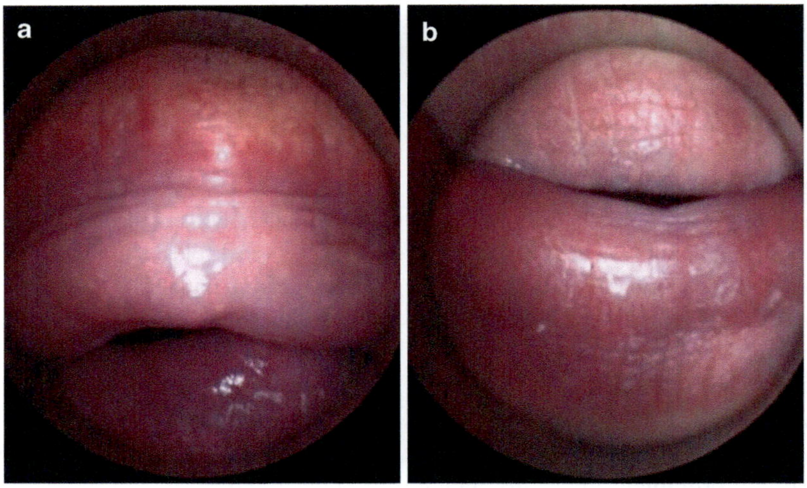

Fig. 8.38 Horizontal mucosal waves (**a**) on the upper lip of a trombonist (downstream type) and (**b**) on the lower lip of a trombonist (upstream type) (© Mauersberger 2016)

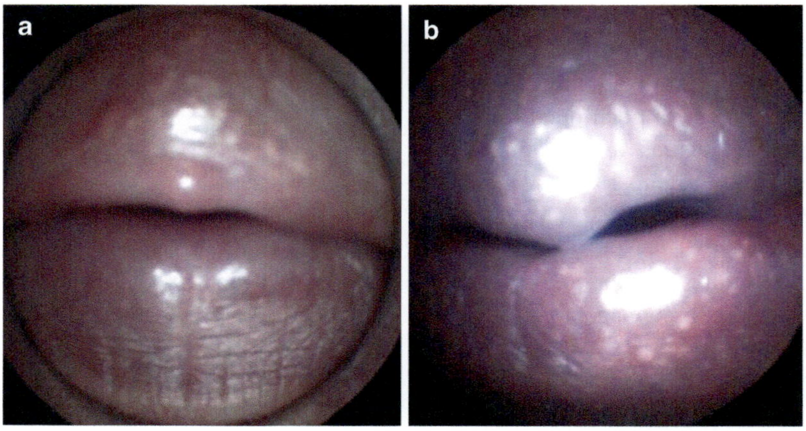

Fig. 8.39 Functional mucosal distensions of the upper lip (**a**) in the middle, swinging towards the examiner in the sagittal plane, and (**b**) right paramedian, swinging downwards into the oral fissure in the frontal plane (© Mauersberger 2016)

Bernoulli suction and should not necessarily be evaluated as pathological (see Fig. 8.39).

Kymography

In kymographic images (Figs. 8.40, 8.41, 8.42, 8.43, 8.44, and 8.45), the upper lip is displayed on the right and the lower lip on the left side.

Vibration Phases

Analogous to stroboscopic observations, opening, closing, open and closed phases can also be distinguished by kymographic examinations (see Fig. 8.40). This phase classification of lip vibration cycles is based on the kymographic analysis of vocal fold vibrations by Gall and Hanson (1973) and by Švec's research group (Böhme and Gross 2001; Švec et al. 1999; Švec and Šram 2002).

Additionally, onset, steady-state and offset phases may be distinguished, since each individual lip vibration is captured separately by this high-speed line scanning technique. During tone onset (see Fig. 8.41), lip vibration amplitudes increase. A constant amplitude during the blown

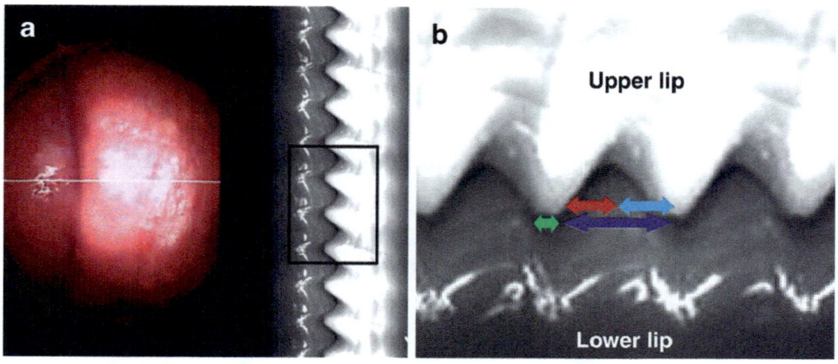

Fig. 8.40 (**a**) Opening, closing, open and closed phases of the lip vibration cycle, observed in a trumpeter (247 Hz, H3, mezzo forte); (**b**) detailed image enlargement rotated 90° to the left: red arrow, opening phase; blue arrow, closing phase; purple arrow, open phase; green arrow, closed phase (© Mauersberger 2016)

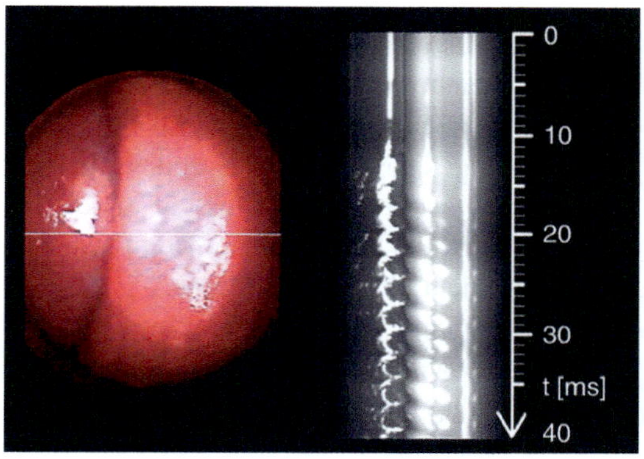

Fig. 8.41 Onset phase of a trumpeter (© Mauersberger 2016)

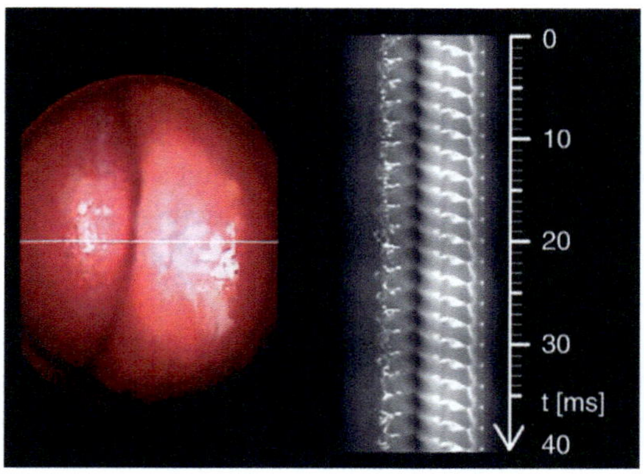

Fig. 8.42 Steady-state phase with low amplitudes (494 Hz, H4, mezzo forte) of a trumpeter (© Mauersberger 2016)

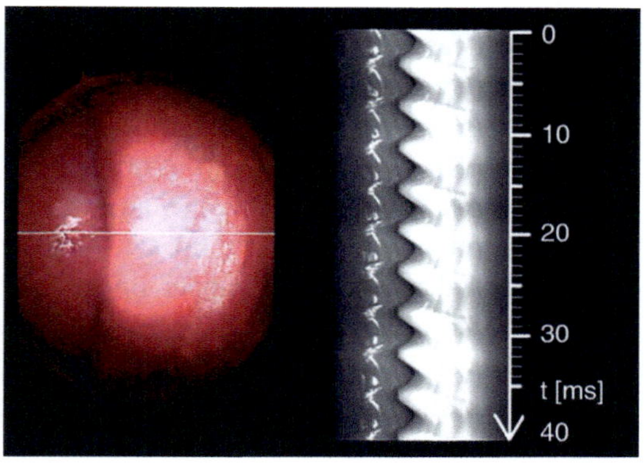

Fig. 8.43 Steady-state phase with large amplitudes (247 Hz, H3, mezzo forte) of a trumpeter (© Mauersberger 2016)

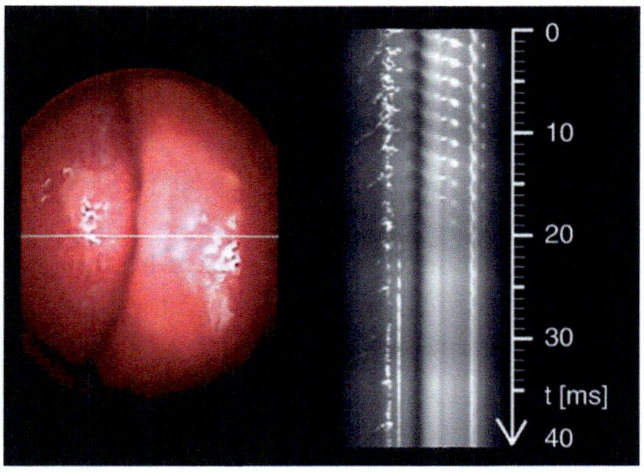

Fig. 8.44 Offset phase of a trumpeter (© Mauersberger 2016)

tone characterises the steady-state phase (see Figs. 8.42 and 8.43). The amplitude varies due to the frequency (see Figs. 8.42 and 8.43). During the offset phase (see Fig. 8.44), the blown tone ends as a result of the decreasing lip vibration amplitudes.

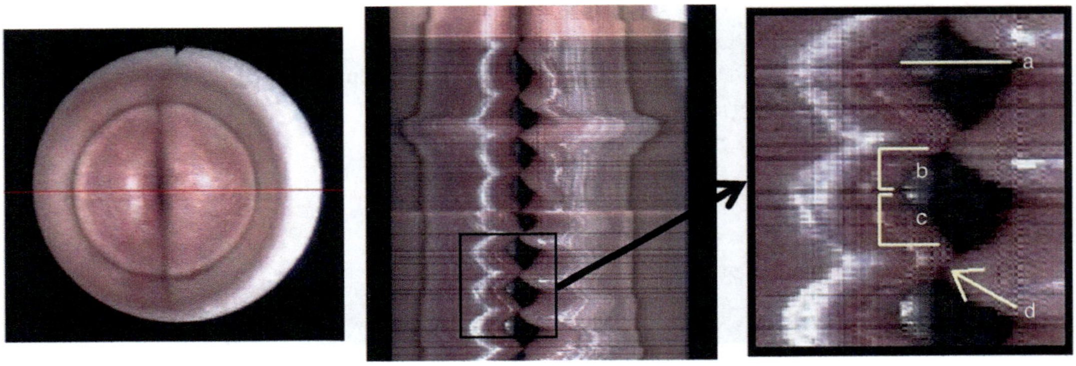

Fig. 8.45 Colour strobe kymography of a trombonist's lips. Left image, photograph of lips with recording line; middle image, reconstructed colour strobe kymography; right image, detailed enlargement of middle image; *a* maximal lip opening; *b* opening phase; *c* closing phase; *b* + *c* open phase; *d* closed phase (© Mauersberger 2016)

Amplitude Measurements

Single lip vibration amplitudes can be measured by a multistep evaluation algorithm with rpSzene® software (rpSzene® version 8.0 (2006–2010)/Rehder/Partner GmbH/Hamburg) (Mauersberger 2016). Vibrations of the lower lip are partially overlaid by vibrations of the upper lip in most brass players (downstream type; see e.g. Figs. 8.40, 8.41, 8.42, 8.43, and 8.44). Therefore, lower lip vibrations of downstream-type players are only partly visible and mostly not measurable.

As with the singer's vocal folds (Schutte and Seidner 2005), there is a negative correlation between pitch and amplitude of the upper lip in brass players: the higher the frequency played, the smaller the amplitudes of the upper lip and vice versa. In addition, the amplitudes vary with intensity: the louder the tone played, the larger the amplitudes of the upper lip and vice versa (Mauersberger 2016).

Methodological limitations may be found in cases of significant overlapping of the lower lip by the upper lip (extreme downstream type) or of the upper lip by the lower lip (extreme upstream type). High-frequency tones that are played in pianissimo may have very small amplitudes (<0.1 mm), which are not measurable (Mauersberger 2016).

8.4.6.6 Conclusions

Kymography and stroboscopy are non-invasive imaging techniques for detailed real-time functional analyses of lip vibrations. They allow the brass musician to play his or her own instrument. By using a mouthpiece with lateral bore hole, fixed guiding sleeve, attached endoscope and camera, image artefacts and loss of air can be avoided so that the lips are examined in near-real brass instrument playing conditions.

One advantage of kymography over stroboscopy is that each individual lip vibration can be examined along a predetermined line (kymography, high-speed line scanning). In contrast to high-speed recordings of lip vibrations (e.g. Bromage et al. 2005, 2010; Bromage 2007; Chick et al. 2005; Stevenson et al. 2009; Newton et al. 2008; Boutin et al. 2015), the volume of accumulated data is considerably lower in kymography. The sampling rates of lip vibrations are similar (7.200 lines per second in kymography (Mauersberger 2016), compared with 2000 (Newton et al. 2008)–11,025 (Boutin et al. 2015) frames per second in high-speed recordings of lip vibrations).

Stroboscopic examinations are more suitable for pictorial, descriptive representations than for measurements and statistical analyses of lip vibrations. Stroboscopic cameras are much less expensive than kymographic cameras and are therefore used more often in clinical practice. With special software, a colour strobe kymographic image can be derived and reconstructed from a stroboscopic video sequence of the lips (see Fig. 8.45) in the same way as for the vocal folds (see Nawka 2012). For this purpose, a previously defined recording line is extracted from consecutive single images of the stroboscopic video sequence (see left image of Fig. 8.45). The single images are then placed one below the other in chronological order (see middle image of Fig. 8.45).

This is an inexpensive alternative to real-time kymography (where a separate kymographic camera is needed), because only one camera is necessary for both stroboscopy and kymography.

Ideally, kymography and stroboscopy should be complemented by further diagnostic methods to evaluate the brass player's embouchure: a non-invasive morphological lip examination is carried out clinically and sonographically (mainly for evaluation of the orbicularis oris muscle). The lower end of the vocal tract with the larynx can be studied by common phoniatric techniques (e.g. laryngoscopy, stroboscopy, kymography, acoustic signal analyses, rating scales).

In clinical practice and outpatient departments for musicians medicine, embouchure investigations of brass players are closely related to insurance, legal and economic aspects relevant to professional liability: for accident and illness coverage and for professional liability insurances, the question of (in)capacity to work largely depends on these embouchure evaluations. In the context of rehabilitation programmes and litigation, those examinations can provide valuable information to judge brass musicians (in)capacity to perform (e.g. assessment of post-traumatic (Satchmo's syndrome), post-operative or strain-induced (embouchure dystonia) alterations of the lips). Therefore, stroboscopic and kymographic studies of lip vibrations are recommended for routine use in musicians medicine consultations.

Case Study 8.4: Stroboscopy of the Lips
Three herniated discs cause cervical myelocompression and a discrete right hemisyndrome. The lip vibrations are mostly uncoordinated. One can see irregular high-frequency fluttering and trembling of the upper lip with markedly reduced amplitudes. Normal cycles are rare. Additionally, an insufficient lip closure with uncontrollable salivation can be observed.

8.4.7 Instrumental Methods for Assessment of Laryngeal Phonatory Function

Philippe Dejonckere

8.4.7.1 Introduction

The voice laboratory can be considered an essential tool for the assessment and treatment evaluation of voice patients and for clinical research on voice disorders.

Several specific questions may be answered from the information obtained in the voice laboratory:

- Is a given voice or voice function measurement to be considered as normal (within normal limits) or pathological?
- If the voice or voice function is to be considered pathological, how severe is the alteration?
- Which aspects or mechanisms of voice production are concerned with the voice disorder? How does the primary (medical) aetiology or lesion explain the components of voice production that are perceived or analysed as deviant (e.g. by limiting vocal fold closure or by eliciting irregular vibrations related to vocal fold asymmetry), and how do they account for the patient's complaints (e.g. voice fatigue or compensation mechanisms)? Is a measure specific for a certain nosologic entity (diagnostics in a narrower sense)? However, as a rule, no acoustic parameter may be considered as pathognomonic for a specific medical aetiological diagnosis.
- What is the result of a comparison of voice production at two or more times (e.g. before and after therapy) or in two or several situations or voicing conditions (spontaneously vs. louder, or during an Isshiki manoeuvre or when applying a defined therapeutic technique)? Have the changes returned the voice to normal function as indicated by voice measurement (Dejonckere 2000)?

8.4.7.2 A Prerequisite: Recording a Voice Sample

Audio recording is the most important basic requisite for voice quality assessment. Once a high-quality recording has been made, it can be stored and remains available—as a document—for performing additional investigations at a later time, as, e.g. blind perceptual evaluation by a panel or sophisticated acoustic analyses (Titze 1995). A sampling frequency of at least 20,000 Hz is recommended. The recordings should ideally be made in a sound-treated room, but a quiet room, with ambient noise permanently <45 dB(A), is acceptable when a head-mounted microphone at close distance from the mouth is used (Sramkova et al. 2015). When recording voice, it is also recommended to record the background sound during the time when the examined subject is silent and determine the ambient noise level of the recording—this level should optimally be at least 10 dB lower than the sound level of the quietest voice signals to ensure quality measurements (Sramkova et al. 2015). Svec and Granqvist (2010) provide technical guidelines for selecting microphones for human voice production research (frequency response and range, dynamic range, directionality). The mouth-to-microphone distance needs to be held constant; Titze (1995) has recommended less than 10 cm (preferably 3–4 cm). A (miniature) head-mounted microphone offers a clear advantage. Off-axis positioning (45–90° from the mouth axis) reduces aerodynamic noise from the mouth in speech (Watson 1994; Sataloff 1997). Contact microphones or accelerometers, being directly in touch with the neck, work well in high-noise environments (Svec et al. 2005). Suppressing background noise and voices from other people (e.g. pupils, children) is a major issue for voice dosimetry and long-term monitoring. Sound pressure levels (SPLs) of speech can be estimated from skin vibration of the neck with acceptable accuracy when the subjects are individually calibrated. The accelerometer is totally selective and non-apparent, well suited for F0 monitoring and to some extent for SPL after adequate calibration, whereas the microphone (headset) is not completely selective, always (to some extent) visible, but it allows qualitative analysis (e.g. harmonics-to-noise ratio, singer's formant). Contactless microphones are wired or wireless. A *wireless microphone* contains a *transmitter* that sends the audio as a radio or optical signal rather than via a cable. Voice dosimeters and portable voice monitors use also accelerometers (Hunter and Titze 2010).

For routine clinical purposes, different voice/speech materials can be used.

An example of protocol for standard recording:

- /a:/ at (spontaneous) comfortable pitch/loudness, recorded 3× in order to evaluate variability of quality (Speyer et al. 2003)
- /a:/ slightly louder, in order to evaluate the possible change in quality (plasticity) and the slope of the regression line frequency/sound pressure level (Dejonckere 1998; Dejonckere and Lebacq 2001)
- A single sentence or a short standard passage

Phonetic selection can be useful, e.g. a short sentence with:

- Constant voicing (no voiceless sounds and to be spoken without interruption)
- No fricatives

Such sentences (e.g. 'We mow our lawn all year') can be analysed by the computer program for sustained vowels, and as it contains no articulation noise, there is no biasing of harmonics-to-noise computations. Computation of percentage voiceless (normal in this case is 100%) is useful for neurological voices or spasmodic dysphonia (Dejonckere 2006b; Dejonckere et al. 2012b). Further, it allows easy determination of the mean habitual fundamental speaking frequency.

Another example of a criterion for phonetic selection could be a multiplication of voice onsets, as they are critical in disturbed voices (Revis et al. 2000). Such criteria are not language-linked.

A standard reading passage should also be recorded, whenever possible. Two classic and often-used reading passages for English-speaking persons are 'the Rainbow Passage' (a phonetically selected passage including all the speech sounds of English) and 'Marvin Williams' (an all-voiced passage) (Sataloff 1997). Removal of non-voiced segments is possible a posteriori for acoustic analysis (Maryn et al. 2010a).

Long-term monitoring of voice as well as voice dosimetry has become an important issue particularly within the field of professional voice diseases. Voice dosimetry (by means of a 'voice accumulator') is a basic concept for measuring voice loading, which is the mechanical stress inflicted on the voice organ when intensively speaking or singing. It can be used, e.g. for defining 'at-risk' occupations. Long-term monitoring (by means of a 'portable voice lab') gives insight into the subject's vocal behaviour, e.g. in working environment (Manfredi and Dejonckere 2016; Cantarella et al. 2014).

8.4.7.3 Aerodynamics

Aerodynamic analysis of voice production includes measurement of airflow, air pressure and their relationships during phonation. By using appropriate instrumentation, a number of derived measurements can provide information of vocal efficiency.

Phonation Airflow

The simplest aerodynamic parameter of voicing is the maximum phonation time (MPT) in seconds. It consists of the prolongation of an /a:/, for as long as possible after maximal inspiration and at spontaneous, comfortable pitch and loudness. It is one of the more widely used clinical measures in voice assessment, worldwide (Hirano 1989). A prior demonstration is necessary, and three trials are required, the longest being selected for comparison to norm (Neiman and Edeson 1981). As it is an 'extreme' performance, it has been shown to be very sensitive to learning and fatigue effects. Further, in good voices, the duration of 'apnoea' (>45 s) can become the limiting factor, rather than the available air. Children show significant lower values of MPT than adults, as their lung volume is smaller (Kent et al. 1987). A reduction of possible bias—e.g. supportive respiratory capabilities compensating for poor membranous vocal fold closure—is possible by computing the ratio: averaged phonation airflow or phonation quotient (PQ) = vital capacity (ml)/MPT (s).

Vital capacity (VC) is defined as 'the volume change at the mouth between the position of full inspiration and complete expiration'. It can be measured in a reliable way by using a hand-held spirometer (Rau and Beckett 1984). VC depends, in normal subjects, on anthropometric factors and is, e.g. quite strongly correlated with height (Morris et al. 1992). It is also sensitive to lung disease. As VC is not directly related to voice quality, it is meaningful to take it in account, certainly if children are investigated.

The mean airflow rate can also be measured by using a pneumotachograph. This consists of a hand-held mouth tube (possibly connected to a mask) within which is placed a fine mesh wire screen in order to create a small resistance to airflow. This resistance results in a pressure difference across the screen that can be measured with a differential pressure transducer; the pressure difference increases with the flow. This device provides a direct measurement of the mean airflow rate (ml/s) for sustained phonation over a comfortable duration, usually 2–3 s, at the habitual pitch and intensity level, following habitual inspiration. Pathophysiological backgrounds and normative values have been reported by Hirano (1981, 1989), Verdolini (1994), Colton and Casper (1996) and Woo et al. (1987, 1994).

The averaged phonation airflow considerably varies among normal subjects, and there is a large overlapping range of values in normal and dysphonic subjects. This limits the value for diagnostic purposes (Schutte 1980). Nevertheless, when comparing glottal function before and after surgical intervention or non-surgical voice training techniques, airflow measurement may be useful in monitoring therapeutic effects (Schutte 1992), e.g. in case of paralytic dysphonia (Hirano et al. 1968; Fritzell et al. 1974; Murry and Bone 1978), or when microlaryngeal phonosurgery has been performed (Woo et al. 1994). The method is especially useful for demonstrating changes in a single test subject over time.

For comparisons (pre-/post-treatment), it is recommended to use the same kind of technique (PQ or mean airflow rate measured by a pneumotachograph).

Several dedicated devices are commercially available (e.g. the Phonatory Aerodynamic System PAS 6600 KayPENTAX, Montvale, NJ, USA) (Zraick et al. 2012). They propose various protocols, including an estimation of voicing efficiency.

Flow Glottography

Flow glottography (FLOG) consists of an inverse filtering of the oral airflow waveform. The basic tool is a high-frequency pressure transducer incorporated within an airtight Rothenberg mask (Rothenberg 1973). The inverse filtering procedure removes the resonant effects of the vocal tract and produces an estimate of the waveform produced at the vocal folds (Alku 2011) (Fig. 8.46).

The special advantage of this technique is that it differentiates and, after calibration, quantifies the leakage airflow (the continuous component of the airflow) and the pulsated airflow. Leakage airflow is an important concept: it assumes that there is an opening somewhere along the total length of the vocal folds through which air escapes. In case of leakage airflow, the plateau of the closed phase is offset from the baseline (flow = 0). Calibration is critical for reliable measurements. Flow glottography can also be used to analyse the voice onset (Dejonckere 2006a; Lebacq and Dejonckere 2019). Glottal airflow waveforms can be used for computing open, closing and speed quotients which are related to sound pressure level of the voice (Sapienza et al. 1998).

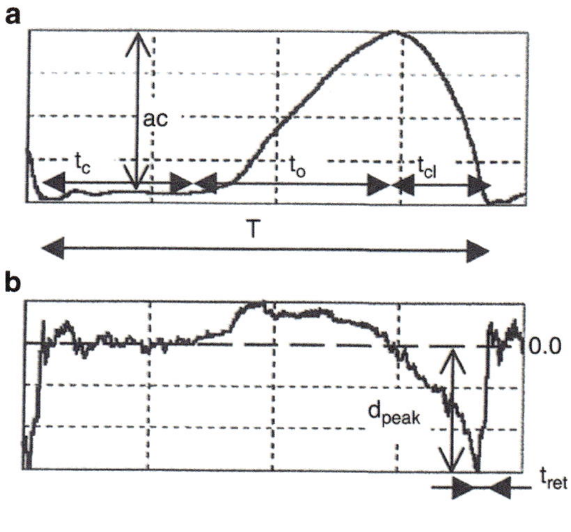

Fig. 8.46 (**a**) Flowglottogram obtained from a normal subject by inverse filtering, showing the closed time (t_c), the opening time (t_o) and the closing time (t_{cl}). In this case there is no dc flow (complete closure without leakage). (**b**) First derivative of the flowglottogram. d_{peak} is the negative peak amplitude of the derivative, at the moment of glottal closure. t_{ret} is the return phase, i.e. the time during which the derivative returns to the zero level after the instant of the negative peak. (From Alku 2011 with kind permission from Springer Nature 2018)

Subglottal Air Pressure

Measurements of subglottal air pressure made by using oesophageal balloons or pressure transducers and transglottal catheters, or by tracheal puncture, are semi-invasive or invasive and limited to research situations. An accurate estimation of subglottal pressure can be obtained by measuring the intra-oral air pressure produced during the repeated pronunciation of /pVp/ syllables (i.e. a vowel between two plosive consonants). A thin catheter is introduced into the mouth through the labial commissure, sealed by the lips, and not occluded by the tongue. If there is no closure of the vocal folds, the intra-oral air pressure should be similar to the pressure elsewhere in the respiratory tract. During the production of a voiceless consonant, the vocal folds are abducted and should not impose any significant obstruction to the airflow from the lungs. Thus, the pressure behind the lips is the same everywhere and reflects the pressure available to drive the vocal folds if they were to vibrate (Rothenberg 1982; Baken and Orlikoff 2000). This technique also allows an approach to the phonation threshold pressure (PTP), the minimum pressure required to initiate phonation (Titze 1992a). Pressure is usually reported in pascal units: 1 Pa is equal to 1 Newton/m^2. 1 kPa is 10 cm of H_2O.

Efficiency of Phonation

Together with airflow and vocal intensity, subglottal air pressure can be used to estimate the efficiency of phonation. Obviously, reduced efficiency is expected to induce voice fatigue. Vocal efficiency is defined as the ratio of the acoustic power to the aerodynamic power and can be estimated by dividing the radiated sound pressure level of the utterance by the product of the air pressure and the airflow used to produce the utterance (Colton and Woo 1995).

8.4.7.4 Acoustics

Acoustic measures provide in an objective and non-invasive way a lot of information about vocal function. Increasingly, these measures have become available affordably and appear to have succeeded very well in monitoring changes in voice quality across time, e.g. before and after treatment. Acoustic measures reflect the status of vocal function but do not relate specifically to various voice disorders, because basic biomechanical changes resulting in acoustic features can be induced by various types of lesions or dysfunctions.

Visible Speech

Acoustic analysis can first be used to make the voice and speech visible, e.g. in spectrograms (Baken and Orlikoff 2000). This visual representation may be a considerable aid to the perception and description of the voice characteristics. Spectrograms are also useful for comparing normal phonation with phonation characterised by excessive noise. Commercially available software packages provide synchronised displays of the microphone signal and the spectrogram, showing the frequency distribution of acoustical energy over time. A choice can be made between narrowband filtering (frequency resolution, mainly demonstrating fundamental frequency, harmonics, interharmonic and high-frequency noise, subharmonics) and broadband filtering (temporal resolution, mainly demonstrating periodicity, but also formant location). Voice characteristics such as SPL, fundamental frequency and formant central frequency can also be displayed over time for analysis of singing voice. Visualising of fast Fourier transform (FFT) graphics (power spectrum) is usually possible, as well as long-time average spectra (LTAS). When visible speech is provided simultaneously with the voice sound, the inter-rater consistency of the perceptual quality evaluation significantly increases (Martens et al. 2007).

Acoustic Parameters

Acoustic analysis can also provide precise numerical values for many voice parameters, from averaged fundamental frequency to sophisticated calculations for noise components or tremor features. Factor analysis allows the large number of acoustic parameters to be reduced to a limited number of clusters (Dejonckere et al. 1996):

- Short-term fundamental frequency perturbation
- Short- or medium-term amplitude perturbation and voiceless segments
- Harmonics-to-noise ratio
- Long-term frequency and amplitude modulation
- Very long-term amplitude variation
- Subharmonics
- Tremor

Perturbation measures (in period and amplitude), as well as the harmonics-to-noise computations on a sustained vowel (/a:/) at comfortable frequency and intensity, appear as the most robust measures and seem to determine the basic perceptual elements of voice quality: grade, roughness and breathiness. Nevertheless, correlations with perceptual data remain usually moderate (Dejonckere et al. 1996; Wolfe et al. 1997). There are, however, arguments for combining voice samples from both continuous speech and sustained vowels in acoustic analysis of dysphonic voices (Maryn et al. 2010a). A considerable variety of mathematically based measures of perturbation has been developed. Clinically, they have led to the near universal clinical use of 'jitter' and 'shimmer' as important measurements for distinguishing normal from pathological voices (Fourcin and Abberton 2008). Jitter is computed as the mean difference between the periods of adjacent cycles divided by the mean period. It is thus an F0 (fundamental frequency)-related measurement (Fig. 8.47).

For shimmer, a similar computation is made on peak-to-peak amplitudes. Voice breaks must always be excluded. For pathological voices, the coefficients of variation of jitter and shimmer for

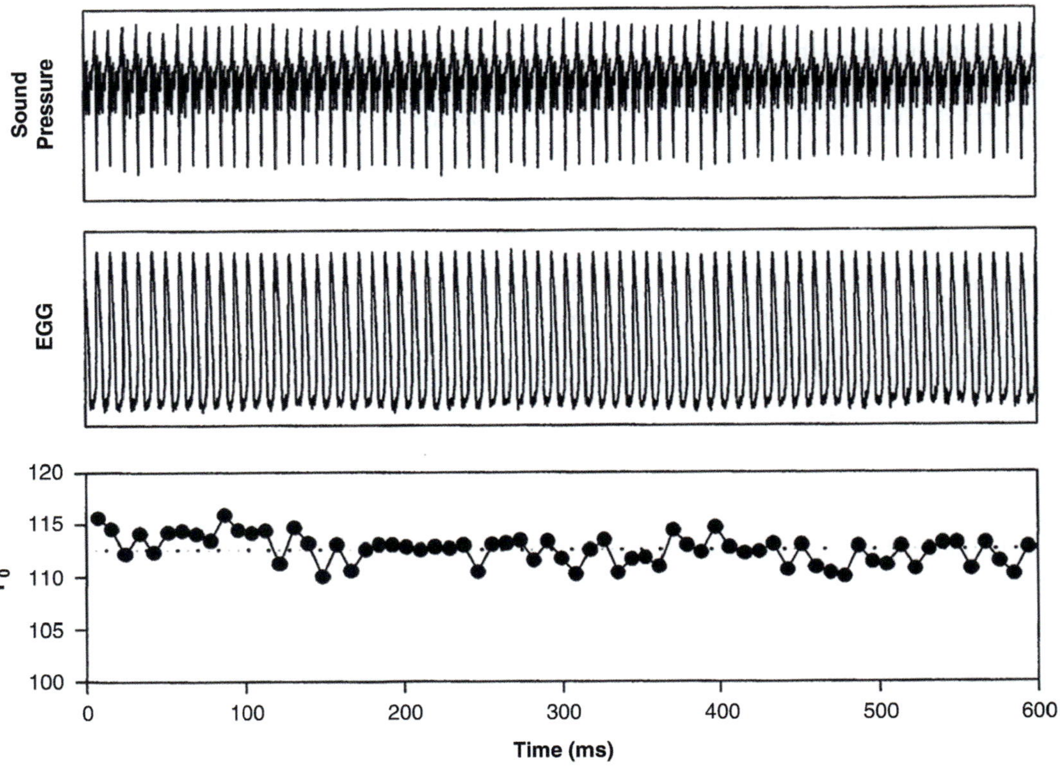

Fig. 8.47 Normal male voice, sustained /a:/: microphone signal, electroglottogram and F0 plot across time. Normal voice is characterised by slight (<1%) random variation of fundamental frequency. In most cases of pathology, this aperiodicity (jitter) increases. (From Dejonckere 2010 with kind permission from Springer Nature 2018)

a sustained /a/ are in the order of 20–30% for successive single trials as well as trials on different days (Speyer et al. 2004a). A general limitation is that the analysis programmes employed for acoustic analysis (and particularly for period identification) cannot (or not in a reliable way) analyse strongly aperiodic acoustic signals. Perturbation measures less than about 5% have been found to be reliable (Titze and Liang 1993), and only 'quasi-periodic' voices are suited to perturbation analysis. Therefore, visual control of the period of definition of the microphone signal is always necessary: even in regular voices, a strong harmonic or subharmonic may account for erratic values. However, recent work having recourse to realistic synthesised deviant voices with controlled jitter and noise has shown that improved acoustic programmes, using more reliable algorithms, could validly transgress the 5% limit (Manfredi et al. 2011, 2012; Dejonckere et al. 2011, 2012a). Alternatives from the field of non-linear dynamics, such as the coefficient of Lyapunov, have been proposed for analysing 'chaotic' or 'bifurcated' signals (Yu et al. 2000). For substitution voices, voicing quantification has also proven to be more relevant than period perturbation (Dejonckere et al. 2012c).

For signal-to-noise ratio computations (NNE (normalised noise energy), HNR (harmonics-to-noise ratio), cepstrum peak, etc.), there is currently insufficient standardisation of the optimal algorithm(s), as well as insufficient knowledge about normative values, for widely spread clinical use. The harmonics-to-noise ratio has also been found to be a parameter less suited for demonstrating the effects of therapy (Speyer et al. 2004b).

Rhinophonia is a particular resonance characteristic of the voice. It may be present without a concomitant articulation disorder. Acoustic nasometry provides objective measurements by (schematically) computing the ratio between nasal and whole voice (nasal + oral) sound pressure levels (Dejonckere and van Wijngaarden 2001).

An important application of acoustic measurements is pre- and post-treatment comparisons within patients (Brockmann-Bauser and Drinnan 2011). Thus, some combined measures have been proposed, such as the 'Dysphonia Severity Index' (DSI) (Wuyts et al. 2000) and the 'Acoustic Voice Quality Index' (AVQI) (Maryn et al. 2010b). The DSI is based on the weighted combination of a selected set of voice measurements: highest frequency, lowest intensity, maximum phonation time and jitter (%). The AVQI is a multivariate acoustic measure consisting of a weighted combination of six time- and frequency-domain metrics.

Phonetography/Voice Range Profile

Basically, the phonetogram plots the dynamic range (dBA) as a function of fundamental frequency range (Hz), documenting the extreme possibilities of voice. These extremes are of importance for professional voice users, especially singers (Schultz-Coulon 1990), but they must be interpreted with care (Titze 1992b) because the acoustic energy is related to spectral distribution. Normative values for children and teachers have been defined by Heylen et al. (2002).

Computerised systems make possible real-time measurement and display of fundamental frequency versus SPL and also of quality parameters such as jitter, within the whole voice area. Jitter results in various colour gradations, showing specific altered zones or register boundaries (Fig. 8.48).

Such computerised systems can also provide range profiles of current speech, possibly coupled with provocation tests, such as the task of reading at a controlled, louder intensity. These profiles are expected to be relevant for occupational voice users.

The highest and lowest frequencies and the softest intensity (dB A at 30 cm) seem most sensitive to changes in voice quality (Heylen et al. 1998; Van de Heyning et al. 1996; Wuyts et al. 2000; Speyer et al. 2003), the latter being related to phonation threshold pressure (Titze 1992a, b). The measurement of the lowest frequency allows the computation of the fundamental frequency range. Such a 'three-point range profile' can be obtained without completing a (time consuming) whole voice range profile (Dejonckere et al. 2001). However, as these three points represent 'extreme' performances, they are, as are MPT and CV, very sensitive to learning and fatigue effects.

8.4.7.5 Electroglottography

Electroglottography (or electrolaryngography) (EGG) is a method for monitoring vocal fold contact, rate of vibration and perturbation of regularity during voice production (Fig. 8.49a, b).

The major advantage of electroglottography is that it does not interfere with the physiological processes of speaking or singing. The signal originates from two electrodes lightly placed on the speaker's neck at the level of the thyroid cartilage. Pitch extraction from the EGG waveform is particularly reliable—as long as there is at least partial vocal fold contact during the vibration cycle—because the waveform is unaffected by vocal tract resonances and environment noise (Fourcin et al. 1995; Dejonckere 1996). The EGG signal has been used to compute period and amplitude perturbation parameters (Fourcin and Abberton 2008; Hosokawa et al. 2014) and even as a predictor of laryngeal electromyography (Mayes et al. 2008).

The main applications of EGG are:

- Fundamental frequency computations (range, regularity, distribution, display across time, cross plots, etc.), as long as there is a vocal fold contact
- Voice onset time
- Pre- and post-phonatory laryngeal gestures
- Closed phase information (hyper- vs. hypokinetic adduction)
- Voice range profile of spontaneous speech (falsetto excluded)
- Triggering of a stroboscopic light source

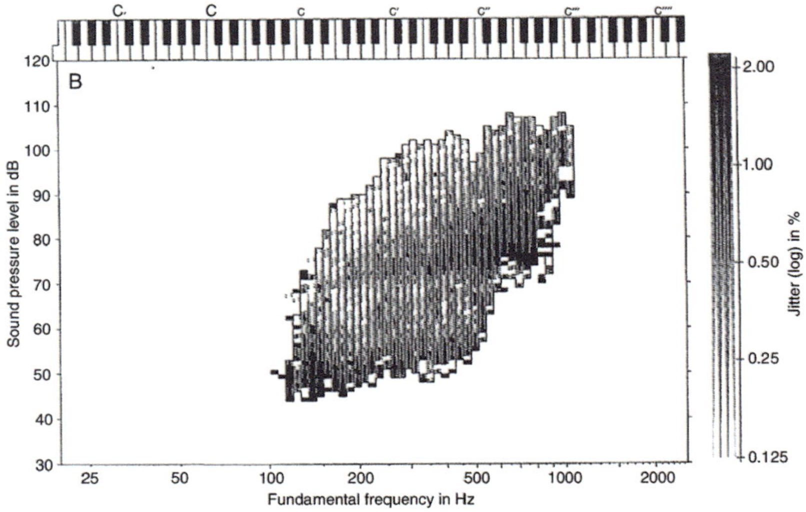

Fig. 8.48 Computerised phonetogram (voice range profile), with a grey scale indicating the amount of jitter (normal female voice). The more jitter, the darker the area. Horizontal axis: fundamental frequency in Hz (or musical tones on a keyboard). Vertical axis: sound pressure level, measured at 30 cm (dB A). This plot combines information about extreme possibilities of voice as well as on an aspect of voice quality. (From Dejonckere 2010 with kind permission from Springer Nature 2018)

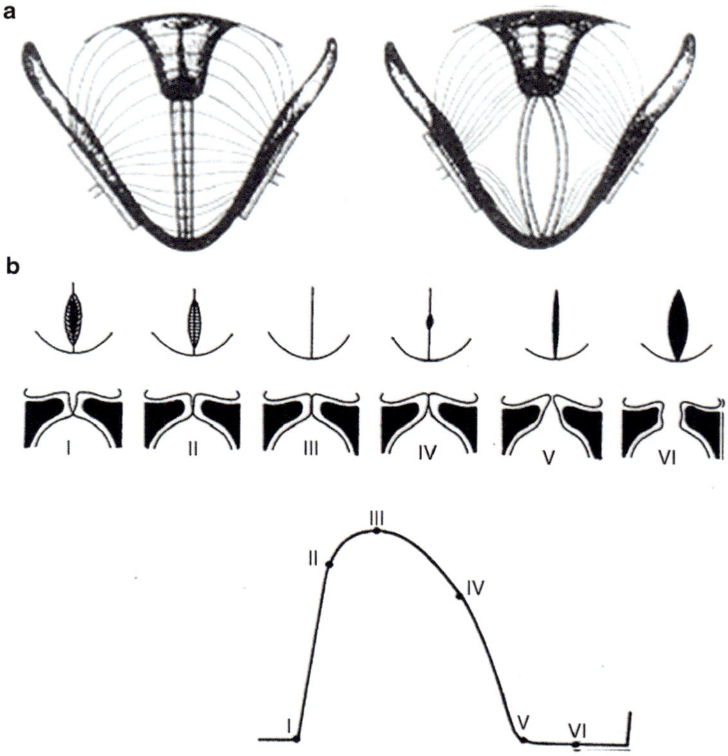

Fig. 8.49 Basic principle of electroglottography (or electrolaryngography). (**a**) Top: Schematic view of current paths across the larynx, as occurring in EGG during vocal fold vibration (left, glottis closed; right, glottis open). (**b**) Bottom: Schematic electroglottographic waveform with the corresponding laryngoscopic view and a frontal section through the midportion of the glottis. Point III corresponds to minimal trans-neck impedance, which is at maximum closure of the glottis. Points I and III can always be identified with certitude on the EGG signal. (From Dejonckere 2010 with kind permission from Springer Nature 2018)

8.4.7.6 Electromyography

Electromyography (EMG) is an electrophysiological investigation of neuromuscular function. Main indications are mobility disorders (especially reduced mobility) (Sataloff et al. 2005). Neuromuscular pathological conditions in laryngeal muscles do not basically differ from neuromuscular pathological conditions in other muscles, so it is recommended that these investigations be performed in cooperation with a clinical neurophysiologist (Blitzer 1995; Dejonckere 1987; Dejonckere et al. 1988; Munin et al. 2000). In a supine patient with the neck extended, the cricothyroid muscle is reached by inserting the electrode off the midline close to the inferior border of the thyroid cartilage. The thyroarytenoid muscle is approached by insertion of a concentric needle electrode through the cricothyroid ligament. The needle electrode is then angled cranially 45° and laterally 20° to an approximate depth of 1.5–2 cm (Fig. 8.50).

In normal situations, the EMG signal in the vocalis muscle typically precedes (around 100–500 ms) the sound emission ('prephonatory tuning') (Fig. 8.51).

It is also possible to explore the posterior cricoarytenoid muscle (curved needle/manual rotation of the larynx or via indirect laryngoscopy with a specific needle-holder), but this is not without danger. Furthermore, this muscle is innervated by the same recurrent laryngeal nerve as the thyroarytenoid muscle but another branch of it. A classical indication for laryngeal EMG is the differential diagnosis between peripheral neurogenic and mechanical (ankylosis) reduction of vocal fold mobility. Such a question may arise, e.g. in the case of blunt and penetrating external laryngeal trauma (Schaefer 2014). The objectivity of EMG provides an additional medicolegal value. In case of unilateral vocal fold paralysis, predictors of poor prognosis for functionally meaningful recovery include fibrillation potentials (Fig. 8.52), positive sharp waves and absent or reduced voluntary motor unit potentials (Misono and Merati 2012).

Large polyphasic potentials reflect partial denervation and collateral regeneration (Fig. 8.53).

However after a few months, paradoxical reinnervation may perturb the actual functional prognostic value of EMG. If dedicated coated injection needles are used, EMG can be used for monitoring botulinum injections in vocal muscles. Laryngeal EMG hypercontractility during voice rest has been considered as typical in patients with Parkinson's disease and vocal complaints (Zarzur et al. 2014).

Contraindications for laryngeal EMG are the presence of dyspnoea (e.g. in a bilateral paralysis in adduction) and anticoagulant medication. Extreme care is mandatory in children. Compli-

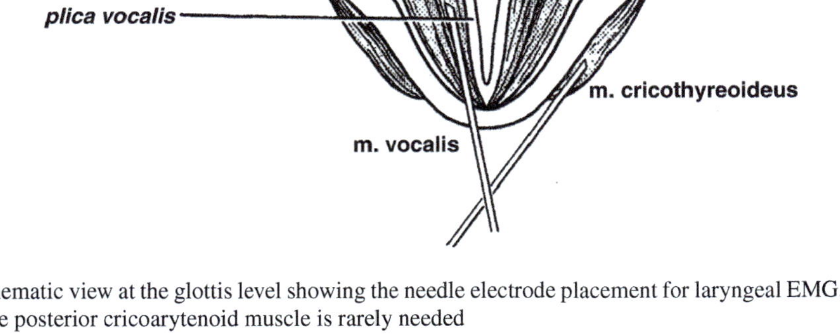

Fig. 8.50 Schematic view at the glottis level showing the needle electrode placement for laryngeal EMG. The selective approach of the posterior cricoarytenoid muscle is rarely needed

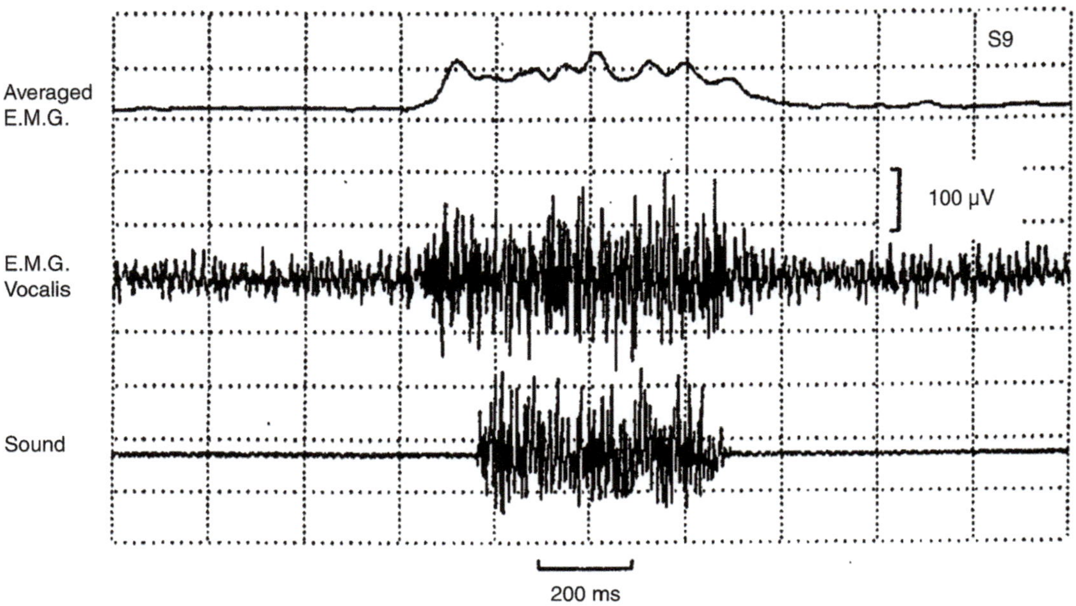

Fig. 8.51 Normal subject. The electrical activity in the vocalis muscle typically increases before the start of the vocal emission (usually 100–500 ms)

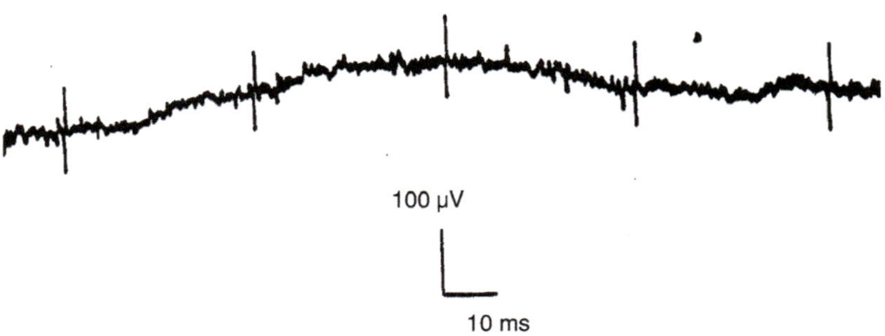

Fig. 8.52 Pathological spontaneous activity (fibrillation potentials) in the vocalis muscle after complete denervation. Fibrillation potentials may appear as soon as 5–6 days after denervation and remain present for several years

cations are rare (vocal fold haemorrhage). An evidence-based review has been provided by Sataloff et al. (2004).

Currently the possibility of temporary injection medialisation of a paralysed vocal fold has reduced the need of a prognostic parameter. However, in future, EMG will become indispensable in context of surgical reinnervation (Dejonckere 2010).

Remark

This section is based on a more detailed book chapter (Dejonckere 2010).

8.4.8 Voice Loading Tests

Tamás Hacki

8.4.8.1 Vocal Load Capacity and Vocal Loading

Vocal load capacity, which refers mainly to how long and how loud one can use the voice, is a crucial component of the phonatory ability of effective communicators. In comparison with hoarseness, which is only one of the numerous symptoms of dysphonia, restricted vocal load capacity arises as a result of several symptoms

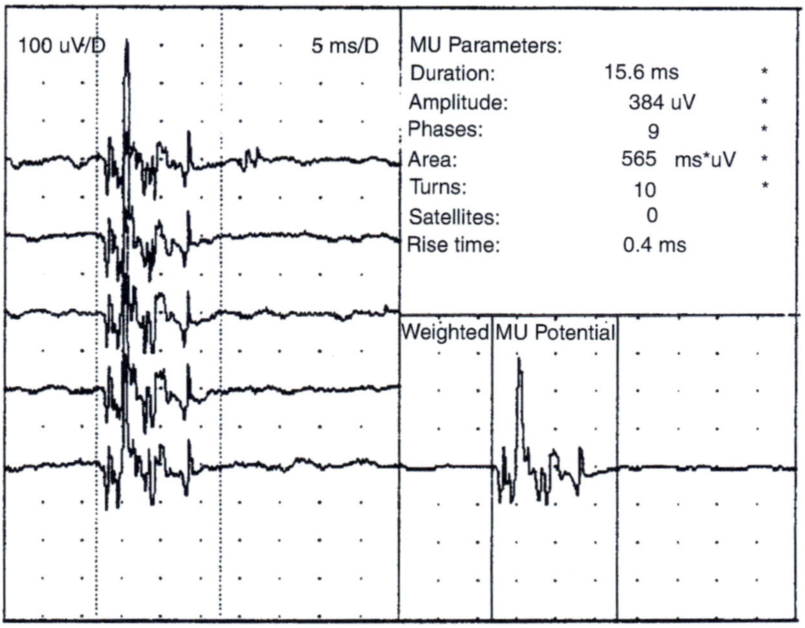

Fig. 8.53 Polyphasic motor unit potential in the vocalis muscle with increased duration and amplitude. Partial peripheral nerve lesion. Sprouting collaterals from intact motor units newly innervate denervated motor units but have a lower conduction velocity

(Hacki 1996). For this reason, vocal load capacity is an important aspect of clinical assessment and voice research.

The load capacity of the phonatory system depends upon many factors, all of which are considered to be risk factors and which may be summarised as follows:

- Physiological factors
  - Constitution of the vocal organ
  - General physical condition
  - Illnesses
- Physical factors
  - Physical environment
  - Room acoustics (attenuation; resonance)
  - Speaking distance
  - Room climate, humidity
- Psychological factors
  - Personality; psychological constitution
  - Psychological condition or state
- Social factors
  - Social environment
  - Work-related stress
  - Conversation partner (supportive; inhibiting)

In addition to general risk factors, several factors influence vocal performance immediately, for example, the current condition of the voice generators (mucosa, muscles) and respiratory structures, the respiratory and vocal technique employed at the time and the status of the patient's recovery from vocal loading. Recovery techniques include periods of rest lasting several hours as well as rapid recovery methods (such as relaxation techniques during speech).

Vocal loading is the long-term, intensive demand beyond the normal use to which the vocal organ is accustomed. The principal vocal load is the voiced aspect of spoken language. Articulation of unvoiced speech components seems to be secondary. (Complaints about vocal strain usually point towards laryngeal and respiratory fatigue.) Figure 8.54 shows the physiological processes that occur during phases of vocal loading.

When one is aware of the general and immediately influential factors, the physiological processes during vocal loading (see above) as well as the many presenting symptoms, it should be clear that testing the consequences of vocal loading

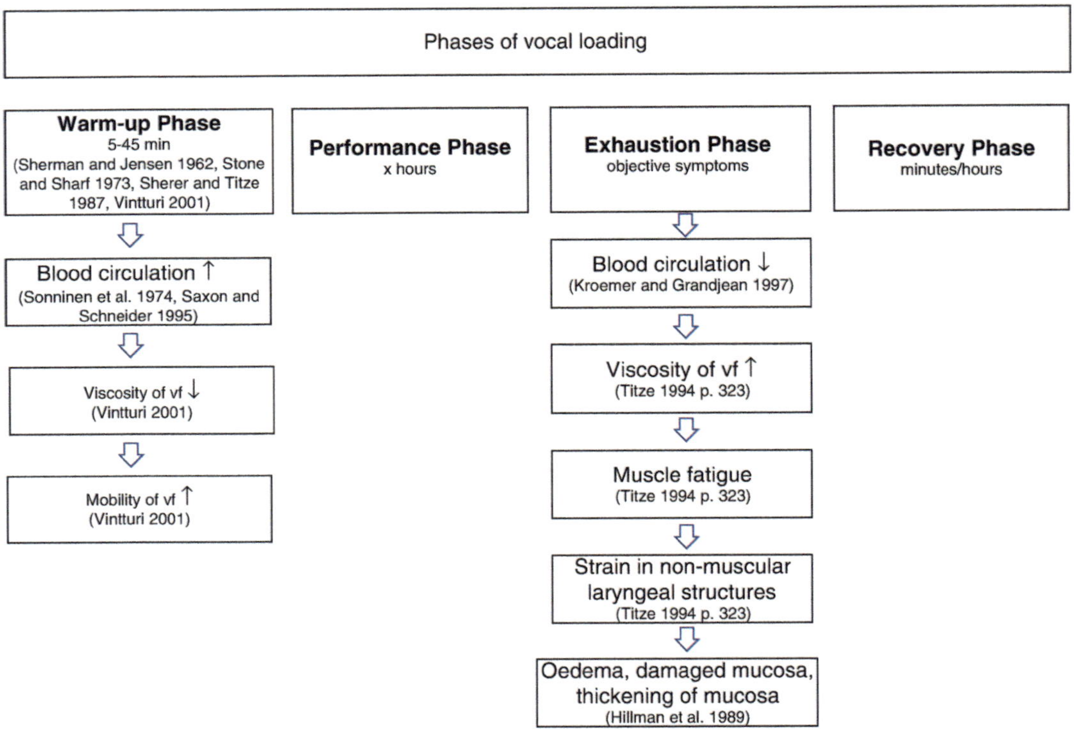

Fig. 8.54 Phases of vocal loading and their impact on vocal fold tissue. *vf* vocal folds (Hillman et al. 1989; Kroemer and Grandjean 1997; Saxon and Schneider 1995; Sherer and Titze 1987; Sherman and Jensen 1962; Sonninen et al. 1974; Stone and Scharf 1973; Titze 1994; Vintturi 2001)

and ascertaining the load capacity of the voice are complicated tasks.

8.4.8.2 Measurement of Voice Performance or Vocal Loading 'In Vivo' and the Necessity for Vocal Load Testing

Voice performance during a working day can be recorded and analysed by using a recording device. The 'voice accumulator' of Beukers et al. (1995) measures the sound pressure level of the voice in dB(A).[1] The Ambulatory Phonation Monitor (APM) (KayPENTAX) enables the gathering and analysis of numerous vocal parameters (intensity, pitch, phonation time, etc.). Useful information about voice function and the subjective perception of the speaker can be gathered by recording (the voice) before and after a vocal load lasting several hours combined with the use of questionnaires (Laukkanen and Kankare 2006). Patients who complain about vocal fatigue generally visit their physicians hours or days after a significant vocal strain, such as teaching sessions or weekend seminars. A doctor can partially reconstruct the complaints on the basis of the history; however, key symptoms may no longer be present (e.g. acute organic alterations such as hyperaemia, surrounding oedema, damage to respiratory and laryngeal function such as glottal hypertonus, and not least, acute voice symptoms). Patients who have already had in- or outpatient treatment for vocal complaints often ask their physician if they are able to resume their vocally demanding work. This question can be best answered by conducting vocal loading tests. Such tests are also necessary when giving out medical advice on vocal abilities.

8.4.8.3 Vocal Loading Tests

What form can a vocal loading test take? Risk factors, such as poor room acoustics or a poor climate within a room, particular work and stress

[1]A-weighting provides reduced low-frequency sensitivity compared with C-weighting.

situations (see Sect. 5.1 in Volume 1) or a vocal load of long duration, cannot be reproduced in the test situation. So how can a test be of practical value and how can the patient be supervised during the test? The creators of vocal loading tests must ensure that tests can be performed by most individuals and are comparable among individuals. Many different approaches to vocal loading tests were taken in the 1970s and early 1980s, featuring various speaking durations (20–45 min) and speech intensities (65–80 dB(A)), with and without surrounding background noise, with different mouth-microphone distances (20–50 cm) and with and without supplementary measurements (e.g. galvanic skin response, respiratory investigations, electromyography (EMG) or audio recording) (Wendler and Seidner 1996). Siegert (1987) made a recommendation for the Union of the European Phoniatricians (UEP) of a speaking duration of 20 min, target sound pressure level of 75–80 dB(A) and 30 cm distance from the microphone. The test should be conducted in the acoustic conditions of a living room. Laukkanen et al. (2004) used a text of 45 min duration, target level of 70 dB(A) and 40 cm mouth-microphone distance. In addition to these measurement parameters, the participants were asked to report their subjective symptoms before, during and after the test.

The first version of Seidner's Alternation Test ('Wechsler test') had a mouth-microphone distance of 50 cm and a 15-min duration. The second version (Seidner 2012) used a 30 cm mouth-microphone distance and 10-min duration, and this latter version proved to be more practical. In the first version, the participant reads a simple text at 70 dB(A) for 5 min and then increases to 75 dB(A) for a further 5 min, before finally returning to 70 dB(A) for 5 min. In the later version, the level varies minute by minute from 75 to 80 dB(A[1]), etc. The person being tested is notified on a monitor when his voice level is dropping below the desired value. A computer displays the following data on a graph: time course of sound level, percentage of lower deviation in sound level and time course of voice frequency. Laryngoscopy and assessment of the voice quality should take place before and immediately after vocal loading. Observation of the patient during the tests is particularly important: breathing, tension, complaints about abnormal sensations, etc. This test is recommended for the assessment of vocal capability and monitoring of therapy and as the basis for expert opinion.

Hacki (1996) developed the following test procedure: the participant phonates the vowel series u:-e:-i:-o:-a: for 20 min with a mouth-microphone distance of 30 cm. The required sound pressure level is 80 dB(C). Use of the dB(C) weighting, rather than dB(A), is to ensure that no artificial difference in output level is generated between low- and high-pitched voices. The reasons for phonating a vowel series are to test phonation more than articulation and to avoid the requirement that the person being tested concentrates on the reading of a text (they can instead monitor the sound level with an on-screen level indicator). The vowel series should be recited in a speaking voice manner, rather than in a singing voice. The output graph should display the average vocal output (expressed as energy-equivalent average level, LeqT) in real time (*X*-axis, time; *Y*-axis, sound pressure level, dB(C)) over 20 min. This value allows a comparison of the intra- and interindividual output. Laryngoscopy, stroboscopy, measurement of the average speaking frequency and an auditory assessment of voice quality (e.g. using GRBAS) (Hirano 1981) should be made before and after vocal loading. The participant should be observed during vocal loading, to ensure that he correctly follows the procedure. A questionnaire designed to measure the level of the patient's motivation and (emotional and physical) sensation during phonation should be completed after the test. Questionnaires determine the duration of any similar feelings of exertion in their daily life compared with that they felt after the test (more than 3 h would be a general indication of low-level or no pathology). Output curves from the above procedure can be classified as normal or pathological (Fig. 8.55) (Kramer et al. 1999). Normal output values (LeqT) for young participants are an average of 79 dB(C), with the lower range not below 75 dB(C) (Pabst et al. 1998). Values indicating pathology vary significantly: Kramer et al. (1998) found that voice

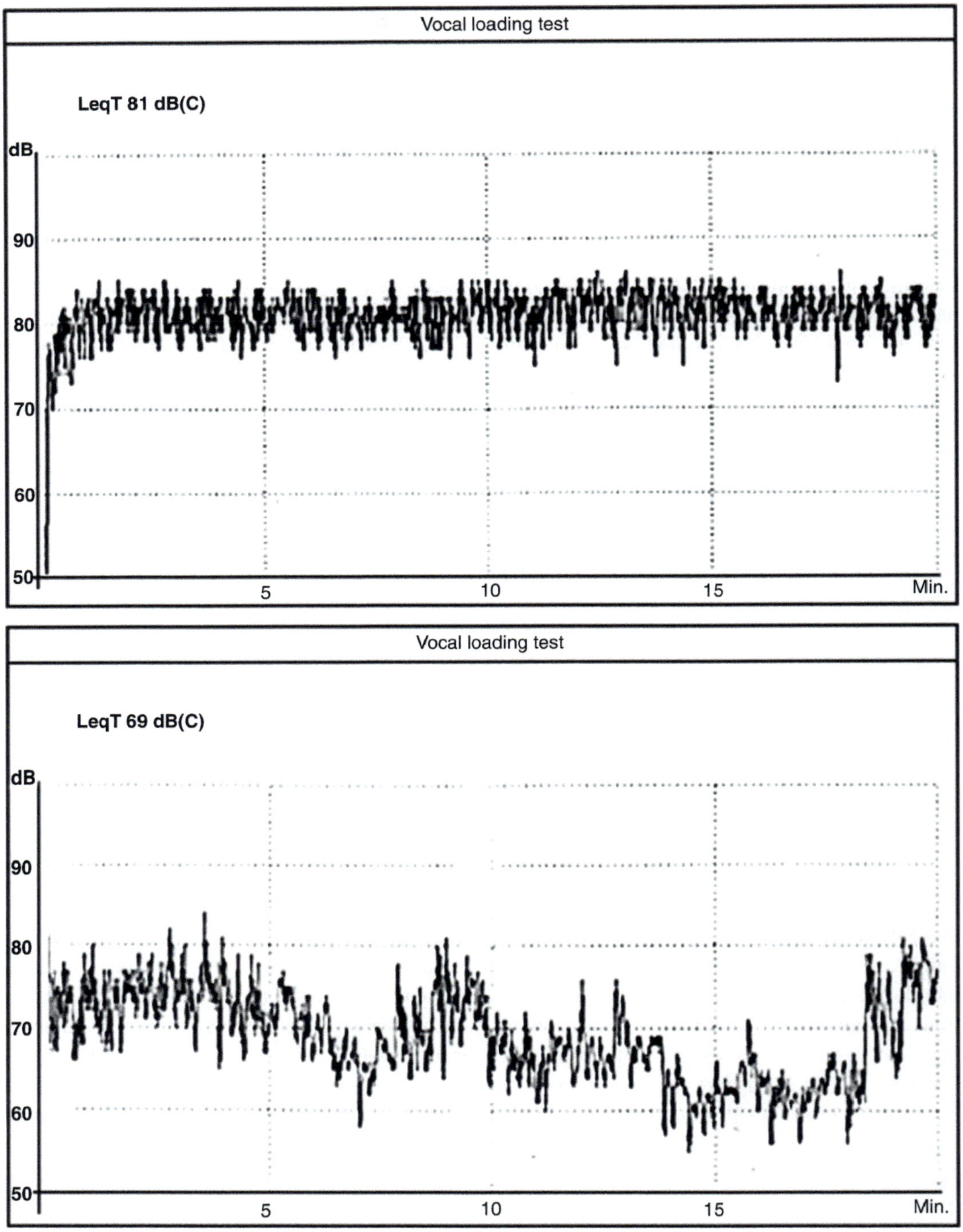

Fig. 8.55 Two types of vocal output curve (ordinate, [dB(C)]; abscissa, time [20 min]). (Taken from seven presented in Kramer et al. 1999). Above, normal homogeneous progress with warm-up phase during the first 2 min. The averaged effort (LeqT) is above average at 81 dB(C). Below, abnormal time course with total power of 69 dB(C) LeqT, indicative of pathology

patients who had undergone 3 weeks of voice rehabilitation had LeqT values under 70 dB(C) (averages of 67.1 dB(C) and 69.1 dB(C) for women and men, respectively). The LeqT values of 40.7% of patients had improved (in comparison with measurements taken on the initial visit to the clinic), and 15.7% had worsened.

8.4.8.4 Symptoms of Voice Strain

Kitzing (1981) and Seidner (2012), among others, report an elevated average speaking pitch as a typical symptom following vocal strain. Pabst et al. (1998) found an increase in the average pitch of the speaking voice of 0.7 semitones among women with normal voices (F) and 1.3 semitones in men with normal voices (M) following a 20-min vocal load at a target level of 80 dB(C). The average intensity of the speaking voices increased by 3.1 dB(A) and 3.5 dB(A) for women and men, respectively.

From our own general clinical experience after vocal loading: we take an increase in speaking pitch of more than four semitones as a sign of overly high muscle tension. Lowered speaking pitch can also be a sign of speech pathology: in such patients, we see hyperaemia or occasionally mild oedema on the edge of the vocal folds after vocal strain. A hyper- or hypotonic vibration patterns (on stroboscopy) and increase in glottal insufficiency (compared with the initial findings) are taken as a sign of intense vocal demand.

Patients claim that the effects of vocal load emerge in the resting phase. Vintturi et al. (2001) therefore investigated the effects of post-loading rest on many different parameters of phonation. Jilek et al. (2004) found that several voice parameters become worse 60 min after a vocal load of 20 min at 80 dB(C), and Echternach et al. (2013) registered deterioration in Dysphonia Severity Index (DSI) scores 60 min after vocal load. These results raise the question of the best time point after vocal loading for investigations to be made.

The motivation for a patient to undergo a vocal loading test is an essential and highly influential factor. Those people who themselves want to have their vocal ability tested are very differently motivated from those who are required to undergo such an examination (e.g. for questions relating to their retirement or pension). People with the latter motivation can be more easily convinced to exert vocal strain if it is made clear that only a vocal load test will provoke their reported vocal exhaustion and other symptoms.

8.4.8.5 Summary

Because of the complexity of the issues and the variety of symptoms of vocal strain, voice loading tests only have diagnostic value in the hands of experienced practitioners. Even here, there is a reasonable case for seeking further test improvement and appropriate standardisation.

8.4.9 The Usefulness of Computed Tomography and Magnetic Resonance Imaging in Investigation of the Vocal Tract

Katarzyna Karmelita-Katulska and
Matthias Echternach

8.4.9.1 Introduction

The mechanism of voice and speech production is a topic of interest for many disciplines such as linguistics, neurology, psychology, physiology and especially phoniatrics. Traditionally, for characterisation of voice and speech acoustics, the vocal tract shape has been studied with radiographic techniques (X-ray), but this method has certain limitations because of the ionising radiation. Radiographic studies (X-ray, computed tomography (CT)) have generally focused on bony structures (skull base, hyoid bone, etc.). MRI (magnetic resonance imaging) can clearly image the soft tissues relevant to voice and speech production (glottis, velum, lips, etc.). Nowadays, especially CT and MRI have a special role in imaging the dysfunction and certain pathologies at all stages of the voice production system, i.e. the lungs, the larynx and the vocal tract.

8.4.9.2 Computed Tomography

Coronal radiography and simple tomography have been used for years to observe changes in the larynx in many pathological states, but CT has become fast enough to replace these techniques. With the advent of multi-detector CT (MDCT), high-resolution reformatted coronal images are now routinely available (Baum et al. 2000; Lell et al. 2004). The advent of MDCT scanners has enabled the acquisition of images of the larynx during phonation as one volume image, and coronal reconstruction of the volume images makes it possible to observe changes in the vocal folds during phonation (Jun et al. 2005) (see Fig. 8.56a, b).

The limit of slice thickness allowing optimal imaging of the larynx is so far 1 mm. Minimal slice thickness is necessary to obtain sufficient image quality of multiplanar reformations, which require longer scan times and pose the risk of severe motion artefacts. MDCT allows an almost isotropic volume dataset to be acquired within an acceptable time interval (≤10 s) (Jun et al. 2005). This is necessary for the most common scanning technique of the larynx during phonation and the Valsalva manoeuvre to show pathology of motion

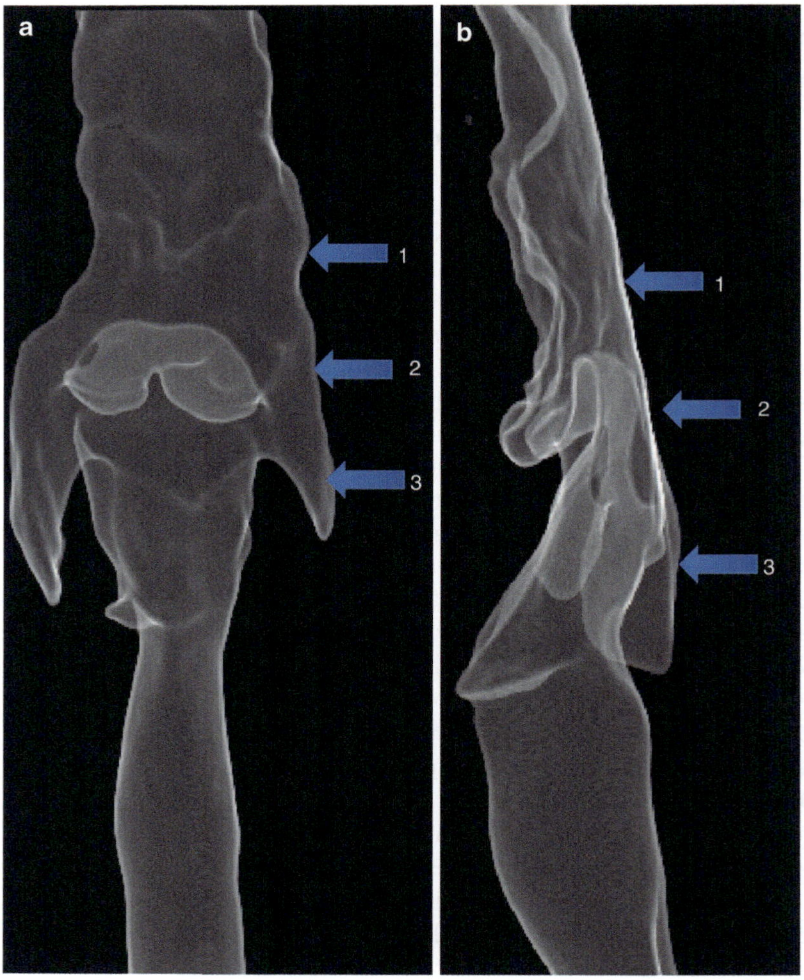

Fig. 8.56 CT volume rendering (VR) air reconstruction normal larynx. (**a**) Coronal view; (**b**) lateral view. The spaces area of the larynx: (1) supraglottal space, (2) transglottal space, (3) subglottal space

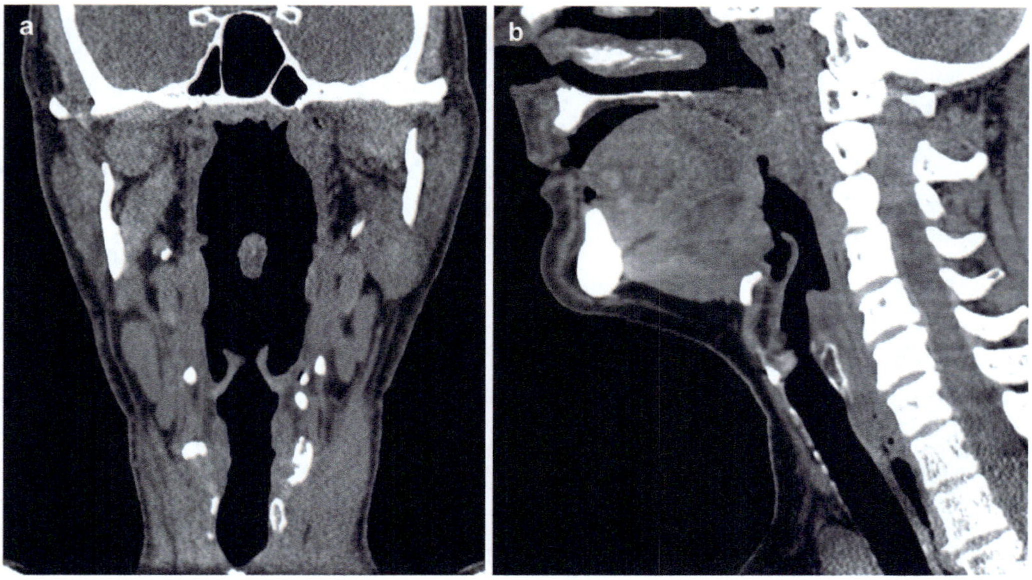

Fig. 8.57 (**a**) Coronal reconstructed CT image of the larynx during normal breathing shows the larynx at the level of the vocal cords; (**b**) sagittal reconstructed CT image of the larynx during phonation of /a/

in the vocal folds (Fig. 8.57a, b) (Bum-Soo et al. 2008). This capability might help in identifying the correct diagnosis of vocal fold palsy (Yumoto et al. 2004). However, radiology is mostly used in order to exclude other pathologies in the recurrent nerve area.

8.4.9.3 Magnetic Resonance Imaging

In contrast to CT technology, magnetic resonance imaging (MRI) is a common medical imaging technique with no known health risks. A further advantage of this technology is the high quality and resolution of soft tissues (Kim et al. 2009). Since the vocal tract consists of soft tissue walls, this technology can be considered superior for imaging the vocal tract. However, a significant drawback of using MRI in voice- and speech-related studies is the long scanning time. Therefore, in recent years, great focus has been placed on the aspect of acceleration (Scott et al. 2014). Up to now, it is possible to record an entire three-dimensional dataset of the vocal tract within 11 s for analysis (Echternach et al. 2011). However, recent experiments have shown the possibility of an acceleration up to 1.3 s per vocal tract.

Nowadays, by using dynamic real-time two-dimensional MRI, the vocal tract can be analysed for functional aspects, such as voice and speech production as well as swallowing (Echternach et al. 2012). Owing to its greater representation of soft tissues, tongue, velum, lips and larynx movements are of crucial interest. Changes in vocal tract shape are of relevance for voice production concerning changing resonatory properties of the vocal tract and for vocal tract voice source interactions. Furthermore, such speech articulatory aspects as constriction and closure gestures of the tongue tip and the tongue body can also be analysed. MRI movements of laryngeal inner structures such as the vocal folds become a challenge, but vertical

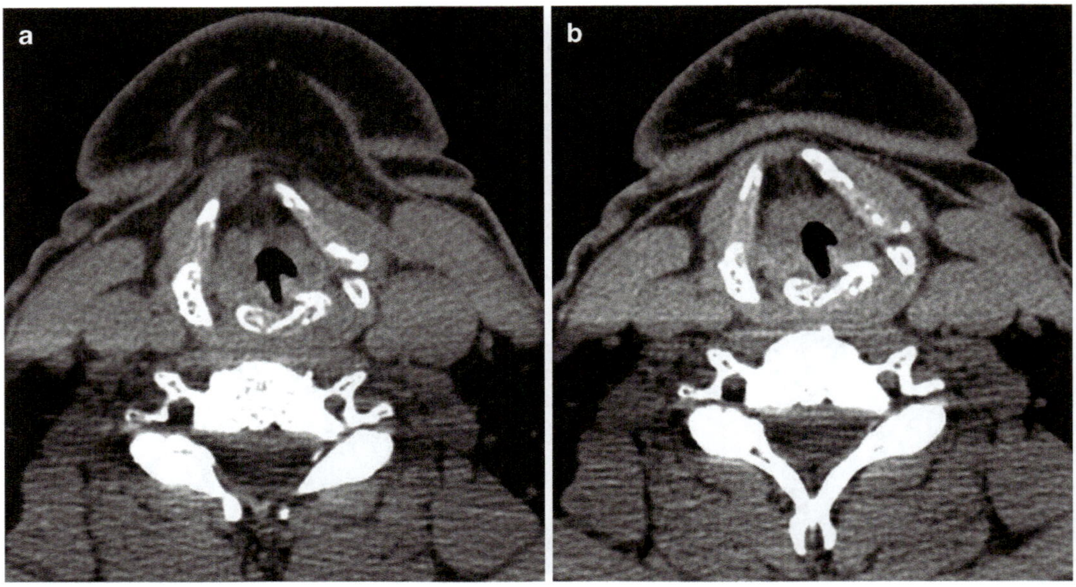

Fig. 8.58 (**a**) Sagittal image of a cine sequence during phonation (oe); (**b**) axial image

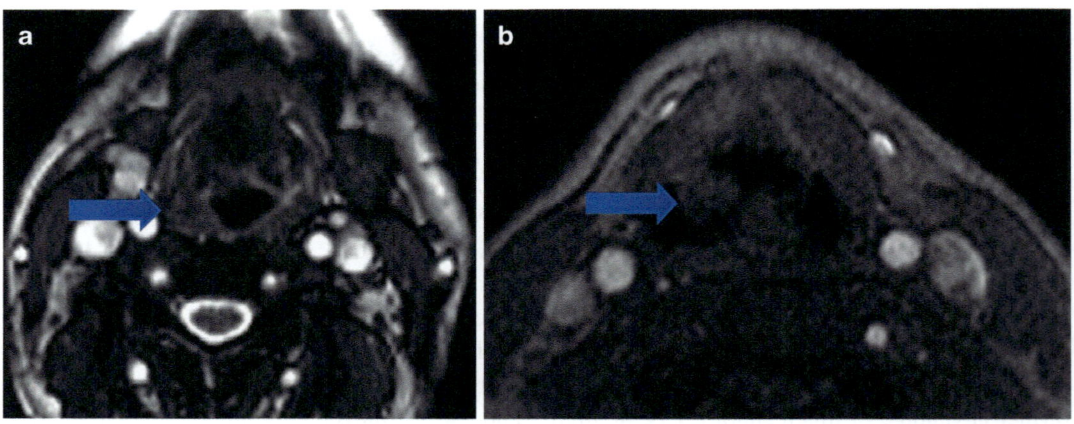

Fig. 8.59 (**a**) Axial view T2-weighted image of the larynx during normal breathing; (**b**) during phonation—on both vocal cords, small fibrotic lesions are marked by arrows

movements of the larynx can be observed during the production of some vowels and other speech sounds (Fig. 8.58a, b).

It should be mentioned, however, that all these recordings are performed from the supine position, which could have a major effect on both articulation and swallowing owing to gravitational forces. In contrast to speech, the vocal tract shape during singing is not considered so much influenced by the position (Traser et al. 2013). The study of the air space of the throat and larynx during obstruction, such as in sleep apnoea, and the study of patients with a deficit of voice/speech function before and after reconstructive surgery of the larynx are important in clinical practice (Fig. 8.59a, b). There are many challenges for

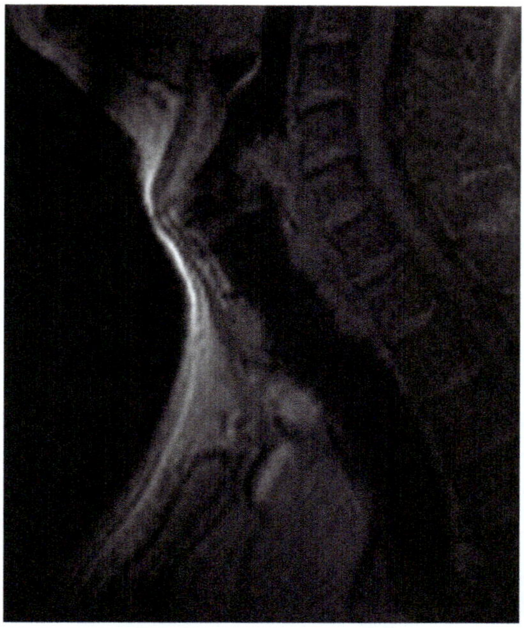

Fig. 8.60 Sagittal T1-weighted images (cine sequence) during swallowing

MRI of the vocal tract, such as respiration, swallowing and voice and speech movements, which require motion-insensitive imaging. All used sequences must be less sensitive to susceptibility artefacts (Fig. 8.60). Imaging during speech processes or in non-cooperative patients demands ultrafast imaging.

8.4.9.4 Three-Dimensional Imaging

In recent years, three-dimensional (3D) imaging of the upper airway during sustained sound production has emerged as a promising research tool in voice production as a means to capture the full geometry of the vocal tract. As a result, these models provide improved information on the visualisation of morphological and anatomical aspects and are useful for partial measurements of the vocal tract shape in different conditions. From these 3D-MRI data, calculations of resonance can be performed on 3D printouts (Fig. 8.61) or from estimations from area functions (Echternach et al. 2015). Furthermore, this material can be used for mathematical vocal tract modelling. From MRI images, it is possible to reconstruct the vocal tract shape and volume, as well as the shape and the dimension of the nasal tract, when the velum is lowered. In addition, the shape of the oral, pharyngeal and nasal cavities can be visualised. Three-dimensional high-resolution MRI, especially with parallel imaging of the upper airway, has provided valuable insights into vocal tract shaping as well as the data for the modelling of voice and speech production in different languages (Ventura et al. 2011). As a result, these computational models provide valuable information for the enhanced visualisation of morphological and anatomical aspects and are useful for partial measurements of the vocal tract shape in different conditions (Fig. 8.62). Potential use of this information can be found in medical and therapeutic applications as well as in acoustic articulatory voice and speech modelling (Baer et al. 1991).

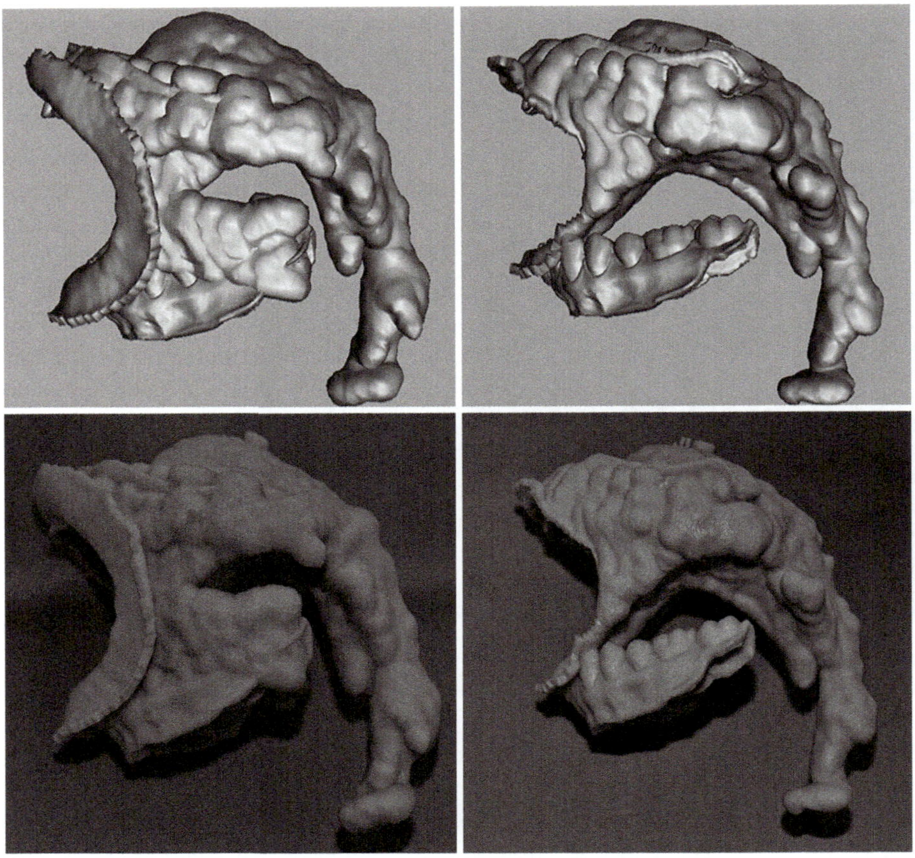

Fig. 8.61 Segmented vocal tract models from the MRI material (upper row, left, pitch C6, and right, pitch G6) and photographs of the 3D print outs (lower row, left, pitch C6, and right, pitch G6, respectively) (Reprinted with permission from Echternach M, Birkholz P, Traser L et al (2015) Articulation and vocal tract acoustics at soprano subject's high fundamental frequencies. J Acoust Soc Am 137(5):2586–2596. Copyright (2015), Acoustic Society of America). The models show the mouth on the left side. The models end at the glottal level. From these models resonatory properties of the vocal tract can be calculated

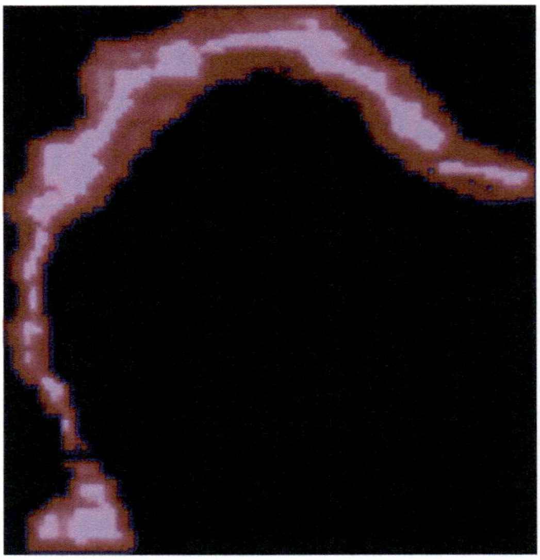

Fig. 8.62 High-resolution MRI 3D after reconstruction using parallel imaging and computer modelling of the upper airway. The shape of airspace during phonation

8.4.10 Ultrasound in Phoniatrics and Sonographic Examination of the Larynx

Wolfgang Angerstein

8.4.10.1 Ultrasound in Phoniatrics

Ultrasound application to living tissues has many advantages: it is harmless (no X-ray exposure) and non-invasive, therefore repeatable as often as necessary. Moreover, it is relatively simple and does not cause any discomfort for the patient. Therefore, it is well suited especially for children, even for small babies. And finally, it is relatively inexpensive compared with other imaging techniques such as CT or MRI.

Nowadays, mostly B-mode scans are used. In these two-dimensional images, different tissue densities are represented by different brightness grades (B = brightness) on the ultrasound screen. When a B-mode image is moved across the screen with constant velocity and the ultrasound transducer is always kept in the same place without being moved, a one-dimensional TM (time motion)-mode image results. Thus, B-mode lines in temporal order are continuously visible on the screen over the course of time.

By dividing the screen into two halves, B-mode may be combined with TM-mode. The TM-mode registers movement amplitudes of defined points at the surface of living tissues (e.g. vocal folds, epiglottis, tongue) over a period of time. The exact location of these surface points may be chosen with a cursor in the corresponding B-mode image during simultaneous recording of B- and TM-mode on the same screen.

Today, mainly high-resolution ultrasound probes with 7.5 or 19 MHz are used, either as linear array or as convex 90° resp. 100° sectorial scanners. In phoniatrics, the sonographic imaging mainly focuses on functional disturbances (dysfunctions) rather than on morphological alterations (see Table 8.13).

Table 8.13 Ultrasound in phoniatrics: spoken articulation, articulation for brass instrument playing, phonation, sucking, swallowing

Organ/region	Ultrasound technique
Lips	B-mode, colour duplex
Tongue	B-mode, TM-mode
Lateral hypopharyngeal walls, upper oesophageal sphincter	B-mode, TM-mode
Pseudoglottis (ructus)	B-mode, TM-mode
Larynx:	
Skeleton (ectolarynx), hyoid bone	B-mode
Vocal folds/vestibular folds (endolarynx)	Colour duplex, B-mode, TM-mode
Cervical veins (hyperfunctional dysphonia)	Colour duplex

8.4.10.2 Ultrasound Investigations of the Larynx

Sonographic Examination of the Larynx

The application of ultrasound to the larynx can be traced back to 1959; the first publications appeared in the 1960s (Beach and Kelsey 1969; Bordone-Sacerdote and Sacerdote 1965; Mensch 1964; Minifie et al. 1968). Sonographic examinations of the larynx are called echolaryngography, echoglottography, ultrasonoglottography, ultrasonic glottography or ultrasound glottography. The aim is an examination and documentation especially of the vocal folds but also of the ventricular folds. Their vibratory patterns during phonation can be observed and analysed. Furthermore, movements of the epiglottis, the vocal folds and the arytaenoid cartilages are visible.

Sonographic visibility of these structures is nevertheless limited by ossification of the thyroid cartilage (Bozzato et al. 2007): since the ultrasound beam is absorbed by ossified thyroid cartilage, a complete extinction of the sonographic signal or artefacts may result. Fortunately, this problem does not appear in children, because

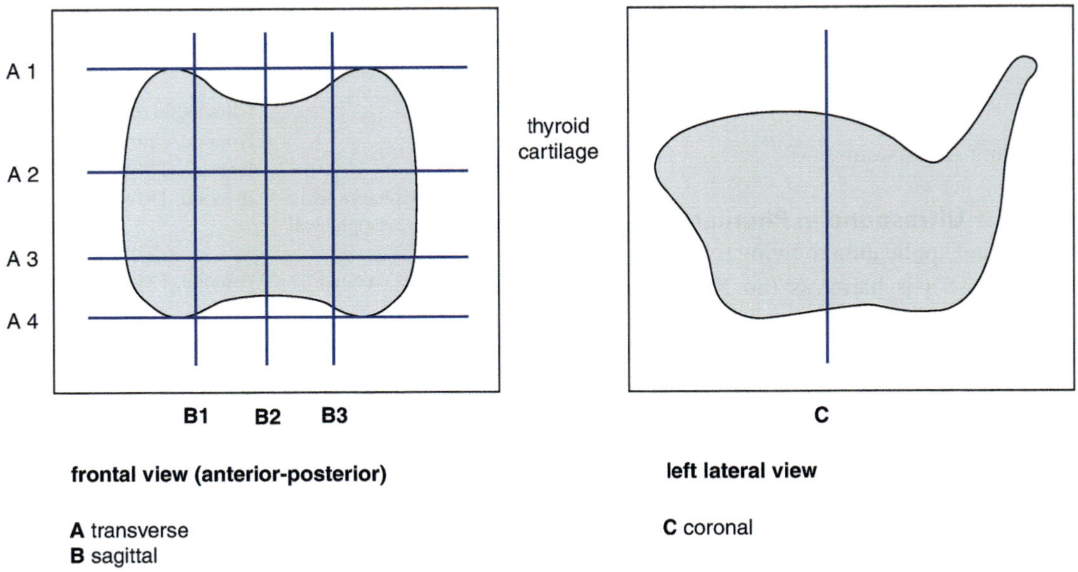

Fig. 8.63 Possible sectional planes for sonographic examination of the larynx

their thyroid cartilage is not yet calcified (Friedman 1997; Garel et al. 1990, 1992; Grunert et al. 1989; Raghavendra et al. 1987). Moreover, conventional transoral or transnasal laryngoscopy is often problematic in children. Therefore, sonographic examination of the larynx (especially the vocal folds) may be a non-invasive alternative to check hoarseness and other voice abnormalities in children. In grown-ups, echolaryngography may be helpful if the larynx is hard to examine by conventional endoscopy (e.g. in patients with a strong gag reflex, with increased pharyngeal or laryngeal muscle tension or with panic attacks). Moreover, irritations of the pharynx or larynx due to endoscopy can be avoided by sonographic imaging. Although the image resolution is not as good as in MRI or CT scans, sonography of the larynx can sometimes serve as a harmless screening method even if the thyroid cartilage is already calcified.

Examples of B- and TM-mode sonography are numerous (Arruti and Poumayrac 2010; Böhme 1988a, 1989; Gomaa et al. 2013; Miles 1989; Murlewska et al. 1992; Ooi 1992; Valente et al. 1996; Zappia and Campani 2000).

The patients are usually examined when in a supine position (alternatively, they sometimes may be reclined, with their neck well extended). Since the thyroid cartilage serves both as anatomical landmark and as acoustic window (facilitating sound transmission), the ultrasound transducer is usually placed horizontally parallel to the upper margin of the thyroid cartilage (A1 in Fig. 8.63) or approximately 2 cm below the thyroid notch (A2 in Fig. 8.63) with a slight caudal inclination, thus producing transverse B-mode scans of the supraglottal and glottal regions. The scanner is then continuously moved down along the midline of the thyroid cartilage. If the scanner is placed horizontally about 1 cm below the thyroid prominence (A3 in Fig. 8.63), the ultrasound beam has an anterior-posterior direction and corresponds to the horizontal level of the vocal folds.

For transverse B-mode scans, the probe may also be positioned horizontally at the ventral side of the neck with an inclination of 30–45° against the surface of the skin. The ultrasound beam is directed upwards through the ligamentum conicum, thus hitting the caudal surface of the glottis, coming from down below in a caudo-cranial direction (A4 in Fig. 8.63, see also Fig. 8.64).

Sagittal B-mode scans of the larynx in anterior-posterior direction are possible through the midline (midsagittal planes, B2 in Fig. 8.63) or through the right and left part of the thyroid cartilage (B1 and B3 in Fig. 8.63). The ultrasound

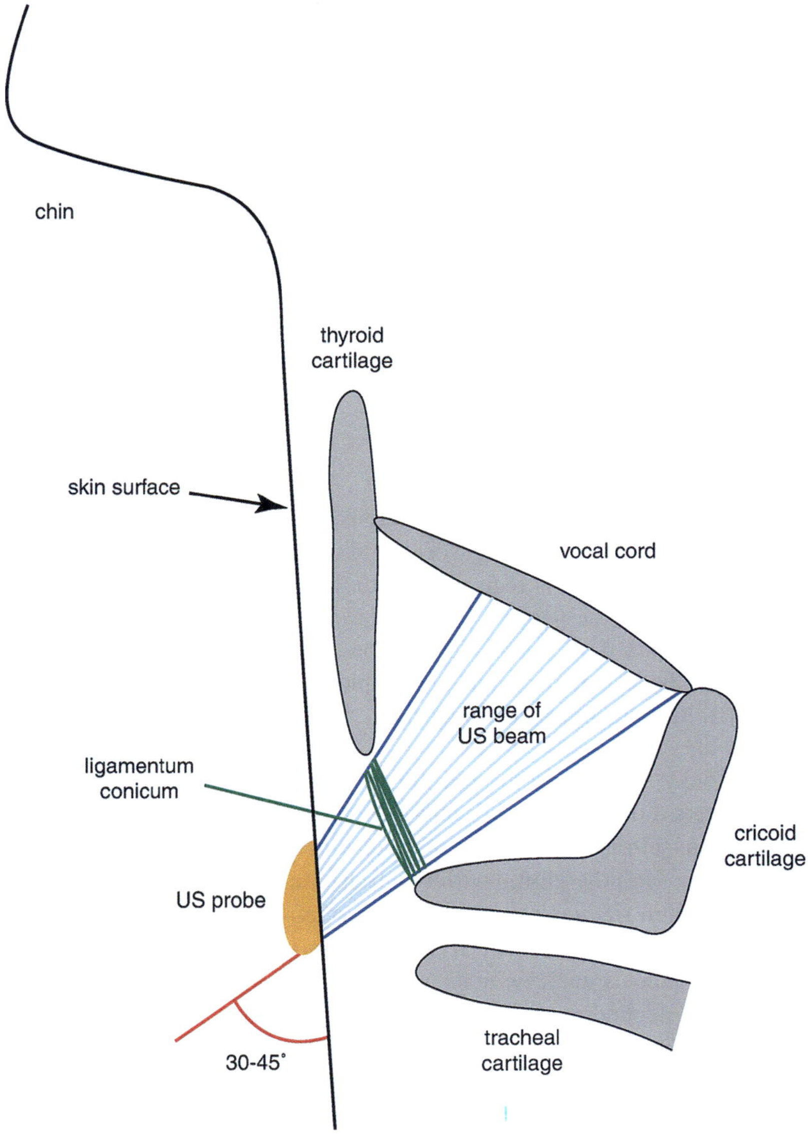

Fig. 8.64 Transverse ultrasound scanning of the glottis through the ligamentum conicum (left lateral view)

transducer is in a vertical position. In paramedian planes (B1 and B3 in Fig. 8.63), with a slight latero-medial inclination of the scanner, the recurrent laryngeal nerve may sometimes be seen as a linear structure behind or below the thyroid lobe.

For coronal B-mode scans of the glottis, the ultrasound probe is positioned vertically along the side of the neck (C in Fig. 8.63). The ultrasound beam is directed perpendicularly to the glottis, against the central parts of the thyroid cartilage and against the surface of the neck.

Movements of the vocal folds may also be observed with simultaneous B- and TM-mode registration in coronal planes. Simultaneous B- and TM-mode registration in sagittal planes shows vertical movements of the epiglottis during swallowing or phonation; simultaneous B- and TM-mode registration in transverse planes along the upper margin of the thyroid cartilage (A1 in Fig. 8.63) shows horizontal epiglottal movements.

Doppler Techniques in Larynx Investigation

By using ultrasonic Doppler techniques, voice alterations and vibratory patterns of the vocal folds during phonation can be observed. Thus, Doppler monitoring may increase the sensitivity of laryngeal B-mode examinations.

The Doppler technique rests on the principle that an echo reflected from a moving structure will be shifted in frequency in proportion to the velocity of the moving structure. At the glottal level, the Doppler frequency shift is produced by a reflection of the ultrasonic beam from the surface of the vibrating vocal folds during phonation.

The following Doppler techniques may be applied:

Pulsed Wave (PW) Method (with One Transducer)

Ultrasound pulses are emitted by a transducer and reflected by the vibrating vocal folds. The reflected signal (echo) is registered by the same transducer. Thus, the time-varying displacement of the vocal folds during phonation may be calculated with the Doppler formula as Doppler frequency shift of the reflected ultrasound.

Continuous Wave (CW) Method (with Two Transducers, a Transmitter and a Receiver)

Continuous ultrasound waves are transmitted laterally through the glottis with two transducers matched in frequency and located on opposite sides of the larynx. One transducer emits the ultrasound signal, which is frequency-modulated depending on vocal fold velocity and displacement during phonation. Only when the glottis is closed, the ultrasound signal is transmitted through the larynx. The ultrasonic beam passing through the vibrating vocal folds is periodically interrupted whenever the glottis is open during the vibratory cycle. This interruption depends on the fact that the acoustic impedance of air is much smaller than that of the vocal folds, and the frequency of the ultrasonic beam changes with the variations of the contact area of the vocal folds. Thus, the second transducer receives altered ultrasound waves with a frequency shift, the Doppler signal.

Duplex Sonography (Transverse B-Mode Scans Combined with PW Doppler)

Duplex sonography (Böhme 1991; Schindler et al. 1990) allows an identification of the glottis even when the vocal folds are not visible in B-mode scans: during phonation, a typical Doppler frequency shift signal may be recorded that is reflected from the surface of the vibrating vocal folds. This pulsed Doppler spectrum has a positive amplitude (above the horizontal baseline), when the vibrating vocal folds are moving towards the Doppler probe. When the vibrating vocal folds are moving away from the Doppler probe, the pulsed Doppler spectrum has a negative amplitude (below the horizontal baseline). The pulsed Doppler spectrum (also called echo Doppler sonogram) shows a fundamental frequency, upper harmonics and formants in the course of time during phonation. Depending on the sample volume (which can be chosen arbitrarily), defined segments of the vocal folds may be examined. Dysphonic voices are characterised by aperiodic echo Doppler sonograms: the more dysphonic the patient, the more structures of the pulsed Doppler spectrum disappear. Also, a time difference between the onset of positive and negative pulsed Doppler spectra may occur.

Colour Duplex Sonography (Colour-Coded Transverse B-Mode Scans Combined with PW Doppler)

This method detects a time difference between the onset of positive and negative pulsed Doppler spectra (Böhme 1992). When the vibrating vocal folds move towards the Doppler probe, the images are red. When they move away from the Doppler probe, the scans are dark blue. When the velocity of the vocal fold vibrations increases, the colour turns from red to orange or yellow. When the velocity decreases, the colour turns from dark blue to light blue or green. By colour Doppler imaging, vibrations of the glottal and supraglottal mucosa may be observed (Tsai et al. 2008), the effective vibration length of the vocal folds can

be measured (Hsiao et al. 2002), and the vocal fold mucosal wave velocity can be calculated (Hsiao et al. 2001; Shau et al. 2001).
A thorough sonographic laryngeal examination takes between 15 min (without Doppler) and 30 min (including Doppler).

Critical Evaluation of Laryngeal Doppler Sonography

Compared with other imaging techniques for analysing vibratory patterns of the vocal folds (e.g. stroboscopy, high-speed line scanning, kymography), the spatial and temporal resolution of laryngeal Doppler sonography is not yet satisfying and needs to be improved. The same is true for voice analyses: so far the accuracy of the echo Doppler sonogram is also not satisfying (Böhme 1991; Schindler et al. 1990). Compared with conventional acoustic voice analyses (e.g. jitter, shimmer, sonography, spectrography), the pulsed Doppler spectrum is still less precise, not so reliable and therefore less meaningful in clinical routine.

At the moment, laryngeal Doppler sonography is limited to screening tests. It may also give additional, supplementary information in combination with conventional diagnostic techniques. In order to become useful for routine clinical examinations of laryngeal function and voice quality, further development and research is needed.

8.4.10.3 Pseudoglottis of Laryngectomised Patients

By simultaneous recording of midsagittal or transverse B-mode and corresponding TM-mode images, vibrations of the pseudoglottis during a laryngeal ructus phonation can be observed (Böckler et al. 1988; Böhme 1988b). The ultrasound probe is positioned vertically in the midline (for midsagittal scans) or horizontally (for transverse scans) at the ventral side of the neck, right below the chin and just above the tracheostoma.

During ructus phonation of different vowels, mucosal vibrations in the pharyngo-oesophageal (PE) segment are clearly visible below the root of the tongue, both in B-mode and in TM-mode scans. Each vowel has a typical, easily reproducible sonographic pattern in the TM-mode. The length of the pseudoglottis (12–18 mm) can be determined in B-mode images by distinguishing vibrating from non-vibrating mucosal tissues of the PE segment between the base of the tongue and the upper oesophagus. The mucosal vibration rates of the pseudoglottis may be determined by counting the maxima of their vibratory amplitudes in TM-mode images. Alternatively, light and dark vertical stripes caused by vibrating mucosal tissues may be counted in the TM-mode images. These sonographic vibration rates of the PE segments (42–74 Hz) are in very good accordance with the fundamental frequencies of the simultaneously recorded ructus speech sounds (44–75 Hz).

By applying special software to the B-mode scans, surface contours of the vibrating mucosal tissues can be marked interactively image by image. When these surface contours are extracted and afterwards sampled in temporal order, a pseudo-3-dimensional (pseudo-3D) reconstruction of the pseudoglottis results. The vibrating mucosal tissues can be analysed over the course of time, since the extracted B-mode contours are lined up along a temporal axis. Thus, pseudoglottal vibrations lasting for several seconds may be summarised in one illustration.

Since ultrasound beams are reflected by implanted voice prostheses, vibrations of the pseudoglottis during ructus phonation can only be observed without voice prosthesis!

8.4.10.4 Cervical Venous Congestion in Hyperfunctional Dysphonia

The flow of blood through the veins of the neck is dependent upon:

- Intra-pulmonary or intrathoracic changes in pressure synchronous with breathing on inspiration and expiration (pathological thoracic breathing or poorly coordinated respiration and phonation in hyperfunctional vocalisation can contribute to reduced blood flow in the jugular vein!)
- The heartbeat (physiological changes in the axis of the heart and relative position of the heart valves during systole and diastole)

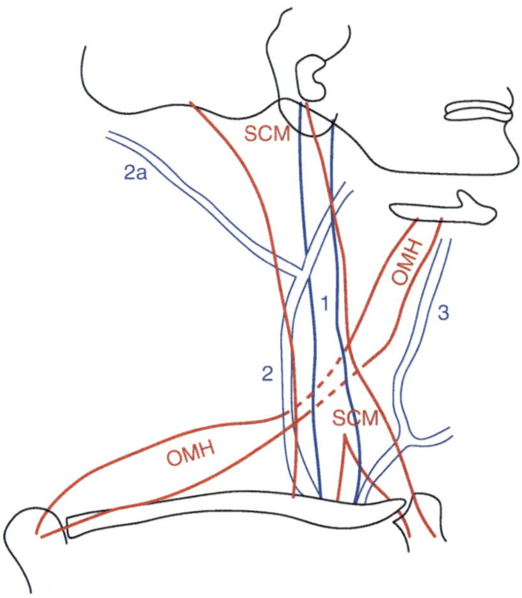

Fig. 8.65 This figure shows a schematic drawing of the topographic-anatomical relationships between the jugular veins, musculus sternocleidomastoideus and musculus omohyoideus. (Modified from Lanz and Wachsmuth 1955: Practical Anatomy). (1) V. jugularis interna; (2) V. jugularis externa [2a = V. jugularis externa posterior]; (3) V. jugularis anterior; *SCM* M. sternocleidomastoideus; *OMH* M. omohyoideus. (Copyright with kind permission from Springer Science and Bus Media BV)

Neck veins that are blocked and therefore engorged owing to strained, hyperfunctional vocalisation were described as early as 1920. This type of enlarged neck veins was not only observed in patients with hyperfunctional dysphonia but also often in woodwind and brass instrument musicians.

The cause of jugular vein distension is a distinct contraction (tension) in the sternocleidomastoid and omohyoid muscles. Figure 8.65 shows a scheme of the topographic-anatomical relationships between the jugular veins and both these muscles. The thin walls of the neck veins are easily 'squeezed' owing to these muscles' abnormal contraction, which can lead to an enormous reduction in blood circulation in the cervical veins.

The largest neck vein, the vena jugularis interna, is most easily seen on ultrasound imaging (Angerstein et al. 1993a, b). The large-calibre vena jugularis externa can also usually be displayed, especially when it is blocked and engorged through hyperfunctional vocalising. A blocked vena jugularis anterior can occasionally be displayed by using sonography.

Identification of the veins in the neck is made much simpler by using the Valsalva manoeuvre (voiceless pressing) which significantly enlarges the lumen of the vein. Dilated, swollen neck veins are then significantly easier to locate. The veins on the right side of the neck are, as a rule, wider and therefore easier to recognise and investigate than those on the left. The vena jugularis interna is also positioned slightly more laterally from the arteria carotis communis on the right side than the left vein, which often overlies the artery.

The ultrasound monitor should be divided vertically in the centre line: the right side should show B-mode sectional images of the lumen of the veins; the left side should show synchronous intravenous blood flow over time (i.e. the Doppler shift frequency spectrum of the speed of the blood flow). 'Pulsed wave' (PW) Doppler signals are also used here. Depiction of the veins of the neck by using B-mode sonography with a simultaneous PW Doppler spectrum is called duplex ultrasonography. Colour-coding these signals ('colour duplex sonography') has several benefits:

- Identification of the veins is easier (especially in children).
- The direction of blood flow (away from or towards the transducer) is discernible.
- Changes in the speed of blood flow can be visualised with colour gradation.

High-resolution 7.5 MHz linear transducers are used in colour duplex sonography of the jugular vein (5 MHz is also acceptable but the resolution is better with 7.5 MHz transducers). The investigation can be performed with the patient sitting or lying supine with the head rotated 10–15° to the opposite side. One advantage of the supine position is that the jugular veins have a higher filling state and are therefore easier to locate. The seated position (with upright upper body), however, has the advantage of being the usual position in which phonation takes place (vocalisation only occasionally takes place when in a supine position!). To avoid compression of the thin-walled veins of the neck, the transducer should be pressed onto the skin of the neck as lightly as possible. A large standoff distance (approx. 5 mm) by using a sufficient amount of ultrasound gel is absolutely necessary. The Doppler probe is held over the surface of the skin at an angle of 10–45° so that the ultrasonic checking is in the antero-caudal plane. The transducer is moved from a ventral position parallel to the course of the vein being investigated (e.g. the vena jugularis interna). The arteria carotis communis and musculus sternocleidomastoideus are useful 'landmarks' to help find the vena jugularis interna. Ideally, the veins should be shown in both longitudinal and cross sections, i.e. in two planes, though it is often only possible to show them longitudinally. The head and body position should vary as little as possible during the investigation in order to minimise any position-related changes of the blood flow in the jugular veins.

The so-called Doppler gate (the locally defined area of measurement inside the lumen of the vessel) should be adjusted to the individual vessel diameter. The size of the gate and the angle between the direction of blood flow and the gate should be kept as constant as possible throughout the entire investigation. This angle varies interindividually from 30° to 45°. The best possible quality of pulsed Doppler signals can be achieved by using a low repetition frequency of the B-mode images (0–2 images per second).

Common current signals of the jugular vein can be heard during Doppler sonography, the main one of which is a low-frequency breath-like noise, synchronous with breathing, which sounds similar to a humming ('venous hum') or the howling wind. This current noise is caused by respiration-dependent pressure changes in the veins of the neck, in which fluctuations in blood flow of 10–15% occur synchronously with breathing.

An investigation of jugular vein distension by colour duplex sonography takes 10–15 min for one side of the neck, depending on how visible the veins and the quality of the Doppler blood flow signal are.

By using colour Doppler one sees a clear reduction in venous blood flow of an average 74% (up to 90% in some individual cases!) in hyperfunctional vocalisation, and the thin-walled veins of the neck can more than double in diameter in comparison with the initial values during calm breathing without phonation. Following successful logopaedic treatment of hyperfunctional dysphonia, the blood flow in the jugular veins normalises, and the diameter during phonation reduces by at least 50%! In participants with healthy voices (with no hypertonic tension of the musculus sternocleidomastoideus or omohyoideus), blood flow in the veins of the neck during physiological phonation can reduce by approximately 10% in comparison with initial values during calm breathing without phonation. Such changes of venous blood flow and diameter can be monitored during the course of therapy non-invasively and without exposure to radiation by using colour duplex sonography. Because it is non-invasive and does not require exposure to radiation, colour duplex sonography is also suitable for visualising biofeedback (hyperfunctional versus relaxed vocalisation).

8.5 Estimation of Psychosocial and Psychobehavioural States

Charley Adams and Susanne Cook

8.5.1 Introduction

Sheehan (1970) developed the iceberg metaphor to describe stuttering because, like an iceberg, most of the problem of stuttering is not perceived by the listener. For example, soon after children begin to stutter, they may observe the reactions of others and realise that something is wrong. By the time they reach school, they may experience victimisation and bullying from classmates. These childhood experiences can activate emotional responses, which over time can bring fear and shame. In addition to thoughts and emotions surrounding stuttering, unseen to the listener are the increased effort to speak, as well as anticipation of stuttering (Jackson et al. 2015). The speech interruptions experienced by listeners are typically a fraction of the overall problem of stuttering. This section explores correlations between stuttering, personality traits and psychosocial factors, as well as their diagnostic and treatment implications. The following personality traits and psychosocial factors will be discussed: perfectionism, avoidance, neuroticism, anxiety, self-esteem and stigma. Suggestions for assessment in each of these domains will be provided.

8.5.2 Perfectionism

Johnson, Van Riper and Starkweather, among others, all believed that there was a correlation between stuttering and perfectionism (see Brocklehurst et al. 2015). Intolerance of imperfection may lead to feelings of low self-esteem and depression (Burns 1980). Because stuttering is seen by society as flawed (imperfect) speech, people who stutter may perceive fluent speech as perfect. Some research indicates that people who stutter are more perfectionist than people who do not (Amster 1995). Fear of stuttering (imperfect speech) can lead to verbal or situational avoidance behaviour (Adriaensens et al. 2015). Reducing perfectionism through cognitive-behavioural therapy is correlated with a reduction in the percentage of syllables stuttered (Klein and Amster 2004). Or, put another way, the less the participants focused on (or valued) more fluent speech, the more fluent their speech was.

Amster (1995) theorised that children with perfectionist tendencies are less likely to outgrow stuttering, regardless of therapy. People with perfectionist tendencies set unreasonably high standards for themselves or others (Hollender 1965). Brocklehurst et al. (2015) concluded that identifying the perfectionism profile of an adult who stutters is clinically relevant.

Perfectionism in light of stuttering can be assessed via the Frost Multi-dimensional Perfectionism Scale (FMPS; Frost et al. 1990). This inventory consists of 35 questions measuring the four subscales of perfectionism (concern over mistakes and doubts about actions, excessive concern with parents' expectations and evaluation, excessively high personal standards, concern with precision, order and organisation).

8.5.3 Avoidance Behaviour

Avoidance is a key factor in stuttering (Bloodstein and Bernstein-Ratner 2008; Shapiro 2011). Adults who stutter and who perceive stuttered speech as imperfect are more likely to engage in error avoidance behaviour (Brocklehurst et al. 2015). One extreme subset of people who stutter are those who stutter covertly, such that no overt behaviour can be detected and the person who stutters is able to pass as fluent (Constantino et al. 2017; Douglass et al. 2019). Douglass et al. (2019) refer to covert stuttering as 'an attempt to harness the able-bodied privileges that come with fluent speech' (p. 4). In their quest for fluency, adults who stutter may encounter increased cognitive demands (Brocklehurst et al. 2015). For those who stutter covertly, the easiest way to mitigate the risk of stuttering is to minimise exposure to talking situations (Guitar 2019). The upside might be an oversized vocabulary, allowing for split-second word changing as the person who stutters navigates the minefield of problem words and sounds. The downside, however, can be a reduced or absent social agenda, limited participation in occupational interactions and few if any meaningful conversations (Yaruss and Quesal 2004).

Avoidance as it relates to stuttering can be assessed via the Overall Assessment of the Speaker's Experience of Stuttering (OASES; Yaruss and Quesal 2006, see Sect. 8.1), the Wright & Ayre Stuttering Self-Rating Profile (WASSP, Wright & Ayre 2000) as well as by the Perception of Stuttering Inventory (PSI; Woolf 1967). The OASES-A (adult version) consists of 100 questions on a 5-point Likert scale to examine the overall impact of the stuttering on a person's life. It addresses the areas of (1) general information, (2) reactions to stuttering, (3) communication in daily situations and (4) quality of life. The PSI consists of 60 statements about stuttering. The person completing the questionnaire checks the statements that are applicable to him or her. Nineteen statements of this questionnaire relate to avoidance, for example, 'avoid talking to people in authority' or 'choosing a job or hobby because little speaking would be required'. The WASSP includes four items related to avoidance, such as avoiding certain words or specific situations (Wright & Ayre 2000).

8.5.4 Neuroticism

Neuroticism as a trait of personality describes negative responses to frustration, threat and loss (Lahey 2009), and is associated with reduced happiness and life satisfaction (Zhang et al. 2020). The five-factor model (Digman 1990; McCrae and John 1992) was developed to describe and outline personality differences. The NEO-Five Factor Inventory (NEO-FFI; Costa and McCrae 1992) was developed as a brief but reliable assessment of the five factors of personality: extroversion, neuroticism, openness to experience, conscientiousness and agreeableness. Iverach et al. (2010) used the NEO-FFI to look for personality trends among people who stutter. Results revealed high scores in the stuttering group for neuroticism, as well as low scores for conscientiousness and agreeableness in comparison to the standard scores.

Bleek et al. (2011) replicated Iverach et al.'s (2010) study with the addition of a control group matching for age and gender. Bleek et al. (2011) were able to confirm the elevated neuroticism scores for the stuttering group, but rather than finding lower scores for conscientiousness and agreeableness, they found significantly higher scores for those same two traits. These results strengthened the finding that neuroticism as a personality trait is more common among people who stutter than people who do not. One year later, Bleek et al. (2012) correlated both higher neuroticism scores and lower extroversion scores from the NEO-FFI with higher impact ratings on the OASES-A, further strengthening the personality trait of neuroticism as elevated in the stuttering population. Jafari et al. (2014) compared people who stutter with people who do not stutter by using the NEO-FFI, and found scores for conscientiousness to be significantly higher in the experimental than the control group. Significantly higher neuroticism scores for the control group could only be obtained after the four female participants were removed from each group. The authors suspect that their small sample size kept them from achieving significance of elevated neuroticism for the full cohort (Jafari et al. 2014).

The NEO-FFI can be used to assess personality traits, including neuroticism, as part of stuttering assessment for adults.

8.5.5 Anxiety

Rachman (2004) defines anxiety as a feeling of apprehension, as the tense, unsettling anticipation of a threatening but vague event. In a study of 132 children who stutter (mean age 11;8) and their mothers, Eggers, Millard and Kelman (2022) found that clinically elevated anxiety levels were more common in children who stutter than in the general population. Spielberger (1966, 1972) draws a distinction between 'state' anxiety and 'trait' anxiety. State anxiety is situation-specific, temporary and typically brief. Trait anxiety refers to an individual's inherent level of anxiety and reflects the different ways in which people interact with the world. Blood et al. (1994) demonstrated heightened state anxiety levels (as determined by salivary cortisol levels) in people who stutter during high stress situations versus age-matched controls who do not stutter. Davis et al. (2007) found that in three out of four speaking situations, adolescents who persisted in stuttering had higher levels of state anxiety than fluent control speakers. Lei, Sasisekaran, and Nguyen-Feng (2024) observed that adults who stutter and have high social trait anxiety tend to experience higher negative affect, lower positive affect, and greater stuttering severity compared to those with low social trait anxiety. Several evaluation tools have demonstrated consistently that trait anxiety levels in adults who stutter are higher than those of adults who do not stutter. Examples include the Trait Anxiety Questionnaire (Craig et al. 2003); Inventory of Interpersonal Situations (IIS; Kraaimaat et al. 2002) and the Cognitive Anxiety Scale (DiLollo et al. 2003). Ezrati-Vinacour and Levin (2004) found that while trait anxiety is not correlated with stuttering severity, state anxiety is; those who present with severe stuttering experience greater state anxiety than those whose stuttering is diagnosed as mild. On the basis of their research, Ezrati-Vinacour and Levin (2004) contend that anxiety is a personality trait of people who stutter.

Anxiety may be assessed with the State-Trait Anxiety Inventory (Spielberger 1983), the Erickson S-24 Scale (Erickson 1969; Andrews and Cutler 1974) and the Speech Situation Checklist (SSC; Brutten and Vanryckeghem 2007; Vanryckeghem 2007; Vanryckeghem and Brutten 2007).

8.5.6 Self-Esteem

Self-esteem is defined as 'an individual's positive or negative evaluation of himself or herself' (Smith et al. 2014). Shames and Rubin (1986) reported that the most common attitudes expressed by people who stutter are anxiety, helplessness, victimisation and low self-esteem. Some recent studies examined the relation between stuttering and self-esteem in children and adolescents. In their preliminary study of self-esteem, stigma and disclosure in adolescents who stutter (ages 13–18), Blood et al. (2003) found that the participants had positive self-esteem. The majority of the adolescents did not experience a negative impact of stuttering on their lives but would rarely or never discuss the topic of stuttering.

Zückner (2011) examined the self-esteem of 171 German children who stutter (ages 8–16). He found that children who stutter scored significantly higher as a group for self-esteem than fluent controls. The data for the children who stutter, however, showed a steady decline in self-esteem beginning at the age of 8. In another study, Davis et al. (2002) found that children who stutter were less popular than their non-stuttering peers, and were also less likely to be nominated as a leader. Klompas and Ross (2004) investigated the impact of stuttering on the lives of South African adults. Most participants felt that stuttering had affected their self-esteem and self-image, and their stuttering had evoked strong emotions within them. In his analysis of speech attitude of children who stutter, Boey (2010) found that a higher stuttering severity was associated with a more negative speech attitude.

In summary, a relation between self-esteem and stuttering seems to exist; however, the reviewed studies do not provide consistent results. As part of stuttering assessment, self-esteem can be evaluated with the Self-Esteem Questionnaire (DuBois et al. 1996) and the Rosenberg Self-Esteem Scale (RSES; Rosenberg 1965).

8.5.7 Stigma

Public stigma involves the negative cognitive, affective and behavioural reactions of members of the public to individuals with stigmatised conditions, in the form of stereotypes, prejudice and discrimination (Corrigan and Watson 2002). Public stigma for stuttering is well-documented; Kalinowski et al. (1996) found that people who stutter are often believed to possess several negative or undesirable personality characteristics, including being introverted, shy, anxious, nervous, quiet, tense, guarded, fearful, embarrassed and frustrated. Examples can also be found in pop culture. Bushey and Martin (1988) found numerous examples in children's literature, and Johnson (2008) found negative stereotypes of stuttering on television and in films. People who stutter are more likely to be the victims of teasing and bullying than people who do not stutter (Evans et al. 2008). Many believe that people who stutter may not be qualified for jobs that place a premium on oral communication (Gabel et al. 2004).

Self-stigma refers to the process of internalising public stigma (Corrigan et al. 2009). When a population is the victim of discrimination and stereotyping, those messages can over time begin to inhabit the beliefs of individuals within that population. For people who stutter, those messages include such adjectives as stupid, crazy, incompetent, foolish—and worse. This can ultimately impinge on decision making; participation in activities that include a fair amount of speaking, whether social, recreational or occupational, can become targets for avoidance (Daniels et al. 2006). Johnson et al. (2024) found that children as young as 10 years old can experience stuttering self-stigma, with its impact increasing during adolescence, a critical period for identity development. Notably, all stages of self-stigma were linked to negative outcomes related to stuttering, with later stages serving as stronger predictors, consistent with the progressive model of self-stigma.

The Self-Stigma of Stuttering Scale (4S; Boyle 2013) can be used to evaluate the experience of stigma associated with stuttering. An adapted version of the 4S scale for children, the Childhood Self-Stigma of Stuttering Scale (Child 4S) has been developed by Johnson et al. (2024).

8.5.8 Discussion and Conclusion

This section has explored correlations between stuttering, personality traits and behaviour such as perfectionism, avoidance, neuroticism, anxiety, self-esteem and stigma. The research highlighted indicates that these are features that are more common within the stuttering population than in their fluent cohorts. In addition to assessment of overt stuttering severity (such as with the SSI-4; Riley 2009) and the impact of stuttering (such as with the OASES; Yaruss and Quesal 2006), information gathered from administration of the assessments referred to in this article could also provide information for treatment for stuttering. For example, if the Frost Multidimensional Perfectionism Scale (FMPS; Frost et al. 1990) is administered and perfectionist tendencies are indicated, a cognitive-behavioural approach (CBT) may be selected in order to address perfectionism. Likewise, if scores on the State-Trait Anxiety Inventory (Spielberger 1983) indicate elevated levels of state anxiety, then mindfulness procedures may be considered for incorporation into or in conjunction with speech therapy. Similarly, if children exhibit high levels of self-stigma, targeted early interventions are essential to mitigate the long-term effects of stuttering-related self-stigma (Johnson et al., 2024).

8.6 Neuroimaging Findings in Stuttering

Katrin Neumann and Nicole E. Neef

8.6.1 Introduction

This section focuses on the neural basis of persistent developmental stuttering and elucidates the link of this speech fluency disorder with morphological and functional brain anomalies, particularly in circuits involved in speech, language and auditory processes. Broca's seminal post-mortem examinations on acquired language disorders, which occurred more than 150 years ago, became the cradle for human brain mapping studies. Since then, the literature has accumulated central knowledge on brain–behaviour relationships, also paving the way for neurological hypotheses on stuttering.

As early as 1927, the American physician Samuel Orton assumed aberrant functional lateralisation of cortical networks as the biological basis of developmental stuttering. Together with Lee Travis, the founding father of the profession of Speech-Language Pathology in America, he postulated a neurophysiological model according to which incomplete development of hemispheric dominance should lead to inefficient activation of motor control regions, which in turn produce prolongations, repetitions and blockages at the level of speech production (Orton 1927, 1928; Travis 1931, 1978). However, empirical studies of the structural and functional features in the brains of people who stutter did not begin until the mid-1980s. Since then, the development and application of modern neuroimaging methods have revolutionised our understanding of the pathophysiology of stuttering.

Although the early model proposed by Orton and Travis was not supported by experimental data, the idea that atypical brain processing for speech somehow plays a role in stuttering has received ongoing attention over the years. Neuroscientific hypotheses for the genesis of stuttering include altered hemisphere dominance structure, an imbalance between ventral and dorsal language network functioning, basal ganglia dysfunction, disconnection of parts of speech-language networks, altered cerebral timing in language networks, impaired sensorimotor integration—all of which seem plausible given the complex and interwoven cognitive, linguistic and sensorimotor processes required for speech production (Neumann and Foundas 2018). The generation of speech fluency requires ongoing dynamic interactions between auditory, somatosensory and speech motor neuron networks.

Before the neuroimaging era, the main source of data on mechanisms underlying language came from lesion studies: damaged brain regions were associated with compromised functions. The advent of modern neuroimaging brought about great advantages. Measurements nowadays can be performed non-invasively in subjects with normal psychological and physiological responses. Because neuroimaging is not limited to a region that has been damaged, but is able to explore 'normal' or compensatory cognitive, sensory and motor processing functions, it can identify functional specialisation in circuits that preserve functionality by cognitive or neuronal reorganisation (Neumann and Euler 2010).

The past 25 years of neuroimaging have given unprecedented insights into the brain's signatures of developmental stuttering. While neuroimaging is no tool to clarify and diagnose developmental stuttering, imaging findings have (1) caused a paradigm shift towards classifying stuttering as a neurodevelopmental speech disorder, (2) elucidated neural signatures of stuttering as a trait, i.e. permanent cerebral characteristics, and as a state, i.e. a transiently occurring functional impairment, (3) detected markers of persistence and spontaneous recovery, (4) provided neurobiologically based explanations for treatment effects and (5) motivated novel therapeutic strategies. Here, we briefly summarise robust imaging findings on stuttering as derived from studies with adults and children who stutter. In addition, we outline actual and potential neuromodulatory attempts to treat stuttering.

8.6.2 Paradigm Shift in the Attribution of Causes of Stuttering

Neuroimaging studies uncovered brain differences between people who stutter and fluent speakers. Such findings called the previous view on the causes of stuttering into question. As a result, it is no longer acceptable to attribute childhood traumata or an overly anxious personality to the causes of stuttering (Chang 2011). Instead, explanatory accounts shifted from a psychogenic to a neurogenic explanation of the disorder, a rationale further supported by the proven heritability (see Sect. 6.4). It is essential to note that some neuroimaging findings strongly support the viewpoint of a primary neurological dysfunction of genetic origin as the cause of stuttering. However, for other findings, it remains to be determined whether they are causal or a mere reflection of experience-dependent processes that follow the appearance of persistent stuttering (Connally et al. 2018).

8.6.3 Neural Signatures of the Stuttering Trait and State

Morphological and functional brain anomalies implicate the sensory, motor and premotor cortices, inferior frontal gyrus (IFG), supplementary motor area (SMA), basal ganglia, cerebellum and connecting white matter tracts (for reviews, see Chang and Guenther 2020; Craig-McQuaide et al. 2014; Neef and Chang 2024, Watkins et al. 2016). Implicated structures do not autonomously control specific speech functions, e.g. the IFG does not produce words and utterances on its own, but involved neural populations are intra- and interconnected and form overlapping and segregated dynamic circuits and networks to drive the speech system. For example, the left IFG together with posterior temporal and middle temporal regions support the access and retrieval of words (Price 2012), while the left inferior frontal sulcus together with preSMA, as part of the cortico-basal ganglia-thalamo-cortical loops, support the planning of speech movements, and the left ventral premotor cortex together with the SMA, as part of the cortico-basal ganglia-thalamo-cortical loops, supports the initiation and production of overlearned motor sequences such as speech patterns (Guenther 2016).

Modern literature on stuttering often differentiates between trait and state of stuttering. 'Trait' in this context refers to the permanent cerebral characteristics, features or qualities that shape individuals' stuttering, which are expressed through their behaviour, speech, actions and feelings; whereas 'state' refers to temporary conditions that alternate with other conditions. Since stuttering fluctuates greatly situationally, it is particularly important to make this distinction while planning neuroimaging studies and interpreting their results.

Stuttering trait signatures predominantly evolve from cross-sectional case–control studies, mainly with adults with long-time experience of stuttering. One characteristic trait marker is the reduced white matter integrity of left hemisphere fibre tracts that connect the frontal articulatory motor and premotor regions with parietal and temporal speech processing hubs (Chang et al. 2008; Connally et al. 2014; Kell et al. 2009; Kronfeld-Duenias et al. 2016; Neef et al. 2015a, 2017; Sommer et al. 2002; Watkins et al. 2008). Further frequent observations are reduced activity of the *left* pre-central gyrus and posterior superior temporal gyrus combined with increased *right* frontal and parietal activity (Belyk et al. 2015). In contrast, stuttering state, i.e. signatures of the functional impairment itself, evolve from experiments testing brain activity within people who stutter under disfluent and fluency-enhancing conditions, such as speaking to the beat of a metronome or speaking together with another speaker (chorus speaking). The stuttering state during overt speaking involves the left IFG pars opercularis and the right IFG pars orbitalis, pre-central gyrus, precuneus and the bilateral preSMA/SMA (Belyk et al. 2015). Another appraoch that offered deeper insights into the neural causes of stuttering was a sophisticated network analysis of stroke-induced brain lesions leading to acquired stuttering. This analysis linked stuttering to key deep brain structures, including the putamen, amygdala, and claustrum and their functional connectivity (Theys et al. 2024), highlighting these regions as critical hubs in the neural network underlying stuttering.

Theories link neuroimaging findings with possible explanations of why stuttering occurs. The most noted accounts discuss stuttering to result from (1) abnormal cerebral lateralisation, (Brown et al. 2005, Demirel et al. 2024) (2) abnormal sensorimotor integration and (3) abnormal basal ganglia function (Alm 2004, Chang and Guenther 2020; Watkins et al. 2016) and (4) more recently from hyperactive action inhibition circuits (Metzger et al. 2018; Neef et al. 2017; Neef et al. 2023).

8.6.4 Markers of Persistence

Because developmental stuttering has a high rate of spontaneous recovery with up to 75% of initially affected children (Yairi and Ambrose 2013), it is desirable to find early markers of persistence in order to predict prognosis and triage treatment. These crucial aims can be addressed with cross-sectional brain investigations that compare persistent stuttering cases with assisted recovery cases in adulthood (Kell et al. 2009), with longitudinal investigations during development (Chow et al. 2017, Chow et al. 2023) or therapy (Watkins et al. 2016) or with large population-based prospective cohort investigations from foetal life until young adulthood (Koenraads et al. 2019, 2020).

Persistence and unassisted recovery in adulthood are associated with a reduced grey matter volume in the anterior dorsal left IFG pars opercularis (Kell et al. 2009). However, while persistent cases over-activate the right IFG pars orbitalis, i.e. in the Brodmann area (BA) 47/12 while speaking, recovered cases activate in addition to their right IFG the left hemisphere homologue. These findings imply that a neural marker of persistence is a grey matter deficit in the left IFG, while a neural marker of spontaneous repair is the additional functional recruitment of the left orbitofrontal cortex (Kell et al. 2009). Furthermore, persistent adult stuttering is linked to altered auditory-to-motor coupling and somatosensory feedback integration via frontoparietal and frontotemporal speech regions (Kell et al. 2018; Neumann et al. 2018). Unlike persistence, recovery is associated with normalised cortical-to-cortical sensorimotor processing but a functional uncoupling of the obviously dysfunctional caudal superior cerebellum from the rest of the speech production network by the left orbitofrontal cortex (BA 47/12) (Kell et al. 2018).

Only few laboratories set out for a longitudinal investigation of stuttering during development. *Structural* brain data from children aged 3 to 10 years revealed that persistence relates to a reduced cortical thickness in left motor and lateral premotor cortical regions (Garnett et al. 2018). This observation is in line with an earlier cross-sectional study that found, in addition, a smaller grey matter volume of the bilateral IFG (Beal et al. 2013). A recent population-based study also confirms the grey matter deficit in the left inferior frontal gyrus and SMA (Koenraads et al. 2019) and reports a grey matter deficit in the left superior frontal grey matter (Koenraads et al. 2020). In summary, *structural* imaging findings in children imply a primary deficit in left frontal brain hubs of speech motor control, consistent with findings in adults with persistent stuttering (Craig-McQuaide et al. 2014; Kell et al. 2009; Watkins et al. 2016).

Functional brain data of children can predict stuttering persistence. A feasible approach is resting-state scanning, particularly for young children because it is not required to engage them in a speech task. During resting-state functional magnetic resonance imaging (rs-fMRI), participants lie quietly in the MR scanner without doing anything. With rs-fMRI it is possible to study intrinsic networks of the brain. Such intrinsic networks arise from the correlated spontaneous neuronal activity of local and distant brain regions and likely reflect actual structural connections (Deco et al. 2013). Analysis of the brains' spontaneous activity at rest revealed at least seven distinct networks that can be attributed to distinct functional systems. For example, the sensory and motor cortices cluster separately from visual areas, limbic areas and the association cortex (Yeo et al. 2011). One of the more studied intrinsic networks is the so-called default mode network. This consists of a set of brain regions that become active during wakeful rest and are deactivated when solving tasks.

In children, whole-brain intrinsic network connectivity analyses link persistence of stuttering to anomalous functional connectivity within the default mode network and between the default mode network and task-positive networks that become active during solving tasks, i.e. the frontoparietal network (involved in sustained attention and problem-solving, working memory-related) and the dorsal attention network (involved in solving attention-demanding tasks) (Chang et al. 2018). Altered network organisations support the view of developmental stuttering as a system-level disorder. Specifically, it is assumed that stuttering is not caused by local brain abnormalities, but by altered dynamics of neural networks involved in speech processing. Longitudinal studies with children who stutter provide the first evidence that developmental trajectories of functional and structural brain changes during maturation are broadly affected. Involved are not only sensorimotor integration and speech motor control but attentional, cognitive and emotional systems. This finding holds even when leveraging big data from the Human Connectome Project and the Adolescent Brain Cognitive Development (Rutherford et al. 2021).

8.6.5 Treatment Effects

To date, only a few research groups have investigated the neuroplasticity potential of intensive stuttering interventions in longitudinal studies (Table 8.14). Existing studies evaluated mainly the neural reorganisation after intensive fluency

Table 8.14 Structural and functional brain responses to treatment and unassisted recovery in adulthood

Study	Number of participants (age range)	Method *Task*	Place *Intervention*	Time	Post-treatment outcome
De Nil et al. (2001)	13 AWS and 10 AWNS (20–45)	Functional PET *Overt reading* *Covert reading* *Verb generation*	Toronto, CA Fluency shaping	3-week intensive 1-year maintenance	• Increased cerebellar activation during reading after therapy • Decreased to normal activation after 1 year • Gradual decrease of activity for verb generation
De Nil et al. (2004)	13 AWS (20–40) 10 AWNS (19–34)	Functional PET *Overt reading* *Covert reading*	Toronto, CA Fluency shaping	3-week intensive 1-year maintenance	• Changes in activation lateralisation • Reduction in over-activation in the primary motor cortex
Neumann et al. (2003, 2005)	9 AWS (24–41) 16 AWNS (19–51)	Functional MRI *Overt reading* *Semantic decision*	Kassel, DE Fluency shaping	3-week intensive	• Widespread left-lateralised frontal and bilateral temporal activation • Increased activation of the anterior cingulum, insula and putamen was related to reduced stuttering
	5 AWS (19–41)			2-year follow-up after 1–2 years maintenance program	• Over-activations slightly reduced and still more right-sided together with slightly increased stuttering • Left-frontal deactivations over 2 years, unchanged by therapy
Kell et al. (2009)	13 AWNS (23–44) 13 AWSa (18–39) 13 AWSr (16–65)	Functional MRI *Overt reading* *Covert reading* Structural MRI *GM, WM*	Kassel, DE Fluency shaping	3-week intensive 1-year maintenance	• AWSa: re-lateralised activity to the left hemisphere with reduced over-activation right frontoparietal including the frontal operculum • AWSr: long-term repair engaged left BA47/12 • AWSr: less left inferior frontal structural anomalies
Kell et al. (2018)					• AWSa: reduced hyper-connectivity between SMG and prefrontal cortex and increased functional connectivity between articulatory motor cortex and aSTG • AWSr: additionally decoupled the superior cerebellum from the rest of the speech production network by left BA 47/12 activity
Neumann et al. (2018)		*Overt reading with modulated prosody*			• Normalised left IFG activity together with normalised prosody
Korzeczek et al. (2021)	28 AWNS (14–52) 22 AWS+ (14–57) 18 AWS– (26–47)	Functional MRI *Resting-state*	Kassel, DE Fluency shaping	3-week intensive 1-year maintenance	• AWS+: strengthened resting-state connectivity of the dorsal laryngeal motor cortex with the left IFG and the right pSTG
Neef et al. (2021)		Structural MRI *WM*	Kassel, DE Fluency shaping	3-week intensive 1-year maintenance	• AWS+: no changes in laryngeal motor cortices' white matter connections

(continued)

Table 8.14 (continued)

Study	Number of participants (age range)	Method *Task*	Place *Intervention*	Time	Post-treatment outcome
Lu et al. (2012, 2017)	13 AWNS (24) 15 AWS+ (24) 13 AWS- (29)	Functional MRI *Resting-state* *Overt reading* Structural MRI *GM*	Beijing, CN Repeat/read two-syllable words to train voicing patterns and phonological awareness	7-day intensive	• Reduced cerebellum rs-fMRI connectivity • Unchanged left IFG rs-fMRI connectivity • Increased left ventral IFC/insula task activity • Unchanged cortical thickness • Cerebellum may reorganise the functional architecture of speech-language processes
Toyomura et al. (2015)	10 AWNS (22–23) 10 AWS (20–31)	Functional MRI *Overt reading*	Tokyo, JP Metronome Speaking	8-week 15 min per day 5 days per week	• No difference between groups • Basal ganglia and cerebellum are involved in improved speech fluency due to external triggers

aSTG—anterior superior temporal gyrus, AWNS—adults who do not stutter, AWS—adults who stutter, AWSa—assisted recovery, AWSr—spontaneous recovery, AWS+—with therapy, AWS-—without therapy, GM—grey matter, pSTG—posterior superior temporal gyrus, SMG—supramarginal gyrus, WM—white matter shaping therapy (see Sect. 10.2). Fluency shaping is an all-encompassing speech restructuring method that requires individuals to change their whole speech patterns, that is, to speak slowly with gentle onsets of phonation and only slight contacts of the constrictions formed by the lips, teeth, palate, tongue, pharynx and larynx during articulation, while keeping the voice on. First studies report local and distributed brain activity changes in the left IFG, the right orbitofrontal cortex (BA 47/12) which compensates for the left IFG, the cerebellum and basal ganglia, and a re-lateralisation of frontal activity (Neumann et al. 2003; De Nil et al. 2004, 2001). Observed re-lateralisation is interpreted as normalisation of brain activity because left frontal brain structures that show reduced activity before treatment show increased activity after treatment, while right orbitofrontal structures in the BA 47/12 that are hyperactive before treatment have reduced hyperactivity after treatment (Kell et al. 2009; Neumann et al. 2003, 2005; De Nil et al. 2004). Furthermore, cumulating evidence relates fluency shaping treatment to a strengthened interaction between brain structures that support auditory-to-motor mapping. In particular, treatment strengthens the speech-specific functional connectivity between the articulatory motor cortex and the auditory anterior superior temporal gyrus (Kell et al. 2009, 2018; Neumann et al. 2018). In this vein, spontaneous resting-state functional connectivity was also strengthened after treatment. Especially, connectivity increased between the left laryngeal motor cortex and the speech planning left IFG pars opercularis and between the left laryngeal motor cortex and the auditory feedback processing right posterior superior temporal gyrus (Korzeczek et al. 2021). Other studies show that stuttering treatment regulates cerebellar activity, which might be related to sequencing and subsyllabic sound structure (Lu et al. 2012). Finally, basal ganglia and cerebellar structures seem to integrate external timing cues while enhancing speech fluency (Kell et al. 2009; Neumann et al. 2003; Toyomura et al. 2015).

The few existing studies are often based on small samples and replication studies are needed to gain a consistent picture. For example, the findings of one of the early intervention studies (Neumann et al. 2003, 2005), which also included longitudinal measurements after a 2-year follow-up (Neumann et al. 2003), were partially replicated with a novel sample (Kell et al. 2009, 2018; Neumann et al. 2018). This replication provided strong support for the view that hyperactive right-frontal areas, in particular the over-activation of the right orbitofrontal cortex (BA 47/12), likely reflect compensatory activity. This interpretation is supported by two observations. First, before therapy, BA 47/12 activity was negatively correlated with stuttering severity, and secondly, fluency-shaping therapy reduced right BA 47/12 hyperactivity and increased activity within left cortical speech network hubs. It seems that therapy nearly normalised brain activity possibly owing to vitalised auditory-motor and somatosensory feedback processes (Fig. 8.66, Table 8.14). Thus, these and other treatment studies (Table 8.14) demonstrate neural changes following fluency shaping therapy.

However, fluency-shaping programmes are not the only approach to treat stuttering. Besides this speech motor intervention that reshapes laryngeal, articulatory or respiratory speech patterns as a whole, common further stuttering interventions consist of (1) speech motor interventions that aim at modifying exclusively stuttering events, (2) feedback and technology interventions which use, e.g. delayed auditory feedback to enhance fluency, or visual feedback to support speech motor interventions, (3) behavioural modification interventions or (4) cognitive interventions improving psychological well-being, self-confidence and self-conception. Most studies tested neurofunctional correlates of brain reorganisation for fluency shaping, metronome speaking and auditory feedback interventions. However, the neurobiological foundation of an intervention-induced relief from stuttering induced by other approaches, such as stuttering modification and the cognitive-behaviour inter-

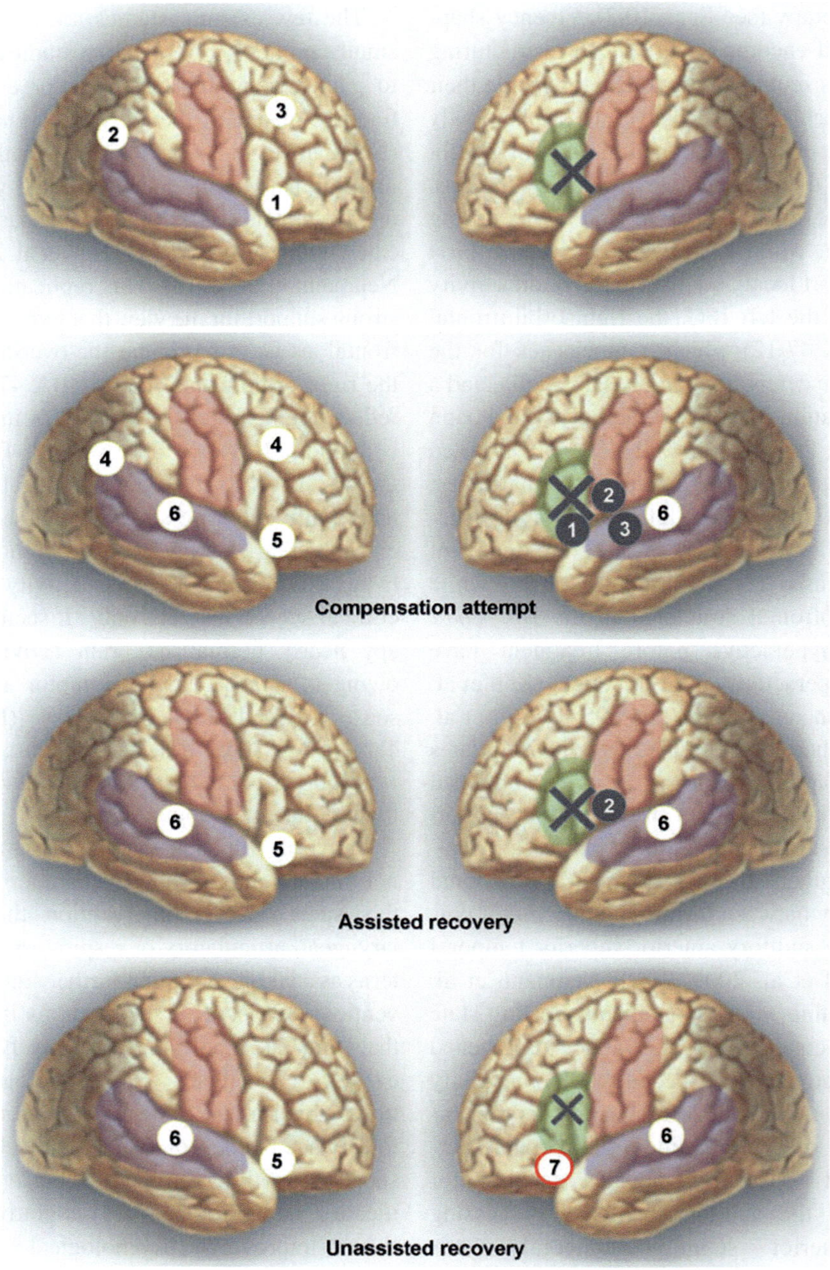

Fig. 8.66 Schematic overview of speech production in fluent speakers and males who stutter. (**a**) (Top, 2 figures) During talking, non-stuttering subjects activate the left inferior frontal cortex (green; speech planning and executive control of speech), bilateral superior temporal cortex (lavender: phonological perception and auditory feedback) and the bilateral speech motor cortex (light pink). In contrast, people who stutter have structural deficits in left-frontal structures (cross) and over-activate right-hemispheric areas, especially the frontal operculum (1), the temporo-parietal junction (2) and the dorsolateral prefrontal cortex (3) during speaking. (**b**) (Bottom, 6 figures) Functional correlates of stuttering: left anterior insula (1), articulatory motor cortex (2) and planum polare (3) close to the anatomical anomalies (grey cross). Recruitment of right-hemispheric dorsal language systems (4) and orbitofrontal BA 47/12 (5) partly reduces symptom severity (compensation attempt). Therapy restricts over-activation to the ventral language network including right BA 47/12 (5) and bilateral auditory cortex (6), and nearly normalises perisylvian function. Unassisted recovery in adulthood additionally involves left BA 47/12 (7) and is associated with less left inferior frontal structural anomalies. (Modified from Kell CA, Neumann K, von Kriegstein K et al. (2009) How the brain repairs stuttering. Brain 132:2747–2760 by permission of Oxford University Press)

vention (Menzies et al. 2016), would be worth studying.

Taken together, it becomes evident that neuroimaging studies provide the opportunity to test the neurobiological basis of treatment effects (Ingham et al. 2018). Moreover, reports noticeably reconcile theories and models of stuttering (Neumann and Foundas 2018). The above-named intervention studies opened the window towards a better understanding of treatment effects and paved the way for novel rationally-designed treatments. Future studies should also take into account that stuttering is a heterogeneous disorder, with possible subtypes, and that—as not all results have been replicated (e.g. Lu et al. 2012 vs. Lu et al. 2017)—further replication studies are needed.

8.6.6 Novel and Potential Therapeutic Strategies

Early neurological attempts to improve persistent developmental stuttering involve (so-far unsuccessful) pharmacological trials (see Sect. 10.6). More recent strategies explore brain stimulation techniques. But strikingly, such stimulation attempts would be impossible without the essential insights gained from neuroimaging studies, which support accumulating knowledge about the potential neurophysiological basis of stuttered speech.

Transcranial direct current stimulation (tDCS) is a non-invasive stimulation of the brain via electrodes placed on the scalp (Nitsche and Paulus 2000). The application of such tDCS, specifically for 20 min with 1-mA anodal tDCS over the left IFG, combined with choral and metronome-timed speaking, results in a higher reduction of stuttering than choral and metronome-timed speaking without tDCS (Chesters et al. 2018). In contrast, a single tDCS session revealed no significant effect (Chesters et al. 2017). Notably, the montage of the stimulating anodal electrode was derived from previous neuroimaging studies. The anodal electrode covered the left IFG, ventral premotor and sensorimotor cortex. Recalling the above-mentioned functional and structural imaging findings, the left IFG appears to be a critical site because it has a reduced grey matter volume in affected children and adults and is less active during stuttering, and IFG stimulation demonstrably improves the outcome of speech fluency training. The authors suggest that future studies should test the feasibility of combining tDCS with conventional clinical interventions. It is a low-cost, low-maintenance technique that might improve therapeutic efficacy, boost outcomes and prevent relapses (Chesters et al. 2018). Indeed, a randomised, double-blind, sham-controlled clinical trial was recently performed to investigate the effects of combined tDCS and delayed auditory feedback (DAF, see Sect. 10.5) intervention. Fifty participants were randomly assigned to two groups, where participants either received six sessions of DAF combined with anodal tDCS or of DAF combined with a sham tDCS. In the anodal tDCS group, the proportion of stutter-typical disfluencies and stuttering severity were reduced significantly, indicating that anodal tDCS when combined with DAF may enhance stuttering reduction effects at least for 6 weeks following the intervention (Moein et al. 2022).

Deep brain stimulation (DBS) is an invasive stimulation via electrodes implanted mainly into subcortical structures, i.e. subthalamic nucleus, globus pallidus, nucleus accumbens, thalamus and cerebellum. DBS is accepted for treatment of movement disorders such as essential tremor and Parkinson's disease and has been experimentally tested to treat dystonia, Tourette syndrome and depression. Neurogenic speech disfluencies have been shown to either worsen (in the majority of cases reported in the literature) or improve owing to uni- or bi-lateral DBS of the globus pallidus internus (GPi), the subthalamic nucleus (STN) or the ventral intermediate nucleus (VIM) of the thalamus in patients with Parkinson's disease, obsessive–compulsive disorder, dystonia, essential tremor, Tourette syndrome or similar diseases. However, in a female with persistent developmental stuttering from childhood who underwent DBS in the left VIM because of essential tremor of her right upper extremity, stutter-typical disfluencies were reduced both in frequency and duration (Maguire et al. 2012). This result encouraged researchers to apply DBS for the first time in a patient with severe stuttering as an investigational treatment, with encouraging results (Kell et al. in press).

8.7 Transcranial Magnetic Stimulation and Stuttering

Martin Sommer and Nicole E. Neef

8.7.1 Introduction

Neural networks drive our behaviour. These are built of neural ensembles that encode information via excitatory and inhibitory neural activity. Transcranial magnetic stimulation (TMS) can test or interact with these two neural principles without injury. In this way, this technique can directly inform us about brain functions in health and disease. Abundant TMS studies have given unprecedented insights into the cortical organisation of the human brain. To mention a few, mapping the motor cortex shows that it resembles Penfield's motor homunculus (Wassermann et al. 1992); stimulating finger movements demonstrates that the primary motor cortex establishes a modular architecture of neural populations that organise complex voluntary movements such as grasping (Gentner and Classen 2006); interfering with motor skill acquisition indicates that the consolidation of novel motor skills engages the primary motor cortex (Muellbacher et al. 2002). To date, TMS is often combined with other neuroimaging techniques such as PET (Strafella 2016) and fMRI (Bestmann et al. 2008), EEG (Hallett et al. 2017) or deep brain stimulation (Ni et al. 2018). Future research will employ biologically informed network analyses to determine the interaction between brain stimulation and brain networks and possibly path the way towards novel diagnostic, monitoring and treatment approaches (Bestmann and Feredoes 2013; Jannati et al. 2021).

8.7.2 Transcranial Magnetic Stimulation (TMS)

The human scalp and skull have a high electrical resistance, which impairs direct electrical stimulation. TMS indirectly induces an electric current in the brain: a copper-wire stimulation coil delivers a rapidly changing magnetic field, which can easily penetrate the scalp. In turn, it induces an electrical current in the cortical area underneath the coil (Barker et al. 1985). As the induced magnetic field falls off steadily with increasing distance from the stimulation coil, TMS primarily activates neurons in the superficial cortex rather than deeper structures.

8.7.2.1 Single, Paired and Repetitive TMS

Single-pulse TMS is a helpful tool for assessing the integrity of the corticospinal tract. Typically, a TMS pulse over the motor cortex induces a muscle twitch in the target muscle, which can be quantified in amplitude and latency. See Fig. 8.67

Paired-pulse TMS designates two pulses delivered sequentially, usually through the same coil. In a classical paradigm a TMS pulse over the motor cortex induces a muscle twitch in the target muscle. It is preceded by a weaker TMS pulse that only acts cortically. The weaker pulse modulates the muscle jerk induced by the stronger pulse. The direction of induced modulation depends on the interstimulus interval. Thus, paired-pulse TMS allows assessment of inhibitory and facilitatory circuits within the primary motor cortex (Kujirai et al. 1993). This has gained popularity in movement disorders, e.g. in focal dystonia. Remarkably, botulinum toxin injections into peripheral muscle influence the balance of inhibition and facilitation within the motor cortex (Gilio et al. 2000).

Repetitive TMS (rTMS) designates a series of TMS pulses. rTMS affects the cortical area underneath the coil:

- either by transiently blocking its function during stimulation ('functional lesion'),
- or by modulating its excitability during and for some time after the end of stimulation.

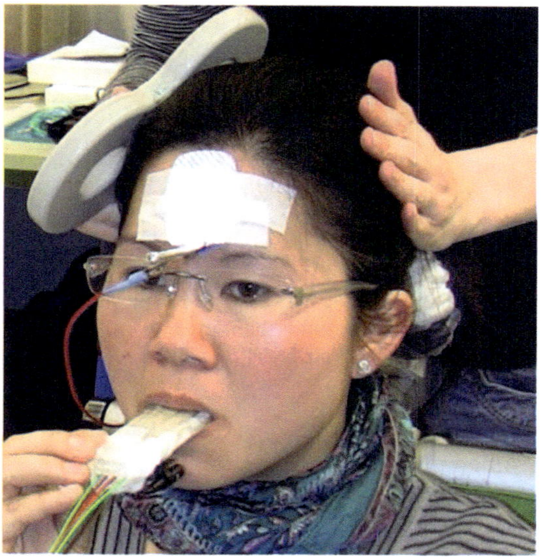

Fig. 8.67 The photograph illustrates the set-up we used for recording motor evoked potentials from either side of the tongue after unilateral stimulation of the tongue motor representation. Note four electrodes (2x2) and a microphone attached to a custom-build spoon-like device. With kind permission of the test person (© Sommer 2024)

8.7.3 TMS and Speech

rTMS can interfere with speech production. If delivered over the primary motor cortex, it activates articulators that impede proper speech. If delivered in a region anterio-lateral to the primary motor cortex, it induces speech distortions, interruptions, slowing or cessation, likely by disturbing speech planning in the inferior frontal gyrus (Stewart et al. 2001).

8.7.4 TMS and Stuttering

To date, only a few laboratories have set out to study the neural basis of stuttering with TMS. Early investigations studied motor cortex excitability of hand muscles (Sommer et al. 2003, 2009, 2019; Alm et al. 2013; Busan et al. 2013, 2020) and how TMS interferes with synchronous finger tapping in adults who stutter (Neef et al. 2011a). Hand muscle activity can easily be stimulated and recorded. This contrasts to speech muscle TMS, where TMS pulses have to be applied to the lateral-anterior surface of the head close to subcutaneous facial nerves. The stimulation of those peripheral nerves can induce discomfort or even pain. Furthermore, recordings from the tongue are tricky, owing to salivation and nearly inaccessibility during natural speaking. Still, existing studies link altered excitability patterns with persistent developmental stuttering (Neef et al. 2011b, 2015a, b; Barwood et al. 2013; Vidaković et al. 2015; Busan et al. 2016; Whillier et al. 2018).

Specifically, single-pulse TMS reveals a decreased asymmetry of excitation in adults who stutter, consistent with long-standing theories of a decreased hemispheric specialisation (Sommer et al. 2019). In addition, paired-pulse TMS indicates reduced intracortical facilitation and, to a lesser extent, a reduced intracortical inhibition in adults with persistent developmental *stuttering* (*AWS*) (Neef et al. 2011b). We examined speech preparation in detail, thereby expanding the pioneering magneto-encephalographic work of Salmelin and co-workers (2000). We used TMS over the tongue motor representation to study the phase of immediate speech preparation. To do this, we recorded motor evoked potentials (MEPs) over the cortical representation of the tongue. The magnitude of these potentials is considered a measure of cortical excitability, which is amplified by speech. We were able to show that this amplification, which occurs primarily in the left hemisphere of the brain, is absent in people with stuttering (Neef et al. 2015b).

The primary motor cortex is a fertile target for TMS because EMG recordings provide easy-to-quantify read-out measures of motor cortex excitability. Probing the integrity of other cortical regions needs different read-out measures. One possibility is to combine TMS with EEG. Busan et al. (2019) recorded EEG activity while applying single TMS pulses to the supplementary motor area (SMA), a crucial cortical region of the motor network involved in voluntary movement control. Early post-TMS EEG activity (160–150 ms) was reduced in the bilateral SMA, left pre-central and right parietal regions in adults who stutter compared with fluent controls. Contrastingly, later post-TMS EEG activity (260–460 ms) was increased in right temporal and frontal regions. It is assumed that the first part of such TMS-evoked EEG signals indicates the excitability of the stimulated site. The following spatio-temporal distribution over the scalp is assumed to correspond to the spread of activation to other brain regions due to connectivity (Hallett et al. 2017). Accordingly, persistent developmental stuttering relates to a reduced initiation of SMA activity. Moreover, the compromised spreading activation towards the left premotor cortex implies a disconnection from speech motor control sites, and the later-evolving hyperconnectivity with right temporal and frontal regions unfolds the spatio-temporal pattern of jeopardised network dynamics in stuttering.

8.7.5 Direct Current Stimulation Add-On to Stuttering Therapy

With another well-established type of non-invasive brain stimulation, transcranial direct current stimulation (tDCS), a study from Oxford indicates that external neurostimulation in the form of transcranial direct current stimulation over the left hemispheric motor cortex of adults who stutter can enhance the success of speech techniques over a few weeks (Chesters et al. 2018). External neurostimulation can alter the excitability of the stimulated superficial brain area for some time (Nitsche and Paulus 2000). It is possible that this at least partially compensates for the disturbance of speech preparation.

8.7.6 Conclusion

Non-invasive brain stimulation is a tool for studying the (patho)physiology of the motor system. Modulations of cortical excitability may provide functional improvement, mainly when administered during behavioural training.

Acknowledgements This contribution incorporates research carried out with support of the Deutsche Forschungsgemeinschaft. The authors are deeply grateful for the continued support of Walter Paulus, M.D., from the Department of Clinical Neurophysiology, University Medical Center Göttingen.

8.8 Neurological Examination in Stutterers/Clutterers

Barbara Maciejewska

8.8.1 Introduction

Stuttering is characterised by involuntary prolongations, repetitions and pauses that disrupt the flow of speech. There are two main types of stuttering: developmental and acquired.

Developmental stuttering (DS) is a speech impairment that severely affects an individual's ability to produce speech fluently. DS affects many children from the ages of 2 to 6 years, with a prevalence of about 2–5% (Yairi and Ambrose 2013; Etchell et al. 2018). About 80% of children with DS regain fluency at the end of this period. The rest, nearly 1% of the adult population, will be affected by persistent developmental stuttering (PDS).

Acquired stuttering (AS) is stuttering with an onset occurring once the language is developed. Acquired neurogenic stuttering (NS) is a much rarer disorder, generally occurring during adulthood in individuals without any previous speech disorders (Cruz et al. 2018). Strokes and traumatic brain injury are the more frequently reported causes of acquired stuttering, followed by neurodegenerative diseases, toxic substances and poisoning, or they may even be of psychogenic origin.

A variety of theories about the origin of stuttering and corresponding treatment approaches has been proposed. In ancient Greece, theories referred to dryness of the tongue. In the nineteenth century, abnormalities of the speech apparatus were thought to cause stuttering. Later, stuttering was primarily thought to be a psychogenic disorder (Buchel and Sommer 2004). Research on the nature of stuttering has produced an extensive amount of data over the years. No doubt a conceptual transformation of the background of stuttering is being observed. This has been a total paradigm shift in recent years—from a nervous or emotional condition to a neurological one that is at least partly genetic. A consensus is growing that stuttering is a neurological condition in AS as well as in DS—though its exact nature is not certain and the mechanisms behind the speech disturbances and the speech initiation problems are still not clear. Genetic and neurobiological approaches are now most common in assessing abnormalities in the structure or function of the central nervous system (CNS) thought to cause stuttering.

Studies performed in patients with DS have identified the involvement of several CNS structures: the right frontal operculum, right frontal parafalcine region, right motor cortex and supplemental right motor cortex, right inferior temporal gyrus and right superior temporal gyrus, right cerebellar hemisphere, left cingulate gyrus, left temporal lobe, left rolandic operculum, left prefrontal cortex, left sensorimotor cortex, basal ganglia (ventrolateral nucleus of the thalamus, mesothalamus and left caudate nucleus) as well as a disturbance in dopaminergic activity (hyperdopaminergic states or a change in D1/D2 receptor ratio in the striatum). Decreased fibre coherence, as observed with DTI, has been shown in persistent developmental stutterers compared with a fluent control group (Buchel and Sommer 2004; Ludlow and Loucks 2003; Charoensook and Maguire 2017; Maguire et al. 2000, 2004). This has been confirmed by many functional and structural imaging tools used to investigate cortical and subcortical brain differences between stuttering and non-stuttering individuals. Earlier studies were done with positron emission tomography (PET); now most current studies have been based on functional magnetic resonance imaging (fMRI), magneto-encephalography (MEG) or diffusion tensor imaging brain scans (DTI) (Ludlow and Loucks 2003).

AS can occur in association with multiple pathologies of the central nervous system. The lesion site is also heterogeneous. There are case reports of stuttering in focal and diffuse lesions, unilateral and bilateral, cortical and subcortical lesions; the lesion site may be located in both hemispheres, brainstem and cerebellum (Etchell et al. 2018; Cruz et al. 2018; Daroff et al. 2016; Lundgren et al. 2010; Penttilä and Korpijaakko-Huuhka 2015; Jankovic 2016; Connally et al. 2014). AS has been reported following lesions in almost all parts of the human brain. Published medical reports report that the frontal lobe, the thalamus and the basal ganglia are commonly involved in AS. Lesions of the primary language cortex do not produce stuttering (Saeedi Borujeni et al. 2016). In fact, AS after neurological damage has already been described in patients after stroke or traumatic brain injury, and in patients with epilepsy, multiple sclerosis, Parkinson, corticobasal ganglionic degeneration, dementia, hypoxic ischaemic encephalopathy and pharmacological iatrogenesis (Sahin et al. 2005). Moreover, the neurological nature of AS is confirmed by reports that it is an early symptom of Landau–Kleffner syndrome, following West Nile virus, aseptic meningitis or symptoms of late onset Tay Sachs disease or progressive supranuclear palsy (PSP) (Tütüncüoğlu et al. 2002; Mickail et al. 2011; Grim et al. 2015).

Diseases leading to stuttering are mentioned in Sects. 6.4 and 7.1.

8.8.2 Neurogenic Background of Stuttering

To understand the neurological examination in stuttering it is important to discuss its possible neurogenic background. It is worth mentioning that the lesions associated with stuttering rarely involve the primary speech and language regions in the left hemisphere (Broca's area, the temporal planum, insula or Wernicke's area). Lesions usually involve other structures, such as the basal ganglia, which may modulate activity in the specific primary speech and language regions. As a result, stuttering may reflect an instability or loss of control in brain function, rather than a loss of function—which makes stuttering similar to some other motor control disorders such as tremor and dystonia.

Most studies indicate that the central control abnormalities in stuttering are not due to a disturbance in one particular brain region but rather to a system dysfunction that interferes with rapid and dynamic processing for speech production (Ludlow and Loucks 2003); thus, the timing of neural activity in different regions may be abnormal.

Studies of relationships among brain regions during normal speech and in persons who stutter suggest that DS involves not only brain regions responsible for motor planning and execution, but also regions that have a role in the processing of sensory feedback (Cruz et al. 2018). As a result, DS may be associated with an imbalanced neural network for speech processing that is not limited to speech production, but also affects cortical responses during speech perception (Halag-Milo et al. 2016). Acquired stuttering (AS) usually appears as a result of lesions following certain injuries or diseases of the nervous system.

In Alm's (2004) review, stuttering seems to result from lesions in the basal ganglia and their circuits, because the basal ganglia provide internal timing cues that are important for subsequent movements of the speech apparatus. Further, Levine and MacDougall (2016) propose that word-initial repetitions are produced because the first component of a word is generated outside the basal ganglia, whereas the normal motor progression to the next sequence is prevented because the basal ganglia subsequently fail to provide the necessary cue for the upcoming movements. The main functions of the basal ganglia (BG) in motor control are to facilitate certain speech control movements while inhibiting competing movements (Jankovic 2016). The basal ganglia are involved in several facets of psychomotor behaviour. Anatomically, this group of nuclei is mainly involved in a closed corticobasal ganglia-thalamus-cortical loop.

Some studies provide evidence of a dysfunctional hyperdopaminergic state of the thalamocortical pathways underlying speech motor control in stuttering. Evidence that stuttering can improve, worsen or recur following deep brain stimulation for other indications emphasises the role of the BG in stuttering (Levine and MacDougall 2016). As a result, examination of the motor function is crucial to diagnosing the neurological background of stuttering.

In addition, lesions in the thalamus may cause stuttering indirectly by disrupting the transmission of signals from the basal ganglia to the cortex, because the role of the thalamus is to relay information to cortical regions. In a recently published review, neural circuits related to disfluency in developmental stuttering DS were shown to contain both an auditory-motor cortical loop, guided by the sensory cortex, which enables speech motor planning and execution, and a basal ganglia-thalamocortical loop, guided by the cerebellum, which provides the initiation and timing of speech sequences (Chang et al. 2019).

Theys et al. (2013) indicate that stroke-induced neurogenic stuttering is not associated with neural dysfunction in one specific brain area but can occur following one or more lesions throughout the corticobasal ganglia cortical network. It is suggested that the onset of neurogenic stuttering may result from a disintegration of neural functions necessary for fluent speech.

Although the mentioned theories seem interesting and promising, it is still difficult to determine the affected neural pathway of stuttering because lesions in one structure may disrupt the function of others. So if some neurological abnormality is found, it is difficult to interpret in which way it may be related to the symptoms of stuttering. The latest study suggested a common neural substrate across a variety of aetiologies. Analyses of neuroanatomical substrate of stuttering - using case reports from the published literature of acquired neurogenic stuttering following stroke and of adults with persistent developmental stuttering - showed that lesion locations were functionally linked to a common network centred around the left corpus callosum, including the claustrum, the amygdala transition area and other neighbouring areas (Theys et al. 2024). Of the many theories, data accounts of stuttering provide support for a crucial role of the basal ganglia. In addition, analyses highlighted involvement of the claustrum and amygdalostriatal transition area. The claustrum is typically not reported as a separate area in studies and models of speech production and its function is still poorly understood (Niu et al. 2022).

Key Points

- There are widespread abnormalities in the structural architecture and functional organisation of the brains of adults and children who stutter.
- Stuttering may reflect an instability or loss of control of brain function rather than a loss of function.
- The exact neurological deficit that causes stuttering is still unknown.

8.8.3 Neurological Examination and Distinguishing the Forms of Stuttering

Contrary to many theories of the possible neurological areas affected in stuttering, the results of neurological examination are usually normal. A routine neurological examination may uncover no abnormal results, preventing identification of the localisation of the neurological deficit in patients with DS. However, the neurological examination could be very important in AS if disfluency is a part of neurological syndrome or neurodegenerative or vascular disease.

Acquired stuttering often differs in some way from 'typical' stuttering. Some characteristics may be helpful in distinguishing forms of stuttering (DS vs. AS) (Cruz et al. 2018):

1. Disfluencies occur in grammatical words at a similar rate of occurrence as in substantive words.
2. Repetitions, prolongations and blocks occur in all positions of words in the sentence.
3. There is a consistency in stuttering behaviour across speech tasks.
4. The speaker does not appear overly anxious about the stuttering behaviour.
5. Secondary symptoms, such as facial grimacing, fist clenching and eye blinking, are rarely observed.
6. An adaptation effect is not observed.

However, these criteria have been questioned. Currently, it is generally accepted that the presence of these criteria favours the diagnosis of acquired neurogenic stuttering, but their presence is not necessary to establish the diagnosis. Thus, the most important distinctive features between DS and NS are:

- Medical history—the age of onset of stuttering, stuttering after neurological damage.
- Neurological examination—some neurological abnormalities in respect of speech fluency (Roth et al. 2015). Coexisting neurological symptoms, such as tremor, bradykinesia, limb paralysis and brisk reflexes, stemming from different brain injuries/lesions can lead to different presentations of co-morbid symptomatology.
- Characteristics of the speech problems—forms of disfluency. A concept of fluency is a relevant dimension. AS frequently shows different accompanying speech dysfluencies, such as aphasia, dysarthria or apraxia (Krishnan and Tiwari 2011). AS frequently co-occurs with aphasia and dysarthria as shown by König (2009). She found that 75% of 60 patients with neurogenic stuttering showed accompanying speech disorders, and 50% of the patients had aphasia. For some diseases (Tourette's syndrome, autism, ADHD), palilalia is the most suitable term to describe the disorder. Some patient suffering from Parkinson's disease or with apraxia of speech may have severe dysfluencies, so the phoniatrist should be able to recognise repetitions, pauses, palilalia, prolongations, akinetic mutism and other disfluensies of speech impairment (McNeil 2008).

This aspect is also discussed in Sect. 7.1.

To sum up, the circumstances of AS onset are usually related to a neurological episode, and often to other neurological signs or symptoms that may exist. Moreover, AS may present as the first symptom (forerunner) of a neurological episode; in DS no neurological episode, signs or symptoms are observed.

Thus, the importance of the diagnostic interview and examination of stutterers should be emphasised. Useful aspects are as follows:

- At what age were the present disfluencies demonstrated for the first time?
- Is there a family history of stuttering?
- Has there been any neurological episode?
- Are there any neurological signs or symptoms?
- Do neurological symptoms create any neurological syndromes?

Key Points
- The neurological examination results in DS are usually normal.
- The main purpose of a neurological examination in case of stuttering is to find if there are more neurological problems/symptoms than stuttering.
- The most important distinctive feature between DS and AS remains.
  - Medical history and the age of onset.
  - Neurological examination—the doctor should look for coexisting characteristic symptoms and try to find neurological deficits to confirm or refute the hypothesis of acquired neurological disease.
  - Characteristics of the speech problems—forms of disfluency.

To identify neurological problems, examination should cover most of the nervous tracts, which include the cortex, subcortical white matter, basal ganglia, brainstem, cerebellum, spinal cord, peripheral nerves, neuromuscular junction and muscles. The neurological examination consists of the following six subdivisions:

1. Mental status.
2. Cranial nerves.
3. Motor exam.
4. Reflexes.
5. Coordination and gait.
6. Sensory exam.

8.8.4 Cognitive Function

The cognitive assessment should include the following: *orientation* and global attention, *attention*, *memory*, language and speech. Generalised impaired attention and cooperation are relatively non-specific abnormalities that can occur in many different focal brain lesions, in diffuse abnormalities such as dementia or encephalitis, and in behavioural or mood disorders. An in-depth examination of this sphere includes a mental status examination. The Mini Mental State Exam (MMSE) actually ascertains cognition, which is a cortical function, and such global assessment of higher functions can be a useful tool. Neurodegenerative diseases such as Parkinson disease (PD) or Huntington disease (HD), as well as post-vascular incidences (stroke) or conditions after meningitis, are often connected with a mental poor condition, dementia and language problems. Neurogenic stuttering frequently occurs with aphasia and dysarthria, as shown by König (2009). Tani and Sakai (2011) also report that different brain injuries lead to different presentations of co-morbid symptomatology—aphasia, dysarthria or apraxia, which can exist separately from neurogenic stuttering. The incidence of neurogenic stuttering following stroke is 5.3%, and an aphasia most frequently co-occurs in neurogenic stuttering following stroke (Theys et al. 2011). Amnestic aphasia, Broca's aphasia, conduction aphasia and Wernicke's aphasia are the most common types of aphasia associated with stuttering-like dysfluencies (Lundgren et al. 2010).

It is important to consider what the core of neurogenic stuttering is, and which dysfluencies are related to aphasia. The new guidelines for analysis of neurogenic stuttering from aphasic features have provided fruitful advice on how to assess which dysfluencies are related to aphasia and which to stuttering (Penttilä and Korpijaakko-Huuhka 2015). However, more research in the area of neurogenic stuttering is needed, especially for developing valid and reliable methods that take into account co-occurring speech and language deficiencies and communicative demands in various discourses.

Table 8.15 Types of communication symptom accompanying neurogenic stuttering (NS) or that overlap with or mimic stuttering (Mendez 2018; Cruz et al. 2018; Lundgren et al. 2010; Duffy 2013)

Type of disfluency	Features of speech pathologies
Cluttering vs. neurogenic stuttering (NS)	In cluttering—rapid speech rate; loss of dysfluencies, word and phrase repetitions, unfinished words and utterances In NS—speech rate rather slow or normal stuttering mostly observed initially in words, then continued involuntary repetition of sounds
Palilalia vs. neurogenic stuttering (NS)	In palilalia—involuntarily repetitions of patient's own words In NS—repetition of word initial sounds, especially initial consonants, also syllable and part-of-word repetitions
Echolalia vs. neurogenic stuttering (NS)	In echolalia—involuntarily repetition of others' utterances In NS—it does not exist
Apraxia of speech (AOS) vs. neurogenic stuttering (NS)	In AOS—motor speech planning deficit with laboured initiation and production, as well as with compensatory efforts to correct phonological errors In NS—there is no variation in the error patterns as in AOS, which makes the speech sound effortful
Dysarthria	In dysarthria—difficult or unclear articulation of speech that is otherwise linguistically normal. Speech may be deformed-slurred, slow and difficult to understand. Phrase repetitions or unfinished words may be observed and difficulty in controlling the pitch, loudness, rhythm and voice qualities of speech coexist

Apraxia of speech (AOS) (Bailey et al. 2017)—a condition described either as a phonological, motor or cognitive disorder (Kent 2000)—sometimes manifests together with NS, although speech features in AOS are often difficult to distinguish from those of stuttering behaviour (Lundgren et al. 2010; McNeil 2008; Theys et al. 2011; Myers et al. 2012; Kikuchi et al. 2008). It is not uncommon for individuals with neurogenic stuttering to experience several other types of communication impairment. These may include (Cruz et al. 2018; Mendez 2018)

- Aphasia—complete or partial impairment in language comprehension, formulation, and use.
- Dysarthria—mistakes in the production of speech sounds, that make the individual's speech intelligible, unclear articulation of speech.
- Apraxia of speech—a speech disorder, corresponding to a neurological impairment of the capacity to programme the positioning and sequencing of muscle movements for the volitional production of phonemes.
- Palilalia—a complex speech disorder, an involuntary repetition of semantically appropriated words or sentences, usually with an increasing rapidity and decreasing loudness.
- Anomia—difficulty in finding the appropriate word to use, inability to produce names for objects or events.

A description of these impairments is presented in Table 8.15.

Key Points
- The patient's general appearance and performance are indicators of neurological and mental health.
- The Mini Mental State Exam (MMSE), a cortical function and global assessment of higher functions, can be a useful tool.
- Neurogenic stuttering accompanies speech disorders—aphasia, dysarthria or apraxia—which can exist separately from neurogenic stuttering.

8.8.5 Motor Function

Motor examination consists of several different components: strength, tone, reflexes, involuntary movements, posture. Abnormalities in all elements can be observed separately from speech disfluency.

Stuttering after stroke, head trauma, neurosurgical procedures or meningitis and that caused by cerebral palsy (Grant et al. 1999) can exist together with paresis or paralysis of the limbs or even one-sided hemiparesis. NS may be associated with subcortical lesions and be secondary to neurodegenerative diseases, especially when the basal ganglia circuit is affected (such as in PD or Wilson Disease) (Brabo et al. 2014; Alm and Risberg 2007; Daroff et al. 2016). As a result, many extrapyramidal symptoms are possible to detect in NS. Bradykinesia, as well as the increased muscle tone called rigidity, is observed in PD and Parkinsonian syndromes—disorders most likely to mimic idiopathic Parkinson's disease (CBD, corticobasal degeneration; DLB, dementia with Lewy bodies; IPD, idiopathic Parkinson's disease; MSA, multiple system atrophy; PEP, post-encephalitic Parkinsonism; PSP, progressive supranuclear palsy). In post-stroke stuttering, spasticity due to corticospinal tract dysfunction can be present. On the other hand, decreased muscle tone co-exists with HD and cerebellar pathologies. Involuntary movements due to dysfunction of the basal ganglia such as tremor, chorea, dystonia, tics of the limbs or tongue, throat or larynx are a part of neurological syndromes in HD, Stuttering:Wilson disease, facial dystonias and Tourette syndrome (McNeil 2008; Daroff et al. 2016; Jankovic 2016).

Key Point

- Increased tone is either pyramidal (spasticity) or extra-pyramidal (rigidity).

8.8.6 Reflexes

Reflexes test the intactness of the spinal reflex arc and presence of superior inhibitions. In stuttering they can be either normal (developmental stuttering), reduced (cerebral diseases) or increased (multiple sclerosis, post-stroke or post-injury stuttering). Deep tendon reflexes may be diminished by abnormalities in muscles, sensory neurons, lower motor neurons and the neuromuscular junction; acute upper motor neuron lesions; and mechanical factors, such as joint disease. Abnormally increased reflexes are associated with upper motor neuron lesions. Pathological reflexes indicating damage to the pyramidal tract should be tested (the *Babinski sign*, as well as a number of Babinski-like responses such as *Rossolimo,* Oppenheim from the lower limbs, and the *Sterling sign* and *Hoffman sign* from the upper limbs). They can coexist in stuttering after stroke or post-cerebral traumas.

Key Point

- Deep tendon reflexes can be influenced by age, metabolic factors, such as thyroid dysfunction or electrolyte abnormalities, and the anxiety level of the patient.

8.8.7 Coordination

Good coordination depends on intact position–sense pathways, lower motor neurons, upper motor neurons, the basal ganglia and the cerebellum. *Appendicular ataxia* is usually caused by lesions of the cerebellar hemispheres and associated pathways, while *truncal ataxia* (see Romberg Test and Gait in Sect. 8.8) is often caused by damage to the midline cerebellar vermis and associated pathway. When stuttering is a result of cerebellar diseases, incoordination, clumsiness and tremor are often observed, because the cerebellum is responsible for smoothing out and refining voluntary movements. Other main signs of cerebellar disease are dysarthria, nystagmus, incoordination and hypotonia of muscles. The main tests include the Heel-to-Shin test, the Finger-to-Nose test and Rapid Alternating Motions (Van Borsel 2014).

8.8.8 Gait and Balance

Neurogenically acquired post-stroke stuttering, stuttering after head trauma or meningitis or in PD, HD and cerebral lesions, can exist together with posture, gait and balance abnormalities. Some balance tests such as Romberg's Test, the walking test, the stepping test may be unable to be done in the neurological disorders mentioned (Van Borsel 2014). Gait involves multiple sensory and motor systems. These include vision, proprioception, lower motor neurons, upper motor neurons, basal ganglia, the cerebellum and higher-order motor planning systems in the association cortex; so it is obvious to test this function in stuttering. Different abilities are assessed: general posture, stability, how high the feet are raised off the floor, the trajectory of leg swing and whether there is *circumduction* (an arced trajectory in the medial to lateral direction), leg stiffness and degree of knee bending, arm swing, the tendency to fall or swerve in any particular direction, rate and speed, the difficulty initiating or stopping gait, and any involuntary movements that are brought out by walking or *tandem gait* by asking the patient to walk a straight line while touching the heel of 1 ft to the toe of the other with each step.

8.8.9 Sensory Function

Neurogenic stuttering can be associated with different pathologies of the central nervous system. The lesion site is also heterogeneous. Somatosensory deficits can be caused by lesions in peripheral nerves, nerve roots, the posterior columns or anterolateral sensory systems in the spinal cord or brainstem, the thalamus or sensory cortex. This is why the examination to detect any loss of sensation and to localise the lesion is needed. There are five main modalities of sensation to test for, and these are light touch, pinprick and temperature (superficial), vibration and joint position (deep). Tests should be performed on all extremities, as well as on the face and trunk, with the patient's eyes closed or covered.

8.8.10 Cranial Nerves

The cranial nerve (CN) examination reflects the function of the brainstem. NS and the pathological function of the nerves are observed in the course of diseases such as vascular diseases, neurodegenerative processes, inflammation of the spinal cord and brain and post-traumatic lesions. Moreover, abnormal cranial nerve examination results should alert the clinician to the possibility not only of central nervous system disease but also of significant systemic illness.

Abnormalities of the cranial nerves may affect one or more of the cranial nerves, and identification of these abnormalities may aid in the localisation of a central nervous system lesion, or suggest a more diffuse process such as meningitis, or the presence of a systemic disease such as diabetes, sarcoidosis, myasthenia gravis, Guillain-Barré, vasculitis and others. More common diseases that can affect the function of CNs are cerebral tumours (basal frontal tumours, pontocerebellar tumours), vascular diseases, inflammation of the CNS and head injuries.

A description of the CNs and their function are presented in Table 8.16.

Key Points

- Abnormalities of the cranial nerves may affect inflammation of the facial nerve (VII), which may result in *Bell's palsy*, or affect more of the cranial nerves in multiple sclerosis.
- Twelve pairs of cranial nerves exit the brainstem; seven are concerned with communication or swallowing.

If any abnormalities are found upon neurological examination, a more detailed neurological diagnostic process is needed. The patient should consult a neurologist. Some extra examination may be crucial for diagnosis (brain imaging by magnetic resonance imaging (MRI), *magnetic resonance angiography* (MRA), magnetic resonance spectroscopy (MRS), specific single-photon emission computed tomography (SPECT), ultrasound of the brain, oncogene antibodies, **blood and urine tests, electromyography, biopsy of the liver or muscle tissue or advanced cognitive tests**).

A number of antipsychotic agents, calcium channel blocking agents and cholinergic and anticonvulsant drugs have been investigated as possible treatments. Although some medications have been tried for stuttering, no drugs have been proved yet to help the problem (Van Borsel 2014;

Table 8.16 CNs and their function and main symptoms of injury (Daroff et al. 2016; Duffy 2013)

Cranial nerve	Function	Associated brain region	Symptoms seen after injury
I olfactory nerve	Distinguishing between smells	Telencephalon-olfactory bulb	Anosmia
II optic nerve	Visual field, visual acuity, pupillary light reflex	Diencephalon–optic chiasma	Anopsia, blindness
III, IV and VI ophthalmic, trochlear, abducens nerves	Control eye movement	Midbrain Pons/medulla junction	Strabismus Abnormal localisation of the eyeball Double vision Large pupil
V trigeminal nerve	Sensory input to the face, mouth, tongue Masticatory movements	Pons	Impairment of the face—hypaesthesia Dropped jaw, asymmetrical chewing
VII facial nerve	Innervates the muscles of facial expression, the submandibular and lacrimal glands, and taste in the anterior two-thirds of the tongue	Pons/medulla junction	Facial paralysis/paresis
VIII vestibulocochlear nerve	Hearing and balance	Pons/medulla junction	Deafness Disequilibrium Nystagmus
IX glossopharyngeal nerve	Taste in the posterior third of the tongue and sensation in the pharynx. The gag reflex	Medulla oblongata	Choking Dysphagia
X vagus nerve	Innervation of the pharyngeal and laryngeal muscles and forms the efferent limb of the gag reflex. Its lesions include dysarthria and dysphagia	Medulla oblongata	Hoarseness Dysphagia Dyspnoea
XI accessory nerve	Innervation of the muscles of the larynx, the trapezius and sternocleidomastoid muscles—neck muscle movements Movement of the uvula and the levator palatini through its cranial root	Medulla oblongata Spinal cord	Weakened turning of the neck
XII hypoglossal nerve	Tongue muscles movements	Medulla oblongata	Deviation of the tongue towards the side of lesion

Sechi et al. 2006). However, in some cases, treatment of neurological disease may control and stop the progression of acquired neurogenic stuttering or other speech dysfluencies.

As a result, treatment of AS is based on the traditional strategies used in DS, namely a specific and individualised intervention by speech therapy. A combination of multiple speech techniques is most often used. Sometimes anti-anxiety drugs and therapy, and **cognitive behavioural therapy (CBT), are useful.** Improvement in psychosocial factors (activity and participation, positive affect on speech and general condition) are found.

Complex treatment may not eliminate all stuttering, but it can teach skills that help in:

- Improving speech fluency.
- Developing effective communication.
- Participating fully in school, work and social activities.

8.8.11 Conclusions

1. Neurological examination should be a part of medical assessment of patients with stuttering. The main goal of the neurological examination in the case of stuttering is to understand better the condition in general, to generate a relevant diagnosis and to exclude additional neurological diseases.

2. Thanks to neurological examination, it is possible:
   (a) To see if there are more neurological problems/symptoms than stuttering.
   (b) To exclude or confirm additional neurological diseases (sometimes coexistent symptoms are so characteristic that the neurological diagnosis is obvious).
   (c) To confirm, refute or modify the initial hypotheses of acquired disease and causation derived from the medical history.
3. AS can be associated with different pathologies of the central nervous system. The lesion location is heterogeneous.
4. Different diseases and other types of communication problems accompany acquired neurogenic stuttering that may overlap with and mimic stuttering, leading to such kinds of speech disfluency as dysarthria, aphasia, apraxia of speech and dysglossia.
5. Brain imaging with the ability to map damage networks is becoming increasingly important in diagnostics.
6. Treatment has to be based on the patient's individual needs. Treatment primarily should be planned on the basis of the nature of the actual speech problem, in relation to the person's resources and additional problems (Theys et al. 2024).

References

Adams MR (1977) A clinical strategy for differentiating the normally nonfluent child and the incipient stutterer. J Fluen Disord 2(2):141–148

Adriaensens S, Beyers W, Struyf E (2015) Impact of stuttering severity on adolescents' domain-specific and general self-esteem through cognitive and emotional mediating processes. J Commun Disord 58:43–57

Alku P (2011) Glottal inverse filtering analysis of human voice production—a review of estimation and parameterization methods of the glottal excitation and their applications. Sadhana 36(5):623–650. https://www.ias.ac.in/article/fulltext/sadh/036/05/0623-0650. Accessed 14 Apr 2019

Alm PA (2004) Stuttering and the basal ganglia circuits: a critical review of possible relations. J Commun Disord 37(4):325–369. https://doi.org/10.1016/j.jcomdis.2004.03.001. PMID: 15159193

Alm PA, Risberg J (2007) Stuttering in adults: the acoustic startle response, temperamental traits, and biological factors. J Commun Disord 40(1):1–41

Alm PA, Karlsson R, Sundberg M et al (2013) Hemispheric lateralization of motor thresholds in relation to stuttering. PLoS One 8(10):e76824

Altenmüller E, Jabusch HC (2006a) Neurologische Erkrankungen bei Musikern. Med Welt 57:569–575

Altenmüller E, Jabusch HC (2006b) Focal dystonia in musicians: from phenomenology to therapy. Adv Cogn Psychol 2(2–3):207–220

Altenmüller E, Jabusch HC (2008) Apollos Fluch—Musikerdystonien. InFo Neurologie Psychiatrie 5:46–53

Ambrose NG, Yairi E (1999) Normative disfluency data for early childhood stuttering. J Speech Lang Hear Res 42(4):895–909

Amster BJ (1995) Perfectionism and stuttering. In: Starkweather C, Peters H (eds) Stuttering: proceedings of first world congress on fluency disorders, vol II. Nijmegen University Press, Nijmegen, pp 540–543

Andrews G, Cutler J (1974) Stuttering therapy: the relation between changes in symptom level and attitudes. J Speech Hear Disord 39(3):312–319

Angerstein W, Klajman S, Neuschaefer-Rube C et al (1993a) Badanie sonograficzne szybkości przepływu krwi w zyle szyjnej wewnetrznej w hyperfunkcjonalnej dysfonii dzieciecej. (Sonographic imaging of internal jugular venous blood flow in juvenile hyperfunctional dysphonia). Otolaryngol Pol 47(3):264–269

Angerstein W, Wein B, Klajman S (1993b) Duplexsonographie der V. jugularis interna bei hyperfunktioneller Dysphonie. Sprache-Stimme-Gehör 17(1):31–34

Arcier AF, Vernay A (1994) Observation clinique: lésions musculaires labiales liées au jeu de cuivres. Médecine des Arts 8:14–19

Aronson A, Bless D (2009) Clinical voice disorders. Thieme, New York

Arruti A, Poumayrac M (2010) Ecografia laringea: una técnica alternativa en la valoración de la encrucijada aero-digestiva. Rev Imagenol 14(1):30–36

Awan SN, Roy N, Zhang D et al (2016) Validation of the Cepstral Spectral Index of Dysphonia (CSID) as a screening tool for voice disorders: development of clinical cutoff scores. J Voice 30(2):130–144

Baer T, Gore JC, Gracco LC et al (1991) Analysis of vocal tract shape and dimensions using magnetic resonance imaging: vowels. J Acoust Soc Am 90(2):799–828

Bailey DJ, Blomgren M, DeLong C et al (2017) Quantification and systematic characterization of stuttering-like disfluencies in acquired apraxia of speech. Am J Speech Lang Pathol 26(2S):641–648

Baken RJ, Orlikoff R (2000) Clinical measurement of speech and voice. Singular Thomson Learning, San Diego

Barker AT, Jalinous R, Freeston IL (1985) Non-invasive magnetic stimulation of human motor cortex [letter]. Lancet 1(8437):1106–1107

Barkley RA, Edwards G (2006) Diagnostic interview, behavior rating scales, and the medical examination. In: Barkley RA (ed) Attention-deficit hyperactivity disorder: a handbook for diagnosis and treatment, 3rd edn. The Guilford Press, New York, pp 337–368

Barwood CHS, Murdoch BE, Goozee JV et al (2013) Investigating the neural basis of stuttering using transcranial magnetic stimulation: preliminary case discussions. Speech Lang Hear 16:18–27

Bassich C, Ludlow C (1986) The use of perceptual methods for assessing voice quality. J Speech Hear Disord 51(2):125–133

Baum U, Greess H, Lell M et al (2000) Imaging of head and neck tumors—methods-CT, spiral-CT, multislice-spiral-CT. Eur J Radiol 33(3):153–160

Bayley N (2006) Bayley scales of infant and toddler development, 3rd edn (Bayley-III). Administration manual, Harcourt, San Antonio

Bayley N (2014) Bayley scales of infant and toddler development, 3rd edn (Bayley-III). Pearson Assessment, Frankfurt/Main (German version: Reuner G, Rosenkranz J (eds))

Beach JL, Kelsey CA (1969) Ultrasonic Doppler monitoring of vocal-fold velocity and displacement. J Acoust Soc Am 46(4b):1045–1047

Beal DS, Gracco VL, Brettschneider J et al (2013) A voxel-based morphometry (VBM) analysis of regional grey and white matter volume abnormalities within the speech production network of children who stutter. Cortex 49:2151–2161

Beilby JM, Byrnes ML, Meagher EL et al (2013) The impact of stuttering on adults who stutter and their partners. J Fluen Disord 38(1):14–29

Belyk M, Kraft SJ, Brown S (2015) Stuttering as a trait or state—an ALE meta-analysis of neuroimaging studies. Eur J Neurosci 41:275–284

Bestmann S, Feredoes E (2013) Combined neurostimulation and neuroimaging in cognitive neuroscience: past, present, and future. Ann N Y Acad Sci 1296(1):11–30

Bestmann S, Ruff CC, Blankenburg F et al (2008) Mapping causal interregional influences with concurrent TMS-fMRI. Exp Brain Res 191(4):383–402

Beukers R, Bierens E, Kingma H et al (1995) Voice load as measured by the voice accumulator. Folia Phoniatr Logop 47(5):252–261

Bishop DV, Adams C (1990) A prospective study of the relationship between specific language impairment, phonological disorders and reading retardation. J Child Psychol Psychiatry 31(7):1027–1050

Bleek B, Montag C, Faber J et al (2011) Investigating personality in stuttering: results of a case control study using the NEO-FFI. J Commun Disord 44(2):218–222

Bleek B, Reuter M, Yaruss JS et al (2012) Relationships between personality characteristics of people who stutter and the impact of stuttering on everyday life. J Fluen Disord 37(4):325–333

Bless DM, Baken RJ (1992) Assessment of voice. J Voice 6(2):95–97

Blitzer A (1995) Laryngeal electromyography. In: Rubin JS et al (eds) Diagnosis and treatment of voice disorders. Igaku-Shoin, New York, pp 316–326

Blood GW, Blood IM, Bennett S et al (1994) Subjective anxiety measurements and cortisol responses in adults who stutter. J Speech Hear Res 37(4):760–768

Blood GW, Blood IM, Tellis GM et al (2003) A preliminary study of self-esteem, stigma, and disclosure in adolescents who stutter. J Fluen Disord 28:143–159

Bloodstein O, Bernstein-Ratner N (2008) A handbook of stuttering, 6th edn. Delmar, Clifton Park

BMA (Ärztl. Sachverständigenrat beim Bundesministerium für Arbeit u. Sozialordnung) (2002) Druckschädigung der Nerven. Merkblatt zur Berufskrankheit Nr. 2106 der Anlage zur Berufskrankheitenverordnung (BKV): Bundesarbeitsblatt 11(62)

Böckelmann I, Schneyer B (2009) Arbeitsbedingte Belastungen und Erkrankungen von Musikern. Arbeitsmed Sozialmed Umweltmed 4:237–242

Böckler R, Wein B, Klajman S et al (1988) Die Ultraschalluntersuchung der Pseudoglottis bei Kehlkopflosen. HNO 36(3):115–118

Boey R (2000) Stotteren: Detecterenenmeten (Stuttering: detection and measurement). Garant, Leuven

Boey R (2010) Communication attitude of stuttering children. In: Conference presentation on the 2nd European symposium on fluency disorders, Antwerp, April 23, 2010

Boey RA, Wuyts FL, Van de Heyning PH et al (2007) Characteristics of stuttering-like disfluencies in Dutch-speaking children. J Fluen Disord 32(4):310–329

Böhme G (1988a) Echolaryngographie—Ein Beitrag zur Methode der Ultraschalldiagnostik des Kehlkopfes. Laryngol Rhinol Otol 67(11):551–558

Böhme G (1988b) Ultraschalldiagnostik der phonatorischen Leistungen des Laryngektomierten. Laryngol Rhinol Otol 67(12):651–656

Böhme G (1989) Ein klinischer Beitrag zur Ultraschalldiagnostik des Kehlkopfes (Echolaryngographie). Laryngol Rhinol Otol 68(9):510–515

Böhme G (1991) Duplexsonographie des Kehlkopfes: 1. Bewegungsanalyse intralaryngealer Strukturen. Otorhinolaryngol Nova 1(6):338–342

Böhme G (1992) Duplexsonographie des Kehlkopfes: 2. Farbkodierte Bewegungsanalyse intralaryngealer Strukturen. Otorhinolaryngol Nova 2(1):43–45

Böhme G, Gross M (2001) Stroboskopie und andere Verfahren zur Analyse der Stimmlippenschwingungen. Median, Heidelberg

Boone D (1993) The Boone voice program for children, 2nd edn. Pro-Ed, Austin

Boone DR, McFarlane SC, Von Berg SL (2005) The voice and voice therapy, 7th edn. Allyn & Bacon, Boston

Borch DZ, Sundberg J, Lindestad PÅ et al (2004) Vocal fold vibration and voice source aperiodicity in 'dist' tones: a study of a timbral ornament in rock singing. Logoped Phoniatr Vocol 29(4):147–153

Bordone-Sacerdote C, Sacerdote G (1965) Investigations on the movement of the glottis by ultrasounds. Paper presented at the 5th international congress on audiology, Liège, 7–14 Sept 1965, Paper Nr. A 42, p 4
Bosshardt HG (2008) Stottern (Stuttering). Hogrefe, Göttingen
Bosshardt HG (2010) Frühintervention bei Stottern. Behandlungsansätze für Kinder im Vorschulalter (Early intervention for stuttering. Treatment approaches for preschool children). Hogrefe, Göttingen
Bough D, Heuer RJ, Sataloff RT et al (1996) Intrasubject variability of objective voice measures. J Voice 10(2):166–174
Boutin H, Fletcher N, Smith J et al (2015) Relationships between pressure, flow, lip motion, and upstream and downstream impedances for the trombone. J Acoust Soc Am 137(3):1195–1209
Boyle MP (2013) Assessment of stigma associated with stuttering: development and evaluation of the self-stigma of stuttering scale (4S). J Speech Lang Hear Res 56(5):1517–1529
Bozzato A, Zenk J, Gottwald F et al (2007) Der Einfluss der Schildknorpelossifikation bei der Larynxsonografie. Laryngol Rhinol Otol 86(4):276–281
Brabo NC, Minett TSC, Ortiz KZ (2014) Fluency in Parkinson's disease: disease duration, cognitive status and age. Arq Neuropsiquiatr 72(5):349–355
Brocklehurst PH, Drake E, Corley M (2015) Perfectionism and stuttering: findings of an online survey. J Fluen Disord 44:46–62
Brockmann-Bauser M, Drinnan MJ (2011) Routine acoustic voice analysis: time to think again? Curr Opin Otolaryngol Head Neck Surg 19(3):165–170
Bromage S (2007) Visualisation of the lip motion of brass instrument players, and investigations of an artificial mouth as a tool for comparative studies of instruments. PhD thesis, University of Edinburgh, Edinburgh. https://www.era.lib.ed.ac.uk/handle/1842/1966. Accessed 9 Feb 2018
Bromage S, Campbell M, Gilbert J (2005) Experimental investigation of the open area of the brass player's vibrating lips. In: Proceedings of the forum acusticum, Budapest, 29 August–2 September 2005. OPAKFI, Budapest, pp 729–734
Bromage S, Campbell M, Gilbert J (2010) Open areas of vibrating lips in trombone playing. Acta Acust Acust 96(4):603–613
Brown S, Ingham RJ, Ingham JC et al (2005) Stuttered and fluent speech production: an ALE meta-analysis of functional neuroimaging studies. Hum Brain Mapp 25(1):105–117. https://doi.org/10.1002/hbm.20140. PMID: 15846815; PMCID: PMC6871755
Brundage SB, Ratner NB, Boyle MP, Eggers K, Everard R, Franken MC, Kefalianos E, Marcotte AK, Millard S, Packman A, Vanryckeghem M, Yaruss JS (2021) Consensus guidelines for the assessments of individuals who stutter across the lifespan. Am J Speech Lang Pathol 30(6):2379–2393. https://doi.org/10.1044/2021_AJSLP-21-00107. Epub 2021 Sep 13. PMID: 34516299; PMCID: PMC9132036
Brutten G, Vanryckeghem M (2007) Behavior assessment battery for school-age children who stutter. Plural, San Diego
Buchel C, Sommer M (2004) What causes stuttering? PLoS Biol 2(2):159–163
Bumiller OE (1936) Antwort zu Frage 25 im "Fragekasten": Lippenverletzungen durch Blasinstrument. Dtsch Zahnärztl Wschr 39:295
Bum-Soo K, Kook JA, Young HP et al (2008) Usefulness of laryngeal phonation CT in the diagnosis of vocal cord paralysis. Am J Roentgenol 190(5):1376–1379
Burns DD (1980) The perfectionist's script for self-defeat. Psychol Today 14(6):34–52
Busan P, D'Ausilio A, Borelli M et al (2013) Motor excitability evaluation in developmental stuttering: a transcranial magnetic stimulation study. Cortex 49(3):781–792
Busan P, Del Ben G, Bernardini S et al (2016) Altered modulation of silent period in tongue motor cortex of persistent developmental stuttering in relation to stuttering severity. PLoS One 11(10):e0163959
Busan P, Del Ben G, Russo LR et al (2019) Stuttering as a matter of delay in neural activation: a combined TMS/EEG study. Clin Neurophysiol 130(1):61–76
Busan P, Del Ben G, Tantone A et al (2020) Effect of muscular activation on surrounding motor networks in developmental stuttering: a TMS study. Brain Lang 205:104774. https://doi.org/10.1016/j.bandl.2020.104774
Bushey T, Martin R (1988) Stuttering in children's literature. Lang Speech Hear Serv Sch 19(3):235–250
Byrd C, Werle D, Coalson G et al (2020) Use of monolingual English guidelines to assess stuttering in bilingual speakers: a systematic review. J Monoling Biling Speech 2(1):1–23
Campos FG (2005) Trumpet technique. Oxford University Press, Oxford, p 51
Cantarella G, Iofrida E, Boria P et al (2014) Ambulatory phonation monitoring in a sample of 92 call center operators. J Voice 28(3):393.e1–393.e6. https://doi.org/10.1016/j.jvoice.2013.10.002
Carding PN, Horsley IA (1992) An evaluation of voice therapy in non-organic dysphonia. Eur J Disord Commun 27(2):137–148
Carlo E, Watson J (2003) Disfluencies of 3- and 5-year old Spanish-speaking children. J Fluen Disord 28(1):37–53
Chang S-E (2011) Using brain imaging to unravel the mysteries of stuttering. Cerebrum 2011:12. PMID: 23447781
Chang S-E, Guenther FH (2020) Involvement of the cortico-basal ganglia-thalamocortical loop in developmental stuttering. Front Psychol 10:3088. https://doi.org/10.3389/fpsyg.2019.03088
Chang S-E, Erickson KI, Ambrose NG et al (2008) Brain anatomy differences in childhood stuttering. NeuroImage 39:1333–1344

Chang S-E, Angstadt M, Chow HM et al (2018) Anomalous network architecture of the resting brain in children who stutter. J Fluen Disord 55:46–67
Chang SE, Garnett EO, Etchell A et al (2019) Functional and neuroanatomical bases of developmental stuttering: current insights. Neuroscientist 25(6):566–582
Charoensook J, Maguire GA (2017) A case series on the effectiveness of lurasidone in patients with stuttering. Ann Clin Psychiatry 29(3):191–194
Chesters J, Watkins KE, Möttönen R (2017) Investigating the feasibility of using transcranial direct current stimulation to enhance fluency in people who stutter. Brain Lang 164:68–76
Chesters J, Möttönen R, Watkins KE (2018) Transcranial direct current stimulation over left inferior frontal cortex improves speech fluency in adults who stutter. Brain 141:1161–1171
Chick J, Bromage S, Campbell M (2005) Transient behaviour in the motion of the brass player's lips. In: Proceedings of the Forum Acusticum, Budapest, 29 August–2 September 2005. OPAKFI, Budapest, pp 753–775
CHILDES (2014) Child language data exchange system. http://childes.talkbank.org/. Accessed 1 June 2014
Chow HM, Chang SE (2017) White matter developmental trajectories associated with persistence and recovery of childhood stuttering. Hum Brain Mapp 38(7):3345–3359. https://doi.org/10.1002/hbm.23590. Epub 2017 Apr 8. PMID: 28390149; PMCID: PMC5632574
Chow HM, Garnett EO, Koenraads SPC, Chang SE (2023) Brain developmental trajectories associated with childhood stuttering persistence and recovery. Dev Cogn Neurosci 60:101224. https://doi.org/10.1016/j.dcn.2023.101224. Epub 2023 Feb 26. PMID: 36863188; PMCID: PMC9986501
Cohen SM, Jacobson BH, Garrett CG et al (2007) Creation and validation of the Singing Voice Handicap Index. Ann Otol Rhinol Laryngol 116(6):402–406
Cohen SM, Statham M, Rosen CA et al (2009) Development and validation of the Singing Voice Handicap Index-10. Laryngoscope 119(9):1864–1869
Coleman C, Yaruss JS (2014) A comprehensive view of stuttering: implications for assessment and treatment. Perspectives 15(2):75–80
Colton RH, Casper JK (1996) Understanding voice problems. Williams & Wilkins, Baltimore
Colton RH, Woo P (1995) Measuring vocal fold function. In: Rubin JS et al (eds) Diagnosis and treatment of voice disorders. Igaku-Shoin, New York, pp 290–315
Connally EL, Ward D, Howell P et al (2014) Disrupted white matter in language and motor tracts in developmental stuttering. Brain Lang 131:25–35
Connally EL, Ward D, Pliatsikas C et al (2018) Separation of trait and state in stuttering. Hum Brain Mapp 39:3109–3126
Constantino CD, Manning WH, Nordstrom SN (2017) Rethinking covert stuttering. J Fluency Disord 53:26–40
Conture EG (1997) Evaluating childhood stuttering. In: Curlee RF, Siegel GM (eds) Nature and treatment of stuttering: new directions. Allyn & Bacon, Boston, pp 237–256
Conture EG (2001) Stuttering: its nature, diagnosis and treatment. Allyn & Bacon, Boston
Cook S (2013) Fragebogen zur psychosozialen Belastung durch das Stottern für Kinder und Jugendliche (Questionnaire on the psychosocial burden of stuttering for children and adolescents). LOGOS Interdisziplinär 21(2):97–105
Cook S, Howell P (2015) Children's and parents' perspectives about the psychosocial impact of stuttering and stuttering-related bullying. In: St. Louis KO (ed) Stuttering meets stereotype, stigma, and discrimination, 1st edn. West Virginia University Press, Morgantown, pp 274–283
Corrigan PW, Watson AC (2002) The paradox of self-stigma and mental illness. Clin Psychol (New York) 9(1):35–53
Corrigan PW, Larson JE, Rüsch N (2009) Self-stigma and the "why try" effect: impact on life goals and evidence-based practices. World Psychiatry 8(2):75–81
Costa PT, McCrae RR (1992) Revised NEO Personality Inventory (NEO-PIR) and NEO Five Factor Inventory (NEO-FFI) professional manual. Psychological Assessment Resources, Odessa
Craig A, Hancock H, Tran Y et al (2003) Anxiety levels in people who stutter: a randomized population study. J Speech Lang Hear Res 46(5):1197–1206
Craig-McQuaide A, Akram H, Zrinzo L et al (2014) A review of brain circuitries involved in stuttering. Front Hum Neurosci 8:884. https://doi.org/10.3389/fnhum.2014.00884
Cruz C, Amorim H, Beça G et al (2018) Neurogenic stuttering: a review of the literature. Rev Neurol 66(2):59–64
Curlee RF (1999) Identification and case selection guidelines for early childhood stuttering. In: Curlee RF (ed) Stuttering and related disorders of fluency, 2nd edn. Thieme Medical, New York, pp 1–21
Curlee RF (2007) Identification and case selection guidelines for early childhood stuttering. In: Conture EG, Curlee RF (eds) Stuttering and related disorders of fluency, 3rd edn. Thieme, New York, pp 3–22
Dacakis G, Davies S, Oates JM et al (2013) Development and preliminary evaluation of the transsexual voice questionnaire for male-to-female transsexuals. J Voice 27(3):312–320
Dale PS (1991) The validity of a parent report measure of vocabulary and syntax at 24 months. J Speech Hear Res 34(3):565–571
Damsté PH (1966) Les vibrations des cordes vocales compares aux vibrations des levres d'un trombonist. J Fr Otorhinolaryngol Chir Maxillofac 4:395–396

Daniels DE, Hagstrom F, Gabel RM (2006) A qualitative study of how African American men who stutter attribute meaning to identity and life choices. J Fluen Disord 31(3):200–215
Daroff RB, Jankovic J, Mazziotta JC et al (2016) Diagnosis of neurological disease. In: Daroff RB, Jankovic J, Mazziotta JC et al (eds) Bradley's neurology in clinical practice, 7th edn. Elsevier, London, pp 1–8
Davis S, Howell P, Cooke F (2002) Sociodynamic relationships between children who stutter and their non-stuttering classmates. J Child Psychol Psychiatry 43(7):939–947
Davis S, Shisca D, Howell P (2007) Anxiety in speakers who persist and recover from stuttering. J Commun Disord 40(5):398–417
De Bodt MS, Van de Heyning PH, Wuyts FL et al (1996) The perceptual evaluation of voice disorders. Acta Otorhinolaryngol Belg 50(4):283–291
De Bodt MS, Wuyts FL, Van de Heyning PH et al (1997) Test-retest study of the GRBAS scale: influence of experience and professional background on perceptual rating of voice quality. J Voice 11(1):74–80
De Krom G (1995) Some spectral correlates of pathological breathy and rough voice quality for different types of vowel fragments. J Speech Hear Res 38(4):794–811
De Nil LF, Kroll RM, Houle S (2001) Functional neuroimaging of cerebellar activation during single word reading and verb generation in stuttering and nonstuttering adults. Neurosci Lett 302:77–80
De Nil LF, Kroll RM, Lafaille SJ et al (2004) A positron emission tomography study of short- and long-term treatment effects on functional brain activation in adults who stutter. J Fluen Disord 28:357–380
Deco G, Ponce-Alvarez A, Mantini D et al (2013) Resting-state functional connectivity emerges from structurally and dynamically shaped slow linear fluctuations. J Neurosci 33:11239–11252
Dejonckere PH (1987) EMG of the larynx. Press Productions, Liège
Dejonckere PH (1996) Electroglottography: a useful method in voice investigation. In: Pais-Clemente M (ed) Voice update. Excerpta Medica/Elsevier, Amsterdam, pp 29–33
Dejonckere PH (1998) Effect of louder voicing on acoustical measurements in dysphonic patients. Logoped Phoniatr Vocol 23(2):79–84
Dejonckere PH (2000) Perceptual and laboratory assessment of dysphonia. Otolaryngol Clin N Am 33(4):731–750
Dejonckere PH (2006a) Aerodynamic and acoustic voice measurements. In: Benninger MS, Murry T (eds) The performer's voice. Plural Publishing, San Diego
Dejonckere PH (2006b) Critères acoustiques de fluence pour l'évaluation des dysphonies spasmodiques. In: Klein-Dallant C (ed) Paris, pp 157–166
Dejonckere P (2010) Assessment of voice and respiratory function. In: Remacle M, Eckel HE (eds) Surgery of larynx and trachea, vol 11. Springer-Verlag, Berlin. https://doi.org/10.1007/978-3-540-79136-2_2
Dejonckere PH, Lebacq J (2001) Plasticity of voice quality: a prognostic factor for outcome of voice therapy? J Voice 15(2):251–256
Dejonckere PH, van Wijngaarden HA (2001) Retropharyngeal autologous fat transplantation for congenital short palate: a nasometric assessment of functional results. Ann Otol Rhinol Laryngol 110(2):168–172
Dejonckere PH, Knoops P, Lebacq J (1988) Evoked muscular potentials in laryngeal muscles. Acta Otolaryngol Belg 42(4):494–501
Dejonckere PH, Obbens C, de Moor GM et al (1993) Perceptual evaluation of dysphonia: reliability and relevance. Folia Phoniatr 45(2):76–83
Dejonckere PH, Remacle M, Fresnel-Elbaz E et al (1996) Differentiated perceptual evaluation of pathological voice quality: reliability and correlations with acoustic measurements. Rev Laryngol Otol Rhinol 117(3):219–224
Dejonckere PH, Crevier L, Elbaz E et al (2000) Clinical implementation of a multidimensional basic protocol for assessing functional results of voice therapy. In: Jahnke K, Fischer M (eds) Proceedings of the 4th EUFOS Congress, Berlin, pp 561–565
Dejonckere PH, Bradley P, Clemente P et al (2001) A basic protocol for functional assessment of voice pathology, especially for investigating the efficacy of (phonosurgical) treatments and evaluating new assessment techniques. Guideline elaborated by the Committee on Phoniatrics of the European Laryngological Society (ELS). Eur Arch Otorhinolaryngol 258(2):77–82
Dejonckere PH, Schoentgen J, Giordano A et al (2011) Validity of jitter measures in non-quasi-periodic voices. Part I: perceptual and computer performances in cycle pattern recognition. The effect of noise. Logoped Phoniatr Vocol 36(2):70–77
Dejonckere PH, Giordano A, Schoentgen J et al (2012a) To what degree of voice perturbation are jitter measurements valid? A novel approach with synthesized vowels and visuo-perceptual pattern recognition. Biomed Signal Process Control 7(1):37–42
Dejonckere PH, Neumann KJ, Moerman MB et al (2012b) Tridimensional assessment of adductor spasmodic dysphonia pre- and post-treatment with botulinum toxin. Eur Arch Otorhinolaryngol 269(4):1195–2003
Dejonckere PH, Moerman MB, Martens JP et al (2012c) Voicing quantification is more relevant than period perturbation in substitution voices: an advanced acoustical study. Eur Arch Otorhinolaryngol 269(4):1205–1212
Demirel B, Chesters J, Connally EL et al (2024) No evidence of altered language laterality in people who stutter across different brain imaging studies of speech and language. Brain Commun 6(5):fcae305. https://doi.org/10.1093/braincomms/fcae305. PMID: 39346021; PMCID: PMC11430911
Digman JM (1990) Personality structure: emergence of the five-factor model. Annu Rev Psychol 41(1):417–440

DiLollo A, Manning WH, Neimeyer RA (2003) Cognitive anxiety as a function of speaker role for fluent speakers and persons who stutter. J Fluen Disord 28(3):167–186

Dilling H, Mombour W, Schmidt MH (2008) Internationale Klassifikation psychischer Störungen, 6th edn. Hans Huber, Bern

Donnet A, Dessi P, Koeppel MC (1996) Le syndrome de Satchmo. Presse Med 25(4):173

Douglass JE, Constantino C, Alvarado J et al (2019) Qualitative investigation of the speech-language therapy experiences of individuals who covertly stutter. J Fluen Disord 61(1):9–26

DuBois DL, Felner RD, Brand S et al (1996) Early adolescent self-esteem: a developmental-ecological framework and assessment strategy. J Res Adolesc 6(4):543–579

Duffy RJ (2013) Motor speech disorders, 3rd edn. Elsevier, London, pp 95–335

Echternach M, Sundberg J, Baumann T et al (2011) Vocal tract area functions and formant frequencies in opera tenors' modal and falsetto registers. J Acoust Soc Am 129(6):3955–3963

Echternach M, Markl M, Richter B et al (2012) Dynamic real-time magnetic resonance imaging for the analysis of voice physiology. Curr Opin Otolaryngol Head Neck Surg 20(6):450–457

Echternach M, Richter B, Traser L et al (2013) Veränderung der stimmlichen Leistungsfähigkeit durch verschiedene Stimmbelastungstests. (Change of vocal capacity due to different vocal loading tests). Laryngo-Rhino-Otol 92(1):34–40

Echternach M, Birkholz P, Traser L et al (2015) Articulation and vocal tract acoustics at soprano subject's high fundamental frequencies. J Acoust Soc Am 137(5):2586–2596

Eggers K (2010) What is normal dysfluency and why measure it? Belgium. Seminar presented at the convention of the International Association of Logopedics and Phoniatrics, 4 October 2010, Athens

Eggers K, Van Eerdenbrugh S, Byrd C (2019) Speech disfluencies in bilingual Yiddish-Dutch speaking children. Clin Linguist Phon 34(6):576–592

Eggers K, Millard SK, Kelman E (2022) Temperament, anxiety, and depression in school-age children who stutter. J Commun Disord. 97:106218. https://doi.org/10.1016/j.jcomdis.2022.106218. Epub 2022 May 4. PMID: 35597191

Epstein R, Hirani SP, Stygall J et al (2009) How do individuals cope with voice disorders? Introducing the Voice Disability Coping Questionnaire. J Voice 23(2):209–217

Erickson RL (1969) Assessing communication attitudes among stutterers. J Speech Hear Res 12(4):711–724

Etchell A, Civier O, Ballard KJ et al (2018) A systematic literature review of neuroimaging research on developmental stuttering between 1995 and 2016. J Fluen Disord 55:6–45

Evans D, Healey CE, Kawai N et al (2008) Middle school students' perceptions of a peer who stutters. J Fluen Disord 33(3):203–219

Eysholdt U (2014) Heiserkeit: biomechanik und quantitative laryngoskopie. HNO 62(7):541–552

Eysholdt U, Lohscheller J (2008) Phonovibrogramm: stimmlippendynamik in einem Bild. HNO 56(12):1207–1212

Ezrati-Vinacour R, Levin I (2004) The relationship between anxiety and stuttering: a multidimensional approach. J Fluen Disord 29(2):135–148

Fang-Ling L, Matteson S (2014) Speech tasks and interrater reliability in perceptual voice evaluation. J Voice 28(6):725–732

Flesch J (1925) Berufs-Krankheiten des Musikers. Ein Leitfaden der Berufsberatung für Musiker, Musikpädagogen, Ärzte und Eltern. Kampmann, Celle, pp 82–113

Fourcin A, Abberton E (2008) Hearing and phonetic criteria in voice measurement: clinical applications. Logoped Phoniatr Vocol 33(1):35–48

Fourcin A, Abberton E, Miller D et al (1995) Laryngography. Eur J Disord Commun 30:101–115

Friedman EM (1997) Role of ultrasound in the assessment of vocal cord function in infants and children. Ann Otol Rhinol Laryngol 106(3):199–209

Fritzell B, Hallen O, Sundberg J (1974) Evaluation of Teflon injection procedures for paralytic dysphonia. Folia Phoniatr 26(6):414–421

Frost RO, Marten P, Lahart C et al (1990) The dimensions of perfectionism. Cognit Ther Res 14(5):449–468

Frucht SJ (2009) Embouchure dystonia—portrait of a task-specific cranial dystonia. Mov Disord 24(12):1752–1762

Frucht SJ, Fahn S, Greene PE et al (2001) The natural history of embouchure dystonia. Mov Disord 16(5):899–906

Fussi F (2005) La voce del cantante, vol III. Omega, Torino

Gabel RM, Blood GW, Tellis GM et al (2004) Measuring role entrapment of people who stutter. J Fluen Disord 29(1):27–49

Gall V, Hanson J (1973) Bestimmung physikalischer Parameter der Stimmlippenschwingungen mit Hilfe der Larynxphotokymographie. Folia Phoniatr 25:450–459

Gall V, Gall D, Hanson J (1971) Larynx-Fotokymografie. Arch klin exp Ohr-, Nas- u Kehlk Heilk 200(1):34–41

Garel C, Legrand I, Elmaleh M et al (1990) Laryngeal ultrasonography in infants and children: anatomical correlation with fetal preparations. Pediatr Radiol 20(4):241–244

Garel C, Contencin P, Polonovski JM et al (1992) Laryngeal ultrasonography in infants and children: a new way of investigating. Normal and pathological findings. Int J Pediatr Otorhinolaryngol 23(2):107–115

Garnett EO, Chow HM, Nieto-Castañón A et al (2018) Anomalous morphology in left hemisphere motor and premotor cortex of children who stutter. Brain 141:2670–2684

Gelfer MP, Pazera JF (2006) Maximum duration of sustained /s/ and /z/ and the s/z ratio with controlled intensity. J Voice 20(3):369–379
Gentner R, Classen J (2006) Modular organization of finger movements by the human central nervous system. Neuron 52(4):731–742
Gerratt B, Kreiman J, Barroso NA et al (1993) Comparing internal and external standards in voice quality judgments. J Speech Hear Res 2(36):14–20
Ghirardi AC, Ferreira LP, Giannini SP et al (2013) Screening index for voice disorder (SIVD): development and validation. J Voice 27(2):195–200
Gilio F, Curra A, Lorenzano C et al (2000) Effects of botulinum toxin type A on intracortical inhibition in patients with dystonia. Ann Neurol 48(1):20–26
Gillam RB, Logan KJ, Pearson NA (2009) TOCS: test of childhood stuttering. Pro-Ed, Austin
Glascoe FP, Dworkin PH (1995) The role of parents in the detection of developmental and behavioral problems. Pediatrics 95(6):829–836
Godino-Llorente JI, Osma-Ruiz V, Saenz-Lecho N et al (2010) The effectiveness of the glottal to noise excitation ratio for the screening of voice disorders. J Voice 24(1):47–56
Gomaa MA, Hammad MS, Mamdoh H et al (2013) Value of high resolution ultrasonography in assessment of laryngeal lesions. Otolaryngol Pol 67(5):252–256
Gould J, Waugh J, Carding P et al (2012) A new voice rating tool for clinical practice. J Voice 26(4):e163–e170
Grant AC, Biousse V, Cook AA et al (1999) Stroke associated stuttering. Arch Neurol 56(5):624–627
Grim KK, Phillips GD, Renner DR (2015) Dysarthria and stutter as presenting symptoms of late-onset Tay-Sachs disease in three siblings. Mov Disord Clin Pract 2(3):289–290
Groner S, Walden T, Jones R (2016) Factors associated with negative attitudes toward speaking in preschool-age children who do and do not stutter. Contemporary issues in communication science and disorders. Contemp Issues Commun Sci Disord 43:255–267
Gross M (1985) Larynxfotokymographie. Sprache Stimme Gehör 9:112–113
Grunert D, Stier B, Klingebiel T et al (1989) Ultraschalldiagnostik des Larynx mit Hilfe der Computersonographie. Laryngol Rhinol Otol 68(4):236–238
Guenther FH (2016) Neural control of speech. MIT Press, Cambridge
Guitar B (2013) Stuttering: an integrated approach to its nature and treatment, 4th edn. Lippincott Williams & Wilkins, Baltimore
Guitar B (2019) Stuttering: an integrated approach to its nature and treatment, 5th edn. Lippincott Williams & Wilkins, Baltimore
Guttormsen LS, Yaruss JS, Næss KAB (2021) Parents' perceptions of the overall impact of stuttering on young children. Am J Speech Lang Pathol 30(5):2130–2142. https://doi.org/10.1044/2021_AJSLP-20-00113
Hacki T (1996) Die Dysphonie und ihre Diagnostik. LOGOS 4(4):255–261
Halag-Milo T, Stoppelman N, Kronfeld-Duenias V et al (2016) Beyond production: brain responses during speech perception in adults who stutter. Neuro Image Clin 11:328–338
Hallett M, Di Iorio R, Rossini PM et al (2017) Contribution of transcranial magnetic stimulation to assessment of brain connectivity and networks. Clin Neurophysiol 128(11):2125–2139
Hammarberg B (2000) Voice research and clinical needs. Folia Phoniatr Logop 52(1–3):93–102
Haynes WO, Moran MJ, Pindzola RH (2006) Communication disorders in the classroom: an introduction for Professionals in School Settings, 4th edn. Jones & Bartlett Learning, Burlington, pp 267–269
Helmholtz H (1875) On the sensations of tone as a physiological basis for the theory of music. Longmans, Green and Co., London, p 146
Herbst CT, Oh J, Vydrová J et al (2015) DigitalVHI-a freeware open-source software application to capture the Voice Handicap Index and other questionnaire data in various languages. Logoped Phoniatr Vocol 40(2):72–76
Heylen L, Wuyts F, Mertens F et al (1998) Evaluation of the vocal performance of children using a voice range profile index. J Speech Lang Hear Res 41(2):232–238
Heylen L, Wuyts FL, Mertens F et al (2002) Normative voice range profiles of male and female professional voice users. J Voice 16(1):1–7
Hillman RE, Holmberg EB, Perkell JS et al (1989) Objective assessment of vocal hyperfunction: an experimental framework and initial results. J Speech Hear Res 32:373–392
Hirano M (1974) Morphological structure of the vocal cord as a vibrator and its variations. Folia Phoniatr 26(2):89–94
Hirano M (1981) Clinical examination of voice. In: Arnold GE et al (eds) Disorders of human communication, vol 5. Springer, Wien
Hirano M (1989) Objective evaluation of the human voice: clinical aspects. Folia Phoniatr 41(2–3):89–144
Hirano M, Koike Y, von Leden H (1968) Maximum phonation time and air usage during phonation. Folia Phoniatr 20(4):185–201
Hogikyan ND, Sethuraman G (1999) Validation of an instrument to measure "voice-related quality of life" (VRQOL). J Voice 13(4):557–569
Hollender MH (1965) Perfectionism. Compr Psychiatry 6(2):94–103
Hosokawa K, Ogawa M, Hashimoto M et al (2014) Statistical analysis of the reliability of acoustic and electroglottographic perturbation parameters for the detection of vocal roughness. J Voice 28(2):263.e9–263.e16. https://doi.org/10.1016/j.jvoice.2013.07.005
Hsiao TY, Wang CL, Chen CN et al (2001) Noninvasive assessment of laryngeal phonation function using color Doppler ultrasound imaging. Ultrasound Med Biol 27(8):1035–1040

Hsiao TY, Wang CL, Chen CN et al (2002) Elasticity of human vocal folds measured in vivo using color Doppler imaging. Ultrasound Med Biol 28(9):1145–1152

Hunter EJ, Titze IR (2010) Variations in intensity, fundamental frequency and voicing for teachers in occupational versus nonoccupational settings. J Speech Lang Hear Res 53(4):862–875

Ingham RJ, Ingham JC, Euler HA et al (2018) Stuttering treatment and brain research in adults: a still unfolding relationship. J Fluen Disord 55:106–119

Isogai Y (1994) X-ray stroboscopy and laryngostrobography. In: Proceedings of the 3rd international symposium on phonosurgery, Kyoto, 26–28 June 1994. International Association of Phonosurgeons, pp 238–239

Iverach L, O'Brian S, Jones M et al (2010) The five factor model of personality applied to adults who stutter. J Commun Disord 43(2):120–132

Jackson ES, Yaruss JS, Quesal RW et al (2015) Responses of adults who stutter to the anticipation of stuttering. J Fluen Disord 45:38–51

Jacobson BH, Johnson A, Grywalski C et al (1997) The Voice Handicap Index (VHI): development and validation. Am J Speech Lang Pathol 6:66–70

Jafari R, Shahbodaghi R, Ashayeri H et al (2014) The five factor model of personality and stuttering. Procedia Soc Behav Sci 127:307–310

Jankovic J (2016) Parkinson disease and other movement disorders. In: Darrof RB, Jankovic J, Mazziotta J et al (eds) Bradley's neurology in clinical practice, 7th edn. Elsevier, London, pp 1422–1460

Jannati A, Ryan MA, Kaye HL et al (2021) Biomarkers obtained by transcranial magnetic stimulation in neurodevelopmental disorders. J Clin Neurophysiol 39:135. https://doi.org/10.1097/WNP.0000000000000784

Jilek C, Marienhagen J, Hacki T (2004) Vocal stability in functional dysphonic versus healthy voices at different times of voice loading. J Voice 18(4):443–453

Johnson J (2008) The visualization of the twisted tongue: portrayals of stuttering in film, television and comic books. J Pop Cult 41(2):245–261

Johnson W, Boehmler RM, Dahlstrom WG et al (1959) The onset of stuttering. University of Minnesota Press, Minneapolis

Johnson DM, Hapner ER, Klein AM et al (2014) Validation of a telephone screening tool for spasmodic dysphonia and vocal fold tremor. J Voice 28(6):711–715

Johnson CA, Gerwin KL, Tichenor SE et al (2024) Evaluating stuttering self-stigma and its relationship to adverse impact in children and adolescents with the child stuttering self-stigma scale. J Speech Lang Hear Res 67(9):2920–2934. https://doi.org/10.1044/2024_JSLHR-24-00069

Jones R, Eggers K, Zengin-Bolatkale H (2020) Temperamental and emotional processes. In: Zebrowski P, Anderson J, Conture E (eds) Stuttering: characteristics, assessment, and treatment, 4th edn. Thieme Medical Publishers, New York. Chapter in review

Jones R, Eggers K, Zengin-Bolatkale H (2022) Temperamental and emotional processes. In: Zebrowksi P, Anderson J, Conture E (eds) Stuttering and related disorders of fluency, 4th edn. Thieme Medical, New York, pp 78–91

Jun BC, Kim HT, Kim HS et al (2005) Clinical feasibility of the new technique of functional 3D laryngeal CT. Acta Otolaryngol 125(7):774–778

Kalinowski J, Stuart A, Armson J (1996) Perceptions of stutterers and nonstutterers during speaking and nonspeaking situations. Am J Speech Lang Pathol 5(2):61–67

Karnell M, Melton S, Childes J et al (2007) Reliability of Clinician-Based (GRABAS and CAPE-V) and Patient-Based (V-RQOL and IPVI) documentation of voice disorders. J Voice 21(5):576–590

Kaufman AS, Kaufman NL (1983) Kaufman assessment battery for children. American Guidance Service, Circle Pines, MN

Kaufman AS, Kaufman NL (2004) Kaufman-assessment battery for children, 2nd edn (KABC-II). AGS Publications, Circle Pines, MN

Kell CA, Neumann K, von Kriegstein K et al (2009) How the brain repairs stuttering. Brain 132:2747–2760

Kell CA, Neumann K, Behrens M et al (2018) Speaking-related changes in cortical functional connectivity associated with assisted and spontaneous recovery from developmental stuttering. J Fluen Disord 55:135–144

Kell CA, Warneke N, Zentsch V et al. (in press) Left thalamic stimulation for developmental stuttering. Manuscript under review at J Fluency Disord.

Keller T (2014) ROC-Analysen. http://www.acomed-statistik.de/roc-kurve.html. Accessed 1 June 2014

Kent RD (2000) Research on speech motor control and its disorders: a review and prospective. J Commun Disorder 33(5):391–427

Kent RD, Kent JF, Rosenbek JC (1987) Maximum performance tests of speech production. J Speech Hear Disord 52(4):367–387

Kikuchi Y, Umezaki T, Uehara T et al (2008) A case of multiple system atrophy-parkinsonian type with stuttering- and palilalia-like dysfluencies and putaminal atrophy. J Fluen Disord 57:51–58

Kim YC, Narayanan SS, Nayak KS et al (2009) Accelerated 3D MRI of vocal tract shaping using compressed sensing and parallel imaging. Proc IEEE Int Conf Acoust Speech Signal Process 34:389–392

Kitzing P (1981) Veränderung der Sprechstimmlage bei Dysphoniepatienten in Zusammenhang mit Stimmbelastung. HNO-Praxis 6:215

Klein ER, Amster BJ (2004) The effects of cognitive behavioral therapy with people who stutter. In: Packmann A, Meltzer A, Peters H (eds) Theory, research, and fluency disorders: proceedings of the fourth world congress of fluency disorders. Nijmegen University Press, Nijmegen, pp 154–160

Kliegman RM, Stanton BF, St. Geme JW et al (eds) (2011) Nelson textbook of pediatrics, 19th edn. Elsevier, Philadelphia

Klompas M, Ross E (2004) Life experiences of people who stutter, and the perceived impact of stuttering on quality of life: personal accounts of South African individuals. J Fluen Disord 29(4):275–305

Koenraads SPC, Marroun HE, Muetzel RL et al (2019) Stuttering and gray matter morphometry: a population-based neuroimaging study in young children. Brain Lang 194:121–131

Koenraads SPC, van der Schroeff MP, van Ingen G et al (2020) Structural brain differences in pre-adolescents who persist in and recover from stuttering. Neuroimage Clin 27:102334. https://doi.org/10.1016/j.nicl.2020.102334

König K (2009) Möglichkeiten und Grenzen in der Behandlung neurogenen Stotterns. Entwicklung, Evaluation und Anwendung eines Erhebungsinstrumentes (Possibilities and limits in the treatment of neurogenic stuttering. Development, evaluation and application of a survey tool). Dissertation. Technische Universität Dortmund, Dortmund

Korzeczek A, Primaßin A, von Gudenberg AW et al (2021) Fluency shaping increases integration of the command-to-execution and the auditory-to-motor pathways in persistent developmental stuttering. NeuroImage 245:118736. https://doi.org/10.1016/j.neuroimage.2021.118736

Kraaimaat FW, Vanryckeghem M, Van Dam-Baggen R (2002) Stuttering and social anxiety. J Fluen Disord 27(4):319–331

Kramer H, Doleschal J, Hacki T et al (1998) Verbesserung der Stimmbelastbarkeit durch stationäre Rehabilitationsmaßnahmen. In: Gross M (ed) Aktuelle phoniatrisch-pädaudiologische Aspekte 1997/98, vol 5. Median Verlag von Killisch Horn GmbH, Heidelberg, pp 76–79

Kramer H, Pérez Álvarez JC, Hacki T (1999) Stimmleistungscharakterisierende Kurventypen im Stimmbelastungstest. In: Gross M (ed) Aktuelle phoniatrisch-pädaudiologische Aspekte 1998/99, 6th edn. Median Verlag von Killisch-Horn GmbH, Heidelberg, pp 75–79

Kreiman J, Gerratt B, Precoda K et al (1992) Individual differences in voice quality perception. J Speech Hear Res 6(35):512–520

Kreiman J, Gerratt B, Kempster G et al (1993) Perceptual evaluation of voice quality: review, tutorial, and a framework for future research. J Speech Hear Res 2(36):21–40

Krishnan G, Tiwari S (2011) Revisiting the acquired neurogenic stuttering in the light of developmental stuttering. J Neurolinguistics 24(3):383–396

Kroemer KHE, Grandjean E (1997) Fitting the task to the human, 5th edn. Taylor & Francis, London

Kronfeld-Duenias V, Amir O, Ezrati-Vinacour R et al (2016) Dorsal and ventral language pathways in persistent developmental stuttering. Cortex 81:79–92

Kujirai T, Caramia MD, Rothwell JC et al (1993) Corticocortical inhibition in human motor cortex. J Physiol 471:501–519

Lahey BB (2009) Public health significance of neuroticism. Am Psychol 64(4):241–256

Landau AR (2011) Experiences and expectations of children who stutter and their significant others. Unpublished master's dissertation. University College London, London

Landeck E (1974) Lippenläsionen bei Blechblasinstrumentalisten. Derm Mschr 160:762–765

Lanz T, Wachsmuth W (1955) Praktische Anatomie. Ein Lehr- und Hilfsbuch der anatomischen Grundlagen ärztlichen Handelns Vol. 1, Part 2: Hals. Springer, Berlin, pp 28–33, 204–205, 469

de Langen-Müller U, Kiese-Himmel C, Neumann K et al (equal authorship) (2012) Diagnostik von (umschriebenen) Sprachentwicklungsstörungen, 1st edn. Peter Lang, Frankfurt am Main

Laukkanen AM, Kankare E (2006) Vocal loading-related changes in male teachers' voices investigated before and after a working day. Folia Phoniatr Logop 58(4):229–239

Laukkanen AM, Järvinen K, Artkoski M et al (2004) Changes in voice and subjective sensations during a 45-min vocal loading test in female subjects with vocal training. Folia Phoniatr Logop 56(6):335–346

Laver J (1980) The phonetic description of voice quality. British Library Catalogue in Publication Data. Cambridge University Press, Cambridge

Laver J, Hiller S, Mackenzie Beck J (1992) Acoustic waveform perturbation and voice disorders. J Voice 6(2):115–126

Law J, Boyle J, Harris F et al (2000) The feasibility of universal screening for primary speech and language delay: findings from a systematic review of the literature. Dev Med Child Neurol 42(3):190–200

Lebacq J, DeJonckere PH (2019) The dynamics of voice onset. Biomed Signal Process Control 49:528–539

Leclercq AL, Suaire P, Moyse A (2017) Beyond stuttering: speech disfluencies in normally fluent French-speaking children at age 4. Clin Linguist Phon 32(2):166–179

Lee L, Stemple J, Glaze L et al (2004) Quick screen for voice and supplementary documents for pediatric voice disorders. Lang Speech Hear Serv Sch 35(4):308–319

Leech KA, Bernstein Ratner N, Brown B et al (2017) Preliminary evidence that growth in productive language differentiates childhood stuttering persistence and recovery. J Speech Lang Hear Res 60(11):3097–3109

Lei X, Sasisekaran J, Nguyen-Feng VN (2024) The experience of stuttering in everyday life among adults who stutter: the impact of trait social anxiety and the social situations. J Fluency Disord 80:106061. https://doi.org/10.1016/j.jfludis.2024.106061

Lell MM, Gress H, Hothorn T et al (2004) Multiplanar functional imaging of the larynx and hypopharynx with multislice spiral CT. Eur Radiol 14(12):2198–2205

Leno L (1971) Lip vibration characteristics of the trombone embouchure in performance. Instrumentalist 25:56–62

Leno L (1974) Lip vibration characteristics of the trombone embouchure in performance. Brass Bulletin 7(1):7–41

Leno L (1995) Eine Studie von (sic) Lippenvibrationen mit Highspeed-Fotographie. Schallstück 16:14–18

Leno L (2009) Lip vibration of trombone embouchures. Part1: http://www.youtube.com/watch?v=CoxnhjLMVBo&feature=channel_page. Part2: http://www.youtube.com/watch?v=UHq7vCihaXg&feature=channel_page. Part3: http://www.youtube.com/watch?v=gmBDG_wAeS4&feature=channel_page. Accessed 6 Dec 2016

Levine AB, MacDougall KW (2016) New-onset stutter after electrode insertion in the ventrocaudalis nucleus for face pain. World Neurosurg 90:703.e7–703.e10. https://doi.org/10.1016/j.wneu.2016.02.085

Likert R (1932) A technique for the measurement of attitudes. Arch Psychol 140:1–55

Lindestad PÅ, Södersten M, Merker B et al (2001) Voice source characteristics in Mongolian "throat singing" studied with high-speed imaging technique, acoustic spectra, and inverse filtering. J Voice 15(1):78–85

Liu S, Hayden GF (2002) Maladies in musicians. South Med J 95(7):727–734

Loock F, Lorenz M (1981) Berufskrankheiten und Berufsunfähigkeiten bei Bläsern. Arbeitshygienische Beratungsstelle der Theater und Orchester der DDR (Berlin Ost). Arbeitsmedizinische Informationen für Theater und Orchester 4:12–16

Lu C, Chen C, Peng D et al (2012) Neural anomaly and reorganization in speakers who stutter. Neurology 79:625–632

Lu C, Zheng L, Long Y et al (2017) Reorganization of brain function after a short-term behavioral intervention for stuttering. Brain Lang 168:12–22

Luchsinger R (1949) Die Stroboskopie des Kehlkopfes. In: Luchsinger R, Arnold GE (eds) Lehrbuch der Stimm- und Sprachheilkunde. Springer, Wien, pp 30–36

Ludlow CL, Loucks T (2003) Stuttering: a dynamic motor control disorder. J Fluen Disord 28(4):273–295

Luiz D, Barnard A, Knosen N et al (2006) Griffiths Mental Development Scales—extended revised: 2 to 8 years (GMDS-ER 2-8). Administration and Analysis Manual. http://www.hogrefe.co.uk/clinical-and-educational/child-development/gmds-er-2-8.html. Accessed 15 Nov 2016

Lundgren K, Helm-Estabrooks N, Klein R (2010) Stuttering following acquired brain damage: a review of the literature. J Neurolinguistics 23(5):447–454

Ma EP, Yiu EM (2001) Voice activity and participation profile: assessing the impact of voice disorders on daily activities. J Speech Lang Hear Res 44(3):511–524

MacWhinney B (1995) The CHILDES project: tools for analyzing talk, 2nd edn. Erlbaum, Mahwah

Maguire GA, Riley GD, Franklin DL et al (2000) Risperidone for the treatment of stuttering. J Clin Psychopharmacol 20(4):479–482

Maguire GA, Yu BP, Franklin DL et al (2004) Alleviating stuttering with pharmacological interventions. Expert Opin Pharmacother 5(7):1565–1571

Maguire GA, Ngo J, Fonsworth PK et al (2012) Alleviation of developmental stuttering following deep brain stimulation of the ventral intermediate nucleus of the thalamus. Am J Psychiatry 169(7):759–760

Maneiro F (2014) Ruptura del músculo orbicular de los labios en un músico de viento (syndrome de Satchmo), a propósito de un caso. (Rupture of the orbicular oris muscle in a wind instrument player SATCHMO Syndrome). About a particular case. Med Segur Trab 60:779–785

Manfredi C, Dejonckere PH (2016) Voice dosimetry and monitoring, with emphasis on professional voice diseases: critical review and framework for future research. Logoped Phoniatr Vocol 41(2):49–65

Manfredi C, Giordano A, Schoentgen J et al (2011) Validity of jitter measures in non-quasi-periodic voices, Part II: the effect of noise. Logoped Phoniatr Vocol 36(2):78–89

Manfredi C, Giordano A, Schoentgen J et al (2012) Perturbation measurements in highly irregular voice signals: performances/validity of analysis software tools. Biomed Signal Process Control 7(4):37–42

Manning WH (2010) Clinical decision making in the diagnosis and treatment of fluency disorders, 3rd edn. Delmar, Clifton Park

Martens JW, Versnel H, Dejonckere PH (2007) The effect of visible speech in the perceptual rating of pathological voices. Arch Otolaryngol Head Neck Surg 13(2):178–185

Martin D (1942) Lip vibrations in a cornet mouthpiece. J Acoust Soc Am 13:305–308

Maryn Y, Corthals P, Van Cauwenberge P et al (2010a) Toward improved ecological validity in the acoustic measurement of overall voice quality: combining continuous speech and sustained vowels. J Voice 24(5):540–555

Maryn Y, De Bodt M, Roy N (2010b) The Acoustic Voice Quality Index: toward improved treatment outcomes assessment in voice disorders. J Commun Disord 43(3):161–174

Mauersberger R (2016) Lippenschwingungen und Stimmgebung bei Blechbläsern. Inauguraldissertation. Heinrich-Heine-Universität Düsseldorf, Düsseldorf

Mayes RW, Jackson-Menaldi C, DeJonckere PH et al (2008) Laryngeal electroglottography as a predictor of laryngeal electromyography. J Voice 22(6):756–759

McCrae RR, John OP (1992) An introduction to the five-factor model and its applications. J Pers 60(2):175–215

McGrew KS (2005) The Cattell-Horn-Carroll theory of cognitive abilities: past, present, and future. In: Flanagan DP, Harrison PL (eds) Contemporary intellectual assessment: theories, tests, and issues, 2nd edn. Guilford, New York, pp 136–181

McNeil MR (2008) Clinical management of sensorimotor speech disorders, 2nd edn. Thieme, New York, pp 249–268

Mendez MF (2018) Non-neurogenic language disorders: a preliminary classification. Psychosomatics 59(1):28–35
Mensch B (1964) Analyse par exploration ultrasonique du mouvement des cordes vocales isolées. Comptes rendus des séances de la Société de Biologie et de ses filiales 158 = A. 116, No. 7–12. Centre National de la Recherche Scientifique/Société de Biologie. Paris, Masson 1964, pp 2295–2296 (séance du 12 décembre 1964)
Menzies R, O'Brian S, Lowe R et al (2016) International Phase II clinical trial of CBTPsych: a standalone Internet social anxiety treatment for adults who stutter. J Fluen Disord 48:35–43
Metzger FL, Auer T, Helms G et al (2018) Shifted dynamic interactions between subcortical nuclei and inferior frontal gyri during response preparation in persistent developmental stuttering. Brain Struct Funct 223:165–182
Mickail N, Klein NC, Cunha BA (2011) West Nile virus aseptic meningitis and stuttering in woman. Emerg Infect Dism 17(8):1567–1568
Michaelis R (2004) Das Grenzsteinprinzip als Orientierungshilfe für die pädiatrische Entwicklungsbetrachtung. In: Schlack HG (ed) Entwicklungspädiatrie. Marseille, München, pp 123–129
Miles KA (1989) Ultrasound demonstration of vocal cord movements. Br J Radiol 62(741):871–872
Miller J, Andriacchi K, Nockerts A (2011) Assessing language production using SALT software: a clinician's guide to language sample analysis. SALT Software LLC, Middleton
Minifie FD, Kelsey CA, Hixon TJ (1968) Measurement of vocal fold motion using an ultrasonic Doppler velocity monitor. J Acoust Soc Am 43(5):1165–1169
Misono S, Merati AL (2012) Evidence-based practice: evaluation and management of unilateral vocal fold paralysis. Otolaryngol Clin N Am 45(5):1083–1108
Moein N, Mohamadi R, Rostami R et al (2022) Investigation of the effect of delayed auditory feedback and transcranial direct current stimulation (DAF-tDCS) treatment for the enhancement of speech fluency in adults who stutter: a randomized controlled trial. J Fluency Disord 72:105907. https://doi.org/10.1016/j.jfludis.2022.105907. Epub 2022 Apr 30. PMID: 35689904
Moreti F, Ávila ME, Rocha C et al (2012) Influence of complaints and singing style in singers voice handicap. J Soc Bras Fonoaudiol 24(3):296–300
Morris S, Jawad MSM, Eccles R (1992) Relationships between vital capacity, height and nasal airway resistance in asymptomatic volunteers. Rhinology 30(4):259–264
Muellbacher W, Ziemann U, Wissel J et al (2002) Early consolidation in human primary motor cortex. Nature 415(6872):640–644
Munin MC, Murry T, Rosen CA (2000) Laryngeal electromyography. Otolaryngol Clin N Am 33(4):759–770
Murlewska A, Gryczynski M, Gadzicki M (1992) Badania ultrasonograficzne krtani. Otolaryngol Pol 46(3):238–245
Murry T, Bone RC (1978) Aerodynamic relationships associated with normal phonation and paralytic dysphonia. Laryngoscope 88(1):100–109
Myers FL, Bakker K, St Louis KO (2012) Disfluencies in cluttered speech. J Fluen Disord 37(1):9–19
Natke U, Sandrieser P, Pietrowsky R et al (2006) Disfluency data of German preschool children who stutter and comparison children. J Fluen Disord 31(3):165–176
Nawka T (2012) Untersuchung des Schwingungsablaufs der Stimmlippen. In: Seidner W, Nawka T (eds) Handreichungen zur Stimmdiagnostik. XION medical, Berlin, pp 75–98
Nawka T, Verdonck-de Leeuw IM, De Bodt M et al (2009) Item reduction of the voice handicap index based on the original version and on European translations. Folia Phoniatr Logop 61(1):37–48
Neef NE, Jung K, Rothkegel H et al (2011a) Right-shift for non-speech motor processing in adults who stutter. Cortex 47(8):945–954
Neef NE, Paulus W, Neef A et al (2011b) Reduced intracortical inhibition and facilitation in the primary motor tongue representation of adults who stutter. Clin Neurophysiol 122:1802–1811
Neef NE, Anwander A, Friederici AD (2015a) The neurobiological grounding of persistent stuttering: from structure to function. Curr Neurol Neurosci 15(9):63. https://doi.org/10.1007/s11910-015-0579-4
Neef NE, Hoang TN, Neef A et al (2015b) Speech dynamics are coded in the left motor cortex in fluent speakers but not in adults who stutter. Brain 15(138):712–725
Neef NE, Anwander A, Bütfering C et al (2017) Structural connectivity of right frontal hyperactive areas scales with stuttering severity. Brain 141:191–204
Neef NE, Primaßin A, von Gudenberg AW et al (2021) Two cortical representations of voice control are differentially involved in speech fluency. Brain Commun 3:fcaa232. https://doi.org/10.1093/braincomms/fcaa232
Neef NE, Chang SE (2024) Knowns and unknowns about the neurobiology of stuttering. PLoS Biol 22(2):e3002492. https://doi.org/10.1371/journal.pbio.3002492. PMID: 38386639; PMCID: PMC10883586
Neef NE, Angstadt M, Koenraads SPC, Chang SE (2023) Dissecting structural connectivity of the left and right inferior frontal cortex in children who stutter. Cereb Cortex 33(7):4085–4100. https://doi.org/10.1093/cercor/bhac328. PMID: 36057839; PMCID: PMC10068293
Neiman GS, Edeson B (1981) Procedural aspects of eliciting maximum phonation time. Folia Phoniatr 33(5):285–293
Neumann K, Keilmann A, Rosenfeld J et al (2009) Leitlinien der Deutschen Gesellschaft für Phoniatrie und Pädaudiologie zu Sprachentwicklungsstörungen bei Kindern (gekürzte Fassung). Kindh Entwickl 18(4):222–231

Neumann K, Euler HA (2010) Neuroimaging in stuttering. In: Guitar B, McCauley R (eds) Treatment of stuttering: established and emerging interventions. Lippincott, Williams & Wilkins, Baltimore, pp 355–377

Neumann K, Foundas AL (2018) From locations to networks: can brain imaging inform treatment of stuttering? J Fluen Disord 55:1–5

Neumann K, Euler HA, von Gudenberg AW et al (2003) The nature and treatment of stuttering as revealed by fMRI a within- and between-group comparison. J Fluen Disord 28:381–410

Neumann K, Preibisch C, Euler HA et al (2005) Cortical plasticity associated with stuttering therapy. J Fluen Disord 30:23–39

Neumann K, Holler-Zittlau I, van Minnen S et al (2011) Katzengoldstandards in der Sprachstandserfassung. Sensitivität-Spezifität des Kindersprachscreenings (KiSS). HNO 59(1):97–109

Neumann K, Euler HA (2013) Kann ein Sprachstandsscreening zwischen Sprachförder- und Sprachtherapiebedarf trennen? In: Redder A, Weinert S (eds) Sprachförderung und Sprachdiagnostik—interdisziplinäre Perspektiven. Waxmann, Münster, pp 297–321

Neumann K, Euler HA, Schneider P et al (2015) An instrument for a universal screening for stuttering in preschoolers. Procedia Soc Behav Sci 193:322

Neumann K, Euler HA, Bosshardt HG et al (2016) Pathogenese, Diagnostik und Behandlung von Redeflussstörungen: Evidenz- und konsensbasierte S3-Leitlinie (Pathogenesis, diagnosis, and treatment of speech fluency disorders: evidence- and consensus-based S3 guideline). AWMF-Registernummer 049-013. Deutsche Gesellschaft für Phoniatrie und Pädaudiologie (ed) (Version 1). http://www.awmf.org/leitlinien/detail/ll/049-013.html

Neumann K, Euler HA, Kob M et al (2018) Assisted and unassisted recession of functional anomalies associated with dysprosody in adults who stutter. J Fluen Disord 55:120–134

Neumann K, Euler H, Zens R et al (2019) 'Spontaneous' late recovery from stuttering: dimensions of reported techniques and causal attributions. J Commun Disord 81:105915. https://doi.org/10.1016/j.jcomdis.2019.105915

Newton MJ, Campbell M, Gilbert J (2008) Mechanical response measurements of real and artificial brass player's lips. J Acoust Soc Am 123:14–20

Ni Z, Kim SJ, Phielipp N et al (2018) Pallidal deep brain stimulation modulates cortical excitability and plasticity. Ann Neurol 83(2):352–362

Niimi S, Miyaji M (2000) Vocal fold vibration and voice quality. Folia Phoniatr Logop 52(1–3):32–38

Nitsche MA, Paulus W (2000) Excitability changes induced in the human motor cortex by weak transcranial direct current stimulation. J Physiol 527:633–639

Niu M, Kasai A, Tanuma M et al (2022) Claustrum mediates bidirectional and reversible control of stress-induced anxiety responses. Sci Adv 8(11):eabi6375. https://doi.org/10.1126/sciadv.abi6375. Epub 2022 Mar 18. PMID: 35302853; PMCID: PMC8932664

Oertel M (1878) Über eine neue "laryngostroboskopische" Untersuchungsmethode des Kehlkopfes. Zbl med Wiss 16:81–82

Oertel M (1895) Das Laryngo-Stroboskop und die laryngo-stroboskopische Untersuchung. Arch Laryngol Rhinol 3:1–16

Ohlsson AC, Andersson EM, Södersten M et al (2012) Prevalence of voice symptoms and risk factors in teacher students. J Voice 26(5):629–634

Onslow M, Lowe R, Jakšić SJ, Franken MC, Hearne A, Uijterlinde I, Eggers K (2023) The Fifth Croatia Stuttering Symposium: Part III. Mental health and early stuttering. J Fluency Disord. 77:106000. https://doi.org/10.1016/j.jfludis.2023.106000. Epub 2023 Aug 2. PMID: 37586168

Ooi LLPJ (1992) B-mode real-time ultrasound assessment of vocal cord function in recurrent laryngeal nerve palsy. Ann Acad Med Singapore 21(2):214–216

Orton ST (1927) Studies in stuttering. Arch Neuro Psychiatry 18:671–672

Orton ST (1928) A physiological theory of reading disability and stuttering in children. N Engl J Med 198:1045–1052

Pabst F, Seiler R, Hacki T (1998) Zur Beurteilung der Sprechstimmleistungen nach Stimmbelastungstest mittels Stimmfeldmessung. In: Gross M (ed) Aktuelle phoniatrisch-pädaudiologische Aspekte 1997/98, vol 5. Median Verlag von Killisch Horn GmbH, Heidelberg, pp 73–75

Papsin BC, Maaske LA, Mc Grail JS (1996) Orbicularis oris muscle injury in brass players. Laryngoscope 106(6):757–760

Paulsen F (2010) Mundhöhle. In: Zilles K, Tillmann B (eds) Anatomie. Springer, Berlin, pp 424–425

Pellowski MW, Conture EG (2002) Characteristics of speech disfluency and stuttering behaviors in 3- and 4-year-old children. J Speech Lang Hear Res 45(1):20–34

Penttilä N, Korpijaakko-Huuhka AM (2015) New guidelines for assessing neurogenic stuttering. Procedia Soc Behav Sci 193:310–313

Perkins WH (1980) Stuttering disorders: current therapy of communication disorders. Thieme-Stratton, New York

Pernambuco LA, Espelt A, Magalhaes HV et al (2016a) Screening for voice disorders in older adults (Rastreamento de Alteracoes Vocais em Idosos-RAVI)-Part I: validity evidence based on test content and response processes. J Voice 30(2):246.e9–246.e16

Pernambuco LA, Espelt A, Magalhaes HV et al (2016b) Screening for voice disorders in older adults (Rastreamento de Alteracoes Vocais em Idosos-RAVI)-Part II: validity evidence and reliability. J Voice 30(2):246.e19–246.e27

Pertijs MAJ, Oonk LC, Beer de JJA et al (2014) Clinical guideline stuttering in children, adolescents and adults. NVLF, Woerden

Petermann F, Macha T (2005) Psychologische Tests für Kinderärzte. Hogrefe, Göttingen
Phyland DJ, Oates J, Greenwood KM (1999) Self-reported voice problems among three groups of professional singers. J Voice 13(4):602–611
Planas J (1982) Rupture of the orbicularis oris in trumpet players (Satchmo's syndrome). Plast Reconstr Surg 69(4):690–693
Planas J (1988) Further experience with rupture of the orbicularis oris in trumpet players. Plast Reconstr Surg 81(6):975–981
Plante E, Vance R (1994) Selection of preschool language tests: a data-based approach. Lang Speech Hear Serv Sch 25(1):15–24
Prendergast S, Lartz M, Fiedler B (2002) Ages of diagnosis, amplification, and early intervention of infants and young children with hearing loss: findings from parent interviews. Am Ann Deaf 147(1):24–30
Price CJ (2012) A review and synthesis of the first 20 years of PET and fMRI studies of heard speech, spoken language and reading. NeuroImage 62:816–847
Pruszewicz A (1992) Foniatria kliniczna. (Clinical phoniatrics). PZWL, Warsaw
Qiu Q, Schutte HK (2006) A new generation videokymography for routine clinical vocal-fold examination. Laryngoscope 116(10):1824–1828
Rachman S (2004) Anxiety, 2nd edn. Psychology Press Ltd, Sussex
Raes JP, Clement PA (1996) Aerodynamic measurements of voice production. Acta Otorhinolaryngol Belg 50(4):293–298
Raghavendra BN, Horii SC, Reede DL et al (1987) Sonographic anatomy of the larynx, with particular reference to the vocal cords. J Ultrasound Med 6(5):225–230
Rau D, Beckett RL (1984) Aerodynamic assessment of vocal function using hand-held spirometers. J Speech Hear Disord 49(2):183–188
Raven J, Raven JC, Court JH (2004) Manual for Raven's progressive matrices and vocabulary scales. Updated. Harcourt Assessment, San Antonio, TX
Reinhardt DS (1973) The encyclopedia of the pivot system for all cupped mouthpiece brass instruments: a scientific text. Colin, New York
Revis J, Barberis S, Giovanni A (2000) Définition d'une mesure temporelle de l'attaque vocale. Rev Laryngol Otol Rhinol 121(5):291–296
Ricci-Maccarini A, De Maio V, Murry T et al (2013) Development and validation of the children's voice handicap index-10 (CVHI-10). J Voice 30(1):120–126
Rice ML, Smolik F, Perpich D et al (2010) Mean length of utterance levels in 6-month intervals for children 3 to 9 years with and without language impairments. J Speech Lang Hear Res 53(2):333–349
Riley GD (2009) Stuttering severity instrument for children and adults (SSI-4), 4th edn. Pro-Ed, Austin
Riley GD, Riley J (1989) Physician's screening procedure for children who may stutter. J Fluen Disord 14(1):57–66
Rocha M, Yaruss JS, Rato JR (2020) Stuttering impact: a shared perception for parents and children? Folia Phoniatr Logop 72(6):478–486. https://doi.org/10.1159/000504221
Rosen CA, Murry T (2000) Voice Handicap Index in singers. J Voice 14(3):370–377
Rosen CA, Lee AS, Osborne J et al (2004) Development and validation of the Voice Handicap Index-10. Laryngoscope 114(9):1549–1556
Rosenberg M (1965) Society and the adolescent self-image. Princeton University Press, Princeton
Roth CR, Cornis-Pop M, Beach WA (2015) Examination of validity in spoken language evaluations: adult onset stuttering following mild traumatic brain injury. NeuroRehabilitation 36(4):415–426
Rothenberg M (1973) A new inverse filtering technique for deriving the glottal airflow during voicing. J Acoust Soc Am 53(6):1632–1645
Rothenberg M (1982) Interpolating subglottal pressure from oral pressure. J Speech Hear Disord 47(2):218–224
Rozanski VE, Rehfuess E, Bötzel K et al (2015) Aufgabenspezifische Dystonie bei professionellen Musikern—Ein systematisches Review zur Bedeutung des intensiven Musizierens als Risikofaktor. Dtsch Arztebl Int 112:871–877
Rutherford S, Angstadt M, Sripada C et al (2021) Leveraging big data for classification of children who stutter from fluent peers. bioRxiv. https://doi.org/10.1101/2020.10.28.359711
Saad Merouwe S, Bertram R, Eggers K (2024) Speech disfluencies in bilingual Lebanese children who do and do not stutter. Am J Speech Lang Pathol 1–20. https://doi.org/10.1044/2024_AJSLP-23-00311. PMID: 38889203
Saeedi Borujeni MJ, Esfandiary E, Almasi Dooghaee M (2016) Childhood neurogenic stuttering due to bilateral congenital abnormality in globus pallidus: a case report and review of the literature. Iran J Child Neurol 10(4):75–79
Sahin HA, Krespi Y, Yilmaz A et al (2005) Stuttering due to ischemic stroke. Behav Neurol 16(1):37–39
SALT Software (2014) Computerized language sample analysis. http://www.saltsoftware.com/. Accessed 1 June 2014
Salmelin R, Schnitzler A, Schmitz F et al (2000) Single word reading in developmental stutterers and fluent speakers. Brain 123:1184–1202
Sandrieser P, Schneider P (2015) Stottern im Kindesalter (Stuttering in childhood), 4th edn. Thieme, Stuttgart
Sapienza CM, Stathopoulos ET, Dromey C (1998) Approximations of open quotient and speed quotient from glottal and EGG waveforms: effects of measurement criteria and sound pressure level. J Voice 12(1):31–43
Sataloff RT (1997) Professional voice. Singular Publishing Group, San Diego
Sataloff RT (2005a) Clinical assessment of voice. Plural Publishing, San Diego
Sataloff RT (2005b) Professional voice: the science and art of clinical care. Plural Publishing, San Diego

Sataloff RT, Mandel S, Mann EA et al (2004) Practice parameter: laryngeal electromyography (an evidence-based review). J Voice 18(2):261274

Sataloff RT, Mandel S, Heman-Ackah YD et al (2005) Laryngeal electromyography, 2nd edn. Plural Publishing, San Diego

Saxon KG, Schneider CM (1995) Vocal exercise physiology. Singular Publishing Group, San Diego

Schaefer SD (2014) Management of acute blunt and penetrating external laryngeal trauma. Laryngoscope 124(1):233–244

Schindler O, Gonella ML, Pisani R (1990) Doppler ultrasound examination of the vibration speed of vocal folds. Folia Phoniatr 42(5):265–272

Schneider-Stickler B, Knell C, Aichstill B et al (2012) Biofeedback on voice use in call center agents in order to prevent occupational voice disorders. J Voice 26(1):51–62

Schönhärl E (1960) Die Stroboskopie in der praktischen Laryngologie. Thieme, Stuttgart

Schultz-Coulon HJ (1990) Stimmfeldmessung. Springer, Berlin

Schuppert M, Altenmüller E (2000) Berufsspezifische Erkrankungen bei Musikern. Orchester 48:24–29

Schutte HK (1980) The efficiency of voice production. Thesis. University of Groningen, Groningen

Schutte HK (1992) Integrated aerodynamic measurements. J Voice 6(2):127–134

Schutte HK, Seidner W (2005) Physiologische Grundlagen. In: Wendler J et al (eds) Lehrbuch der Phoniatrie und Pädaudiologie, 4th edn. Thieme, Stuttgart, p 80

Scott AD, Wylezinska M, Birch MJ et al (2014) Speech MRI: morphology and function. Phys Med 30(6):604–618

Sechi G, Cocco GA, D'Onofrio M et al (2006) Disfluent speech in patients with partial epilepsy: beneficial effect of levetiracetam. Epilepsy Behav 9(3):521–523

Seidner W (2012) Messung der stimmlichen Belastbarkeit. In: Seidner W, Nawka T (eds) Handreichungen zur Stimmdiagnostik. XION GmbH, Berlin

Seidner W, Eysholdt U (2005) Stimme—Diagnostik. In: Wendler J et al (eds) Lehrbuch der Phoniatrie und Pädaudiologie, 4th edn. Thieme, Stuttgart, pp 115–116

Shames H, Rubin R (1986) Stuttering then and now. Merrill Publishing, Columbus

Shapiro DA (2011) Stuttering intervention: a collaborative journey to fluency freedom, 2nd edn. Pro-Ed, Austin

Shau YW, Wang CL, Hsieh FJ et al (2001) Noninvasive assessment of vocal fold mucosal wave velocity using color Doppler imaging. Ultrasound Med Biol 27(11):1451–1460

Sheehan JG (1970) Stuttering: research and therapy. Harper & Row, New York

Sherer RC, Titze IR (1987) The abduction quotient related to vocal quality. J Voice 1(3):246–251

Sherman D, Jensen R (1962) Harshness and oral reading time. J Speech Hear Res 27:172–177

Siegert C (1987) Recommendation for a standard tolerance test. Union of European Phoniatricians, annual bulletin, pp 46–47

Simberg S, Sala E, Laine A et al (2001) A fast and easy screening method for voice disorders among teacher students. Logoped Phoniatr Vocol 26(1):10–16

Singer K (1926) Berufskrankheiten der Musiker. Systematische Darstellung ihrer Ursachen, Symptome und Behandlungsmethoden. Hesse, Berlin, pp 130–131

Sloper P, Turner S (1994) Families of teenagers with Down's syndrome: parent, child and sibling adaptation. Final report to ESRC. University of Manchester & Hester Adrian Research Centre, Manchester

Smith ER, Mackie DM, Claypool HM (2014) Social psychology. Psychology Press, New York

Snijders JT, Tellegen PJ, Laros JA (1989) Snijders-Oomen Non-Verbal Intelligence Test: SON-R 5.5-17. Manual and research report. Wolters-Noordhoff, Groningen

Sommer M, Koch MA, Paulus W et al (2002) Disconnection of speech-relevant brain areas in persistent developmental stuttering. Lancet 360:380–383

Sommer M, Wischer S, Tergau F et al (2003) Normal intracortical excitability in developmental stuttering. Mov Disord 18(7):826–830

Sommer M, Knappmeyer K, Hunter EJ et al (2009) Normal interhemispheric inhibition in persistent developmental stuttering. Mov Disord 24(5):769–773

Sommer M, Omer S, Wolff von Gudenberg A et al (2019) Hand motor cortex excitability during speaking in persistent developmental stuttering. Front Hum Neurosci 13:349. https://doi.org/10.3389/fnhum.2019.0034

Sonninen A, Damsté PH, Jol J et al (1974) Microdynamics in vocal fold vibration. Acta Otolaryngol 78:1–6

Speyer R, Wieneke GH, van Wijck-Warnaar I et al (2003) Effects of voice therapy on the voice range profiles of dysphonic patients. J Voice 17(4):544–556

Speyer R, Wieneke GH, Dejonckere PH (2004a) The use of acoustic parameters for the evaluation of voice therapy for dysphonic patients. Acta Acust United Acust 90(3):520–527

Speyer R, Wieneke GH, Dejonckere PH (2004b) Documentation of progress in voice therapy: perceptual, acoustic and laryngostroboscopic findings pretherapy and posttherapy. J Voice 18(3):325–339

Spielberger CD (1966) Anxiety and behavior. Academic Press, New York

Spielberger CD (1972) Conceptual and methodological issues in anxiety research. In: Spielberger CD (ed) Anxiety—current trends in theory and research, 2nd edn. Academic Press, New York

Spielberger CD (1983) Manual for the State-Trait-Anxiety Inventory (STAI). Consulting Psychologists Press, Palo Alto

Šram F, Švec J (2000) Die Tonerzeugung beim Spielen von Blasinstrumenten. In: Pahn J et al (eds) Sprache und Musik: Beiträge der 71. Jahrestagung der Deutschen Gesellschaft für Sprach- und Stimmheilkunde. Zeitschrift für Dialektologie und Linguistik: Beihefte;

Heft 107. Berlin, 12–13 März 1999. Steiner, Stuttgart, pp 155–159

Šram F, Švec J, Schutte HK (1998) Possibilities for use of videokymography in laryngologic and phoniatric practice. In: Dejonckere PH, Peters HFM (eds) Communication and its disorders: a science in progress: proceedings of the 24th congress of the International Association of Logopedics and Phoniatrics, Amsterdam, 23–27 August 1998. University press, Nijmegen, pp 256–259

Sramkova H, Granqvist S, Herbst CT et al (2015) The softest sound levels of the human voice in normal subjects. J Acoust Soc Am 137(1):407–418

Stes R, Boey R (1997) D.I.S. Detectie instrument voor Stotteren (Detection instrument for stuttering). CIOOS-vzw, Antwerp

Stevenson S, Campbell M, Bromage S (2009) Motion of the lips of brass players during extremely loud playing. J Acoust Soc Am 125:152–157

Stewart L, Walsh V, Frith U et al (2001) TMS produces two dissociable types of speech disruption. NeuroImage 13:472–478

Stone R, Scharf D (1973) Vocal change associated with the use of atypical pitch and intensity levels. Folia Phoniatr Logop 25:91–103

Story BH, Titze I (1995) Voice simulation with a body-cover model of the vocal folds. J Acoust Soc Am 97(2):1249–1260

Stotterfonds (2019) Screening lijststotteren (Sreening list stuttering). https://www.stotteren.nl/ouders/screeningslijst-voor-stotteren-sls.html. Accessed 23 Jan 2022

Strafella AP (2016) TMS-PET and the dopaminergic system [Conference abstract]. Clin Neurophysiol 127(3):e45. https://doi.org/10.1016/j.clinph.2015.11.145

Sullivan WG (1989) Repair of ruptured orbicularis oris in trumpet players. Plast Reconstr Surg 83:578

Sung MW, Kim KH, Koh TY et al (1999) Videostrobokymography: a new method for the quantitative analysis of vocal fold vibration. Laryngoscope 109(11):1859–1863

Švec JG, Granqvist S (2010) Guidelines for selecting microphones for human voice production research. Am J Speech Lang Pathol 19(4):356–368

Švec JG, Schutte HK (1996) Videokymography: high-speed line scanning of vocal fold vibration. J Voice 10(2):201–205

Švec JG, Schutte HK (2012) Kymographic imaging of laryngeal vibrations. Curr Opin Otolaryngol Head Neck Surg 20(6):458–465

Švec J, Šram F (2002) Kymographic imaging of the vocal fold oscillations. In: Hansen JHL, Pellom B (eds) Proceedings of the 7th international conference on spoken language processing, Denver, CO, 16–20 Sept 2002. Center for Spoken Language Research, Boulder, pp 957–960

Švec JG, Šram F (2011) Videokymographic examination of voice. In: Ma EPM, Yiu EML (eds) Handbook of voice assessments. Plural Publishing, San Diego, pp 129–146

Švec J, Šram F, Schutte HK (1999) Videokymografie: nová vysokofrekvenční metoda vyšetřování kmitů hlasivek. (Videokymography: a new high-speed method for the examination of vocal-fold vibrations). Otorinolaryngologie a Foniatrie (Praha) 48:155–162

Švec J, Titze IR, Popolo P (2005) Estimation of sound pressure levels of voiced speech from skin vibration of the neck. J Acoust Soc Am 117(3 Pt 1):1386–1394

Švec JG, Šram F, Schutte HK (2007) Videokymography in voice disorders: what to look for? Ann Otol Rhinol Laryngol 116(3):172–180

Švec JG, Šram F, Schutte HK (2009) Videokymography. In: Fried MP, Ferlito A (eds) The larynx, vol 1, 3rd edn. Plural Publishing, San Diego, pp 253–274

Svenning A, Panzarino R, Vanryckeghem M, Vestner T (2021) Life partners' perceptions of the emotional, speech disruptive, and attitudinal correlates of stuttering. J Fluency Disord 67:105821. https://doi.org/10.1016/j.jfludis.2020.105821

Tani T, Sakai Y (2011) Analysis of five cases with neurogenic stuttering following brain injury in the basal ganglia. J Fluen Disord 36(1):1–16

Tellegen P, Laros J (1993) The construction and validation of a nonverbal test of intelligence: the revision of the Snijders-Oomen test. Eur J Psychol Assess 9(2):147–157

Tellegen PJ, Laros JA (2005) Fair assessment for children from cultural minorities: a description of the SON-R non-verbal intelligence tests. In: Kopcanová D (ed) Quality education for children from socially disadvantaged settings. Commission of UNESCO, Bratislava, pp 50–73

Tellegen PJ, Winkel M, Wijnberg-Williams BJ et al (1998) Snijders-Oomen Non-Verbal Intelligence Test. SON-R 2.5-7. Manual and research report. Swets Test Publishers, Lisse

Tellegen PJ, Winkel M, Wijnberg-Williams BJ et al (2009) Snijders-Oomen Non-Verbal Intelligence Test. SON-R 2.5-7. Manual and research report. Hogrefe, Göttingen

The Stuttering Foundation (2010) Stuttering: straight talk for teachers. 3rd edn. Publication no 0125. www.stutteringhelp.org/sites/default/files/Migrate/teacher_book_2010.pdf. Accessed 7 Mar 2021

The Stuttering Foundation (2020) Physician's checklist for referral. https://www.stutteringhelp.org/checklist-referral. Accessed 23 Jan 2022

Theys C, van Wieringen A, Sunaert S et al (2011) A one year prospective study of neurogenic stuttering following stroke: incidence and co-occurring disorders. J Commun Disord 44(6):678–687

Theys C, De Nil L, Thijs V et al (2013) A crucial role for the cortico-striato-cortical loop in the pathogenesis of stroke-related neurogenic stuttering. Hum Brain Mapp 34(9):2103–2112

Theys C, Jaakkola E, Melzer TR et al (2024) Localization of stuttering based on causal brain lesions. Brain 147(6):2203–2213. https://doi.org/10.1093/brain/awae059. PMID: 38797521; PMCID: PMC11146419

Tillmann B (1997) Farbatlas der Anatomie Zahnmedizin-Humanmedizin. Thieme, Stuttgart, p 98
Titze IR (1992a) Phonation threshold pressure—a missing link in glottal aerodynamics. J Acoust Soc Am 91(5):2926–2935
Titze IR (1992b) Acoustic interpretation of the voice profile (phonetogram). J Speech Hear Res 35(1):21–34
Titze IR (1994) Principles of voice production. Prentice Hall, Englewood Cliffs
Titze IR (1995) Workshop on acoustic voice analysis: summary statement. National Center for Voice and Speech, The University of Iowa, Denver
Titze IR, Liang H (1993) Comparison of Fo extraction models for high precision voice perturbation measurements. J Speech Hear Res 36(6):1120–1133
Titze IR, Lemke J, Montequin D (1997) Populations in the US workforce who rely on voice as a primary tool of trade: a preliminary report. J Voice 11(3):254–259
Toyomura A, Fujii T, Kuriki S (2015) Effect of an 8-week practice of externally triggered speech on basal ganglia activity of stuttering and fluent speakers. NeuroImage 109:458–468
Traser L, Burdumy M, Richter B et al (2013) The effect of supine and upright position on vocal tract configurations during singing—a comparative study in professional tenors. J Voice 27(2):141–148
Travis LE (1931) Speech pathology. Appleton-Century, New York
Travis LE (1978) The cerebral dominance theory of stuttering: 1931–1978. J Speech Hear Disord 43(3):278–281
Tsai CG, Shau YW, Liu HM et al (2008) Laryngeal mechanisms during human 4-kHz vocalization studied with CT, videostroboscopy, and color Doppler imaging. J Voice 22(3):275–282
Tumanova V, Backes N (2019) Autonomic nervous system response to speech production in stuttering and normally fluent preschool-age children. J Speech Lang Hear Res 62(11):4030–4044
Tumanova V, Conture EG, Lambert EW et al (2014) Speech disfluencies of preschool-age children who do and do not stutter. J Commun Disord 49:25–41
Tumanova V, Choi D, Conture EG et al (2018) Expressed parental concern regarding childhood stuttering and the test of childhood stuttering. J Commun Disord 72:86–96
Tütüncüoğlu S, Serdaroğlu G, Kadoğlu B (2002) Landau-Kleffner syndrome beginning with stuttering: case report. J Child Neurol 17(10):785–788
Unger J, Schuster M, Hecker DJ et al (2016) A generalized procedure for analyzing sustained and dynamic vocal fold vibrations from laryngeal high-speed videos using phonovibrograms. Artif Intell Med 66(C):15–28
Valente T, Farina R, Minelli S et al (1996) Anatomia ecografica della laringe e delle strutture perilaringee. Radiol Med 91(3):231–237
Van Borsel J (2014) Acquired stuttering: a note on terminology. J Neurolinguistics 27(1):41–49
Van de Heyning PH, Remacle M, Cauwenberge PV et al (1996) Research work of the Belgian study group on voice disorders. Acta Otorhinolaryngol Belg 50(4):321–386
Van Eerdenbrugh S, Eggers K (2020) Knowledge about and referral of stuttering by general practitioners and pediatricians. Poster presented at the Flemish Federations of Speech, Language Pathologists, Ghent
Vanryckeghem M (2007) Behavior assessment battery: evidence-based approach to the assessment and treatment of children who stutter. In: Proceedings of 5th world congress on fluency disorders (International Fluency Association), Dublin, Ireland 2007: research, treatment and self-help in fluency disorders: new horizons, pp 209–214
Vanryckeghem M, Brutten G (2001) The Behavior Assessment Battery: a research pathway. J Fluen Disord 26:349–352
Vanryckeghem M, Brutten GJ (2007) Communication attitude test for preschool and kindergarten children who stutter (KiddyCAT). Plural Publishing, San Diego
Vanryckeghem M, Brutten G (2018) The Behavior Assessment Battery for adults who stutter. Plural, San Diego
Ventura S, Diamantino F, João M et al (2011) Imaging of the vocal tract based on magnetic resonance techniques. In: Ranchordas A et al (eds) Computer vision, imaging and computer graphics. Theory and applications. Springer, Heidelberg, pp 146–157
Verdolini K (1994) Voice disorders. In: Tomblin JB et al (eds) Diagnosis in speech-language pathology. Singular Publishing Group, San Diego, pp 247–306
Verduyckt I, Remacle M, Jamart J et al (2011) Voice-related complaints in the pediatric population. J Voice 25(3):373–380
Verduyckt I, Morsomme D, Remacle M (2012) Validation and standardization of the Pediatric Voice Symptom Questionnaire: a double-form questionnaire for dysphonic children and their parents. J Voice 26(4):e129–e139
Vidaković MR, Schönwald MZ, Jurić T et al (2015) Evaluation of corticobulbar and corticospinal excitability in developmental stuttering: the navigated transcranial magnetic stimulation study. Brain Stimul 8:317–318
Vilkman E (2004) Occupational safety and health aspects of voice and speech professions. Folia Phoniatr Logop 56(4):220–253
Vintturi J (2001) Studies on voice production. Academic dissertation. Medical Faculty of the University of Helsinki, Helsinki
Vintturi J, Alku P, Lauri ER et al (2001) The effects of post-loading rest on acoustic parameters with special reference to gender and ergonomic factors. Folia Phoniatr Logop 53(6):338–350
Wechsler D (2003) The Wechsler Intelligence Scale for children, 4th edn. The Psychological Corporation, San Antonio, TX

Wechsler D (2012) Wechsler Preschool and Primary Scale of Intelligence–IV (WPPSI-IV). The Psychological Corporation, San Antonio, TX (German version; Petermann F, Daseking M, 2018)

Wechsler D (2014) Wechsler Intelligence Scale for Children, 5th edn (WISC-V). Pearson, Bloomington, MN (German version: Petermann F, 2017)

Walther C (2009) Wie erleben stotternde Kinder ihr Sprechen? Eine empirische Untersuchung (How do children who stutter experience their speech? An empirical investigation). Forum Logopädie 23(2):24–28

Walther C (2015) Lebensqualität stotternder Kinder—ein Instrument für Vier bis Siebenjährige (Quality of life of children who stutter—a tool for four to seven year olds). Sprachtherapie aktuell: Schwerpunktthema: Aus der Praxis für die Praxis (Speech therapy current: main topic: from practice for practice) 2(2): e2015-13. https://doi.org/10.14620/stadbs151013

Ward D (2006) Stuttering and cluttering: frameworks for understanding and treatment. Psychology Press, Hove

Wassermann EM, McShane LM, Hallett M et al (1992) Noninvasive mapping of muscle representations in human motor cortex. Electroencephalogr Clin Neurophysiol 85(1):1–8

Watkins KE, Smith SM, Davis S et al (2008) Structural and functional abnormalities of the motor system in developmental stuttering. Brain 131:50–59

Watkins KE, Chesters J, Connally EL (2016) The neurobiology of developmental stuttering. In: Hickok G, Small S (eds) Neurobiology of language. Academic Press, Amsterdam, pp 995–1004

Watson C (1994) Database management of the voice clinic and laboratory. J Voice 3:99–106

Welsch U (2006) Lehrbuch histologie, 2nd edn. Urban & Fischer, München, pp 338–339

Wendler J, Seidner W (1996) Lehrbuch der Phoniatrie und Pädaudiologie. Thieme, Stuttgart

Wendler J, Anders LC, Krüger H (1986) Classification of voice qualities. J Phon 14:483–488

Whillier A, Hommel S, Neef NE et al (2018) Adults who stutter lack the specialised pre-speech facilitation found in non-stutterers. PLoS One 13(10):e0202634. https://doi.org/10.1371/journal.pone

Wilken D (2009) Brass embouchures. Chapter 1 of 6 http://www.youtube.com/user/wilktone#p/u/0/aNfZpapmLIg. Chapter 2 of 6 http://www.youtube.com/user/wilktone#p/u/1/VFi5g1tqHhE. Chapter 3 of 6 http://www.youtube.com/user/wilktone#p/u/2/AfoeACB6bA4. Chapter 4 of 6 http://www.youtube.com/user/wilktone#p/u/3/gkIi6YXy8CI. Chapter 5 of 6 http://www.youtube.com/user/wilktone#p/u/4/KVa7spYJXvY. Chapter 6 of 6 http://www.youtube.com/user/wilktone#p/u/5/ImJoiuyfJ5Y. Accessed 6 Dec 2016

Wilson DK (1987) Voice problems of children, 3rd edn. Williams & Wilkins, Baltimore

Wilson JA, Webb A, Carding PN et al (2004) The VoiSS and the VHI: a comparison of structure and content. Clin Otolaryngol 29(2):169–174

Wittenberg T, Tigges M, Mergell P et al (2000) Functional imaging of vocal fold vibration: digital multislice high-speed kymography. J Voice 14(3):422–442

Wolfe V, Fitch J, Martin D (1997) Acoustic measures of dysphonic severity across and within voice types. Folia Phoniatr Logop 49(6):292–299

Woo P, Colton RH, Shangold L (1987) Phonatory air flow analysis in patients with laryngeal disease. Ann Otol Rhinol Laryngol 96(5):549–555

Woo P, Casper J, Colton R et al (1994) Aerodynamic and stroboscopic findings before and after microlaryngeal phonosurgery. J Voice 8(2):186–194

Woolf G (1967) The assessment of stuttering as struggle, avoidance, and expectancy. Br J Disord Commun 2(2):158–171

World Health Organization (1971) The economics of health and disease. WHO Chron 25:20–24

World Health Organization (2011) International statistical classification of diseases and related health problems, 10th revision, edition 2010. http://www.who.int/classifications/icd/en/. Accessed 1 June 2014

Wright L, Ayre A (2000) WASSP: wright & ayre stuttering self-rating profile. Winslow Press Ltd., Bicester, Oxon. 20 p. ISBN: 0836882757

Wuyts FL, De Bodt MS, Molenberghs G et al (2000) The dysphonia severity index. An objective measure of vocal quality based on a multiparameter approach. J Speech Hear Res 43(3):796–809

Yairi E (1997) Disfluency characteristics of childhood stuttering. In: Curlee RF, Siegel GM (eds) Nature and treatment of stuttering: new directions, 2nd edn. Allyn and Bacon, Boston

Yairi E (2007) Subtyping stuttering I: a review. J Fluen Disord 32(3):165–196

Yairi E, Ambrose NG (2005) Early childhood stuttering. Pro-Ed, Austin

Yairi E, Ambrose NG (2013) Epidemiology of stuttering: 21st century advances. J Fluen Disord 38(2):66–87

Yairi E, Seery CH (2015) Stuttering: foundations and clinical applications, 2nd edn. Pearson, Essex

Yaruss JS (2007) Application of the ICF in fluency disorders. Semin Speech Lang 28(4):312–322

Yaruss JS, Quesal RW (2004) Stuttering and the international classification of functioning, disability, and health (ICF): an update. J Commun Disord 37(1):35–52

Yaruss JS, Quesal RW (2006) Overall assessment of the Speaker's experience of stuttering (OASES): documenting multiple outcomes in stuttering treatment. J Fluen Disord 31(2):90–115

Yaruss JS, Quesal RW (2016) Overall assessment of the speaker's experience of stuttering. Stuttering Therapy Resources, McKinney

Yeo BTT, Krienen FM, Sepulcre J et al (2011) The organization of the human cerebral cortex estimated by intrinsic functional connectivity. J Neurophysiol 106:1125–1165

Yu P, Ouaknine M, Giovanni A (2000) Intérêt clinique du calcul des coefficients de Lyapunov pour l'analyse objective des dysphonies. (Clinical significance of calculating the coefficients of Lyapunov in the objective assessment of dysphonia). Rev Laryngol Otol Rhinol 121(5):301–305

Yumoto E, Oyamada Y, Nakano K et al (2004) Three-dimensional characteristics of the larynx with immobile vocal fold. Arch Otolaryngol Head Neck Surg 130(8):967–974

Zappia F, Campani R (2000) La laringe: studio ecografico anatomico e funzionale. Radiol Med 99:138–144

Zarzur AP, de Campos DA, Cataldo BO et al (2014) Laryngeal electromyography as a diagnostic tool for Parkinson's disease. Laryngoscope 124(3):725–729

Zeller HJ (1985) Therapieempfehlungen bei Beschäftigungsneuropathien und Beschäftigungsneurosen von Blechbläsern. Arbeitshygienische Beratungsstelle der Theater und Orchester der DDR (Berlin Ost). Arbeitsmedizinische Informationen für Theater und Orchester 8:1–8

Zhang D, Huebner ES, Tian L (2020) Longitudinal associations among neuroticism, depression, and cyberbullying in early adolescents. Comput Hum Behav 112:1–9

Zraick RI, Smith-Olinde L, Shotts LL (2012) Adult normative data for the KAYPentax Phonatory Aerodynamic System Model 6600. J Voice 26(2):164–176

Zückner H (2011) Self-esteem of children and adolescents who stutter—impact on speech behaviour and stuttering experience. Sprache-Stimme-Gehör 35(2):E77–E86

Zur KB, Cotton S, Kelchner L et al (2007) Pediatric Voice Handicap Index (pVHI): a new tool for evaluating pediatric dysphonia. Int J Pediatr Otorhinolaryngol 71(1):77–82

9 Prevention of Speech Fluency Disorders

Patricia Sandrieser and Sabine Van Eerdenbrugh

9.1 Guidance on Stuttering for Parents of Children Who Stutter

Patricia Sandrieser

9.1.1 Introduction

Counselling of the parents, and in many cases the stuttering child itself, is one of the main responsibilities of speech-language therapists and trained physicians who deal with children who stutter (Lutermann 2008, cited in ASHA 2020). Everyone can understand the significance of the first counselling session after performing the assessment but this is only a small part of the therapeutic liability: if the family decides to engage in therapy, counselling remains an ongoing process. Furthermore, depending on the age of the child, every therapist must be prepared to deal with their questions and concerns. Therefore, the speech-language therapist must be trained to provide child and parents with educational information as well as the use of counselling to help them to express their feelings, beliefs, worries or prejudices. The application of the well-known 'International Classification of Functioning, Disability and Health', ICF (WHO 2001) requires—apart from the phenomenon 'stuttering' at the level of body structures—taking into consideration aspects of participation in activities, as well as contextual factors and the personal and environmental situation.

Counselling is an integral part of every therapeutic process. ASHA's special interest group dealing with fluency and fluency disorders lists 'counselling' as one of the special topics they deal with (ASHA 2020), and the German guidelines on stuttering also refers to the importance of continued counselling (Neumann et al. 2017). The impact of counselling depends on a variety of factors; this section deals with the various aims of counselling in different stages of escorting a stuttering child and its family from the moment of the diagnosis onwards.

9.1.2 The Different Aims of Counselling

Counselling children who stutter and their parents has different aims, depending on the setting and the moment it is offered (i.e. directly after the assessment or during therapy). Directly after performing the stuttering assessment (see Sect. 8.1),

P. Sandrieser (✉)
Catholic Clinic Koblenz Montabaur, Koblenz, Germany
e-mail: p.sandrieser@kk-km.de

S. Van Eerdenbrugh
Thomas More College of Applied Sciences, Antwerp, Antwerp, Belgium
e-mail: sabine.vaneerdenbrugh@thomasmore.be

A. am Zehnhoff-Dinnesen et al. (eds.), *Phoniatrics II*, European Manual of Medicine,
https://doi.org/10.1007/978-3-031-25175-7_9

the speech-language therapist has the obligation to inform the whole family concerning the diagnosis. The aim of this first counselling is to provide them with information and to give them the opportunity to ask questions and to express their concerns. The major aim is to enable them to decide about the next steps that should be taken, such as the question whether therapy should start immediately in a very young child, and if therapy is requested which programme to choose (Neumann et al. 2017). Flasher and Fogle (2012) call this step an informational counselling.

During therapy, counselling pursues different goals: at the beginning, it builds the information base required for the therapeutic process, and during therapy it is necessary to keep all parties involved well-informed. It is one of the cornerstones in clinical reasoning to ensure that the therapist takes this responsibility seriously (Beushausen 2020). Sandrieser and Schneider (2015) emphasise that adequate counselling on the duties and responsibilities at the beginning of the therapeutic process leads to a decrease in break-ups during therapy and to a better outcome. The precondition is that therapists explain the proceedings in the chosen approach and make sure that everybody receives the chance to query and to ask for adjustment if they feel that it would be impossible to perform the designated role. For example, if a family knows that their daily-life routine will not offer the possibility to spare daily and reliably a specific amount of time, adjustments will need to be made to allow obligatory time for the exercise.

This careful evaluation of the different aims, needs, skills and capabilities should lead to an agreement at the beginning of the therapeutic process. Very often, the method of Eric Berne's transaction analysis (Berne 2000) is used here: the bilateral work contract that emphasises an agreed goal of therapy and the responsibilities of every participant. The younger the children are, the more responsibility is taken by the parents and the therapist, but even young children have to be made aware they can speak out if they feel overburdened.

In addition, counselling offers the possibility of referring to the feelings, beliefs and attitudes of parents and child. This element of counselling is called personal adjustment counselling (Flasher and Fogle 2012). It requires that the therapists reflect on their own feelings, attitudes and the prerequisites concerning stuttering therapy. Speech-language therapists are well-trained in this reflection as part of their education. More details can be found in the book by Flasher and Fogle 'Counselling Skills for Speech-Language Pathologists and Audiologists' (2012).

Some therapists acquire additional qualifications that enable them to enhance the offer of counselling, e.g. systemic or cognitive-behavioural approaches. Ethical objectives demand that these approaches, in the context of speech-language therapy, are connected only to issues concerning stuttering. If psychotherapy seems appropriate, e.g. if an anxiety disorder reinforces the moments of stuttering or enhances avoidance behaviour, the family must be counselled that a multidisciplinary approach is necessary.

The goal of counselling, at the end of the therapeutic process, is for the child and its family to become independent of the therapist. The family members should be able to act with a feeling of self-efficacy concerning the issue of stuttering (Manning 2001). At best, they could counsel those in the child's environment. At the end of the stuttering therapy, informational counselling provides information on the course of action in the case of relapse or the need for consolidation.

Speech-language therapists must be aware of their own limitations concerning the counselling process. Ethical objectives demand speaking frankly about professional limitations (e.g. not being able to offer all recommended therapy approaches) or cultural constraints. It is important that the therapist asks for background information on family beliefs about stuttering (e.g. the assumed cause of the disorder or the role of therapists in the family's society). In some societies, therapists and doctors are viewed as healers, and in these it seems to be inappropriate for the family to enrol in a therapeutic process in a form of an 'assistant'.

Counselling has the aim of informing and aiding the stuttering children and their parents with regard to their social or cultural background, their resources and their individual needs.

The ongoing counselling process should improve the well-being of the involved parties and the outcome of the therapy.

9.1.3 Post-Assessment Counselling

Following the initial assessment, the most important content of the first counselling session is the summary of the results, and in most cases the confirmation of the parents' or caregiver's assumption that the disfluency in their child's speech is not part of the normal speech-language-development (see Sect. 8.1.1). The parents need prompt and easy access to basic principles on how to deal with the situation. Crucial information includes:

- Confirmation of the diagnosis.
- Aetiology of stuttering.
- Rate of spontaneous remissions and the inability to predict the chance of remission for a single child.
- Known risk factors of persistency (for an overview see Lattermann 2011).
- Recommended therapy approaches (for an overview see Neumann et al. 2017 and Sect. 9.2).
- Setting, access and costs of therapy (if necessary information about time of waiting).

Stuttering is still a disorder that attracts a lot of prejudices (e.g. the assumption that it is the parents' fault, that the educational style or a traumatic experience is responsible or that persons who stutter tend to behave in a certain way, are more sensitive or less stable than their non-stuttering peers). The therapist should address these opinions and comment in a supportive and professional manner.

Furthermore, the therapist has to provide an opportunity for the parents to ask questions and to express concerns. Frequent topics are:

- Has there been a possibility to prevent stuttering?
- If the family remembers a profound or dramatic incident around the beginning of stuttering (e.g. birth of a sibling, mother started working, entering kindergarten, an accident or hospitalisation). Did this event cause stuttering?
- How can the disposition be called genetic if there are no other family members known to stutter?
- Should we change the daily routine to stabilise fluent speech?

Fortunately, much research has been done and we have proven knowledge that should be passed to parents in an appropriate communication style and while facing the parents at eye level (Beushausen 2020). The German guidelines offer a 'patients' version' with basic information, suggestions and an overview of recommended approaches, and of approaches that are advised not to be accepted (AWMF 2020).

The parents should come to realise that:

- Every child who stutters does not have to learn how to talk fluently—they already speak fluently most of the time. Fluency breaks down in certain circumstances owing to a frailty. Therefore, it is not helpful to advise them to 'think hard/to breathe deeply/to think before speaking' or to punish them or ask them to repeat the stuttered word.
- A child is not in charge and cannot decide when there is a moment of stuttering. Unspecific advice to 'try harder/to concentrate' bears the risk of reinforcing secondary behaviour (see Sect. 8.1.3.3).
- There exists no therapeutic approach that can promise to 'cure' every child. Therapists who promise to cure a specific person are not trustworthy (Bloodstein and Bernstein Ratner 2008).
- Secondary behaviour is learned behaviour and a sign of a disadvantageous problem-solving strategy towards stuttering. Learned behaviour can be changed—this means that a therapist cannot promise to heal stuttering, but to give the prospect that secondary behaviour can diminish—and in most cases the secondary behaviour is more noticeable in social contexts than the stuttering itself.

- 'Wait and see' can be an appropriate response if the onset of stuttering was not long ago or if there is no secondary behaviour, no sign of avoidance and no constraint in the participation of everyday-life situations (WHO 2001; Sandrieser and Schneider 2015; Neumann et al. 2017).

9.1.4 Counselling During Therapy

Every speech-language therapist is aware that parents need cautious guidance through therapy. At the beginning, the information-focused counselling is important, to enable them to decide on the continuing procedure (Beushausen 2020). Later, they need space to express their feelings, concerns and beliefs that are connected to stuttering. The therapist serves as a counterpart to reflect the child's and its parents' own situation. In this secure environment (Katz-Bernstein 1996), they learn to change their attitudes and beliefs, to gain self-confidence in dealing with the situation and to protect the child from inappropriate reactions.

Parents should be aware that:

- Situational circumstances (excitement, time-pressure, high linguistic level) can impinge on the symptomatology of stuttering (see e.g. the model by Packman and Attanasio 2010). After a long period in the last century of indirect therapies that counselled the parents to reduce challenging and exciting situations, we came to understand that even the establishment of many tranquil situations is not a guarantor of enhancing long-term fluency. It can be relieving to create calm or undemanding linguistic situations, but the parents must not expect to 'teach' the child thereby to speak fluently. Most parents understand the comparison that though children with asthma may benefit from a stay at the seaside, a three-week vacation by the sea will not heal asthma; nor is it ethically justifiable to advise parents to move to the sea to supress asthma symptoms.
- We distinguish between direct and indirect therapeutic effects. For example, the use of games with a low linguistic level will in most cases lead to a decrease in moments of stuttering in this situation, which is therefore called a direct therapeutic effect. The relief of having an appointment for the first diagnostic and counselling session can lead to various changes in parental behaviour towards the stuttering child, and may also be responsible for a decrease in symptomatology. This is called an indirect therapeutic effect. The model by Packman and Attanasio (2010) is quite helpful in explaining the reactions following therapeutic intervention.
- Children who stutter should be treated like children who do not stutter. Challenges are the key to achieving the next level of development—on a linguistic, communicative, motoric and social-emotional level. Parents cannot prevent their getting into situations with competition, time-pressure, excitement and even excessive demands. Instead of steering clear of these situations, it turns out to be more promising to strengthen the child and to invest energy in informing those in the child's environment about appropriate reactions. As long as there is no solid proof that children with more routine in their daily lives, with less media-consumption, with slower-speaking mothers or with caring fathers tend to recover more often, therapists can only reveal the correlation of trigger factors and moments of stuttering. But they should not claim that interaction style or educational style was the cause of stuttering and that changing them will be the cure of stuttering (Neumann et al. 2017). However, if parents recognise the correlation of certain situations and their impact on the moments of stuttering, they might be motivated to try to change something in the families` routine and to observe whether the potential positive outcome of this adjustment is worthwhile and justifies being maintained.
- Mental reactions towards stuttering, such as anger, worry or impatience, are to be expected and should be taken seriously. For example, it seems inappropriate ethically to advise parents not to pay attention to the moments of stuttering but only to the content—it is well known and comprehensible that stuttering leads to irritation in the audience (Sandrieser and Schneider 2015). In an outcome-orientated

proceeding, the therapist asks the parents which fears trigger their reactions and what kind of support they need in order to stay calmer when they listen to their stuttering child.

- Getting in touch with other affected families can relieve both parents and children. Parents must be informed about self-help organisations and their valuable engagement—on a personal and also a social level.
- The development of stuttering varies. Recovery rates change over time and the older the child gets, the longer the stuttering persists, the smaller is the chance of recovery.
- If there is a decrease in stuttering at the end of therapy, this is not necessarily a sign of a complete remission—the literature shows that some children show stages with fewer or no symptoms. Ultimate recoveries can only be stated after at least 12 months without symptoms and while using no technique or avoidance behaviour.

9.1.5 Counselling Instead of Therapeutic Intervention

Some families decide that they do not want therapeutic intervention, but wait and hope for a spontaneous recovery. Other families feel that the burden of stuttering weighs less than any form of therapeutic intervention. In this case, they should be offered counselling concerning specific situations (e.g. beginning of school) or recurring situations (e.g. increase of stuttering in conflicts with siblings or peers). They need information about the possibilities of participating in therapy later, and should be informed about services of self-help organisations and appropriate literature, such as the parental guiding booklet from Natke-Verlag available in German and English (Schneider 2013, 2017; Schneider and Kohmaescher 2017).

9.1.6 Counselling the Child

We know that children who stutter are aware that there is a change in their speech (Boey et al. 2009)—even if younger children often don't know the word 'stuttering' and many children don't seem to be concerned about this phenomenon. Children who are referred to diagnostic procedures are a sub-group: They show (or their environment shows) reactions towards stuttering such as unfavourable coping strategies and difficulties in different social contexts.

The first step to building a reliable relationship is to inform the child in an age-appropriate way why it occurs. Ethical principles (Beushausen 2020) demand that they be taken seriously and that signs of stress during therapy be thoroughly monitored by the therapist.

The younger the children are, the more likely they will recover spontaneously (Neumann et al. 2017). The older they are, the more likely a persistent stuttering is, and the more situations they have to manage on their own, in which they are forced to struggle with prejudices or awkward responses to their stuttering. School is an environment with a high risk of being humiliated or treated unfairly—by peers but also by teachers (Bennecken and Spindler 2002; Wieser 2002).

Even with the best support and therapy, some children who stutter will remain stuttering. Therefore, fluency cannot be the only goal offered in therapy. The reduction of avoidance behaviour or secondary behaviour, conquering fears concerning speaking and building self-esteem as a competent speaker are equal aims.

The child should come to realise that:

- Stuttering is not their fault. Its aetiology is genetic—like allergies. It occurs in every language—even sign-language (Boyes Braem 1990).
- Stuttering is not linked to intelligence and is not an expression of a psychological defect.
- Stuttering can be exhausting and annoying. If children are irritated, they can get consolation from their parents and support by therapists.
- No therapy can promise healing for every single child, but therapy can enhance fluency and help to gain control over stuttering.
- A child who stutters can achieve everything that another child can—stuttering should not be a limitation at school or in private situations.

- A person who stutters can be expected to be treated respectfully.

Older children must also be aware that therapy does not work like a miracle—everybody involved has to engage and work hard; relapses are frequent and not necessarily a sign of failure.

Many (older) children benefit from encounters with other persons who stutter. Group-therapy can be helpful in mastering a technique and some self-help organisations offer meetings for teenagers and young adults.

9.1.7 Summary

The goal of this section was to give an overview of the guidance for children who stutter and their parents. Counselling is an ambitious task and requires knowledge about stuttering as well as a therapeutic education to deal with persons in distress—sometimes over a long period of time. Speech-language therapists are prepared, besides their ability to offer treatment approaches, to provide information and to use counselling techniques to facilitate the changing of attitudes and beliefs and to broaden the level of self-confidence in dealing with a deficit that can affect the core of human beings: verbal communication.

9.2 Early Intervention for Speech Fluency Disorders

Sabine Van Eerdenbrugh

9.2.1 Early Intervention and Stuttering

Early intervention can have two meanings. It either refers to

> intervention initiated at the initial stages of an illness or a disorder if this illness or disorder evolves gradually," or it refers to "intervention initiated at a young age of an individual"—Chanen and Thompson (2018) p. 133

To apply the correct meaning of early intervention to stuttering, it is necessary to understand the onset of stuttering and the early stages (evolution) of stuttering.

Young children from 3 to 6 years who do not stutter gradually become aware during those years of what stuttering is (Ezrati-Vinacour et al. 2001). Preschool children who stutter are usually aware that stuttering has an impact on their speech (Langevin et al. 2010; Vanryckeghem et al. 2005). Vanryckeghem et al. (2005) investigated the attitude towards speech with the KiddyCAT in 63 children from 3 to 6.5 years who did not stutter and in 45 children who stuttered. Children who did not stutter had significantly lower scores (and so a more positive attitude) than children who stuttered. When grouping the 3-to-4-year-old children and the 5-to-6-year-old children, the mean scores on the KiddyCAT between those who stuttered and those who did not also significantly differed, implying that even young children who stutter often have a more negative attitude towards their speech than peers who do not stutter. In large cohort studies in which also children who stutter aged 3–5 years participated (Briley and Ellis 2020; McAllister 2016), significantly more signs of difficulties in emotional, social and behavioural development and lower well-being were observed in preschool children who stuttered than in peers who did not stutter.

Early stuttering, that is, stuttering in young children, differs significantly from stuttering in older children, adolescents and adults. Stuttering in older children, adults and adolescents is often accompanied by social anxiety, negative emotions and subsequent secondary behaviour such as avoiding words or situations or movements which are thought to be helpful during a word struggle. In preschool children, stuttering usually is not yet accompanied by pronounced emotional and cognitive behaviour. Subsequently stuttering treatment for preschool children is significantly different from that for older children and adults. The most important difference is that, in general, preschool children who stutter often achieve great treatment success related to fluency (e.g. Jones et al. 2005; de Sonneville-Koedoot et al.

2015). It is, however, difficult to ignore the proportion of children who recover naturally, as they possibly accumulate in the success of early stuttering intervention. But it cannot be denied that even without this group of children who recover naturally, the treatment success in preschool children who stutter is still high.

Ideally, children who will recover with or without treatment and those who will not are identified at the early stages of stuttering, soon after stuttering onset. According to a review of Sugathan and Maruthy (2020), four factors are statistically related to stuttering recovery at 1 year post-onset: phonological abilities, articulatory rate, change in the pattern of dysfluencies and the trend in stuttering severity in the year after stuttering onset. Singer et al. (2020a) found that children who recovered were usually younger at stuttering onset, had less severe stuttering pre-treatment, and had better speech sound and language skills than children whose stuttering persisted. Girls and children without family members who stutter were also more likely to recover. In addition, Singer et al. (2020b) found that a less optimal attention span was related to stuttering recovery. In the study of Reilly et al. (2013), predictors for recovery included gender, stuttering incidence in the family, language skills, temperament, quality of life of the child and non-verbal cognition. The predictive power of these factors, however, was low, which means that these factors cannot be considered clinically relevant. The findings from Reilly et al. strengthened the findings of Yairi et al. (1996). For example, in the study of Yairi et al. (1996, p. 69), a family incidence of stuttering applied to the majority of children who did not recover but not for all of them. In clinical terms, however, the Speech and Language Therapist (SLT) would not withhold treatment from a child who stutters without a relative who stutters.

Predicting recovery with or without treatment is not yet possible at a level that makes clinical sense. We know that a large group of children recover naturally from stuttering within 4 years after stuttering onset (Yairi and Ambrose 1999). For a long time, waiting for natural recovery to occur was the recommended approach. Carey et al. (2020) conducted a study in which 16 children who stutter were observed for 19.4 months after stuttering onset. It became clear that natural recovery only occurred in one child (6.3%) within the first 19.4 months after onset. This supports the findings of Yairi and Ambrose that 6% of 84 preschool children who stuttered recovered 12–17 months after stuttering onset without treatment or with minimal treatment advice.

The low natural recovery rate of preschool children in the first year after stuttering onset, the growing awareness of preschool children about their stuttering, the significant negative impact of stuttering on emotional, social and behavioural development and well-being throughout the life span, and the high treatment success rate in preschool children make waiting for natural recovery to occur no longer the accepted approach. SLTs need to observe the evolution of the stuttering actively during the first weeks and months after stuttering onset if they decide treatment should not be initiated straight away. Initiating treatment timely (within the first year after stuttering onset) is essential if the speech does not show signs of improvement to avoid negative consequences in the preschool child who stutters.

9.2.2 Early Intervention for Stuttering

Early intervention often starts with a period of active monitoring, as discussed above. When the SLT decides it is necessary to start stuttering treatment, it can be provided in various ways. The treatment approaches that are discussed here are (1) the Restart-DCM Programme; (2) the Parent–Child Interaction (PCI) Approach; (3) the Lidcombe Programme; (4) the Mini-KIDS Programme and (5) the Westmead Programme.

9.2.2.1 The Restart-DCM Programme

The Restart-DCM Programme (Franken and Putker-de Bruijn 2007) is based on the multifactorial Demands and Capacities Model (DCM; e.g. Starkweather et al. 1990). The DCM claims that the balance between the demands of communicative situations and the capacities of children who stutter is disturbed. The aim of the programme is to achieve a balance between the demands and the capacities. This balance is established by reducing the demands and training the child's capacities to meet the expectations of the communicative situations. A favourable balance, i. e. positive changes in the motoric, linguistic, socio-emotional or cognitive functioning of a preschool child who stutters and his environment, leads to more fluent speech.

The treatment approach always starts by addressing the environment of the child, mainly to reduce the demands that the environment imposes on communicative situations in which the child is involved. Decreasing the demands is established by counselling and by training the parents, the child and the wider environment including siblings, teachers and significant others. This is mainly done by parents who model slower more relaxed speech, with pauses between utterances, parallel talk, description of the child's emotions and appropriate turn-taking. These are temporary intervention strategies. By reducing the demands, the child can practise speaking more fluently or even without stuttering. If a child continues to stutter even though demands have been successfully reduced, explicit training of relevant capacities of the child is added to the programme while the reduced demands are maintained in the communicative situations.

Assessment of the language, speech and oral-motor skills of the child and the parent–child interaction is necessary to make a comprehensive evaluation of the child to find out the strong and weak(er) skills. The parent–child interaction is observed during a play session that is video-recorded to assess and formulate demands in the four domains (linguistic, cognitive, motoric and emotional). This videorecording is also used to determine the severity and types of stuttering. An initial parent treatment session is organised straight after the assessment. Parents then express their concerns, receive general information about stuttering and about the assessment of their child (psycho-education). At the end of this treatment session, parents realise that stuttering arises from congenital (inherited) factors as well as developmental factors and environmental factors, and these can worsen or ameliorate stuttering. Parents know that they are never the cause of their child's stuttering. During the next treatment sessions, child and parent both are present. Parents learn also about *special times*, during which skills are practised: first parent skills (to lower demands), further in treatment also child skills (to strengthen capacities). Special times are 15 min per day (at least 5 times/week) in which parents give their child their undivided attention. Parents make notes in the *logbook* (when and how long the special times went on for, how fluent a child was, additional observations, ...). The aim of special times is to create a fluency-enhancing environment.

Demands and capacities differ for each child and family. Therefore, treatment only focuses on those demands and capacities that are potentially causing a problem for the stuttering (demands) or for promoting fluent speech (capacities). Several demands and capacities are related to emotional or cognitive aspects. Treatment includes dealing with emotions and cognitions about stuttering of child and family. Criteria to end the treatment include (1) normal-fluent speech or incidental mild dysfluencies, (2) parents' implementation of a fluency enhancing environment and (3) the parents', the child's and the SLT's acceptance of the child's speech.

9.2.2.2 The Palin Parent–Child Interaction Approach

The Palin PCI Approach (Botterill and Kelman 2010; Millard et al. 2008, 2009) is, like the Restart-DCM programme, based on the premise that stuttering is a heterogeneous, multifactorial condition and that linguistic, physiological, environmental and emotional aspects influence its onset and development.

The Palin PCI Approach focuses on adjusting the interaction between parents and children to maximise the child's fluency and confidence in order to become a competent communicator. The goal of the programme is for the parents to develop their knowledge about stuttering, to increase confidence about managing their child's stuttering and to reduce their concern about it.

The assessment focuses on existing and lacking interaction strategies in the child-parent dyads. Not all strategies are necessary to be implemented for each family. Psychological and emotional factors, related to stuttering, are included in the treatment. Both parents are required to attend the clinic-based sessions if possible. SLTs provide interaction, family and child strategies during six clinic-based treatment sessions. Interaction strategies include reducing parental speech rate, following the child's lead in play and using simplified language. Examples of family strategies are assisting in managing anxiety and children's emotions, building confidence, and setting boundaries and routines. If necessary, that is if the stuttering does not decline, direct child strategies may also need to be implemented. Direct strategies include desensitisation, turn-taking, increasing the frequency and duration of pauses and using easy onset. Parents and children are asked to have *Special Times* at home to practise these strategies. Video recordings of the Special Times, conducted at the clinic and at home, facilitate identification of correct implementation of the strategies.

9.2.2.3 The Lidcombe Programme

The Lidcombe Programme (e.g. Jones et al. 2005; Onslow et al. 2003, 2024) is not based on a specific theory or model. It is a behavioural programme that aims to achieve (near) zero levels of stuttering and has been extensively trialled since its development. The programme consists of *Stages 1* and *2*. The goal of *Stage 1* is to achieve (near) zero levels of stuttering; the goal of *Stage 2* is to maintain the (near) zero levels of stuttering. Parents are prepared to respond adequately if relapse occurs.

Throughout the programme, progress is visualised by severity ratings, assigned weekly by the SLT and daily by the parents, after they receive the necessary training from the SLT. Severity ratings are scores from 0 (for no stuttering) to 10 (extremely severe stuttering). Psycho-education, referring to information about stuttering, stuttering onset and stuttering development, is provided to the children and parents if and as they need this. If a child is teased or bullied, SLTs will take the appropriate measures. Other stuttering-related emotions or cognitions are addressed before they become a problem or concern.

The Lidcombe Programme is directed to the child even though parents are intensely involved in the treatment. The child practises each day to speak without or with very limited stuttering for 10–15 min during *practice sessions*. Parents are shown how they can organise these practice sessions and how they can provide verbal contingencies. Verbal contingencies are verbal feedback, provided for the stutter-free speech during the daily practice sessions and provided occasionally during everyday conversations throughout the day. When the child responds well to the verbal contingencies and parents provide them correctly and adequately, parents also provide verbal contingencies for stuttering to their child. The verbal contingencies for stuttering, however, are given significantly less frequently than verbal contingencies for stutter-free speech.

Initially, the practice sessions give children the opportunity to practise talking without stuttering during playful activities that require communication between child and parent. The likelihood of stutter-free speech occurring during the practice sessions needs to be high and can be established by choosing activities that match the child's language level and interest. Verbal contingencies, mainly reinforcement for stutter-free speech and occasional verbal contingencies for stuttering, give the preschool child who stutters direction to easy flowing, stutter-free speech.

Not all children progress similarly through the programme (Goodhue et al. 2010; Hayhow 2009) and individualising is necessary (Van Eerdenbrugh et al. 2018). The stuttering of each child differs, but family dynamics also differ. Individualising is necessary for the verbal contingencies (types and frequency) and organisation of practice sessions (types of activities, timing, ...).

9.2.2.4 The Mini-KIDS Programme

The Mini-KIDS Programme is not based on a specific theory or model. It is based on the techniques of stuttering modification (Van Riper 1973) and consists of three or four stages, depending on the age and progress of the child (Waelkens 2018; Schneider et al. 2023). During assessment, emotions and cognitions are assessed in parent and child. The aim of desensitising techniques is to change negative emotions and cognitions towards stuttering (e.g. anxiety). The treatment stages consequently follow each other. In stage 1, *Desensitisation*, the SLT uses pseudo-stuttering as a means of desensitising the child and parent for the child's stuttering. Depending on the tolerance of parent and child towards pseudo-stuttering, this stage can take more time. The goal of this stage is that the child is not afraid of stuttering. Stage 2, *Identification*, is only included in the programme for 4-to-6-year-old children (not for younger children). The child talks with pseudo-stuttering and describes the type (e.g. 'long word' = prolongation, 'frog word' = repetition, 'stuck word' = block) and the quality (e.g. 'hard' = for tense sounds, 'soft' for relaxed sounds) of the stuttering. Parents also use pseudo-stuttering in their speech when talking to the child. Parents and child have daily practice sessions at home. Stage 3, *Modification*, is only necessary for children who still stutter with tense prolongations or blocks at this point in the treatment process. The child learns to morph the tense stuttering moments into relax stuttering moments. Parents and child have daily practice sessions or they practise in natural conversations at home. In stage 4, *Generalisation*, there are two scenarios: (1) the child continues to use the modification techniques if necessary and wanted in other than practice situations. The child does this with an internal locus of control; that is, he wants to use the technique, he thinks about how to use the technique and he decides when to use the technique; (2) the child does not need the technique as the stuttering moments have disappeared. In both cases, the levels of stuttering are (near) zero. Parents know that relapse can occur and know what to do in case it does. If necessary, triggers for stuttering can be worked on during treatment if they prevent the stuttering to morph to normal disfluencies or mild stuttering. When the SLT concludes that the stuttering has reached (near) zero levels of stuttering, the *Follow-up phase* commences in which the programme's defined (near) zero levels of stuttering are maintained.

The stages in the treatment are individualised to each child and family. Not all techniques are introduced to all children and parents, and stages can take more or less time depending on the progress and needs of the child and family.

9.2.2.5 The Westmead Programme

The three factor model (Packman 2012) provides support for the main mechanism of the Westmead Programme (Trajkovski et al. 2006, 2009, 2011, 2019). This model assumes that the variability of stress in words (linguistic stress) can be a trigger for stuttering. The other two factors in the model besides *triggers* are *impaired neurological processing of spoken language* and *modulators* that influence the thresholds at which moments of stuttering are triggered (e.g. a fearful response to a specific communicative situation). The Westmead Programme uses syllable-timed speech to reduce or eliminate the linguistic variability and to help stabilise the speech motor system during speech.

The SLT manages negative feelings and cognitions about the stuttering during the treatment process when and if necessary. Psychoeducation about stuttering is provided during the first treatment sessions. The programme consists of two stages (Andrews et al. 2023). In *Stage 1*, (near) zero levels of stuttering are achieved; in *Stage 2*, the (near) zero levels of stuttering, achieved in Stage 1, are maintained. Children learn to use syllable-timed speech (or 'robot talking'). This refers to saying words in rhythmic beats. A sentence like 'the dinosaurs are drinking from the water' becomes 'the-di-no-saurs-are-drin-king-from-the-wa-ter', pronounced with one syllable per beat. The SLT models syllable-timed speech for the child and the parent. Video demonstrations of syllable-timed speech are available on the Australian Stuttering Research Centre website. Syllable-timed speech practice starts with short utterances in a low speech rate, then moves to simple conversations. Picture books or games are suited to elicit this practice. Using simple activities is essential to reduce the cognitive load for the child. At the end of Stage 1, the speech rate, pitch and intonation have increased to normal. Parents implement four to six practice sessions per day in which they and their child use syllable-timed speech, each session lasting 5–10 min.

It may be necessary to use verbal reinforcement or non-verbal rewards to encourage the child to use the syllable-timed speech. When the practice sessions are correctly implemented during the day, syllable-timed speech will also occasionally be introduced in everyday conversations. It is important that the total duration of using syllable-timed speech is limited to 1 hour per day to avoid 'overtreating' the child.

Each day, parents record the severity of the stuttering of their child throughout the day (not during practice sessions) with a scale from 0 (no stuttering) to 10 (extremely severe stuttering). The SLT guides parents to use the severity rating scale in a reliable way. This is essential given that the planning and progress of treatment depend on the severity ratings. The length of the Stage 1 differs for each family. For example, some children learn syllable-timed speech more easily, are more compliant or the stuttering responds better to the treatment than others; some parents learn syllable-timed speech more easily or can implement the practice sessions more smoothly than others.Stage 2 takes about a year with two treatment sessions in the clinic 4 weeks apart, two with 8 weeks apart, and two with 16 weeks apart. Syllable-timed speech is slowly withdrawn to avoid relapse.

An overview of the five stuttering treatment approaches discussed in this section is given in Table 9.1.

9.2.3 Summary

Different treatment approaches exist to treat preschool children who stutter. They all install temporary low-demanding communicative situations at certain moments during treatment in order to promote speech that flows more easily (stutter-free speech or very mild stuttering).

Table 9.1 Overview of five stuttering treatment programmes

	Underlying model	Main underlying mechanism(s)	Individualising	Responding to cognitions and emotions
The restart-DCM Programme	Multifactorial model (DCM)	Lowering environmental demands Increasing child's capacities	Only those demands and capacities that are potentially triggering the stuttering (demands) or promoting fluent speech (capacities)	Treatment includes dealing with emotions and cognitions about stuttering of child and family
Palin PCI approach	Multifactorial model	Adjusting parent–child interaction	Only the interaction strategies that are necessary for a family	Psychological and emotional factors related to stuttering are addressed during treatment
The Lidcombe Programme		Verbal contingent responses Practice sessions for stutter-free speech	Individualising of the verbal contingencies (types and frequency) and practice sessions (types of activities, timing, ...) to meet the needs of the child and family	Psycho-education is provided for the child and parent at the start. Other stuttering-related emotions or cognitions are openly discussed
The mini-KIDS Programme		Desensitisation, stuttering modification	Only the techniques that are necessary for the child and family	During assessment, emotions and cognitions are assessed in parent and child. Desensitisation aims at changing negative emotions and cognitions towards stuttering
The Westmead Programme	Three-factor model	Syllable-timed speech	Individualising of the practice sessions, depending on the skills and compliance of child and parent	Psycho-education about stuttering is provided during the first treatment sessions. The SLT deals with negative feelings and cognitions when and if necessary

DCM Demands Capacities Model, *PCI* Parent–Child Interaction

Two treatment approaches, the Restart-DCM Programme and the Palin PCI Approach, mainly focus on changing the environment of the child. If necessary, they include direct strategies with the child at the end of treatment if strategies for the environment seem unsatisfactory. The three other treatment approaches, i. e. the Lidcombe Programme, the Mini-KIDS Programme and the Westmead Programme, mainly or initially focus on the child's speech. In the Lidcombe Programme, the child is given the opportunity to practise stutter-free speech and verbal contingencies accompany the stutter-free speech. In the Mini-KIDS Programme, children learn to morph the stuttering moments into normal disfluencies or relaxed stuttering moments. In the Westmead Programme, syllable-timed speech allows children to speak without stuttering within a more stabilised speech motor system. In these three direct approaches, the low-demanding communicative situations are limited to the daily practice sessions and generalise to the everyday conversations of the child.

References

Andrews C, Trajkovski N, O'Brian S et al (2023) The Westmead Program treatment guide. https://www.uts.edu.au/research/australian-stuttering-research-centre/resources/westmead-program

ASHA (American Speech-Language-Hearing Association) (2020) About special interest group 4, fluency and fluency disorders. https://www.asha.org/sig/04/about-sig-4/#vision. Accessed December 2020

AWMF (Arbeitsgemeinschaft der Wissenschaftlichen Medizinischen Fachgesellschaften) (2020) Leitlinien-Detailansicht. Redeflussstörungen, Pathogenese, Diagnostik und Behandlung (guideline detail view. Speech fluency disorders, pathogenesis, diagnosis and treatment). https://www.awmf.org/leitlinien/detail/ll/049-013.html. Accessed Dec 2020

Bennecken J, Spindler L (2002) Mobbing und Stottern: Zur schulischen situation stotternder kinder (mobbing and stuttering; on the situation in schools concerning children who stutter). Forum Logopädie 6:6–11

Berne E (2000) Die Transaktionsanalyse in der Psychotherapie (transaction analysis in psychotherapy). Junfermann, Paderborn

Beushausen U (ed) (2020) Therapeutische Entscheidungsfindung in der Sprachtherapie (clinical reasoning in speech-language therapy). Ernst Reinhard Verlag, Munich

Bloodstein O, Bernstein Ratner N (2008) A handbook on stuttering, 6th edn. Thomson Delmar, New York, NY

Boey RA, Van de Heyning PH, Wuyts FL et al (2009) Awareness and reactions of young stuttering children aged 2–7 years old towards their speech disfluency. J Commun Disord 42(5):334–346

Botterill W, Kelman E (2010) Palin parent-child interaction therapy. In: Guitar B, McCauley R (eds) Treatment of *stuttering*: established and emerging interventions. Williams & Wilkins, Baltimore MD. http://downloads.lww.com/wolterskluwer_vitalstream_com/sample-content/9780781771047_Guitar/samples/Chapter05.pdf

Boyes Braem P (1990) Einführung in die Gebärdensprache und ihre Erforschung (Introduction to sign-language and its research). Signum Verlag, Hamburg

Briley PM, Ellis C (2020) Behavioral, social, and emotional well-being in children who stutter: the influence of race-ethnicity. Logoped Phoniatr Vocol 46(4):171–179

Carey B, Onslow M, O'Brian S (2020) Natural recovery from stuttering for a clinical cohort of pre-school children who received no treatment. Int J Speech Lang Pathol 23(1):48–56

Chanen AM, Thompson KN (2018) Early intervention for personality disorder. Curr Opin Psychol 21:132–135

de Sonneville-Koedoot C, Stolk E, Rietveld T et al (2015) Direct versus indirect treatment for preschool children who stutter: the restart randomized trial. PLoS One 10(7):E0133758. https://doi.org/10.1371/journal.pone.0133758

Ezrati-Vinacour R, Platzky R, Yairi E (2001) The young child's awareness of stuttering-like disfluency. J Speech Lang Hear Res 44(2):368–380

Flasher LV, Fogle PT (2012) Counselling skills for speech-language pathologists and audiologists, 2nd edn. Delmar, New York NY

Franken M-C, Putker-de Bruijn D (2007) RESTART-DCM method. https://nedverstottertherapie.nl/wp-content/uploads/2016/07/RESTART-DCM.Method.-English.pdf

Goodhue R, Onslow M, Quine S et al (2010) The Lidcombe program of early stuttering intervention: mothers' experiences. J Fluen Disord 35:70–84

Hayhow R (2009) Parents' experiences of the Lidcombe program of early stuttering intervention. Int J Speech Lang Pathol 11(1):20–25

Jones M, Onslow M, Packman A et al (2005) Randomised controlled trial of the Lidcombe program of early stuttering intervention. BMJ 331(7518):659–661

Katz-Bernstein N (1996) Das Konzept des "safe place"—ein Beitrag zur Praxeologie integrativer Kinderpsychotherapie (the concept of "safe place"—a contribution to the practice of integrated psychotherapy with children). Theorie und Praxis 2:111–141

Langevin M, Packman A, Onslow M (2010) Parent perceptions of the impact of stuttering on their preschoolers and themselves. J Commun Disord 43(5):407–423

Lattermann C (2011) Frühkindliches Stottern: Abwarten oder sofort behandeln? (early stuttering: to treat immediately or wait and see?). Forum Logopädie 2(25):6–11

Lutermann D (2008) Counseling for professional service delivery. https://www.asha.org/Practice-Portal/Professional-Issues/Counseling-For-Professional-Service-Delivery/. Accessed 5 July 2021

Manning W (2001) Clinical decision-making in fluency disorders, 2nd edn. Singular Thomson Learning, Vancouver

McAllister J (2016) Behavioural, emotional, and social development of children who stutter. J Fluen Disord 50:23–32

Millard SK, Nicholas A, Cook FM (2008) Is parent-child interaction therapy effective in reducing stuttering? J Speech Lang Hear Res 51:636–650

Millard SK, Edwards S, Cook FM (2009) Parent-child interaction therapy: adding to the evidence. Int J Speech Lang Pathol 11:61–76

Neumann K, Euler HA, Bosshardt HG et al (2017) Stottern und Poltern: Entstehung, Diagnose und Behandlung. In: Die Leitlinie zu Redeflussstörungen (stuttering and cluttering. Aetiology, diagnosis and treatment. The guidelines concerning fluency disorders). Peter Lang, Frankfurt

Onslow M, Attanasio J, Harrison E (2003) Parents talk about the Lidcombe program. In: Onslow M, Packman A, Harrison E (eds) The Lidcombe program of early stuttering intervention: a clinician's guide. Pro-Ed, Austin TX, pp 193–206

Onslow M, Webber M, Harrison E et al (2024) The Lidcombe Program treatment guide. https://www.uts.edu.au/research/australian-stuttering-research-centre/resources/lidcombe-program

Packman A (2012) Theory and therapy in stuttering: a complex relationship. J Fluen Disord 37(4):225–233

Packman A, Attanasio J (2010) A model of the mechanisms underpinning early intervention for stuttering. In: Seminar presentation at the annual convention of the American speech-language and hearing association, November 18-19 2010, Philadelphia PA

Reilly S, Onslow M, Packman A et al (2013) Natural history of stuttering to 4 years of age: a prospective community-based study. Pediatrics 132(3):460–467

Sandrieser P, Schneider P (2015) Stottern im Kindesalter: 4. Aufl (Stuttering in childhood), 4th edn. Thieme, Stuttgart

Schneider P (2013) Stottern bei Kindern erfolgreich bewältigen (managing stuttering in children successfully). Natke, Neuss

Schneider P (2017) Moje Dziecko sie jaka. Co mogezrobic? (My child stutters—what can I do?) Centrum Logopedyczne, Katowice

Schneider P, Kohmaescher A (2017) My child stutters—what can I do? Natke, Neuss

Schneider P, Kohmaescher A, Sandrieser P (2023) KIDS: A Modification Approach in Stuttering Therapy for School Children (Chapter 7). In Dialogue Without Barriers: A Comprehensive Approach to Dealing with Stuttering. Agere Aude Foundation for Knowledge and Social Dialogue

Singer CM, Hessling A, Kelly EM et al (2020a) Clinical characteristics associated with stuttering persistence: a meta-analysis. Speech Lang Hear Res 63(9):2995–3018

Singer CM, Walden TA, Jones RM (2020b) Attention, speech-language dissociations, and stuttering chronicity. Am J Speech Lang Pathol 29(1):157–167

Starkweather CW, Gottwald SR, Halfond MM (1990) Stuttering prevention: a clinical method. Prentice Hall, Hoboken, NJ

Sugathan N, Maruthy S (2020) Predictive factors for persistence and recovery of stuttering in children: a systematic review. Int J Speech Lang Pathol 23(4):359–371

Trajkovski N, Andrews C, O'Brian S et al (2006) Treating stuttering in a preschool child with syllable timed speech: a case report. Behav Change 23(4):270–277

Trajkovski N, Andrews C, Onslow M et al (2009) Using syllable timed speech to treat preschool children who stutter: a multiple baseline experiment. J Fluen Disord 34(1):1–10

Trajkovski N, Andrews C, Onslow M et al (2011) A phase II trial of the Westmead program: syllable-timed speech treatment for preschool children who stutter. Int J Speech Lang Pathol 13(6):500–509

Trajkovski N, O'Brian S, Onslow M et al (2019) A three-arm randomized controlled trial of Lidcombe program and Westmead program early stuttering interventions. J Fluen Disord 61:105708. https://doi.org/10.1016/j.jfludis.2019.105708

Van Eerdenbrugh S, Packman A, O'Brian S et al (2018) Challenges and strategies for speech-language pathologists using the Lidcombe program for early stuttering. Am J Speech Lang Pathol 27(3S):1259–1272

Van Riper C (1973) The treatment of stuttering. Prentice Hall, Hoboken, NJ

Vanryckeghem M, Brutten GJ, Hernandez LM (2005) A comparative investigation of the speech-associated attitude of preschool and kindergarten children who do and do not stutter. J Fluen Disord 3(4):307–318

Waelkens V (2018) Mini-KIDS: stottertherapie bij jonge kinderen (2–6 jaar) (Mini-KIDS: treatment for stuttering in young children (2–6 years)). Acco, Leuven

WHO (World Health Organization) (2001) International classification of functioning, disability and health. WHO, Geneva

Wieser E (2002) Zur Bedeutung von Scham bei stotternden menschen (the meaning of shame in people who stutter). Dissertation. Leopold-Franzen-Universität, Innsbruck

Yairi E, Ambrose NG (1999) Early childhood stuttering I: persistency and recovery rates. J Speech Lang Hear Res 42(5):1097–1112

Yairi E, Ambrose NG, Paden EP et al (1996) Predictive factors of persistence and recovery: pathways of childhood stuttering. J Commun Disord 29(1):51–77

Rehabilitation and Prognosis of Speech Fluency Disorders

10

Susan Block, Sibylle Brosch, Ashley Craig, Kurt Eggers, Harald Euler, Dobrinka Georgieva, Matt Jason V. Llamas, Gerald A. Maguire, Stephanie Wong, and J. Scott Yaruss

10.1 Fundamentals of Stuttering Treatment

Sibylle Brosch, J. Scott Yaruss, and Dobrinka Georgieva

Stuttering is a communication disorder affecting 4–8% of children at some point during early childhood (Bloodstein et al. 2021; Yairi and Ambrose 2013), though some recent studies put the incidence even higher (Reilly et al. 2009). Roughly 75% of young children who start to stutter in the preschool years will ultimately stop stuttering (Yairi and Ambrose 2013; Smith and Weber 2016; Neumann et al. 2017). The purpose of the diagnostic evaluation is therefore to determine which child is likely to stop stuttering naturally and which child is more likely to continue to stutter (and who would, as a result, be in need of

Harald Euler has died before the publication of this book.

Supplementary Information The online version contains supplementary material available at https://doi.org/10.1007/978-3-031-25175-7_10.

S. Block (✉)
School of Allied Health, Discipline of Speech Pathology, La Trobe University, Melbourne, VIC, Australia
e-mail: s.block@latrobe.edu.au

S. Brosch
Section Phoniatrics & Pedaudiology ENT Department , University of Ulm, Ulm, Germany
e-mail: sibylle.brosch@uniklinik-ulm.de

A. Craig
John Walsh Centre for Rehabilitation Research, University of Sydney, Royal North Shore Hospital, St Leonards, NSW, Australia
e-mail: a.craig@sydney.edu.au

K. Eggers
Department of Rehabilitation Sciences, Faculty of Medicine and Health Sciences, Ghent University, Ghent, Belgium
e-mail: kurt.eggers@ugent.be

H. Euler
Department of Phoniatrics and Pediatric Audiology, University Hospital Münster, University of Münster, Münster, Germany
e-mail: Harald.Euler@ukmuenster.de

D. Georgieva
Research Center Medical University - Plovdiv, Plovdiv, Bulgaria
e-mail: Doby_logo@abv.bg

M. J. V. Llamas
UCR School of Medicine, Los Angeles, CA, USA
e-mail: mllam006@medsch.ucr.edu

G. A. Maguire
Department of Psychiatry, University of California, Irvine School of Medicine, Irvine, CA, USA
e-mail: gerald.maguire@ucr.edu

S. Wong
Pacific Grove Hospital, Riverside, CA, USA
e-mail: swong053@ucr.edu

J. S. Yaruss
Communicative Sciences and Disorders, Michigan State University, East Lansing, MI, USA
e-mail: jsy@msu.edu

A. am Zehnhoff-Dinnesen et al. (eds.), *Phoniatrics II*, European Manual of Medicine,
https://doi.org/10.1007/978-3-031-25175-7_10

intervention). Unfortunately, there is no single specific test that can determine this. Simply waiting would delay treatment for those who need it.

Several predisposing factors can help in the selection of which children are likely to need treatment (Yairi and Ambrose 2013; Smith and Weber 2017b). These include, among others, the presence of a family history of stuttering, a longer time since the onset of stuttering, differences in the children's speech and language skills (language or phonological delay/maturation of the speech motor system's capacities) and a high degree of reactivity to stuttering. The more risk factors that are present, the more confident a clinician can be in making a recommendation in favour of intervention.

The importance of early diagnosis and intervention lies in the fact that the longer a child stutters the more the chance of acquiring fluent speech decreases (Bloodstein 2008, 2021; Yairi and Ambrose 1999). However, speech development may serve as a protective factor or catalyst for recovery (Hollister et al. 2017; Leech et al. 2017).

If after a careful clinical investigation there are no signs of stuttering or reports of stuttering from parents or other caregivers, no formal intervention with the child is likely to be needed. Counselling with parents, however, may be recommended (Fig. 10.1).

In this context, it is important to explore what the parents' exact expectations are, what their judgment of the linguistic peculiarities of their child is and, if required, to alter or cutback possibly unrealistic or over-critical perceptions. If the clinical picture does not show clear stuttered dysfluencies, supervision with regular checks every 6 months can be recommended. At the same time, a systematic exchange with the persons the child relates to most closely should take place (Schulze and Johannsen 1986; Johannsen 1996). Therapy should be started if the stuttering persists after a period of 6–12 months. There should be no delay if several risk factors for persistent stuttering are present, such as long-term symptoms with loss of control, increased effort or avoidance behaviour or both (Neumann et al. 2017).

Parental counselling might address the parents' way of talking (how fast, how sophisticated), communication behaviour, clarification

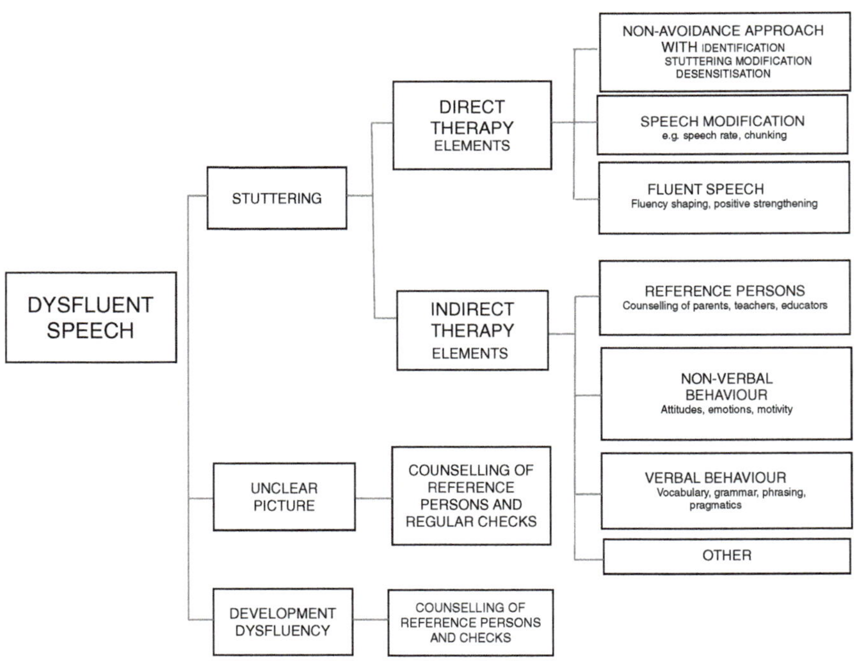

Fig. 10.1 Diagnostic pathway and therapeutic elements used in the therapy of stuttering children. (Compiled by S. Winkler in Brosch and Winkler (2008), with permission of Georg Thieme Verlag KG © Georg Thieme Verlag KG)

and acceptance of therapeutic goals, handling of stuttering and any reaction it elicits, information on the symptoms of stuttering, on differentiation between favourable and non-favourable symptoms and the re-transition of stuttering into more fluent speech and reduction of concerns.

Another vital therapeutic aspect in the treatment of stuttering children should be the counselling and information of educators and teachers. Here, the following topics are relevant: handling of stuttering in kindergarten and at school, symptoms of stuttering (above all avoidance behaviour), advantages and disadvantages through stuttering at school and handling of teasing (Brosch and Winkler 2008). Notably, there is no uniform agreement as how best to treat youngsters who stutter, and many clinicians advocate different approaches (Onslow et al. 2003; Jones et al. 2005). Still, research shows that the success rates from all of these different therapy approaches are quite similar—and all quite high (de Sonneville-Koedoot et al. 2015).

One of the primary goals of therapy for young children who stutter is to help them recover from stuttering. Clinicians have choices about how to pursue this goal: It may be accomplished through operant conditioning therapy, as is seen in the Lidcombe programme (Onslow et al. 2003; Johnson et al. 2024). It may also be accomplished through a combination of approaches that may involve changes to the child's environment and changes to the child's speech (de Sonneville-Koedoot et al. 2015; Millard et al. 2009; Yaruss et al. 2006). Independent of the assessment of stuttered speech, the child's speech development, perceptive faculties, general motor control and cognitive abilities should be considered. Such therapy is generally provided by a speech- language pathologist. In rare cases, a psychologist may be consulted.

Many speech-language pathologists begin with a period of less-direct therapy, in which they work with parents to identify aspects of the child's communication environment that may make it harder for the child to maintain fluent speech. Common examples include a rapid pace of communication by those in the child's environment, competition for talking time with siblings and peers, frequent interrupting, and a high demand on the child to speak quickly and precisely. Reducing these and other communicative stressors can help to improve speech fluency, and for many children, this appears to be all that is necessary (Packman et al. 1996; Yaruss et al. 2006).

The shorter the period between onset of stuttering and therapeutic intervention, the better the prognosis (Smith and Weber 2016; Shenker and Santayana 2018) (see Sect. 9.2). Speech therapists who specialise in stuttering are capable of treating children at any age with adequate, playful, but thoroughly direct methods. It is not the child's age that is decisive for therapy onset, but the individual symptoms, such as the presence of physical tension and blocks, and the time course of the dysfluencies (Brosch and Winkler 2008). It might be absolutely appropriate to start stuttering therapy younger than the age of 3, by using non-avoidance concepts. The children are confronted with stuttering by means appropriate for their age and so taboos are broken. They may learn that dysfluencies are as useful for communicative situations as 'smooth speech'. These concepts are based on the pioneering work of Van Riper (1971, 1982) and Dell (2001) and all aim at restitution from tense and strenuous symptoms to a looser, smoother kind of conversation. This process helps children learn to speak with more ease. These more-direct approaches to therapy might include specific changes to the child's speech, such as reduction in the child's speaking rate or in the physical tension that may be present during stuttered or fluent speech. Concurrent with all of these potential changes in the speech of the child and those in the environment is an emphasis on showing the child that stuttering is acceptable. This helps to support the development of healthy, appropriate attitudes towards speaking and communicating, and diminishes the likelihood of negative consequences if the child should continue to stutter.

Young children frequently regain completely fluent speech.

An overview of five stuttering treatment approaches for early intervention is given in Sect. 9.2.

Often a realistic therapeutic option is to help people learn to speak more easily and with less physical tension, and fewer secondary reactions or avoidance. A further option, apart from the non-avoidance concept—in particular for preschool children—should be the strengthening and consolidation of easier yet still natural ways of speaking. Very young children do have the chance to integrate a slightly changed model of speech in their natural way of talking. In this context, suitable methods are those concerning rate and modification of speech, e.g. using pauses. One therapeutic goal is to reduce stuttering events and to modify existing symptoms into loose repetitions. Some children additionally need intervention in the areas of joyful speech and capacity to communicate in general. Dependent of the child's age, a non-avoidance approach (address stuttering and break taboos, be aware of stuttering, modify stuttering) and speech modification (strengthening of fluent speech) are appropriate for school-age children.

Parental counselling is a central element in working with stuttering children. Parents are an important model, not only in their speech and communication, but in particular also in their attitude towards the disturbance of speech. They should develop a stress-free attitude towards stuttering so that they are able to accept a relatively easy, light stuttering as therapeutic goal. Nevertheless, some young children who stutter will continue to stutter. The focus of therapy must be adapted to account for this. The goals of treatment must then expand from simply focusing on fluency to addressing also the potential negative consequences that can accompany stuttering (Yaruss et al. 2012). Put simply, stuttering can be an embarrassing experience. It can be uncomfortable for the speaker to experience that moment of having difficulty saying words, and it can be emotionally painful for children to endure the negative responses of listeners. This can result in significantly negative reactions to stuttering on the part of the speaker, difficulties in communicating in key situations, and an overall adverse impact on the child's quality of life. Treatment of stuttering for older children must therefore take all of these aspects of the broader stuttering disorder into account.

A recent interdisciplinary, evidence- and consensus-based clinical practice guideline (Neumann et al. 2017) has shown that there is strong evidence for any particular treatment approach in preschool children; for children aged 6–12, there is no solid evidence for the efficacy of any specific treatment; and, for adolescents and adults, there is good evidence for speech restructuring methods such as fluency shaping. Treatment results should always be monitored by follow-up examinations.

One way of describing these aspects of therapy is through the terminology of the World Health Organization's *International Classification of Functioning, Disability and Health* (ICF). In a comprehensive approach to stuttering therapy, clinicians address the impairment (i.e. the observable speech dysfluencies), the speaker's negative reactions to stuttering, the reactions of those in the speaker's environment, and the impact of stuttering on the speaker's overall quality of life (Yaruss and Quesal 2004; Tichenor and Yaruss 2019b). Addressing the impairment involves enhancing the child's fluency through the so-called speech modification strategies, such as a slower speaking rate, increased pausing and reduced reducing physical tension. Addressing negative reactions involves various cognitive therapy methods, including desensitisation, cognitive restructuring and acceptance therapies. Educating those in the child's environment helps to reduce stigma, and reducing the adverse impact involves generalising gains into real-world settings. Together, these aspects of therapy help children overcome the burden of their stuttering disorder so they can communicate effectively and say what they want to say, regardless of whether or how much they stutter.

Hence, the focus on therapy should not only be to increase ease of speaking. Further important goals must also be the capacity to communicate with comfort and authenticity, where speaking is adapted to different situations, and the joy of talking in general—all of which helps to reduce the pressure and thus has a positive effect on achieving fluency.

10.2 Therapeutic Concepts: Evidence-Based Strategies for Treating Stuttering

Harald A. Euler and Katrin Neumann

10.2.1 Eminence-Based Treatment of Stuttering

In the stirring movie *The King's Speech*, speech therapist Lionel Logue, played by Geoffrey Rush, gave an impressive and moving performance that helped the king make public speeches relatively fluid. Was Logue a good therapist for the treatment of stuttering? He seemed to have had enough clients requesting his services after setting up a private practice in 1926, and when a British duke seeks treatment from an Australian therapist with a foreign accent, the reputation by the standards of his time must have been very good (Duchan 2012). But how effective were his treatments with his other clients? He claimed that he could cure stuttering in about 3 months (Bowen 2011), a claim that would rather disqualify a current speech therapist. With empathy and enthusiasm, he used elocutionist techniques, that is, speech training for actors: articulation, inflection, accent, reading verse, good voice and proper gestures. However, the particular composition of his treatment components is unknown, as he has never published his method(s), let alone his results. Thus, even though he was extraordinarily successful in the treatment of dysfluencies, he took his therapeutic insights to the grave and did not promote the discipline of stuttering treatment. If a current speech therapist were to attempt to emulate Logue, in the case she could reconstruct what his treatment typically and accurately consisted of, she would use an eminence-based treatment ('stuttering therapy according to Logue'), also known as assertion-based treatment (Nye et al. 2013). However, for the advancement of the practice of stuttering treatment, with all due respect to Logue, evidence-based treatment is required.

10.2.2 Evidence-Based Treatment of Stuttering in Research

Although the reliance on solid evidence is not new to science, since the end of the last century, evidence-based treatment has become a movement with a name tag (Sackett et al. 1996) that permeates most areas of health intervention. With the publication of a special issue of the *Journal of Fluency Disorders* in 2003 (Ingham 2003; Onslow 2003a), the movement soon reached the scientific discourse on stuttering and has slowly permeated the practice of stuttering treatment. Slowly, because—as the physicist Max Planck noted (Planck 1948)—a paradigm shift is usually not a change within people but requires a new generation to adopt the new idea.

Evidence-based treatment requires that a good or the best treatment be chosen, whereby the quality of treatment is defined by the evidence, not by personal opinion ('opinion-based') or by reference to a scientific authority ('eminence-based'). Good evidence usually comes as numbers, e.g. significance level and effect size, collected according to the standards of rigorous empirical science. Moreover, the evidence is more convincing if it has been replicated by other researchers. Quantifiability and reproducibility are therefore basic criteria.

In the medical field, there exist classifications of evidence levels, ranging from an upper level of a meta-analysis of randomised controlled trials, to an intermediate level of well-designed treatment studies, to the lowest level of case reports or personal clinical experience. The American Speech-Language-Hearing Association (ASHA) has endorsed the principle of evidence-based research and practice (Robey 2004). A treatment consisting of interactions between therapist and patient cannot meet the same standards of evidence as a pharmaceutical treatment. For example, a randomised placebo psychotherapy is difficult or even unethical to implement. Bloodstein et al. (2021) have outlined which criteria a stuttering treatment must fulfil in order to be called successful. Some of these 12 criteria are so general that they apply to every treatment, but some are specific to the treatment of stuttering. Hardly any treatment is able to meet all 12 criteria satisfactorily.

10.2.2.1 Twelve Criteria for a Stuttering Treatment to Be Called Successful

1. **Effectiveness in a Sufficiently Large and Representative Sample** It is a well-known phenomenon in a variety of scientific disciplines that subsequent studies with larger samples and more rigorous methods report smaller effects than initial reports with less rigorous methods and smaller samples (Jennions and Møller 2002). There is no agreement on the question of how large an effect must be. The significance of the reduction in dysfluency (*p* value) may be misleading for large samples, where statistical significance can be achieved with small and clinically meaningless improvements. A better index of clinical significance is the effect size, which is usually given as Cohen's *d* for within-subject comparisons (Cohen 1988). By convention, an effect size above $d = 0.20$ is considered a small effect, above $d = 0.80$ a large one. Reports on effect sizes have become a methodological standard because this measure is clinically meaningful and allows comparisons between studies, for example in meta-analyses.

   Reporting percentages may also be of value, but not just the percentage of persons who have improved, because a small improvement may neither be significant nor clinically meaningful. Rather, the percentage reduction from pre-therapy measures to outcome measures is required. This criterion of relative reduction raises the question of the absolute success criterion: how many dysfluencies are still considered to be within the range of normal, fluent speech, because some dysfluencies also occur in persons who do not stutter? Unfortunately, the requirements here vary between 0% stuttered syllables (%SS) and 3.65% (Bothe et al. 2006b). For a longer-term success criterion, the 3% limit seems to be most accepted. Given this criterion, the relative percentage of improvement is a problematic measure. For example, a reduction from 20%SS to 10%SS represents a solid 50% relative reduction but does not come close to the required fluency criterion.
2. **Objective and Subjective Assessment of Stuttering** As an objective measure, the %SS, or alternatively the percentage of consecutive intervals of a few seconds containing a dysfluency, should be counted by a third person who is preferably blind to when the sample was taken, and the agreement with an independent fourth person should be checked (Cordes et al. 1992). The subjective measure could simply be a rating of the severity of stuttering, or better, a comprehensive assessment by the person who stutters (PWS), such as the OASES (Overall Assessment of the Speaker's Experience of Stuttering) questionnaire (see point 9 below).
3. **Adequate Speech Samples and Repeated Assessments** When assessing stuttering, it should be considered that dysfluencies vary with time and situation. Therefore, repeated speech samples should be taken, preferably in different speaking situations. For example, before treatment the correlation between %SS in three dialogic speech situations on the one hand and scripted speech (reading) on the other hand was only $r = 0.43$, while the correlations between three different dialogic speech situations (talk with therapist; calling an unknown person by telephone; interviewing passers-by) were considerably higher (Euler and Wolff von Gudenberg 2000). Dialogic speech frequently allows word substitutions, but reading does not. It is therefore advisable to include scripted speech for clients who can read, as recom-

mended in the Stuttering Severity Instrument, for example (SSI-4; Riley 2009).

4. **Transfer of Improvement to Situations Outside the Treatment Setting** This requirement is so obvious that it requires no further comment.
5. **Long-Term Follow-up Assessment** Because a relapse into stuttering often occurs, especially in the first weeks or months after treatment, the treatment gain must be shown to persist. Reports of improvements from before treatment to immediately after treatment are therefore no longer state of the art, and they are particularly annoying when therapists present selected clients in the mass media. How 'long-term' is defined has not yet been agreed upon, but 1 year after the last treatment intervention is the minimum time. This means that if a treatment consists of an intensive treatment phase followed by a maintenance phase, which may include refresher courses for example, the last refresher course would be the last clinical intervention.

A convenient procedure is to make the follow-up assessment by telephone call. Because some treated clients speak more fluently when they are called overtly, i.e. when they know that their speech is being examined for dysfluencies (Andrews and Craig 1982), a covert call may be indicated. However, the question is whether competence (*can* she or he?) or performance (*does* she or he?) is the treatment goal. In my opinion, competence (control) is what has to be aspired to, because this is a realistic treatment goal that can be achieved. For example, if people need glasses for good vision, they do not have to wear them all the time, but can decide for themselves when and where they put them on. Likewise, if a PWS is equipped with a speaking technique that avoids or reduces stuttering, it is up to the person when to use this technique. The PWS may well decide to resort to the aid in situations of communicative demand, but not, for example, speaking at home with the children. Gaining control over one's dysfluencies is a realistic and sufficient criterion for success, not the unrealistic goal of a complete and lasting cure (Cooper 1987).

6. **Treatment Control Conditions** Fluency gains after treatment could be partially due to two factors:
   (a) During treatment, spontaneous recovery might have occurred regardless of the treatment, which is most likely to happen in children.
   (b) Owing to increased familiarity, the second assessment might be more relaxed for the client than the first assessment before the start of treatment. For this reason, a wait-control group is often used. The fluency gain in adult wait-controls is usually small (Andrews et al. 1980) and not significant (Euler and Wolff von Gudenberg 2000). Direct prospective comparisons between two treatments are possible but difficult to implement and thus rare (Bothe et al. 2006a; Herder et al. 2006).
7. **Speech Naturalness** The speech of the client ought to sound natural and spontaneous to a listener. The naturalness of speech is most often rated by non-professional listeners on a single 9-point scale (Martin et al. 1984). Even after a speech-restructuring treatment that intentionally starts with unnatural-sounding slow speech, the speech naturalness after the treatment is rated better than before the treatment (Euler et al. 2009) owing to the elimination or reduction of unnatural-sounding speech blocks. However, the speech naturalness of treated PWS is still rated worse than the speech naturalness of people who do not stutter (Franken et al. 1992).
8. **Freedom from Necessity to Monitor One's Speech** The ideal stuttering treatment should not require the client to continue monitoring his or her speech after the end of the treatment. However, the need for *occasional* monitoring is the best that can be achieved in most adult or adolescent clients with devel-

opmental stuttering and with the most promising behavioural treatments, regardless of whether the previous treatment consisted of some kind of fluency shaping or of dysfluency shaping (stuttering modification).

9. **Improvement in the Quality of Life** The treatment of stuttering must not only reduce dysfluencies but should also eliminate negative emotions associated with stuttering, such as social anxieties, and have a positive effect in everyday communication situations. Menzies et al. (2008) report that speech restructuring alone, i.e. without a special cognitive-behaviour therapy package to treat social anxieties, has no impact on social anxiety. However, several of the prolonged/smooth speech treatment approaches listed in the review by Bothe et al. (2006a) do not support this claim (Bothe et al. 2006a, p. 327). Our own research also contradicts this finding (Euler et al. 2016). We administered the comprehensive questionnaire OASES (Yaruss and Quesal 2006) to a large sample of adolescents and adults who had been treated with fluency shaping in the Kassel Stuttering Therapy, and found that the improvements in everyday communication situations, including negative emotions, showed even larger effect sizes than the improvements in dysfluency reductions. OASES has been translated into a variety of languages and is the first choice for assessing the impact of stuttering treatment on affective reactions, communication difficulties and on the speaker's quality of life.
10. **Drop-outs Must Be Reported** Clients who do not finish treatment are more likely to be those with unsatisfying treatment effects than clients who stay until the end of treatment. Therefore, real drop-outs must be indicated. Those clients who discontinue treatment for reasons obviously unrelated to the effects of treatment effects (e.g. change of residence, illness, death) should not be considered as real drop-outs.

    A related problem concerns missing data (no-shows) in cases where repeated assessments are made after treatment. In the study by Euler and Wolff von Gudenberg (2000) assessments were made before and after intensive treatment, and then after 6 months, 1 year, 2 years and 3 years. When comparing 'regular shows' (clients with complete data set) with 'irregular shows' (clients with at least one missing follow-up assessment), the irregular group stuttered 2%SS more (%SS averaged over all assessment points) than the regular. This suggests that a client who comes for follow-up assessment less reliably, or is more difficult to reach than a client with easy access, is more likely to be a person for whom treatment has been less effective. The inclusion of no-shows in the data set may therefore inflate the effectiveness indicators of the treatment.
11. **The Method Must Be Effective When Done by Any Professional Qualified in the Treatment of Stuttering** Obviously, a guru treatment method that works only when applied by privy insiders cannot spread and is of little help for the long-term advancement of stuttering treatment. Instead, the evidence-based treatment must be clearly described in a treatment manual so that any professional can repeat the treatment if it is performed with manual fidelity.
12. **The Treatment Must Remain Effective Even if it is no Longer New** This criterion refers to the well-known Hawthorne effect and the so-called decline effect (Schooler 2011): a new and innovative treatment is usually more effective than the same type of treatment when it is no longer original but has become routine. Unfortunately, this effect often occurs in the treatment of stuttering, because new forms of therapy are constantly emerging, while methodologically rigorous studies of the treatment effect are rare, even in Anglo-Saxon countries where empirical approaches to phenomena of human behaviour are highly valued.

10.2.2.2 What Is the Available Evidence for Successful Stuttering Treatments?

Several problems arise when the evidence of good stuttering treatments is to be presented.

1. To the author's knowledge, only a few comparative efficacy studies (effectiveness under optimal clinical conditions) or effectiveness studies (effectiveness under conditions in the field), i.e. studies designed to compare a treatment with one or several alternatives, have been done to quantify the relative effectiveness of the treatments. From these few studies, no coherent picture of the comparative effectiveness of treatments can be derived. However, there are two retrospective evaluations described below, one of which (Euler et al. 2014) allows a limited number of multiple comparisons.
2. Treatments are usually not pure, with a single element, but come in different packages of components. Therefore, meta-analyses are often limited to comparable treatment approaches, and statements can often only be made about components of treatments that have proven to be effective.
3. Treatments must be tailored to the age of the clients. How fine-grained the age groups should be is controversial. It is undisputed that the treatment of children of pre-school or school age who need one parent as co-therapist represents a specific client population, which must be treated and evaluated separately from the adults. Should the treatment of adolescents differ from that of adults? In the Kassel Stuttering Therapy data files, which have existed for 20 years with a large number of documented treatment cases, there are hardly any differences between adolescents and young adults in terms of treatment effects, but other stuttering specialists might not share this opinion.
4. Some professionals disapprove of the standard evidence requirements, and this refusal is often based on general philosophical-anthropological assumptions. It may be argued that a person cannot be cast into numbers; or that the 'whole person' must be seen (a goal that is psychologically completely impossible!); or that the persons who stutter are so different from each other, with individual configurations of the causes of their stuttering, that they cannot be grouped for statistical analyses. Proponents of multiple determinants of the origin of stuttering (early home environment; childhood trauma; sociological and cultural factors; personality differences; high parental speaking demands, etc.) often seem to disregard the repeated and consistent findings over decades of behavioural genetics about stuttering (Fagnani et al. 2011; Kraft and Yairi 2012) from different research groups: that stuttering has a high heritability of from 70% to 84%. Of the remaining variance, *little or none is due to shared environmental influences*, that is, influences that can be expected to make siblings alike compared with same-age children from other families.

The remaining 30% to about 16% of the variance is unexplained and, apart from measurement error, is attributed to non-shared (by siblings) environmental experiences. However, because in behavioural genetics everything outside the genome is considered as environment, these individual experiences may be more strongly rooted in inner-individual processes of the complicated developmental dynamics of embryology and the resulting physiological and brain-forming cascades than in different individual social environments after birth. In any case, the message from behavioural genetics is clear: developmental stuttering is originally caused by some genetic mechanisms, and it is not originally caused by early social or language interactions between family members and the young child, as these interactions can be considered shared environment influences that have repeatedly proven to be of little or no importance. The latter statement does not dispute the possibility that early parent–child verbal interactions can be effective in the *secondary* prevention of stuttering (Gottwald 2010) or in reducing or eliminating stuttering, as is the case with the Lidcombe programme (Harrison and Onslow 2010).

5. Publications in languages other than English are hardly visible in the international scientific community. Meta-analyses and systematic reviews do not normally include non-English publications on treatment effects, with the commendable exception of Herder et al. (2006), and may therefore not be as comprehensive as is desirable. However, for various reasons, therapists for stuttering (e.g. logopaedists, speech-language pathologists, clinical linguists) in non-English speaking countries often do not read English publications and therefore are only used to publications in their native language. Stuttering-researchers in non-English speaking countries, on the other hand, might refrain from publications in English in order to address readers in their own language.

Meta-analyses and Comprehensive Reviews The results of three meta-analyses (Andrews et al. 1980; Herder et al. 2006; Nippold 2011) and two comprehensive reviews (Bothe et al. 2006a; Neumann et al. 2017) provide information about established treatment effects. The meta-analysis of Andrews et al. (1980) is listed here despite its age. With this inclusion I should like to pay homage to the authors, because this study was not only the first meta-analysis on the treatment effects of stuttering, but one of the very early meta-analyses ever. Understandably, most of the 42 studies discussed there do not meet the current methodological criteria. For example, only relatively short-term effects were reported (average effect size $d = 1.3$), study sample sizes were generally small (median = 14, range $n = 3$ to $n = 100$), and no study involved children under 8 years of age. In terms of results, treatments based on the training of slowed speech or soft syllable onset or both were superior to other types of treatment such as attitude changes and airflow techniques.

The meta-analysis by Herder et al. (2006) covered behavioural stuttering treatments, but the publication is of limited value because 8 of the 12 included studies, many of them with relatively small sample sizes, reported only short-term effects. It is well known that a variety of techniques can temporarily reduce stuttering (Bloodstein et al. 2021), but the required evidence is long-term effectiveness. It is therefore not surprising that Herder et al. (2006) report a conclusion reminiscent of the Dodo's in Alice's Adventures in Wonderland ('Everybody won …'): all therapies are equally effective. The same criticism can be made of the meta-analysis by Nye et al. (2013) on stuttering interventions in children and adolescents between 2 and 18 years of age, where 5 of the 9 studies included reported only short-term effects. One longer-term study included in both meta-analyses (Ryan and Ryan 1995) had at 14 months follow-up with a sample so small ($n = 11$) that only very large differences would have been detectable. No wonder that the two treatments compared (Delayed Auditory Feedback [DAF] and General Increase in Length of Utterances [GILCU]) proved to be equally effective.

A tentative conclusion may be drawn from the three meta-analyses. The best evidence is provided for treatments that contain speech-restructuring components of slowed/smooth speech for adolescents and adults, and the Lidcombe programme for pre-school children. This conclusion is in accordance with the resumé of the comprehensive review by Bothe et al. (2006a). These authors summarise that

> response-contingent principles are the predominant feature of the most powerful treatment procedures for young children who stutter. The most powerful treatments for adults, with respect to both speech outcomes and social, emotional or cognitive outcomes, appear to combine variants of prolonged speech, self-management, response contingencies and other infrastructural variables
> Bothe et al. (2006a, p. 321)

In a companion paper on the effects of pharmacological treatments, Bothe et al. (2006b) conclude that these treatments cannot be recommended at present because the effects on dysfluency reductions and on social and emotional benefits are unreliable and too small compared with the relatively frequent negative side effects.

A remarkable feature of the more recent reviews (Bothe et al. 2006a, b; Herder et al. 2006; Neumann et al. 2017; Nye et al. 2013) is the small number of studies that met the desired methodological quality criteria. In the analysis by Herder et al. (2006), 375 studies met the inclusion criteria, but only 12 of them (3.2%) met the quality criteria. In the Bothe et al. (2006b) study about non-pharmacological treatments published between 1970 and 2005, 39 out of 162 articles (24%) passed the quality criteria; in the analysis by Nye et al. (2013), 9 of 312 studies (2.9%). As described above, the majority of the studies in these meta-analyses were concerned with short-term treatment effects. What is required is methodologically sound and solid evidence-based treatment research, particularly for children (Nippold 2011), that meets modern standards, rather than single case studies, simple pre-post studies or nice descriptions of new treatments without supportive data.

Most of the studies reported are carried out under good or optimal conditions, that is, in well-controlled institutional contexts (often referred to as 'efficacy' studies). Whether positive treatment effects are actually transferred to daily life (Langevin and Kully 2003) is another question but is of great importance for PWS seeking the best available treatment.

For younger children, the Lidcombe programme (Harrison and Onslow 2010) has the most solid published evidence and is therefore recommended (Guitar and McCauley 2010). For older children, adolescents and adults there are two types of treatment that are the most popular and probably the most effective: (1) speech restructuring and (2) stutter restructuring approaches. The former has various labels, most often fluency shaping, the latter most often stuttering modification, non-avoidance, Van Riper approach, or 'Iowa' therapies. In speech restructuring, an attempt is made to teach a new type of speech pattern (initially slowed speech, easy syllable onset, continuous phonation) that is incompatible with stuttering events. Stutter restructuring aims at the stuttering event itself in order to escape from the dysfluency block swiftly and easily ('fluent stuttering') by using various techniques (for example, cancellation, pull-out, preparatory set).

There is ample evidence for the effectiveness of fluency shaping, but little for stuttering modification (Prins and Ingham 2009); but there are also exceptions (Blomgren et al. 2005; Kohmäscher et al. 2023; Natke et al. 2010), although Iowa therapies, which were the forerunners of stuttering modification, were considered the only professionally accepted treatment of stuttering for many decades of the twentieth century (Johnson 1955). The lack of evidence for the effectiveness of stuttering modification might have two reasons: (1) the treatment goal of stuttering modification is not the numerical reduction of dysfluencies, but the nature of the stuttering event; (2) stuttering modification has the emancipatory goal, apart from easing disturbing speech blocks, to depathologise stuttering ('non-avoidance'): don't be afraid to stutter or even be ashamed of it.

Retrospective Client Evaluations Asking people who stutter about their previous experiences with treatments has several advantages:

1. Most adult PWS have undergone different treatments in their biography and can therefore make comparisons.
2. The clients compare the effectiveness of treatments in everyday practice, not when administered under particularly well-controlled conditions (efficacy).
3. With the exception of the most recent treatments, the clients can assess the long-term effectiveness. There are of course also drawbacks of such studies. For example, when people are asked about the treatments they received in their childhood decades ago, they cannot include treatments that were not available then. To the knowledge of the author, there are two retrospective client evaluation studies that complement the meta-analyses and comprehensive reviews reported above.

Euler et al. (2014) used a questionnaire to ask 88 PWS various questions about their past stuttering treatments (231 single treatment cases of the 5 more popular treatments in Germany). The central questions were the effectiveness of, and the satisfaction with, each treatment received in the past (5-point rating scale). Two types of treatment (fluency shaping and stuttering modification) received favourable ratings; the other three treatments (breathing regulation, hypnosis, unspecified logopaedic treatment) received unfavourable ratings. The differences between the two effective treatments were not significant, nor were the differences between the three less-effective treatments. However, the effectiveness gap between the two effective and the three rather ineffective treatments were large. As expected, the ratings of effectiveness and satisfaction were highly correlated. The typical therapy biography of a PWS begins in childhood with an unspecified logopaedic treatment administered extensively in single and individual sessions, and this is unfortunately the most frequently prescribed treatment for stuttering in Germany. 'Unspecified' here refers to the fact that the treatment components used varied considerably between logopaedists and were usually combinations of components rather than an evidence-based standard treatment with a generally known name. Intensive treatments were superior to extensive treatments, and group treatments superior to individual treatments. An ethological analysis was consistent with the ratings: fluency shaping and stuttering modification were most often the last or only treatment, as one would expect from effective treatments, whereas the other treatments were more often followed by another treatment.

Another retrospective treatment evaluation has been reported by Yaruss et al. (2002), probably with a less representative sample of PWS (attendants of a conference of the National Stuttering Association). Because these authors report their data in a different format (grouped data), the two retrospective studies are not directly comparable. However, the respondents in the Yaruss et al. (2002) study reported more favourable experiences with stuttering modification than with fluency shaping approaches.

If fluency shaping and stuttering modification are best assessed by PWS themselves, the question arises of the combination of both approaches, as most clearly suggested by Guitar (2006). Clients may have different preferences, some preferring 'fluency', i.e. a speech restructuring approach; others 'freedom', i.e. a stuttering modification approach (Venkatagiri 2009). A possible intervention strategy would be to start with fluency shaping and to supplement this treatment with a stuttering modification add-on for those patients with unsatisfactory success. If both approaches, fluency shaping and stuttering modification, were applied in a randomised controlled trial with a sufficiently large sample, insights into differential therapy indications could be gained. However, there is no evidence for the superiority of such a combined approach, let alone data on differential indications.

10.2.3 Evidence-Based Treatment of Stuttering in Practice

In the practice of treating stuttering, resources are usually so limited that only minimal evidence criteria can be met. The most important criterion is the best-practice strategy of administering a treatment with proven effectiveness with high manual fidelity. The second criterion is that a dysfluency measure (for example, percentage of stuttered syllables, or an SSI-4 stuttering severity score for speech restructuring approaches: an assessment of the severity of the stuttering events for stuttering restructuring approaches) should be taken on at least three time-points, namely before the start of treatment, at the end of treatment and 12 months after the last treatment intervention. Audio recordings with at least 500 syllables at these assessment points are advisable. The speech sample 12 months after the last intervention can be done by telephone. The third criterion is to obtain self-reports by the clients. If a lengthy questionnaire such as the OASES is considered too time-consuming, at least a simple overall numerical severity rating of stuttering and a rating of the impact of stuttering in everyday life should be taken on all three occasions.

In this context an insight from psychotherapy is worth heeding. When asked about the effects of therapy, the greatest effects are reported by the therapists themselves. Less rosy effects are reported by patients, and the least effects are seen by the friends or family members of the patients (Dineen 1999). Therefore, a statement of a therapist such as 'I have had good experience with my therapy' is worthless unless it is grounded on evidence, which means numbers rather than impressions.

10.2.4 Conclusion and Recommendations

Progress in science is achieved not only by new ideas and new methods, but also by a dispassionate disposal, or at least a benign neglect, of theories and methods that have not provided solid and robust empirical evidence. The same can be said of the treatment of stuttering. There is no need for new and seemingly attractive treatment proposals, but more and better evidence of the effectiveness of existing or novel treatments. For this reason, the majority of stuttering treatments that fill the books on stuttering are not mentioned in this section. There may indeed be good treatments that have been overlooked, but what counts under the banner of evidence-based stuttering therapy is not how good a treatment appears to be or even is, but what evidence has been provided for the effectiveness of the treatment.

10.3 Treatment for Stuttering Across the Lifespan

J. Scott Yaruss

10.3.1 Introduction

Stuttering is a neurodevelopmental communication condition that can affect all aspects of an individual's life (Tichenor and Yaruss 2019b; Yaruss and Quesal 2004). On the surface, stuttering involves disruption in the forward flow of speech, or speech dysfluencies, which can interfere with a person's ability to produce speech smoothly (Bloodstein et al. 2021). Examples of such dysfluencies include repetitions of parts of words ('li-li-like this'), prolongations of sounds ('lllllike this') or complete blockages when no sound is produced ('l----ike this'). Importantly, such behaviours occur inconsistently in people's speech: People who stutter may appear to speak fluently at some times or in some situations yet experience significant stuttering at other times or in other situations (Yaruss 1997; Constantino et al. 2016). Speech dysfluencies may be accompanied by other physical behaviours, such as physical tension or struggle in the speech muscles or elsewhere (Tichenor et al. 2017) or avoidance of words or speaking situations (Plexico et al. 2009a; Jackson et al. 2015; Tichenor and Yaruss 2018; Tichenor and Yaruss 2019a). These dysfluencies and associated behaviour can lead to negative emotional and cognitive reactions, such as anxiety and shame, as a speaker copes with the speaking difficulties (Blumgart et al. 2010; Iverach and Rapee 2014), and these reactions in turn can lead to functional communication problems and adverse impact on the person's quality of life (Yaruss and Quesal 2004; Craig et al. 2009).

Stuttering begins in early childhood, typically between the ages of 2½ and 4 years (Yairi and Ambrose 2014). Many young children go through a period of stuttering during their development (Ambrose and Yairi 1999; Reilly et al. 2013), though most of these children—roughly 75–80%—stop stuttering (Yairi and Ambrose 1999). It appears that early treatment can help some young children completely overcome stuttering, so that they do not continue to stutter into adulthood (de Sonneville-Koedoot et al. 2015). Unfortunately, differentiating between natural recovery and assisted recovery is a significant challenge, so it is difficult to determine the true success rates for therapy. Ultimately, roughly 20% of children who start to stutter are at risk of continuing to do so into the school-age years. For these older children, adolescents and adults, stuttering typically becomes a chronic condition. Overall, roughly 1% of the population as a whole stutters, with minimal apparent differences between cultures, societies or languages (Bloodstein et al. 2021).

There is no single treatment approach that is effective for all people who stutter. Different approaches appear to have value for different individuals, but there is considerable disagreement in the field about appropriate treatment strategies and the value and validity of supporting data for various treatments (Bloodstein 1993). The field of fluency disorders has, somewhat belatedly, entered the age of evidence-based practice, but the literature base for many therapy approaches is sorely lacking. Many commonly used approaches have little or no research support, though this is due to a lack of studies rather than to studies indicating a lack of efficacy. Thus, consideration of each individual speaker's performance throughout the therapy process becomes particularly important. This is in keeping with the principles of evidence-based practice; however, the lack of published evidence for many approaches highlights the value of ongoing data collection and evaluation by individual clinicians.

This section presents a high-level overview of different approaches to treating stuttering across the lifespan. Importantly, the goals and procedures of treatment for stuttering depend upon the age of the person being treated, in part because complete recovery from stuttering is common in pre-school children but uncommon in school-age children, adolescents and adults. As noted above, there are numerous opinions about which approach is best for each age group; no attempt is made here to promote one approach over another, or to evaluate the literature base for any single approach. Instead, the goal is to provide a survey of commonly described approaches as a springboard for future exploration of the efficacy and appropriateness of different approaches for helping individuals who stutter.

10.3.2 Assessment of Stuttering

Before discussion of treatment approaches, it is important to acknowledge the value of a comprehensive diagnostic evaluation. Without such assessment, it is impossible to determine the appropriateness of therapy or the specific goals that such therapy should address. As with treatment, the goals and procedures of the diagnostic evaluation differ depending upon the speaker's age.

For younger children, the primary goal of the evaluation is to determine whether the child is likely to recover from stuttering or is at risk of developing persistent or chronic stuttering. Current theories of stuttering highlight the fact that multiple aspects of a child's development contribute to the onset of stuttering (Smith and Weber 2017a), and a considerable body of research has explored a range of potential risk factors that indicate an elevated risk for ongoing stuttering (Yairi et al. 1996; Walsh et al. 2018). The more risk factors that are detected during a diagnostic evaluation, the more likely it is that a child will need therapy to increase the chance of recovery. Examples of common risk factors include a family history of stuttering, due to a genetic predisposition (Kraft and Yairi 2012); a relatively long time since the onset of stuttering (though there is debate about just how long is relatively long); and difficulties with other aspects of speech or language development. Clinicians are therefore encouraged to conduct a thorough evaluation of a child's overall speech and language skills and gather a complete case history in order to assess the presence of such risk factors before making a recommendation for therapy.

For children older than approximately age 7, the likelihood of recovery diminishes significantly (Yairi and Ambrose 1999), though later recovery is possible (Howell et al. 2008). For school-age children, adolescents and adults, a comprehensive evaluation is still needed, but the focus of the evaluation may shift from attempts to identify potential causal factors or risk predictors towards the evaluation of the adverse impact of stuttering on the person's life (Yaruss and Quesal 2006; Yaruss and Quesal 2016). A person in this age range who is experiencing adverse impact is in need of therapy; a person who is not experiencing adverse impact may not need (or want) intervention, even if observable stuttering remains.

10.3.3 Treatment of Stuttering

As indicated above, stuttering treatment goals differ, depending upon the client's age. For a preschool or young school-age child, there is fairly uniform agreement within the field that at least one of the key goals will be a reduction in observable speech dysfluencies and the development of easier speech. Still, there are differences of opinion about how this might be achieved and about whether other goals (such as improved communication attitudes) should also be included (Onslow and Yaruss 2007; Onslow and Millard 2012). Although there is overlap between approaches, treatment for early childhood stuttering can generally be divided into three categories: less-direct therapy, more-direct therapy and operant conditioning therapy. (Note that some authors only differentiate between 'indirect' and 'direct' approaches, classifying operant conditioning therapy as an example of 'direct' treatment (de Sonneville-Koedoot et al. 2015).)

- In **less-direct therapy**, clinicians help parents, caregivers and others in the environment to support the child's development of typically fluent speech through modifications to the child's communication environment that reduce demands or stressors that might increase stuttering (Yaruss et al. 2006; Kelman and Nicholas 2008; de Sonneville-Koedoot et al. 2015; Yaruss and Reardon-Reeves 2017). Examples of common modifications include reductions in parental speaking rates or increased pausing during conversational interactions, modelling of easier ways of speaking, and a reduction in requirements that the child speak a certain way or at a certain time. Such therapy is largely parent-administered: typically, parents are taught how to make these communication modifications during therapy sessions, then they are instructed to use these altered speaking styles with their child at home or in other speaking situations, particularly at times when communication demands are high.
- **More-direct therapy** involves specifically teaching children to modify their own speech, just as may be done with older children, adolescents or adults (Yaruss and Reardon-Reeves 2017). Common adjustments include reductions in the child's rate of speech or overall pace of communication, as well as reductions in physical tension during both fluent and stuttered speech. Importantly, both less-direct and more-direct approaches may involve activities designed to reduce or prevent the development of negative communication attitudes by the child or family (Logan and Yaruss 1999). Such therapy includes messages designed to help the child learn that it is acceptable to have difficulty when speaking and that stuttering is not something to fear. These messages of acceptance can be provided alongside therapy designed to help the child develop typically fluent speech.
- **Operant conditioning therapy** (Onslow et al. 2001) involves teaching parents to provide verbal contingencies to support fluent speech or correct stuttered speech. Operant therapy does not specifically require the parents to use or model any different type of communication pattern. Instead, parents are encouraged to support the child's natural fluency abilities through praise of fluency and occasional, gentle correction of stuttering. As with less-direct approaches to therapy, the treatment is parent-administered: parents are taught how to provide contingencies during therapy during sessions, then they are encouraged to use the contingencies with their children during home practice sessions.

Research on the efficacy of early childhood stuttering therapy is uneven. Numerous studies have demonstrated the efficacy of operant therapy (Jones et al. 2005; Miller and Guitar 2009); fewer studies have addressed the efficacy of less-direct or more-direct approaches (Yaruss et al. 2006; Millard et al. 2009; de Sonneville-Koedoot et al. 2015). Importantly, however, a randomised controlled trial comparing a less-direct with a more-direct treatment approach demonstrated nearly identical outcomes (de Sonneville-Koedoot et al. 2015), suggesting that clinicians have a number of viable options to consider when selecting a particular treatment approach for young children who stutter.

For older children, adolescents and adults there is greater disagreement about the appropriate procedures and outcomes for therapy (Nippold 2012; Yaruss et al. 2012): some practitioners focus therapy primarily on the observable features of stuttering, while others focus on reducing the overall impact of stuttering on the person's life *in addition to* reducing observable speech disruptions. Either way, clinicians should ensure that the goals they select for their clients are consistent with the speakers' own goals for themselves and their communication, for research has shown that different people who stutter have different goals in treatment (Yaruss et al. 2002; Tichenor and Yaruss 2019a).

One way of considering the broad range of possible procedures and outcomes of stuttering therapy is to employ the structure of the World Health Organization's International Classification of Functioning, Disability, and Health (ICF) (WHO 2001). The present author has adapted the ICF framework to the stuttering disorder (Yaruss and Quesal 2004; Tichenor and Yaruss 2019b), both for the assessment of stuttering treatment outcomes (Yaruss and Quesal 2006, 2016) and for the development of a comprehensive approach to treatment (Yaruss 2007; see also Reardon-Reeves and Yaruss 2013). In brief, the ICF explains that people experience health problems through an impairment in body function or structure and the resulting activity limitations or participation restrictions, which may be mediated by personal and environmental contexts. As applied to stuttering, one can define the impairment in body function as the underlying sensation, often referred to as a 'loss of control' (Perkins 1990), that speakers report immediately before an observable disruption in speech (Tichenor and Yaruss 2018, 2019b; Jackson et al. 2019). The activity limitations and participation restrictions refer to the difficulties that people who stutter experience with functional communication (e.g. engaging in conversations) and the adverse impact on quality of life referred to at the beginning of this section (Craig et al. 2009; Koedoot et al. 2011). In this view, personal context includes the speech dysfluencies that may be observable to a listener, as well as concomitant struggle behaviour and physical tension (Tichenor et al. 2017). Other personal reactions may include avoidance of speaking and word substitution as speakers attempt to prevent an overt moment of stuttering behaviour from becoming apparent (Lowe et al. 2017), as well as negative emotional and cognitive features of stuttering, including anxiety, shame and low self-esteem (Boyle 2015; Iverach et al. 2017). Finally, the environmental context includes the reactions of those in the speaker's environment, such as discrimination and societal stigma and bullying, which have been shown to be commonly experienced by people who stutter across all ages (Hugh-Jones and Smith 1999; St. Louis 2011; Blood and Blood 2016; Boyle 2018).

By using the ICF framework, it is possible to identify some aspects of therapy as being focused on reducing or preventing the occurrence of speech disruptions that result from the impairment in body function. These have been described as 'fluency shaping', 'fluency enhancing', 'speech modification' and 'speech restructuring' techniques (Blomgren 2010, 2013). Examples include reducing speaking rates, increasing pausing, or minimising physical tension that might lead to moments of overt stuttering, through the use of strategies such as light articulatory contacts. Aspects of therapy focused on reducing the behavioural reactions include the so-called stuttering modification strategies (Van Riper 1973), which involve helping a speaker learn to modify physical tension before, during or after stuttering, so instances of stuttering are less disruptive to speech production. Aspects of therapy focused on reducing affective and cognitive reactions include counselling strategies for minimising anxiety and shame surrounding stuttering. This can be accomplished through cognitive therapy approaches, such as cognitive-behavioural therapy, acceptance and commitment therapy, mindfulness approaches, systematic desensitisation, exposure therapy and the like (Menzies et al. 2009; Beilby et al. 2012; Kelman and Wheeler 2015; Scheurich et al. 2019). Aspects of therapy focused on reducing activity limitations and participation restrictions involve helping speakers generalise their speaking strategies and attitudinal improvements in real-world situations, so they can speak more freely, participate more actively, and experience less adverse impact in their daily lives.

Nearly all therapy approaches involve generalisation strategies, though this remains a challenging aspect of the therapy process: Many people who stutter report that they have an easier time achieving success in managing stuttering and communication attitudes within the therapy setting but much greater difficulty in everyday situations (Yaruss et al. 2002). One of the key reasons for this difficulty is the environmental context, for people who stutter live in an environment that does not understand and is largely unaccepting of their communication difficulties (St. Louis 2011). Through treatment, self-advocacy and the work of stuttering support and self-help organisations (Yaruss et al. 2007), people who stutter can learn to educate others about stuttering and thereby create a more understanding and accepting environment that ultimately helps them communicate more freely in their daily lives.

In addition to these commonly used aspects of therapy for stuttering, many other approaches have been tried, including delayed auditory feedback and masking devices, medications, hypnosis, psychoanalysis, relaxation, biofeedback and more (Bloodstein 1993). In general, evidence in support of these alternative treatments is lacking, with improvements in speech being temporary, though there are promising signs in recent medication trials (Maguire et al. 2010). Even with traditional therapy approaches, however, relapse is common (Craig 1998), and maintenance of the therapeutic gains requires ongoing practice, monitoring and vigilance. Although improvements in speech fluency and communication attitudes are definitely possible, it appears that relatively few school-age children, adolescents or adults who stutter report a complete disappearance of stuttering behaviour and associated negative reactions, either with or without treatment (Finn et al. 2005; Neumann et al. 2019; Tichenor and Yaruss 2020). Therefore, additional research is needed to develop appropriate treatments for people who stutter—and in particular to identify which treatments might be most appropriate for which individual speakers.

In part because of the lack of success that many people who stutter have experienced in formal treatment, a strong self-help and support movement has developed (Trichon and Tetnowski 2011), with both children and adults who stutter consistently reporting improvements in communication and attitudes following participation in stuttering support (Yaruss et al. 2002; Trichon and Tetnowski 2011; Byrd et al. 2016, 2018; Tichenor and Yaruss 2019a). There has also been a growing focus on viewing stuttering through the lens of neurodiversity, with an emphasis on complete acceptance of stuttering, both by the individual speaker and by society as a whole (Campbell et al. 2019). Clinicians should be aware that not all people who stutter will want to change their speech behaviour and that increased fluency may not be the primary focus of an individual's therapy. Therefore, speech-language therapists should be certain not to exacerbate societal or personal stigma by focusing too much on observable speech disruptions (Tichenor and Yaruss 2019a). Instead, they should follow the guidance of their clients to identify appropriate treatment outcomes for individual speaker.

10.3.4 Summary

Stuttering is a complex communication condition that can have significant and lasting consequences for a person's life. It appears that early intervention can help young children who stutter overcome the challenge associated with stuttering and achieve complete recovery from the observable behaviour and resulting adverse consequences. Although this becomes less likely as stuttering continues into the school-age years, appropriate speech therapy and self-help experiences can help people who stutter learn to speak more easily, reduce their own negative reactions to stuttering and create a supportive and accepting environment, so that they can say what they want to say without being held back by the fact that they may stutter when they talk.

10.4 Basic Knowledge of Psychological Approaches in Stuttering

Kurt Eggers

10.4.1 Introduction

In the Section on stuttering assessment (see Sect. 8.1), we stated that although overt speech dysfluencies are the most characteristic symptom of stuttering, the diagnosis should not only focus on the overt symptoms, but also on a number of covert aspects such as underlying cognitions and emotions associated with stuttering, and the impact that stuttering has on the client's day-to-day functioning. The same thing can be said for the treatment of stuttering.

Sheehan (1970) used the iceberg metaphor to describe stuttering, with only a small part of the iceberg above the waterline, i.e. the overt symptoms, and a much bigger part below referring to the covert aspects, including fear, shame, guilt and anxiety. Flattening the top of the iceberg will only cause the iceberg to rise again, so, just eliminating overt symptoms will cause relapse after a short time. Consequently, if treatment is only focused on the top of the iceberg by stuttering modification or fluency shaping techniques, one could argue that the whole stuttering problem is not effectively addressed (Guitar 2013). Therefore, addressing the covert aspects should form an integral part of any stuttering treatment, especially in people who have been stuttering for a long period of time and where covert aspects—most likely—will have developed further.

Several authors have described how the covert aspects are not only a consequence of the overt symptomatology but can also increase the overt stuttering severity (Conture 2001; Eggers and Heselmans 2024; Jones et al. 2020). Blood (1995) described that covert aspects, i.e. cognitive and affective reactions, are due to the subjective evaluations made by a person who stutters while experiencing speech interruptions. Van Riper (1982) stated how these covert aspects can be narrowed down to different types of fear/anxiety: fear for social punishment, for listener loss, for loss of self-control, for being stigmatised as a person who stutters (for more information about (self-)stigma, see Leahy and Eggers 2023). In stuttering, similar psychological mechanisms are involved, as can be seen in anxiety disorders. Individuals anticipate future danger, experience negative feelings and bodily symptoms, have low sense of self-efficacy to exercise control over their stressors, try to avoid fearful situations, and experience severe impairment in their daily functioning (Maniadaki 2017). This anxiety is caused and maintained by cognitive biases such as preferentially allocating attention towards the anticipation of stuttering (Lowe et al. 2016; McAllister et al. 2015).

There is a reasonable degree of consensus that children, adolescents and adults who stutter are at greater risk than population statistics would predict of experiencing and exhibiting behaviour that is characteristic of social anxiety, also referred to as social phobia (Craig et al. 2003; Craig and Tran 2014; Eggers et al. 2022; Iverach et al. 2016; Onslow et al. 2023; Smith et al. 2014). The co-existence of stuttering and anxiety has implications for assessment (see Sect. 8.1) and therapy, and has led to the development of a number of therapy programmes that incorporate strategies to manage or reduce anxiety associated with stuttering (e.g. Harley 2018; Kelman and Wheeler 2015; Menzies et al. 2019). Furthermore, it seems logical to conclude that psychological approaches that are typically being used to address anxiety in order to change dysfunctional beliefs and avoiding behaviour, such as cognitive-behavioural approaches, can also be applied for stuttering therapy (e.g. Boey 2010; Reddy et al. 2010).

So, in addition to direct therapy (working with the client on overt stuttering symptoms) and indirect therapy (working with the environment of children to create a fluency-enhancing environment), speech language therapists should also incorporate and apply psychology-based therapy components in their treatment of people who stutter, particularly in older children and adults. Such psychology-based therapies include cognitive-behavioural therapy, personal construct therapy, narrative therapy, mindfulness, and acceptance and commitment therapy.

Finally, some might question if speech language therapists should be dealing with counselling aspects of people who stutter, or if working with emotions and cognitive change should be addressed by psychologists (Manning 2010). If clients are experiencing chronic life-adjustment problems, it is evident that referral to other professionals, such as counsellors and psychologists, is the most appropriate choice. Although communication disorders often result in serious problems on many levels, in most cases we are not working with people who have chronic life-adjustment problems. The vast majority of the people who stutter are ordinary people experiencing a normal reaction (i.e. emotions of stress and anxiety) to a very difficult communication problem (Luterman 2001). We agree with Manning's viewpoint that a comprehensive treatment should include client and family counselling, and that trying to achieve behavioural change in the absence of cognitive restructuring is a recipe for relapse. Hence, speech-language therapists specialised in working with stuttering must be trained in applying some of these psychology-based treatments.

10.4.2 Cognitive (Behavioural) Therapy

Cognitive-behavioural therapy (CBT) is a form of psychological treatment, developed by Beck in the 1950s, that has been found to be effective for a range of problems including depression and anxiety disorders (Beck 2011). Numerous research studies suggest that CBT leads to significant improvement in the client's functioning and quality of life. CBT is based on the cognitive model, stating that the way in which individuals perceive a situation is more closely related to their reaction and interpretation of the situation than the situation itself. This can be helpful because it makes the world more predictable, but can also lead to errors. Beck stated that some people develop systematic, unhelpful biases in the way they interpret information, resulting in patterns of negative/unhelpful thinking. One of the core principles is that people can learn better ways of coping with these psychological adversities by efforts to change one's thinking patterns actively. This is done by identifying, evaluating and changing one's automatic thoughts, assumptions and core beliefs. Strategies to do so include (a) recognising one's distortions in thinking that are creating problems (e.g. catastrophising, mind reading, all-or-nothing thinking) and re-evaluating them in light of reality; (b) gaining a better understanding of the behaviour and motivation of others; (c) using problem-solving skills to cope with difficult situations and (d) learning to develop a greater sense of confidence in one's own abilities.

The fact that people who stutter often feel anxious about specific (speaking) situations can be linked to negative/unhelpful thoughts or predictions of what is going to happen in these situations. These predictions can be about the stuttering itself ('I am sure I will stutter in that situation'), listener reactions ('People will start laughing') or how they will be perceived by others ('They will think I am incompetent'). Treatment gives clients insight into the link between their (automatic) thoughts, feelings and behavioural responses, focuses on problem-solving skills and aims to create more flexible thinking patterns.

CBT has been positively implemented in treatment for both individuals (e.g. Boey 2010; Blood 1995; Eggers 2020; Menzies et al. 2008) and groups (Fry et al. 2009) for stuttering, as well as in a stand-alone internet treatment for social anxiety in stuttering (Menzies et al. 2019). Different variants of this approach, such as Ellis's Rational emotive behaviour therapy (Ellis 2004), have also been successfully applied to the management of stuttering (Grossman 2020; Moleski and Tosi 1976).

10.4.3 Personal Construct Therapy

Personal construct therapy (PCT) was developed by Kelly (1955) and first applied to stuttering by Fransella (1970). Kelly considered each person as a scientist, engaged in a continuous process of hypothesising about one's environment and seeking evidence to test that understanding in terms of how it guides future events and behaviour (DiLollo et al. 2002; Manning 2010). The 'person-as-scientist' anticipates events, shapes behaviour accordingly, thus reducing uncertainty. The result of construing actions leads to the development of personal constructs. Kelly's idea of constructive alternativism states that all our present perceptions are open to question and reconsideration. Even the most obvious occurrences of everyday of life might appear totally transformed if we were inventive enough to construe them differently. Constructive alternativism states that there is always another way of construing events (Dalton 1983).

In stuttering therapy, PCT can be used to explore different ways one can talk (e.g. varying loudness, speed and pitch). Checking out the variety of ways or alternatives open to clients is part of the process of loosening constructs. In addition, when clients stutter, they can move beyond the feeling that there is only one way to speak, i.e. with a stutter. Loosening construing can lead to being able to make more choices, and ultimately to exercise better control in managing (stuttering) behaviour (Stewart and Birdsall 2001).

PCT has been implemented with people who stutter of different age ranges (Hayhow and Levy 1993; Shapiro 2011), offering a psychological framework to alter the clients' perception of himself with regard to his stuttering, and to the world in which he and his stuttering exists (Ward 2006). Both improvements in fluency, as well as decreases in anxiety have been reported (Botterill and Cook 1987).

10.4.4 Narrative Therapy

The application of PCT to stuttering has received widespread attention in Britain but much less in other countries, such as the United States. DiLollo et al. (2002) attribute this to the complexity of Kelly's (1955) theory, assessment that tends to be time-consuming and the lack of collaboration between psychologists and speech-language therapists. An alternative treatment approach, adhering to the theoretical principles of a personal construct view, has gained considerable momentum is narrative therapy.

Narrative therapy (NT) has its origins in social constructionism, recognising that people construct their lives and identities socially and culturally, through language, discourse and communication (Ryan et al. 2015). NT was developed in the 1980s (White 2000, 2007; White and Epston 1990) and is based on the idea that people understand their lives through their 'storying' of lived experience. NT begins with the narrative as told by the client; for people who stutter, this is often the stuttering-saturated narrative of how stuttering is central in the life of the client (Leahy et al. 2012). The process continues with externalising the problem through externalising conversations, assisting the client to separate the problem from oneself. In doing so, clients gain insight in and realise that the person is not the problem, but the problem is the problem. This implies that people who stutter make a shift from a 'stutterer'-perspective to a 'stuttering'-perspective. Through specific questioning techniques (e.g. outcome-, account-, possibility-, circulation- and re-description questions), clients are invited to map the influence of the problem on their personal life and relationships and to 'rewrite and re-author their stories' to one that fits with their hopes, values and dreams.

NT can contribute to the long-term maintenance of more fluent speech (DiLollo et al. 2002), has been identified as a possible means of addressing the impact of stuttering on the person who stutters, and has been introduced as, e.g. a core component of the Irish intervention programme 'Free to Stutter...Free to Speak' (Ryan et al. 2015).

10.4.5 Mindfulness- and Acceptance-Based Therapy

Mindfulness-based interventions (Kabat-Zinn 1996) and acceptance and commitment therapy (ACT; Harris 2009) have been developed relatively recently and are sometimes labelled as 'third-wave behaviour therapies', which also include, e.g. Dialectical Behaviour Therapy or Metacognitive Therapy. All of these therapies generally share an emphasis on acceptance and mindfulness (Merwin et al. 2019). Mindfulness and acceptance are closely related concepts. Mindfulness, described as intentionally focusing one's attention on the experiences occurring at the present moment in a non-judgmental and accepting way (Baer and Krietemeyer 2006), can be contrasted with states of mind in which attention is focused elsewhere, such as a preoccupation with memories or worries. Mindfulness results in decreased avoidance, increased emotional and attentional regulation, and acceptance. Acceptance can be described as willingness to experience a wide range of unwanted/unpleasant sensations, cognitions or emotional states without attempting to avoid, escape or terminate them.

Both professionals (e.g. Gregory 2003; Guitar 2013) and clients (e.g. Plexico et al. 2009a, b) have emphasised the importance of acceptance for the successful management of stuttering. Recent findings suggest that increased acceptance and less avoidance of stuttering are related to adaptive coping skills and increased quality of life among people who stutter (Plexico et al. 2009a, b). Mindfulness may be used as a valuable means for facilitating acceptance of stuttering-related behaviour, thoughts and feelings among people who stutter.

Different authors have described how these principles can be applied to the management of stuttering (e.g. Cheasman et al. 2015). Boyle (2011) concludes that the integration of mindfulness training and stuttering treatment appears practical and worthy of exploration and that mindfulness strategies adapted to stuttering may help in the management of cognitive, affective and behavioural challenges associated with stuttering.

10.4.6 Summary

The goal of this section was to provide doctors with an overview of the psychological approaches that are frequently being used by speech-language therapists in the overall management of stuttering, aimed at addressing its covert aspects, i.e. normal cognitive (irrational or dysfunctional thoughts and beliefs) and affective (social anxiety and avoidance behaviour) reactions to the experience of stuttering. These include approaches such as cognitive therapy, personal construct therapy, narrative therapy and mindfulness- and acceptance-based approaches. By no means did we have the intention to provide an all-encompassing overview of all treatments, and others used are, e.g. solution-focused brief therapy and dialectical therapy. They are applied by speech-language therapists in a counselling context, i.e. for the purpose of support or (re)education for behavioural problems not associated with mental illness (Crowe 1997). In case of chronic life-adjustment problems, referral to other professionals such as counsellors and psychologists is evident.

10.5 Assistive Technology Used in the Treatment of Stuttering

Ashley Craig

10.5.1 Introduction

The treatment of stuttering has been dominated by behavioural, speech and psychological approaches, with the treatment modality largely dependent on the theoretical basis believed to cause the stuttering (Tran et al. 2011). For example, early theories assumed stuttering had a psychogenic basis, that is, the dysfluency was caused by underlying psychological deficits such as unconscious neurotic and psychosexual processes (Bloodstein et al. 2021; Glauber 1958). Others believed stuttering was caused by chronically high levels of anxiety, as argued by the approach-avoidance conflict or anticipatory-struggle theories, where stuttering was believed to occur owing to learned anxieties about speaking or from subconscious personality factors

(Sheehan 1958). Treatments developed on the basis of these types of theory were principally psychotherapy-based (Bloodstein et al. 2021). Psychologically based treatments alone have not proved to be effective in significantly reducing stuttering severity, though they may have some benefit for improving psychological reactions to the stuttering such as social anxiety (Bloodstein et al. 2021; Menzies et al. 2008). In contrast, contemporary theories have argued that stuttering is a result of dysfunction in the speech sensory-motor control neural system with an inherited predisposition (Bloodstein et al. 2008, 2021; Ludlow and Loucks 2003).

Notwithstanding the above, it is important to note that any elevated psychopathology associated with the disorder (such as elevated trait or social anxiety or depressive mood) is believed to be the result of negative reactions to the distress of living with the fluency disorder (Tran et al. 2011; Craig and Tran 2014). Consequently, more recent treatment approaches have targeted both speech/stuttering and psychological aspects of the disorder, with speech re-training and behavioural-contingent strategies, which have been found to be significantly effective in reducing stuttering and improving psychological states such as anxiety (Bothe et al. 2006a; Craig and Tran 2006).

It has been recognised that clinicians have under-utilised technology in the treatment of stuttering (Packman and Meredith 2011). However, internet and world-wide web technology is now used by people who stutter, especially for access to educational resources concerning the nature and management of stuttering (Packman and Meredith 2011). Furthermore, technology used in the treatment of stuttering by speech pathologists, psychologists and others, has increased over the past 30–40 years or so, as described by Larry Molt (2019) in an excellent online resource. This section will summarise and briefly explore technology used in the treatment of stuttering, with special attention given to the efficacy of technology that utilises electromyography (EMG) feedback in combination with speech re-training and behaviour modification strategies to treat stuttering.

10.5.2 Overview of Technology Used in the Treatment of Stuttering

Molt (2019) provided a thorough breakdown of the types of technology used to help people who stutter to manage their disfluency. He classified types of technologies into the following:

- Devices that alter speech motor patterns. These include technology that alters a speech production pattern, such as a fork placed under the tongue, or the Idehara 'Stutter-Cure' appliance, which consists of a palatal prosthesis similar to an orthodontic retainer, fitted into the mouth, against the hard palate (Van Riper 1973). The device includes a whistle, used to enhance continuous airflow when speaking, a factor known to reduce stuttering and increase fluency (Craig and Tran 2006). The person who stutters (PWS) is encouraged to maintain a whistling noise while speaking. There is little or no evidence of the efficacy of such devices; though if a PWS uses continuous airflow, fluency improves (Craig et al. 1996).
- Devices that provide feedback of physiological mechanisms. These for example include devices that provide feedback on respiratory, speech muscle and articulation timing. These types of technology have been used to help the PWS in identifying and altering speech production processes as part of therapy (Molt 2019). Physiological processes targeted include feedback on respiratory function, speech muscle EMG activity and feedback of phonatory/articulatory production and timing. An example of a respiratory device is called the 'Breathing Monitor', included in the 'Dr. Fluency' computerised stuttering treatment program (Friedman et al. 1999). The Breathing Monitor provides real-time feedback on respiratory flow, which can be used in training the PWS to regulate breathing; first without speech, followed by exercises involving breathing plus speech of graded complexity, beginning with single syllables and moving on to more complex speech, all the time maintaining appropriate air production. The CAFET (Computer Aided Fluency

Establishment Trainer) device also provides feedback on the quality of voice onsets (Goebel 1994). Speech muscle feedback technology and its usefulness will be discussed in more detail below, given that a controlled trial has been conducted testing its efficacy (Craig et al. 1996).

- Devices that provide information on timing of speech, for example, in which the PWS is required to speak in time with a metronome. Metronome technology was widely used for the treatment of stuttering in the 1960s to 1980s, with wearable devices such as the Pacemaster. There is limited support for effectiveness (Berman and Brady 1973). A major problem was the unnatural sound of metronome speech produced, even if it improved fluency.
- Devices that alter speech feedback to the PWS. These include altered auditory feedback (AAF), including masked auditory feedback (MAF), delayed auditory feedback (DAF) and frequency-altered feedback (FAF), and combinations of these. MAF devices were popularised by the Edinburgh Masker (Dewar et al. 1979). The Edinburgh Masker uses a throat microphone (held by an elastic strap), a small control unit attached to a belt or carried in a pocket, and a headphone set. Masking is activated by vocalisation detected by the microphone, and masking stops when the PWS stops speaking. One problem for the Edinburgh Masker is the issue of having to wear a microphone around the neck, as well as when the PWS has non-vocalised or silent stuttering, as for example, in a stuttering block. Further, there is little or no evidence for the efficacy of MAF approaches. AAF devices are discussed in more detail directly below.

10.5.3 Altered Auditory Feedback

The use of AAF devices such as DAF in the treatment of stuttering has been prevalent since the mid-twentieth century (Bloodstein et al. 2021; Ingham 1984; Packman and Meredith 2011). DAF became popular when evidence that delaying the feedback of a person's speech reduced stuttering frequency (Ingham 1984). DAF mostly slows speech rate, and research has found that the same effect can be achieved by asking the PWS to slow down their speech without DAF (Bloodstein et al. 2021; Packman and Meredith 2011). FAF involves feedback of altered frequency of the speech of a PWS (Stuart et al. 2004; Casa Futura Technologies 2015). AAF devices have been widely used in the treatment of stuttering with commercial AAF products available (Bakker 2006; Bloodstein et al. 2021) that employ masking, DAF and FAF. One example is the SpeechEasy device that employs DAF and AAF. The SpeechEasy device is believed to help reduce stuttering because the person using the device hears their voice slightly delayed and at a different pitch. Their voice is therefore perceived as the voice of someone else, and this effect helps to reduce stuttering frequency. This phenomenon is called choral speech, i.e. talking in unison, and this effect is well known to reduce stuttering and induce fluency (Kalinowski and Saltuklaroglu 2003). Evidence does exist for the efficacy of SpeechEasy in reducing stuttering, especially when reading but less so when speaking in a conversation (Foundas et al. 2013; Stuart et al. 2004). Another similar device is a small unobtrusive ear device called the SmallTalk, a device that also employs AAF, DAF and FAF and that comes with headphones and microphones (see Casa Futura Technologies (2015) for the website on their technology). The efficacy of AAF devices has been investigated with mixed findings (Foundas et al. 2013; Gallop and Runyan 2012; Packman and Meredith 2011; Pollard et al. 2009).

10.5.4 Electromyography Feedback

Electromyography (EMG) feedback (Craig and Cleary 1982; Craig et al. 1996) is designed to help the person who stutters to control speech muscle activity associated with their stuttering behaviour by teaching them (a) to reduce muscle activity/tension to low levels before speaking with a computer-based speech muscle activity biofeedback; (b) to lower overall levels of muscle tension in the face while speaking; (c) to learn to control speech muscle tension, called EMG mastery, in the absence of the computer biofeedback; (d) to help them raise their levels of confidence, increase their sense of control over their speech and stuttering, and raise their levels of self-esteem. EMG biofeedback therapy attempts to train the PWS to become aware of and to control tension in their speech muscles.

EMG biofeedback utilises at least two EMG channels in a biomonitoring system (Craig et al. 1996), consisting of a computer feedback and electrodes attached to various speech muscles, providing immediate and sensitive feedback of muscle activity. Silver–silver chloride electrodes are attached to speech muscles on the PWS's face in muscles such as the zygomaticus, levator anguli oris, depressor anguli oris muscle sites and superior and inferior obicularis oris muscles. A grounding electrode is usually placed near the active biofeedback site. Figure 10.2 shows the process of treating the EMG activity signals so they can be understood by the PWS, allowing learning to occur. A typical biofeedback device comprises the EMG amplifier unit, recording and reference electrodes, electrode cables and a PC with a stereo microphone port. The PC screen displays the EMG waveforms, their power spectrum and a meter to measure muscle contraction levels by using various feedback forms such as audio/visual formats (see http://www.neuromotionphysio.com/about/our-equipment/ for a typical EMG feedback system setup).

Training begins on a specific muscle and then learning is transferred to other speech muscles, once control at the first site has been learnt. In a controlled trial (Craig et al. 1996), the PWS were taught to raise and lower their muscle tension without speaking by using visual or auditory biofeedback. When achieved, a hierarchy system was initiated, commencing with repeating simple one-syllable words and progressing to more complex, multi-syllabic words, then on to conversational speech. Fluency skills should be reinforced by behavioural modification strategies, such as reward, assignments and telephone calls. EMG signal-based games can also be played to maintain interest and reinforce EMG mastery. Follow-up should occur regularly (Craig et al. 1996).

Evidence suggests that EMG biofeedback is best delivered in a behavioural modification programme (Craig and Cleary 1982; Craig et al. 1996). Controlled trials (Craig et al. 1996; Hancock et al. 1998) have shown that EMG biofeedback can be effective in reducing stuttering when in a combined therapeutic programme that includes airflow techniques, a regimen of achievable behavioural goals, assessment of behavioural outcomes, rewards, transfer and

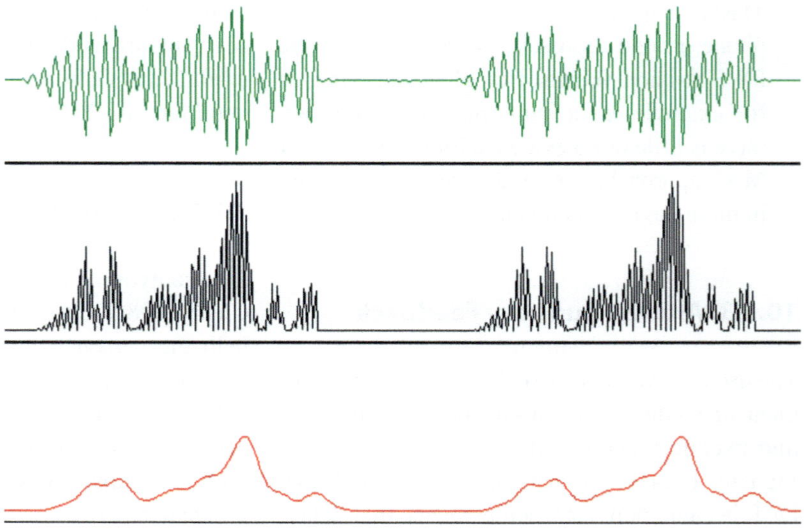

Fig. 10.2 Raw electromyography activity in the upper trace, rectified EMG activity in the middle trace and smoothed activity in the bottom trace that is used in the biofeedback. The EMG signal is amplified, filtered and processed so that it can be sensibly displayed to the PWS by means of visual or auditory feedback. (With kind permission of Brian Kaminski at Advancer Technologies)

maintenance procedures, and that employs behavioural assignments to reinforce skills, and cognitive behavioural therapy techniques to address anxiety and social fears. A replication study also found benefits, but to a lesser extent than in the original trials (Block et al. 2004; Craig et al. 1996; Hancock et al. 1998); however, this study has been criticised because it did not utilise response-cost strategies (Bothe et al. 2006a). EMG feedback is currently rarely used for the treatment of stuttering.

10.5.5 Conclusions and Implications

Technology is being used for the treatment of stuttering. While many stuttering people I know say that devices such as those discussed above are helpful and enhance their ability to communicate verbally, the efficacy of most devices has a long way to go before gold standard evidence is available for any device currently in use. It should be understood that technology is always a component of a therapy package, and it is best that the technology is not the sole component. It is also crucial that principles of treatment should be adhered to by clinicians to ensure that stuttering treatment effectiveness is optimised. These include (a) taking a comprehensive diagnosis by using a behavioural approach (e.g. measuring stuttering frequency and speech rate) as well as psychological measures (e.g. social anxiety); (b) clinicians' conducting therapy in a professional, caring and accepting manner, working on developing a positive relationship with the PWS; (c) gaining the support of family and friends to assist the PWS in self-managing; (d) employing appropriate response cost methods, such as effective rewards and negative reinforcements, whatever the age of the PWS; (e) encouraging the PWS to learn relaxation strategies and to be sure they are engaging in frequent pleasant life events; (f) encouraging self-responsibility and self-management; (g) employing follow-up and anti-relapse strategies (Craig et al. 2011; Craig and Tran 2006; Tran et al., 2021).

10.6 Basic Principles in Stuttering Medication Treatment

Matt Jason V. Llamas, Stephanie Wong, and Gerald A. Maguire

10.6.1 Introduction

Childhood-onset fluency disorder, also known as stuttering, is a neurodevelopmental disorder characterised by disturbances of normal speech. Although current treatments focus on non-pharmacological techniques, the potential use of medications as a treatment for stuttering is still being investigated today. Fortunately, recent advances in the neurophysiology of stuttering have helped guide pharmacological inquiry. Over the last few decades, various different classes of medication have been investigated, but increasing bodies of evidence suggest that medications with dopamine-blocking activity (e.g. olanzapine) have been most effective in reducing stuttering symptoms for various individuals. It is theorised that these medications are efficacious because stuttering may be associated with an overactive pre-synaptic dopamine system, which may disrupt the selection, initiation and execution of motor sequences necessary for fluent speech production. However, medications in this class may be associated with adverse side effects that may limit utility in certain individuals. This section will review basic principles regarding the neuropharmacological treatment of stuttering, and discuss the potential therapeutic benefits of these medications if delivered in an interdisciplinary care model involving speech-language pathologists and other healthcare professionals.

Stuttering is present in every culture of recorded history, yet to this day, the underlying mechanism is still not fully understood. It appears the causes of stuttering are varied, as different studies have shown that genetic components, autoimmune factors (e.g. paediatric autoimmune neuropsychiatric disorders associated with streptococcal infections (PANDAS)) and other aetiologies may result in similar physical symptomatic presentations (Alm 2020). As per the DSM-5, stuttering is defined as disturbances in the normal fluency and time patterning of speech that are inappropriate for the individual's age, persist over time, and are characterised by frequent and marked occurrences of one (or more) of the following: sound and syllable repetitions, prolongations, broken words, audible and silent blocking, and circumlocutions (American Psychiatric Association (APA) 2013). Motor movements such as eye blinks, tics, tremors of the lips or face, and jerking of the head may accompany stuttering as well (APA 2013). The degree to which these symptoms manifest may vary with the situation, but the fearful anticipation associated with it only makes dysfluency worse. The resulting stigma and shame associated with stuttering can often be a disabling feature of this condition, limiting one's ability to engage in social functions and causing functional impairments in one's academic or professional life.

It is well-established that stuttering is often coexistent with other neuropsychiatric conditions that are amenable to pharmacological treatment (Maguire et al. 2020). Evidence suggests that individuals who stutter have an increased risk of developing social anxiety, which often begins in adolescence and continues throughout adulthood (Smith et al. 2014). Adults who stutter also have a twofold increase in mood disorders and a threefold increase in personality disorders when compared with controls (Shugart et al. 2004). Stuttering in adults has been associated with a lower quality of life, occupational and educational barriers, and difficulties with access to high-quality treatment plans (Iverach et al. 2009b; Koedoot et al. 2011). Therefore, as with the standard of care for other neuropsychiatric conditions such as depression, social anxiety and attention-deficit hyperactivity disorder (which are often comorbid with stuttering), it is important to consider utilising a biopsychosocial model of interdisciplinary care and employ different healthcare professionals with complementary skills and knowledge to deliver optimised therapy for those who stutter.

10.6.2 Aetiology of Stuttering

Historically, stuttering was considered secondary to physical abnormalities of the larynx and tongue; however, surgical and chemical treatments specifically targeting these anatomical areas did not improve symptoms. In the 1930s, stuttering science and interdisciplinary treatment and evaluation was off to a good start when Samuel Orton, an MD, and Lee Edward Travis, a PhD and speech-language pathologist, together conceptualised stuttering as a brain abnormality. They suggested that stuttering could be a manifestation of incomplete cerebral dominance of speech (Orton 1927; Travis 1931), leading to enlightened theories regarding the aetiology of stuttering. However, subsequent research went down a different path. It was here that the medical profession largely abandoned the stuttering community by not pursuing the biological underpinning of stuttering until it was resurrected decades later. Thoughts based on psychoanalytical theory dominated the treatment of neuropsychiatric disorders for some time, and stuttering was unfortunately included. Writings as recent as the 1960s described stuttering as an unconscious neurotic need fulfillment with unresolved oral conflict during one's early parent and child interactions (Barbara 1963). This theory did little but further the stigma of stuttering. Today, several theories have been proposed that have attempted to explain the structural basis of stuttering, such as theories of cerebral lateralisation, hemispheric conflict and white matter dissociation (Alm 2020), but one established interpretation linking stuttering to alterations in functions of the cortico-basal ganglia-thalamocortical loop serves as the target of emerging pharmacological treatments.

10.6.3 The Cortico-Basal Ganglia-Thalamocortical Loop

Malfunction of the cortico-basal ganglia-thalamocortical loop (CBGTC loop) was first implicated by the German physicians Shali and

Shilder in the 1920s and later expounded upon in future studies (Alm 2020). As stated in the name, the loop involves connections between the cerebral cortex (i.e. premotor, motor and somatosensory cortex; supplementary motor area (SMA)); the basal ganglia (i.e. putamen, globus pallidus (GP), substantia nigra (SNr)); the thalamus, and back to the cerebral cortex (Chang and Guenther 2020).

Various steps are involved in the production of speech. The initiation of sound involves communication between the areas of the cerebral cortex involved in movement planning and execution, and the basal ganglia, specifically the putamen, which is primarily associated with motor planning. Components of the basal ganglia, most notably the globus pallidus (GP) and the substantia nigra (SNr), simultaneously excite the correct motor programme and inhibit the competing motor programmes in order to produce a specific sound (Chang and Guenther 2020). In addition, the basal ganglia have been associated with making sound production more 'automatic'. Early on in development (roughly before the age of 3), input from the pre-supplementary motor area (pre-SMA) in the cerebral cortex is essential for learning how to pronounce the individual phonemes of a word (i.e. pet). However, as a person matures and repeatedly practices the pronunciation of the individual phonemes, there is less reliance on the pre-SMA and more control via the CBGTC loop. When this occurs, the production of sound becomes more 'automatic', with less emphasis on the individual phonemes (Chang and Guenther 2020).

Given the CBGTC loop's significant involvement in the production of speech, three theories have been proposed relating to the development of persistent developmental stuttering (PDS). They are: (1) Impairment within the basal ganglia proper, (2) Impairment of the connections between the cortex, basal ganglia and thalamus, and (3) Impairment in cortical processing (Chang and Guenther 2020). Impairment within the basal ganglia proper can lead to the development of stuttering, as the basal ganglia are involved with both exciting and inhibiting the cerebral cortex during the production of sound. Excitation of the cerebral cortex occurs via a direct pathway and results in the activation of the correct motor programme to produce the specific sound needed; inhibition of the cerebral cortex occurs via an indirect pathway and suppresses competing motor programmes that would inhibit the production of the specific sound required (Chang and Guenther 2020). If either the direct pathway or the indirect pathway is underactive, stuttering may occur. Additionally, imaging has also implicated the basal ganglia's involvement in stuttering. A study by Giraud et al. (2008) found that activity in the striatum during speech was positively correlated with the severity of stuttering, and this relationship generally disappeared after intensive therapy. Another study by Lu et al. (2010) discovered increased grey matter volume concentrated in the left putamen of adults who stuttered compared with adults who did not stutter.

Furthermore, it is theorised that there are two loops of speech that affect speech production, one of which may be implicated in the development of stuttering. There is an 'inner loop' that runs through a part of the basal ganglia called the striatum, which is in charge of timing and spontaneous speech, and an 'outer loop' that bypasses the striatum, which is associated with singing and chorus reading. A study by Wu et al. (1997a) found that abnormally low function of the left striatum led to low activity in the left cortical speech areas, whereas fluency induced through techniques such as chorus reading showed increased activity the same areas equal to that in normal controls. This suggests that stuttering may be due to a defect in the inner subcortical speech loop, specifically in the striatum, whereas induced fluency would activate the outer cortical speech loop and bypass the defective striatum leading to normal speech. It was further discovered that the decreased activity of the striatum in patients who stutter may be associated with an overactive pre-synaptic dopamine system (Wu et al. 1997b), which may explain why dopamine-antagonist medications have shown efficacy in the treatment of stuttering.

Consequences of impaired connections between the cortex, basal ganglia and thalamus have also been demonstrated in neuroimaging results in children with stuttering (CWS). The connection between the cortex and the striatum in the left hemisphere is essential to speech production, and in CWS neuroimaging has shown that there is less structural connectivity between the left putamen and several cortical regions of the left hemisphere (Chang and Guenther 2020). Additionally, other studies have revealed that in CWS there is a decreased growth rate in white matter in the thalamic region, which connects the prefrontal cortical areas with the cortico-basal ganglia-thalamocortical loop (Chow and Chang 2017).

Lastly, if there is cortical processing within the cerebral cortex, generally the language-dominant left hemisphere is damaged and associated with an increased risk for the development of persistent developmental stuttering (PDS) (Chang and Guenther 2020). Structural brain differences between adults who stutter versus fluent speakers have revealed that persons who stutter have a decreased thickness of the left ventral motor cortex and the ventral premotor cortex, which is associated with components involved in the articulation of speech (i.e. larynx, tongue, jaw and lips). If the left hemisphere is impaired, greater white matter tract development within the right hemisphere has been seen as a compensatory mechanism, resulting in increased right hemispheric involvement during speech production (Chang and Guenther 2020).

In summary, various components of the cortico-basal ganglia-thalamocortical loop have been proposed to be involved with the development of persistent developmental stuttering (PDS): (1) Deficits within the basal ganglia proper, (2) Impairment of the connections between the cortex, basal ganglia and thalamus, and (3) Deficits in cortical processing. However, it is important to note that the functions of the CBGTC loop are highly dependent on the tight regulation of dopamine activity. Therefore, many medications that have been shown to have the strongest modulating effect on stuttering, target dopaminergic receptors.

10.6.4 Pharmacological Treatment of Stuttering

10.6.4.1 Dopaminergic Medications

Over the last five decades, the effects of a variety of pharmacological agents on persons who stutter have been evaluated, but usually in very limited trials. However, recurrent and replicated evidence suggests that medications with dopamine-modulating activity have been most effective in reducing stuttering symptoms, perhaps owing to their effects on the CBGTC loop.

Haloperidol was one of the early medications to be studied. In a 1976 double-blind crossover study by Rosenberger et al. (1976), it was found to have a significant effect on reducing the proportion of time subjects were dysfluent, but not on the number of dysfluencies per minute . Four years later, another study revealed that haloperidol helped reduce stuttering blocks in two individuals, by potentially increasing brain activity in cortical speech areas (Wood et al. 1980). Yet, despite these findings, haloperidol is generally not recommended as a first-line treatment for stuttering. Its association with potential adverse side effects such as movement disorders impedes its widespread utility. Nevertheless, haloperidol, a pure D2 receptor antagonist, illuminated the path for further, better tolerated, pharmacological approaches to stuttering.

Risperidone, another dopamine-modulating agent, was investigated next. At doses from 0.5 to 2 mg/day, it was shown to increase activity in both the striatum and cortical speech areas, significantly decreasing the severity of stuttering in some affected individuals (Maguire et al. 2000). However, while risperidone is generally well-tolerated, it can increase blood levels of the hormone prolactin, leading to side-effects such as sexual dysfunction, galactorrhoea, amenorrhoea and gynaecomastia.

After the positive data from haloperidol and risperidone, Stager set forth to determine if manipulating the neurotransmitter serotonin, which mediates mood and anxiety, would modulate similar effects. She utilised the medication *paroxetine*, an SSRI, and compared it to *pimozide*, which acts on dopamine. The study showed that pimozide improved stuttering symptoms, but paroxetine did not (Stager et al. 2005). Such findings further supported the growing understanding that stuttering can be pharmacologically affected via the dopamine system. Pimozide is an older generation dopamine blocker, and although still used for Tourette's Syndrome, carries with it certain side-effects such as anxiety, blurred vision and even depression (Blotch et al. 1997) that limit its usage as treatment (Stager et al. 2005).

Fortunately, newer second-generation dopamine-blocking agents were developed beyond haloperidol and pimozide that bypassed the prolactin hormone effects of risperidone. Medications such as *olanzapine* pose a lower risk of motor side-effects and are generally better tolerated than first-generation medications for the treatment of stuttering. *Olanzapine* has been one of the more commonly prescribed medications worldwide since its introduction in 1996. It acts as a dopamine antagonist to D2 receptors in the mesolimbic pathway and works similarly on serotonin 5HT2a receptors in the frontal cortex. At doses from 2.5 to 5 mg/day, olanzapine has been shown to be more effective than placebo at reducing stuttering symptoms for some individuals (Maguire et al. 2004). In a randomised, double-blind, placebo-controlled trial, olanzapine was statistically superior to placebo in reducing stuttering symptoms, as judged by a 22% reduction in the subjective stuttering scale of olanzapine vs. <1% reduction by placebo (Maguire et al. 2004). A more recent 2013 single-blind, randomised control trial by Shaygannejad et al. (2013) compared the effects of olanzapine with those of haloperidol and concluded that olanzapine does have better impact in controlling stuttering symptoms than haloperidol and may be a potential leading pharmacological choice for the treatment of stuttering. However, olanzapine's use is limited owing to its association with metabolic side effects such as weight gain, lipid elevation and potential diabetes (Tran et al. 1997; Maguire et al. 2004). Olanzapine has also been noted to induce down-regulation of postsynaptic GABA-A receptors (Farnbach-Pralong et al. 1998), suggesting that direct-action GABA-A agonists may possess potential benefit in the treatment of stuttering.

Other studies have considered alternative *atypical anti-psychotics* as potential treatment options. A recent case report demonstrated *ziprasidone* to be an effective and well-tolerated medication for persons who stutter (Munjal et al. 2018), but further research is warranted. Additional case reports propose that *asenapinemay* improves fluency in generally well-tolerated doses of 5–10 mg (Maguire et al. 2011); however, just as for ziprasidone, randomised placebo-controlled trials are needed to investigate further the use of this medication in stuttering treatment.

Aripiprazole is a unique medication that acts as a *partial agonist* of D2 and 5HT1a receptors and is approved for the treatment of many conditions including Tourette's syndrome. There are case reports that suggest aripiprazole's efficacy in stuttering, and when compared with other dopamine agents, it tends to be associated with fewer metabolic side effects (Hoang et al. 2017; Tran et al. 2008). However, further research is required to elucidate fully aripiprazole's potential role in stuttering therapy.

Lurasidone is a relatively new dopamine antagonist medication with a unique pharmacological profile. It is approved in children and adolescents for schizophrenia (13–17 years old) as well as bipolar depression (10–17 years old). A small open-label study of lurasidone in seven patients showed improvement in all areas of stuttering as rated by the Subjective Screening of Stuttering (SSS) scale. Two patients were scored as 'very much improved' and five as 'much improved' in the Clinical Global Impression (CGI) Scale, and they all reported improvement in subjective symptoms. Advantages include less sedation and lower risk of metabolic side effects including weight gain and lipid elevations (Charoensook and Maguire 2017); however, more studies need to be performed to determine its true potential utility in stuttering.

10.6.4.2 Other Medications

Several other classes of medication have also been investigated in stuttering, but in limited trials: GABA receptor agonists were studied owing to their known anxiolytic effects, which may potentially reduce stuttering symptoms; however, placebo-controlled studies have revealed that these agents only reduce anxiety in the short-term, fail to improve fluency in stuttering and demonstrate no benefits when compared with placebo (Brady 1991).

Pagoclone, a *selective GABA-A partial agonist*, was theorised to have downstream effects on dopamine and potentially show efficacy in the treatment of stuttering. It underwent the largest clinical trial of stuttering treatment to date; however, it appeared to decrease stuttering only by lowering social anxiety levels and showed limited efficacy on the primary outcome of fluency (Maguire et al. 2010). Pagoclone did show strong placebo response in the trial and was likely under-dosed; however, further development from the company that held the rights to pagoclone did not materialise.

Anti-depressants such as *selective serotonin re-uptake inhibitors* (SSRIs) and *tricyclic antidepressants* (TCAs) have shown little benefit for the treatment of stuttering. *Paroxetine*, an antidepressant medication that decreases the re-uptake of serotonin (SSRI), exhibited no clinical response in stuttering (Stager et al. 1997). Similarly, tricyclic antidepressants such as *clomipramine* and *desipramine* showed minimal short-term improvements in fluency, although clomipramine did exhibit superior improvement than desipramine on self-reported scales of fluency (Gordon et al. 1995; Stager et al. 1995).

Clonidine is an *α-receptor agonist* shown to be effective in controlling signs and symptoms of Tourette's syndrome. Therefore, it was hypothesised that it may be an effective treatment for stuttering. Unfortunately, a well-designed study failed to show any difference between clonidine and placebo for objective measures of stuttering (Althaus et al. 1995).

Calcium channel blockers such as *verapamil* and *nimodipine* have also shown limited efficacy in stuttering in separate studies (Brumfitt and Peake 1988; Brady et al. 1990; Maguire et al. 1994); however, no additional research has materialised.

Lastly, supplementation with *thiamine* or *vitamin B1* has also been considered as a possible treatment for stuttering. In a 1951 study by Hale, thiamine was postulated to help regulate CNS metabolism in the brain and therefore correct for any neurological imbalances that could result in stuttering. In this double-blind study, each child received either 30 mg of thiamine or a placebo for 1 month, and then the opposite for a second month. At the end, observable speech was seen to improve by 80% in 2–3-year-olds; 50% in 4-year-olds; little improvement in 5-year-olds and no improvement in 7–8-year-olds (Hale 1951). Interestingly, however, these results are similar to what we know is the spontaneous recovery rate of stuttering for children, so it is difficult to say whether thiamine had a direct effect on fluency. It is also important to note that this study never disclosed the number of children tested nor provided any objective measurements for stuttering to assess fluency. While this does not entirely invalidate the study, it limits the results of this study significantly. Therefore, a modern study investigating thiamine supplementation in stuttering is warranted.

Regardless of the medication, one should always consult a medical doctor before considering medication treatment of stuttering to review all potential risks and benefits.

10.6.5 Non-pharmacological Treatment of Stuttering

Non-pharmacological treatments may range anywhere from non-invasive therapies to maximally invasive strategies. One of the more common and established non-pharmacological treatments of stuttering is speech therapy. The Lidcombe programme is a behavioural treatment programme developed for early stuttering in children under the age of 6 that utilises operant training principles. The parent primarily responds when the child speaks without stuttering and limits their responses when the child speaks with stuttering.

In 2005, Jones et al. conducted a randomised controlled trial to evaluate the effects of the Lidcombe programme as an early stuttering intervention. They found a significant difference in stuttering frequency 9 months after randomisation of children who participated in the Lidcombe programme versus those who did not (Jones et al. 2005).

Speech therapy has also been shown to act on areas of the brain involved in stuttering. In persistent developmental stuttering (PDS), there is decreased activation of the left hemisphere, but speech therapy can correct this hypo-activation. Additionally, white matter tract development within the right hemisphere has been seen as a compensatory mechanism in people who stutter, and speech therapy can decrease this compensatory over-action, ultimately restoring a left-dominant network for speech production. It is important to note that in order for these effects to be maintained, continuous refresher therapies need to be in place (Maguire et al. 2020).

Other non-pharmacological therapeutic interventions, such as cognitive behavioural therapy (CBT), have also been utilised in the treatment of stuttering, especially given its association with social anxiety and anxiety-related disorders (Maguire et al. 2020). The co-occurrence of anxiety disorders and stuttering generally predicts poor outcomes in speech programmes, and thus, anxiety should be adequately managed. In 2008, Menzies et al. conducted a clinical trial of CBT combined with speech therapy and found that while CBT did not have a significant impact on stuttering frequency, CBT itself did reduce anxiety and avoidance of regular speaking situations (Menzies et al. 2008).

Lastly, interventional forms of treatment and different forms of neuromodulation have also been evaluated as non-pharmacological management of stuttering (Maguire et al. 2020). Transcranial direct current stimulation (tDCS) to the left inferior frontal cortex has been studied in those who stutter because this region is underactive in them. The implementation of tDCS involves a daily administration of a1 mA anodal tDCS for 20 min over the left inferior frontal cortex combined with such behavioural therapy interventions as choral speech and metronome-timed speech (Maguire et al. 2020). In a 2018 study, Chesters et al. found that 1 week after tDCS intervention, there was a significant reduction in stuttering frequency, which was maintained in reading ability at 6 weeks. However, pre-intervention baseline levels of stuttering returned in conversations (Chesters et al. 2018).

Other techniques, such as repetitive transcranial magnetic stimulation (rTMS) and deep brain stimulation (DBS), have also been studied as forms of treatment for stuttering. rTMS utilises large magnets outside of the skull to modify the brain's electrical activity. In people who stutter, rTMS has been used to modify timed neural integration in intra-cortical motor networks in order to increase the understanding of dynamics within the brain during stuttering (Busan et al. 2019). On the other hand, deep brain stimulation involves inserting programmed electrodes into the brain and emitting electrical pulses to regulate brain activity. Maguire et al. (2012) published the first case of DBS treatment for developmental stuttering, and this was replicated in France the following year (Thiriez et al. 2013).

10.6.6 Future Directions

Future directions in the treatment of stuttering include further research of medications as monotherapies in larger, randomised-control trials. More studies are also needed to address stuttering in adolescents, since some approved medications do not include research into this population. Lastly, additional studies need to be conducted that combine pharmacological treatment with speech therapy. Speech therapy should always be initiated in persons who stutter; however, if medications and speech therapy are both effective separately, perhaps their therapeutic effects will be synergistic when combined.

Approaching comprehensive therapy in a manner similar to that applied in other neuropsychiatric conditions, by utilising the biopsychosocial model and employing multidisciplinary care (speech therapy, psychotherapy and pharmacotherapy) will possibly result in improved outcomes to those who stutter. As physicians, psychiatrists are the most practised in facilitating interdisciplinary care and are well-poised to partner phoniatric physicians, speech-language pathologists and psychologists to ensure the most comprehensive, optimised care for our stuttering community. Further research involving such interdisciplinary models of care in stuttering treatment is warranted.

10.7 Prognosis of Stuttering

Susan Block

This section presents information relating to prognosis of stuttering for consideration at various stages of the treatment process—when deciding whether to commence treatment, when evaluating progress and when considering discharge from treatment. Factors impinging on prognosis will also be discussed.

10.7.1 Definition of Prognosis

Prognosis is generally described as

> foreseeing, predicting, or estimating the probability or risk of future conditions
> Moons et al. (2009, p. 338)

In a medical sense this usually means the course of an illness. However, this is not always straightforward, especially in the case of stuttering, as the course of the problem or treatment can be affected by the individual's history, experience, age, sex, symptoms, amount and type of treatment and many other factors. Moons et al. (2009) propose that factors to consider in researching prognosis include outcomes with regard to progression of the disorder and the resultant quality of life. Reports regarding quality of life, in particular the relationship between speech-related anxiety and social phobia, and their impact on relapse or fluency maintenance concur (e.g. Iverach et al. 2018; Iverach and Rapee 2014).

10.7.2 Importance of Prognosis

The issue of prognosis is a topic frequently raised by clients of all ages, and their families, upon presentation for assessment of their stuttering. The queries may relate to the amount of treatment required, the time it will take, as well as the cost, and in the case of a child, whether they are likely to grow out of stuttering. The answers to these questions are important not only for the client, but also for the clinician and the healthcare providers and funders. Who will do best in treatment, where should limited money be best spent, how much treatment time is required, how much is available? Answers to these questions are not always straightforward.

10.7.3 Issues for Consideration in Prognosis of Stuttering

What are we evaluating? Speech outcome is only one aspect of successful treatment. Onslow (2021) provides a discussion of the role of Evidence-Based Practice in stuttering treatment. He contends that it is not a replacement for common sense (p. 132). Consequently, information from both the client and the speech pathologist has importance. Thus, when considering prognosis, we need to consider more than fluency alone or the amount of stutter-free speech after treatment. Relapse and quality of life are also vital considerations when assessing treatment success. Similarly, the goals of each individual undertaking treatment are important. If these and the thoughts or feelings of each person undertaking treatment are not addressed, the individual is unlikely to consider treatment a success whether they are fluent or not. In a recent report by Yandeau et al. (2021), the feedback from a child who had experienced treatment was that the key contributor to success for him was that the treatment was enjoyable.

10.7.3.1 Natural Recovery of Stuttering

Defining natural recovery and establishing its occurrence with confidence is complex and at times confusing, Einarsdottir et al. (2020) and Onslow (2021) discuss these issues and also the limitations of much of the data that has been presented: problems with definition and measurement in particular. As a result, data reports have varied widely, depending on the measurements used. Early data from Yairi and Ambrose (1999) suggest a recovery rate in young children of 73.8%. Similarly, Månsson (2000) reports recovery as 71.4%. In their report of routine screening of 3-year-olds in Hokkaido in Japan, Shimada et al. (2018) found that of the 2274 children who were screened, 1.4% were stuttering (20 boys and 12 girls). Of those, 82.8% appeared to have recovered 6 months later.

In contrast, in their prospective studies Reilly et al. (2009, 2013) reported the findings of a large prospective study of young children at the time of onset of stuttering. There were 181 children confirmed as stuttering by 4 years. Their data indicate the cumulative incidence of stuttering onset by 4 years of age was 11.2%. The children who stuttered displayed better receptive and expressive language skills, as well as better non-verbal intelligence scores, than the control fluent children. Only 9 of 142 children (6.3%) who were stuttering at age 4 years had recovered from stuttering within 12 months. The predictive factors of recovery at onset were higher levels of maternal education, male sex and twinning.

Howell and Davis (2011) examined seven predictors considered to be related to the persistence of stuttering, as well as recovery, by the teenage years. The only predictor of recovery they found was initial severity (at age 8 years).

In their review of factors related to onset and prediction, Nang and Ciccone (2016) concluded that there was evidence supporting both a family history of stuttering and age as being common factors in stuttering onset and persistence in young children. In children who are older at onset, persistence is higher (p. 96). They discuss the relationship or difference between a predictive factor and a prognostic indicator in stuttering. Similarly, Adolfsson and Steineck (2000) propose that prognostic indicators might not necessarily predict treatment outcomes. Thus, when discussing prognosis with clients, it is important to clarify whether they are referring to the likelihood of persistence without treatment, or to successful treatment outcome.

Singer et al. (2020) in their meta-analysis identified risk factors for persistence of stuttering in children under 6 years.

> Children who persist, compared to children who eventually recover, (a) were more likely to be male; (b) begin stuttering at a later age; (c) have known family histories of stuttering (persistent and/or recovered); (d) produce higher stuttering frequencies; and (e) perform lower on measures of speech sound accuracy, expressive language, and receptive language
> Singer et al. (2020, p. 3005)

It is evident that there are some common findings and some inconsistencies in the literature about natural recovery. Most recently, in reviewing the literature about natural recovery, Onslow (2021) concludes:

> findings suggest that, after onset during the early years of life, around two-thirds to three-quarters of children will recover naturally at some later time.
> Onslow (2021, p. 66)

10.7.3.2 Anxiety

Social anxiety as a consequence of stuttering in adults and adolescents has been well-described (Gunn et al. 2014; Iverach et al. 2009a, b, 2011a, b, 2018; Iverach and Rapee 2014; Menzies et al. 1999; Smith et al. 2014). To promote better long-term fluency outcome in adults who stutter, and thus to prevent stuttering relapse, St Clare et al. (2008) reported the development of a tool to measure unhelpful thoughts and beliefs of speech-related anxiety about stuttering (UTBAS). This has subsequently been revised by Iverach et al. (2011a). In 2009, Menzies et al. published a tutorial on Cognitive Behaviour Therapy to equip speech pathologists better with information to manage the people with whom they were working and who presented with speech-related anxiety. Further, Menzies et al. (2016) reported favourably on the development and use of an internet-based self-administered program for social anxiety for adults who stutter.

In their systematic review of treatments for adults who stutter, Brignell et al. (2020)

concluded that there was evidence that adding a psychological intervention, in this case Cognitive Behaviour Therapy (CBT), to the stuttering treatment, as described in Menzies et al. (2009), enhanced well-being in adults who stutter:

> The group that received CBT treatment experienced substantial and sustained improvements in psychological measures that were consistent with clinical advantages in global psychiatric functioning.
> Menzies et al. (2009, p. 7)

10.7.3.3 Predictors in Adolescents and Adults

Hancock and Craig (1998) presented data on a cohort of 77 children aged 9–14 years, 12 months after treatment. The only pre-treatment factor that predicted stuttering outcome a year after treatment was its severity. However, they also reported that those who were less anxious (i.e. had lower trait anxiety scores) immediately post-treatment may have had poorer fluency outcomes. The authors suggested this may be due to less concern about and adherence to practice, resulting in a potential for decreased likelihood of fluency maintenance. Reporting similar findings for a group of 54 German adolescents, Cook et al. (2013) found that the only predictor of outcome following intensive stuttering treatment was pre-treatment severity.

Andrews and Craig (1988) studied the outcome of a group of adults who had speech restructuring post-treatment and concluded that those who maintained their fluency better were those who demonstrated normal attitudes to communication, an internal locus of control and mastery of the techniques. In a replication of aspects of the work of Andrews and Craig, Block et al. (2006) concluded from their larger cohort study that only severity (mastery of techniques) was the discerning factor.

10.7.4 Evaluation of Outcome

10.7.4.1 Measurement of Stuttering

Accurate and representative measurement of outcome or performance can be difficult. Indeed, in their introductory text, Shipley and McAfee (2019) discuss the benefits of an authentic assessment approach (p. 8), which allows evaluation across time and in a range of settings. Earlier, Onslow et al. (2008), in their tutorial for clinicians, discussed how to evaluate evidence of treatment results appropriately. Later in 2019, Onslow and Lowe (2019) described six guidelines for trials of early stuttering intervention. One of these is the use of a continuous measure of stuttering (or whatever the primary outcome is deemed to be). However, how to measure stuttering itself has been the topic of recent discussion. Most of the discussion has centred on the use of severity rating scales vs. counts of stuttering (see Onslow et al. 2018; O'Brian et al. 2020).

While there is evidence that speech restructuring in adults results in a decrease in stuttering of ~50% (Brignell et al. 2020), there is concern about the lack of evidence on sufficient long-term follow up and relapse information. Nevertheless, however stuttering is measured, it is clear that only measuring the amount or severity of stuttering is inadequate if an accurate reflection of the nature and impact of the stuttering is to be accurately ascertained.

10.7.4.2 Measurement of Impact of Stuttering

Stuttering has been shown to have an impact not only on the well-being of the person who stutters (Iverach et al. 2009a, b), but also on their potential educational performance (O'Brian et al. 2011), occupational attainment (Klein and Hood 2004) and general quality of life (Onslow 2021). A range of measures have been used to evaluate this impact. These include the UTBAS (Unhelpful Beliefs About Stuttering) (St Clare et al. 2008), UTBAS-6 (ASRC 2020), Fear of Negative Evaluation (Leary 1983), OASES (Overall Assessment of the Speaker's Experience of Stuttering) (Yaruss and Quesal 2006), WASSP (Wright and Ayre Stuttering Self-Rating Profile) (Wright et al. 1998) and SCAS (Spence Child Anxiety Scales) (Spence 1998). More recently, the (SCESS) scale (Satisfaction with Communication in Everyday Speaking Situations) (Karimi et al. 2018) was devised to overcome the difficulty of a lack of a common primary outcome for use in meta-analyses in stuttering research evaluation. It has potential for use in regular clinical outcome evaluation as well.

10.7.4.3 International Classification of Functioning (ICF)

The ICF is an international classification of health and health-related conditions that was developed by the World Health Organization (WHO) in 2001. It encompasses the domains of impairment, activity, participation and restriction.

In considering outcome evaluation in stuttering, it would seem appropriate to consider whether the outcome has resulted in decreased impairment and restriction or increased activity and participation. Evaluation of these domains presents some challenges.

Mendes et al. (2015) describe the use of an Ambulatory Phonation Monitor (APM; KayPENTAX 2011) to measure the amount spoken over 3 consecutive days by three adults who stutter. The APM and use of a diary to record speaking situations enabled clinically relevant information to be obtained, which could provide a more comprehensive assessment of the communication profile of adults who stutter. This is a small step in considering any increase or change in the ICF domains of participation and activity. It also conforms to the requirement of Shipley and McAfee (2019) for an authentic approach to evaluation of one aspect of stuttering impact at any stage of the treatment process. The lack of information regarding measurement of changes in activity and participation of those who stutter after treatment makes this an area that should receive increased focus in future research. While there are scales that address avoidance etc., measurement of such aspects in the real world remains lacking.

10.7.4.4 Factors That Can Affect Outcome

Common sense dictates that there are factors that can affect treatment outcome and that these will vary for each individual. Whereas the main prognostic indicators are generally intrinsic or related to the client, other factors affecting outcome may relate to the speech pathologist. These include ensuring:

- Provision of treatment that has a strong evidence base.
- Provision of sufficient treatment.
- Provision of maintenance and relapse management.
- Troubleshooting with the client why transfer of fluency may not be happening, and then providing additional strategies.
- Inclusion of anxiety treatment/management where indicated.
- Provision of a range of tasks and activities to maintain motivation.
- Monitoring transfer and maintenance.
- Consistent and continual speech measurement to evaluate change.

10.7.5 Summary

There is evidence on which children are likely to continue stuttering without treatment (Nang and Ciccone 2016; Jones et al. 2000). They are those who are male, have a family history of stuttering, start to stutter later, possibly have lower scores on speech sound accuracy, as well as for expressive and receptive language, and as is most widely reported, greater stuttering severity than those who stop stuttering spontaneously. Similarly, data on treatment outcome indicate that children who have a greater severity of stuttering require more treatment time (Jones et al. 2000).

Cook et al. (2013) investigated pre-treatment factors that would predict outcome of treatment in children and adolescents who had undergone an intensive programme of treatment. Again, stuttering severity was the only pre-treatment factor that predicted post-treatment stuttering severity. However, it is also noteworthy that these authors found that psychosocial impact also related to more positive fluency outcome.

Similar to the findings on children and adolescents, adults who have a more negative outcome in terms of amount of stuttering post-treatment are those with a higher pre-treatment stuttering severity (Andrews and Craig 1988; Hancock and Craig 1998; Block et al. 2005).

Irrespective of the amount of stuttering present, it is important that we also consider factors such as changes in participation and activity, as well as quality of life, for all those with whom we work. Further research into the means of doing so is essential to ensure comprehensive treatment provision and maximal outcome.

References

Adolfsson J, Steineck G (2000) Prognostic and treatment-predictive factors: is there a difference? Prostate Cancer Prostatic Dis 3:265–268

Alm PA (2020) Streptococcal infection as a major historical cause of stuttering: data, mechanisms, and current importance. Front Hum Neurosci 14:389–408

Althaus M, Harry JF, Ruud B et al (1995) Lack of effect of clonidine on stuttering in children. Am J Psychiatry 152(7):1087–1089

Ambrose NG, Yairi E (1999) Normative disfluency data for early childhood stuttering. J Speech Lang Hear Res 42(4):895–909

Andrews G, Craig A (1982) Stuttering: overt and covert measurement of the speech of treated subjects. J Speech Hear Disord 47(1):96–99

Andrews G, Craig A (1988) Prediction of outcome following treatment for stuttering. Br J Psychiatry 153:236–240

Andrews G, Guitar B, Howie P (1980) Meta-analysis of the effects of stuttering treatment. J Speech Hear Disord 45(3):287–307

APA (American Psychiatric Association) (2013) DSM-5: diagnostic and statistical manual of mental disorders, 5th edn (Proposed Revision): childhood onset fluency disorder. www.dsm5.org. Accessed 7 Dec 2020

ASRC (Australian Stuttering Research Centre) (2020) Unhelpful thoughts and beliefs about stuttering (UTBAS) scales. University of Technology Sydney, Sydney. (uts.edu.au)

Baer RA, Krietemeyer J (2006) Overview of mindfulness- and acceptance-based treatment approaches. In: Baer RA (ed) Mindfulness-based treatment approaches: clinician's guide to evidence base and applications. Elsevier Academic Press, Amsterdam, pp 3–17

Bakker K (2006) Technical support for stuttering treatment. In: Bernstein Ratner N, Tetnowski J (eds) Current issues in stuttering research and practice. Lawrence Erlbaum Associates, Mahwah, pp 205–237

Barbara DA (1963) The psychotherapy of stuttering. Curr Psychiatr Ther 3:114–123

Beck JS (2011) Cognitive behavior therapy: basics and beyond, 2nd edn. The Guilford Press, New York

Beilby JM, Byrnes ML, Yaruss JS (2012) Acceptance and commitment therapy for adults who stutter: psychosocial adjustment and speech fluency. J Fluen Disord 37(4):289–299

Berman PA, Brady JP (1973) Miniaturized metronomes in the treatment of stuttering: a survey of clinician's experiences. J Behav Ther Exp Psychiatry 4(2):117–119

Block S, Onslow M, Roberts R et al (2004) Control of stuttering with EMG feedback. Adv Speech Lang Pathol 6:100–106

Block S, Onslow M, Packman A et al (2005) Treatment of chronic stuttering: outcomes from a student training model. Int J Lang Commun Disord 40:455–466

Block S, Onslow M, Packman A et al (2006) Connecting stuttering management and measurement: IV. Predictors of outcome for a behavioral treatment for stuttering. Int J Lang Commun Disord 41(4):395–406

Blomgren M (2010) Stuttering treatment for adults: an update on contemporary approaches. Semin Speech Lang 31(4):272–282

Blomgren M (2013) Behavioral treatments for children and adults who stutter: a review. Psychol Res Behav Manag 6:9–19

Blomgren M, Roy N, Callister T et al (2005) Intensive stuttering modification therapy: a multidimensional assessment of treatment outcomes. J Speech Lang Hear Res 48(3):509–523

Blood GW (1995) A behavioral-cognitive therapy program for adults who stutter: computers and counseling. J Commun Disord 28:165–180

Blood GW, Blood IM (2016) Long-term consequences of childhood bullying in adults who stutter: social anxiety, fear of negative evaluation, self-esteem, and satisfaction with life. J Fluen Disord 50:72–84

Bloodstein O, Bernstein-Ratner N (2008) A handbook on stuttering (6th ed.). New York: Thomson Delmar Learning

Bloodstein O (1993) Stuttering: the search for a cause and cure. Allyn & Bacon, Boston

Bloodstein O, Bernstein Ratner N, Brundage SB (2021) A handbook on stuttering. Plural Publishing

Blotch M, Stager S, Braun A et al (1997) Pimozide-induced depression in men who stutter. J Clin Psychiatry 58(10):433–436

Blumgart E, Tran Y, Craig A (2010) Social anxiety disorder in adults who stutter. Depress Anxiety 27(7):687–692

Boey R (2010) Sociaal cognitieve gedragstherapie voor stotteren: adolescenten en volwassenen (Social cognitive behavioral therapy for stuttering: adolescents and adults). VVL, Belsele

Bothe AK, Davidow JH, Bramlett RE et al (2006a) Stuttering treatment research 1970–2005: I. Systematic review incorporating trial quality assessment of behavioral, cognitive, and related approaches. Am J Speech Lang Pathol 15(4):321–341

Bothe AK, Davidow JH, Bramlett RE et al (2006b) Stuttering treatment research 1970–2005: II. Systematic review incorporating trial quality assessment of pharmacological approaches. Am J Speech Lang Pathol 15(4):342–352

Botterill W, Cook F (1987) Personal construct theory and the treatment of adolescent dysfluency. In: Rustin L, Purser H, Rowley D (eds) Progress in the treatment of fluency disorders. Taylor & Francis, London, pp 147–165

Bowen C (2011) Lionel Logue: a pioneer in speech-language pathology. The ASHA Leader. https://leader.pubs.asha.org/doi/10.1044/leader.FTR1.16022011.10. Accessed 28 Jan 2022

Boyle MP (2011) Mindfulness training in stuttering therapy: a tutorial for speech-language pathologists. J Fluen Disord 36:122–129

Boyle MP (2015) Identifying correlates of self-stigma in adults who stutter: further establishing the construct validity of the self-stigma of stuttering scale (4S). J Fluen Disord 43:17–27

Boyle MP (2018) Enacted stigma and felt stigma experienced by adults who stutter. J Commun Disord 73:50–61

Brady JP (1991) The pharmacology of stuttering: a critical review. Am J Psychiatry 148(10):1309–1316

Brady JP, McAllister TW, Price TR (1990) Verapamil in stuttering. Biol Psychiatry 27(6):680–681

Brignell A, Krahe M, Downes M et al (2020) A systematic review of interventions for adults who stutter. J Fluen Disord 64:105766. https://doi.org/10.1016/j.jfludis.2020.105766

Brosch S, Winkler S (2008) Diagnostics and therapy of stuttering children [in German]. Laryngorhinootologie 87(7):511–518

Brumfitt SM, Peake MD (1988) A double-blind study of verapamil in the treatment of stuttering. Br J Disord Commun 23(1):35–40

Busan P, Del Ben G, Russo LR et al (2019) Stuttering as a matter of delay in neural activation: a combined TMS/EEG study. Clin Neurophysiol 130(1):61–76

Byrd C, Chmela K, Coleman C et al (2016) An introduction to camps for children who stutter: what they are and how they can help. Perspectives 1(4):55–69

Byrd CT, Gkalitsiou Z, Werle D et al (2018) Exploring the effectiveness of an intensive treatment program for school-age children who stutter, Camp Dream. Speak. Live: a follow-up study. Semin Speech Lang 39(5):458–468

Campbell P, Constantino CD, Simpson S (eds) (2019) Stammering pride and prejudice: difference not defect. J & R Press, Guildford

Casa Futura Technologies (2015) Technology for treating stuttering and Parkinson's speech. http://casafuturatech.wpengine.com/smalltalk-anti-stuttering-device/. Accessed 1 Feb 2022

Chang SE, Guenther FH (2020) Involvement of the cortico-basal ganglia-thalamocortical loop in developmental stuttering. Front Psychol 10:3088. https://doi.org/10.3389/fpsyg.2019.03088

Charoensook J, Maguire GA (2017) A case series on the effectiveness of lurasidone in patients with stuttering. J Clin Psychopharmacol 29(3):191–194

Cheasman C, Simpson S, Everard R (2015) Acceptance and speech work: the challenge. Procedia Soc Behav Sci 193:72–81

Chesters J, Möttönen R, Watkins KE (2018) Transcranial direct current stimulation over left inferior frontal cortex improves speech fluency in adults who stutter. Brain 141(4):1161–1171

Chow HM, Chang SE (2017) White matter developmental trajectories associated with persistence and recovery of childhood stuttering. Hum Brain Mapp 38(7):3345–3359

Cohen J (1988) Statistical power analysis for the behavioral sciences, 2nd edn. Lawrence Erlbaum, Hillsdale

Constantino CD, Leslie P, Quesal RW et al (2016) A preliminary investigation of daily variability of stuttering in adults. J Commun Disord 60:39–50

Conture EG (2001) Stuttering: its nature, diagnosis and treatment. Allyn & Bacon, Boston

Cook S, Donlan C, Howell P (2013) Stuttering severity, psychosocial impact and lexical diversity as predictors of outcome for treatment of stuttering. J Fluen Disord 38:124–133

Cooper EB (1987) The chronic perseverating stuttering syndrome: incurable stuttering. J Fluen Disord 12(6):381–388

Cordes AK, Ingham RJ, Frank P et al (1992) Time-interval analysis of interjudge and intrajudge agreement for stuttering event judgments. J Speech Hear Res 35(3):483–494

Craig A (1998) Relapse following treatment for stuttering: a critical review and correlative data. J Fluen Disord 23(1):1–30

Craig AR, Cleary PJ (1982) Reduction of stuttering by young male stutterers using EMG feedback. Biofeedback Self Regul 7(3):241–255

Craig A, Tran Y (2006) Fear of speaking: chronic anxiety and stuttering. Adv Psychiatr Treat 12(1):63–68

Craig A, Tran Y (2014) Trait and social anxiety in adults with chronic stuttering: conclusions following meta-analysis. J Fluen Disord 40:35–43

Craig A, Hancock K, Chang E et al (1996) A controlled clinical trial for stuttering in persons aged 9 to 14 years. J Speech Hear Res 39(4):808–826

Craig A, Hancock K, Tran Y et al (2003) Anxiety levels in PWS: a randomized population study. J Speech Lang Hear Res 46:1197–1206

Craig A, Blumgart E, Tran Y (2009) The impact of stuttering on the quality of life in adults who stutter. J Fluen Disord 34(2):61–71

Craig A, Blumgart E, Tran Y (2011) Resilience and stuttering: factors that protect people from the adversity of chronic stuttering. J Speech Lang Hear Res 54(6):1485–1496

Crowe TA (1997) Counseling: definition, history, rationale. In: Crowe TA (ed) Applications of counseling in speech-language pathology and audiology. Williams & Wilkins, Baltimore, pp 3–39

Dalton P (1983) Psychological approaches to the treatment of stuttering. In: Dalton P (ed) Approaches to the

treatment of stuttering. Imprint Routledge, London, pp 106–135
de Sonneville-Koedoot C, Stolk E, Rietveld T et al (2015) Direct versus indirect treatment for preschool children who stutter: the RESTART randomized trial. PLoS One 10(7):1–17
Dell C (2001) Therapie für das stotternde Schulkind. Übersetzt und bearbeitet von Andreas Starke (Therapy for the stuttering schoolchild. Translated and edited by Andreas Starke), 3rd edn. Demosthenes, Jena
Dewar A, Dewar AD, Austin WTS et al (1979) The long-term use of an automatically triggered auditory feedback masking device in the treatment of stammering. Br J Disord Commun 14(3):219–229
DiLollo A, Neimeyer RA, Manning WH (2002) A personal construct psychology view of relapse: indications for a narrative therapy component to stuttering treatment. J Fluen Disord 27(1):19–42
Dineen T (1999) Manufacturing victims. Constable Press, London
Duchan JF (2012) Historical and cultural influences on establishing professional legitimacy: a case example from Lionel Logue. Am J Speech Lang Pathol 21(4):387–396
Eggers K (2020) Addressing cognitions and emotions in people who stutter using Beck's cognitive therapy. Two-day workshop presented at Dilgem Istanbul, Turkey
Eggers K, Heselmans I (2024) Delay frustration in children who do and do not stutter: A preliminary study. J Commun Disord 107:106403. https://doi.org/10.1016/j.jcomdis.2023.106403. Epub 2023 Dec 10. PMID: 38101316
Eggers K, Millard SK, Kelman E (2022) Temperament, anxiety, and depression in school-age children who stutter. J Commun Disord 97:106218. https://doi.org/10.1016/j.jcomdis.2022.106218. Epub 2022 May 4. PMID: 35597191
Einarsdottir J, Crowe K, Kristinsson S et al (2020) The recovery rate of early stuttering. J Fluen Disord 64:105764. https://doi.org/10.1016/j.jfludis.2020.105764
Ellis A (2004) Rational emotive behavior therapy: it works for me—it can work for you. Prometheus Books, Amherst
Euler HA, Wolff von Gudenberg A (2000) Die Kasseler Stottertherapie (KST). Ergebnisse einer computergestützten Biofeedbacktherapie für Erwachsene (The Kassel therapy of stuttering (KST). Results of a computer-based biofeedback therapy for adults). Sprache Stimme Gehör 24(2):71–79
Euler HA, Wolff von Gudenberg A, Jung K et al (2009) Computergestützte Therapie bei Redeflussstörungen: Die langfristige Wirksamkeit der Kasseler Stottertherapie (KST) (Computer-assisted therapy for speech disfluency: the long-term effectiveness of the Kassel Stuttering Therapy (KST)). Sprache Stimme Gehör 33(4):193–201
Euler HA, Lange BP, Schroeder S et al (2014) The effectiveness of stuttering treatments in Germany. J Fluen Disord 39(1):1–11
Euler HA, Anders C, Merkel A et al (2016) Mindert eine globale Sprechrestrukturierungwie die Kasseler Stottertherapie (KST) stotterbegleitende negative Emotionen? (Can an integrative speech restructuring treatment reduce stuttering-related negative emotions?). Logos 24(2):84–94
Fagnani C, Fibiger S, Skytthe A et al (2011) Heritability and environmental effects for self-reported periods with stuttering: a twin study from Denmark. Logoped Phoniatr Vocol 36(3):114–120
Farnbach-Pralong D, Bradbury R, Copolov D et al (1998) Clozapine and olanzapine treatment decreases rat cortical and limbic GABAA receptors. Eur J Pharmacol 349(2–3):R7–R8
Finn P, Howard R, Kubala R (2005) Unassisted recovery from stuttering: self-perceptions of current speech behavior, attitudes, and feelings. J Fluen Disord 30(4):281–305
Foundas AL, Mock JR, Corey DM et al (2013) The SpeechEasy device in stuttering and nonstuttering adults: fluency effects while speaking and reading. Brain Lang 126(2):141–150
Franken MC, Boves L, Peters HFM et al (1992) Perceptual evaluation of the speech before and after fluency shaping stuttering therapy. J Fluen Disord 17(4):223–241
Fransella F (1970) Stuttering: not a symptom but a way of life. Br J Disord Commun 5:22–29
Friedman A, Fetterman E, Jolson Y (1999) Dr. fluency computerized stuttering treatment program User's guide (version 2.3). Speech Therapy Systems Ltd, Jerusalem
Fry J, Botterill W, Pring T (2009) The effect of an intensive group therapy program for young adults who stutter: a single subject study. Int Speech Lang Pathol 11:12–19
Gallop RF, Runyan CM (2012) Long-term effectiveness of the SpeechEasy fluency-enhancement device. J Fluen Disord 37(4):334–343
Giraud AL, Neumann K, Bachoud-Levi AC et al (2008) Severity of dysfluency correlates with basal ganglia activity in persistent developmental stuttering. Brain Lang 104(2):190–199
Glauber IP (1958) The psychoanalysis of stuttering. In: Eisenson J (ed) Stuttering; a symposium. Harper & Row, New York, pp 71–120
Goebel MD (1994) CAFET Program. Annandale Fluency Clinic, Annandale
Gordon CT, Cotelingam GM, Stager S et al (1995) A double-blind comparison of clomipramine and desipramine in the treatment of developmental stuttering. J Clin Psychiatry 56(6):238–242
Gottwald SR (2010) Stuttering prevention and early intervention: a multidimensional approach. In: Guitar B, McCauley R (eds) Treatment of stuttering: established and emerging interventions. Lippincott, Williams & Wilkins, Philadelphia, pp 118–140

Gregory HH (2003) Stuttering therapy: rational and procedures. Allyn & Bacon, Boston
Grossman HL (2020) Rational emotive behavior therapy for stuttering (REBT). Webinar presented for the Stuttering Foundation
Guitar B (2006) Stuttering: an integrated approach to its nature and treatment, 3rd edn. Lippincott, Williams & Wilkins, Baltimore
Guitar B (2013) Stuttering: an integrated approach to its nature and treatment, 4th edn. Lippincott, Williams & Wilkins, Baltimore
Guitar B, McCauley R (2010) An overview of treatments for preschool stuttering. In: Guitar B, McCauley R (eds) Treatment of stuttering: established and emerging interventions. Lippincott, Williams & Wilkins, Philadelphia, pp 56–62
Gunn A, Menzies RG, O'Brian S et al (2014) Axis I anxiety and mental health disorders among stuttering adolescents. J Fluen Disord 40:58–68
Hale L (1951) A consideration of thiamin supplement in prevention of stuttering in preschool children. J Speech Hear Dis 16(4):327–333
Hancock K, Craig A (1998) Predictors of stuttering relapse one year following treatment for children aged 9 to 14 years. J Fluen Disord 23(1):31–48
Hancock K, Craig A, Campbell K et al (1998) Two to six year controlled trial stuttering outcomes for children and adolescents. J Speech Lang Hear Res 41(6):1242–1252
Harley J (2018) The role of attention in therapy for children and adolescents who stutter: cognitive behavioral therapy and mindfulness-based interventions. Am J Speech Lang Pathol 27(3S):1139–1151
Harris R (2009) ACT made simple. New Harbinger Publications, Oakland
Harrison E, Onslow M (2010) The Lidcombe program for preschool children who stutter. In: Guitar B, McCauley R (eds) Treatment of stuttering: established and emerging interventions. Lippincott, Williams & Wilkins, Philadelphia, pp 118–140
Hayhow R, Levy C (1993) Working with stuttering: a personal construct approach. Winslow Press, Bicester
Herder CL, Howard C, Nye C et al (2006) Effectiveness of behavioral stuttering treatment: a systematic review and meta-analysis. Contemp Issues Commun Sci Disord 33:61–73
Hoang JL, Patel S, Maguire GA (2017) Case report of aripiprazole in the treatment of adolescent stuttering. Ann Clin Psychiatry 2(1):64–65
Hollister J, Van Horne AO, Zebrowski P (2017) The relationship between grammatical development and disfluencies in preschool children who stutter and those who recover. Am J Speech Lang Pathol 26(1):44–56
Howell P, Davis S (2011) Predicting persistence of and recovery from stuttering by the teenage years based on information gathered at age eight. J Dev Behav Pediatr 32(3):196–205
Howell P, Davis S, Williams R (2008) Late childhood stuttering. J Speech Lang Hear Res 51(3):669–687
Hugh-Jones S, Smith PK (1999) Self-reports of short- and long-term effects of bullying on children who stammer. Br J Educ Psychol 69(2):141–158
Ingham R (1984) Stuttering and behavior therapy. College-Hill Press, San Diego
Ingham JC (2003) Evidence-based treatment of stuttering: I. Definition and application. J Fluency Disord 28(3):197–207
Iverach L, Rapee RM (2014) Social anxiety disorder and stuttering: current status and future directions. J Fluen Disord 40:69–82
Iverach L, O'Brian S, Jones M et al (2009a) Prevalence of anxiety disorders among adults seeking speech therapy for stuttering. J Anxiety Disord 23(7):928–934
Iverach L, Jones M, O'Brian S et al (2009b) Screening for personality disorders among adults seeking speech treatment for stuttering. J Fluen Disord 34(3):173–186
Iverach L, Menzies RG, Jones M et al (2011a) Further development and validation of the unhelpful thoughts and beliefs about stuttering (UTBAS) scales: relationship to anxiety and social phobia among adults who stutter. Int J Lang Commun Disord 46(3):286–299
Iverach L, Menzies RG, O'Brian S et al (2011b) Anxiety and stuttering: continuing to explore a complex relationship. Am J Speech Lang Pathol 20(3):221–232
Iverach L, Jones M, McLellan LF et al (2016) Prevalence of anxiety disorders among children who stutter. J Fluen Disord 49:13–28
Iverach L, Rapee RM, Wong QJJ et al (2017) Maintenance of social anxiety in stuttering: a cognitive-behavioral model. Am J Speech Lang Pathol 26(2):540–556
Iverach L, Jones M, Lowe R et al (2018) Comparison of adults who stutter with and without social anxiety disorder. J Fluen Disord 56:55–68
Jackson ES, Yaruss JS, Quesal RW et al (2015) Responses of adults who stutter to the anticipation of stuttering. J Fluen Disord 45:38–51
Jackson ES, Rodgers NH, Rodgers DB (2019) An exploratory factor analysis of action responses to stuttering anticipation. J Fluen Disord 60:1–10
Johnson G, Onslow M, Carey B et al. (2024) Lidcombe Program telehealth treatment for children 6–12 years of age: A Phase II trial. J Fluency Disord 80:106057. https://doi.org/10.1016/j.jfludis.2024.106057. Epub 2024 Apr 7. PMID: 38613876
Jennions MD, Møller AP (2002) Relationships fade with time: a meta-analysis of temporal trends in publication in ecology and evolution. Proc Biol Sci 269(1486):43–48
Johannsen HS (1996) Prävention und Frühtherapie bei kindlichem Stottern (Prevention and early treatment of infantile stuttering). Forum Logopädie 6:5–9
Johnson W (ed) (1955) Stuttering in children and adults: thirty years of research at the University of Iowa. University of Minnesota Press, Minneapolis
Jones M, Onslow M, Harrison E et al (2000) Treating stuttering in young children: predicting treatment time in the Lidcombe program. J Speech Hear Res 43:1440–1450

Jones M, Onslow M, Packman A et al (2005) Randomised controlled trial of the Lidcombe programme of early stuttering intervention. Br Med J 331(7518):659–661

Jones R, Eggers K, Zengin-Bolatkale H (2020) Temperamental and emotional processes. In: Zebrowski P, Anderson J, Conture E (eds) Stuttering: characteristics, assessment, and treatment, 4th edn. Thieme Medical Publishers, New York

Kabat-Zinn J (1996) Full catastrophe living. Piatkus, London

Kalinowski J, Saltuklaroglu T (2003) Choral speech: the amelioration of stuttering via imitation and the mirror neuronal system. Neurosci Biobehav Rev 27(4):339–347

Karimi H, Onslow M, Jones M et al (2018) The satisfaction with communication in everyday speaking situations (SCESS) scale: an overarching outcome measure of treatment effect. J Fluen Disord 58:77–85

KayPENTAX (2011) Lincoln Park, New Jersey, United States of America. Ambulatory Phonation Monitor (APM), Model 3200. http://www.kayelemetrics.com/index.php?option=comproduct&view=product&Itemid=3&controller=product&cid%5B%5D=9&task=prodetails

Kelly GA (1955) The psychology of personal constructs. Norton, New York

Kelman E, Nicholas A (2008) Practical intervention for early childhood stammering: Palin PCI approach. Speechmark Publishing, Milton Keynes

Kelman E, Wheeler S (2015) Cognitive behaviour therapy with children who stutter. Procedia Soc Behav Sci 193:165–174

Klein JF, Hood SB (2004) The impact of stuttering on employment opportunities and job performance. J Fluen Disord 29(4):255–273

Koedoot C, Bouwmans C, Franken MC et al (2011) Quality of life in adults who stutter. J Commun Disord 44(4):429–443

Kohmäscher A, Primaßin A, Heiler S et al (2023) Effectiveness of stuttering modification in school-age children who stutter: a randomized clinical trial. J Speech Lang Hear Res 66(11):4191–4205

Kraft SJ, Yairi E (2012) Genetic bases of stuttering: the state of the art, 2011. Folia Phoniatr Logop 64(1):34–47

Langevin M, Kully D (2003) Evidence-based treatment of stuttering: III. Evidence-based practice in a clinical setting. J Fluen Disord 28(3):219–236

Leahy M, Eggers, K (2023) Fluency, disorders of fluency, and dysfluency. In K. Eggers & M. Leahy (Eds.), Clinical cases in fluency disorders (pp. 1–10). Routledge, London

Leahy MM, O'Dwyer M, Ryan F (2012) Witnessing stories: definitional ceremonies in narrative therapy with adults who stutter. J Fluen Disord 37:234–241

Leary MR (1983) A brief version of the fear of negative evaluation scale. Pers Soc Psychol Bull 9:9371–9375

Leech KA, Bernstein Ratner N, Brown B et al (2017) Preliminary evidence that growth in productive language differentiates childhood stuttering persistence and recovery. J Speech Lang Hear Res 60(11):3097–3109

Logan KJ, Yaruss JS (1999) Helping parents address attitudinal and emotional factors with young children who stutter. Contemp Issues Commun Sci Disord 26:69–81

Lowe R, Menzies R, Packman A et al (2016) Assessing attentional biases with stuttering. Int J Lang Commun Disord 51:84–94

Lowe R, Helgadottir F, Menzies R et al (2017) Safety behaviors and stuttering. J Speech Lang Hear Res 60(5):1246–1253

Lu C, Peng D, Chuansheng C et al (2010) Altered effective connectivity and anomalous anatomy in the basal ganglia-thalamocortical circuit of stuttering speakers. Cortex 46(1):49–67

Ludlow CL, Loucks T (2003) Stuttering: a dynamic motor control disorder. J Fluen Disord 28(4):273–295

Luterman DM (2001) Counseling persons with communication disorders and their families, 4th edn. Pro-Ed, Austin

Maguire GA, Riley G, Hahn R et al (1994) Nimodipine in the treatment of stuttering. ASHA J 36:51

Maguire GA, Riley G, Franklin D et al (2000) Risperidone for the treatment of stuttering. J Clin Psychopharmacol 20(4):479–482

Maguire GA, Riley G, Franklin D et al (2004) Olanzapine in the treatment of developmental stuttering: a double-blind, placebo-controlled trial. Ann Clin Psychiatry 16(2):63–67

Maguire G, Franklin D, Vatakis NG et al (2010) Exploratory randomized clinical study of pagoclone in persistent developmental stuttering: the EXamining Pagoclone for peRsistent dEvelopmental Stuttering Study. J Clin Psychopharmacol 30(1):48–56

Maguire GA, Franklin D, Kirsten J (2011) Asenapine for the treatment of stuttering: an analysis of three cases. Am J Psychiatry 168(6):651–652

Maguire GA, Ngo J, Fonsworth PK et al (2012) Alleviation of developmental stuttering following deep brain stimulation of the ventral intermediate nucleus of the thalamus. Am J Psychiatry 169(7):759–760

Maguire GA, Nguyen DL, Simonson K et al (2020) The pharmacological treatment of stuttering and its neuropharmacologic basis. Front Neurosci 14:158. https://doi.org/10.3389/fnins.2020.00158

Maniadaki K (2017) Let's talk about stuttering in a journal of child psychology. J Child Psychol 1(1):1–2

Manning WH (2010) Clinical decision making in the diagnosis and treatment of fluency disorders, 3rd edn. Delmar, Clifton Park

Månsson H (2000) Childhood stuttering: incidence and development. J Fluen Disord 25(1):47–57

Martin RR, Haroldson SK, Triden KA (1984) Stuttering and speech naturalness. J Speech Hear Res 49(1):53–58

McAllister J, Kelman E, Millard S (2015) Anxiety and cognitive bias in children and young people who stutter. Procedia Soc Behav Sci 193:183–191

Mendes L, Dacakis G, Block S et al (2015) A novel approach for measuring social participation in adults who stutter. J Fluen Disord 44:88–95

Menzies RG, Onslow M, Packman A (1999) Anxiety and stuttering: exploring a complex relationship. Am J Speech Lang Pathol 8(1):3–10

Menzies RG, O'Brian S, Onslow M et al (2008) An experimental clinical trial of a cognitive-behavior therapy package for chronic stuttering. J Speech Lang Hear Res 51(6):1451–1464

Menzies RG, Onslow M, Packman A et al (2009) Cognitive behavior therapy for adults who stutter: a tutorial for speech language pathologists. J Fluen Disord 34(3):187–200

Menzies R, O'Brian S, Lowe R et al (2016) International phase II clinical trial of CBTPsych: a standalone internet social anxiety treatment for adults who stutter. J Fluen Disord 48:35–43

Menzies RG, Packman A, Onslow M et al (2019) In-clinic and standalone internet cognitive behavior therapy treatment for social anxiety in stuttering: a randomized trial of iGlebe. J Speech Lang Hear Res 62(6):1614–1624

Merwin R, O'Rourke S, Ives L et al (2019) Chapter 16—Third-wave cognitive-behavioral therapies for the treatment of anxiety among children and adolescents. In: Compton SN, Villabø MA, Kristensen H (eds) Pediatric anxiety disorders. Academic Press, Cambridge, pp 335–357

Millard SK, Edwards S, Cook FM (2009) Parent-child interaction therapy: adding to the evidence. Int J Speech Lang Pathol 11(1):61–76

Miller B, Guitar B (2009) Long-term outcome of the Lidcombe program for early stuttering intervention. Am J Speech Lang Pathol 18(1):42–49

Moleski R, Tosi DJ (1976) Comparative psychotherapy: rational-emotive therapy versus systematic desensitization in the treatment of stuttering. J Consult Clin Psychol 44:309–311

Molt L (2019) A brief historical review of assistive devices for treating stuttering. https://www.mnsu.edu/comdis/isad8/papers/molt8/molt8.html. Accessed 26 Aug 2019

Moons K, Royston P, Vergouwe Y et al (2009) Prognosis and prognostic research: what, why, and how? Br Med J 338:b375. https://doi.org/10.1136/bmj.b375

Munjal S, Schultheis G, Ferrando S (2018) Ziprasidone for the treatment of stuttering. J Clin Psychopharmacol 38(4):404–405

Nang C, Ciccone N (2016) Stuttering prognosis and predictive factors of treatment outcome: a review. J Clin Pract Speech Lang Pathol 18(2):94–99

Natke U, Alpermann A, Heil W et al (2010) Langzeiteffekte der Intensiv-Modifikation Stottern (IMS) (Long-term effects of intensive modification of stuttering (IMS)). Sprache Stimme Gehör 34(3):155–164

Neumann K, Euler HA, Bosshardt HG et al (2017) The pathogenesis, assessment and treatment of speech fluency disorders. Dtsch Arztebl Int 114(22–23):383–390

Neumann K, Euler HA, Zens R et al (2019) "Spontaneous" late recovery from stuttering: dimensions of reported techniques and causal attributions. J Commun Disord 81:105915. https://doi.org/10.1016/j.jcomdis.2019.105915

Nippold MA (2011) Stuttering in school-age children: a call for treatment research. Lang Speech Hear Res Schools 42(2):99–101

Nippold MA (2012) When a school-age child stutters, let's focus on the primary problem. Lang Speech Hear Serv Sch 43(4):549–552

Nye C, Vanryckeghem M, Schwartz JB et al (2013) Behavioral stuttering interventions for children and adolescents: a systematic review and meta-analysis. J Speech Lang Hear Res 56(3):921–932

O'Brian S, Jones M, Packman A et al (2011) Stuttering severity and educational attainment. J Fluen Disord 36:86–92

O'Brian S, Heard R, Onslow M et al (2020) Clinical trials of adult stuttering treatment: comparison of percentage syllables stuttered with self-reported stuttering severity as primary outcomes. J Speech Lang Hear Res 63(5):1387–1394

Onslow M (2003a) Evidence-based treatment of stuttering: IV. Empowerment through evidence-based treatment practices. J Fluen Disord 28(3):237–245

Onslow M (2003b) Overview of the Lidcombe program. In: Onslow M, Packman A, Harrison E (eds) The Lidcombe program of early stuttering intervention: a clinician's guide. Pro-Ed, Austin

Onslow M (2021) Stuttering and its treatment—eleven lectures. www.uts.edu.au/ASRC/resources

Onslow M, Lowe R (2019) After the RESTART trial: six guidelines for clinical trials of early stuttering intervention. Int J Lang Commun Disord 54(4):517–528

Onslow M, Millard S (2012) Palin parent child interaction and the Lidcombe program: clarifying some issues. J Fluen Disord 37(1):1–8

Onslow M, Yaruss JS (2007) Differing perspectives on what to do with a stuttering preschooler and why. Am J Speech Lang Pathol 16(1):65–68

Onslow M, Menzies RG, Packman A (2001) An operant intervention for early stuttering: the development of the Lidcombe program. Behav Modif 25(1):116–139

Onslow M, Packman A, Harrison E (eds) (2003) The Lidcombe program of early stuttering intervention: a clinician's guide. Pro-Ed, Austin

Onslow M, Jones M, O'Brian S et al (2008) Defining, identifying, and evaluating clinical trials of stuttering treatments: a tutorial for clinicians. Am J Speech Lang Pathol 17(4):401–415

Onslow M, Jones M, O'Brian S et al (2018) Comparison of percentage of syllables stuttered with parent-reported severity ratings as a primary outcome measure in clinical trials of early stuttering treatment. J Speech Lang Hear Res 61(4):811–819

Onslow M, Lowe R, Jakšić SJ et al. (2023) The Fifth Croatia Stuttering Symposium: Part III. Mental health and early stuttering. J Fluency Disord 77:106000. https://doi.org/10.1016/j.jfludis.2023.106000. Epub 2023 Aug 2. PMID: 37586168

Orton S (1927) Studies in stuttering: introduction. AMA Arch Neurol Psych 18(5):671–672
Packman A, Meredith G (2011) Technology and the evolution of clinical methods for stuttering. J Fluen Disord 36(2):75–85
Packman A, Onslow M, Richard F et al (1996) Syllabic stress and variability: a model of stuttering. Clin Linguist Phonet 10(3):235–263
Perkins WH (1990) What is stuttering? J Speech Hear Disord 55(3):370–382
Planck M (1948) Wissenschaftliche Selbstbiographie (Scientific autobiography). Verlag Johann Ambrosius Barth, Leipzig
Plexico LW, Manning WH, Levitt H (2009a) Coping responses by adults who stutter. Part I. Protecting the self and others. J Fluen Disord 34:87–107
Plexico LW, Manning WH, Levitt H (2009b) Coping responses by adults who stutter. Part II. Approaching the problem and achieving agency. J Fluen Disord 34:108–126
Pollard R, Ellis JB, Finan D et al (2009) Effects of the SpeechEasy on objective and perceived aspects of stuttering: a 6-month Phase 1 clinical trial in naturalistic environments. J Speech Lang Hear Res 52(2):516–533
Prins D, Ingham RJ (2009) Evidence-based treatment and stuttering-historical perspective. J Speech Lang Hear Res 52(1):254–263
Reardon-Reeves NA, Yaruss JS (2013) School-age stuttering therapy: a practical guide. Stuttering Therapy Resources, McKinney
Reddy RP, Sharma MP, Shivashankar N (2010) Cognitive behavior therapy for stuttering: a case series. Indian J Psychol Med 32:49–53
Reilly S, Onslow M, Packman A et al (2009) Predicting stuttering onset by the age of 3 years: a prospective, community cohort study. Pediatrics 123(1):270–277
Reilly S, Onslow M, Packman A et al (2013) Natural history of stuttering to 4 years of age: a prospective community-based study. Pediatrics 132(3):460–467
Riley GD (2009) SSI-4. Stuttering severity instrument, 4th edn. Pro-Ed, Austin
Robey RR (2004) Levels of evidence. The ASHA Leader. https://leader.pubs.asha.org/doi/full/10.1044/leader.FTR2.09072004.5. Accessed 29 Jan 2022
Rosenberger PB, Wheelden JA, Kalotkin M (1976) The effect of haloperidol on stuttering. Am J Psychiatry 133(3):331–334
Ryan BP, Ryan BVK (1995) Programmed stuttering treatment for children: comparison of two establishment programs through transfer, maintenance, and follow-up. J Speech Hear Res 38(1):61–75
Ryan F, O'Dwyer M, Leahy MM (2015) Separating the problem and the person: insights from narrative therapy with people who stutter. Top Lang Disord 35:267–274
Sackett DL, Rosenberg WM, Gray JA et al (1996) Evidence-based medicine: what it is and what it isn't. BMJ 312(7023):71–72
Scheurich JA, Beidel DC, Vanryckeghem M (2019) Exposure therapy for social anxiety disorder in people who stutter: an exploratory multiple baseline design. J Fluen Disord 59:21–32
Schooler JW (2011) Unpublished results hide the decline effect. Nature 470(7335):437. https://doi.org/10.1038/470437a
Schulze H, Johannsen HS (1986) Stottern bei Kindern im Vorschulalter. Theorie, Diagnostik, Therapie (Stuttering in preschool children. Theory, diagnostics, therapy). Phoniatrische Ambulanz der Universität Ulm, Ulm
Shapiro DA (2011) Stuttering intervention: a collaborative journey to fluency freedom, 2nd edn. Pro-Ed, Austin
Shaygannejad V, Khatoonabadi SA, Shaifiei B et al (2013) Olanzapine versus haloperidol: which can control stuttering better? Int J Prev Med 4(Suppl 2):S270–S273
Sheehan JB (1958) Conflict theory of stuttering. In: Eisenson J (ed) Stuttering; a symposium. Harper & Row, New York, pp 121–166
Sheehan JG (1970) Stuttering: research and therapy. Harper & Row, New York
Shenker RC, Santayana G (2018) What are the options for the treatment of stuttering in preschool children? Semin Speech Lang 39(4):313–323
Shimada M, Toyomura A, Fujii T et al (2018) Children who stutter at 4 years of age: a community-based study. J Fluen Disord 56:45–54
Shipley K, McAfee J (2019) Assessment in speech-language pathology: a resource manual, 6th edn. Plural Publishing, San Diego
Shugart Y, Mundorff J, Kilshaw J et al (2004) Results of a genome-wide linkage scan for stuttering. Am J Med Genet 124A(2):133–135
Singer C, Hessling A, Kelly E et al (2020) Clinical characteristics associated with stuttering persistence: a meta-analysis. J Speech Lang Hear Res 63(9):2995–3018
Smith A, Weber C (2016) How stuttering develops: the multifactorial dynamic pathways theory. J Speech Lang Hear Res 60(9):2483–2505
Smith A, Weber C (2017a) How stuttering develops: the multifactorial dynamic pathways theory. J Speech Lang Hear Res 60(9):2483–2505
Smith A, Weber C (2017b) Childhood stuttering—where are we and where are we going? Semin Speech Lang 37(4):291–297
Smith KA, Iverach L, O'Brian S et al (2014) Anxiety of children and adolescents who stutter: a review. J Fluen Disord 40:22–34
Spence SH (1998) A measure of anxiety symptoms among children. Behav Res Ther 36(5):545–566
St Clare T, Menzies R, Onslow M et al (2008) Unhelpful thoughts and beliefs linked to social anxiety in stuttering: development of a measure. Int J Lang Commun Disord 44(3):338–351
St. Louis KO (2011) The Public Opinion Survey Of Human Attributes-Stuttering (POSHA-S): summary framework and empirical comparisons. J Fluen Disord 36(4):256–261
Stager S, Ludlow C, Gordon CT et al (1995) Fluency changes in persons who stutter following a double

blind trial of clomipramine and desipramine. J Speech Lang Hear Disord 38(3):516–525

Stager S, Calis K, Grothe D et al (1997) A double-blind trial of pimozide and paroxetine for stuttering. In: Hulstijn H, Peters HFM, Van Lieshout PHHM (eds) Speech production: motor control, brain research, and fluency disorders. Elsevier, Amsterdam, pp 379–382

Stager S, Calis K, Grothe D et al (2005) Treatment with medications affecting dopaminergic and serotonergic mechanisms: effects on fluency and anxiety in persons who stutter. J Fluen Disord 30(4):319–335

Stewart T, Birdsall M (2001) A review of the contribution of personal construct psychology to stammering therapy. J Constr Psychol 14:215–225

Stuart A, Kalinowski J, Rastatter MP et al (2004) Investigations of the impact of altered auditory feedback in-the-ear devices on the speech of people who stutter: initial fitting and four-month follow-up. Int J Lang Commun Disord 39(1):93–113

Thiriez C, Roubeau B, Ouerchefani N et al (2013) Improvement in developmental stuttering following deep brain stimulation for Parkinson's disease. Parkinsonism Relat Disord 19(3):383–384

Tichenor S, Yaruss JS (2018) A phenomenological analysis of the experience of stuttering. Am J Speech Lang Pathol 27(3S):1180–1194

Tichenor SE, Yaruss JS (2019a) Group experiences and individual differences in stuttering. J Speech Lang Hear Res 62(12):4335–4350

Tichenor SE, Yaruss JS (2019b) Stuttering as defined by adults who stutter. J Speech Lang Hear Res 62(12):4356–4369. https://doi.org/10.1044/2019_JSLHR-19-00137

Tichenor SE, Yaruss JS (2020) Recovery and relapse: perspectives from adults who stutter. J Speech Lang Hear Res 63(7):2162–2176

Tichenor S, Leslie P, Shaiman S et al (2017) Speaker and observer perceptions of physical tension during stuttering. Folia Phoniatr Logop 69(4):180–189

Tran P, Hamilton S, Kuntz AJ et al (1997) Double-blind comparison of olanzapine versus risperidone in the treatment of schizophrenia and other psychotic disorders. J Clin Psychopharmacol 17(5):407–418

Tran N, Maguire GA, Franklin D et al (2008) Case report of aripiprazole for persistent developmental stuttering. J Clin Psychopharmacol 28(4):470–472

Tran Y, Blumgart E, Craig A (2011) Subjective distress associated with chronic stuttering. J Fluen Disord 36(1):17–26

Tran Y, Blumgart E, Craig A (2021) Situational embarrassment and its relationship to social anxiety in adults who stutter. Journal of Speech, Language and Hearing Research 64:3759–3768.

Travis LE (1931) Speech pathology; a dynamic neurological treatment of normal speech and speech deviations. D. Appleton and Company, New York

Trichon M, Tetnowski J (2011) Self-help conferences for people who stutter: a qualitative investigation. J Fluen Disord 36(4):290–295

Van Riper C (1971) The nature of stuttering. Prentice Hall, Englewood Cliffs

Van Riper C (1973) The treatment of stuttering, 2nd edn. Prentice-Hall, Englewood Cliffs

Van Riper C (1982) The nature of stuttering, 2nd edn. Prentice Hall, Englewood Cliffs

Venkatagiri HS (2009) What do people who stutter want—fluency or freedom? J Speech Lang Hear Res 52(2):500–515

Walsh B, Usler E, Bostian A et al (2018) What are predictors for persistence in childhood stuttering? Semin Speech Lang 39(4):299–312

Ward D (2006) Stuttering and cluttering: frames for understanding and treatment. Psychology Press, Hove

White M (2000) Reflections on narrative practice. Dulwich Centre Publications, Adelaide

White M (2007) Maps of narrative practice. Norton, New York

White M, Epston D (1990) Narrative means to therapeutic ends. Norton, New York

WHO (World Health Organization) (2001) International classification of functioning, disability, and health. World Health Organization, Geneva. www.who.int/classifications/icf/en/

Wood F, Stump D, McKeehan A et al (1980) Patterns of regional cerebral blood flow during attempted reading aloud by stutterers both on and off haloperidol medication: evidence for inadequate left frontal activation during stuttering. Brain Lang 9(1):141–144

Wright L, Ayre A, Grogan S (1998) Outcome measurement in adult stuttering therapy: a self-rating profile. Int J Lang Commun Disord 33(Suppl):378–383. https://doi.org/10.3109/13682829809179455

Wu JC, Riley GD, Maguire G et al (1997a) PET scan evidence of parallel cerebral systems related to treatment effects: FDG and FDOPA PET scan findings. In: Hulstijn W, Peters HFM, van Lieshout P (eds) Speech production: motor control, brain research, and fluency disorders. Elsevier, Amsterdam, pp 329–339

Wu JC, Maguire GA, Riley G et al (1997b) Increased dopamine activity associated with stuttering. Neuroreport 8(3):767–770

Yairi E, Ambrose NG (1999) Early childhood stuttering I: persistency and recovery rates. J Speech Lang Hear Res 42(5):1097–1112

Yairi E, Ambrose NG (2013) Epidemiology of stuttering: 21st century advances. J Fluency Dis 38(2):66–87

Yairi E, Ambrose N (2014) A longitudinal study of stuttering in children. J Speech Lang Hear Res 35(4):755–760

Yairi E, Ambrose NG, Paden EP et al (1996) Predictive factors of persistence and recovery: pathways of childhood stuttering. J Commun Disord 29(1):51–77

Yandeau E, Carey B, Onslow M (2021) The Lidcombe program: a client report 7 years post-treatment. Speech Lang Hear 25(4):492–497. https://doi.org/10.1080/2050571X.2021.1923304

Yaruss JS (1997) Clinical implications of situational variability in preschool children who stutter. J Fluen Disord 22(3):187–203

Yaruss JS (2007) Application of the ICF in fluency disorders. Semin Speech Lang 28(4):312–322
Yaruss JS, Quesal RW (2004) Stuttering and the international classification of functioning, disability and health (ICF): an update. J Commun Dis 37(1):35–52
Yaruss JS, Quesal RW (2006) Overall assessment of the speaker's experience of stuttering (OASES): documenting multiple outcomes in stuttering treatment. J Fluen Disord 31(2):90–115
Yaruss JS, Quesal RW (2016) Overall assessment of the speaker's experience of stuttering. Stuttering Therapy Resources Inc., McKinney
Yaruss JS, Reardon-Reeves NA (2017) Early childhood stuttering therapy: a practical guide. Stuttering Therapy Resources Inc., McKinney
Yaruss JS, Quesal RW, Reeves L et al (2002) Speech treatment and support group experiences of people who participate in the National Stuttering Association. J Fluen Disord 27(2):115–134
Yaruss JS, Coleman C, Hammer D (2006) Treating preschool children who stutter: description and preliminary evaluation of a family-focused treatment approach. Lang Speech Hear Serv Schools 37(2):118–136
Yaruss JS, Quesal RW, Reeves L (2007) Self-help and mutual aid groups as an adjunct to stuttering therapy. In: Conture EG, Curlee RF (eds) Stuttering and related disorders of fluency, 3rd edn. Thieme Medical Publishers, New York, pp 256–276
Yaruss JS, Coleman CE, Quesal RW (2012) Stuttering in school-age children: a comprehensive approach to treatment. Lang Speech Hear Serv Sch 43(4):536–548

Part III

Literacy Development Disorders

Editor
Antoinette am Zehnhoff-Dinnesen

Lectors
Mirela Duranovic, Anja Fiori,
Ben Maassen, and Rudolf Reiter

Basics of Literacy Development Disorders

11

Anja Fiori, Ben A. M. Maassen,
Barbara Maciejewska, Rudolf Reiter, Georg Romer,
and Bozena Wiskirska-Woznica

11.1 Definition and Epidemiology of Developmental Literary Disorders

Rudolf Reiter and Ben A. M. Maassen

11.1.1 Introduction

Reading and spelling disorders represent a distinct impairment in the development of reading skills and the frequently related orthographic abilities. In later childhood and at an adult age, the course of the disorder is highly variable with many adults with reading disorder reading too slowly to function in a literate society, and the orthography could also remain deficient (Ferrer et al. 2015).

11.1.2 Definition of Developmental Literacy Disorders

According to the fifth Edition of the Diagnostic and Statistical Manual of Mental Disorders (DSM-5) (American Psychiatric Association 2013), the term 'dyslexia' is avoided, but is mentioned in a note:

> *Dyslexia* is an alternative term used to refer to a pattern of learning difficulties characterized by problems with accurate or fluent word recognition, poor decoding, and poor spelling abilities. If dyslexia is used to specify this particular pattern of difficulties, it is important also to specify any additional difficulties that are present, such as difficulties with reading comprehension or math reasoning
> (DSM-5; paragraph Specific Learning Disorder; 315.00 (F81.0): With impairment in reading)

Dyslexia thereby can be categorised under 'Specific Learning Disorder', comprising diffi-

Anja Fiori and Ben A. M. Maassen shared first authorship.

A. Fiori (✉)
Münster Department of Health MDH, Münster University of Applied Science, Muenster, Germany
e-mail: fiori@fh-muenster.de

B. A. M. Maassen
Department Neurosciences/BCN, Center for Language and Cognition, University of Groningen Medical Center, Groningen, The Netherlands
e-mail: b.a.m.maassen@rug.nl

B. Maciejewska · B. Wiskirska-Woznica
Department and Clinic of Phoniatrics and Audiology, Poznan University of Medical Sciences, Poznan, Poland
e-mail: barbaramaciejewska@ump.edu.pl

R. Reiter
Department of Otolaryngology, Section for Phoniatrics and Paedaudiology, University HNO Clinic, Ulm, Germany
e-mail: rudolf.reiter@uniklinik-ulm.de

G. Romer
Klinik fuer Kinder- und Jugendpsychiatrie, -psychosomatik, und -psychotherapie, University Muenster, Muenster, Germany
e-mail: georg.romer@ukmuenster.de

A. am Zehnhoff-Dinnesen et al. (eds.), *Phoniatrics II*, European Manual of Medicine,
https://doi.org/10.1007/978-3-031-25175-7_11

culties in learning and using academic skills, and more specifically inaccurate or slow and effortful word reading, difficulties with spelling and difficulty understanding the meaning of what is read.

For professionals in the educational rather than the psychiatric field, the following definition is better applicable to their practice:

> Dyslexia is a specific learning disability that is neurobiological in origin. It is characterised by difficulties with accurate and/or fluent word recognition and by poor spelling and decoding abilities. These difficulties typically result from a deficit in the phonological component of language that is often unexpected in relation to other cognitive abilities and the provision of effective classroom instruction. Secondary consequences may include problems in reading comprehension and reduced reading experience that can impede growth of vocabulary and background knowledge.
>
> Lyon et al. (2003, p. 2)

According to ICD-10 (International Statistical Classification of Diseases and Related Health Problems), the reading or spelling disorder belongs to the group of distinct impairments in the development of scholastic skills (World Health Organization 2019). The main characteristic is a specific and significant impairment in the development of reading or spelling skills. Reading comprehension, written word recognition, oral reading and performance of tasks requiring reading may all be affected.

Dyslexia is considered a life-long condition. At the skill level, however, selective progress can be made, in most cases because of specific training. Specific reading disorders are frequently associated with spelling disorders and often remain in adulthood, even after some progress in reading has been made. Developmental disorders in language development or speech, e.g. phonological or morphological skills or awareness, can precede dyslexia (Rothou and Padeliadu 2019; Schaadt and Männel 2019; Volkmer et al. 2019). During the school-age period, associated emotional and behavioural disturbances are common (Dilling and Freyberger 2012). Dyslexia cannot be explained by intellectual/mental development, low mental age, inadequate schooling, deficient hearing or visual abilities, or by neurological or psychiatric disturbances; however, these factors do play a role in determining the severity of the reading and spelling difficulties. It is assumed that this specific performance disturbance, occurring in all linguistic communities, is genetically rooted (Schleider 2009; Warnke et al. 2004).

11.1.3 Diagnostic Criteria for Developmental Literacy Disorders

The presence of a reading or spelling disorder, isolated spelling disorder or isolated reading disorder is commonly detected when the reading performance or spelling performance is well below the level that would have been reached by others of similar age, class or intelligence. For diagnosis in the early stages of reading, acquisition of diagnostic criteria varies among countries, but a European study on more than 2000 children spanning a large range of orthographic complexity, highlights on a persistent delay, i.e. after at least 1.5 years of reading instruction, in reading fluency of 1.25 standard deviations below the age and educational level norm group (Landerl et al. 2013). In later years in primary and secondary school, and higher education, persistence is generally assumed, unless there are clear indications of educational deprivation. Reading or spelling skills must be seriously behind, in the lowest 10% on several tasks, and in addition, the criterion is added that reading skills are below that needed to cope with the demands of everyday life, which is thus impaired or endangered.

The German dyslexia (LRS) Guidelines (2015) suggest a less stringent limit (from 1.0 SD below the average of the class standard, the age norm or the level of reading performance) if the evidence from the clinical investigation and the results of the psychometric procedures indicate reading or spelling difficulties associated with lowered intelligence (Schulte-Körne and Galuschka 2015).

11.1.4 Epidemiology of Developmental Literacy Disorders

Reading and spelling disorders are the more commonly occurring distinct developmental disturbances with prevalence from approximately

3% (Schulte-Körne 2010) to 7% (Suchodoletz 2006; Warnke et al. 2004; Snowling and Melby-Lervåg 2016). Depending on the age, a disturbance in reading or spelling can be found in 3.3–24.2% of 8-year-olds, about 6% of 12-year-olds and 3.1–6.4% of young adults (Hasselhorn and Schuchardt 2006; Sun et al. 2013; Snowling and Hulme 2012; Fluss et al. 2008; Schulte-Körne 2010). However, it should be noted that all of the diagnostic criteria are subject to a certain amount of arbitrariness. Boys are more frequently affected than girls by a factor of almost two (Katusic et al. 2001; Lewis et al. 1994; Rutter et al. 2004; Berninger et al. 2008). Distribution of reading skills in the population is continuous, and the 'cut-offs' used to define a person as 'dyslexic' are arbitrary (e.g. Pennington 2006). Transparency of the orthography to be learnt is an important determiner of prevalence, and dyslexia tends to occur with other disorders, including specific language impairment (Boada and Pennington 2006; Kalashnikova et al. 2019; Adlof and Hogan 2018).

11.2 Symptomatic Profile of Developmental Dyslexia

Anja Fiori and Ben A. M. Maassen

11.2.1 What Are the Typical Symptoms of Developmental Dyslexia?

According to its definition, developmental dyslexia is a learning difficulty resulting in deficient reading fluency, reading accuracy, decoding or spelling that is not due to overall or specific poor cognitive functions and not due to lack of education. Reading difficulties persist despite appropriate intervention, and developmental dyslexia is a life-long condition (Munzer et al. 2020). Developmental dyslexia has a negative impact on general scholastic achievement. Although the main symptoms are well-defined, persons with developmental dyslexia can exhibit a broad variety of individual symptomatic constellations and a high variability in degree of involvement (Munzer et al. 2020). These individual profiles have to be differentiated carefully diagnostically if intended to serve as basis of individualised intervention programmes.

> Dyslexia is still a clinical diagnosis, with no definitive biochemical or neuroimaging markers, and there is no one test that can diagnose it. Diagnosis is based on history, observation, and psychological assessment.
>
> Munzer et al. (2020, p. 38)

The high symptomatic variability results partly from the fact that literacy acquisition is a very complex developmental domain that is influenced by many different factors. One reason for assessing individual symptomatic constellations is that difficulties change over the course of time owing to aspects of education and experience in literacy.

11.2.2 Dyslexia in Different Languages and Cultures

From an international point of view, general classification into subtypes or stages should be handled with care: languages vary with regard to their orthographic regularity as well as prevailing educational methods in different cultural contexts. There are series of studies and reviews showing that orthographic transparency (Borleffs et al. 2019; Ziegler and Goswami 2005, 2006) and educational history (Perfetti and Harris 2013) leave a developmental footprint characterising the reading processes of an individual.

11.2.3 Developmental Models of Literacy

For a general understanding of changing symptomatic profiles, it is helpful to consider developmental models of literacy as proposed by Frith (1980), Günther (1986) and Scheerer-Neumann (2001a, b). Such models, as shown in Sect. 12.5, are helpful in assigning specific difficulties of dyslexic children to broadly accepted stages of literacy development.

11.2.4 Prevailing Symptoms in Different Stages of Acquisition

Concerning the modality of reading, difficulties in accuracy and fluency prevail in early stages, i.e. the child makes many mistakes reading single words or short sentences, or it takes long to decode even simple, highly frequent words. Furthermore, children with developmental dyslexia often show difficulties in automatisation of the reading process: skills in automatised recognition of known words or smaller lexical units. Automatisation in letter-to-letter-decoding, which implies knowledge and highly automatised processing of letter-to-sound (or grapheme-phoneme) correspondence, lies at the base of these difficulties. As a consequence, difficulties in fluency are a life-long symptom. In later stages of reading development, difficulties in text comprehension and fast capturing of contents are described as sequelae of the slow word decoding process.

In the modality of spelling, young writers often exhibit problems in learning to produce words in their correct phonetic form (correct sequence of letters) in early stages. These can range from the complete inability to write down any of the required letters, to the deletion, rearrangement or exchange of single letters or letter strings. In later stages of development, orthographic mistakes (breaches of orthographic rules, which require deviation from the alphabetic principle) prevail. Independent from their skills in applying the alphabetic principle, at this later stage, children vary with respect to their ability to learn and store in memory larger orthographic units (Bekebrede et al. 2009). For a substantial subgroup, administering orthographic knowledge to their spelling is the main challenge.

11.2.5 Types of Dyslexia and Prevailing Symptoms

The discussion about the role of a general phonological or orthographic deficit in developmental dyslexia, given mainly in the Anglo-American literature, goes back to the 1990s. Then Castles and Coltheart (1993) distinguished specific difficulties in learning the alphabetic principle, with an underlying deficit in phonological awareness from troubles in learning orthographic rules. Both difficulties can be involved simultaneously, but different profiles of degree of involvement are the rule rather than the exception.

In addition, several symptomatic constellations, besides a combination of reading and spelling difficulties, have been described (Klicpera et al. 2013; Warnke et al. 2004).

11.2.5.1 Severe Spelling Disorders: Difficulties in Learning Orthographic Rules

There are children who mainly experience problems with spelling, whereas reading abilities are less affected. Depending on the orthographic transparency of the language, children with severe spelling disorders can make many orthographic mistakes, especially in phonetically irregular words. Often, pre-school deficits in phonological awareness as well as verbal working memory (repeating pseudo-words) have been described and interpreted as causal factors. Klicpera et al. (2013) give a critical view on the criteria to classify isolated spelling disorders in ICD 10; if reading difficulties are an exclusion criterion, it would be impossible to find isolated spelling disorders, at least in German children.

11.2.5.2 Severe Reading Disorders

These children mainly experience reading difficulties, whereas spelling abilities are less affected. Different forms of reading difficulty can be distinguished (Klicpera et al. 2013; Warnke et al. 2004; Hulme and Snowling 2014):

- **Difficulties in Reading Fluency** Most children and adults with dyslexia primarily experience difficulties with reading fluency, which can be accompanied by more or less severe difficulties with reading accuracy. Dyslexic children lag behind their peers in measures of reading speed. Reading can be described as slow and halting. This specific difficulty becomes evident not only when the child is presented with single words, but especially when presented with sentences as well as small texts in reading assessments. Though many children usually learn to read correctly, reading fluency remains stably below average in further development, and continues to be the main problem during adulthood.

- **Difficulties in Reading Accuracy** During the early stages of reading acquisition, reading accuracy can be the main problem, partly because reading fluency needs time to develop. Some children struggle much harder with correct grapheme-to-phoneme association than others, and go through a protracted phase of making many mistakes in reading aloud. At later stages, their specific difficulties may remain noticeable especially for uncommon, complicated words such as loanwords or in tasks including decoding of longer pseudo-words.
- **Difficulties in Reading Comprehension** According to the simple view of reading (SVR), reading comprehension is the product of decoding and linguistics, which is oral language comprehension (Hoover and Gough 1990). Isolated difficulties in reading comprehension without decoding difficulties are to be diagnosed as language, not reading impairment. On the other hand, a decoding deficit hampers the motivation of the child, and the amount of practice—up to a factor of 50—in reading texts, such that poor reading comprehension generally is the consequence. In addition, since language development of literate children develops for a large part through reading texts, vocabulary especially tends to stay behind in dyslexic children, and some of them—not necessarily those with poor oral language comprehension of fluent text reading—suffer from a tendency to understand only explicitly given textual information and an inability to gather implicit information or to interpret reflexive or referring phrases or words. For these children, context information is not helpful for decoding words. While their memory capacity tends to be normal, analogue deficits in auditory comprehension are most likely to be the underlying cause. A relation to impaired language development can be assumed.
- **Hyperlexia** This is characterised by a striking discrepancy between extraordinary fluency and the inability to capture the contents of sentences or texts. Hyperlexia can be considered a combination of excellent decoding abilities and (very) poor text comprehension, irrespective of the text being presented in written or spoken form. Hyperlexia is often found in children with autistic disorders.

11.2.6 Multifactorial Profile of Dyslexia

In the recent literature, models for developmental disorders such as dyslexia are probabilistic and multifactorial, rather than deterministic and focused on a single cause (e.g. Pennington 2006). The implication is that multiple factors together determine the symptomatic profile of dyslexia, such that for diagnosis and treatment a dimensional rather than a categorical approach is warranted. Thus, the extent to which different aspects of literacy skills—such as decoding, reading accuracy and fluency, spelling, reading comprehension—are affected, as well as the extent and severity of possible co-morbidities—such as ADHD, language, phonological and speech disorder—can vary tremendously.

Several authors argue that pure, clearly distinguishable subtypes of dyslexia are unlikely to be found; diagnosis needs to focus on describing traits, which give the most sensible starting point for deriving specific measures of remediation. According to this multiple deficit approach (Pennington 2006; Pennington et al. 2012; Ring and Black 2018), an alternative to subdividing dyslexia into subtypes is to take a dimensional approach in which all subskills are diagnosed on a continuous scale, and individuals are diagnosed in terms of (relative) strengths and weaknesses.

11.3 Aetiology and Pathogenesis Including Genetics of Developmental Dyslexia

Georg Romer and Barbara Maciejewska

11.3.1 Introduction

Developmental literacy disorders, commonly referred to as developmental dyslexia (DD), represent a specific developmental learning disability with a complex multi-factorial aetiology. This corresponds with complex developmental trajectories in the acquisition process of reading and spelling skills. These developmental trajectories have their origin in early childhood, long before school age, and are intrinsically interwoven. The specific functions and skills involved in this acquisition process of reading and spelling encompass the auditory as well as the visual system, both in perception and information processing.

Some of the relevant basic functions in auditory perception and processing include the capacity to discriminate acoustic sounds in rapid sequences, the ability to discriminate similar language sounds such as 'b' and 'p', auditory short-term memory and the presence of so-called phonological awareness (Raskind et al. 2000; Schulte-Körne 2002). Phonological awareness refers to the ability to hear, discriminate and manipulate phonemes, i.e. the smallest units of sound that can differentiate meaning. For example, the spoken word 'fat' can be separated into three distinct phonemes, /f/, /æ/ and /t/, and by exchanging the first sound into /k/, one can hear and understand the word 'cat'.

Relevant basic functions in visual perception and processing encompass the stability of gaze fixation, the discrimination of rapidly changing stimuli with low contrast, as well as the decoding of graphic and lexical units. Dyslexic individuals have been found to need more time than normal readers when analysing written syllables and to use more eye saccades during this task, which is assumed to reflect their reduced capacity to capture lexical units from written information. In other words, they are assumed to depend more on analysing the meaning of words from graphic units (graphemes, i.e. syllables) than from lexical units (entire words). From the observation of a high familial concordance of dyslexia, a strong heredity component has long been postulated. However, familial concordance by itself does not prove heredity, as members of the same family share both genes and environment. In the following sections, the aspects of nature vs. nurture in the development of dyslexia as well as the current understanding of the specific neurobiological dysfunctions in the aetiology and pathogenesis of dyslexia are depicted.

11.3.2 Genetics

Developmental dyslexia does not just occur randomly within the population. The disorder is a highly heritable as it tends to run in families. Familial clustering in dyslexia was recognised a few years after the first description of the disorder (Schumacher et al. 2007). Children with familial history of dyslexia constitute a common risk group and tend to have around a 45% chance to develop a reading disorder (Snowling and Melby-Lervåg 2016). In the Snowling et al. study (2003), the development of 56 children at family risk of dyslexia was followed from the age of 3 years 9 months to 8 years. In the high-risk group, 66% had reading disabilities at age 8 years compared with 13% in a control group from similar, middle-class backgrounds. An individual's risk of being affected increased when other family members are affected: 9% of control children had a sibling or parent with some form of reading problem, compared with 34% of children with DD (Rutter and Yule 1975). Gilger et al. (1996) observed that 20–33% of siblings of affected individuals, with unaffected parents, are themselves also affected, and this increased to 54–63% if either parent was also affected, and 76–78% if both parents were affected. The sibling recurrence risk of DD, i.e. the probability of an individual being affected with DD given a sibling is already affected (regardless of parental affection status), is estimated at 43–60% (Scerri and Schulte-Körne 2010). The family risk of dyslexia, as the dyslexia itself, is continuous (Snowling et al. 2003; Maciejewska et al. 2013).

Children with a familial history of dyslexia exhibit under-activation during phonological processing in the bilateral occipito-temporal and left temporo-parietal areas, as well as in the cerebellum (Raschle et al. 2014). They also show disruption in the left frontal brain regions during auditory processing (Raschle et al. 2014). Dębska et al. (2016), who tested Polish-speaking preschoolers and first-graders, reported similar results. Children with a familial history of dyslexia show reduced activation of many brain regions, including the left occipito-temporal cortex. For this particular region, reduced activation was observed only among pre-schoolers in the familial risk group.

The presence of a familial history of dyslexia and reading impairment can change and interfere with normal phonological brain network reorganisation (Łuniewska et al. 2019). Typical readers without risk for dyslexia have already activated structures responsible for phonological processing at the beginning of literacy. This group shows reduced brain activation over time during phonological processing, perhaps due to automatisation of phonological skills. Children who develop reading impairment present a delay in the development of phonological structures, such as the bilateral superior temporal gyri, left middle temporal gyrus, right insula and right frontal cortex, where we observe time and group interaction. Children with familial dyslexia also have abnormally delayed auditory event-related potentials (ERPs). Abnormal findings may not reflect only maturational lag but also more fundamental processing deficiencies (Maciejewska et al. 2013; Leppänen and Lyytinen 1997).

11.3.2.1 Findings from Twin Studies

With such a strong familial basis for DD, twin studies have been employed to evaluate the genetic components underlying its aetiology. Studies with large enough twin cohorts are particularly informative for estimating the relation between genetic and environmental factors causing a specific condition. For this, the concordant occurrence of the condition in monozygotic (MZ) co-twins is compared with the respective concordant occurrence in dizygotic (DZ) co-twins. To illustrate this, the following two extreme hypotheses are explained by Olson (2002): if one assumes that dyslexia is entirely caused by genes, MZ co-twins of dyslexic individuals should be dyslexic as well by 100%, as they share all their genes, whereas DZ co-twins should be dyslexic by a rate of approximately 50% as 'they share about half of their segregating genes on average' (Olson 2002). If one assumes that dyslexia is entirely caused by environmental factors, MZ co-twins of dyslexic individuals should also be dyslexic by 100%, given that the twins have been raised in the same family. However, the same concordance rate should be found in DZ co-twins of dyslexic individuals. From the difference in the phenotypical concordance rates between MZ and DZ twin pairs, the relation of genetic versus environmental causation can be estimated. From these types of twin studies, there is evidence of a strong impact of heritability in developmental dyslexia. The retarded acquisition of spelling skills has been found to be more genetically determined (genetic impact of 50–70% vs. 30–50% environmental influences) than the retarded acquisition of reading skills (50–60% vs. 40–50% environmental influences) (Olson 2002; Schulte-Körne et al. 2006; Warnke 2007). Furthermore, specific partial skills that are relevant for reading and spelling differ in their degree of genetic determination (see Table 11.1).

Twin- and family-based studies have shown that DD is highly familial and also heritable and complex, involving multiple risk factors, both genetically and environmentally (Scerri and Schulte-Körne 2010).

11.3.2.2 Findings from Molecular Genetics

Some independent linkage studies have been performed in the search for DD susceptibility genes. As a result, nine DD risk loci from DYX1 to DYX9 on eight different chromosomes have been mapped (1p36-p34, 2p16-p15, 3p12-q13, 6p22 and 6q13-16.2, 11p15.5, 15q21.3, 18p11.2 and Xq27.3) (cytogenetic location: p-shorter arm of the chromosome, q-longer arm of chromosome, and the number of chromosome on which the

Table 11.1 Heritability vs. environment estimates for specific tasks involved in the acquisition of reading and spelling (based on Olson 2007)

Task	Heritability estimate (%)	Environment estimate (%)
Word recognition	54	46
Phonological decoding	71	29
Orthographic coding	67	33
Phoneme deletion[a]	72	28

[a] The ability to identify how a word would sound if one sound were omitted

gene can be found). There are DD-candidate genes to the brain structure and function. Moreover the involvement of several genes spanning these regions in the aetiology of DD has been reported so far (Scerri and Schulte-Körne 2010; Mascheretti et al. 2017).

As Mascheretti et al. (2017) have written in their cross-sectional and interdisciplinary study: 'Apart from these DYX loci, other genes implicated in other disorders, before being examined for DD, have also been associated with reading (dis)ability, that is, *FOXP2*, *CNTNAP2*, *DOCK4* and *GTF2I* on chromosome 7, *GRIN2B* and *SLC2A3* on chromosome 12, *ATP2C2* and *CMIP* on chromosome 16, *PCNT*, *DIP2A*, *S100B* and *PRMT2* on chromosome 21'. Dyslexia-susceptibility genes probably affect neuronal migration, neurite outgrowth, cortical morphogenesis and ciliary structure and function (Mascheretti et al. 2017). Despite the recognition of a strong genetic component in the aetiology of developmental dyslexia, we are far from understanding the molecular mechanisms involved in this heritability. A number of gene loci and regions have been reported to be relevant. However, these findings have not been replicated convincingly. As the authors of a recent European multi-national study, with the largest to date cross-lingual cohort comprising 900 dyslexic individuals from 8 countries, conclude, 'we did not find any marker or haplotype that was significantly associated with either case–control status or quantitative measurements of word-reading or spelling in the meta-analysis of all eight countries combined. Like [sic] in other neurocognitive disorders, our findings underline the need for larger sample sizes to validate possibly weak genetic effects' (Becker et al. 2014). Findings from molecular genetics suggest that there is no specific 'dyslexia gene'. Dyslexia is probably not caused by a single gene, but by a combination of genetic traits. The traits also may be expressed differently among different people, because of their mediating or enhancing influence on other genes. The multi-factorial mechanisms to be involved in the heritability of DD. The model of heritability is unknown, but is not Mendelian (Snowling et al. 2003; Schumacher et al. 2007; Maciejewska et al. 2013; Habib 2000).

In summary, there is strong evidence that heritability plays a major role in the aetiology of DD. Although the field is immature, the role of genetics in DD is rapidly growing and much has been learned regarding the possible downstream effects of DD risk genes on the brain structure, function and circuitry (Mascheretti et al. 2017). However, it cannot entirely explain its phenotypic occurrence. Despite the successful characterisation of DD-susceptibility genes, we are far from understanding the molecular aetiological pathways underlying the development of reading (dis)ability.

There are several reasons for children at family risk of dyslexia possibly experiencing more risks than children not at risk in the preschool years. For example, parents with dyslexia spend less time reading for pleasure than adults who are not dyslexic, and children carrying a genetic risk of dyslexia may evoke less literacy-related (and hence oral language) input from their caregivers than those who do not carry a familial risk (Dilnot et al. 2017).

No specific dyslexia gene has been identified. If DD forms are differentiated by particular disabilities in specific skills contributing to the complex process of acquiring spelling and reading, the influence of heredity differs between particular forms. Performing joint genetic and neuroimaging studies in humans seems to be an emerging strategy to link DD-candidate genes to the brain structure and function. Imaging data provide a background for complex neurobehavioural disorders and have been extensively used to investigate morphological, structural and functional brain abnormalities in DD (see Sects. 11.4 and 11.3.3).

11.3.3 Neurobiology: Findings from Neuroanatomical Studies

It has been shown that learning to read changes the brain network and language system (Łuniewska et al. 2019). The phonological brain network undergoes reorganisation during the first 2 years of formal education. The brain regions mainly involved in speech perception and processing are located in the temporal lobe of the left hemisphere, where Wernicke's speech area is also located (see Fig. 11.1a, b). Specific regions responsible for partial functions can be localised separately. For instance, the function of assigning speech sounds to literal information can be localised in the supramarginal gyrus and the gyrus temporalis superior (Price et al. 1996), whereas the functions of detecting words as meaningful entities and naming of pictures, colours and letters can be localised in the posterior parts of the gyrus temporalis inferior (Price and Friston 1997).

In post-mortem anatomical and histological studies, a number of differences between dyslexic and normal control brains have been demonstrated, including reduced left–right asymmetry of the planum temporal (Galaburda and Kemper 1979; Altarelli et al. 2014) as well as anomalies

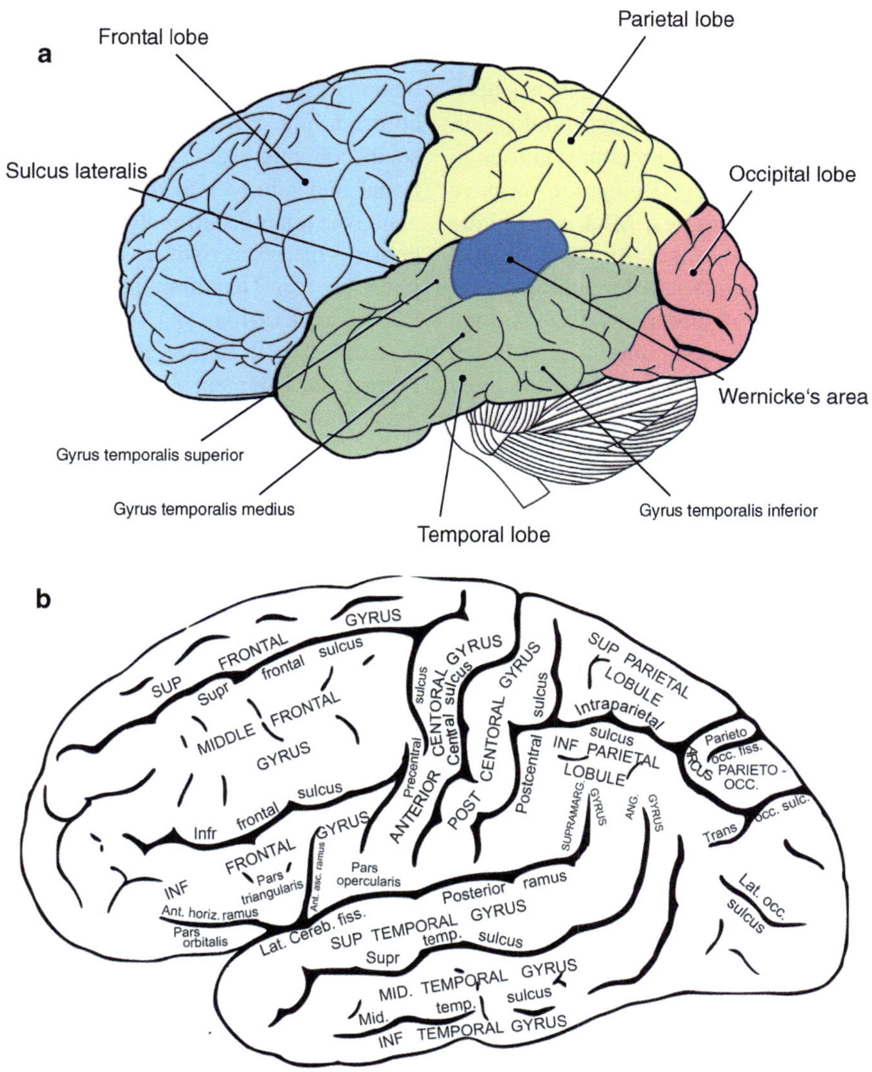

Fig. 11.1 (**a**) Lateral surface of the left cerebral hemisphere, viewed from the side; the temporal lobe, where Wernicke's speech area is located, is shown. (Adapted from Henry Vandyke Carter, Public domain, via Wikimedia Commons). (**b**) Lateral surface of the left cerebral hemisphere, viewed from the side; the parietal lobe with the supramarginal gyrus is shown. (Henry Vandyke Carter, Public domain, via Wikimedia Commons)

of cell migration in the temporal cortex in the left perisylvian regions appearing as atypical cell formations (so-called molecular layer ectopias or neuronal ectopias) and cell dysplasia (Galaburda et al. 1985). Owing to small samples and possible comorbidity biases, these neuroanatomical findings cannot fully explain the role of neurobiological deficits in developmental dyslexia. However, they underline the importance of neuronal deficits at a structural level. Furthermore, they appear to be quite compatible with findings from EEG and neuroimaging studies, which elucidate the neurobiological correlates of dyslexia at the functional level.

Magnetic resonance imaging (MRI) has been extensively used to investigate morphological, structural and functional brain abnormalities in DD patients (see Fig. 11.1). Being non-invasive and allowing in vivo studies, MRI is a unique and valuable tool for disentangling tissue modifications and functional (re)organisation in developmental such disorders as DD. Among different MRI-based techniques, voxel-based morphometry (VBM) is used to quantify grey and white matter volumes, while diffusion tensor imaging (DTI), which probes water diffusivity at the micron scale, detects alterations in white matter (WM) structure and indirectly in the architecture of fibre pathways (Vandermosten et al. 2012a). DTI allows the structural identification of white matter tracts (Mascheretti et al. 2017; Vandermosten et al. 2012b). Finally, functional MRI (fMRI) detects brain activations during cognitive and sensory tasks, and when at rest.

Results of imaging studies on pre-reading children at risk for DD are in agreement with results found for children with DD, suggesting that neural alterations in DD predate reading onset, reflect the differential developmental trajectory of reading brain networks, and may serve as early biomarkers of risk for DD (Mascheretti et al. 2017). Most findings support the importance of neural deficits in brain regions for the aetiology of dyslexia. Apart from neuroanatomical studies, imaging–genetics studies in DD could be a way to investigate this further.

11.3.4 Environmental Influences

There is no doubt a child's school achievement is influenced by environmental factors. Generally, low socio-economic status and a poor school environment are associated with a higher risk of poor reading performance. However, low socio-economic status, as well as poor reading performance due to a disadvantaged educational environment, is not regarded as developmental dyslexia. Only when a specific learning disability in reading and spelling can be identified in spite of an otherwise normal intellectual performance and an adequate educational milieu, should DD be diagnosed. Environmental risk factors tend to co-occur, e.g. low parental educational and low socioeconomic status, or low parental educational and family risk. As expected, there is a negative relationship between risks and outcomes—the more risks a child experiences, the poorer is their 'readiness for learning' in school (Dilnot et al. 2017).

According to Dilnot et al. (2017), the home literacy environment (storybook exposure, frequency of story reading, number of children's books in the home and adult author checklist) is an important predictor of reading readiness. The home literacy environment has been found to be associated with early reading and may at least in part mediate the effects of socioeconomic status (Sénéchal and LeFevre 2002, 2014). The second crucial factor is general child health including premature birth, birth complications, hearing problems, visual problems, physical difficulties, significant accidents.

11.3.5 Further Scientific Approaches to Aetiology: Imaging–Genetics and Gene–Environment Interaction in DD

Increasing numbers of studies have evaluated imaging–genetics integration as well as gene–environment interaction in DD. The results are still not sufficient to unravel the complexity of the reading circuit, owing to heterogeneous study designs and data processing. Nevertheless, neuroimaging and genetics and gene–environment research have substantially enhanced understanding of the mechanisms underlying atypical reading development and DD. By using imaging techniques, it is established, for example, that:

- CNTNAP2 is associated with structural brain connectivity and brain activation in BA7, BA44 and BA21 during language processing tasks in healthy individuals.
- GRIN2B is negatively correlated with dorsolateral prefrontal cortex activity during working-memory-related tasks.
- DCDC2 is associated with individual differences in cortical thickness.
- There are associations between DCDC2-READ1 and brain activation in the left antero-inferior parietal lobe and in the right lateral occipital temporal gyrus during reading tasks.

Performing joint genetic and neuroimaging studies in humans, where the association between genotypes and brain phenotypes can be tested, is an emerging strategy to link DD-candidate genes to brain structure and function. Despite neuroimaging techniques playing a fundamental part in explaining the role of genes in the aetiology of complex cognitive functions such as reading and writing, the complexity of the reading process is still far from being completely understood.

There is some evidence that children select specific environments as a result of genotype (Peterson and Pennington 2015). Even at preschool age, children who later develop dyslexia avoid being read to and spend less time looking at books than their siblings who will not develop the disorder (Scarborough et al. 1991). At school age, they read many fewer words per year than children who are not affected (Cunningham and Stanovich 1998). But 'if the environment is enriched for literacy development as we assume it is among better educated parents, [persistent] deficits in reading are more likely to be driven by genotype' (Pennington and Smith 2009).

Vanderauwera et al. (2019) have proposed a relationship between paternal educational level and a specific white matter pathway that is important for reading, aiming to guide future research that can determine processes underlying this relationship. The relation between socio-economic status (SES), quantified by paternal educational level, reading of the offspring and the structure of white matter pathways in the left hemisphere, as derived from DTI-based tractography analyses, has been shown. The results demonstrated a relation between word reading, SES quantified by paternal educational level, and fractional anisotropy (FA) within the left dorsal AF segment and the left ventral UF.

11.3.6 Summary and Clinical Implications

Developmental dyslexia is understood as a specific disability in particular brain functions leading to impaired reading acquisition. It is classified as a neurodevelopmental disorder that runs in families. Dyslexia is the outcome of multiple risk factors (Catts and Petscher 2022, Dilnot et al. 2017, Thompson et al. 2015). All findings mentioned show that neuroimaging, genetic research and environment have substantially enhanced the understanding of the mechanisms underlying developmental dyslexia (Mascheretti et al. 2017). Family risk of dyslexia is thus best conceptualised, not purely as a proxy for genetic risk, but as reflecting gene–environment interplay. The imaging–genetics approach and gene–environment interaction are promising ways to unravel new insights behind the pathophysiology of reading (dis)ability.

The potential plasticity of brain development allows compensation to a large degree, given early detection of this disability and a supportive educational environment, including training programmes specifically devised for dyslexic children. A profound knowledge of the specific developmental precursors of an impaired acquisition of reading and spelling skills, such as deficits in phonological awareness and visual attention, can substantially permit early detection and preventive measures in preschool educational and therapeutic settings.

11.4 Neurocognitive Background and Theories Concerning Dyslexia

Barbara Maciejewska,
Bozena Wiskirska-Woznica,
and Ben A. M. Maassen

11.4.1 Developmental Dyslexia: Specific Reading Disability

Developmental dyslexia (DD), or specific reading disability, is defined as a type of learning disorder characterised by the inability to acquire typical reading and writing skills, despite unimpaired fluid intelligence and adequate educational opportunities. Most commonly, in clinical practice, a consultation is provoked in the first two years of primary school because of difficulties with written language (Habib 2021). The disorder is observed in children who, despite conventional classroom experience, fail to attain the language skills of reading, writing and spelling commensurate with their intellectual abilities (Tschentscher et al. 2019; Prestes and Feitosa 2016). DD as a neurodevelopmental disorder is contributed to by multiple neural and cognitive factors and activities (Moreau et al. 2018; Hancock et al. 2017; Nicolson and Fawcett 2019). These include linguistic processes (phonological, semantic and morphological; syntactic and pragmatic) as well as visual and auditory decoding processes (related to sensory and higher-level processes). Together, they facilitate the establishment of fixed associations between the spoken and written equivalents of words. So, complex connections between language, writing and reading are part of what confronts a child in learning to read (Perfetti and Harris 2013).

11.4.2 The Neurobiological Basis of Dyslexia

Developmental dyslexia is a heterogeneous disorder whose main cause is still unknown. However, for more than a century, scientists have focused their attention on the neurobiological basis of language and reading. The notion of the role of neurobiological factors in dyslexia is contained in the definition—dyslexia is understood as a cognitive disability of constitutional origin. Over the last twenty years, scientific findings in neuroscience and neuroimaging supported our understanding of dyslexia as a neurological disorder, aiming at some coherence between diverse theories (Habib 2021).

Many brain areas are engaged in reading and writing processes (Danelli et al. 2013; Dronkers and Ogar 2004; Bloom et al. 2013; Kershner 2015). These include visual and hearing pathways, the occipital lobe with the primary and secondary visual areas, the temporal lobe with the primary and secondary auditory areas and posteriori speech area (Wernicke's area) in the left hemisphere, the temporo-parieto-occipital junction with supramarginal and angular gyri, the insula, the frontal lobes with premotor and motor areas as well as Broca's area, and finally the non-neo-cortical structures of cerebellum, pyramidal and extrapyramidal tracts, and the limbic system responsible for the analysis of intonation, melody, rhythm. What is interesting is that the brain areas involved in reading/language skills seem to change during development. As a result children, adolescents and adults use their brains differently during a simple reading task.

Many evaluations of dyslexic brains (post mortem and neuroimaging) have revealed neuroanatomical as well as neurophysiological differences from brains of normal readers. Most neuroscientific research has investigated abnormalities in DD at the cerebral cortex level and treat dyslexia as a dysfunction in cortical connectivity (for review, see Vandermosten et al. 2012b). However, there is also evidence of dyslexia-related alterations in subcortical regions (e.g. in the left auditory thalamus-medial geniculate body MGB) and auditory brainstem (Tschentscher et al. 2019). Independent studies using functional brain imaging identified brain substrates of different linguistic forms of dyslexia (Habib 2021). The findings of such research have become the origin of neuronal basis of dyslexia (Eckert et al. 2003; Wajuihian 2011, 2012).

11.4.2.1 Abnormal Morphology of Dyslexics' Brains

Research has linked abnormal morphology of certain brain areas to DD. A detailed review of the neurobiology of DD has resulted from past autopsy studies and current structural imaging studies (computed tomography—CT and magnetic resonance imaging—MRI). However, anatomically atypical structures of the brain are not limited to a single area. At the very beginning, examination of post-mortem brains showed several histological differences in dyslexics. The analysis of cortical pathology demonstrated the presence of subtle cortical malformations, cortical scars, dyslaminations and ectopias (Bloom et al. 2013; Galaburda 1993; Stein 2001). Specifically, dyslexia has been linked to neurobiological abnormalities in Broca's area, the angular gyrus, the planum temporale (PT) and the surrounding perisylvian cortex, the lateral/medial geniculate nucleus of the thalamus, the occipital cortex and the corpus callosum. Of these, the region of the planum temporale, corpus callosum and arcuate fasciculus have received the most attention from researchers, as it is believed to play a pivotal role in the neurolinguistic deficits typically reported in dyslexia (Bloom et al. 2013; Kershner 2015). Substantial malformations in brain areas such as the corpus callosum (CC), planum temporale, thalamus and cortex can be found in Wajuihian's papers (2011, 2012) on DD.

Eckert et al. (2003) measured and analysed the inferior frontal gyrus, cerebellum, insula, caudate, corpus callosum, left temporal lobe and thalamus. Bloom et al. (2013) examined the planum temporale in *dyslexic* brains, as did *Galaburda* et al. (1985), and found that planum temporale asymmetry was altered in children with DD. The function of the PT, as demonstrated by functional imaging, may be related to acoustic processing, phonological decoding and language tasks (also see below).

11.4.2.2 Brain Networks Involved in Dyslexia

A major development in brain imaging research has been observed because of new tools for investigating not only structure but also function and network connections. Being non-invasive and allowing in vivo studies, magnetic resonance imaging (MRI) has been used to investigate different abnormalities in DD patients such as morphological, structural and functional ones. Voxel-based morphometry (VBM) is used to quantify grey- and white-matter volumes. Altered grey-matter density has been identified in several areas of the brain (left temporal and parietal regions, the fusiform gyrus, lingual gyrus, temporo-parieto-occipital junction, frontal lobe, planum temporale, inferior temporal cortex, caudate, thalamus and cerebellum, the right parietal lobe: Mascheretti et al. 2017). Altered white-matter density was found in the bilateral temporal and frontal lobes, in the left cuneus and arcuate fasciculus, and in the right precuneus and cerebellum. Functional MRI (fMRI) investigates the brain areas activated while performing specific cognitive and sensory, phonological and semantic tasks, such as integration of letters and speech, visual perception and attention, and working memory and auditory tasks. fMRI is an important tool used to understand the pathophysiology of dyslexia. Altered activations were found in subjects with dyslexia in the following areas: the left hemispheric temporo-parietal regions (Brodman's areas 20, 21, 37, superior and middle temporal gyrus, operculum, supplementary motor area) and the bilateral frontal and occipital areas (Brodman's areas 44, 45, and inferior and middle frontal gyrus, visual areas and extrastriate cortex) (Mascheretti et al. 2017). Diffusion tensor imaging (DTI) detects alterations in white-matter structure and in the neuronal fibre pathways. Changes in dyslexics have been localised in bilateral tracts within the frontal, temporal, occipital and parietal lobes, in the superior longitudinal fasciculus, in the left superior corona radiata, in the left centrum semiovale, in the left inferior frontal gyrus and temporo-parietal white matter, in the left middle and inferior temporal gyri, in the left arcuate fasciculus and in the corpus callosum (Mascheretti et al. 2017).

As a result, the major recent development in cognitive neuroscience has been the identification of a range of neural networks that develop in early childhood (Nicolson and Fawcett 2019; Moreau et al. 2018). Current research suggests that the neurobiological substrate of dyslexia involves the dysfunction of a multi-dimensional circuitry of at least three left hemispheric neuronal networks. This circuitry involves:

- The posterior occipito-temporal network (ventral circuit, including the visual word form area), which responds rapidly in word identification.
- The posterior temporo-parietal network (dorsal circuit, containing the angular gyrus, the supra-angular gyrus and Wernicke's Areas), which has been linked to phoneme level word analysis, and is associated with slow decoding.
- The anterior network of the inferior frontal gyrus (IFG) including Broca's area (appears to be associated with fine-grained, speech-gestural (articulatory), phonological recording and functions in silent reading and naming) (Moreau et al. 2018; Pugh et al. 2001).

Multiple neuroimaging studies show under-activation in dyslectics during reading-related tasks, in the left posterior temporo-parietal and occipito-temporal regions of the cortex, but increased activation of the left and right inferior frontal gyri (IFG). Such hyperactivation of the anterior reading network is a type of compensatory strategy—dyslectics use memorisation of the structure of the words to read, not phonological skills as do normal readers; this explains why they over-engage in frontal brain regions (Moreau et al. 2018; Hoeft et al. 2011). Because of these compensatory processes, it is possible to overcome dysfunctions in the left posterior cortical areas subserving phonological and orthographic processes (Moreau et al. 2018; Pugh et al.; Hoeft et al. 2011; Sanfilippo et al. 2019). Functional neuroimaging studies of dyslexia have focused mainly on identifying the neural correlates of dyslexia, but have also identified neural systems that could mediate successful remediation. Greater right prefrontal activation during a reading task that demands phonological awareness and white-matter organisation in the right superior longitudinal fasciculus (including the arcuate fasciculus) can significantly predict future reading gains in dyslexia. These findings identify right prefrontal brain mechanisms that may be critical for reading improvement in dyslexia and that may differ from typical reading development (Sanfilippo et al. 2019). Moreover, the changes in brain activity are the same regardless of the mother tongue (Dębska et al. 2016). Habib, in his article on the neurological basis of developmental dyslexia, cites recent research on the role of the cerebellum in dyslexia, indicating that there are no specific differences in the cerebellum in dyslexic individuals compared to normal readers: 'the cerebellum is the best biomarker of developmental dyslexia'. Although there are studies of the cerebellum in people with dyslexia that have generally found no significant specific differences in the morphology and function of the organ compared to normal readers, however, functional connectivity studies provide positive findings regarding the cerebellum (Habib 2021).

11.4.2.3 Subcortical Structures

Recent evidence points towards sensory thalamus dysfunctions: dyslexics show reduced responses in the left auditory thalamus during speech processing in contrast to neurotypical readers. Studies have revealed that dyslexics have reduced white-matter connectivity in a cortico-thalamic auditory pathway between the left auditory motion-sensitive planum temporale (mPT) and the left medial geniculate body (MGB)—left mPT-MGB connectivity. The reconstruction of the fibre structures between the mPT and the MGB revealed that dyslexics have less fibre connectivity in the left hemisphere of the brain than people from the control group. In contrast, the controls showed very strong fibre connectivity between mPT and MGB, particularly those who performed extremely well in the reading test (Tschentscher et al. 2019).

In summary:

- Increasingly, data show that persons with developmental dyslexia have structural and functional dysfunctions in the cerebral cortex, as well as in the cerebellum and subcortical structures. These differences between dyslexic and typical readers need to be interpreted with caution regarding the direction of causality: differences in structure and function of the brain could be the cause as well as the consequence of the dyslexia. Not only compensatory processes, but also poorer development of the visual word form area, could very well be the consequence of reading difficulties, rather than the cause.

- Decreased activity of the left hemisphere in the linguistic temporo-parietal area can be observed in dyslexics, while activity is increased in the frontal lobes. Disturbances point to disruption of left-hemispheric connections and poor synchronisation of reading/writing areas.
- Dyslexics show reduced responses in the left auditory thalamus (medial geniculate body, MGB) during speech processing in contrast to neurotypical readers.

11.4.3 Current Explanatory Theories of Dyslexia

No doubt DD is a complex, high-order phonological-linguistic processing deficit, rather than a visual or audiological letter recognition one. Reading involves extracting linguistic information from the visual code that represents speech (Prestes and Feitosa 2016). A range of impairments has been reported to be associated with dyslexia, and diverse theories and mechanisms have been proposed to account for the neurological aspects of the condition and linguistic defects related to it. Many different concepts and models have been created as the main dyslectic theory. These include deficits in several modalities as well as in cross-modal functions. Some of them are not strong or have been queried, such as cognitive deficit theories of dyslexia, selective attention, associative learning, cross-modal transfer, serial-order processing, and both pattern analysis and rule learning (Vellutino et al. 2004). The magnocellular theory, the temporal processing deficit hypothesis, the left-mini-neglect syndrome, and the role of the parietal lobe have also been strongly disputed. Most recently, studies have produced strong support in some individuals with dyslexia for deficits in spatial and auditory attention (Ruffino et al. 2014), visual magnocellular-dorsal pathway deficits (Gori et al. 2015), deficits in cerebellar functions (Van Ermingen et al. 2013) and deficits in inter-hemispheric processing (Welcome and Joanisse 2014). The present predominant view is that dyslexia is a multifactorial disorder (Pennington et al. 2012), with a deficit in the phonological domain predominating (Prestes and Feitosa 2016).

11.4.3.1 Phonology and Its Role in Developmental Dyslexia

A vital component in the development of phonological representations is the awareness of individual speech sounds. Phonological awareness is the ability to detect, process and manipulate the sound structure of words.

Reading and spelling both require phonological skills, and in their turn foster phonological skills and phonological awareness. The latter plays an important role in children's ability to create grapheme-to-phoneme correspondence (Pennington et al. 2012). This ability at the age of 4–5 years precedes reading, and rapidly develops during the initial stages of reading acquisition (age 6–9 in most school systems). The most influential cause of difficulties in learning to read is the failure to acquire phonological awareness and skills in alphabetic coding. There is a large body of evidence indicating that the domain of the relationship between graphemes and phonemes is crucial to learning reading and writing. The learning of reading and writing demands complex levels of phonological knowledge: it requires the proper representation of the smallest sound elements of the language (phonemes), a good ability of reflecting on these elements, and knowledge that such sounds may be represented by different graphemes (Prestes and Feitosa 2016; Hebert et al. 2018).

The main competing theories of developmental dyslexia, based on phonological coding, are on phonological, allophonic and hearing deficits.

Phonological Deficit Theory This postulates that the reading difficulties are attributable to problems in phonological processing, that is, deconstructing a word into separate, constituent sounds (Nicolson and Fawcett 2019). Phonological awareness is characteristically deficient (or lacking) in reading-disabled readers who, as a consequence, have difficulty mapping the alphabetic characters of print onto the spoken word (Pugh et al. 2001). There are three specific brain regional neuronal networks identified within phonological circuitry (posterior dorsal, posteriori ventral and anterior region) (Moreau et al. 2018; Pugh et al. 2001; Dennis and Thompson 2013; Boets 2014).

Manifestations of this phonological deficit have been observed in, and measured through, three aspects of phonological processing: phonological awareness (PA), verbal short-term memory (the part of our memory system that makes use of the so-called phonological loop) and lexical retrieval of the phonological representation of items (pictures, colours, digits and letters as measured by rapid automatic naming [RAN]) (Landerl and Willburger 2010; Leinenger 2014).

Allophonic Theory According to this theory, dyslexic individuals present change on speech perception—they do not integrate the allophonic characteristics into phonemic characteristics during speech perception development (Noordenbos and Serniclaes 2015). As a result, phonological dyslexia seems to be a specific disability of speech perception that is characterised by the use of allophonic units, rather than phonemic ones (allophonic perception) (Serniclaes et al. 2004).

Auditory Deficit Theory The auditory experience is the typical sensorial route that allows children to acquire the phonological representations required to learn the skill of grapheme decoding. According to this theory, auditory deficits during early development disrupt the development of phonological perception and phoneme categorisation. The phonological deficit would be a secondary deficit to a more elementary auditory deficit (Prestes and Feitosa 2016). Speech stimuli are acoustic signals, so a deficit in auditory temporal processing may lead to difficulty in processing consonants—short acoustic elements (Banai and Kraus 2006). The findings on alterations in auditory processing and speech perception, and their relationships with reading, writing and phonological awareness have different interpretations depending on the theoretical assumptions.

11.4.3.2 Delayed Neural Commitment (DNC): A Network Perspective

The explanation for DD has recently been connected with neuronal networks. A neuronal network perspective is increasingly common owing to major developments in brain imaging research in the past decade. In particular, Diffusion Tensor Imaging (DTI) in combination with fMRI are tools to investigate structure and function at the network level. DTI has allowed the identification of white-matter tracts and yielded the identification of intrinsic connectivity networks. As a result, much cognitive neuroscience research has been focused on the identification of neural networks that develop in early childhood (Nicolson and Fawcett 2019).

The Delayed Neural Commitment (DNC) framework could explain the neural background of developmental dyslexia and provide an important link to the development of networks for language and speech. The main issue is delayed development of neural networks because of a widely understood minimal brain dysfunction. According to DNC theory, dyslexic children take longer than non-dyslexics to build (and to rebuild) the neural networks that underpin the acquisition of reading. DNC explains not only the delay in development of specific skills and of automaticity, but also the delays both in constructing new neural circuits (as required for executive function and for internalised speech) and in bypassing or eliminating the previous, less efficient neural circuits. The neural anomaly generally leads to slower and more effortful processing, difficulties with multi-tasking, and makes habits and new skills less strong. According to Nicolson and Fawcet (2019), DNC is a very broad framework, thereby providing a natural and immediate explanation for many other frameworks (such as phonological deficit, double deficit, phonological access, speech rhythm deficit, visual processing deficit, auditory temporal deficit, automatisation deficit, magnocellular deficit, cerebellar deficit and procedural learning deficit), and thus is able to bring together both the learning framework and a temporal accuracy perspective.

11.4.4 Concluding Remarks

Undoubtedly, reading processes are crucial for an individual's neurocognitive development. DD is a multifactorial disorder, with a wide range of associated behavioural symptoms that cannot be explained by a single deficit. This is why there is still the need for efforts towards building an integrative theory to explain dyslexia. Unfortunately, the main problem now is the so-called wait-to-fail approach to dyslexia diagnosis. In spite of so many theories, interventions are typically not early enough. Rather than wait until age 8 or 9 to diagnose and treat dyslexia, parents, teachers and clinicians should look for predictors of dyslexia in children as early as preschool.

References

Adlof SM, Hogan TP (2018) Understanding dyslexia in the context of developmental language disorder. Lang Speech Hear Serv Sch 49(4):762–773

Altarelli I, Leroy F, Monzalvo K et al (2014) Planum temporale asymmetry in developmental dyslexia: revisiting an old question. Hum Brain Mapp 35(12):5717–5735

American Psychiatric Association (2013) Diagnostic and statistical manual of mental disorders, 5th edn. American Psychiatric Publishing, Arlington

Banai K, Kraus N (2006) Neurobiology of (central) auditory processing disorder and language-based learning disability. In: Musiek FE, Chermak GD (eds) Handbook of (central) auditory processing disorder: auditory neuroscience and diagnosis. Plural Publishing, San Diego, pp 89–116

Becker J, Czamara D, Scerri T et al (2014) Genetic analysis of dyslexia candidate genes in the European cross-linguistic NeuroDys cohort. Eur J Hum Genet 22(5):675–680

Bekebrede JI, Van der Leij A, Share DL (2009) Dutch dyslexic adolescents: phonological-core variable-orthographic differences. Read Writ 22(2):133–165

Berninger VW, Nielsen KH, Abbott RD et al (2008) Gender differences in severity of writing and reading disabilities. J Sch Psychol 46(2):151–172

Bloom JS, Garcia-Barrera MA, Miller CJ et al (2013) Planum temporale morphology in children with developmental dyslexia. Neuropsychologia 51(9):1684–1692

Boada R, Pennington BF (2006) Deficient implicit phonological representations in children with dyslexia. J Exp Child Psychol 95(3):153–193

Boets B (2014) Dyslexia: reconciling controversies within an integrated developmental perspective. Trends Cogn Sci 18(10):501–503

Borleffs E, Maassen BAM, Lyytinen H et al (2019) Cracking the code: the impact of orthographic transparency and morphological-syllabic complexity on reading and developmental dyslexia. Front Psychol 9:2534. https://doi.org/10.3389/fpsyg.2018.02534. Accessed 4 Sep 2010

Castles A, Coltheart M (1993) Varieties of developmental dyslexia. Cognition 47(2):149–180

Catts HW, Petscher Y (2022). A cumulative risk and resiliencemodel of dyslexia. Journal of Learning Disabilities, 55(3), 171–184.

Cunningham AE, Stanovich KE (1998) The impact of print exposure on word recognition. In: Metsala JL, Ehri LC (eds) Word recognition in beginning literacy. Erlbaum, Hillsdale, pp 235–263

Danelli L, Berlingeri M, Bottini G et al (2013) Human brain mapping. Neural intersections of the phonological, visual magnocellular, and motor/cerebellar systems in normal readers: implications for imaging studies on dyslexia. Hum Brain Mapp 34(10):2669–2687

Dębska A, Łuniewska M, Chyl K et al (2016) Neural basis of phonological awareness in beginning readers with familial risk of dyslexia—results from shallow orthography. NeuroImage 132:406–416

Dennis E, Thompson P (2013) Mapping connectivity in the developing brain. Int J Dev Neurosci 31(7):525–542

Dilling H, Freyberger H (2012) Taschenführer ICD-10 Klassifikation psychischer Störungen (Pocket guide ICD-10 classification of mental disorders), 6th edn. Huber, Bern

Dilnot J, Hamilton L, Maughan B, Snowling MJ (2017) Child and environmental risk factors predicting readiness for learning in children at high risk of dyslexia. Dev Psychopathol 29(1):235–244

Dronkers N, Ogar J (2004) Brain areas involved in speech production. Brain 127(7):1461–1462

Eckert MA, Leonard CM, Richards TL et al (2003) Anatomical correlates of dyslexia: frontal and cerebellar findings. Brain 126(2):482–494

Ferrer E, Shaywitz BA, Holahan JM et al (2015) Achievement gap in reading is present as early as first grade and persists through adolescence. J Pediatr 167(5):1121–1125

Fluss J, Ziegler J, Ecalle J et al (2008) Prevalence of reading disabilities in early elementary school: impact of socioeconomic environment on reading development in 3 different educational zones. Arch Pediatr 15(6):1049–1057

Frith U (1980) Unexpected spelling problems. In: Frith U (ed) Cognitive processes in spelling. Academic Press, London, pp 495–515

Galaburda AM (1993) Neuroanatomic basis of developmental dyslexia. Neurol Clin 11(1):161–173

Galaburda AM, Kemper TL (1979) Developmental dyslexia: four consecutive patients with cortical anomalies. Ann Neurol 6(2):94–100

Galaburda AM, Sherman GF, Rosen GD et al (1985) Developmental dyslexia: four consecutive patients with cortical anomalies. Ann Neurol 18(2):222–233

Gilger JW, Hanebuth E, Smith SD et al (1996) Differential risk for developmental reading disorders in the offspring of compensated versus noncompensated parents. Read Writ 8(5):407–417

Gori S, Cecchini P, Bigoni A et al (2015) Magnocellular-dorsalpathway and sub-lexical route in developmental dyslexia. Front Hum Neurosci 8:460. https://doi.org/10.3389/fnhum.2014.00460

Günther KB (1986) Ein Stufenmodell der Entwicklung kindlicher Lese- und Schreibstrategien (A step-by-step model for developing children's reading and writing strategies). In: Brügelmann H (ed) ABC und Schriftsprache (ABC and written language). Libelle, Konstanz

Habib M (2000) The neurological basis of developmental dyslexia. An overview and working hypothesis. Brain 123:2373–2399

Habib M (2021). The Neurological Basis of Developmental Dyslexiaand Related Disorders: A Reappraisal of the Temporal Hypothesis, Twenty Yearson. Brain Sci. 11(6):708. https://doi.org/10.3390/brainsci11060708. PMID:34071786; PMCID: PMC8229928.

Hancock R, Pugh KR, Hoeft F (2017) Neural noise hypothesis of developmental dyslexia. Trends Cogn Sci 21(6):434–448

Hasselhorn M, Schuchardt K (2006) Lernstörungen-Eine kritische Skizze zur Epidemiologie (Learning disabilities—a critical sketch on epidemiology). Kindheit Entwicklung 15:208–215

Hebert M, Kearns DM, Hayes JB et al (2018) Why children with dyslexia struggle with writing and how to help them. Lang Speech Hear Serv Sch 49(4):843–863

Hoeft F, McCandliss BD, Black JM et al (2011) Neural systems predicting long-term outcome in dyslexia. Proc Natl Acad Sci U S A 108(1):361–366

Hoover W, Gough P (1990) The simple view of reading. Read Writ 2(2):127–160

Hulme C, Snowling MJ (2014) The interface between spoken and written language: developmental disorders. Philos Trans R Soc B 369:20120395. https://doi.org/10.1098/rstb.2012.0395. Accessed 4 Sep 2010

Kalashnikova M, Goswami U, Burnham D (2019) Delayed development of phonological constancy in toddlers at family risk for dyslexia. Infant Behav Dev 57:101327. https://doi.org/10.1016/j.infbeh.2019.101327. Accessed 4 Sep 2021

Katusic SK, Colligan RC, Barbaresi WJ et al (2001) Incidence of reading disability in a population-based birth cohort, 1976–1982, Rochester, Minn. Mayo Clin Proc 76(11):1081–1092

Kershner JR (2015) A mini-review: toward a comprehensive theory of dyslexia. J Neurol Neurosci:1–6. https://doi.org/10.21767/2171-6625.S10013

Klicpera C, Schabmann A, Gasteiger-Klicpera B (2013) Legasthenie—LRS (dyslexia), 4th edn. Reinhardt UTB, Munich

Landerl K, Willburger E (2010) Temporal processing, attention, and learning disorders. Learn Individ Differ 20(5):393–401

Landerl K, Ramus F, Moll K et al (2013) Predictors of developmental dyslexia in European orthographies with varying complexity. J Child Psychol Psychiatry 54(6):686–694

Leinenger M (2014) Phonological coding during reading. Psychol Bull 140(6):1534–1555

Leppänen PH, Lyytinen H (1997) Auditory event-related potentials in the study of developmental language-related disorders. Audiol Neurootol 2(5):308–340

Lewis C, Hitch GJ, Walker P (1994) The prevalence of specific arithmetic difficulties and specific reading difficulties in 9- to 10-year-old boys and girls. J Child Psychol Psychiatry 35(2):283–292

Łuniewska M, Chyl K, Dębska A et al (2019) Children with dyslexia and familial risk for dyslexia present atypical development of the neuronal phonological network. Front Neurosci 13:1287. https://doi.org/10.3389/fnins.2019.01287

Lyon GR, Shaywitz SE, Shaywitz BA (2003) A definition of dyslexia. Part I defining dyslexia, comorbidity, teachers' knowledge of language and reading; a definition of dyslexia. Ann Dyslexia 53(1):1–14

Maciejewska B, Wiskirska-Woźnica B, Świdziński P et al (2013) Evaluation of auditory event-related potentials (ERPs) in children with the familial dyslexia. Otorynolaryngology 12(1):34–41

Mascheretti S, De Luca A, Trezzi V et al (2017) Neurogenetics of developmental dyslexia: from genes to behavior through brain neuroimaging and cognitive and sensorial mechanisms. Transl Psychiatry 7(1):e987. https://doi.org/10.1038/tp.2016.240

Moreau D, Stonyer JE, McKay NS et al (2018) No evidence for systemic white matter correlates of dyslexia: an activation liklihood estimation meta-analysis. Brain Res 1683:36–47

Munzer T, HussainK SN (2020) Dyslexia: neurobiology, clinical features, evaluation and management. Transl Pediatr 9(Suppl 1):S36–S45

Nicolson RI, Fawcett AJ (2019) Development of dyslexia: the delayed neural commitment framework. Front Behav Neurosci 13:112. https://doi.org/10.3389/fnbeh.2019.00112

Noordenbos MW, Serniclaes W (2015) The categorical perception deficit in dyslexia: a meta-analysis. Sci Stud Read 19(5):340–359

Olson RK (2002) Dyslexia: nature and nurture. Dyslexia 8:143–159

Olson RK (2007) Genes, environment, and dyslexia. The 2005 Norman Geschwind Memorial Lecture. Ann Dyslexia 56:205–238

Pennington BF (2006) From single to multiple deficit models of developmental disorders. Cognition 101(2):385–413

Pennington BF, Smith SD (2009) Gene x environment interactions in reading disability and attention-deficit/hyperactivity disorder. Dev Psychol 45(1):77–89

Pennington BF, Santerre-Lemmon L, Rosenberg J et al (2012) Individual prediction of dyslexia by single versus multiple deficit models. J Abnorm Psychol 121(1):212–224

Perfetti CA, Harris LN (2013) Universal reading processes are modulated by language and writing system. Lang Learn Dev 9(4):296–316

Prestes MRD, Feitosa MAG (2016) Theories of dyslexia: support by changes in auditory perception. Psic Teor e Pesq Brasilia 32:1–9

Price CJ, Friston KJ (1997) The temporal dynamics of reading: a PET study. Proc R Soc Lond B Biol Sci 264(1389):1785–1791

Price CJ, Wise RJS, Warburton EA et al (1996) Hearing and saying: the functional neuro-anatomy of auditory word processing. Brain 119(3):919–931

Pugh KR, Mencl WE, Jenner AR et al (2001) Neurobiological studies of reading and reading disability. J Commun Disord 34(6):479–492

Raschle NM, Stering PL, Meissner SN et al (2014) Altered neuronal response during rapid auditory processing and its relation to phonological processing in prereading children at familial risk for dyslexia. Cereb Cortex 24:2489–2501

Raskind WH, Hsu L, Berninger VW et al (2000) Familial aggregation of dyslexia phenotypes. Behav Genet 30(5):385–396

Ring J, Black J (2018) The multiple deficit model of dyslexia: what does it mean for identification and intervention? Ann Dyslexia 68(2):104–125

Rothou KM, Padeliadu S (2019) Morphological processing influences on dyslexia in Greek-speaking children. Ann Dyslexia 69(3):261–278

Ruffino M, Gori S, Boccardi D et al (2014) Spatial and temporal attention in developmental dyslexia. Front Hum Neurosci 8:331. https://doi.org/10.3389/fnhum.2014.00331

Rutter M, Yule W (1975) The concept of specific reading retardation. J Child Psychol Psychiatry 16(3):181–197

Rutter M, Caspi A, Fergusson D et al (2004) Sex differences in developmental reading disability: new findings from 4 epidemiological studies. JAMA 291(16):2007–2012

Sanfilippo J, Ness M, Petscher Y et al (2019) Reintroducing dyslexia: early identification and implications for pediatric practice. Pediatrics 146(1):e20193046. https://doi.org/10.1542/peds.2019-3046

Scarborough HS, Dobrich W, Hager M (1991) Preschool literacy experience and later reading achievement. J Learn Disabil 24:508–511

Scerri TS, Schulte-Körne G (2010) Genetics of developmental dyslexia. Eur Child Adolesc Psychiatry 19:179–197

Schaadt G, Männel C (2019) Phonemes, words, and phrases: tracking phonological processing in preschoolers developing dyslexia. Clin Neurophysiol 130(8):1329–1341

Scheerer-Neumann G (2001a) Rechtschreibschwäche im Kontext der Entwicklung (Spelling difficulties in the context of development). In: Naegele I, Valtin R (eds) LRS – Legasthenie in den Klassen 1–10. Handbuch der Lese- und Rechtschreibschwierigkeiten. Vol 1: Grundlagen und Grundsätze der Lese-Rechtschreib-Förderung (Dyslexia in grades 1–10. Handbook of reading and spelling difficulties, vol 1: Fundamentals and principles of reading and spelling support). Beltz, Weinheim, pp 58–77

Scheerer-Neumann G (2001b) Förderdiagnostik beim Lesenlernen (Funding diagnostics when learning to read). In: Naegele I, Valtin R (eds) LRS – Legasthenie in den Klassen 1–10. Handbuch der Lese- und Rechtschreibschwierigkeiten Vol 2: Schulische Förderung und außerschulische Therapien (LRS) (Dyslexia in grades 1–10. Handbook of reading and spelling difficulties, Vol 2: School support and extracurricular therapies). Beltz, Weinheim, pp 70–86

Schleider K (2009) Lese- und Rechtschreibstörungen (Reading and spelling disorders). UTB Profile: Ernst Reinhardt Verlag, Munich, pp 79–83

Schulte-Körne G (2002) Neurobiologie und Genetik der Lese-/Rechtschreibstörung (Legasthenie): Zum aktuellen Stand der Ursachenforschung, der diagnostischen Methoden und der Förderkonzepte. Winkler, Bochum

Schulte-Körne G (2010) The prevention, diagnosis, and treatment of dyslexia. Dtsch Arztebl Int 107(41):718–726

Schulte-Körne G, Galuschka K (2015) Diagnostik und Behandlung von Kindern und Jugendlichen mit Lese- und/oder Rechtschreibstörung. S3-Leitinie AWMF-Register-Nr. 028-044. https://www.bvl-legasthenie.de/images/static/pdfs/Leitlinien/LF_Leitlinie.pdf. Accessed 12 Jul 2020

Schulte-Körne G, Warnk A, Remschmidt H (2006) Zur Genetik der Lese-Rechtschreib-Schwäche. Z Kinder Jugendpsychiatr Psychother 34(6):435–444

Schumacher J, Hoffmann P, Schmäl C et al (2007) Genetics of dyslexia: the evolving landscape. J Med Genet 44(5):289–297

Sénéchal M, LeFevre JA (2002) Parental involvement in the development of children's reading skill: a five-year longitudinal study. Child Dev 73(2):445–460

Sénéchal M, LeFevre J (2014) Continuity and change in the home literacy environment as predictors of growth in vocabulary and reading. Child Dev 85:1535–1551

Serniclaes W, Van Heghe S, Mousty P et al (2004) Allophonic mode of speech perception in dyslexia. J Exp Child Psychol 87(4):336–361

Snowling MJ, Hulme C (2012) Annual research review: the nature and classification of reading disorders—a commentary on proposals for DSM-5. J Child Psychol Psychiatry 53(5):593–607

Snowling MJ, Melby-Lervåg M (2016) Oral language deficits in familial dyslexia: a meta-analysis and review. Psychol Bull 142(5):498–545

Snowling MJ, Gallagher A, Frith U (2003) Family risk of dyslexia is continuous: individual differences in the precursors of reading skill. Child Dev 74:358–373

Stein J (2001) The magnocellular theory of developmental dyslexia. Dyslexia 7(1):12–36

Suchodoletz W (2006) Therapie der Lese-Rechtschreib-Störung (LRS): traditionelle und alternative Behandlungsmethoden im Überblick (Therapy of dyslexia (LRS): traditional and alternative treatment methods at a glance), 2nd edn. Kohlhammer, Stuttgart

Sun Z, Zou L, Zhang J et al (2013) Prevalence and associated risk factors of dyslexic children in a middle-sized city of China: a cross-sectional study. PLoS One 8(2):e56688. https://doi.org/10.1371/journal.pone.0056688. Accessed 4 Sep 2021

Thompson PA, Hulme C, Nash HM et al (2015) Developmental dyslexia: predicting individual risk. J Child Psychol Psychiatry 56(9):976–987

Tschentscher N, Ruisinger A, Blank H et al (2019) Reduced structural connectivity between left auditory thalamus and the motion-sensitive planum temporale in developmental dyslexia. J Neurosci 39(9):1720–1732

Van Ermingen MM, Grade M, Pape NJ et al (2013) Distinct neural signatures of cognitive subtypes of dyslexia with and without phonological deficits. NeuroImage 2:477–490

Vanderauwera J, van Setten ERH, Maurits NM et al (2019) The interplay of socio-economic status represented by paternal educational level, white matter structure and reading. PLoS One 14(5):e0215560. https://doi.org/10.1371/journal.pone.0215560

Vandermosten M, Boets B, Wouters J et al (2012a) A qualitative and quantitative review of diffusion tensor imaging studies in reading and dyslexia. Neurosci Biobehav Rev 36(6):1532–1552

Vandermosten M, Boets B, Poelmans H et al (2012b) A tractography study in dyslexia: neuroanatomic correlates of orthographic, phonological and speech processing. Brain 135(3):935–948

Vellutino FR, Fletcher JM, Snowling MJ et al (2004) Specific reading disability (dyslexia): what have we learned in the past four decades? J Child Psychol Psychiatry 45(1):2–40

Volkmer S, Schulte-Körne G, Galuschka K (2019) Die Rolle der morphologischen Bewusstheit bei Lese- und Rechtschreibleistungen (The role of morphological awareness in reading and spelling performance). Z Kinder Jugendpsychiatr Psychother 47(4):334–344

Wajuihian SO (2011) Neurobiology of developmental dyslexia: Part 1: a review of evidence from autopsy and structural neuro-imaging studies. S Afr Optom 70(4):191–202

Wajuihian SO (2012) Neurobiology of developmental dyslexia: Part 2: a review of magnetic resonance imaging (MRI) studies of the corpus callosum. S Afr Optom 71(1):39–45

Warnke A (2007) Umschriebene Entwicklungsstörung des Lesens und der Rechtschreibung. In: Herpertz-Dahlmann B, Resch F, Warnke A, Schulte-Markwort M (eds) Entwicklungspsychiatrie– Biopsychologische Grundlagen und die Entwicklung psychischer Störungen, 2nd edn. Schattauer, Stuttgart, pp 534–569

Warnke A, Hemminger U, Plume E (2004) Lese-Rechtschreib-Störungen. Leitfaden Kinder- und Jugendpsychotherapie (Reading and writing disorder. A guide to child and adolescent psychotherapy). Hogrefe, Göttingen

Welcome S, Joanisse M (2014) Individual differences in white matter anatomy predict dissociable components of reading skill in adults. NeuroImage 96:261–275

World Health Organization (2019) ICD-10. https://icd.who.int/browse10/2019/en#/F80-F89. Accessed 12 Jul 2020

Ziegler JC, Goswami U (2005) Reading acquisition, developmental dyslexia, and skilled reading across languages: a psycholinguistic grain size theory. Psychol Bull 131(1):3–29

Ziegler JC, Goswami U (2006) Becoming illiterate in different languages: similar problems, different solutions. Dev Sci 9:429–453

12 Diagnosis and Differential Diagnosis of Literacy Development Disorders

Tahany Abdul Karim Al-Sayed Ahmed, Doris-Eva Bamiou, Nicole Campbell, Mirela Duranovic, Anja Fiori, Mona Hegazi, Christiane Kiese-Himmel, Barbara Maciejewska, David Moore, Katrin Neumann, Georg Romer, Tony Sirimanna, Esther Strittmatter, and Dagmar Weise

12.1 Cognitive, Auditory, Linguistic and Psychomotor Stages of Literacy Acquisition in Normal Individuals of Different Ages

Christiane Kiese-Himmel

12.1.1 Background to Literacy Acquisition

Young children who enter elementary school have to acquire formal symbolic modes of literacy (and numeracy) among other aspects such as alphabetic knowledge, notation system, orthography, sentence semantics, style and writing composition (see Stone et al. 2013). This requires many prerequisites, and in this respect, the development of literacy starts long before school entry (e.g. Hayes 2016), proceeds gradually and continues through adult life.

The onset of this development is mainly defined by the healthy auditory channel of an infant allowing him or her access to auditory information of spoken language in its environment (e. g. Kenner et al. 2017), especially to prosodic information (e.g. supra-segmental, spectral shape, amplitude modulation, phonetic contrasts, rhythm), which help to build up phonological awareness, meaningful units of oral language and listening comprehension. Hence, the acquisition

T. Abdul Karim Al-Sayed Ahmed (✉)
ENT & Audiology, COSMOMID CA Clinic, Salmyia, Kuwait

D.-E. Bamiou
University College London, National Hospital for Neurology and Neurosurgery, London, UK
e-mail: d.bamiou@ucl.ac.uk

N. Campbell
University of Southampton, Southampton, UK
e-mail: N.G.Campbell@soton.ac.uk

M. Duranovic
Department of Speech and Language Pathology, University of Tuzla, Tuzla, Bosnia and Herzegovina

A. Fiori
Muenster Department of Health MDH, University of Applied Science, Muenster, Germany
e-mail: fiori@fh-muenster.de

M. Hegazi
ENT Department, Ain Shams University, Cairo, Egypt

C. Kiese-Himmel
Phoniatrics/Pediatric Audiological Psychology, University Medical Center, Goettingen, Germany
e-mail: c.kiese@med.uni-goettingen.de

A. am Zehnhoff-Dinnesen et al. (eds.), *Phoniatrics II*, European Manual of Medicine,
https://doi.org/10.1007/978-3-031-25175-7_12

of literacy is a developmental continuum starting early in the life of a child with perception and segmentation of the speech stream of those around him or her and even before babies are born, they hear the language spoken around them.

There are many interrelated prerequisites, and as an aside, these interrelationships are also crucial for early identification of literacy difficulties. Reading difficulties are associated with phonological processing deficits (Siegel 1993) and, to a lesser extent, with visual-perceptive deficits (originally regarded as causal in the 1960s and 1970s, e.g. Rosen 1965; Guthrie and Goldberg 1972). Many poor readers have difficulties in phonological skills such as phoneme awareness, phoneme discrimination, phoneme identification, phonological working memory or encoding temporal order (processing of serial order). Phonological deficits at kindergarten age may be predictive of later poor reading (Olofsson and Niedersoe 1999). However, deficits in phonological processing are only present in some individuals, while others show deficits in vocabulary, morphological learning or in visual attention (Le Jan et al. 2011). For children with developmental language disorders 'letter identification' has proved to be a more accurate predictor of poor word reading and the neurodevelopmental disorder 'dyslexia' according to a recent study by Alonzo et al. (2020).

In the following sections, precursors most important for the mechanisms and the development of literacy in schoolchildren aged 6–10 years old are presented. This applies both to monolingual and bilingual children who are growing up. Understanding children's literacy is realising how their individual cognitive, perceptual (especially listening, linguistic and psychomotor) skills develop, and how these structures change with increasing age (see Berk 2013; Brooks and Kempe 2012). All of them affect children's ability to learn in school.

12.1.2 What Kinds of Development Occur?

Development of reading and writing interacts with several other areas of development.

12.1.2.1 Intelligence and General Cognitive Development

This is the increase and alteration of various mental abilities and general knowledge from infancy to adolescence and early adulthood. More rapid and efficient perceptual organisation and information processing speed represent a central aspect of great cognitive power. For example, an increase in processing speed is correlated with changes in 'fluid intelligence', one of the two intelligence factors considered by Cattell (1987), which reflects higher mental abilities (e.g. reasoning). The 'Openness-Fluid-Crystallized-Intelligence-Model' (Ziegler et al. 2012) describes how both intelligence constructs interact in the course of development. More

B. Maciejewska
Department and Clinic of Phoniatrics and Audiology, Poznan University of Medical Sciences, Poznan, Poland
e-mail: barbaramaciejewska@ump.edu.pl

D. Moore
Cincinnati Children's Hospital Medical Center, Cincinnati, OH, USA
e-mail: david.moore2@cchmc.org

K. Neumann
Department of Phoniatrics and Pediatric Audiology, ENT Clinic, St. Elisabeth Hospital, University of Bochum, Bochum, Germany
e-mail: Katrin.neumann@rub.de

G. Romer
University Muenster, Klinik fuer Kinder- und Jugendpsychiatrie, -psychosomatik, und –psychotherapie, Muenster, Germany
e-mail: georg.romer@ukmuenster.de

T. Sirimanna
Audiological Medicine and Cochlear Implant Department, Great Ormond Street Hospital, London, UK

E. Strittmatter
Health Care Centre Walstedde Day Hospital, Drensteinfurt, Germany

D. Weise
Abteilung Neuropädiatrie, Universitätsmedizin Göttingen, Göttingen, Germany
e-mail: dweise@med.uni-goettingen.de

openness leads to more learning opportunities, thereby fostering 'fluid intelligence', accompanied by an indirect positive effect on the 'crystallised intelligence' that reflects acquired knowledge by teaching, classroom learning and self-regulated learning.

There exists an overlap between intelligence and 'executive functions' (Engelhardt et al. 2016). The latter are a set of higher-order cognitive abilities, including supervisory functions, which are viewed as the neuropsychological basis of intelligence. They control and regulate, inter alia, domain-specific abilities both verbal and non-verbal. Other components of executive functions are 'working memory' (correlating broadly with 'fluid intelligence'), 'inhibitory control', 'cognitive flexibility' and 'planning ability'.

At about 6–7 years, children begin to reason logically, but still they cannot think abstractly. The 'concrete-operational stage', the third stage of Piaget's 'Theory and Stages of Cognitive Development' (Piaget 1936), marks the beginning of operational thought. Owing to advancing age, children show an improved understanding of relationships; for instance, they can understand (and tell) jokes. According to the Swiss psychologist Jean Piaget, the systematic way of thinking is reached in the final stage of the cognitive development course, in the formal-operational period at the age of approximately 11 years. For details, see Sect. 9.2 in Volume 1.

12.1.2.2 Phonetic and Phonological Development

This development strand comprises a process of organisation of auditory perception and of learning speech sounds to comprehend the meaning of oral language and forming words (see Stoel-Gammon et al. 2024). Children need to be able to segment the phonemes in spoken words, and later, they must be able to segment the phonemes in lexical structures in order to read their graphic forms. The speech sounds that children perceive, and the words that they speak, are always dependent on the linguistic environment in which they grew up, on the interaction with their parents, grandparents, caregivers or peers in social contexts. How babies acquire phonological knowledge via recognition of speech sounds and words from the auditory input is well described by Marylin May Vihman (2014). The ability to track words in a sentence is acquired by the second year of life. Rhyme awareness starts from 24 to 30 months, followed by the production of rhymes approximately 6 months later. By the age of 4 years, the average pre-school child can recognise words with the same initial sound and can blend an omitted sound into a word. She or he uses all vowels and nearly all consonants in her or his native language (phonetic acquisition), but may have some difficulties with consonants at the end of words. In the age range from 3 to 4 years, normally developing children demonstrate phonological awareness (see definition below), syllable awareness (counting, clapping, tapping, blending or segmenting a word into syllables) and other reading-related phonological processing abilities skills.

Wagner and Torgesen (1987) have identified three kinds of reading-related phonological processing abilities: (a) Phonological awareness, (b) Phonological memory and (c) Phonological access to the lexical store.

- **Phonological Awareness**, the ability to detect, comprehend and manipulate sounds and smaller acoustical units in spoken words, is critical for learning written language and reading success—and vice versa, learning to read and other experiences with written language increase phonological awareness. Insofar as it is a bi-directional development, alphabetic literacy development also causes phonological skills. Phonological awareness arises from children's sound play and rhyming games, and in this way children become over the years increasingly sensitive to smaller units of a word.
- **Phonological Working Memory**, which is the ability to recall immediately linguistic units presented orally (temporary storage), is involved in the learning of language, especially in vocabulary acquisition.
- **Phonological Access to the Lexical Store**, which refers to the fact that phonological representations allow access to lexical entries in the mental lexicon of an individual, thus making oral language the base of literacy.

Reading-related phonological processing abilities of English-speaking pre-schoolers are best characterised by a two-factor model of correlated, yet distinct, factors: factor 1: phonological awareness/phonological memory; factor 2: lexical access (Lonigan et al. 2009). In other words, there is still a lack of distinction between phonological awareness and phonological memory at pre-school age. Nevertheless, it should be noted that phonological awareness depends on the nature of the task used (e.g. rhyme detection or phonological discrimination).

At school entry, children start to experience the connection between language at the phonological level (phonemes) and spelling (letter-speech sound or grapheme-phoneme knowledge) by explicit teaching. Against this background, they learn to identify and to write letters and words by the teaching process (see e. g. Melzi and Schick 2024).

12.1.2.3 Linguistic Development

The base of literacy, a decontextualised symbol system for representing oral language, will be gradually formed by spoken language—and spoken language competence is, inter alia, a strong predictor of academic achievement, defined primarily by reading, writing and mathematics.

In typical linguistic development (see e. g. Gleason and Phillips 2024), word comprehension in everyday contexts occurs before word expression, because infants are sensitive to the prosodic, phonetic-phonological and morphological cues in the speech streams of persons around them. At about 10 months of age, infants have up to 10 words in their lexical comprehension store (receptive vocabulary). These are personal names, so-called performatives such as ‘hello’ or ‘bye’, first object names, soon to be followed by context-bound object words (e.g. ‘car’ when hearing a sound of a car), and first action-words (e.g. verbs describing actions or movements). For most children language production starts with pre-linguistic utterances and becomes more focused when their receptive vocabulary contains between 11 and 50 words.

The first word-combinations (two-word stage) typically emerge when the productive vocabulary consists of approximately 50 words—a green light for syntactic development. This proceeds from one-word sentences and simple sentences via compound and complex sentences to a combination of the latter two. The pre-school child can distinguish words of different grammatical forms and of different word endings, e.g. adverbial endings. Irregular plurals emerge. In the further course, the basic rules of grammar will be learned.

A child’s vocabulary must be large enough for recognising words, or for understanding addition and subtraction tasks to solve problems in maths. In the event of weak phonological awareness, children may need to rely especially heavily on their vocabulary (words as constituents of propositions) demonstrating some knowledge of the structure of language. Progressively, children can understand the meaning of connectives (e.g. ‘although’, ‘but’) and the passive forms of speech (i.e. the object of a sentence becomes the subject). They have knowledge of both word order and the correct grammatical structure of a sentence, and they produce increasingly complex syntactic constructions (syntactic awareness). They can take part in conversations or class discussions and expand their narrative skills in understanding and storytelling. They use the articles correctly, the past perfect tense, an irregular comparative/superlative and make conditional inferences with ‘if-then’ sentences. They acquire plenty of abstract words; those with an emotional association are easier to learn. A more pronounced use of complex and sophisticated mental activity (e.g. idioms), an increasing mental lexicon and a more complex grammar can be observed over the primary-school years (see e. g. Guasti 2016, Zukowski and Ratner 2024). Their spatial communication skills increase, and by age 10 most children can follow five commands in row. Children with speech and language difficulties often demonstrate literacy problems (e. g. De Thorne et al. 2006; Murphy et al. 2016; McLeod et al. 2017; Alonzo et al. 2020).

12.1.2.4 Psychomotor Development (See Sect. 9.2 in Volume 1)

This line of development reflects brain maturation and interaction with the external environment to build and improve functional abilities for the development of gross and fine motor skills, balance, movement patterns and coordinated actions. Psychomotor development itself depends on cognitive, perceptual, motor and affective capacities (Cioni and Sgandurra 2013). This is precisely why playing games and playful activities support not only the child's mental, linguistic and emotional-social development, but also his or her psychomotor development, which in turn is a great help for such psychological components as self-knowledge, self-awareness, self-concept.

When the individual developmental motor precursors are biologically mature, a healthy child can initiate motor processes such as fine finger movement, from the ages of 6 to 12 months, and at later stages, from 5 to 6 years for example, handclapping to segment syllables in acoustically decoding words, drawing letters or writing his or her name. Besides such fine motor skills, visual-motor integration, motor planning and cognitive planning underlie the ability of handwriting—another essential skill for a schoolchild and his or her academic progress. Gradually, children learn to identify and to write letters and words in the alphabetic writing system by the teaching process, in Western culture in a linear fashion from left to right. Details for this are provided in a review about handwriting development from Feder and Majnemer (2007). The development of handwriting proficiency comprises two independent features, more specifically measures: quality (legibility) and speed (e.g. Karlsdottir and Stefansson 2002) whereby speed develops in a linear way throughout primary school and continues up to the age of 13–15 years.

Physical activity, engagement in sports or physical education, is clearly related to academic achievement in primary school (Becker et al. 2014). Therefore, physical education is of great importance for pre-school children's psychomotor development (Teixeira Costa et al. 2015), and those responsible for a child's education should offer a variety of situations, learning opportunities and expressive possibilities to encourage his or her development through the use of the body. According to a study published by Kacenelenbogen et al. (2016), young children exhibit slower progression in psychomotor development, especially in language and graphic abilities, when their parents are separated, probably resulting in less time spent playing and moving with them.

Children in mid-childhood (and in adolescence) develop increased global coordination involving arms, hands, fingers, feet. Their movements become increasingly precise and complex, motor performances such as balance, speed or laterality will be refined, the use of precision instruments as well as prolonged endurance and concentration emerge.

12.1.3 Supporting the Developmental Pathway

Read-aloud sessions of caregivers or regular storytelling without a book, but only by speaking voice modulation, exaggerated facial expressions and gestures will greatly benefit the language learning of a child. In the acquisition of language, as well as of reading skills, mother/father-child book reading, or the quality of everyday conversations between parents and children play an important role, especially about past events, when there are no cues in the present immediate environment, so that children have no perceptual information for comprehension. Impact of home parenting environment on cognitive and psychomotor development in children under 5 years was reported by Yang et al. (2021). A study has shown that decontextualised talk of mothers with their 40-month-old child can positively predict children's print skills at 70 months of age (Reese 1995). Giving attention, providing both a demanding and versatile language environment with multiple inputs, and challenging the physical condition will greatly benefit a child in acquiring not only sufficient but proficient skills, in spoken and in written language.

12.2 Academic Stages of Normal Individuals of Different Ages

Tahany Abdul Karim Al-Sayed Ahmed

Enrolment and presence in the educational system are important measures of educational attainment. Gathering information regarding national and international methodology is monitored universally by the United Nations Educational, Scientific and Cultural Organisation (UNESCO), Institute for Statistics (UIS) and other organisations such as the Organisation for Economic Cooperation and Development (OECD 2017), Eurostat (UNESCO-UIS 2011) and OECD/Eurostat/UNESCO Institute for Statistics (2015). The latter two organisations provide guidelines for classifying national education programmes and related qualifications from other OECD countries (such as Australia, Canada, Japan, Europe and the United States), while the UIS collects data from other participating countries according to the International Standard Classification of Education (ISCED). This is the basis for international education statistics; it developed for national statisticians to report data on education to international organisations.

The data reported in Education at a Glance (OECD 2018) as ISCED level (0) programmes may differ from those given in national reports of early childhood education. Foundation (0) Education and care for young children starting from three-, four- and five-year-olds is known by several terms: child care/day care/nursery school/preschool/pre-kindergarten/early education. Early childhood education (ECE) programmes include any type of educational programme that serves children at young ages, designed to stimulate a child's development in all key developmental areas: cognitive, physical and social-emotional, to improve later school performance and to introduce young children to organised instruction outside of the family context.

The first and second stages are the initial formal education, variously called primary/junior/elementary education, and countries have a very similar focus on basic aptitudes in compulsory education provision in school, where children stay in steadily advancing classes until they complete these stages. Primary education is intended to provide students with major skills in reading, writing and mathematics (i.e. literacy and numeracy), and to establish a solid foundation for learning, understanding essential areas of information, particularly personal development, and preparing for lower secondary education.

The third and fourth stages comprise Lower secondary/Middle school education, where students continue the basic programmes started in the primary level, with more focused subjects. The pedagogy is usually aimed at laying the basis for life-long learning and individual development. Education systems may then expand further educational opportunities. Programmes at this level are usually organised around a more subject-orientated curriculum, introducing theoretical concepts across a broad range of subjects.

Finally, **the upper secondary education/**high school level commonly begins at the end of compulsory education. It is characteristically designed to complete secondary education in preparation for tertiary education, to provide skills; entrance recommendations require completion of compulsory education relevant to employment. Programmes at this level offer students more, specialised and in-depth training than in lower secondary education. The content of **post-secondary non-tertiary** education—programmes that are developed to deliver educational practices that build on secondary education and prepare students for the workforce or tertiary education—is broader than that of secondary education, but not as complex as tertiary education (e.g. Vocational school-technical College). **Vocational education and training (VET)** programmes are further divided into two categories (school-based programmes and combined school- and work-based programmes), on the basis of the amount of training provided in school, as opposed to the workplace (OECD 2020). **Tertiary education** (ISCED levels 5 and 6) augments secondary education, providing learning activities in specialised fields of education. It aims at instilling a very broad and deep level of knowledge (OECD 2019) (see Table 12.1, Fig. 12.1).

Table 12.1 The basic educational stages (Adapted from OECD/Eurostat/UNESCO Institute for Statistics (2015). https://doi.org/10.1787/9789264228368-en)

Level/key stage	Age (years)	Programmes			Description	Grades/Years
0/Early years	<1–3	Nursery/infant (e.g. Scandinavia)	Nursery kindergarten from 1 to 5 years (e.g. Germany)		This stage marks the stepping of the child from the comforts of a home to the world outside.	None
0/ Foundation	3–5	Preschool/kindergarten/senior kindergarten/reception			Pre-primary education is designed to support early development in preparation for participation in school and society. It is the first step towards gaining formal education.	None
1	5–7	Primary/elementary/junior	Primary from 6- to 9-year-old Grades from 1 to 4		Primary education builds foundation skills in reading, writing and mathematics, science, social sciences and language primary education and the subjects taught differ from one country to another.	1–3
2	7–11					3–6
3	11–14	Elementary middle school	Secondary/I Ages 10–14 Grades from 5–10		First stage of secondary education building on primary education, typically with a more subject-orientated curriculum.	6–9
4	14–16	Secondary/lower high school	Secondary higher/II Ages 15–18/19	Academic secondary school	The final stage that a child undergoes in a school during adolescence. Here he receives detailed information and knowledge on his preferred subjects.	10–11
5	16–18/19	Upper school/Sophomore/ Senior/high school (USA)/ secondary college (Canada)/ sixth form college (UK)	Grades from 10 to 13 Vocational school-technical college	Ages 10–18/19 Grades from 5 to 13	First stage of tertiary education: Typically shorter, more practical/technical/occupationally specific programmes leading to professional qualifications.	12–13 (UK)
6	18 and above	University			Bachelor or equivalent. Programmes designed to provide intermediate academic or professional knowledge, skills and competence leading to a first tertiary degree or equivalent qualification.	Bachelor's or equivalent level degree
7	22 and above	University—Postgraduate—First level			Theoretically or professionally based content. Providing learning activities in specialised fields of education.	Master's or equivalent level degree
8		University—Postgraduate—Second level			Written work requirements. Two orientation categories: academic and professional.	Doctoral or equivalent level degree

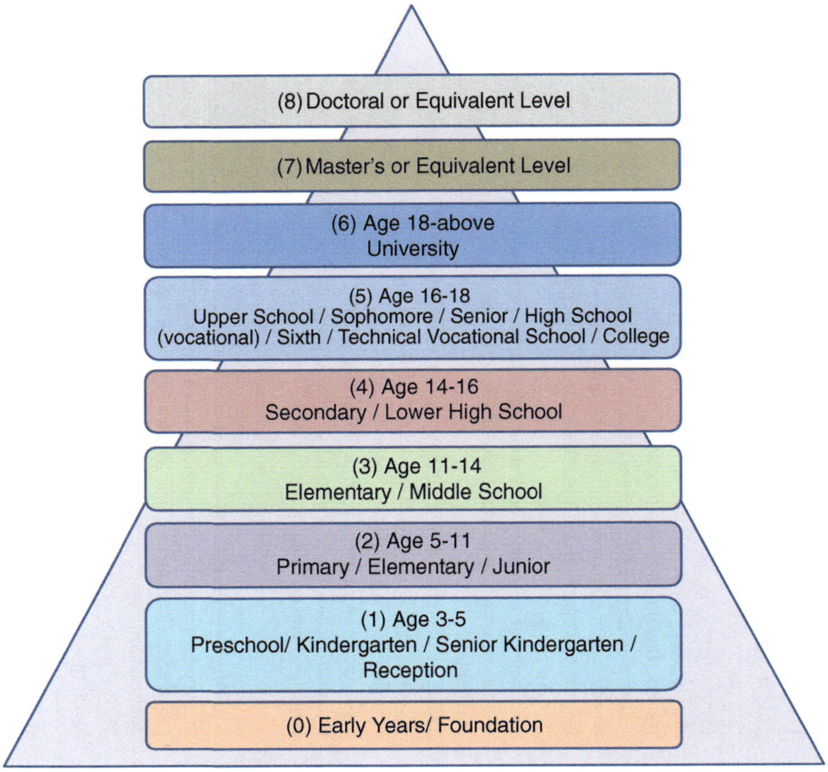

Fig. 12.1 Basic academic stages of normal individuals of different ages (Adapted from OECD/Eurostat/UNESCO Institute for Statistics (2015). https://doi.org/10.1787/9789264228368-en)

12.3 Medical Aspects of Diagnosis of Dyslexia/Dysgraphia

Barbara Maciejewska

12.3.1 Why Is Diagnosis of Developmental Dyslexia/ Dysgraphia a Challenge?

Specific learning disorders (SLD) with impairment in reading can vary between problems in word reading accuracy, reading rate or fluency and reading comprehension, despite normal intelligence, conventional instruction and adequate socio-cultural opportunities.

Reading and writing disorders are found in the category of SLD (Döhla and Heim 2016). SLD with impairment in reading (developmental dyslexia, DDL) can vary from problems in word reading accuracy, reading rate or fluency to reading comprehension. SLD with impairment in written expression (developmental dysgraphia, DDG) is divided into problems with spelling accuracy, grammar and punctuation accuracy and clarity, and organisation of written expression. Developmental dyslexia is a disability present in current international medical classifications: in the International Statistical Classification of Diseases and Related Health Problems (ICD-10) (2019) as F81.0 (as a specific reading disorder) and in the Diagnostic and Statistical Manual of Mental Disorders (DSM5) (2022) under number 315.00.

The current DSM-5 guidelines for learning disability assessments specify that specific learning disorders with impairment in reading (dyslexia), impairment in written expression and impairment in mathematics (dyscalculia) are diagnosed through:

- A clinical review of the individual's developmental, medical, educational and family history
- Reports of test scores and teacher observations
- An evaluation of the individual's response to academic interventions

In DSM 5, the IQ-achievement discrepancy requirement is not present. There are four criteria as follows (A–D):

- Criterion A refers to the key characteristics of SLD (at least one of six symptoms of learning difficulties that have persisted for at least 6 months despite the provision of extra help or targeted instruction).
- Criterion B refers to measurement of those characteristics (the affected academic skills are substantially and quantifiably below those expected for the age and cause impairment in academic, occupational or everyday activities, as confirmed by individually administered standardised achievement measures and comprehensive clinical assessment).
- Criterion C refers to age at onset of the problems (during the school-age years, although possibly not fully manifested until young adulthood in some individuals).
- Criterion D specifies which disorders (Intellectual Disabilities, uncorrected auditory or visual acuity problems, other mental or neurological disorders) or adverse conditions (psychosocial adversity, lack of proficiency in the language of instruction, inadequate instruction) must be ruled out before a diagnosis of SLD can be confirmed.

All four criteria must be met, and the level of functional impact is determined as being mild, moderate or severe (Petretto and Masala 2017).

Some studies report a high correlation between dyslexia and dysgraphia (Ehri 2000). The two basic skills have much in common: their background is the alphabetic system and phoneme-to-grapheme as well as grapheme-to-phoneme correspondence. Many studies have highlighted a connection between phonological processing difficulties and reading and writing disabilities. As a result, the comorbidity rate is high. Depending on the variables studied and the definitions utilised, from 30% to 47% of children with writing problems also have reading problems (Chung and Patel 2015).

However, reading and writing are similar but not symmetric processes. Writing seems to be more demanding than reading and the cognitive and motor requirements for writing differ in some important aspects from those for reading. Unfortunately, the diagnostic process for SLD is complex.

First of all, disabilities should be diagnosed by the team of specialists. Doctors such as psychiatrists, paediatricians, neurologists, audiologists and phoniatricians should cooperate with speech-language pathologists, school psychologists, counselling psychologists, and other learning disability specialists. To diagnose dyslexia or dysgraphia, learning problems that are primarily the result of visual, hearing or motor handicaps; of intellectual disability; of emotional disturbance; or of environmental, cultural or economic disadvantages should be excluded. It should be proved that areas that are included in the definition of dyslexia/dysgraphia are below expectations. Standardised instruments are available as diagnostic aids through a combination of intelligence testing, academic achievement testing, classroom performance, and social interaction and aptitude, aimed at identifying underlying difficulties, and checklists.

The assessment of IQ and the literacy skills, centred around the key areas of reading (single word and at length), writing and spelling, coding/decoding at the single word level, as well as complex tasks such as comprehension, should be done by specialists (for more information see Reid 2016; Duranovic and Smythe 2010; Shaywitz 2005).

Secondly, to date no unique biological marker or specific test for dyslexia/dysgraphia exists. That is why diagnosis should be a result of cooperation of psychologists, audiologists, phoniatricians, child psychiatrists and neurologists, speech therapists, social workers and others. Diagnosis of SLD is usually performed in psychological-educational counselling centres, child psychiatric outpatient centres or in psycho-pedagogical outpatient institutions, depending on the country (Berninger et al. 2015; Moll et al. 2020).

Thirdly, early signs of learning difficulties may appear in the preschool years (e.g. difficulty learning names of letters or counting objects), but they can only be diagnosed reliably after starting formal education. SLD is understood to be a cross-cultural and chronic condition that typically persists into adulthood, albeit with cultural differences and developmental changes in the way the learning difficulties are manifested. For example, in English-speaking countries, children struggle to learn the correspondence between letters and sounds in order to decode single words accurately, whereas adults may have mastered basic decoding skills but read slowly and with effort. By contrast, in countries with a non-alphabetic language or in which the correspondence between speech sounds of one's language and the letters used to represent those sounds is much simpler than in English (e.g. German, Polish and Italian), orthographies are rather transparent (Vellutino et al. 2004) and children with SLD (e.g. dyslexia) master letter-sound correspondence quickly, and both children and adults with SLD struggle with reading fluency (Margari et al. 2013).

Written language is based on mapping between orthographic units (letters) and corresponding phonological units (phonemes). A consistent pattern of differences across languages concerns the size of the phonological and orthographic units on which readers rely for mapping across the two domains (Diamanti et al. 2018). The ability of grapheme-to-phoneme conversion, which is necessary for reading, and the ability of phoneme-to-grapheme conversion, necessary for writing, have to be taught and are part of Phonological Awareness (PA) (Döhla and Heim 2016). Dyslexic/dysgraphic children are poor at PA tasks such as phoneme manipulation (Diamanti et al. 2018). So research suggests that a core phonological deficit (one affecting the representation of phonological elements; Ramus et al. 2003, Vellutino et al. 2004) primarily underlies SLD, especially DDL.

More and more research has provided new information on different languages. There have been suggestions that the aetiology of dyslexia might differ somewhat across languages and writing systems, involving not only metaphonological problems but also, especially in more transparent languages, fluency-related skills or other language and non-language factors (Pugh and Verhoeven 2018). Some cross-linguistic studies have assessed relative impairments in different orthographic systems with comparable materials directly contrasting groups of impaired readers across languages:

- English and German (Landerl and Wimmer 2000).
- English and French (Caravolas et al. 2003).
- English and Hebrew (Katzir et al. 2004).
- English and Greek (Diamanti et al. 2018).

However, the existing evidence is mainly based on studies in children learning to read English (Pugh and Verhoeven 2018). Thus, many questions remain open regarding the extent and severity of reading deficits across languages in different kinds of materials and tasks. Moreover, there is evidence that reading disability is not an 'all-or-nothing' deficiency. Rather, DDL (as well as DDG) should be considered on a continuum starting from 'very slight and mild' to 'very strong and intensive'—the continuum of reading skills (Ellis 2016; Maciejewska et al. 2013a, b). Heterogeneity and identification of different forms of DDL and DDG make the diagnostic process more opaque (Zoccolotti and Friedmann 2010).

What is more, dyslexia frequently occurs with other disorders (Margari et al. 2013; Moll et al. 2020). In the case of dyslexia, co-morbidity is the rule not the exception (Ijeoma and Chinelo 2019). Currently, there is much research presenting comorbidity of dyslexia with other developmental disorders/learning disabilities; dysgraphia/dyscalculia/dyspraxia (Ijeoma and Chinelo 2019). SLD can also co-exist with neurological conditions: anxiety, depression, attention-deficit hyperactivity disorder (ADHD), autism spectrum disorder (ASD) (see Sect. 15.5). The fact has large implications for diagnosis. Finally, in recent years, advances in several areas of neuroscience, neurobiology and neuroimaging have changed the understanding of dyslexia as a neurological disorder (Habib 2021). The disorder continues to be redefined by tightening the links between scientific research and clinical observations in the field of neurodevelopmental disorders. The combination of different data continues to lead to a new understanding of dyslexia and other specific learning disorders with direct implications to the interface of medicine and education (Habib 2021).

12.3.2 Important Diagnostic Data and Risk Groups of Dyslexia—Medical History, Familial Incidence and School Educational History

Medical history is always crucial. Behavioural markers, genes, brain structure/function in dyslexia and dysgraphia are examined increasingly often (Berninger and Richards 2010; McGrath and Stoodley 2019). However, the parents' observations of children's early development are also important, even the most important in some cases. Teachers and sitters should be also asked about the early stages of the child's growth and mental development. There are some aspects that should be remembered during taking a medical history of dysgraphic and dyslexic groups:

1. It should be noted that DDL/DDG is not a problem that can be outgrown. Children with DDL/DDG continue to have reading difficulties. Reading/writing disability is not a temporary deficiency, and its level of severity does not decrease with the passage of time. Learning problems are experienced from childhood into adolescence and adulthood (Thompson et al. 2015), but effective intervention generally has a significant positive effect on reading skills, and accommodation can minimise the impact of dyslexia on daily life (McNulty 2003; Shaywitz et al. 1999).
2. Dysgraphia may manifest in a variety of ways depending on the age at presentation, as neurodevelopment progresses and academic expectations increase (Chung and Patel 2015).
3. Children with dyslexia/dysgraphia may present different symptoms, since developmental disabilities are likely to be a continuum of skills (Maciejewska et al. 2013b).
4. There is evidence of high overlap between symptoms of LD and other neurodevelopmental conditions and mental disorders (Cederlof et al. 2017; Ijeoma and Chinelo 2019). Children with poor reading skills exhibit high rates of attention-deficit/hyperactivity, affective and anxiety disorders, particularly social phobia and generalised anxiety disorder. As result, LD are lifelong disabilities, but symptoms may change with time. Signs of DDL/DDG can be difficult to recognise before a child enters school, but some early clues may indicate a problem.

The early signs of dyslexia include delays in speech and language development, with phonological memory (non-word repetition) and expressive language (naming) skills being particularly affected. These studies highlight the slow development of language (so-called late talkers) in children at risk of dyslexia (Lyytinen et al. 2015; Thompson et al. 2015). Other symptoms to consider are general motor development (clumsiness), evaluation of posture, pencil grip, tremor and writing habits. Once a child reaches school age, dyslexia signs and symptoms may become more apparent so the child's teacher may be the first to notice a problem. Severity varies, but the condition often becomes apparent as a child starts learning to read. It is important to check the history of school education because abandoning the teaching process, inadequate pre-reading experience or incorrect instruction can often lead to poor reading skills and the observed deficiencies can often resemble the effects of basic cognitive deficits. It is thus crucial to distinguish between children whose reading problems are caused primarily by cognitive deficits of biological origin, and those whose reading problems are caused primarily by limitations in pre-reading experience or inadequate instruction (Goldston et al. 2007). Signs and symptoms characteristic of DDL/DDG depending on the age are presented in Table 12.2.

Table 12.2 Common signs and symptoms that a toddler, young child and adolescent may present (adapted from Lyytinen et al. 2015; Reid 2016; Thompson et al. 2015, Dyslexia: Merck Manual Professional Version (2017), Roitsch and Watson 2019)

	Before school	School age	Teens and adults
Dyslexia	Late talking Reversing sounds in words or confusing words that sound alike Problems with articulation Problems remembering or naming letters, numbers and colours Trouble recognising similar words that begin with the same sound Difficulty with rhythm and rhythmic games	Reading below the expected level of age Problems processing and understanding what is heard Difficulty spelling Inability to voice the pronunciation of an unfamiliar word Spending an unusually long time completing tasks that involve reading or writing Difficulty seeing (occasionally hearing) similarities and differences in letters and words Avoiding activities that involve reading Slow reading speed, inaccurate reading, omission of words	Difficulty reading, including reading aloud Slow and labour-intensive reading and writing Problems spelling Avoiding activities that involve reading . Spending an unusually long time completing tasks that involve reading or writing Problem with memorising number facts Trouble learning a foreign language Other neuropsychological problems: Dyscalculia, dyspraxia, ADHD, ASD, anxiety, social phobia
Dysgraphia	An awkward grip when writing Strange and awkward body position when writing Difficulty staying within margins Writing is exhausting, make the child tired = avoidance of writing and drawing tasks	Illegible handwriting Switching between cursive and print Difficulty with word-finding, sentence completion and written comprehension	Difficulty with written organisation of thought Difficulty with written syntax and written grammar that is not duplicated with oral tasks Illegible handwriting

Table 12.3 Significant and prominent risk factors of developmental dyslexia (adapted from Bonifacci et al. 2014; Demonet et al. 2004; Dilnot et al. 2017; Duff et al. 2015; Friend et al. 2008; He et al. 2014; Korat et al. 2013; Liu et al. 2016; Maciejewska et al. 2013b; Reid 2016; Sun et al. 2013; Thompson et al. 2015)

Child health	Home literacy environment	Family stresses	Family history	Socio-economic status
Maternal infectious diseases	Storybook exposure	Bereavement	History of DD in family	Parents' education
Premature birth and birth complications (asphyxia)	Reading stories to or with a child at bedtime	Parental separation	Existing learning problems in siblings	Parents' occupation
Physical difficulties Hearing problems Visual problems	Reading stories to or with a child at bedtime, during the day	Serious illness	Neuropsychiatric diseases in family	
Early health diseases	Number of children's books in the home			
Early significant accidents	Adult author checklist number of books at home			

There are a number of risk factors predicting trouble in learning/writing/reading (Dilnot et al. 2017). Several of them have been found to be associated with pregnancy and labour, so-called prenatal and perinatal factors (Table 12.3). The common SLD risk factors include:

- Premature birth
- Low birth weight
- Hyperbilirubinaemia
- Exposure during pregnancy to drugs, alcohol or nicotine while in the womb
- Infections that may alter brain development in

the foetus
- Infant oxygen deprivation
- Maternal diseases, e.g. high blood pressure

Data about risk factors during pregnancy and labour should be checked, such as pre-term labour, Apgar scale, weight at birth, respiratory problems, hypotrophy, etc. Moreover, familial medical history is important because developmental dyslexia is a strongly hereditary condition.

Family risk in SLD is of great value. It is known that DDL/DDG run in families. The role of genetic factors was already noticed in 1905 by Thomas and Hinshelwood (Blakemore and Frith 2005). Familial incidence of DDL is observed on the basis of multi-generational analyses of the families and especially twins (De Fries and Alacron 1996; Demonet et al. 2004; Maciejewska et al. 2013b). Studies of children and their parents reveal an increased chance of developing a reading disorder when the parents are dyslexic (up to 66%) (Bonifacci et al. 2014). Many children at family risk of dyslexia experience delays and difficulties with speech and language development, and many 'late talkers' have parents who report a history of reading difficulties (Duff et al. 2015). To sum up, a family history of any symptoms and signs in parents, siblings is always needed. Thompson et al. (2015) followed children at high risk of dyslexia from preschool through the early primary years, assessing them from age 3 years and 6 months at approximately annual intervals on tasks tapping cognitive, language and executive-motor skills. They found that family-risk status was a strong predictor of further learning disability at 8 years—a stronger predictor of dyslexia than poor language skills in preschool. Infants at family risk of dyslexia have been shown to experience auditory processing and phonological deficits years before any delays in reading or spelling skills are observed: at-risk infants show differences in novel word-learning (fast-mapping) tasks compared with not at-risk infants (Kalashnikova et al. 2020).

Risk factor for dyslexia is a genetic predisposition. The existing literature suggests a correlation between children's reading skills and those of their parents (Bonifacci et al. 2014, Roitsch and Watson 2019). The prevalence of dyslexia is higher in children with a family history of dyslexia. The risk of dyslexia in first-degree relatives who have this reading and spelling disorder is higher than in the general population. Evidence shows that dyslexia is associated with multiple genes (polygenic inheritance) and has a complex genetic basis (Roitsch and Watson 2019). The genetic profile of dyslexics has been evaluated, and so far nine loci (DYX1-DYX9) have been identified as a candidates for susceptibility to dyslexia, which contain many genes possibly related to DDL (Sánchez-Morán et al. 2018; Liu et al. 2016). No doubt dyslexia is highly familial, but the interpretation of these familial effects is not transparent because of the interplay of genes and environment in contributing to reading skills (Dilnot et al. 2017). The genetic risk might be modulated by the environment because gene–environment correlations are particularly important. Parental education is an important environmental risk factor interacting with gene influence on reading disability according to Friend et al. (2008). The language and pre-literacy environments that parents provide to their children are also environmental factors of strong impact on reading (Korat et al. 2013). It has been found that the mother's education level, the time spent on electronic devices, and the literacy-related activity are associated with developmental dyslexia (Sun et al. 2013; He et al. 2014). Interestingly, the home literacy environment (e.g. print exposure) is one of the more important predictors of reading. The influence of home literacy environment on reading is well established (Dilnot et al. 2017).

The conclusion is clear: it is crucial to offer children the best chances in education from the early years, and there is a great potential for interventions that support parents in providing a rich home literacy environment to help their children with emergent reading skill (Dilnot et al. 2017). Because of the gene– environment correlation, the home literacy environment is an important predictor of reading readiness.

12.3.3 The Battery of Tests Used in Dyslexia

The battery of tests useful for the diagnostic process includes:

- Tests for sensory deficits, audiological and ophthalmological examinations
- Intelligence tests
- Writing and reading tests
- Phonological system tests
- Laterality tests
- Speech tests
- Perception tests
- Psychomotricity tests
- Audiological tests
- Neurological examinations
- Examinations by child and adolescent psychiatrist, if needed

Standardised instruments and diagnostic tests to assess the literacy skills, centred around the key areas of reading (single word and at length), writing and spelling need to be used. They may include coding/decoding at the single word level, as well as complex tasks such as comprehension, phoneme processing, rapid naming, working memory, phoneme discrimination, orthographic lexicon, visual memory, vocabulary, maths, etc. (Duranovic and Mrkonjic 2013; Reid 2016).

However, at the very beginning, all concomitant diseases that may impinge on learning abilities and cognition should be excluded. Uncorrected auditory or visual acuity can impair normal development of language and speech and could cause language and reading deficits. These sensory deficits have to be diagnosed and excluded, because of their lack of specificity. That is why an audiological and ophthalmological evaluation is always useful. To recognise potential organic causes of learning disorders or reading problems, a neurological evaluation is crucial.

Children should be assessed by psychologists and pedagogues for two reasons:

1. To detect delayed development of psychomotor functions, as well as emotional or behavioural deficits that could be considered a cause of poor reading and spelling abilities.
2. To evaluate the development of basic learning processes and cognitive function, and the degree of literacy. For a better diagnosis, the child should go through several sessions with a psychologist, during which their cognitive and emotional potentials are assessed.

After these phono-audiologist functions, oral communication and high-level auditory functions have to be assessed by speech-language therapists, as well as by audiologists and phoniatricians. In their work, Roitsch and Watson (2019) list tests to help in the diagnosis of dyslexia, such as: Comprehensive Test of Phonological Processing (CTOPP); Delis Kaplan Executive Function System (D-KEFS); Gray Oral Reading Test, Fifth Edition (GORT-5); Process Assessment of the Learner, Second Edition; RAN/RAS: Rapid Automatized Naming and Rapid Alternating Stimulus Tests; Test of Word Reading Efficiency, Second Edition (TOWRE-2); Wechsler Individual Achievement Test, Third Edition (WIAT-III); Wide Range Achievement Test 4 (WRAT4); Woodcock Reading Mastery Tests, Third Edition (WRMT –III). However, the ideal test set is constantly being developed and revised.

12.3.4 Audiological Tests in Dyslexia

In addition to the described neurological markers, many studies have already evaluated and assessed the connection between auditory processing and DDL/DDG. Research discusses audiological skills and the link between auditory impairment and phonological deficit (Ramus et al. 2003; Maciejewska et al. 2013a; Döhla and Heim 2016; Ramus and Szenkovits 2008).

The children's behavioural performance of basic sound processing (discrimination of frequency, intensity, onset ramp and tone duration) and more complex auditory pattern recognition, such as metre, rhythm, melody and pitch perception have been tested (Serrallach et al. 2016). Dyslexics perform significantly poorer in almost all categories than the control group. Steinbrink et al. (2014) and Christmann et al. (2015) found abnormal auditory processing skills for dyslexics with respect to temporal, spectral or spectro-temporal deficits. The auditory cortex (AC) is very widely connected with different brain regions, including subcortical, prefrontal and parietal areas, where attentional and default processes are performed. Because of the strong interdependence of such integrated networks (Scheich et al. 2011; Rodriguez-Fornells et al. 2012), difficulties in recognising and interpreting acoustic patterns may arise from dysfunction in the central nervous system and are often associated with language and literacy problems. While in the normal population the prevalence of APD is 2–3%, Hämäläinen et al. (2013) have given an estimate that 30–50% of individuals with dyslexia are affected by auditory problems.

Taking into consideration the latest phonological theory of dyslexia and rapid auditory processing, as well as the fact that in many cases auditory processing disorder (APD) and learning disorders co-occur, clinicians are increasingly using audiological tests (Serrallach et al. 2016). Much research has proven that auditory processing is connected with language-based learning disabilities such as dyslexia. There is increasing evidence that a severe auditory deficit can have a negative influence on phonological skills and therefore affect reading and writing as well. Hence, evaluating the auditory cortex (AC) and auditory processing by audiological tests has become a part of the diagnostic process for LD (Döhla and Heim 2016). Auditory tests for evaluating processing deficits in APD can be applied to dyslexia. In people with APD and dyslexia, it is impossible to point to a single abnormal underlying psychophysiological process. This is why dyslexics present abnormal processing at different levels of the auditory system, including the brainstem or the auditory cortex or both. As a result, no single test is sufficient, but a battery of behavioural and (electro)physiological tests is needed. Furthermore, different instruments with electrophysiological procedures are used.

The following tests can be used to assess auditory processes:

- Behavioural tests
  - Auditory pattern/temporal tests
  - Monaural low redundancy speech tests
  - Binaural/dichotic speech tests
  - Binaural interaction tests
  - Auditory discrimination tests
- Electroacoustic and electrophysiological auditory procedures
  - Electroacoustic measures (oto-acoustic emissions (OAEs), immitance audiometry)
  - Electrophysiological measures (auditory brainstem response (ABR), auditory middle latency response (AMLR), auditory late response (ALR))
  - Cognitive potentials (event-related responses (ERPs), especially mismatch negativity (MMN) and P300 wave/responses)

Behavioural tests allow the checking of deficiencies in one or more of the following areas: auditory pattern recognition, temporal processing (temporal integration, discrimination, ordering and masking), auditory performance with degraded acoustic signals (monaural low redundancy), auditory performance with competing acoustic signals (dichotic test), auditory discrimination and localisation or lateralisation (binaural interaction) (Hämäläinen et al. 2013; Serrallach et al. 2016). These behavioural tests constitute the basis of 'A Screening Test for Auditory Processing Disorders' (SCAN) (Hämäläinen et al. 2013).

Electroacoustic and electrophysiological auditory procedures evaluate the function of the auditory pathways from the cochlea to the cortical levels, and help in the differential diagnosis of a peripheral or central problem in the auditory system. Most of the procedures are objective and independent of behavioural responses (motivation, developmental age, attention, state of arousal, oral motor skills, native language or ability to understand verbal instructions).

For a central disorder of the sound stimuli transformation process, auditory evoked potentials, particularly cognitive ones, may be needed. The event-related potentials (ERPs) are an objective and quantifiable index for evaluating sensory representations in the central nervous system, even for highly complex linguistic stimuli. They have become increasingly popular in the studies of central auditory processing and sound discrimination. Assessment of cognitive potential is still attractive for researchers and is commonly used all the time in the studies of normal development and ageing, as well as their disorders such as developmental language disorders, e.g. SLD and DDL (Baldeweg et al. 1999; Faustmann et al. 2005; Kujala et al. 2007a, b; Lovio et al. 2010; Naatanen 2000; Pakarinen et al. 2013; Vuust et al. 2011).

Mismatch negativity (MMN) is related to changes in different sound features such as pitch, timbre, location of sound source, intensity and rhythm (Vuust et al. 2011). MMN can serve as an index of sensory memory in audition, involuntary attention switch to sound change, and language-specific phoneme traces (Leikin 2002). Moreover, the process of maturation of MMN in children may be observed (Shafer et al. 2000). In the Finnish study by Lyytinen et al. (2015), dyslexic children were assessed from birth to puberty. Their MMN measured at 3–5 days of age presented a significant predictive correlation with reading skills at school age. In fact, MMN is useful in research of central auditory processing (Naatanen et al. 2007). Another longitudinal study starting before primary school age revealed that ERPs to assess responses of AC to unexpected deviations in basic sound features were correlated with phonological processing and letter-naming skills at kindergarten age (Hämäläinen et al. 2015). Similarly, ERPs measured by van Zuijen et al. (2013) were correlated with word reading fluency at primary school age. The amplitudes of MMN in pre-schoolers at risk of dyslexia were smaller for frequency deviants (Maurer et al. 2003) than they were for vowel, vowel duration, consonant and intensity deviants (Lovio et al. 2010; Hämäläinen et al. 2015; van Zuijen et al. 2013; Maurer et al. 2003).

Neural biomarkers for DDL in the AC of children were investigated by Serrallach et al. (2016). The dyslexic group exhibited an abnormal inter-hemispheric asynchrony of the primary auditory-evoked P1-response. Responses to acoustic stimuli were faster on the right side and the P1 peak was enlarged in the right-hemisphere.

A P300 response is treated as proof of resolving a problem ('aha'-wave), a general index of cognition, and an index of awareness, completion of stimulus evaluation, attention (ability to concentrate on a presented stimulus), detecting novelty ('something important has occurred'), and transfer of information to controlled processing or consciousness (Jerger and Musiek 2000; Vlachos et al. 2007). Investigations clearly show that P300 is connected to the speed with which a patient classifies signals, updates memory and allocates attention. The nature of the response can be deformed in many neurological and psychiatric diseases, and disorders with cognitive dysfunction and impairments (weakness of information processing, short-term memory, attention allocation). ERPs are used to investigate language processes and to study language processing because their different components have been found to be sensitive to semantic and syntactic aspects of language processing (Kutas and Federmeier 2000).

The components reflect semantic integration processes (N400) or controlled processes of syntactic reanalysis (P600) during auditory sentence comprehension (Faustmann et al. 2005; Sabisch et al. 2006). N400 is usually regarded as a manifestation of lexical integration and is associated with different aspects of semantic processing (Shaul 2008). The P600 component is triggered by linguistic incongruence and is also associated with searching for words in memory, with processing the words that are syntactically inappropriate, and processing pseudo-words or any irregular words (Shaul 2008). Left anterior negativities (LAN) are observed to be correlated with aspects of syntactic processing. Early left anterior negativities (ELAN) have only been observed for the processing of phrase structure violations, while LAN are observed in correlation with morpho-syntactic violations and sub-categorisation violations (Faustmann et al. 2005).

12.3.5 Neuroimaging and Other Up-to-Date Methods in Dyslexia

The number of reported brain imaging studies involving individuals with and without dyslexia has increased exponentially and findings depend greatly on the imaging modality, acquisition parameters, including use or non-use of tasks, the specific nature of requirements when tasks are performed, and data analysis procedures (Berninger and Richards 2010). There are numerous studies of dyslexia in which neuroimaging and functional neuroimaging modalities have been used to assess linguistic skills by the response of the brain to cognitive challenges. Neuroimaging in dyslexia utilises different modalities, including magnetic resonance imaging (MRI), functional magnetic resonance imaging (fMRI), positron emission tomography (PET), magnetic source imaging (MSI), magnetic resonance spectroscopy (MRS) and magneto-encephalography (MEG) (Vandermosten et al. 2012a). Neuroimaging and functional neuroimaging methods are the most influential tools researchers can use today for neurological studies on dyslexia.

Voxel-based morphometry (VBM) based on MRI—a computational approach to neuroanatomy that measures differences in local concentrations of brain tissue through a voxel-wise comparison of multiple brain images—is the most widely-used automated technique for the analysis of structural brain images (McGrath and Stoodley 2019). A number of brain-imaging studies have found that during reading dyslexics have reduced activation in the major components of the reading and speech-processing system of the left hemisphere of the brain. Neuroscientific studies have provided convincing evidence for a variety of alterations in the brains of dyslexics (Shaywitz et al. 2006; Richlan et al. 2013). Regardless of the language and in spite of different symptoms in language tests, dyslexic readers have very similar activation (reduction) in the word form area of the left hemisphere—a region that plays an important role in understanding whole words (Blakemore and Frith 2005). The most commonly implicated neural correlates for dyslexia involve a reading network that comprises left occipito-temporal regions, left temporo-parietal regions and the left inferior frontal gyrus (Ramus et al. 2018).

Voxel-based morphometry (VBM) studies have also revealed differences in brain structure between controls and children, and between controls and adults with developmental dyslexia. Increases and decreases of grey matter volume (GMV) in group comparisons of developmental dyslexics and good readers constitute a widely distributed set of regions in both left and right hemispheres (Jednoróg et al. 2013; Richardson and Price 2009; Widmann et al. 2012).

McGrath and Stoodley (2019) in their meta-analysis show VBM-reduced grey matter (GM) in dyslexia in the left-hemisphere middle and superior temporal regions, the inferior parietal regions and cerebellum; the right medial and orbital frontal regions; and the caudate bilaterally. Increased GM in dyslexia compared with controls was evident in the left supramarginal gyrus/inferior parietal lobule, the middle temporal gyrus and cerebellum; the right precuneus, supplementary motor area and pre-central gyrus; and the medial frontal regions. The meta-analytical approach provides much more data than a single study. Table 12.4 includes meta-analyses concerning dyslexia and its neural correlates.

The auditory cortex (AC) is also investigated in dyslexia, including Heschl's gyrus (HG), the planum temporale (PT) and the anterior supratemporal gyrus (aSTG). Serrallach et al. (2016) found remarkable differences in gyrification, size and hemispheric asymmetry with regard to the developmental disorder: smaller HG and consequently enlarged PT volumes in the left hemisphere, resulting in considerably smaller left HG/PT ratios than in controls. HG/PT ratios in the right hemisphere were significantly decreased in children with dyslexia.

Diffusion tensor imaging (DTI) tractography is another structural magnetic resonance imaging technique allowing reconstruction and assessment processes during reading. The left arcuate fasciculus plays a crucial role in reading development, as it connects two regions of the reading network, the left temporo-parietal region and the left inferior frontal gyrus, for which atypical functional activation and lower fractional anisotropy values have been reported in dyslexic readers (Vandermosten et al. 2012a, b). Analysis of DTI scans and functional magnetic resonance imaging (fMRI) connectivity scans in children

Table 12.4 Meta-analyses of VBM studies in developmental dyslexia (adapted from Eckert et al. 2016; Linkersdorfer et al. 2012; McGrath and Stoodley 2019; Richlan et al. 2013)

Research	Number of meta-analysed studies	Grey matter reduction
Richlan et al. (2013)	9	– In the right superior temporal gyrus and the left superior temporal sulcus – In left ventral occipito-temporal and left cerebellar regions
Linkersdorfer et al. (2012)	9	– In the left fusiform gyrus (extending into the left inferior temporal gyrus) – Bilateral supramarginal gyrus (right cluster extended to the posterior portion of the superior temporal gyrus) – Bilateral cerebellum (lobule VI)
Eckert et al. (2016)	11	– In left orbitofrontal cortex/inferior frontal gyrus – Left posteriori superior temporal sulcus/middle temporal gyrus – Right cerebellum
McGrath and Stoodley (2019)	15	– In left-hemisphere middle and superior temporal regions, inferior parietal regions – Right medial and orbital frontal regions – The caudate bilaterally – Cerebellum (lobule VI) – Reduced grey matter in the right caudate

with and without dysgraphia or dyslexia was performed by Richards et al. (2015). There were significant differences between the control group and both dysgraphic and dyslexic groups in DTI and functional connectivity. The study revealed that dysgraphia and dyslexia differ in white matter integrity, fMRI functional connectivity and white matter–grey matter correlations. The dysgraphic and dyslexic groups differed on radial diffusivity (RD) in seven left-sided fibre tracts.

There is also a tendency to use different methods together to evaluate the impaired reading process in dyslexia, such as different event-related potentials—MMN, P300, P2, N2 and P300, P600 in dyslexic readers (Leikin 2002; Savill and Thierry 2011) or ERPs and gamma band response (GRB) (Widmann et al. 2012) or neurocognitive and genetic correlation (Nopola-Hemmi et al. 2002). However, many studies suggest that areas that are not typically considered auditory areas play an important role in auditory processing (Blakemore and Frith 2005; Vellutino et al. 2004). Electrophysiological procedures and neuroimaging are both useful in evaluating neural responses to an intense training and intervention in dyslexics (Blakemore and Frith 2005; Shaywitz et al. 2006; Serrallach et al. 2016). ERPs and MRI for morphometry were performed to investigate the anatomy of AC and the whole-head MEG system, to measure and analyse the response of AC to acoustic stimuli. With the rapid advance in technology, researchers today can observe different parts of the brain, bringing new insights into the understanding of learning difficulties. Currently, because of the wide spectrum of tests, neuroimaging and functional neuroimaging techniques, professionals and researchers in medical sciences, psychology, and educational sciences are working hand in hand with the diagnosis, treatment and prevention of dyslexia (McGrath and Stoodley 2019).

12.3.6 Conclusions

1. Diagnosis of developmental dyslexia/dysgraphia is a challenge.
2. Family risk of dyslexia is a strong predictor of reading outcome.
3. Dyslexia and dysgraphia are familial and heritable. Parents should be interviewed by a doctor, psychologist and speech language pathologist to discover the following risk factors:
   (a) Any genetic trait in the family, any history of neuropsychiatric diseases
   (b) Any aggravating circumstances during the mother's pregnancy and labour infectious diseases, difficult vaginal delivery, pre-term birth and neonatal asphyxia

   (c) Disharmonious child psychomotor development, especially a preschool language impairment (late talkers)
4. Medical history is always important. However, be careful because:
   (a) Dyslexia frequently co-occurs with other disorders so symptoms may overlap
   (b) Children can present different symptoms since SLD is a kind of continuum of skills
   (c) Symptoms of DDL/DDG may change with time
5. Because the gene-environment correlation is crucial, the home literacy environment is an important predictor of reading readiness (together with child health).
6. SLDs are diagnosed in educational and clinical settings. The assessment of the literacy skills, centred on the key areas of reading (single word and at length), writing and spelling is crucial. This may include coding/decoding at the single word level as well as complex tasks such as comprehension and should be done by professionals—results of various medical tests are used to exclude those who have neurogenetic/neurological disorders or other conditions with different biological bases for their reading and writing problems (visual, hearing or motor handicaps; intellectual disability; emotional disturbance; environmental, cultural or economic disadvantages).
7. Emerging trends in research of DD include:
   (a) Increased number of genetic studies designed to identify the chromosomal linkage or site for dyslexia gene candidates related to specific dyslexia phenotypes (behavioural expression of an underlying genotype)
   (b) Neuroimaging studies employing many new technologies and methods
   (c) Evaluation of the auditory cortex (AC) and its brain connections
   (d) Tendency to join different methods (electrophysiological such as ERPs and neuroimaging) to create a specified neuroauditory profile for dyslexics

12.4 Estimation of Linguistic, General Cognitive and Academic Developmental Stages

Anja Fiori

12.4.1 Introduction

Several diagnostic aspects have to be taken into account regarding the complex nature of reading and spelling disorders. The central questions are: to what extent does the student's difficulty in reading and writing affect other domains of academic achievement, and the other way round, to what extent do weak general or specific cognitive abilities underlie the dysfunction in literacy? Therefore, depending on the diagnostic goal and the anamnestic information given, a raft of domains in general development of the dyslectic student may be crucial to understanding the specific circumstances of a given case. These are: general achievement in school, general cognitive ability, mathematical ability, speech and language development, as well as attention and concentration deficits, which can occur as a primary comorbidity, or secondarily owing to unease reflecting the excessive demands in literacy (Hendren et al. 2018). For details on attention deficits, compare Sects. 12.7, 12.8 and 15.5 in this textbook; for sensorimotor development, see Sects. 12.1, 12.10 and 15.4 in this textbook; for memory, see Sect. 12.5 in this textbook.

12.4.2 General Achievement in School, General Cognitive Ability

During recent decades, the question of whether developmental dyslexia should be defined in relation to IQ scores has been a matter of constant debate (Gustafson and Samuelsson 1999; Stage et al. 2003; Hoskyn and Swanson 2000; Stanovich 2005). According to the latest edition of the

Diagnostic and Statistical Manual of Mental Disorders (DSM-52013), developmental dyslexia is subsumed under the generic term specific learning disorder (SLD). DSM-5 criteria describe general academic difficulties with deficits in reading or written expression as possible specifiers. To meet diagnostic criteria, students have to show persistent deficits in reading or writing (class norm discrepancy) such as inaccurate or slow and effortful reading, poor spelling or written expression, with a negative impact on their academic achievement, occupational performance or activities of daily living. The earlier intelligence-achievement-discrepancy criterion has been abandoned in DSM-5. As a consequence, the diagnosis of an SLD no longer requires formal intellectual assessment unless a general intellectual deficit is suspected. A further consequence is the possibility of providing special education services for children with specific learning disorders and lower IQ scores. In line with this development, several guidelines for assessing developmental dyslexia no longer recommend intelligence-achievement-discrepancy as a mandatory component of diagnostics (IDA 2009; DGKJP 2015; CDE 2017). Alternatively, the California Dyslexia Guidelines recommend guidance on response to intervention and instruction as a

> collaborative, comprehensive, multi-tiered system for identifying students who are struggling academically and providing them with appropriate interventions…—CDE (2017), p. 45

Fletcher and Miciak (2017) even claim that testing cognitive functions is not helpful in diagnosing specific learning disorders because there is only very limited evidence for their predictive power regarding remedial interventions. They recommend reducing comprehensive testing of cognitive functions in diagnostics in favour of detailed individualised educational assessment with the goal of targeted intervention. According to IDA (2009, p. 2),

> A formal measure of intelligence is not always needed to document average intellectual abilities. For younger children, (…) teacher information about the child's ability to learn orally may indicate average intellectual abilities. For older students or adults, past achievement in school or work may indicate at least average intelligence.

On the other hand, ICD-11 criteria still include the intelligence-achievement-discrepancy as defining developmental dyslexia as a 'developmental learning disorder with impairment in reading' with an impact on prevalence estimates. Should a check of general intelligence appear necessary, the use of non-verbal tests is recommended to avoid confounding with linguistic abilities.

As a consequence of the DSM-5 criteria, a general estimation of academic achievement compared with that of class peers (class norm discrepancy), given by the teachers involved, is helpful for understanding the clinical relevance of the student's difficulties. The central question is: to what extent do the student's difficulties affect his or her everyday life in school? In most school subjects, reading comprehension is increasingly important for collecting technical information and the contents of learning units.

12.4.3 Effects on Academic Achievement and Possible Socio-Emotional Sequelae of Developmental Dyslexia

Hendren et al. (2018) state a general risk for academic struggle and social, emotional and behavioural problems, which is also mentioned as 'emotional challenges in addition to academic challenges' in the California Dyslexia Guidelines (CDE 2017, p. 24), these include anxiety, depression, avoidance, a low academic self-concept and low self-esteem, with secondary behavioural problems often interpreted as reduced motivation, resistance and defiance, which can also lead to family stress. According to Hendren et al. (2018), the reciprocal association of developmental dyslexia with such mental disorders as anxiety and depression, disruptive, impulse-control and conduct disorders, is often underestimated by professionals concerned with developmental dyslexics. Good inter-professional collaboration and a broad view of possible comorbidities is essential for optimal care of affected students.

12.4.4 Developmental Dyslexia and Mathematics

Dyscalculia, or mathematics disorder, is a further frequently reported comorbidity of dyslexia (Fussenegger and Landerl 2006; Peterson and Pennington 2015; Hendren et al. 2018; Peters et al. 2018; Meiri et al. 2019). According to Fussenegger and Landerl (2006), the prevalence of this comorbidity ranges from 42% to 64%, owing to differences in diagnostic material. In consequence, if poor achievement in mathematics is found in dyslexic children, further testing is necessary to differentiate between secondary difficulties in mathematics tasks, due to poor reading comprehension, and a 'real' comorbidity. Hendren et al. (2018) report a comorbidity of approximately 40% for reading and mathematics disorders. More recent research points to shared underlying cognitive functions relevant for both reading and mathematical ability, such as working memory, semantic memory and phonological processes (Ashkenazi et al. 2013), executive function for error monitoring and phonological processing for both reading and arithmetic fluency (Meiri et al. 2019). Meiri et al. point out that general difficulties in attending to instructions and maintaining attention might also account for high comorbidity. A cluster analysis applied to children with SLD points to a relation between mathematical ability and text reading speed: both being associated with cognitive processing (Poletti et al. 2018). According to Hendren et al. (2018, p. 5), these approaches are

> ...promising in recognizing the heterogeneity within R[eading]D[isorder] and M[athematics] D[isorder] themselves as well as adopting a dimensional approach to highlight shared cognitive deficits

12.4.5 Developmental Dyslexia and Language Skills

Frequent comorbidities of developmental dyslexia mentioned by Peterson and Pennington (2015) are language impairment and speech sound disorder, which the authors attribute to similar aetiological and neurocognitive risk factors. They therefore approve of the current diagnostic criteria in DSM-5, which define learning disabilities as an over-arching category Specific Learning Disorder. In general, there is broad consent to the assumption that reading acquisition and reading difficulties may have their foundation in language development (Catts and Hogan 2003; Snowling and Hulme 2012; Hulme and Snowling 2013; Adlof and Hogan 2018). According to Snowling and Hulme (2012, p. 33),

> language and phonological skills are the foundations of literacy development.

As these authors argue, it is crucial to differentiate between decoding and comprehension difficulties in reading, as both show different underlying cognitive deficits and require differential therapeutic approaches shown to be effective by the authors. They conclude that oral language skills, like vocabulary knowledge, grammatical, morphological and pragmatic skills (Hulme and Snowling 2013), are prerequisites of reading comprehension at the text level, and phonological skills and letter knowledge underlie decoding skills in word reading. They clarify that despite this therapeutically relevant distinction they do not assume distinct groups of dyslexics with pure decoding or comprehension difficulties. Adlof and Hogan (2018) discuss the idea of developmental dyslexia as a language-based disorder. In their article, they examine historical and theoretical evidence of a relationship between developmental language disorder and developmental dyslexia. They agree with Snowling and Hulme's view that difficulties in decoding and spelling at the word level can be explained by phonological deficits. For text comprehension, however, these skills are not sufficient; here the understanding of spoken language is fundamental, for which an adequate vocabulary is required, as well as semantic and syntactic processing, inference and discourse. They conclude that developmental language disorder and developmental dyslexia are separate but often comorbid disorders with reciprocal interference. For example, reading disorders can negatively affect vocabulary and syntactic development in the long term, a phenomenon often paraphrased as the Matthew Effect. This view is also taken in the

California Dyslexia Guidelines (CDE 2017, p. 13):

> Spoken language serves as a foundation for the development of written language skills, and written language development also positively affects spoken language development by facilitating growth in various aspects of language, including vocabulary, syntax, and comprehension.

These considerations suggest that good inter-professional collaboration in the treatment and support of affected students is needed, in order to keep all the above aspects in mind and to respond adequately to the individual needs of each student over the course of time.

12.5 Interpretation of Results of Logopaedic/SLP and Pedagogic Examinations

Anja Fiori

12.5.1 Introduction

The aim of the current section is to provide a general understanding of relevant diagnostic aspects and their impact on deriving goals and methods of remediation for dyslexic children or adolescents in their individual stage of development. Specific details on school grades or on particular testing material are not provided, as they are highly dependent on specific language, educational and cultural backgrounds. Thus, they are considered not to be helpful in an international textbook. Furthermore, diagnostics in pre-school children are not addressed here, but in Chap. 14 of this textbook.

The following section summarises different diagnostic approaches that help to attain a complete picture of the strengths and weaknesses of an individual dyslexic student. The general scope of quantitative testing is contrasted with the opportunity to derive individualised treatment opportunities from qualitative diagnostics.

A child's reading and spelling level is usually assessed via standardised and normed tests on literacy (quantitative testing) after difficulties in school have occurred and sensory disorders have been ruled out. Nevertheless, additional diagnostic data in the sense of educational assessment are crucial for deriving therapeutic goals and for the choice of adequate procedures of intervention. A qualitative analysis of spelling mistakes and a description of reading behaviour (referring to fluency, accuracy and comprehension) may generate hypotheses about reading and writing strategies and suggest an allocation of observable reading and spelling abilities to stages of literacy development. Combined with an estimation of specific additional precursor and partial abilities, these data serve as a basis for tailored therapeutic intervention. Thus, the Speech and Language Pathologist or Teacher responsible for remediation or support of dyslexic children or adolescents can derive individual goals of intervention. In addition, it is necessary to describe a baseline as a starting point for therapy, on the basis of careful diagnostics, by which to evaluate therapeutic progress in due course. In their examinations, SLPs as well as pedagogic specialists follow certain diagnostic questions that are formulated in the subheadings of this Section.

12.5.2 How Do the Child's Achievements Compare with Those of His or Her Peers? The Scope of Quantitative Testing

Quantitative testing is crucial for evaluating competence in literacy in terms of a comparison of achievements. The aim is to detect readers or writers achieving below average results compared with a reference group (mainly class-level peers). Achievement is expressed in standard values. Weak results in standardised tests, in combination with school problems, are a strong indicator of dyslexia. Yet, these data are not sufficient for planning a specific intervention (IDA 2009).

Standardised reading and spelling tests provide a range of tasks, depending on the diagnostic goal intended. These may include coding/decoding at the single word level (real words and non-words) as well as complex tasks such as comprehension. Relevant features that reading tests might aim at are reading fluency, reading comprehension, reading accuracy and application of lexical and sublexical reading strategies. Most spelling tests require the child to complete sentences according to word dictation, with word material representing different levels of development. In general, they provide a qualitative analysis of spelling mistakes, complexity varying enormously.

12.5.3 In Which Manner Does the Child Write and Read? Educational Assessment Through Qualitative Description

Educational assessment aims at qualitative analyses of spelling mistakes and reading behaviour.

With reference to spelling, informal testing can be used for qualitative analysis, in addition to standardised test material, as demonstrated by Hebert et al. (2018). Qualitative testing aims at describing and grouping types of spelling mistakes. Individual profiles of spelling help to define core types of mistakes in terms of frequency, to describe strengths and weaknesses of the individual student, as well as suggesting pertinent hypotheses about applied spelling strategies. These data allow the child to be assigned to a specific stage of spelling acquisition.

With reference to reading, formal and informal testing should aim at reading fluency (e.g. words per minute), reading accuracy (counting and analysing reading mistakes) and literal as well as inferential reading comprehension in narrative as well as expository texts (CDE 2017). Again, the aim is to assign reading proficiency to stages of reading development, to describe strengths and weaknesses of the individual student.

12.5.4 What Stage of Reading Acquisition Has the Child Reached? The Purpose of Stage Models

The assignment of the child's reading and spelling performance to a certain stage of development is very central diagnostic information. It enables the practitioner to find appropriate exercises for the child, who is addressed precisely at his or her individual stage of development. In this way, targeted intervention becomes possible without over- or under-challenging the student. Several reference models of reading and spelling acquisition have been developed over the course of time (cf. Günther 1986; Scheerer-Neumann 2001a, b for the German language, Frith 1980; Gehsmann and Templeton 2011 for English). As an example, Scheerer-Neumann distinguishes six stages of spelling development (see Table 12.5) and five stages of reading development (see Table 12.6) that imply mastery of specific strategies of reading and spelling.

Table 12.5 A stage model of spelling development (modified from Scheerer-Neumann (2001a))

Stage, name of strategy	Description of strategy
1. Logographic strategy, before school entry	Knowledge that written words consist of letters, single letter writing, 'words' without relation to their phonological form, reproduction of a few, highly frequent, words (e.g. child's name)
2. Alphabetic strategy (attempt to derive the written form from spoken language)	Sounding phonemes of words and transcription into graphemes via acquisition of phoneme–grapheme correspondence, moving from transcription of only few phonemes to full word transcription Phonologically derived word forms even in familiar irregular words
3. Alphabetic strategy, modified by orthographic and morphematic elements	Modification of purely alphabetic spelling by orthographic elements, first prefixes and suffixes Over-exact articulation accompanying spelling
4. Orthographic strategy	Order of learned orthographic rules depends highly on educational methods Whole-word learning triggered by growing insight in orthographic structures
5. Advanced orthographic competence	Inclusion of syntactic knowledge in orthographic rules
6. Prevailing whole-word retrieval in skilled writers	Automated retrieval of whole words, ability to rely on alphabetic as well as orthographic strategy as required Further growth of written word vocabulary, particularly technical terms and loanwords

Table 12.6 A stage model of reading development (modified from Scheerer-Neumann (2001b))

Stage, name of strategy	Description of strategy
1. Pre-stage	Recognition of symbols, e.g. logos of brands, context enhances recognition
2. Logographic strategy	Whole-word recognition due to visually salient elements such as single letters in specific positions, contextual hints often needed, very small sight vocabulary
3. Alphabetic strategy	Acquisition of first grapheme–phoneme correspondences halting, slow and tedious reading, difficulties in reading long and phonologically complex words, approach to correct word form via repetition and re-composing of sounded elements
4. Lexical strategy	Recognition of grapheme clusters, highly frequent words or parts of words, making use of orthographic units Fluent reading of words and parts of words, few reading mistakes Semantically or syntactically adequate substitution of words, making use of context information to correct mistakes, relevance of context increases
5. Further development	Increasingly automated and flexible application of acquired strategies: In unknown words—Alphabetic strategy In familiar words—Orthographic strategy, expansion of structured sight vocabulary, flexible use of context information

For example, the alphabetical phase can be considered accomplished when the child can easily write out all audible sounds in a word in the correct sequence, even if the spelling does not conform to the orthographic norm. Before reaching this stage it is not sensible to confront the child with orthographic rules that deviate from the alphabetic principle. As a contribution to an international textbook, the description of stages and strategies has to be restricted to a general level, abstaining from giving examples, as these would only be helpful in the context of a specific language. Even assigning strategies to class levels originally proposed by Scheerer-Neumann (2001a, b) does not seem helpful in an overview across languages and cultures. First, reading and writing acquisition is likely to differ substantially, depending on the orthographic regularity of a given language. In addition, the course of development is highly influenced by educational methods and strategies differing from country to country.

> The differences between languages and orthographies also interact with teaching and instruction. (…) Thus, the instruction to apply phonics in order to transform the phonemes into spelling is confusing in English and relatively straightforward in Italian.—Schulte-Körne et al. (2007)

For a detailed analysis of the differences in opaque rather than shallow orthographies on reading acquisition, see Aro (2014). The presented stages can therefore only serve as general qualitative guidelines without being able to provide an internationally valid timeline of development.

12.5.5 Which Routes of Reading and Writing Are Available?

Targeting different routes (sublexical or lexical) of word processing is additionally helpful in determining which approaches to written language the student can draw upon. Regarding the relevance of this differentiation for developmental dyslexia, see Keméný et al. (2018). Appropriate test materials are lists of real words of high frequency (referring to lexical reading or writing), in contrast to pseudowords (i.e. meaningless sequences of syllables such as <vobado> referring to sublexical reading or writing), which can be read aloud or written upon dictation. Some standardised test batteries include these formats of testing. Differences in fluency as well as accuracy can reveal specific difficulties in sublexical (letter-by-letter) or lexical (whole-word) reading or writing that have a differential impact on therapeutic goals.

12.5.6 Are There Any Partial or Precursor Skills That the Child Shows Difficulties in? Essential Precursor Abilities

Additionally, several precursor abilities, considered to be relevant for literacy acquisition, are recommended to be assessed (CDE 2017; IDA 2009, 2017). These are:

- Phonological working memory as a prerequisite for sublexical reading or writing (phonological coding) (Brady 1991)

- Phonological awareness as a prerequisite for applying the alphabetic principle to word decoding and writing words (Stackhouse 1997)
- Rapid naming (RAN) as a prerequisite for recognition and naming of words and highly frequent sublexical units, such as syllables or morphemes (Norton and Wolf 2012)
- Paired associate learning, the ability to link unrelated stimuli via repeated learning assumed to be a prerequisite for word recognition (Hulme et al. 2007)
- Receptive and expressive oral language as 'the foundation of written language' (CDE 2017, p.53)
- Alphabet knowledge
- Grapheme–phoneme and phoneme–grapheme association (IDA 2017)

For more detailed information, refer to Sects. 14.1 and 14.2 in this textbook.

12.6 Neurological Examination

12.6.1 Neurological Examination of Children: Basics

Mona Hegazi, Barbara Maciejewska, Katrin Neumann and Dagmar Weise

12.6.1.1 Introduction

Neurological evaluation is an integral part of the assessment protocol of an abnormal language development of children in cases of suspected neurological disorders or general developmental abnormalities. It includes a parental interview, a general physical examination and a detailed neurological examination. The latter involves an examination of the cranial nerves, the motor and sensory systems and additional neurological tests when necessary. A detailed neurological evaluation reflects the developmental status of the central nervous system and may identify indicators for brain lesions or abnormal cerebral functions. Phoniatricians should know and recognize common neurological symptoms of children and consult neuro-pediatricians when needed.

12.6.1.2 Clinical History with Respect to Neurodevelopmental Disorders

A detailed child's history should include the following information:

- Pregnancy, perinatal and neonatal history: Apgar score, birth weight, prematurity, infections.
- Developmental history: child's age at acquisition of developmental milestones such as social smiling; head control; rolling over; maintaining a sitting position; walking independently; babbling; vocal play and use of first words; phrases and sentences; toilet training; self-feeding and dressing.
- Presence of neurological symptoms or complaints in general: nature, duration, permanent or episodic (e.g. seizure) occurrence; maintained, progressive or resolving course; localization to a specific anatomical region.
- Symptoms related to specific neurological disorders such as cerebral palsy: impaired coordination; muscle tone; spasticity; weakness; tremor; developmental disorders of speech and language; loss of vision or hearing; difficulties in sensation; motor developmental delay, e.g. inability to roll over, sit, crawl or walk; disturbed cognitive functions; seizure; and dysphagia.
- Impact of the diagnosed or suspected neurological disorder on cognition, behaviour and language, the degree to which activities of daily life are compromised and if any medication, treatment or rehabilitation is applied or has been given in the past.
- Family history: parental consanguinity; number and gender of siblings; position in the sequence of children; maternal age at delivery and family history of neurological; systemic and other disorders including hearing loss, developmental language disorders, intellectual disability and dyslexia.

12.6.1.3 General Physical Examination

This should include:

- Height, weight, head circumference and blood pressure.

- General appearance, dysmorphia and skin examination for neurocutaneous lesions.
- Examination of the midline of the back and neck for sacral dimples, tufts of hair or other signs of spinal dysraphism.
- General abdominal and chest examination.

12.6.1.4 Detailed Neurological Examination

General Appearance

- Dysmorphia.
- Body position: supine, symmetrical and with flexion of all limbs.
- Skin exam: neurocutaneous lesions such as cafè-au-lait macules, which may indicate a neurofibromatosis; angiofibrosis or shagreen patches in case of tuberous sclerosis and other mucocutaneous lesions.
- Location of the hair whorl: may signify presence of cerebral malformations.
- Palmar creases: typical for several genetic syndromes such as Down syndrome.
- Midline of the back and neck: exam for sacral dimples, tufts of hair or other signs of spinal dysraphism.
- Unusual body odour: may be present in several neurometabolic disorders (Swaiman 2012; Michelson and Shu 2012; Fenichel 2009).

Spontaneous Position

- A healthy infant lies supine, with flexion of the limbs.
- Muscle tone assessment of limbs and in the head-neck-trunk axis: movements need to be symmetrical (Swaiman 2012; Michelson and Shu 2012; Fenichel 2009).

Skull and Cranial Nerve Examination

- The shape of the skull and the head circumference (microcephaly, macrocephaly, craniosynostosis) and the bulging and tension of the anterior and posterior fontanelle should be assessed at first.
- In infants and young children, squint and nystagmus, pupillary size and reaction to light, extra-ocular movements as well as facial asymmetries and facial mimic should be noted. Temporalis and masseter muscles can be tested during sucking.
- The jaw reflex, glabellar reflex, gag reflex and palmomental reflex need to be evaluated.
- The child's response to a bell or by recalling a whispered word can be observed, and the auropalpebral reflex should be checked (closure of the eye in response to loud noises).
- In older children detailed cranial nerve examination is performed assessing the function of all cranial nerves (I–XII) (Swaiman 2012; Michelson and Shu 2012; Fenichel 2009).

Motor System

- Posture and abnormal movements: opisthotonus, abducted hips or 'frog-sign', myoclonus, cerebellar tremor and choreo-athetotic movements.
- Muscle state: muscle atrophy, pseudohypertrophy (bulky appearance but with weakness) and fasciculations.
- Muscle tone: passive muscle tone is assessed by testing the resistance of passive movements in the joints while the infant is awake and not crying.
- Muscle power: this is tested by observing the response to simple manoeuvres such as retrieving a toy. The following grading system is used for assessing muscle strength according to the Lovett scale:

  - 0 No muscle contraction, no movement
  - 1 Flicker or trace of contraction visible or palpable
  - 2 Active movement without gravity
  - 3 Active movement against gravity
  - 4 Active movement against gravity with some resistance
  - 5 Active muscle contraction against full resistance, normal, full strength (for age).

Reflexes (Movement Automatisms)

Examples are shown in Table 12.7.

Table 12.7 Developmental reflexes and reactions, procedure of elicitation and response onset, integration and significance (based on Fenichel 2009; Zafeiriou 2004; Berger 2007; Blomberg and Dempsey 2011; Goddard 2005)

Reflex	Method of eliciting stimulus	Expected response	Duration	Significance—abnormal indication
Sucking	Touching the baby's mouth or upper lip	Sucking rhythmical movements of the lips	Birth to 1 year	Weak or immature sucking ability or lacking reflex in immature/premature babies; reflex reappears in advanced and diffuse cerebral atrophy
Moro (startle)	With the child in the supine position, apply a loud noise or an unpredictable sudden movement of the baby's body 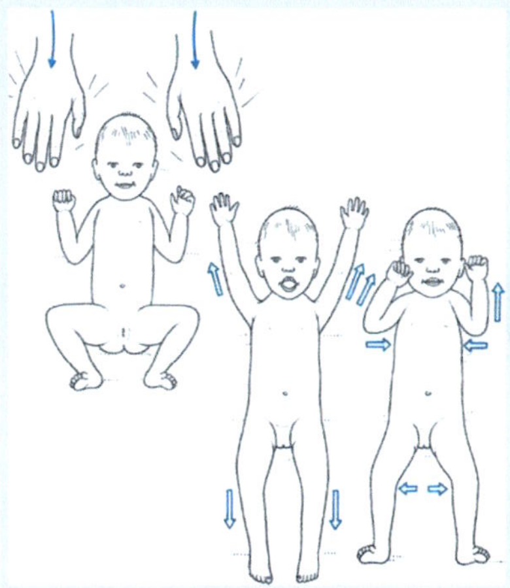	Symmetrical rapid abduction and then extension of the arms with the opening of hands (similar to hugging), legs and head extend; subsequently the shoulders adduct, the elbows and fingers flex	Birth to 4–6 months	Asymmetry may indicate a brain lesion or peripheral nerve injury, e.g. paresis, paralysis
Blinking	Shine bright light in eyes	Eyelids close	From birth on throughout life	Absence indicates pure light sensation
Acoustic blink	Create loud noise around child	Both eyes blink	From birth on throughout life	Absence indicates hearing loss
Flexor withdrawal	With the child supine, and the lower extremities in an extended position, press a stimulus to the sole of the foot	Stimulated limb is withdrawn (hip and knee flexion)	Birth to 2 months	Persistence denotes brain damage such as cerebral palsy
Extensor thrust	With the child supine and the lower extremities in flexed position, apply pressure against the sole of the foot	Reflex extension of the leg muscles	Birth to 2 months	Persistence denotes brain damage such as cerebral palsy

(continued)

Table 12.7 (continued)

Reflex	Method of eliciting stimulus	Expected response	Duration	Significance—abnormal indication
Galant	While the child lies in prone position, stroke along one side of the spine—The dorsal paravertebral skin especially lumbar region 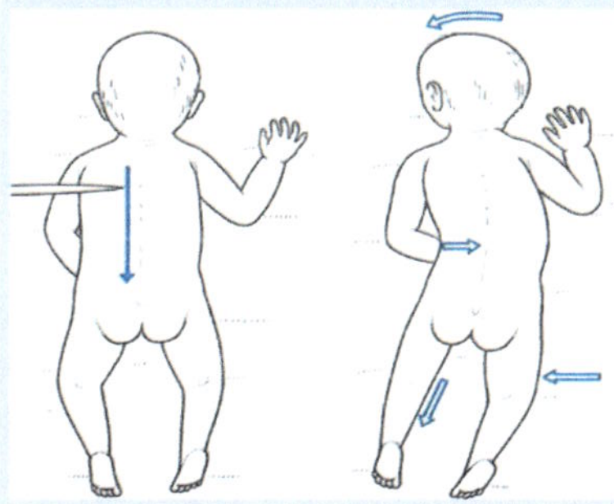	Lateral flexion or outward rotation of the hip towards the irritated side	Birth to 4–6 months	Lack of the reflex—Damage of the spinal cord in thoracic segments Asymmetrical reaction—Pyramid paresis/paralysis
Palmar grasp	Stimulate the skin of the palmar surface of the infant, for example, by placing a finger in the infant's hand 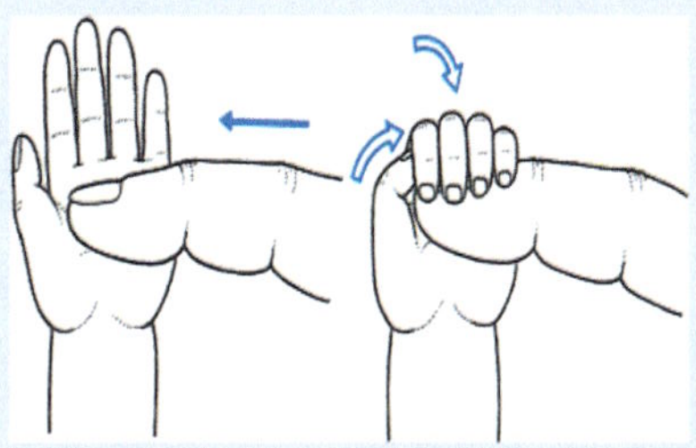	Infants fingers flex around the finger or an object in a grasp	Birth to 5–6 months	Persistence indicates cerebral dysfunction
Plantar grasp	Stroking the sole of the foot	Flexion of the toes and the foot	Birth to 5–6 months	Absence indicates spastic cerebral palsy

(continued)

Table 12.7 (continued)

Reflex	Method of eliciting stimulus	Expected response	Duration	Significance—abnormal indication
Rooting	Touch or stroke the cheek or lips (corner of the mouth) laterally 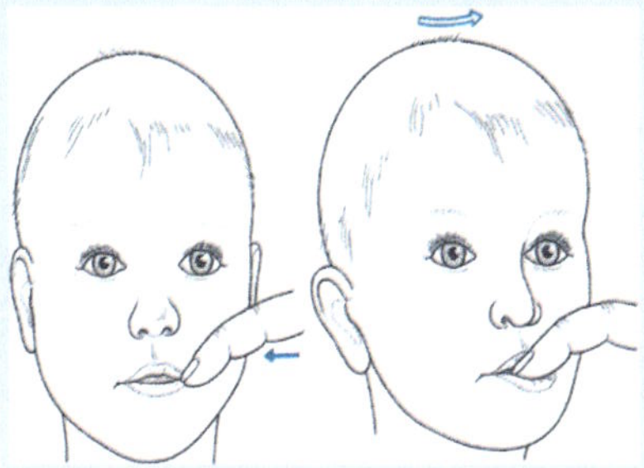	Head and mouth are turned towards the same side touched and a sucking motion is done	Birth to 2 months	Persistence indicates cerebral dysfunction
Placing	Support the child upright, the dorsum of the foot is placed against the edge of the table 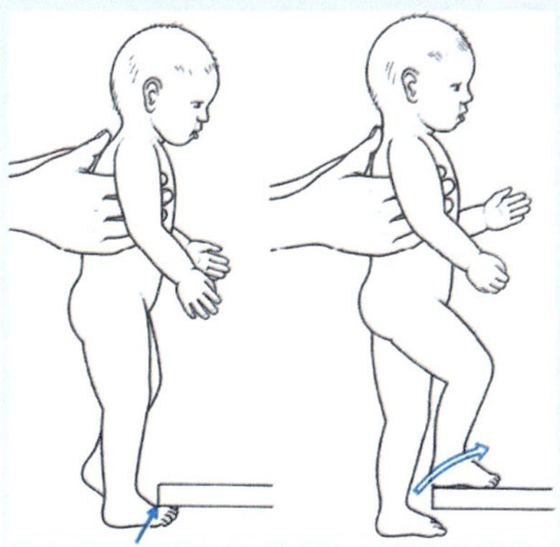	Lifting the leg up (e.g. on the table)	Birth to 3 months	Absence could indicate paresis or breech presentation at birth

(continued)

Table 12.7 (continued)

Reflex	Method of eliciting stimulus	Expected response	Duration	Significance—abnormal indication
Primitive walking/ stepping	The child is held under the arms in vertical position with feet touching a solid surface and then leaned forward and the feet are pressed on the surface 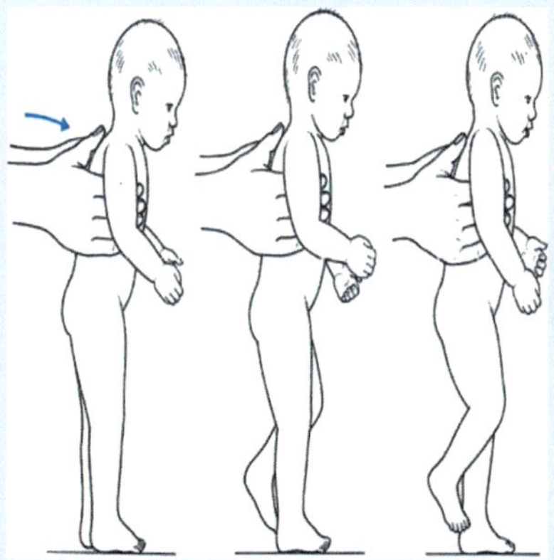	Alternate flexion and extension of the legs (as if walking)—Rhythmical alternating steps	Birth to 3–4 months	Absence could indicate paresis or cerebral palsy
Palmomental reflex	Stroke the thenar eminence in a proximal to distal direction using a sharp object (causing discomfort not pain)	Ipsilateral or bilateral contraction of the mentalis muscle	Birth to 3 months	Reappearance indicates processes that disrupt normal cortical inhibitory pathways and thus affection of frontal lobes (frontal release sign)
Rotation test/dolls's eye/vestibulo-ocular reflex	Rotate child from one side to another	Eyes turn in direction of rotation	Birth to 11–14 days	Vestibular problem or eye muscle paresis
Labyrinthine head righting	While the child is in the vertical position and blindfolded, tilt the child anteriorly, posteriorly or vertically	The head is orientated vertically and is maintained steadily	From birth to 2 months on throughout life	Allows controlling the head position irrespective of gravity

(continued)

Table 12.7 (continued)

Reflex	Method of eliciting stimulus	Expected response	Duration	Significance—abnormal indication
Asymmetrical tonic neck/fencer	With body supine, gently turn the head to one side 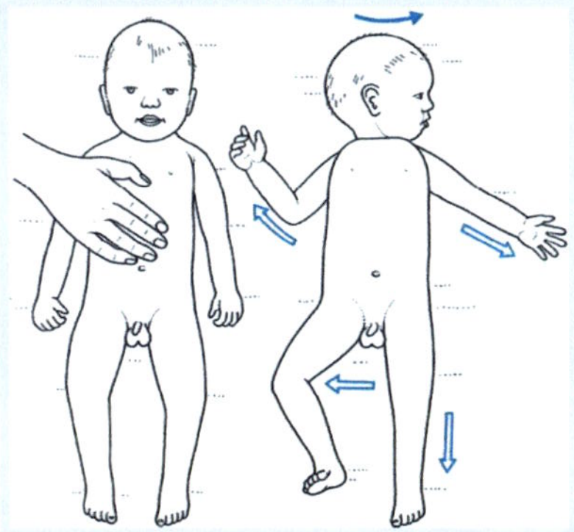	Extension of the limbs on the side of the face and flexing of the arm and leg of the other side (fencing position)	Birth to 6 months	Persistence impedes active rolling and the development of hand-eye coordination; can indicate major cerebral palsy
Symmetrical tonic neck	With a child prone over the examiner's knee or placed in quadruped position on the floor, flex the child's head forwards (tonic neck I) 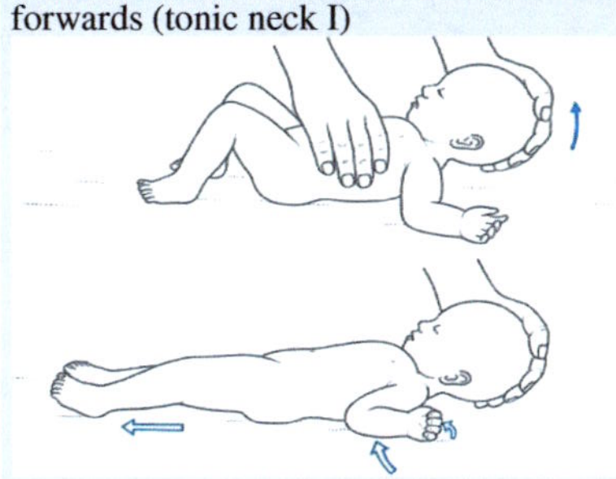 and then extend the head backwards (tonic neck II) (not shown)	Flexion of the infant's head forwards causes flexion of the arms and extension of the legs (tonic neck I) Extension of the head backwards leads to extension of the arms and flexion of the legs (tonic neck II)	From 2/3 months to 6/9 months	Persistence impedes vertical positioning such as crawling on hands and knees, sitting without support

(continued)

Table 12.7 (continued)

Reflex	Method of eliciting stimulus	Expected response	Duration	Significance—abnormal indication
Babinski/plantar reflex	Firmly stroke along the lateral surface of the plantar foot surface from the heel to the fifth toe 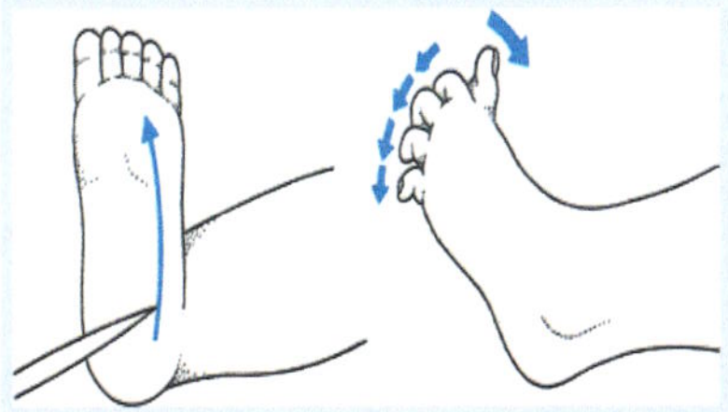	Upward extension (dorsiflexion) of the big toe towards the top of the foot and fanning of the other toes	Up to about 2 years of age	Persistence beyond 2 years indicates upper motor neuron lesion, unilateral persistence—Possible cerebral palsy
Landau reflex	Hold the child horizontally in a prone position in the air 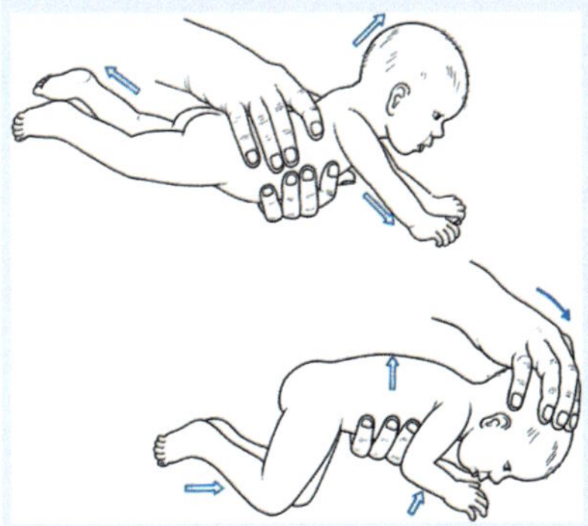	Infant maintains a convex arc position with the head raised and arms extended and spine and hips extended in sequence When the infant's head is flexed by the examiner, the extension of the hips disappears	From 6 months to 2.5 years	The appearance of this reflex breaks up the total flexion pattern seen at birth Failure to integrate means over-reactiveness to stimulation or vestibular problems

(continued)

Table 12.7 (continued)

Reflex	Method of eliciting stimulus	Expected response	Duration	Significance—abnormal indication
Parachute reflex (protective extension reaction forward)	Suspend the baby in the horizontal prone position and then drop him or her a short distance onto a soft surface—Head first; suddenly lower the infant as in falling 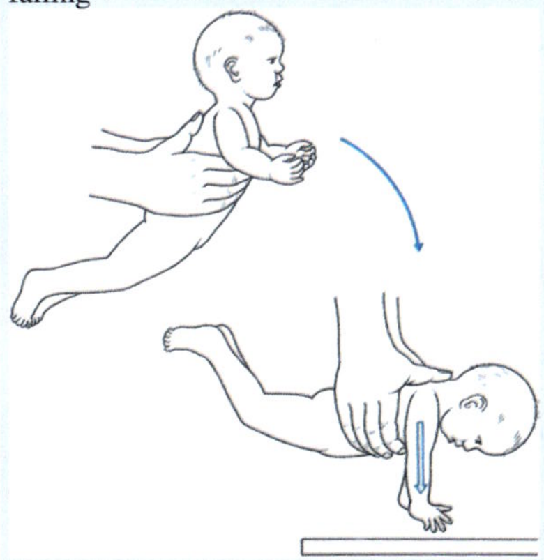	Arms extend and hands open in a defensive mechanism to protect the head	From 8 months on throughout life	Upper extremity pyramidal tract dysfunction, asymmetrical response—Sign of hemiparesis
Neonatal neck righting	With child supine, flex his head and rotate it slowly to one side	The whole body (shoulders, trunk and pelvis) move towards the side to which the head is turned	Birth to 6 months	Early in development the infant uses the reflex for transition between supine, lying on the side and eventually prone positons
Neonatal body righting	With body supine, flex one leg up towards the chest and rotate (adduct) the leg across the body	Infant's body follows the direction of pelvic, move towards the side to which the leg is turned	From 6 to 12 months	Assists the child in rolling between supine and prone It allows rotation of one part of the body before the other, helping sitting and standing from supine position without rolling over to prone
Positive supporting reaction (magnetic reaction)	Place a finger on the sole of the foot	Limb extension that follows the finger as it is withdrawn	Birth to 4–5 months	Consists of those reflex muscular contractions whereby the body is supported against gravity

(continued)

Table 12.7 (continued)

Reflex	Method of eliciting stimulus	Expected response	Duration	Significance—abnormal indication
Negative supporting reactions	Standing Stretch of extensor muscle	Consists of inhibition of the extensor muscles and unfixing of the joints that thus enable the limb to be flexed and moved into a new position (disappearance of positive supporting reaction)	Birth to 4 months	Presence of positive supporting (+) after 8 months is abnormal. Also excessive flexion (−) is abnormal after 4 months
Tonic labyrinthine prone reflex	While child is prone, lift him up to evaluate the presence of flexor tone	Tonic flexion of the body	Birth to 6 months	Persistence impedes normal rolling patterns, balance and gross motor skills
Tonic labyrinthine supine reflex	While child is supine, lift the child to sitting to observe for extensor tone	Tonic retraction of the shoulders and extension of the body	Birth to 6 months	Persistence impedes normal rolling patterns, balance and gross motor skills
Supine or prone lying	While the child lies supine or prone on a tilt board, with arms and legs extended, tilt the board to one side	Righting of head and thorax, abduction and extension of arm and leg on the raised side (equilibrium reaction), protective reaction on the lowered side of board	From 6 months on throughout life	Cerebral cortex dysfunction
Four-foot kneeling	While child is in quadruped position, tilt him to one side	Righting of head and thorax (body flexes on the side of the tilt), abduction and extension of the arm and the legs on the raised side (equilibrium reaction), protective reaction on the lowered side	From 8 months on throughout life	Lacking indicates cerebral cortex dysfunction
Sitting	While child is seated, pull or tilt him to one side		From 10 months on throughout life	Lacking indicates cerebral cortex dysfunction
Kneel standing	While child is in kneel-standing position, pull or tilt him to one side		From 18 months on throughout life	Lacking indicates cerebral cortex dysfunction
Hopping reactions	With child in standing position and held by the arms, move the child backwards, forwards or to one side	Righting of head and thorax, hopping steps in the opposite direction of the tilt to maintain equilibrium	From 18 months on throughout life	Lacking indicates cerebral cortex dysfunction
Optical righting reflex	Hold child with armpit in a suspended position and then change position of the head from side to side	Eyes will move to the same side as head	From 1 to 2 years on throughout life	Lacking indicates cerebral cortex dysfunction

Figures with kind permission from Prof. Lietz (1996)

Newborn and Infant Reflexes (Primitive Reflexes)

The primitive reflexes (also called infantile, infant or newborn reflexes) are a group of motor reflexes found in newborns. These automated movements are mediated at the spinal cord or brainstem levels. They do not require cortical involvement and disappear over time. They develop in utero and are usually present at birth. These reflexes are patterned, consistent and involuntary movements that help to make the baby aware of his or her body and surroundings (Zafeiriou 2004; Berger 2007). They build the fundament for conscious movements.

The roles of primitive reflexes are:

- To assist the birthing process
- To help the newborn to adjust to a life outside the womb when his or her nervous system is not fully developed
- To assist the baby to move and build up motor and cognitive skills

The primitive reflexes can be divided into three groups:

- The multisensory reflex—the Moro reflex (0–4 months).
- Primitive reflexes of position that affect all four limbs include the:
  - Tonic labyrinthine reflex (TLR) (0–6 months)
  - Asymmetrical tonic neck reflex (ATNR) (2–6 months)
  - Symmetrical tonic neck reflex (STNR) (3–6 months)
- Primitive tactile reflexes, triggered by touch and include:
  - The suck-swallow reflex (0–12 months)
  - Stepping/primitive walking (0–2 months)
  - The placing reflex (0–3 months)
  - The palmomental reflex (0–3 months)
  - The palmar reflex (0–4 months)
  - The plantar reflex (0–8 months)
  - The rooting reflex (0–3 months)
  - The Galant reflex (0–6 months)
  - The Babinski reflex (0–18 months)

The primitive reflexes are observed in normal infants in response to particular stimuli, but it is impossible to evoke them in neurologically intact adults. These reflexes disappear owing to the maturation-associated development of the frontal lobes (Mazurkiewicz-Bełdzińska 2017). Gradually, as the primitive reflexes retreat or are integrated, conscious voluntary movements are established. In a typically developing child, paralleled by cortical maturation and myelinisation, most of these reflexes are integrated, i.e. they are replaced by voluntary motor skills, controlled by upper levels of the brain motor processing. They disappear within or after the first year of life and transit to mature responses. If a baby is unable to inhibit the primitive reflexes within the appropriate time window, his or her motor development is delayed, making it more difficult to follow the inborn program. Such a delay is a stumbling block of the brain maturation (Blomberg and Dempsey 2011), causing problems with gross and fine motor coordination and sensory perception (Mazurkiewicz-Bełdzińska 2017; Goddard 2005).

A child may retain the primitive reflexes for some of the following reasons: low birth weight, premature birth, severe illness, trauma or injury in infancy, decreased ability to explore environment in early months.

Postural Reflexes

When the primitive reflexes are integrated, postural reflexes develop. These reflexes ensure the unconscious control of posture, balance and coordination in the active and static individual (Zafeiriou 2004; Berger 2007; Goddard 2005). They are mainly responsible for the reflective maintenance of the body's posture when its position is altered by movement and ensure that the body remains upright and aligned. Because gravity effects on the body trigger these responses, these reflexes usually start to develop after birth. They help in carrying the maturing child through the developmental milestones of head control, rolling, sitting, crawling and standing.

Most of the postural reflexes arise in the midbrain, i.e. they are mediated from a higher cerebral level than the primitive reflexes, and thus their appearance signifies a maturation of the nervous system. The shift from primitive to postural reflexes is a gradual process with some overlap. Usually the postural reflexes are established by the age of 3.5 years. Typically, they are maintained throughout life but may decay with age, allowing the primitive reflexes to reappear (Swaiman 2012; Berger 2007; Blomberg and Dempsey 2011; Goddard 2005).

Postural reflexes are divided into two groups:

- Righting reflexes: for example, neck righting reflex, labyrinthine head righting reflex (LHRR), body righting reflex, Landau reflex (6 months to 2.5 years).
- Equilibrium reactions: parachute reflex (from 8 months on throughout life).

The movement automatisms mentioned above can be checked in three basic positions in infants:

- The supine position (rooting reflex, Moro reflex, ATNR).
- The prone position (Galant reflex, STNR).
- The holding position (Landau reflex, parachute reflex).

Classification of Reflexes According to Integration Centres in the Central Nervous System

These are:

- Infant reflexes: e.g. suck-swallowing, defaecation and urinating reflexes are essential for a newborn's survival immediately after birth; their centres are located in the brainstem and the spinal cord. The reflexes are automatic till the cortex centres take control of these processes.
- Spinal reflexes: they include flexor withdrawal, extensor thrust, crossed extension and the Galant reflex, deep tendon reflexes (the biceps (C5-6), triceps (C6-8), brachioradialis (C5-6), patellar (L2-4) and ankle (L1-2) reflexes) and superficial reflexes (such as the plantar reflex (S1), the superficial abdominal reflex (T7-T12), comprising reflexes of the upper abdominal (T8, 9) and lower abdominal quadrants (T11, 12) and the cremasteric reflex (L1-2)).
- Brainstem reflexes: these reflexes are static-postural reflexes; their persistence denotes delayed CNS maturation. They include the asymmetrical tonic neck reflex (0–6 months), symmetrical tonic neck reflex (0–6 months) and tonic labyrinthine reflex (prone and supine) (0–4 months) (Mazurkiewicz-Bełdzińska 2017).
- Midbrain reflexes: these reflexes, combined with the equilibrium reflexes, enable the child to roll over, to sit up and to get on her or his hands and knees. They include the neck righting reflex (0–6 months), the body righting reflex (6–18 months) and the labyrinthine righting reflex (from 2 months on throughout life).
- Cortical equilibrium reactions: these are movement responses to maintain equilibrium or balance. They include supine and prone lying (from 6 months on throughout life), four-foot kneeling (from 8 months on throughout life), sitting (from 10 months on throughout life), kneel standing (from 15 months on throughout life) and the hopping reflex (from 18 months on throughout life). Maturation of equilibrium reactions brings the individual to the human bipedal stage of motor development. The next higher level of motor activity can be reached only when a proper reaction at the lower level has been created. Therefore, the reflexes are needed to achieve the next higher level of motor activity. Their occurrence indicates normal muscle tone and the body's adaptation in response to changes of the centre of gravity. They emerge together with the postural reaction of righting from 6 months on.

Cerebellar System

The examination of the cerebellar system includes the testing of rapid alternating movements (diadochokinesis), finger-to-nose and heel-to-shin tests as well as the Romberg sign.

Locomotion

Crawling and gait in older children: gait is best assessed by observing the patient walking barefooted with the legs and feet exposed. Pathological examples are circumduction gait (hemiparesis), broad-based ataxic gait (cerebellar disorder), steppage gait (high stepping) (peripheral neuropathy) and waddling gait (myopathy).

Sensory System

- Light touch: tested by pinprick
- Joint position sense (proprioception): measures the child's ability to perceive the position of a joint with his or her vision occluded and minimal external cues, tested by asking the child to replicate a joint position accurately with the opposite extremity or describing the position verbally
- Vibration sense: tested by tuning fork
- Higher cortical functions: examined by two-point discrimination, stereognosis and graphesthesia (see Sect. 11.10, Volume 1)

Additional Diagnostic Tests

See Sects. 9.9, 9.10, 3.1 and 16.22 (Volume 1) for genetic examination; Sects. 11.16, 16.21 and 1.15 (Volume 1) for neuroimaging such as magnetic resonance imaging (MRI) and computed tomography (CT); and Sects. 11.12–11.14 (Volume 1) for metabolic tests and electroencephalography.

12.7 Assessment of Behaviour and Attention of Students with Specific Learning Disorders (SLD) and Interpretation of Results of Neuropsychological Tests

Tahany Abdul Karim Al-Sayed Ahmed and Mirela Duranovic

12.7.1 Neuropsychological Evaluation of SLD

Reading and other neurodevelopmental disorders often co-occur, which is important for both theory and practice. Understanding the nature and causes of comorbidities is the basis for a better understanding of developmental disorders (Moll et al. 2020). Attention-deficit/hyperactivity disorder (ADHD) is the most common disorder that occurs with reading disorder (Maughan and Carroll 2006). The treatment for attention and the intervention for reading have largely independent effects on attention and on aspects of reading fluency (Moll et al. 2020). The results of various studies emphasise the importance of identifying effective multimodal treatments that positively affect the common and unique neuropsychological deficiencies of both disorders in carefully planned clinical trials (Sexton et al. 2012). Therefore, assessment of behaviour and attention for pupils with SLD should be an important aspect of evaluation for appropriate treatment to be given.

Assessment of behaviour and attention for children or adults with SLD must include a variety of evaluation tools for gathering relevant functional, developmental and academic information. It should recognise each child's specific functional difficulties in academic and behavioural spheres, and it is therefore likely to be the most effective way of assessing a child's social and educational needs (Norwich 2014). It may include information provided by the parents and caregivers, and results from tests that may help determine the degree of difficulty and provide a clear understanding of the student's cognitive functioning, highlighting strengths and weaknesses. Primary care must place emphasis on medical examination and interviews in order to obtain relevant demographic information, medical history, family history, nutrition, behavioural, emotional, genetic, neurobiological, environmental and cognitive factors affecting individuals with SLD. Referral procedures to teamwork specialists (e.g. neurologists, psychiatrists, audiologists) and comprehensive testing can be performed by clinical/educational psychologists, or in some countries a speech and language therapist. Psychologists or speech and language therapists undertaking assessments determine that the student has an SLD by using a battery of neuropsychological and psychometric tests (Schneider and Kaufman 2017, see Table 12.8).

A neuropsychological evaluation helps parents, teachers, physicians and therapists to understand a child's processing abilities better, by integrating specialised academic and cognitive

Table 12.8 Commonly used neuropsychological tests for determining specific learning disorders

Domain	Neuropsychological test
Intellectual functioning	Wechsler Adult Intelligence Scale-Revised (WAIS-R; Wechsler 1981) Wechsler Adult Intelligence Scale-III (WAIS-III; Wechsler 1997) Wechsler Adult Intelligence Scale (4th edn) (WAIS-IV; Wechsler 2008) Wechsler Memory Scale (4th edn) (WMS-IV; Wechsler 2009b) Wechsler Intelligence Scale for Children-IV (WISC-IV; Wechsler (2003) Wechsler Intelligence Scale for Children-V (WISC-V; Wechsler (2014) Stanford–Binet Intelligence Scale-IV (Thorndike et al. 1986) Stanford–Binet Intelligence Scales-V (Roid 2003) Kaufman Adolescent and Adult Intelligence Test (KAIT; Kaufman and Kaufman 1993) Reynolds Intellectual Assessment Scales (RIAS; Reynolds and Kamphaus 2003) Differential Abilities Scale (2nd edn) (DAS-II) Elliott (2007)
Academic achievement	The *Wechsler Individual Achievement Test* (3rd edn) *(WIAT-III;* Wechsler 2009a) The Woodcock–Johnson IV *Tests* of *Achievement* (*WJ*-IV ACH; Schrank et al. 2014) KeyMath-3 Diagnostic Assessment (KeyMath-3 DA; Connolly 2008) Differential Ability Scales® (2nd edn) (DAS-II*;* Elliott 2007) Detroit Test of Learning Aptitude (4th edn) (DTLA-4; Hammill 1998) Detroit Tests of Learning Abilities (5th edn) (DTLA-5; Hammill et al. 2018*)* Stanford Diagnostic Mathematics Test-IV (Harcourt Brace Educational Measurement 1996) Process Assessment of the Learner (2nd edn) Diagnostic for Math (PAL-II M; Berninger 2007b) Process Assessment of the Learner (2nd edn) Diagnostic for Reading and Writing (PAL-II RW; Berninger 2007a) Test of Written Language (4th edn) (*TOWL-4;* Hammill *and* Larsen 2009)
Reading	Gray Oral Reading Test-5 (GORT-5; Wiederholt and Bryant 2012) Test of Reading Comprehension (TORC-4; Brown et al. 2008) Nelson Denny Reading Test Forms I & J (NDRT; Fishco 2018) **OWLS II Oral and Written Language Scales II (Carrow-Woolfolk** 2012a) Test of Word Reading Efficiency (2nd edn) (TOWRE-2; Torgesen et al. 2012) Illinois Test of Psycholinguistic Ability-3 (ITPA-3; Hammill et al. 2001) Feifer Assessment of Reading (FAR; Feifer and Gerhardstein Nader 2015) Gary's Silent Reading Test (GRST; Wiederholt and Blalock 2000)
Orthographic short-term and long-term decoding	Test of Orthographic Processing (TOC; Mather et al. 2008) Process Assessment of the Learner (2nd edn) Diagnostic for Reading and Writing (PAL-II RW; Berninger 2007a) Jordan Left-Right Reversal Test-3 (Jordan-3; Jordan 2011) OWLS-II Reading Comprehension (RC) and Written Expression (WE) Hand-Scored Kit (Carrow-Woolfolk 2012b)
Expressive and receptive language	Clinical Evaluation of Language Fundamentals (CELF-5; Wiig et al. 2013) **OWLS II Oral and Written Language Scales II (Carrow-Woolfolk** 2012a) Mullen Scales of Early Learning (Mullen 1995)
Written expression	Test of Written Language (4th edn) (*TOWL-4;* Hammill *and* Larsen 2009) The *Wechsler Individual Achievement Test (3rd edn) (WIAT-III;* Wechsler 2009a) Process Assessment of the Learner (2nd edn) Diagnostic for Reading and Writing (PAL-II RW; Berninger 2007a) OWLS-II Reading Comprehension (RC) and Written Expression (WE) Hand-Scored Kit (Carrow-Woolfolk 2012b) Test of Early Written Language-4 (TEWL-4; Hresko et al. 2012)
Language processing	Boston Naming Test (Kaplan et al. 1983) Multilingual Aphasia Examination (Benton et al. 1994) Boston Diagnostic Aphasia Examination (3rd edn) (BDAE-3; Goodglass et al. 2001) Token Test (De Renzi and Vignolo 1962)

(continued)

Table 12.8 (continued)

Domain	Neuropsychological test
Phonological processing	Comprehensive Test of Phonological Processing *(CTOPP-2;* Wagner et al. 2013) A developmental neuropsychological assessment (NEPSY-II; Korkman et al. 2007) The Woodcock–Johnson Tests of Oral Language (WJ-IV OL; Mather and Wendling 2014a) A Language Processing Skills Assessment-4 (TAPS-4; Martin et al. 2018)
Visuo-spatial processing	the Rey–Osterrieth Complex Figure (ROCF) (Osterrieth 1944; Rey 1941) A developmental neuropsychological assessment (NEPSY-II; Korkman et al. 2007) Delis-Kaplan Executive Function System (D-KEFS; Delis et al. 2001) WAIS Block Design Subtest from the WAIS-III (Wechsler 1997), WAIS-R (Wechsler 1981) Judgement of Line Orientation, measure of visuospatial judgement (Benton et al. 1978) Hooper Visual Organization Test (VOT; Hooper 1958)
Attention/concentration	Conners Performance Test (KCPT; Conners 2015) Conners Continuous Auditory Test of Attention (Conners CATA; Conners 2014a) Digit Span Forward and Reverse from WAIS-III (Wechsler 1997), WMS-IV (Wechsler 2009b) Trail Making Tests (TMT) was developed by Partington and Leiter in 1938 as a divided attention test, and was originally part of the Army Individual Test Battery (Partington and Leiter 1949) and subsequently was incorporated into the Halstead–Reitan Battery (Reitan and Wolfson 1993) Cancellation Tasks (Letter and symbol) (Diller et al. 1974; Gauthier et al. 1989; Geldmacher 1996, 1998; Halligan et al. 1990; Weintraub and Mesulam 1988) Test of Everyday Attention for Children (TEA-Ch; Manly et al. 1998) Test of Variables of Attention (TOVA; Greenberg 1991) Paced Auditory Serial Addition Test (PASAT; Gronwall 1977, Gronwall and Sampson 1974) Integrated Visual and Auditory Continuous Performance Test (IVA + Plus; Sandford and Turner 2004) Tests of continuous performance to assess attention, impulsivity, and vigilance: Conners' Continuous Performance Test (3rd edn) (Conners CPT-3; Conners 2014b) Test of Variables of Attention, Version 9 (TOVA-9; Greenberg et al. 2017)
Verbal learning and memory	Wechsler Memory Scale (4th edn) (WMS-IV; Wechsler 2009b) Logical Memory I and II from WMS-III (Wechsler 1997), WMS-IV (Wechsler 2009b) Verbal Paired-Associates from WMS-IV (Wechsler 2009b) Verbal Memory Index from Wechsler Memory Scale-III (WMS-III; Wechsler 1997) Rey Auditory Verbal Learning Test (AVLT; Rey 1964) California Verbal Learning Test (Delis et al. 1987, 1993) Verbal Selective Reminding Test (VSRT; Buschke 1973) Hopkins Verbal Learning Test (HVLT; Brandt 1991)
Visual learning and auditory memory	Children's Memory Scale (CMS; Cohen 1997) Wechsler Memory Scale–Fourth Edition (WMS-IV; Wechsler 2009b) Visual Reproduction I and II from WMS-IV (Wechsler 2009b) Visual Memory Index from WMS-III (Wechsler 1997) Wide Range Assessment of Memory and Learning (2nd edn) (WRAMAL II; Sheslow and Adams 2003) the Rey–Osterrieth Complex Figure (ROCF) (Osterrieth 1944; Rey 1941) A developmental neuropsychological assessment (NEPSY-II) (Korkman et al. 2007) Nonverbal Selective Reminding Test (NSRT; Fletcher 1985) Continuous Recognition Memory Test (CRM; Hannay and Levin 1988) Block design subtest of the WISC (Wechsler 2014)

(continued)

Table 12.8 (continued)

Domain	Neuropsychological test
Executive functions	Delis-Kaplan Executive Function System (D-KEFS™) (Delis et al. 2001) Kaufman Assessment Battery for Children (KABC-II NU; Kaufman and Kaufman 2018) Wisconsin Card Sorting Test (WCST; Grant and Berg 1948) Children's Category Test (CCT; Boll 1993) Stroop Color and Word Test (SCWT; Stroop 1935) Trail Making Test-B (Partington and Leiter 1949; Reitan and Wolfson 1993) Subtests of Similarities and Block Design from the WAIS-III (Wechsler 1997), WAIS-R (Wechsler 1981) Porteus Maze Test and Intelligence (Porteus 1950) Multiple Errands Test (MET; Shallice and Burgess 1991) A Quick Test of Cognitive Speed (AQT; Wiig et al. 2002) Tests of Cognitive Abilities Woodcock-Johnson IV (WJ-IV-COG; Mather and Wendling 2014b) Behavior Rating Inventory of Executive Functioning (BRIED; Gioia et al. 2000) The *Conners' Teacher Rating Scale* (CTRS; Conners 1969, 1997a, b) Conners' Parent Rating Scales (S; Conners 1997c)
Speed of processing	Simple Response Time task (SRT) and Choice Response Time task (CRT) (Stebbins 2007) Symbol Digit Modalities Test (SDMT; Smith 1973)
Sensory-perceptual functions	Halstead–Reitan Neuropsychological Battery (HRNB; Reitan and Wolfson 1993) Tactual Performance Test and Sensory Perceptual Examination, subtests of HRNB (Reitan and Wolfson 1993)
Motor speed and strength	Computerized Index Finger Tapping (CTAP; Gur et al. 2010) Grooved Pegboard Task, a component of several neuropsychological assessment batteries, including the Wisconsin Neuropsychological Test Battery (Harley et al. 1980; Matthews and Klove 1964), the Repeatable Cognitive-Perceptual-Motor Battery (Kelland et al. 1992; Lewis and Kupke 1992), and the expanded Halstead-Reitan Battery (Heaton et al. 1992) Hand Grip Strength (see Massy-Westropp et al. 2011) Thurston Uni- and bimanual coordination test
Social awareness and skills	Social Language Development Test-elementary (SLDT-E: NU; Bowers et al. 2016), adolescent (SLDT-A: NU; Bowers et al. 2017) Social Responsiveness Scale II (SRS-2; Constantino 2012) The Pervasive Developmental Disorders Screening Test (Siegel 1996) Gilliam Autism Rating Scale (3rd edn) (GARS-3; Gilliam 2013) Asperger Syndrome Diagnostic Scale (ASDS; Myles et al. 2000) Test of Problem Solving (TOPS; Zachman et al. 1984)
Emotional and behavioural functioning	Minnesota Multiphasic Personality Inventory-2-Restructured Form (MMPI-II-RF; Ben-Porath and Tellegen 2008) Millon Scales of Personality-Millon Pre-Adolescent Clinical Inventory (M-PACI; Millon et al. 2005), Millon Adolescent Clinical Inventory (MACI; Millon et al. 1993). Millon Clinical Multiaxial Inventory-IV (MCMI-IV; Millon et al. 2015) Behaviour Assessment Scale for Children (3rd edn) (BASC-3; Reynolds and Kamphaus 2015) Piers-Harris Self-Concept Scale (Piers-Harris 3; Piers et al. 2018) Child Behavior Checklist (Achenbach 2011) Thematic Apperception Test (TAT; Murray 1943) Roberts Apperception Test for Children (McArthur and Roberts 1982) Children's Apperception Test (Bellak and Bellak 1949) The Rotter Incomplete Sentences Blank (Rotter and Rafferty 1950) Projective Drawings (Cummings 1986)
Personality assessment	Minnesota Multiphasic Personality Inventory (MMPI; Hathaway and McKinley 1943) Millon Clinical Multiaxial Inventory-IV (MCMI-IV; Millon et al. 2015) Beck Anxiety Inventory (BAI; Beck and Steer 1990) Beck Depression Inventory (BDI-II; Beck et al. 1996) Rorschach Test (Smith 2011) Thematic Apperception Test (TAT; Murray 1943)

testing. The most important aim of psychometric and neuropsychological assessment is to provide clinicians with a deeper understanding of the heterogeneity of the functional profiles of people with SLD and to help them to define appropriate interventions (Mourea and Waldie 2016). Direct assessment of a student's academic skills (including core reading, writing and maths skills) is anticipated to reveal deficits in the cognitive-linguistic skills, which have been empirically demonstrated to be critical for acquiring the related academic skills (Oakhill et al. 2015). Because research has established the basis for SLD in cognitive/linguistic skill deficits, particularly in the area of reading, such skills are analysed when assessing a student for possible SLD (Stuebing et al. 2015). Multiple cognitive domains include accumulated knowledge, achievement, attention, memory processing, and processing speed, problem solving and reasoning (Miller and Maricle 2019; Schneider and McGrew 2018). Cognitive assessment data provide insights into how a student learns and reasons that he or she is struggling academically (e.g. Sanders et al. 2018). Learning and behaviour may be affected by reduced language and visual/spatial skills, impaired motor co-ordination skills or central auditory processing disorders (CAPD) (de Wit et al. 2018). There is a high correlation between cognitive abilities and processes, and specific academic skills (e.g. Niileksela and Reynolds 2019), see Fig. 12.2.

We can understand SLD as a cross-cultural and chronic condition that typically persists into adulthood, albeit with cultural differences and developmental changes in the way the learning difficulties are manifested. Therefore, during the assessment, we have to take into consideration comorbidities. Comprehensive models of learning disorders should explain isolated learning disorders that affect one learning domain only, and any comorbidity between them (Landerl et al. 2013). Comorbidity can result from overlapping symptoms (when the same behavioural outcome is produced by different cognitive risk factors), which is explained by shared risk factors affecting more than one outcome (Moll et al. 2019b). It is important to note that children with comorbidity have unique underlying factors, in addition to their shared disabilities (Moura et al. 2017). Researchers have found that dyslexia and dyscalculia co-occur in 30% to 70% of children who have either disorder (Willcutt et al. 2013). Rates of comorbidity between reading disorders and other neurodevelopmental disorders range from 11% to 70% for reading and mathematics disorders (Moll et al. 2014); from 20% to 50% for reading and behavioural disorders (e.g. ADHD and conduct disorder; Hendren et al. 2018), and from 9% to 29% for reading disorders

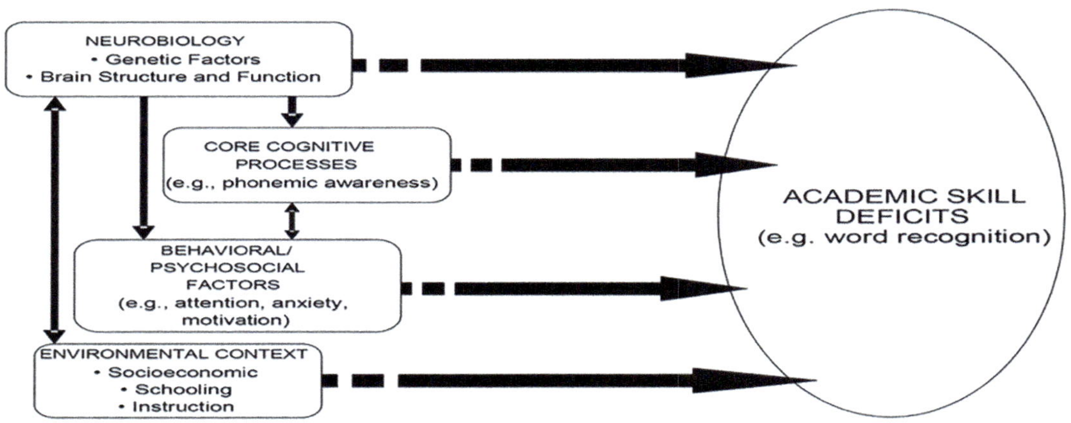

Fig. 12.2 Framework representing different sources of variability that influence academic outcomes in children with learning disabilities (Republished with permission of Guilford Publications, Inc. from Fletcher et al. (2007) Learning disabilities: from identification to intervention (1st edn) Guilford Press, New York NY, p 3; permission conveyed through Copyright Clearance Center, Inc.)

and emotional problems (Margari et al. 2013). From these findings the association between literacy and arithmetic is expected to be in line with recent fMRI findings showing similar neural activation patterns during arithmetic tasks (dot arrays, digits and number words) in children with reading and mathematical difficulties and comorbid problems (Peters et al. 2018). Furthermore, poor performance in mathematical word problems or multiplication fact retrieval can be caused by poor number-processing skills, or a consequence of poor language or reading skills (Moll et al. 2019b).

At the level of SLD students' behaviour outcomes, poor performance may be the result of a lack of self-confidence, social and behavioural problems, which may cause emotional problems, and poor peer relationships relating to their poor learning skills (Cortiella and Horowitz 2014). Manoj et al. (2015) report that 40% of children with SLD are diagnosed with behavioural problems, 30% children are aggressive and 10% are withdrawn. Continued behavioural problems in adults lead to depressive symptoms, somatic complaints, adaptation problems and difficulties in maintaining a permanent job (Alesi et al. 2012). In the UK, a study by Dahle et al. (2011) found more behavioural problems in the group with severe dyslexia than in controls, in all areas measured. In addition, parents reported that more children with dyslexia were anxious and depressed and had social and attention problems than those without. Prior et al. (1999) highlighted the risks of internalising problems, including anxiety, depression and phobias, in pre-adolescent children with mathematical difficulties. Jorm et al. (1986) studied a sample of 453 Australian children, followed over the first 3 years of schooling, and found that at school entry, backward readers had behavioural problems.

In brief, a deep and accurate assessment can help to determine comorbidity conditions in SLD. This provides a defensible basis for measurement and interpretation, and stronger statements regarding probable causal links, so that possibilities for appropriate remediation and logical intervention can be made (Decker et al. 2018).

12.7.2 Interpretation of Results from Neuropsychological Tests

Neuropsychological test results can be conceptualised as therapeutic intervention in determining the goals of assessment.

Test-gathered data, from a comprehensive evaluation of the psychological processes that underlie learning strengths and weaknesses, and other information, contribute towards:

- Making the use of results helpful to clinicians/family/teachers, who collaborate in helping the student/adult understand their condition better and thus increase their level of achievement
- Interpreting student/adult behaviour, their current cognitive, adaptive challenges and supporting positive chances in their life
- Encouraging the student's family/adults to develop realistic expectations of minimally and maximally supportive environments that can be constructed, allowing the child/adolescent to choose the right intervention programme from their known capabilities. (Clarification: some of the families put high expectations on their child's learning.)
- Choosing the proper or suitable programme for intervention (by adults, since children in early education stages cannot decide)
- Providing data from a great number of children, which can help in proactive screening of academic and behavioural performance and early interventions
- Establishing probable causal links and avenues for appropriate remediation and logical intervention
- Guiding more targeted instructional approaches or strategies and interventions
- Managing and informing others of the development of appropriate recommendations regarding curricular modifications and support, remedial techniques, accommodation and compensatory strategies

The monitoring of progress remains an essential component for documenting the effectiveness of interventions and developing revised instructional strategies. Intervention programmes are universally used, with each country using the programme appropriate to its educational system. Over the past few years, two models have emerged as alternatives to ability-achievement discrepancy for identifying SLD. The first, called the Response-to-Intervention (RTI) approach (Special Education Guide 2018), provides the student with different levels of support (base, middle and top), depending on their needs, and the second is called Processing Strengths and Weaknesses (PSW; Hale et al. 2010).

In general, the RTI model (Fig. 12.3) is defined as a preventive model that aims to improve the academic and behavioural performance of all students, as well as to assist them with immediate difficulties (Maier et al. 2016).

RTI is also an early intervention means of providing precise instructional tools for each student to meet and exceed his or her individual targeted growth goals within a culturally responsive learning environment (Wisconsin RTI Center 2017). In the United States, Canada, Brazil and Australia, the RTI programme is one of the key models of preventive-level intervention that has been more effective for learners (Cheung et al. 2016; Fry 2015; Robertson and Pfeiffer 2016).

The RTI programme has emerged as an instructional support with three tiers. It was intended to be a model of instruction monitoring the improvement of all students' academic and behavioural proficiencies through universal screening and organised instruction (Preston et al. 2016). The RTI programme's central objective is to monitor the student's progress towards

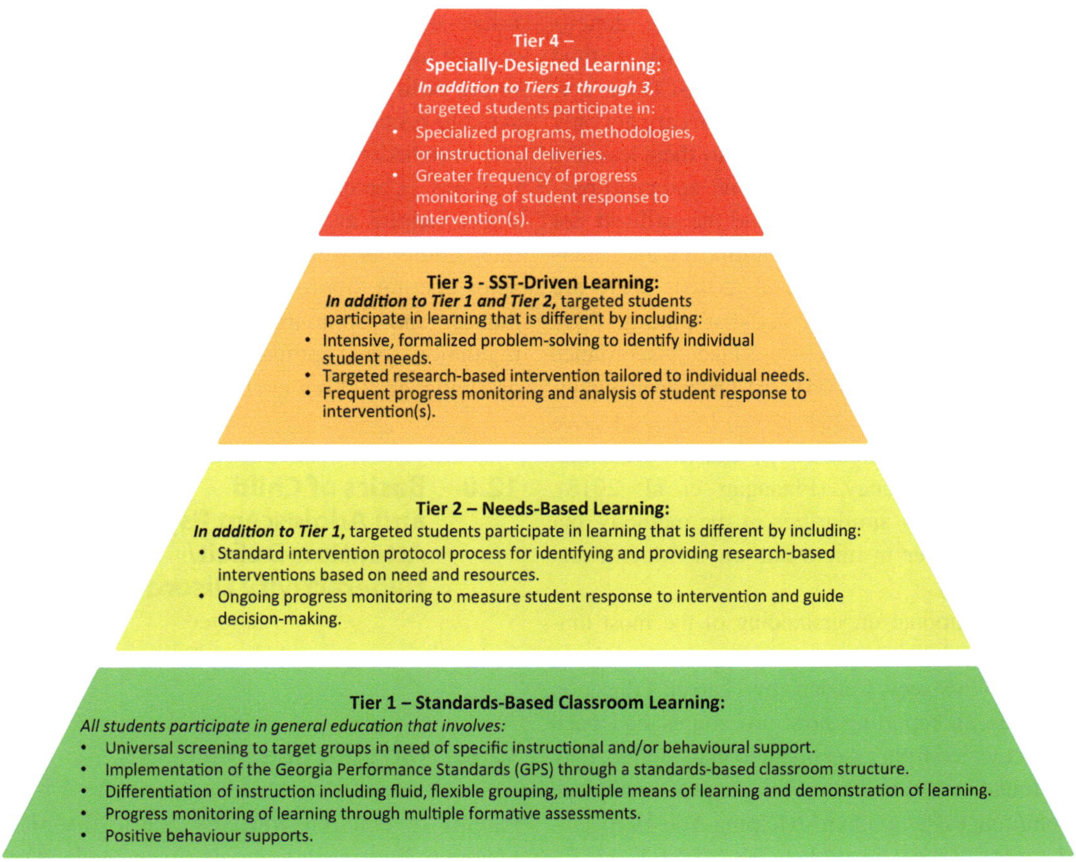

Fig. 12.3 Academic Intervention Pyramid adapted from the Georgia Student Achievement Pyramid of Interventions, with permission from the Georgia Department of Education, Atlanta

decision-making, on the basis of teaching. Information and data are collected through RTI, with emphasis on differences in the learning process and meeting student needs (Harlacher et al. 2015; Maier et al. 2016).

Furthermore, the RTI model is intended to provide targeted intervention to all children, to increase learning and avoid school failure by providing scientifically based intervention to all struggling students, as identified by school staff (Compton et al. 2012). Whenever the student continues to make insufficient improvement after intervention, despite repeated progress-monitoring and curriculum modifications, a comprehensive individualised evaluation may be justified. Therefore, further evaluation of processing strengths and deficits is needed to provide accurate identification (Meteyard and Gilmore 2015).

The other method of intervention, the Pattern of Strengths and Weaknesses (PSW), is to identify underlying cognitive processing deficits directly related to the SLD. The PSW method assumes that an individual with an SLD has certain cognitive processing deficits that are not only causally and predictably linked to their learning difficulties; the results of cognitive and neuropsychological assessments should be utilised for both identifying learning disabilities and intervention planning (Hale et al. 2010). There are currently four major methods of putting PSW into operation: (a) Concordance/discordance (Hale and Fiorello 2004), (b) Discrepancy/consistency (Naglieri 2011), (c) Core-selective (Schultz and Stephens 2015) and (d) Dual discrepancy/consistency (Flanagan et al. 2018). There are many similarities of the methods, but they also differ in important ways (McGill and Busse 2016).

For additional understanding of the most universal intervention programme, case studies of RTI/PSW (Stacey, Caeden) by Pearson Education Inc (2012), reporting how procedures had been implemented from assessment to intervention, may be found by this link http://images.pearsonclinical.com/images/ca/brochures/Helping-You-Help-Students-Succeed/BB3F5450E0EF-A5E57B503879B44E1613/7325_SLD%20Identification%20ezine_CS55_HR-noCrops.pdf.

Finally, we have to consider that the main aim of any intervention is to guarantee people with a learning disorder the right to study, the right to work and the right to well-being, in a learning context, and to support them in developing their potentials, interests and well-being (Petretto et al. 2017). If their problems are not recognised, and suitable programme modifications and supports are not provided, the risk of some disorders, such as depression, anxiety and delinquency, increase for these children; other possible outcomes for individuals with learning disorders who have not received appropriate intervention or help are emotional and behavioural problems, which include low self-esteem and suicide (Nel and Grosser 2016). We need information from all professionals when assessing the patient, investigating the test results, establishing and monitoring intervention programmes; this can be considered an input and output network for the future of the child/adolescent. Developmental science findings indicate that children who experience difficulties 'may be more malleable—and stand to benefit most—in the context of supportive, enriched environmental supports and interventions' (Cantor et al. 2018, p. 9). Additionally, warm, helpful and encouraging student–teacher interactions, as well as other child–adult relationships, permit improvements in school performance and commitment, greater emotional regulation, social aptitude and enthusiasm to take on challenges (Osher et al. 2018).

12.8 Basics of Child and Adolescent Psychiatry: Attention-Deficit/Hyperactivity Disorder

Esther Strittmatter and Georg Romer

12.8.1 Introduction

Parents of children with psychiatric disorders may initially consult a phoniatrician/paedaudiologist owing to anomalies in communication resembling developmental disorders of speech and language, hearing impairment or perception disorders. Therefore, knowledge about the most common diseases in child and adolescent psychiatry is essential for early recognition and therapy of affected children. Marked inattention/hyperactivity may hint at an attention-deficit/hyperactivity disorder; verbal and nonverbal impairment in communication and in social interaction at an autism spectrum disorder; and consistent failure to speak in unfamiliar public settings combined with social phobia at selective mutism.

Phoniatricians/paedaudiologists should be alert to psychiatric disorders such as differential diagnoses of a delay in hearing or speech/language development and immediately refer affected children to a child and adolescent psychiatrist. Early detection improves the effectiveness of therapeutic options and prevents secondary comorbidities and significant social, occupational and academic impairment.

Similarly, children with psychiatric disorders should be referred to phoniatricians/paedaudiologists to exclude hearing impairment and to give support in improving speech/language development.

In this Sect. 3.5 (Volume 1) and the following Sects. 3.6 and 3.7 (Volume 1), some of the more relevant disorders in child and adolescent psychiatry are presented.

12.8.2 Prevalence of Attention-Deficit/Hyperactivity Disorder (ADHD)

As the name of the disorder indicates attention-deficit/hyperactivity disorder (ADHD) presents as a pattern of persistent inattention or hyperactivity and impulsivity that interferes with functioning or development. ADHD is one of the more common disorders in child and adolescent psychiatry. Meta-analysis suggests a pooled prevalence of 5.3% in children and adolescents (Polanczyk et al. 2007) and 2.5% in adults (Simon et al. 2009). The prevalence of ADHD seems to have been stable over the past three decades (Polanczyk et al. 2014). Males are more often affected than females with a male-to-female sex ratio of 2.4:1 in population studies and 4:1 in clinical studies (Polanczyk et al. 2007). Often, comorbid disorders (e.g. oppositional defiant and conduct disorder, anxiety disorders, depressive disorders) occur in individuals with ADHD (Steinhausen et al. 2006). While only 15% of the children with ADHD meet full diagnostic criteria at the age of 25 years, approximately two-thirds will have persistent functional impairment into adulthood (Faraone et al. 2006).

12.8.3 Symptomatology

The core symptoms of ADHD are inattention or hyperactivity-impulsivity (American Psychiatric Association 2013). Typically, the symptoms start in early childhood. However, because of the high variability in behaviour in young children, a valid diagnosis is difficult before the age of 4 years. In preschool children the main manifestations are excessive motor activity and shorter playing time. Sometimes these children are greater risk-takers than their peers and are thus more likely to injure themselves. When their elementary schooling begins, their inattention becomes often more apparent. Often ADHD is associated with learning disorders and poorer academic achievement. Furthermore, impulsive behaviour, affective instability and motor hyperactivity can lead to conflict with parents, teachers and peers. In adolescents hyperactive symptoms manifest as inner restlessness, while inattention persists and is often accompanied by poor planning abilities. School failure and peer rejection may lead to low self-esteem, social disability and secondary comorbidities (e.g. substance abuse). For an overview the main DSM-5 diagnostic criteria are summarised in Table 12.9. They are further exemplified in the case report.

12.8.3.1 Case Study 3.5

On the advice of the child and adolescent psychiatrist, Mrs. Schmidt presents with her 9-year-old son Kevin to the phoniatrician for the purpose of excluding sound conduction and perception disorders. In the waiting room, Kevin is disturb-

Table 12.9 DSM-5 diagnostic criteria for ADHD (modified from American Psychiatric Association 2013)

Inattention	Hyperactivity-impulsivity
(a) Fails to give close attention, makes careless mistakes	(a) Fidgets with or taps hands or feet or squirms in seat
(b) Has difficulty sustaining attention	(b) Leaves seat in situations when remaining seated is expected
(c) Does not seem to listen	(c) Often runs about or climbs in inappropriate situations (in adolescents/adults: Feeling restless)
(d) Fails to finish tasks (e.g. schoolwork)	(d) Unable to play quietly
(e) Has difficulty organising tasks and activities	(e) Often 'on the go', acting as if 'driven by a motor'
(f) Avoids or is reluctant to engage in tasks that require sustained mental effort	(f) Talks excessively
(g) Often loses things	(g) Blurts out an answer before a question has been completed
(h) Easily distracted by extraneous stimuli	(h) Has difficulty waiting his or her turn
(i) Forgetful in daily activities	(i) Often interrupts or intrudes on others
Six or more of the preceding symptoms have been present for at least 6 months	
Yes	Yes

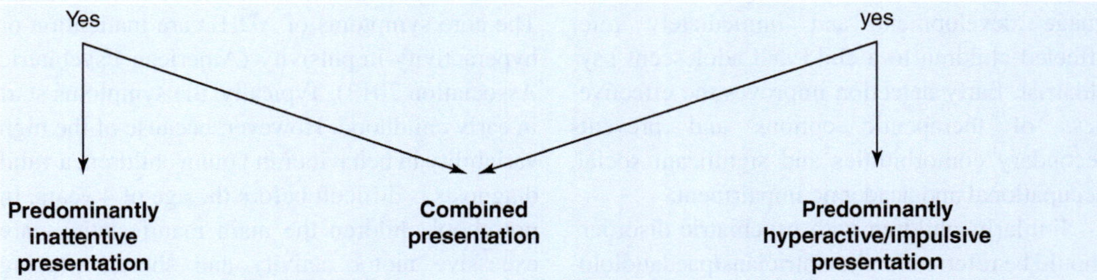

Predominantly inattentive presentation	**Combined presentation**	**Predominantly hyperactive/ impulsive presentation**

ing the other patients by his antics. On entering the doctor's room, Kevin begins to explore his surroundings and without permission starts to finger the doctor's instruments and a personal family picture. When Mrs. Schmidt tells Kevin to sit down, he doesn't appear to hear her. In order to conduct a conversation with the doctor, Mrs. Schmidt takes out a Gameboy to occupy Kevin. Immediately Kevin sits down and begins to play. Mrs. Schmidt complains to the doctor that he often disturbs lessons with his fidgeting, inability to sit still and by leaving his seat. Because Kevin cannot concentrate for more than a few minutes, he does not complete schoolwork (or homework). Furthermore he frequently mislays or loses his school materials. Kevin is often embroiled in conflict with his peers and his mother. At home his room looks a mess. While Kevin is reluctant to do homework or schoolwork, he can play videogames for hours.

12.8.4 Aetiology and Developmental Psychopathology

In 2013, the American Psychiatric Association (APA) has reconceptualised ADHD as a neurodevelopmental disorder in the fifth edition of the *Diagnostic and Statistical Manual of Mental Disorders* (DSM-5) (American Psychiatric Association 2013). ADHD is caused multifactorially. Studies on twins indicate a heritability of ADHD of 70–80% (Larsson et al. 2014). The interaction of several genetic and environmental risk factors leads to epigenetic changes and dysregulation of dopaminergic, noradrenergic and serotonergic monoamine systems. Structural and functional brain imaging studies have shown an under-activation and lower connectivity in frontal, striatal, limbic and cerebellar pathways. Furthermore, total brain volume is 3–5% smaller than normal. The described abnormalities result in a wide range of neurocognitive impairments (e.g. dysregulation of information processing, attention, inhibitory control and reward), which is consistent with the heterogeneity of the disorder (for elaborated review, see Faraone et al. 2015).

12.8.5 Differential Diagnosis

For differential diagnosis, oppositional defiant disorder, specific learning disorder, tic disorders, intellectual disability, reactive attachment disorder, anxiety disorders, depressive disorders and personality disorders should be considered. However, 60–85% of the patients have at least one of the mentioned disorders as a coexisting condition (Steinhausen et al. 2006).

12.8.6 Diagnostics and Treatment

The diagnosis relies on clinical symptoms reported by the patient, the parents or other informants (e.g. teachers). Thus, a structured clinical interview remains the 'gold standard' for diagnosis. The diagnostic criteria are listed in Table 12.9. According to the International Classification of Diseases (ICD-10), the age of onset has to be below 7 years. In contrast, DSM-5 has increased the age of onset from 7 years to 12 years. Validated rating scales help to assess quantitatively the behaviour in different contexts (e.g. at home and at school). A physical examination and laboratory tests should be performed to exclude somatic disorders. Furthermore, impaired hearing (e.g. disturbances of sound conduction and perception) and impaired vision should be excluded.

Although ADHD cannot be cured, several evidence-based treatments exist to reduce impairment and improve quality of life. Meta-analysis has shown that stimulants (methylphenidate, amphetamine) and non-stimulants (atomoxetine, guanfacine) effectively reduce the ADHD core symptoms inattention and hyperactivity-impulsivity (Faraone et al. 2015). In most cases medications are well tolerated, and adverse events are manageable (Cortese et al. 2013). Non-pharmacological treatment approaches (e.g. cognitive behavioural therapy, parent training, parent-child interaction therapy, school-based approach) mainly help to prevent or to improve secondary comorbidities and aim at ameliorating quality of life (Faraone et al. 2015; Sonuga-Barke et al. 2013).

12.8.7 Summary and Clinical Implications

ADHD is a common and impairing disorder in children and adolescents. Each ear, nose and throat specialist/phoniatrician/paedaudiologist should be alert to the disorder when a child presents for the differential diagnosis of an auditory disorder. Children with marked inattention or hyperactivity-impulsivity should be referred to a child and adolescent psychiatrist, as effective treatment options exist that can ameliorate the course of the disease and prevent secondary comorbidities.

12.9 Diagnosis and Differential Diagnostics in Respect of Specific Learning Disorders in Children and Adolescents

Christiane Kiese-Himmel and
Tahany Abdul Karim Al-Sayed Ahmed

12.9.1 Introduction

Verbal and non-verbal learning disorders (e.g. Developmental Visuo-spatial or Developmental Coordination Disorder) present a body of significant persistent learning difficulties and malfunctions that affect some school-age children's abilities to receive, process, analyse, store or (re) produce information efficiently and accurately. This results in poor school performance in the areas of education skills (reading, writing/spelling, mathematics), and sometimes in (serious) educational consequences (e.g. dropping out of school), as well as in unwanted social and emotional consequences that may continue into adulthood (estimated prevalence among adults: around 4%; see Morsanyi et al. 2018, p. 932) including a lower income in later life. According to the internationally used medical manual DSM-5 (American Psychiatric Association (APA) 2013), 'Specific Learning Disorders' (SLDs)—or 'Developmental Learning Disorders' (impairment in reading, mathematics or written expression) as it was recently retitled in the ICD-11 (World Health Organization 2022); are considered as neurodevelopmental conditions (see on this subject, for example Thapar et al. 2017) and thus a clinical diagnosis.

SLDs as an overall diagnosis are common in primary school children, more in males (ratio 2:1 to 3:1; DSM-5: APA 2013) and impede a student's ability to learn or use such specific academic skills as reading, spelling and mathematics. Impairments in these basic skills, sometimes also alternatively named as developmental dyslexia, developmental dysgraphia or developmental dyscalculia, form the over-arching category of SLD. Prevalence varies, depending on age, environmental factors, and especially on the cut-off criterion for the individual result of a domain-specific test. DSM-5 (APA 2013) states the prevalence of SLDs in reading, spelling and mathematics in school-age children belonging to different cultures as being from 5% to 15%. These are characterised by impairments in the following subskills ('specifiers'):

(a) Reading accuracy, reading rate of fluency or reading comprehension
(b) Spelling accuracy, grammar and punctuation accuracy or clarity or organisation of written expression
(c) Number sense, memorisation of arithmetic facts, accurate or fluent calculation or accurate mathematical reasoning

SLDs can occur as an isolated deficit or as combined deficits (mixed type of disorder; e.g. Moll et al. 2014, 2019a) and vary in severity (mild, moderate, severe). The prevalence of the isolated disorders with respect to the comorbidity is approximately the same (Moll et al. 2014), but in general more frequent. From 11% to 70% of children with a deficit in a single learning domain also experience a deficit in another. Therefore, it is quite possible that domain-general cognitive factors, such as executive functions, memory, attention or processing speed, are likely to have an impact on learning in several domains (Moll et al. 2016; Alahmadi 2017; Raddatz et al. 2017; Moll et al. 2019b). Genetic predisposition, epigenetic and environmental factors are implicated in SLDs. In a prospective cross-sectional study with 42 children with cerebral palsy (CP) (mean age: 9 yrs 8 months; SD: 2 yrs 2 months) and 60 children with SLDs (mean age: 10 yrs; SD: 1 yr 7 months) presented about 59% of the children with CP reading, writing or mathematics disorders. Children with CP and learning disorders had a low performance-IQ, normal phonological awareness, and working memory difficulties, whereas children with SLDs showed normal performance-IQ, impaired phonological awareness, and mild working memory difficulties (Micheletti et al. 2024).

Children and adolescents with SLDs typically fail to meet approved grade-level standards in listening comprehension, reading comprehension, basic reading accuracy and reading fluency skills, written expression, mathematical calculations, mathematical problem-solving or arithmetic fact retrieval, despite age-appropriate learning opportunities and instructions (Rosemary 2017; Kelly and Natale 2016). These difficulties must have existed for at least 6 months, despite targeted interventions.

Peters et al. (2018) compared fMRI findings of 9- to 12-year-old children with dyslexia, dyscalculia and their combination while they were performing arithmetical tasks in different formats, and found that all children with SLDs were slower in responding than typically developing children, despite their neural activation patterns being highly similar. We know that poor language definitely affects mathematical ability, from studies showing that individuals with poor language, phonological or literacy skills perform more poorly in aspects of mathematics that depend upon verbal abilities than typically developing controls (e.g. Boets and De Smedt 2010; Moll et al. 2015; Morsanyi et al. 2018). These children usually present difficulties in their early learning years, at an age when complex learning issues are involved, and there are even significant numbers of pre-adolescent children from mainstream schools who show learning difficulties and some adults (De Smedt and Boets 2010).

12.9.2 Basic Method of Assessment

SLDs are not due to a disorder of intellectual development (defined by IQ below 70 in a standardised IQ-test). Further exclusionary criteria are: sensory impairments (e.g. uncorrected visual or hearing acuity), motor disorders, Attention Deficit Hyperactivity Disorder ADHS, neurological disorders, psychiatric or psychosocial adversity (e. g. autism spectrum disorder), emotional disturbance/mood disorders, a lack of availability of education (e. g. school absenteeism), a lack of proficiency in the language of academic instruction or inadequate educational instruction, culture or economic disadvantages (exclusionary criteria) (DSM-5; APA 2013). They can only be diagnosed after formal school education has started and when the difficulties have persisted for at least 6 months despite the provision of academic interventions. Diagnosis is based on the individual's achievement in an individually administered, linguistically appropriate, standardised domain-specific test of high quality in reading, written expression or/and mathematics. SLDs can be supposed if the performance is substantially below what is expected for the student's chronological age (and scholastic achievement), at least one standard deviation (SD) below the average for the student's chronological age (and gender) group—in the presence of normal intellectual functioning, school opportunities and education (DSM-5; APA 2013). Nevertheless, cut-off points for the size of this discrepancy vary between 1 and 2 SDs (e.g. 1.25, 1.5) in practice.

Subsequently, the affected subskills in an impaired domain must be specified (see above). This evaluation has to be completed with a thoroughly documented history of learning problems, contextual variables and educational support, as well as by comprehensive school anamnesis and observer reports by the present teachers and by the parents. Finally, a logically clear and organised diagnostic statement that describes how the diagnosis was achieved (objective information regarding student history, recent educational impact and psycho-educational reports) must be included.

12.9.3 Differential Diagnosis

Children with SLDs often have concomitant disorders. Differential diagnosis of SLD is necessary to distinguish SLD from other disorders, syndromes and factors that can interfere with the acquisition and use of basic learning skills. This is highly important to ensure adequate interventions such as special education services or targeted treatments. A full clinical assessment involves different healthcare professionals, to rule out the exclusionary criteria of an SLD in a stepwise procedure to determine whether there exists only a small, irrelevant overlap between conspicuous features or a real associated disorder. However, it has to be taken into account during the examination that an SLD may aggravate an existing clinical impairment. There are five main steps in differential diagnostics:

1. A standardised intelligence test
2. Physical examinations
3. A neurocognitive evaluation
4. Examining the current developmental status in spoken language
5. Determining the current social-emotional status

(1) Differential diagnosis starts with testing the intelligence, because differential diagnostic criteria are based exclusively on the overall IQ-score, an index of general mental abilities obtained by a *standardised intelligence test in the psychological assessment.* The main diagnostic change in accordance with DSM-5 (APA 2013) is that the IQ-achievement dis-

crepancy criterion (the discrepancy between IQ and the affected learning domain(s)) has been abandoned. However, some psychologists prefer to measure not only the global intellectual capability of a student, but also to map the intelligence profile, including an analysis of strengths and weaknesses in cognitive ability scores (e.g. Moll et al. 2014). On the contrary, Fletcher et al. (2018) postulated differential diagnosis criteria, based exclusively on IQ, which disregard intra-individual differences in skills and performance. These are more predictive of many important social outcomes than any other measurable psychological trait independent of IQ, but especially academic achievement (e.g. Gottfredson 2018).

(2) The next step is a *physical examination for medical conditions* such as sensory impairments in vision or hearing, motor disorders, neurological symptoms or brain dysfunctions (including an electroencephalogram). A family history of learning disabilities (SLD clusters in families), a medical and a full developmental history of the student has to be taken and assessed, psychosocial stressors should be asked for, from the student (e.g. domestic violence, substance use) and from his or her parents (e.g. education, socio-economic status, economic disadvantage, living environment). At this point, it should be mentioned that Roca-Stappung et al. (2017) have provided an electroencephalographic characterisation of subgroups of children with learning disorders.

(3) Research has revealed a number of cognitive skills to be essential factors in academic development and the acquisition of reading, writing and mathematical competence. These skills are cognitive precursors in the individual development. They include executive functioning skills (cognitive-regulating processes), visual and auditory processing (e.g. processing speed, temporal processing, visuospatial/phonological working memory, phonological awareness, phonological processing), which are likely to have an impact on learning in several domains (Kilpatrick 2015; Slot et al. 2016; British Society of Audiology 2017; Raddatz et al. 2017; Knoop-van Campen et al. 2018). From these should be determined in a *neurocognitive evaluation* whether a child has perceptual disabilities, processing impairments, deficits in attention or in short-term-memory. In addition, it should be checked whether an attention-deficit disorder, a mental retardation due to not yet fully developed processing abilities, is also present.

Some clinical and genetic studies have reported extremely high prevalence of SLD and ADHD (82.3%) in comorbid cases (Altay and Görker 2018). This supports the view that both disorders are associated with similar hereditary factors. A study by Morsanyi et al. (2018) reported the performance of 2.421 school children on standardised tests of mathematics, English and IQ over the primary school years from urban and outlying rural schools in Northern Ireland, and analysed this large data set. Difficulties in maths, as well as consistently exceptionally high performance in maths, were equally common in boys and girls. The prevalence of persistent severe difficulties with mathematics was 6%, and 5.7% of school children demonstrated an SLD in mathematics (SLDM). About half of the children exhibiting an SLDM profile from the study had difficulties with English, 20% of those with SLDM showing a language or communication disorder, and some of these children had social, emotional and behavioural difficulties or an ADHD too.

(4) Further, the *current developmental status* in spoken language has to be examined, because there may still exist residual symptoms of a language impairment from early childhood that might be responsible for the diagnosed SLDs.

(5) Social-emotional reasons or performance anxiety can affect academic performance, and SLDs often occur with emotional or behavioural problems or both (e.g. Altay and Görker 2018; Horbach et al. 2020). Hence, such factors need to be ruled out as explanatory condi-

tions for the weaknesses in learning and academic performance. Differential diagnosis of SLDs versus emotional or social-behavioural problems can be very challenging because children with SLDs may have low self-confidence, low self-esteem, a low positive self-concept, and may be anxious. Therefore, it is important to note that children might not be sufficiently cooperative in the psychological/psychiatric examination. Sometimes, they become frustrated, but sometimes they become also quite aggressive.

The study from Morsanyi et al. (2018) confirmed social, emotional and behavioural difficulties in primary school children with SLDs. Rodrigues et al. (2016) showed in a control-group comparison that children with learning disorders had a higher frequency of depressive symptoms varying according to their age, especially so in girls. Mammarella et al. (2016) compared the results of self-report questionnaires on internalising symptoms such as anxiety and depression, for three groups each consisting of 15 children at the ages of 8–11 years: children with non-verbal learning disabilities (NLD); those with reading disabilities (RD), and a typically developing (TD) group. Social anxiety experiences were more frequent in children with learning disabilities than in TD children. Children with RD reported worse depressive symptoms than children with NLD or TD, whereas NLD children claimed more severe anxiety about school and separation than TD children. Visser et al. (2020) found a high rate of psychopathology in a study of 3014 German children from grades 3 and 4 with an SLD in reading, spelling or arithmetic: 28% had depression; 22% conduct disorders; 21% anxiety disorders (and 28% ADHD). Children with a mixed SLD had a broader spectrum of psychopathology than children with an isolated disorder. Finally, Klassen et al. (2013) have shown by meta-analysis that adults with learning disabilities continue to exhibit higher levels of internalising symptoms (anxiety and depression) or co-occurring mental health problems, as Hendren et al. (2018) later summarised in their review regarding reading disorders.

At the end of the differential diagnostic process, performed by an interdisciplinary examiner team, a clinical synthesis has to be performed by evaluating the individual's test results, medical, family and educational history, including school reports. Nonetheless, it must be noted that different approaches to identification of SLD(s) exist.

According to a multiple-deficit models approach, SLDs are associated with several risk factors and result from complex interactions between core deficits that are specific to a given disorder (Hulme and Snowling 2013) and to domain-general risk factors that may be shared between disorders. The evaluation described in this subsection includes testing of reading, spelling and arithmetic abilities, IQ-testing, medical examinations (including audiological and visual), neurocognitive/neuropsychological testing, speech/language evaluation and socio-emotional evaluations. Furthermore, alternative diagnostic criteria may include critical discrepancies within specific achievement areas, an intra-cognitive pattern of discrepancy, and information processing discrepancies (Fiorello et al. 2008; Flanagan et al. 2011). However, a consensus has not yet been reached on the specific deficits underlying the different learning disorders. As a result, the extant empirical research suggests that.

> … school psychologists [are] spending too much time conducting assessments with a low probability of accurately identifying SLD—e.g. Kranzler et al. (2019), p. 207

To conclude, the use of diagnostic criteria and standardised achievement measures can help to determine whether an SLD is of uniform or mixed type. Furthermore, it may be helpful to define the characteristics of spoken and written language, to seek aetiological accounts, and to describe the involvement of environmental factors. The diagnostic challenge is to determine whether the complex disorder 'SLD' is an accompanying symptom, in the sense of attribution to another existing disorder, or an independent disorder based on innate factors. In mastering this very difficult task, the use of multiple indicators meets the statutory requirements for a comprehensive clinical assessment. Additionally, the use of multiple data points allows greater sensitivity in identifying potential academic problems, assessment of a full range of component academic skills and multi-resource data collection (including medical, developmental, educational, and family history and relations, reports of observations in home and school environment, culture-academic difficulties, school achievement tests, intelligence quotient [IQ], neuropsychological evaluations, language status survey, comorbid behavioural symptoms). Last but not least, this might not only be informative but also helpful for future academic interventions and for therapy.

12.10 Differential Diagnostics in Respect of Auditory Processing Disorder

David Moore, Nicole Campbell, Tony Sirimanna and Doris-Eva Bamiou

Auditory processing disorder (APD) is a term used in audiology, speech language pathology (SLP), phoniatric and behavioural paediatric clinics to describe children who have normal audiograms (i.e. tone sensitivity) but difficulty with listening. These children and their caregivers and teachers typically report difficulties with hearing speech in challenging listening environments, and poor comprehension of, or attention to, spoken instructions. For more information, see Sects. 15.2 (Auditory Processing Disorders) and 16.8 (Auditory Processing Tests) in Volume 1.

APD occurs with a number of more widely recognised developmental learning problems of specific language, reading, autism spectrum and attention-deficit/hyperactivity disorders. Secondary issues associated with APD that may be misconstrued as poor behaviour in the classroom include disturbing surrounding children (for clarification of what the teacher has said), not participating in class discussions or responding appropriately, and missing verbal instructions. Learning a new language may also be more challenging. A detailed case history is helpful in differentiating between primary and secondary issues.

Tests of auditory function in childhood developmental learning problems have generally shown a higher than expected incidence of APD (around 50% for both language and reading disorders (Sharma et al. 2009)). This high co-occurrence raises the possibility that the learning problems may be caused, in part, by listening problems; that listening problems may be caused by learning problems; or that both sets of problems are caused by a more general source (a 'neurodevelopmental disorder') (Moore and Hunter 2013). Figure 12.4 offers a schematic representation of the interaction between different developmental disorders. It has long been suggested that language disorders are dependent on a specific auditory timing deficit (the 'temporal processing hypothesis' (Tallal 2004)). In other words, language ability depends on a person's ability to fill in missing 'gaps' (i.e. missed sections in spoken language), which is dependent on good hearing, listening, language, cognition and memory (both short- and long-

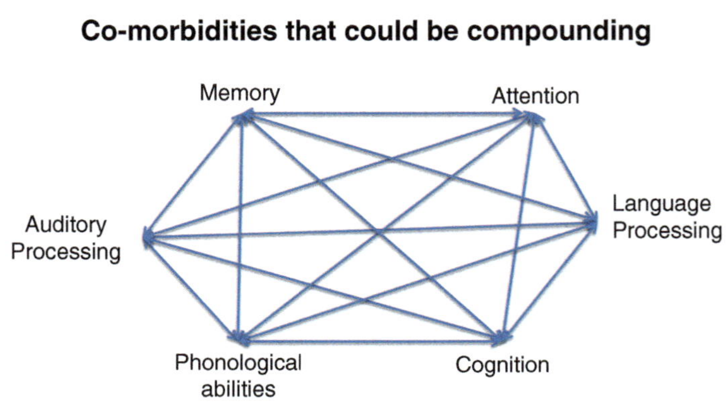

Fig. 12.4 The interaction between different childhood developmental disorders (adapted from Sirimanna 2020, with permission from SAGE Publishing, Thousand Oaks CA)

term); all of which affect the speed at which spoken language is processed; skills that are important for listening and understanding discourse speech. This hypothesis has been controversial, receiving mixed support over many years. One recent study suggested that training-related changes in temporal processing predict, and therefore cause, phonological dyslexia, the most common form of reading disorder; but the task used was not a clearly specific temporal task (Fostick et al. 2014). Nevertheless, the synergy between APD and literacy disorders makes differential diagnosis an important issue for both fields.

Among those primarily interested in APD, there has been a concerted attempt to distinguish listening from other learning problems. In fact, earlier professional guidelines on APD (American Speech-Language-Hearing Association, ASHA 1996) specifically stated that APD should not be diagnosed where there were co-occurring language or other cognitive difficulties. Research has attempted to separate the symptoms of each disorder (Chermak et al. 1999, 2002), but many papers over the last 10 years have shown a high co-occurrence and inter-dependence of cognition and hearing in general (Ronnberg et al. 2011) and among children with APD in particular (Dawes and Bishop 2010; Ferguson et al. 2011; Miller and Wagstaff 2011; Sharma et al. 2009; Tomlin et al. 2015). The American Academy of Audiology (AAA 2010) and the British Society of Audiology (BSA 2011, 2018) both recognise that language and reading problems co-occur with APD, although the AAA guidelines state that (Central C)APD in children is due to 'deficits in the function of the central auditory nervous system (CANS)', while the BSA guidelines state that APD involves 'higher level processing that provides "top-down" modulation of [the auditory system]'. In summary, there is currently no consensus concerning differential diagnosis of APD and developmental language disorders. On the contrary, there is a high but incomplete co-occurrence between these conditions, and suggestions that one may be causally related to the other.

When considering the diagnosis of APD, it is also important to consider other conditions where individuals also present with normal pure tone audiometry thresholds (125–8000 Hz) but report speech perception difficulty, particularly in noise. These are, in addition to language and cognitive aspects as outlined above, other conditions including Hidden Hearing loss (HHL) (Plack et al. 2014; Barbee et al. 2018; Zadeh et al. 2019; Kohrman et al. 2020), Extended High-Frequency Hearing Loss (EHFHL) (Al-Malky et al. 2015; Harrison 2012; Hunter et al. 2020) and Auditory Neuropathy Spectrum Disorder (ANSD) (Rance 2005). HHL requires more sensitive measures, such as otoacoustic emissions, extended high-frequency audiometry, electro-cochleography; identifying early waves within auditory brainstem responses will help to identify subtle cochlear hair-cell and synaptic dysfunction. At this time it is still unclear what the best markers for HHL in humans are. EHFHL is frequently seen in ototoxicity and noise exposure, as well as following early otitis media (Hunter et al. 2020). High-frequency audiometry is a useful adjunct in such cases. Finally, ANSD is a neural disorder affecting one or more of the following; inner hair cells and synapses, auditory nerve, auditory nucleus or brainstem auditory connections. Hearing level in ANSD can span from normal to profound hearing loss. Small numbers of those with ANSD have normal hearing sensitivity but have difficulties with hearing speech when the signal is degraded, e.g. in background noise. Otoacoustic emissions, cochlear microphonics and auditory brainstem response (ABR) are needed to diagnose ANSD.

In summary, when considering the diagnosis for APD, it is also important to take into account other childhood developmental delays that can co-exist, such as language and attention, and at the same time evaluate aspects such as HHL, EHFHL and ANSD which, if suspected, may be ruled out with further audiological testing. The APD MESH Guide (Campbell et al. 2019), an evidence-based APD live resource commissioned by the British Association of Teachers of the Deaf Foundation, offers more information and practical guidance for professionals, those with APD and their families.

References

American Academy of Audiology (AAA) (2010) Guidelines for the diagnosis, treatment, and management of children and adults with central auditory processing disorder. Available via https://audiology-web.s3.amazonaws.com/migrated/CAPD%20Guidelines%208-2010.pdf_539952af956c79.73897613.pdf Accessed 26th Sept 2021

American Psychiatric Association (2013) Attention-deficit/hyperactivity disorder. In: Diagnostic and statistical manual of mental disorders, 5th edition (DSM-5™). American Psychiatric Publishing, Washington, DC, pp 59–65

Achenbach TM (2011) Child behavior checklist. In: Kreutzer JS, DeLuca J, Caplan B (eds) Encyclopedia of clinical neuropsychology. Springer, New York NY

Adlof SM, Hogan TP (2018) Understanding dyslexia in the context of developmental language disorders. Lang Speech Hear Serv Sch 49(4):762–773

Alahmadi NA (2017) Cognitive control in children with learning disabilities: Neuromarker for deficient executive function. Neuroreport 28(11):638–644

Alesi M, Rappo G, Pepi A (2012) Self-esteem at school and self-handicapping in childhood: comparison of groups with learning disabilities. Psychol Rep 111(3):952–962

Al-Malky G, Dawson SJ, Sirimanna T et al (2015) High-frequency audiometry reveals high prevalence of aminoglycoside ototoxicity in children with cystic fibrosis. J Cyst Fibros 14(2):248–254

Alonzo CN, McIlraith AL, Catts HW et al (2020) Predicting dyslexia in children with developmental language disorder. J Speech Lang Hear Res 63(1):151–162

Altay MA, Görker I (2018) Assessment of psychiatric comorbidity and WISC-R profiles in cases diagnosed with specific learning disorder according to DSM-5 criteria. Noro Psikiyatri Ars 55(2):127–134

American Psychiatric Association (APA) (2013) The diagnostic and statistical manual of mental disorders (5th edn) (DSM-5). American Psychiatric Association Publishing, Arlington, VA

American Speech-Language-Hearing Association, ASHA (1996) Central auditory processing: current status of research and implications for clinical practice. Am J Audiol 5(2):41–54

Aro M (2014) Learning to read: the effect of orthography. Academic dissertation. Faculty of Social Sciences of the University of Jyväskylä

Ashkenazi S, Black JM, Abrams DA et al (2013) Neurobiological underpinnings of math and reading learning disabilities. J Learn Disabil 46(6):549–569

Baldeweg T, Richardson A, Watkins S et al (1999) Impaired auditory frequency discrimination in dyslexia detected with mismatch evoked potentials. Ann Neurol 45(4):495–503

Barbee CM, James JA, Danhauer JL et al (2018) Effectiveness of auditory measures for detecting hidden hearing loss and/or cochlear synaptopathy: a systematic review. Semin Hear 39(2):172–209

Beck AT, Steer RA (1990) BAI—manual for the Beck Anxiety Inventory. Psychological Corporation, San Antonio TX

Beck AT, Steer RA, Brown GK (1996) BDI–II - Beck depression inventory-II. Psychological Corporation, San Antonio TX

Becker DR, McClelland MM, Loprinzi P et al (2014) Physical activity, self-regulation, and early academic achievement in preschool children. Early Educ Dev 25(1):56–70

Bellak L, Bellak SS (1949) Children's apperception test. In: CPS Co, Oxford

Ben-Porath YS, Tellegen A (2008) MMPI-2-RF—Minnesota multiphasic personality inventory-2-restructured form. Pearson, San Antonio TX

Benton A, Varney N, Hamsher K (1978) Visuospatial judgment. A clinical test. Arch Neurol 35(6): 364–367

Benton AL, Hamsher KD, Sivan AB (1994) Multilingual aphasia examination. Psychological Assessment Resources Inc., Lutz FL

Berger D (2007) Primitive reflexes and righting reactions. A look through the lens of survival, emotions and memory. https://daveberger.net/daves-articles/primitive-reflexes-and-rightingreactions-a-look-through-the-lense-of-survival-emotions-and-memory/. Accessed 5 May 2018

Berk LE (2013) Child development, 9th edn. Pearson Education, Boston

Berninger VW (2007a) PAL-II Reading and writing - process assessment of the learner (2nd edition) Diagnostic for Reading and Writing. Pearson, San Antonio, TX

Berninger VW (2007b) PAL-II math - process assessment of the learner (2nd edn). Diagnostic for math. Pearson, San Antonio TX

Berninger VW, Richards T (2010) Inter-relationships among behavioral markers, genes, brain and treatment in dyslexia and dysgraphia. Future Neurol 5(4):597–617

Berninger VW, Richards T, Abbott RD (2015) Differential diagnosis of dysgraphia, dyslexia, and OWL LD: behavioral and neuroimaging evidence. Read Writ 28(8):1119–1153

Blakemore SJ, Frith U (2005) The learning brain - lessons for education. Dev Sci 8(6):459–471

Blomberg H, Dempsey M (2011) Movements that heal: rhythmic movement training and primitive reflex integration. BookPal, Coopers Plains

Boets B, De Smedt B (2010) Single-digit arithmetic in children with dyslexia. Dyslexia 16(2):183–191

Boll T (1993) CCT—Children's category test. Pearson, San Antonio TX

Bonifacci P, Montuschi M, Lami L et al (2014) Parents of children with dyslexia: cognitive, emotional and behavioural profile. Dyslexia 20(2):175–190

Bowers L, Huisingh R, LoGiudice CM (2016) SLDT-E: NU: social language development test-elementary. Pro-Ed, Austin TX

Bowers L, Huisingh R, LoGiudice CM (2017) SLDT-A: NU: social language development test-adolescent. Pro-Ed, Austin TX
Brady SA (1991) The role of working memory in reading disability. Haskins Laboratories status report on speech research 105/106:9–22
Brandt J (1991) The Hopkins verbal learning test: development of a new memory test with six equivalent forms. Clin Neuropsychol 5(2):125–142
British Society of Audiology (BSA) (2017) Position statement and practice guidance, auditory processing disorder (APD). Available via http://www.thebsa.org.uk/wp-content/uploads/2017/04/APD-Position-Statement-Practice-Guidance-APD-2017.pdf. Accessed 28th July 2021
Brooks PJ, Kempe V (2012) Language development (BPS textbooks in psychology). Wiley & Sons, Chichester, West Sussex/UK
Brown VL, Jl W, Hammill DD (2008) Test of Reading comprehension (TORC-4). Pro-Ed, Austin TX
British Society of Audiology (BSA) (2011) Position statement: Auditory processing disorder (APD). Available via https://eprints.soton.ac.uk/338076/1/BSA_APD_PositionPaper_31March11_FINAL.pdf. Accessed 26th Sept 2021
British Society of Audiology (BSA) (2018) Position statement and practice guidance: auditory processing disorder (APD). Available via https://www.thebsa.org.uk/wp-content/uploads/2018/02/Position-Statement-and-Practice-Guidance-APD-2018.pdf. Accessed 26th Sept 2021
Buschke H (1973) Selective reminding for analysis of memory and learning. J Verbal Learn Verbal Behav 12:543–550
Campbell N, Grant P, Rosen S et al (2019) Auditory processing disorder (APD) in children. BATOD foundation. Available via http://www.meshguides.org/guides/node/1432. Accessed 26th Sept 2021
Cantor P, Osher D, Berg J et al (2018) Malleability, plasticity, and individuality: how children learn and develop in context. Appl Dev Sci 1:307. https://doi.org/10.1080/10888691.2017.1398649
Caravolas M, Bruck M, Genesee F (2003) Similarities and differences between English- and French-speaking poor spellers. In: Goulandris N (ed) Dyslexia in different languages: cross-linguistic comparisons. Whurr, London, pp 157–180
Carrow-Woolfolk E (2012a) OWLS II—oral and written language scales II, 2nd edn. Pro-Ed, Austin, TX
Carrow-Woolfolk E (2012b) OWLS-II reading comprehension (RC) and written expression (WE) hand-scored kit. Pro-Ed, Austin, TX
Cattell R (1987) Intelligence: its structure, growth and action. Elsevier, Amsterdam
Catts HW, Hogan TP (2003) Language basis of reading disabilities and implications for early identification and remediation. Read Psychol 24(3–4):223–246
CDE (2017) California dyslexia guidelines. California Department of Education, Sacramento, CA
Cederlof M, Maughan B, Larsson H et al (2017) Reading problems and major mental disorders—co-occurrences and familial overlaps in a Swedish nation-wide cohort. J Psychiatr Res 91:124–129
Chermak GD, Hall JW, Musiek FE (1999) Differential diagnosis and management of central auditory processing disorder and attention deficit hyperactivity disorder. J Am Acad Audiol 10(6):289–303
Chermak GD, Tucker E, Seikel JA (2002) Behavioral characteristics of auditory processing disorder and attention-deficit hyperactivity disorder: predominantly inattentive type. J Am Acad Audiol 13(6):332–338
Cheung KC, Mak SK, Sit PS et al (2016) A typology of student reading engagement: preparing for response to intervention in the school curriculum. Stud Educ Eval 48:32–42
Christmann CA, Lachmann T, Steinbrink C (2015) Evidence for a general auditory processing deficit in developmental dyslexia from a discrimination paradigm using speech versus nonspeech sounds matched in complexity. J Speech Lang Hear Res 58(1):107–121
Chung P, Patel DR (2015) Dysgraphia. Int J Child Adolesc Health 8(1):27–36
Cioni G, Sgandurra G (2013) Normal psychomotor development. In: Dulac O, Lassonte M, Sarnat HB (eds) Handbook of clinical neurology 111. Elsevier, Amsterdam, pp 3–15
Cohen M (1997) CMS—Children's memory scale. Pearson, San Antonio TX
Compton DL, Gilbert JK, Jenkins JR et al (2012) Accelerating chronically unresponsive children to tier 3 instruction: what level of data is necessary to ensure selection accuracy? J Learn Disabil 45(3):204–216
Conners CK (1969) A teacher rating scale for use in drug studies with children. Am J Psychiatry 126:884–888
Conners CK (1997a) Conners' rating scales—revised: long form. Multi-Heath Systems, North Tonawanda, NY
Conners CK (1997b) Conners' rating scales—revised: short form. Multi-Heath Systems, North Tonawanda, NY
Conners CK (1997c) Conners' parent rating scales—revised (S). Multi-Heath Systems, North Tonawanda, NY
Conners KC (2014a) Conners CATA - Conners continuous auditory test of attention. Pearson, San Antonio TX
Conners KC (2014b) Conners CPT 3 – Conners' continuous performance test, 3rd edn. Pearson, San Antonio, TX
Conners KC (2015) KCPT—Conners performance test. Pearson, San Antonio TX
Connolly J (2008) KeyMath-3 diagnostic assessment (DA). Pearson, San Antonio, TX
Constantino JN (2012) SRS-2—Social responsiveness scale, 2nd edn. Pearson, Antonio TX
Cortese S, Holtmann M, Banaschewski T et al (2013) Practitioner review: current best practice in the management of adverse events during treatment with

ADHD medications in children and adolescents. J Child Psychol Psychiatry 54(3):227–246
Cortiella C, Horowitz SH (2014) The state of learning disabilities: facts, trends and emerging issues. National Center for Learning Disabilities, New York, NY
Cummings JA (1986) Projective drawings. In: Knoff HM (ed) The assessment of child and adolescent personality. Guildford Press, New York NY, pp 199–244
Dahle AE, Knivsberg AM, Andreassen AB (2011) Coexisting problem behaviour in severe dyslexia. J Res Spec Educ Needs 11(3):162–170
Dawes P, Bishop DV (2010) Psychometric profile of children with auditory processing disorder and children with dyslexia. Arch Dis Child 95(6):432–436
De Fries JC, Alacron M (1996) Genetics of specific reading disability. Ment Retard Dev Disabil Res Rev 2(1):39–47
De Renzi E, Vignolo LA (1962) The token test: a sensitive test to detect receptive disturbances in aphasics. Brain 85:665–678
De Smedt B, Boets B (2010) Phonological processing and arithmetic fact retrieval: evidence from developmental dyslexia. Neuropsychologia 48(14):3973–3981
de Wit E, van Dijk P, Hanekamp S et al (2018) Same or different: the overlap between children with auditory processing disorders and children with other developmental disorders: a systematic review. Ear Hear 39(1):1–19
Decker SL, Strait JE, Roberts AM et al (2018) Cognitive mediators of reading comprehension in early development. Contemp Sch Psychol 22(3):249–257
Delis DC, Kramer JH, Kaplan E et al (1987) The California verbal learning test: research edition, adult version. The Psychological Corporation, San Antonio TX
Delis DC, Kramer JH, Kaplan E et al (1993) The California verbal learning test for children. The Psychological Corporation, San Antonio, TX
Delis DC, Kaplan E, Kramer J (2001) D-KEFS™—Delis Kaplan executive function system™. Pearson, San Antonio, TX
Demonet JF, Taylor MJ, Chaix Y (2004) Developmental dyslexia. Lancet 363(9419):1451–1460
DeThorne LS, Hart SA, Petrill SA et al (2006) Children's history of speech-language difficulties: genetic influences and associations with reading-related measures. J Speech Lang Hear Res 49(6):1280–1293. https://doi.org/10.1044/1092-4388(2006/092)
DGKJP (2015) Deutsche Gesellschaft für Kinder- und Jugendpsychiatrie, Psychosomatik und Psychotherapie e.V. Diagnostik und Behandlung von Kindern und Jugendlichen mit Lese- und/oder Rechtschreibstörung. Evidenz- und konsensbasierte Leitlinie (S3); AWMF-Registriernummer 028-044 (Diagnosis and treatment of children and adolescents with reading and/or spelling disorders. Evidence- and consensus-based guideline (S3); AWMF registration number 028-044)
Diagnostic and Statistical Manual of Mental Disorders (2022), Fifth Edition, Text Revision (DSM-5-TR®) Amer Psychiatric Assn Pub. 1120. ISBN 978-0-89042-576-3
Diamanti V, Goulandris N, Campbell R et al (2018) Dyslexia profiles across orthographies differing in transparency: an evaluation of theoretical predictions contrasting English and Greek. Sci Stud Read 22(1):55–69
Diller L, Ben-Yishay Y, Gerstman LJ et al (1974) Studies in cognition and rehabilitation in hemiplegia. University Medical Center, New York, NY
Dilnot J, Hamilton L, Maughan B et al (2017) Child and environmental risk factors predicting readiness for learning in children at high risk of dyslexia. Dev Psychopathol 29(1):235–244
Döhla D, Heim S (2016) Developmental dyslexia and dysgraphia: what can we learn from the one about the other? Front Psychol 6:2045. https://doi.org/10.3389/fpsyg.2015.02045
Duff FJ, Reen G, Plunkett K et al (2015) Do infant vocabulary skills predict school-age language and literacy outcomes? J Child Psychol Psychiatry 56(8):848–856
Duranovic M, Mrkonjic Z (2013) Procjena disleksije (Dyslexia assessment.). Print-Com, Tuzla Bosnia
Duranovic M, Smythe I (2010) Disleksija (Dyslexia.). Harfo-graf, Tuzla Bosnia
Eckert MA, Berninger VW, Vaden KI et al (2016) Gray matter features of reading disability: a combined meta-analytic and direct analysis approach. eNeuro 3(1):ENEURO.0103-15.2015. https://doi.org/10.1523/ENEURO.0103-15.2015. PMID: 26835509; PMCID: PMC4724065.
Ehri LC (2000) Learning to read and learning to spell: two sides of a coin. Top Lang Disord 20(3):19–36
Elliott CD (2007) DAS-II: differential ability scales, 2nd edn. Pearson, New York, NY
Ellis AW (2016) Reading, writing, and dyslexia: a cognitive analysis. Taylor & Francis Group, Routledge, London, pp 1–8. 62–72
Engelhardt LE, Mann FD, Briley DA et al (2016 Sep) (2016) Strong genetic overlap between executive functions and intelligence. J Exp Psychol Gen 145(9):1141–1159. https://doi.org/10.1037/xge0000195
Faraone SV, Biederman J, Mick E (2006) The age dependent decline of attention-deficit/hyperactivity disorder: a meta-analysis of follow-up studies. Psychol Med 36(2):159–165
Faraone SV, Asherson P, Banaschewski T et al (2015) Attention-deficit/hyperactivity disorder. Nat Rev Dis Primers 1:1–23
Faustmann A, Murdoch BE, Finnigan SP et al (2005) Event-related brain potentials elicited by semantic and syntactic anomalies during auditory sentence processing. J Am Acad Audiol 16(9):708–725
Feder KP, Majnemer A (2007) Handwriting development, competency, and intervention. Dev Med Child Neurol 49(4):312–317
Feifer S, Gerhardstein Nader R (2015) FAR-Feifer assessment of reading. PAR, Lutz, FL

Fenichel GM (2009) Clinical pediatric neurology. A signs and symptoms approach, 6th edn. Elsevier, New York
Ferguson MA, Hall RL, Riley A et al (2011) Communication, listening, cognitive and speech perception skills in children with auditory processing disorder (APD) or specific language impairment (SLI). J Speech Lang Hear Res 54(1):211–227
Fiorello CA, Hale JB, Snyder LE et al (2008) Validating individual differences through examination of converging psychometric and neuropsychological models of cognitive functioning. In: Thurman SK, Fiorello CA (eds) Applied cognitive research to K-3 classroom learning. Routledge, New York, NY, pp 232–254
Fishco VV (2018) NDRT—Nelson Denny Reading Test Forms I & J. Pro-Ed, Austin, TX
Flanagan DP, Alfonso VC, Mascolo JT (2011) A CHC-based operational definition of SLD: integrating multiple data sources and data-gathering methods. In: Flanagan DP, Alfonso VC (eds) Essentials of psychological assessment. Essentials of specific learning disability identification. John Wiley & Sons, New York, NY, pp 233–298
Flanagan DP, Alfonso VC, Sy MC et al (2018) Dual discrepancy/consistency operational definition of SLD: integrating multiple data sources and multipledata-gathering methods. In: Alfonso VC, Flanagan DP (eds) Essentials of specific learning disability identification, 2nd edn. Wiley, Hoboken, NJ, pp 329–430
Fletcher JM (1985) Memory for verbal and nonverbal stimuli in learning disability subgroups: analysis by selective reminding. J Exp Child Psychol 40:244–259
Fletcher JM, Miciak J (2017) Comprehensive cognitive assessments are not necessary for the identification and treatment of learning disabilities. Arch Clin Neuropsychol 32(1):2–7
Fletcher JM, Lyon GR, Fuchs LS et al (2007) Learning disabilities: from identification to intervention, 1st edn. Guilford Press, New York, NY, p 3
Fletcher JM, Lyon GR, Fuchs LS et al (2018) Learning disabilities: from identification to intervention, 2nd edn. Guilford Press, New York, NY
Fostick L, Eshcoly R, Shtibelman H et al (2014) Efficacy of temporal processing training to improve phonological awareness among dyslexic and normal reading students. J Exp Psychol Hum Percept Perform 40(5):1799–1807
Friend A, Defries JC, Olson RK (2008) Parental education moderates genetic influences on reading disability. Psychol Sci 19(11):1124–1130
Frith U (1980) Unexpected spelling problems. In: Frith U (ed) Cognitive processes in spelling. Academic Press, London, pp 495–515
Fry J (2015) Facilitating success in tertiary education for students with specific learning disabilities: a framework for success (DocEd). La Trobe University. Albury-Wodonga, Victoria
Fussenegger B, Landerl K (2006) Dyscalculia and dyslexia: same or different? Sprache Stimme Gehör 30(4):165–170
Gathercole S, Baddeley AD (1993) Working memory and language. Psychology Press, Hove, NY
Gauthier L, Dehaut F, Joanette Y (1989) The Bells test: a quantitative and qualitative test for visual neglect. Int J Clin Neuropsychol 11:49–54
Gehsmann KM, Templeton S (2011) Stages and standards in literacy: teaching developmentally in the age of accountability. J Educ 192(1):5–16
Geldmacher DS (1996) Effects of stimulus number and target-to-distractor ratio on the performance of random array letter cancellation tasks. Brain Cogn 32:405–415
Geldmacher DS (1998) Stimulus characteristics determine processing approach on random array letter-cancellation tasks. Brain Cogn 36:346–354
Gilliam JE (2013) GARS-3—Gilliam Autism Rating Scale, 3rd edn. Pearson, San Antonio, TX
Gioia GA, Isquith PK, Guy SC et al (2000) BRIEF—behavior rating inventory of executive functioning. PAR, Odessa, FL
Gleason JB, Phillips BC (2024) The development of language: An overview and a preview. In: Ch.1 in Gleason JB & Ratner NB (eds.), The development of language, 10th edn. Plural Publishing, Inc., San Diego, CA, pp 1–28
Goddard S (2005) Reflexes, learning and behavior: a window into the child's mind. Fern Ridge Press, Eugene
Goldston DB, Walsh A, Mayfield AE et al (2007) Reading problems, psychiatric disorders, and functional impairment from mid- to late adolescence. J Am Acad Child Adolesc Psychiatry 46(1):25–32
Goodglass H, Kaplan E, Barresi B (2001) BDAE-3—Boston diagnostic aphasia examination, 3rd edn. Lippincott Williams & Wilkins, Philadelphia, PA
Gottfredson LS (2018) G theory: how recurring variation in human intelligence and the complexity of everyday tasks create social structure and the democratic dilemma. In: Sternberg RJ (ed) The nature of human intelligence. Cambridge University Press, New York, pp 130–151
Grant DA, Berg E (1948) A behavioral analysis of degree of reinforcement and ease of shifting to new responses in Weigl-type card-sorting problem. J Exp Psychol 38:404–411
Greenberg LM (1991) TOVA—test of variables of attention. The Tova Company, Los Alamitos, CA
Greenberg L, Holder C, Kindschi CL et al (2017) Clinical manual: TOVA 9—test of variables of attention, version 9. The TOVA Company, Langley, WA
Gronwall DMA (1977) Paced auditory serial addition task: a measure of recovery from concussion. Percept Mot Skills 44:367–373
Gronwall DMA, Sampson H (1974) The psychological effects of concussion. Auckland University Press–Oxford University Press, Auckland
Guasti MT (2016) Language acquisition: The growth of grammar, 2nd edn. The MIT Press, Cambridge, Massachussetts and London, England
Günther KB (1986) Ein Stufenmodell der Entwicklung kindlicher Lese- und Schreibstrategien. In:

Brügelmann (ed) ABC und Schriftsprache. Libelle, Konstanz

Gur RC, Richard J, Hughett P et al (2010) A cognitive neuroscience-based computerized battery for efficient measurement of individual differences: standardization and initial construct validation. J Neurosci Methods 187(2):254–262

Gustafson S, Samuelsson S (1999) Intelligence and dyslexia: implications for diagnosis and intervention. Scand J Psychol 40(2):127–134

Guthrie JT, Goldberg HK (1972) Visual sequential memory in reading disability. J Learn Disabil 5(1):45–50

Habib M (2021) The Neurological Basis of Developmental Dyslexia and Related Disorders: A Reappraisal of the Temporal Hypothesis. Twenty Years on. *Brain Sci 11(6)*:708. https://doi.org/10.3390/brainsci11060708

Hale JB, Fiorello CA (2004) School neuropsychology: a practitioner's handbook. Guildford Press, New York, NY

Hale JB, Alfonso V, Berninger B et al (2010) Critical issues in response-to-intervention, comprehensive evaluation, and specific learning disabilities identification and intervention: an expert white paper consensus. Learn Disabil Q 33(3):223–236

Halligan P, Wilson B, Cockburn J (1990) A short screening test for visual neglect in stroke patients. Int Disabil Stud 12:95–99

Hämäläinen JA, Salminen HK, Leppänen PH (2013) Basic auditory processing deficits in dyslexia: systematic review of the behavioral and event-related potential/ field evidence. J Learn Disabil 46(5):413–427

Hämäläinen JA, Lohvansuu K, Ervast L et al (2015) Event-related potential to tones show differences between children with multiple risk factors for dyslexia and control children before the onset of formal reading instruction. Int J Psychophysiol 95(2):101–112

Hammill DD (1998) DTLA-4 Detroit tests of learning aptitude, 4th edn. Pearson, San Antonio TX

Hammill DD, Larsen SC (2009) TOWL-4—test of written language, 4th edn. Pro-Ed, Austin, TX

Hammill DD, Mather N, Roberts R (2001) ITPA-3—Illinois test of psycholinguistic ability—3. Pro-Ed, Austin, TX

Hammill DD, McGhee RL, Ehrler DJ (2018) DTLA-5: Detroit tests of learning abilities, 5th edn. Pro-Ed, Austin, TX

Hannay HJ, Levin HS (1988) CRM—the continuous recognition memory test: a manual. Neuropsych Resources, Houston, TX

Harcourt Brace Educational Measurement (1996) Stanford diagnostic mathematics test, 4th edn. Pearson, San Antonio, TX

Harlacher JE, Potter JB, Weber JM (2015) A team-based approach to improving core instructional reading practices within response to intervention. Interv Sch Clin 50(4):210–220

Harley JP, Leuthold CA, Matthews CG et al (1980) Wisconsin neuropsychological test battery T-score. Norms for Older Veterans Administration Medical Center Patients. Department of Neurology, University of Wisconsin Medical School, Madison WI

Harrison RV (2012) The prevention of noise induced hearing loss in children. Int J Pediatr 1–13. https://doi.org/10.1155/2012/473541

Hathaway SR, McKinley JC (1943) *MMPI*—Minnesota multiphasic personality inventory. Manual for administration and scoring. University of Minnesota Press, Minneapolis MN

Hayes C (2016) Literacy and communication in the early years. A critical foundation. Critical Publishing, Northwich, UK

He Z, Shao S, Zhou J et al (2014) Does long time spending on the electronic devices affect the reading abilities? A cross-sectional study among Chinese school-aged children. Res Dev Disabil 35(12):3645–3654

Heaton RK, Grant I, Matthews CG (1992) Comprehensive norms for an expanded Halstead-Reitan battery. Psychological Assessment Resources, Odessa, FL

Hebert M, Kearns DM, Baker Hayes J et al (2018) Why children with dyslexia struggle with writing and how to help them. Lang Speech Hear Serv Sch 49(4):843–863

Hendren RL, Haft SL, Black JM et al (2018) Recognizing psychiatric comorbidity with reading disorders. Front Psych 9:101. https://doi.org/10.3389/fpsyt.2018.00101

Hooper HE (1958) VOT—The Hooper Visual Organization Test manual. Western Psychological Services, Los Angeles, CA

Horbach J, Mayer A, Scharke W et al (2020) Development of behavior problems in children with and without specific learning disorders in reading and spelling from kindergarten to fifth grade. Sci Stud Read 24(1):57–71

Hoskyn M, Swanson HL (2000) Cognitive processing of low achievers and children with reading disabilities: a selective meta-analytic review of the published literature. Sch Psychol Rev 29(1):102–119

Hresko W, Herron S, Peak P et al (2012) TEWL-4—test of early written language—4. Pro-Ed, Austin TX

Hulme C, Snowling MJ (2013) The interface between spoken and written language: developmental disorders. Philos Trans R Soc Lond Ser B Biol Sci 369(1634):20120395. https://doi.org/10.1098/rstb.2012.0395

Hulme C, Goetz K, Gooch D et al (2007) Paired associate learning, phoneme awareness and learning to read. J Exp Child Psychol 96(2):150–166

Hunter LL, Monson B, Moore DR et al (2020) Extended high frequency hearing and speech perception implications in adults and children. Hear Res 107922. https://doi.org/10.1016/j.heares.2020.107922

ICD-10 (2019). Available: https://icd.who.int/browse10/2019/en

IDA (2009) Factsheet testing and evaluation. International Dyslexia Association Information Services Committee, Baltimore MD

IDA (2017) Dyslexia assessment: what is it and how can it help? International Dyslexia Association Information Services Committee, Baltimore, MD

Ijeoma AJ, Chinelo U (2019) Dyslexia, neurodevelopmental conditions and comobidity: a rule rather than an exception. Arch Neurol Neurosci 4(2):1–5

International Classification of Diseases Eleventh Revision (ICD-11). Geneva: World Health Organization; 2022. License: CC BY-ND 3.0 IGO

Jednoróg K, Gawron N, Marchewka A et al (2013) Cognitive subtypes of dyslexia are characterized by distinct patterns of grey matter volume. Brain Struct Funct 219(5):1697–1707

Jerger J, Musiek F (2000) Report of the consensus conference on the diagnosis of auditory processing disorder in school-aged children. J Am Acad Audiol 11:464–474

Jordan BT (2011) Jordan-3 Jordan Left-Right Reversal Test, 3rd edn. Academic Therapy Publications, Novato, CA

Jorm AF, Share DL, Matthews R et al (1986) Behaviour problems in specific reading retarded and general reading backward children: a longitudinal study. J Child Psychol Psyc 27(1):33–43

Kacenelenbogen N, Dramaix-Wilmet M, Schetgen M et al (2016) Parental separation: a risk for the psychomotor development of children aged 28 to 32 months? A cross-sectional study. BMC Pediatr 16:89. https://doi.org/10.1186/s12887-016-0621-y

Kalashnikova M, Goswami U, Burnham D (2020) Novel word learning deficits in infants at family risk for dyslexia. Dyslexia 26(1):3–17

Kaplan E, Goodglass H, Weintrab S (1983) The Boston naming test. Lea & Febiger, Philadelphia, PA

Karlsdottir R, Stefansson T (2002) Problems in developing functional handwriting. Percept Mot Skills 94(2):623–662

Katzir T, Shaul S, Breznitz Z et al (2004) The universal and the unique in dyslexia: a cross-linguistic investigation of reading and reading fluency in Hebrew-and English-speaking children with reading disorders. Read Writ 17(7):739–768

Kaufman AS, Kaufman NL (1993) KAIT—Manual: Kaufman adolescent and adult intelligence test. American Guidance Service, Circle Pines, MN

Kaufman AS, Kaufman NL (2018) Kaufman assessment battery for children (2nd edition) Normative update. Pearson, San Antonio, TX

Kelland DZ, Lewis R, Gurevitch D (1992) Evaluation of the repeatable cognitive-perceptual-motor battery: reliability, validity, and sensitivity to diazepam. J Clin Exp Neuropsychol 14:65, abstract

Kelly DP, Natale M (2016) Neurodevelopmental function and dysfunction in the school age child. In: Kliegman S, Game S (eds) Nelson textbook of pediatrics, vol 1, 20th edn. Elsevier, New Delhi, pp 192–199

Keméńy F, Banfi C, Gangle M et al (2018) Print-, sublexical and lexical processing in children with reading and/or spelling deficits: an ERP study. Int J Psychophysiol 130(5):53–62

Kenner BB, Terry NP, Friehling AH et al (2017) Phonemic awareness development in 2.5- and 3.5-year-old children: an examination of emergent, receptive, knowledge and skills. Read Writ 30:1575–1594. Published online: 05 April 2017. https://doi.org/10.1007/s11145-017-9738-0

Kilpatrick DA (2015) Essentials of assessing, preventing, and overcoming reading difficulties. Wiley, Hoboken, NJ

Klassen RM, Tze VM, Hannok W (2013) Internalizing problems of adults with learning disabilities: a meta-analysis. J Learn Disabil 46(4):317–327

Knoop-van Campen CAN, Segers E, Verhoeven L (2018) How phonological awareness mediates the relation between working memory and word reading efficiency in children with dyslexia. Dyslexia 24(2):156–169

Kohrman D, Wan G, Cassinotti L et al (2020) Hidden hearing loss, a disorder with multiple etiologies and mechanisms. Cold Spring Harb Perspect Med 10:1. https://doi.org/10.1101/cshperspect.a035493

Korat O, Arafat SH, Aram D et al (2013) Book reading mediation, SES, home literacy environment, and children's literacy: evidence from Arabic-speaking families. First Lang 33(2):132–154

Korkman M, Kirk U, Kemp S (2007) NEPSY-II: a developmental neuropsychological assessment. Pearson, San Antonio, TX

Kranzler JH, Gilbert K, Robert CR et al (2019) Further examination of a critical assumption underlying the dual-discrepancy/consistency approach to specific learning disability identification. Sch Psychol Rev 48(3):207–221

Kujala T, Aho E, Lepistö T et al (2007a) Atypical pattern of discriminating sound features in adults with Asperger syndrome as reflected by the mismatch negativity. Biol Psychol 75(1):109–114

Kujala T, Tervaniemi M, Schröger E (2007b) The mismatch negativity in cognitive and clinical neuroscience: theoretical and methodological considerations. Biol Psychol 74(1):1–19

Kutas M, Federmeier KD (2000) Electrophysiology reveals semantic memory use in language comprehension. Trends Cogn Sci 4(12):463–470

Landerl K, Wimmer H (2000) Deficits in phoneme segmentation are not the core problem of dyslexia: evidence from English and German children. Appl Psycholinguist 21(02):243–263

Landerl K, Göbel SM, Moll K (2013) Core deficit and individual manifestations of developmental dyscalculia (DD): the role of comorbidity. Trends Neurosci Educ 2(2):38–42

Larsson H, Chang Z, D'Onofrio BM et al (2014) The heritability of clinically diagnosed attention-deficit/hyperactivity disorder across the lifespan. Psychol Med 44(10):2223–2229

Le Jan G, Le Bouquin-Jeannès R, Costet N et al (2011) Multivariate predictive model for dyslexia diagnosis. Ann Dyslexia 61:1–20

Leikin M (2002) Processing syntactic functions of words in normal and dyslexic readers. J Psycholinguist Res 31:145–163

Lewis R, Kupke T (1992) Intermanual differences on skilled and unskilled motor tasks in non-lateralized brain dysfunction. Clin Neuropsychol 6:374–382
Lietz R (1996) Klinisch-neurologische Untersuchung im Kindesalter. Deutscher Ärzte Verlag, Köln
Linkersdorfer J, Lonnemann J, Lindberg S et al (2012) Grey matter alterations co-localize with functional abnormalities in developmental dyslexia: an ALE meta-analysis. PLoS One 7(8):e43122
Liu L, Wang J, Shao S et al (2016) Descriptive epidemiology of prenatal and perinatal risk factors in a Chinese population with reading disorder. Sci Rep 6:36697. https://doi.org/10.1038/srep36697
Lonigan CJ, Anthony JL, Phillips BM et al (2009) The nature of preschool phonological processing abilities and their relations to vocabulary, general cognitive abilities, and print knowledge. J Educ Psychol 101(2):345–358
Lovio R, Näätänen R, Kujala T (2010) Abnormal pattern of cortical speech feature discrimination in 6-year-old children at risk for dyslexia. Brain Res 1335:53–62
Lyytinen H, Erskine J, Hämäläinen J et al (2015) Dyslexia-early identification and prevention: highlights from the Jyväskylä longitudinal study of dyslexia. Curr Dev Disord Rep 2:330–338
Maciejewska B, Wiskirska-Woźnica B, Świdziński P et al (2013a) Assessing auditory processing disorders in children with developmental dyslexia using auditory cognitive event-related potentials. Folia Phoniatr Logop 65(3):129–135
Maciejewska B, Wiskirska-Woźnica B, Świdziński P et al (2013b) Evaluation of auditory event-related potentials (ERPs) in children with the familial dyslexia. Otorynolaryngol 12(1):34–41
Maier MP, Pate JL, Gibson NM et al (2016) A quantitative examination of school leadership and response to intervention. Learn Disabil Res Pract 31(2):103–112
Mammarella IC, Ghisi M, Bomba M et al (2016) Anxiety and depression in children with nonverbal learning disabilities, reading disabilities, or typical development. J Learn Disabil 49(2):130–139
Manly T, Robertson IA, Anderson V et al (1998) TEA-Ch - test of everyday attention for children. Pearson, San Antonio, TX
Manoj KS, Haritha B, Susanta KP (2015) Psychological comorbidity in children with specific learning disorders. J Family Med Prim Care 4(1):21–25
Margari L, Buttiglione M, Craig F et al (2013) Neuropsychopathological comorbidities in learning disorders. BMC Neurol 13(1):198. https://doi.org/10.1186/1471-2377-13-198
Martin N, Brownell R, Hamaguchi P (2018) A language processing skills assessment—4 (TAPS-4). Pro-Ed, Austin TX
Massy-Westropp NM, Gill TK, Taylor AW et al (2011) Hand grip strength: age and gender stratified normative data in a population-based study. BMC Res Notes 4:127
Mather N, Wendling BJ (2014a) WJ-IV-OL—Woodcock-Johnson IV tests of oral language. Houghton Mifflin Harcourt, Boston MA (in Canada via Nelson Education)
Mather N, Wendling BJ (2014b) Woodcock-Johnson IV—tests of cognitive abilities (WJ-IV-COG). Houghton Mifflin Harcourt, Boston MA (in Canada via Nelson Education)
Mather N, Roberts R, Hammill DD et al (2008) Test of orthographic processing (TOC). Pro-Ed, Austin, TX
Matthews CG, Klove H (1964) Instruction manual for the adult neuropsychology test battery. University of Wisconsin Medical School, Madison WI
Maughan B, Carroll J (2006) Literacy and mental disorders. Curr Opin Psychiatry 19:350–354
Maurer U, Bucher K, Brem S et al (2003) Altered responses to tone and phoneme mismatch in kindergartners at familial dyslexia risk. Neuroreport 14(17):2245–2250
Mazurkiewicz-Bełdzińska M (2017) Neurological evaluation—from newborns to teenagers. In: Steinborn B (ed) Neurology of development age, 1st edn. PZWL, Waszawa, pp 68–84
McArthur DS, Roberts GE (1982) Roberts apperception test for children manual. Western Psychological Services, Los Angeles, CA
McGill RJ, Busse RT (2016) When theory trumps science: a critique of the PSW model for SLD identification. Contemp Sch Psychol 1:1–9
McGrath LM, Stoodley CJ (2019) Are there shared neural correlates between dyslexia and ADHD? A meta-analysis of voxel-based morphometry studies. J Neurodev Disord 11(1):31
McLeod S, Crowe K, Masso S et al (2017) Profile of Australian preschool children with speech sound disorders at risk for literacy difficulties. Aust J Learn Diffic 22(1):15–33. https://doi.org/10.1080/19404158.2017.1287105
McNulty MA (2003) Dyslexia and the life course. J Learn Dis 36(4):363–381
Meiri R, Levinson O, Horowitz-Kraus T et al (2019) Altered association between executive functions and reading and math fluency tasks in children with reading difficulties compared to typical readers. Dyslexia 25(3):267–283
Melzi G, Schick AR (2024) Language and Literacy in the School Years. Ch.10. In: Gleason JB, Ratner NB (eds) The development of language, 10th edn. Plural Publishing, Inc., San Diego, CA, pp 335–366
Merck Manual Professional Version (2017) Dyslexia. Available via http://www.merckmanuals.com/professional/pediatrics/learning-and-developmental-disorders/dyslexia. Accessed 8th June 2017
Meteyard J, Gilmore L (2015) Psycho-educational assessment of specific learning disabilities: views and practices of Australian psychologist and guidance counsellors. J Psychol Couns Sch 25(1):1–12
Micheletti S, Galli J, Vezzoli M et al (2024) Academic skills in children with cerebral palsy and specific learning disorders. Dev Med Child Neurol 66(6):778–792. https://doi.org/10.1111/dmcn.15808

Michelson DJ, Shu SK (2012) Cognitive and motor regression. In: Swaiman KF et al (eds) Pediatric neurology: principles and practice, 5th edn. Mosby Elsevier, Philadelphia

Miller DC, Maricle DE (2019) Essentials of school neuropsychological assessment. John Wiley & Sons Inc., Hoboken, NJ

Miller CA, Wagstaff DA (2011) Behavioral profiles associated with auditory processing disorder and specific language impairment. J Commun Disord 44(6):745–763

Millon T, Millon C, Davis R et al (1993) MACI—Millon adolescent clinical inventory. Pearson, San Antonio, TX

Millon T, Tringone R, Millon C et al (2005) M-PACI—Millon pre-adolescent clinical inventory. Pearson, San Antonio TX

Millon T, Grossman S, Millon C (2015) MCMI-IV—Millon clinical multiaxial inventory-IV. Pearson, San Antonio TX

Moll K, Kunze S, Neuhoff N et al (2014) Specific learning disorder: prevalence and gender differences. PloSOne 9(7):e103537. https://doi.org/10.1371/journal.pone.0103537

Moll K, Göbel SM, Snowling MJ (2015) Basic number processing in children with specific learning disorders: comorbidity of reading and mathematics disorders. Child Neuropsychol 21(3):399–417

Moll K, Göbel SM, Gooch D et al (2016) Cognitive risk factors for specific learning disorder: processing speed, temporal processing, and working memory. J Learn Disabil 49(3):272–281

Moll K, Landerl K, Snowling JM et al (2019a) Understanding comorbidity of learning disorders: task-dependent estimates of prevalence. J Child Psychol Psychiatry 60(3):286–294

Moll K, Gangl M, Banfi C et al (2019b) Stability of deficits in reading fluency and/or spelling. Sci Stud Read 24(3):241–251

Moll K, Snowling MJ, Hulme CH (2020) Introduction to the special issue "comorbidities between reading disorders and other developmental disorders". Sci Stud Read 24(1):1–6

Moore DR, Hunter LL (2013) Auditory processing disorder (APD) in children: a marker of neurodevelopmental syndrome. Hear Balance Commun 11(3): 160–167

Morsanyi K, van Bers BMC, McCormack T et al (2018) The prevalence of specific learning disorder in mathematics and comorbidity with other developmental disorders in primary school-age children. Br J Psychol 109(4):917–940

Moura O, Pereira M, Alfaiate C et al (2017) Neurocognitive functioning in children with developmental dyslexia and attention-deficit/hyperactivity disorder: multiple deficits and diagnostic accuracy. J Clin Exp Neuropsychol 39(3):296–312

Mourea D, Waldie KE (2016) Developmental learning disorders: from generic interventions to individualized remediation. Front Psychol 6:2053. https://doi.org/10.3389/fpsyg.2015.02053

Mullen EM (1995) Mullen scales of early learning (AGS edn). American Guidance Service Inc, Circle Pines, MN

Murphy KA, Justice LM, O'Connell AA et al (2016) Understanding Risk for Reading Difficulties in Children With Language Impairment. J Speech Lang Hear Res 59(6):1436–1447. https://doi.org/10.1044/2016_JSLHR-L-15-0110

Murray HA (1943) TAT—Thematic apperception test manual. Harvard University Press, Cambridge MA

Myles B, Simpson R, Jones-Bock S (2000) ASDS—Asperger syndrome diagnostic scale. Pearson, San Antonio, TX

Naatanen R (2000) Mismatch negativity (MMN): perspectives for application. Int J Psychophysiol 37(1):3–10

Naatanen R, Paavilainen P, Rinne T et al (2007) The mismatch negativity (MMN) in basic research of central auditory processing: a review. Clin Neurophysiol 118(12):2544–2590

Naglieri JA (2011) The discrepancy/consistency approach to SLD identification using the PASS theory. In: Flanagan DP, Alfonso VC (eds) Essentials of specific learning disability identification. Wiley, Hoboken NJ, pp 145–172

Nel M, Grosser MM (2016) An appreciation of learning disabilities in the south African context. Learn Disabil 114(1):79–92

Niileksela CR, Reynolds MR (2019) Enduring the tests of age and time: Wechsler constructs across versions and revisions. Intelligence 77:2–15

Nopola-Hemmi J, Myllyluoma B, Voutilainen A et al (2002) Familial dyslexia: neurocognitive and genetic correlation in a large Finnish family. Dev Med Child Neurol 44(9):580–586

Norton ES, Wolf M (2012) Rapid automatized naming (RAN) and reading fluency: implications for understanding and treatment of reading disabilities. Annu Rev Psychol 63:427–452

Norwich B (2014) Categories of special educational needs. In: Florian L (ed) The SAGE handbook of special education, vol 1. Sage, London, pp 55–72

Oakhill J, Cain K, Elbro C (2015) Understanding and teaching reading comprehension: a handbook. Routledge, New York NY

OECD (2017) OECD handbook for internationally comparative education statistics: concepts, standards, definitions and classifications. OECD Publishing, Paris. https://doi.org/10.1787/9789264279889-en. Accessed 20th Sept 2021

OECD (2018) Indicator B2 how do early childhood education systems differ around the world? In: Education at a glance 2018: OECD indicators. OECD Publishing, Paris. https://doi.org/10.1787/eag-2018-15-en. Accessed 20th September 2021

OECD (2019) Education at a glance 2019: OECD indicators. OECD Publishing, Paris. https://doi.org/10.1787/f8d7880d-en. Accessed 20 Sept 2021

OECD (2020) Education at a glance 2020: OECD indicators. OECD Publishing, Paris. https://doi.org/10.1787/69096873-en. Accessed 20 Sept 2021

OECD/Eurostat/UNESCO Institute for Statistics (2015) ISCED 2011 operational manual: guidelines for classifying national education programmes and related qualifications. OECD Publishing, Paris. https://doi.org/10.1787/9789264228368-en. Accessed 20 Sept 2021

Olofsson A, Niedersøe J (1999) Early language development and kindergarten phonological awareness as predictors of reading problems: from 3 to 11 years of age. J Learn Disabil 32(5):464–472. https://doi.org/10.1177/002221949903200512

Osher D, Cantor P, Berg J et al (2018) Drivers of human development: how relationships and context shape learning and development. Appl Dev Sci 1:6. https://doi.org/10.1080/10888691.2017.1398650

Osterrieth PA (1944) Le test de copie d'une figure complexe: contribution a l'étude de la perception et de la memoire [copying a complex figure: contributions to the study of perception and memory]. Arch Psychol (Genève) 30:203–353

Pakarinen S, Teinonen T, Shestakova A et al (2013) Fast parametric evaluation of central speech-sound processing with mismatch negativity (MMN). Int J Psychophysiol 87(1):103–110

Partington J, Leiter R (1949) Partington's pathway test. Psychol Serv Center J 1:11–20

Pearson Education Inc. (2012) Specific learning disability—professional assessments, pdf 7325_SLD Identification ezine_S55_HR-noCrops. Pearson Education, Inc. or its affiliate(s) 7325 3/13. Available via http://images.pearsonclinical.com/images/ca/brochures/Helping-You-Help-Students-Succeed/BB3F5450E0EFA5E57B503879B44E1613/7325_SLD%20Identification%20ezine_CS55_HR-noCrops.pdf, Accessed 12 Sept 2020

Peters L, Bulthé J, Daniels N et al (2018) Dyscalculia and dyslexia: different behavioral, yet similar brain activity profiles during arithmetic. Neuroimage Clin 18:663–674

Peterson RL, Pennington BF (2015) Developmental dyslexia. Ann Rev Clin Psychol 11:283–307

Petretto DR, Masala C (2017) Dyslexia and specific learning disorders: new international diagnostic criteria. J Child Dev Disord 4(19):1–5

Petretto DR, Piras P, Pistis I et al (2017) Disability, learning difficulties and environment: psychology of disability and neuropsychology as basis for the development of a "school for all"? In: Faiferri M, Bartocci S, Pusceddu F (eds) ILS innovative learning spaces. List Laboratorio Internazionale Editoriale, Trento

Piaget J (1936) Origins of intelligence in the child. Routledge & Kegan Paul, London

Piers EV, Shemmassian SK, Herzberg DS (2018) Piers-Harris 3—Piers-Harris self-concept scale, 3rd edn. Western Psychological Services, Los Angeles, CA

Plack JC, Daphne Barker D, Prendergast G (2014) Perceptual consequences of "hidden" hearing loss. Trends Hear 18:1–11

Polanczyk G, de Lima MS, Horta BL et al (2007) The worldwide prevalence of ADHD: a systematic review and metaregression analysis. Am J Psychiatry 164(6):942–948

Polanczyk GV, Willcutt EG, Salum GA et al (2014) ADHD prevalence estimates across three decades: an updated systematic review and meta-regression analysis. Int J Epidemiol 43(2):434–442

Poletti M, Carretta E, Bonvicini L et al (2018) Cognitive clusters in specific learning disorder. J Learn Disabil 51(1):32–42

Porteus D (1950) The Porteus maze test and intelligence. Pacific Books, Palo Alto, CA

Preston A, Wood C, Stecker P (2016) Response to intervention: where it came from and where it's going. Prev School Fail 60(3):173–182

Prior M, Sanson A, Smart D et al (1999) Relationships between learning difficulties and psychological problems in preadolescent children from a longitudinal sample. J Am Acad Child Adolesc Psychiatry 38(4):429–436

Pugh K, Verhoeven L (2018) Introduction to this special issue: dyslexia across languages and writing systems. Sci Stud Read 22(1):1–6

Raddatz J, Kuhn JT, Holling H et al (2017) Comorbidity of arithmetic and reading disorder. J Learn Disabil 50(3):298–308

Ramus F, Szenkovits G (2008) What phonological deficit? Q J Exp Psychol 61(1):129–141

Ramus F, Rosen S, Dakin SC et al (2003) Theories of developmental dyslexia: insights from a multiple case study of dyslexic adults. Brain 126(4):841–865

Ramus F, Altarelli I, Jednoróg K et al (2018) Neuroanatomy of developmental dyslexia: pitfalls and promise. Neurosci Biobehav Rev 8:434–452

Rance G (2005) Auditory neuropathy/dys-synchrony and its perceptual consequences. Trends Amplif 9(1):1–43

Reese E (1995) Predicting children's literacy from mother-child conversations. Cogn Dev 10(3):381–405

Reid G (2016) Dyslexia: a practitioner's handbook, 5th edn. John Wiley & Sons Ltd., Chichester

Reitan RM, Wolfson D (1993) HRNB—The Halstead-Reitan neuropsychological test battery, 2nd edn. Neuropsychology Press, Tucson, AZ

Rey A (1941) L'examen psychologique dans les cas d'encéphalopathie traumatique (the psychological examination of cases of traumatic encephalopathy). Archiv Psychol (Genève) 37:126–139

Rey A (1964) L'examen clinique en psychologie (clinical tests in psychology). Presses Universitaires de France, Paris

Reynolds CR, Kamphaus RW (2003) RIAS—Reynolds intellectual assessment scales. Psychological Assessment Resources Inc, Lutz, FL

Reynolds CR, Kamphaus RW (2015) BASC-3—Behavior assessment system for children, 3rd edn. Pearson, San Antonio, TX

Richards TL, Grabowski TJ, Boord P et al (2015) Contrasting brain patterns of writing-related DTI parameters, fMRI connectivity, and DTI–fMRI con-

nectivity correlations in children with and without dysgraphia or dyslexia. Neuroimage Clin 8:408–421
Richardson FM, Price CJ (2009) Structural MRI studies of language function in the undamaged brain. Brain Struct Funct 213(6):511–523
Richlan F, Kronbichler M, Wimmer H (2013) Structural abnormalities in the dyslexic brain: a meta-analysis of voxel-based morphometry studies. Hum Brain Mapp 34(11):3055–3065
Robertson S, Pfeiffer S (2016) Development of a procedural guide to implement response to intervention (RtI) with high-ability learners. Roeper Rev 38(1): 9–23
Roca-Stappung M, Fernández T, Bosch-Bayard J et al (2017) Electroencephalographic characterization of subgroups of children with learning disorders. PLoS One 12(7):e0179556. https://doi.org/10.1371/journal.pone.0179556
Rodrigues IA, Freire T, Gonçalves TDS et al (2016) Predicting signs of depression in children with specific learning disorder. Rev CEFAC 18:864–875
Rodriguez-Fornells A, Rojo N, Amengual JL et al (2012) The involvement of audio-motor coupling in the music-supported therapy applied to stroke patients. Ann N Y Acad Sci 1252:282–293
Roid GH (2003) Stanford-Binet intelligence scales -V, 5th edn. Riverside Publishing, Itasca, IL
Roitsch J, Watson S (2019) An overview of dyslexia: definition, characteristics, assessment, identification, and intervention. J Sci Educ 7(4):81–86. https://doi.org/10.11648/j.sjedu.20190704.11
Ronnberg J, Rudner M, Lunner T (2011) Cognitive hearing science: the legacy of Stuart Gatehouse. Trends Amplif 15(3):140–148
Rosemary T (2017) Specific learning disorder. In: Sadock BJ, Sadock VA (eds) Kaplan and Sadock's comprehensive textbook of psychiatry (10th edn) Vol. 1. Wolters Kluwer, New Delhi, p 320
Rosen CL (1965) Visual deficiencies and reading disability. J Read 9:57–61
Rotter JB, Rafferty JE (1950) The Rotter incomplete sentences blank. Manual, College Form. The Psychological Corporation, New York, NY
Sabisch B, Hahne A, Glass E et al (2006) Auditory language comprehension in children with developmental dyslexia: evidence from event-related brain potentials. J Cogn Neurosci 18(10):1676–1695
Sánchez-Morán M, Hernández JA, Duñabeitia JA et al (2018) Genetic association study of dyslexia and ADHD candidate genes in a Spanish cohort: implications of comorbid samples. PLoS One 13(10):e0206431. https://doi.org/10.1371/journal.pone.0206431
Sanders EA, Berninger VW, Abbott RD (2018) Sequential prediction of literacy achievement for specific learning disabilities contrasting in impaired levels of language in grades 4 to 9. J Learn Disabil 51(2):137–157
Sandford JA, Turner A (2004) IVA + plus—Integrated visual and auditory continuous performance test administration manual. Brain Train, Richmond, VA
Savill NJ, Thierry G (2011) Electrophysiological evidence for impaired attentional engagement with phonologically acceptable misspellings in developmental dyslexia. Front Psychol 2:139. https://doi.org/10.3389/fpsyg.2011.00139
Scheerer-Neumann G (2001a) Rechtschreibschwäche im Kontext der Entwicklung. In: Naegele I, Valtin R (eds) LRS–Legasthenie in den Klassen 1-10. Handbuch der Lese- und Rechtschreibschwierigkeiten vol 1: Grundlagen und Grundsätze der Lese-Rechtschreib-Förderung. Beltz, Weinheim, pp 58–77
Scheerer-Neumann G (2001b) Förderdiagnostik beim Lesenlernen. In: Naegele I, Valtin R (eds) LRS–Legasthenie in den Klassen 1-10. Handbuch der Lese- und Rechtschreibschwierigkeiten vol 2: Schulische Förderung und außerschulische Therapien. Beltz, Weinheim, pp 70–86
Scheich H, Brechmann A, Brosch M et al (2011) Behavioral semantics of learning and crossmodal processing in auditory cortex:the semantic processor concept. Hear Res 271(1–2):3–15
Schneider WJ, Kaufman AS (2017) Let's not do away with comprehensive cognitive assessments just yet. Arch Clin Neuropsychol 32:8–20
Schneider WJ, McGrew KS (2018) The Cattell–Horn–Carroll theory of cognitive abilities. In: Flanagan DP, McDonough EM (eds) Contemporary intellectual assessment: theories, tests, and issues, 4th edn. The Guildford Press, New York, NY, pp 73–163
Schrank FA, Mather N, McGrew KS (2014) *WJ* IV ACH—Woodcock-Johnson IV tests of achievement. Riverside, Rolling Meadows, IL
Schulte-Körne G, Ludwig KK, el Sharkawy J et al (2007) Genetics and neuroscience in dyslexia: perspectives for education and remediation. Mind Brain Educ 1(4):162–172
Schultz EK, Stephens TL (2015) Core-selective evaluation process: an efficient & comprehensive approach to identify students with SLD using the WJ IV. J Texas Educ Diagn Assoc 44:5–12
Serrallach B, Groß C, Bernhofs V et al (2016) Neural biomarkers for dyslexia, ADHD, and ADD in the auditory cortex of children. Front Neurosci 10:324. https://doi.org/10.3389/fnins.2016.00324
Sexton CC, Gelhorn HL, Bell JA et al (2012) The co-occurrence of reading disorder and ADHD: epidemiology, treatment, psychosocial impact, and economic burden. J Learn Disabil 45(6):538–564
Shafer VL, Morr ML, Kreuzer JA et al (2000) Maturation of mismatch negativity in school-age children. Ear Hear 21(3):242–251
Shallice T, Burgess P (1991) Deficits in strategy application following frontal lobe damage in man. Brain 114:727–741
Sharma M, Purdy SC, Kelly AS (2009) Comorbidity of auditory processing, language, and reading disorders. J Speech Lang Hear Res 52(3):706–722
Shaul S (2008) Event-related potentials (ERPS) in the study of dyslexia. In: Breznitz Z (ed) Brain research

in language. Springer Literacy Studies, Switzerland, pp 51–92

Shaywitz SE (2005) Overcoming dyslexia: a new and complete science-based program for reading problems at any level. Vintage Books, New York, NY

Shaywitz SE, Fletcher JM, Holahan JM et al (1999) Persistence of dyslexia: the Connecticut longitudinal study at adolescence. Pediatrics 104(6):1351–1359

Shaywitz BA, Lyon GR, Shaywitz SE (2006) The role of functional magnetic resonance imaging in understanding reading and dyslexia. Dev Neuropsychol 30(1):613–632

Sheslow D, Adams W (2003) WRAML2—Wide range assessment of memory and learning, 2nd edn. Pearson, San Antonio, TX

Siegel B (1996) World of the autistic child: understanding and treating autistic spectrum disorders. Oxford University Press, New York, NY, p 107

Siegel LS (1993) Phonological processing deficits as the basis of a reading disability. Dev Rev 13(3):246–257. https://doi.org/10.1006/drev.1993.1011

Simon V, Czobor P, Balint S et al (2009) Prevalence and correlates of adult attention-deficit/hyperactivity disorder: meta-analysis. Br J Psychiatry 194(3): 204–211

Sirimanna T (2020) Auditory processing disorder (APD). In: Peer L, Reid G (eds) Special educational needs: a guide for inclusive practice. SAGE Publishing, Thousand Oaks, CA

Slot EM, van Viersen S, de Bree EH et al (2016) Shared and unique risk factors underlying mathematical disability, reading, and spelling disability. Front Psychol 7:803. https://doi.org/10.3389/fpsyg.2016.00803

Smith A (1973) SDMT—Symbol digit modalities test. Western Psychological Services, Los Angeles, CA

Smith SR (2011) Rorschach test. In: Goldstein S, Naglieri JA (eds) Encyclopedia of child behavior and development. Springer, Boston, MA

Snowling MJ, Hulme C (2012) Interventions for children's language and literacy difficulties. Int J Commun Disord 47(1):27–34

Sonuga-Barke EJ, Brandeis D, Cortese S et al (2013) Nonpharmacological interventions for ADHD: systematic review and meta-analyses of randomized controlled trials of dietary and psychological treatments. Am J Psychiatry 170(3):275–289

Special Education Guide (2018) A guide to specific learning disabilities | special education guide. Available via https://www.specialeducationguide.com/disability-profiles/specific-learning-disabilities. Accessed 20th June 2018

Stackhouse J (1997) Phonological awareness: connecting speech and literacy problems. In: Hodson BW, Edwards ML (eds) Perspectives in applied phonology. Aspen CO, Gaithersburg, MD, pp 157–196

Stage SA, Abbott RD, Jenkins JR et al (2003) Predicting response to early reading intervention from verbal IQ, reading-related language abilities, attention ratings, and verbal IQ-word reading discrepancy: failure to validate discrepancy method. J Learn Disabil 36(1):24–33

Stanovich KE (2005) The future of a mistake: will discrepancy measurement continue to make the learning disabilities field a pseudoscience? Learn Disabil Q 28(2):103–106

Stebbins GT (2007) Neuropsychological testing. In: Textbook of clinical neurology, 3rd edn. WB Saunders Company, Chicago, IL

Steinbrink C, Klatte M, Lachmann T (2014) Phonological, temporal and spectral processing in vowel length discrimination is impaired in German primary school children with developmental dyslexia. Res Dev Disabil 35(11):3034–3045

Steinhausen HC, Nøvik TS, Baldursson G et al (2006) Co-existing psychiatric problems in ADHD in the ADORE cohort. Eur Child Adolesc Psychiatry 15(Suppl 1):125–129

Stoel-Gammon C, Velleman S, Menn L (2024) Learning sounds and sound patterns. Ch.3. In: Gleason JB, Ratner NB (eds) The development of language, 10th edn. Plural Publishing, Inc., San Diego, CA, pp 59–92

Stone CA, Silliman ER, Ehren BJ et al (eds) (2013) The handbook of language and literacy: development and disorders, 2nd edn. Guilford Press, New York, NY

Stroop JR (1935) Studies of interference in serial verbal reactions. J Exp Psychol 18:643–662

Stuebing KK, Barth AE, Trahan LH et al (2015) Are child cognitive characteristics strong predictors of responses to intervention? A meta-analysis. Rev Educ Res 85(3):395–429

Sun Z, Zou L, Zhang J et al (2013) Prevalence and associated risk factors of dyslexic children in a middle-sized city of China: a cross-sectional study. PLoS One 8(2):e56688

Swaiman KF (2012) Neurologic examination of the older child. In: Swaiman KF et al (eds) Pediatric neurology. Principles and practice, 5th edn. Mosby Elsevier, Philadelphia

Tallal P (2004) Improving language and literacy is a matter of time. Nat Rev Neurosci 5(9):721–728

Teixeira Costa HJ, Abelairas-Gomez C, Arufe-Giráldez V et al (2015) Influence of a physical education plan on psychomotor development profiles of preschool children. J Hum Sport Exerc 10(1):126–140

Thapar A, Cooper M, Rutter M (2017) Neurodevelopmental disorders. Lancet. Psychiatry 4(4):339–346

Thompson PA, Hulme CH, Nash HM et al (2015) Developmental dyslexia: predicting individual risk. J Child Psychol Psychiatry 56(9):976–987

Thorndike RL, Hagen EP, Sattler JM (1986) Stanford-Binet intelligence scale—IV, 4th edn. Riverside Publishing, Itasca, IL

Tomlin D, Dillon H, Sharma M et al (2015) The impact of auditory processing and cognitive abilities in children. Ear Hear 36(5):527–542

Torgesen J, Wagner R, Rashotte C (2012) TOWRE-2—Test of word reading efficiency, 2nd edn. Pearson, San Antonio, TX

UNESCO-UIS (2011) International standard classification of education. Available via http://uis.unesco.org/en/topic/international-standard-classification-education-isced. Accessed 20 Sept 2021

van Zuijen TL, Plakas A, Maassen BA et al (2013) Infant ERPs separate children at risk of dyslexia who become good readers from those who become poor readers. Dev Sci 16(4):554–563

Vandermosten M, Boets B, Poelmans H et al (2012a) A tractography study in dyslexia: neuroanatomic correlates of orthographic, phonological and speech processing. Brain 135(3):935–948

Vandermosten M, Boets B, Wouters J et al (2012b) A qualitative and quantitative review of diffusion tensor imaging studies in reading and dyslexia. Neurosci Biobehav Rev 36(6):1532–1552

Vellutino FR, Fletcher JM, Snowling MJ et al (2004) Specific reading disability (dyslexia): what have we learned in the past four decades? J Child Psychol Psychiatry 45(1):2–40

Vihman MM (2014) Phonological development, 2nd edn. Wiley-Blackwell, Chichester

Visser L, Kalmar J, Linkersdörfer J et al (2020) Comorbidities between specific learning disorders and psychopathology in elementary school children in Germany. Front Psych 11:292. https://doi.org/10.3389/fpsyt.2020.00292

Vlachos F, Papathanasiou I, Andreou G (2007) Cerebellum and reading. Folia Phoniatr Logop 59(4):177–183

Vuust P, Brattico E, Glerean E et al (2011) New fast mismatch negativity paradigm for determining the neural prerequisites for musical ability. Cortex 47(9):1091–1098

Wagner RK, Torgesen JK (1987) The nature of phonological processing and its causal role in the acquisition of reading skills. Psychol Bull 101:192–212

Wagner R, Torgesen J, Rashotte C et al (2013) CTOPP-2—Comprehensive test of phonological processing. Pro-Ed, Austin, TX

Wechsler D (1981) WAIS-R: manual: Wechsler adult intelligence scale—revised. Harcourt Brace Jovanovich (for) Psychological Corporation, New York, NY

Wechsler D (1997) WAIS–III: Wechsler Adult Intelligence Scale, 3rd edn. Pearson, San Antonio TX

Wechsler D (2003) Wechsler intelligence scale for children-IV (WISC-IV). Pearson, San Antonio, TX

Wechsler D (2008) WAIS-IV: Wechsler Adult Intelligence Scale, 4th edn. Pearson, San Antonio, TX

Wechsler D (2009a) WIAT-III: Wechsler individual achievement test, 3rd edn. Pearson, San Antonio, TX

Wechsler D (2009b) WMS-IV: Wechsler memory scale, 4th edn. Pearson, San Antonio, TX

Wechsler D (2014) WISC-V: Wechsler intelligence scale for children, 5th edn. Pearson, San Antonio, TX

Weintraub S, Mesulam MM (1988) Visual hemispatial inattention: stimulus parameters and exploratory strategies. J Neurol Neurosurg Psychiatry 51:1481–1488

Widmann A, Schröger E, Tervaniemi M et al (2012) Mapping symbols to sounds: electrophysiological correlates of the impaired reading process in dyslexia. Front Psychol 3:60. https://doi.org/10.3389/fpsyg.2012.00060

Wiederholt JL, Blalock G (2000) Gary's silent reading test (GRST). Pro-Ed, Austin, TX

Wiederholt JL, Bryant BR (2012) GORT-5—gray oral reading tests, 5th edn. Pro-Ed, Austin, TX

Wiig EH, Minthon L, Nielsen NP et al (2002) A quick test of cognitive speed (AQT). Pearson, San Antonio TX

Wiig EH, Semel E, Secord WA (2013) Clinical evaluation of language fundamentals (CELF-5). Pearson, San Antonio, TX

Willcutt EG, Petrill SA, Wu S et al (2013) Comorbidity between reading disability and math disability concurrent psychopathology, functional impairment, and neuropsychological functioning. J Learn Disabil 46(6):500–516

Wisconsin RTI Center (2017) A guiding document. Available via https://www.wisconsinrticenter.org/assets/files/rti-guiding-doc.pdf Accessed 19 Dec 2017

World Health Organization (2019) ICD-11 International Classification of Diseases. 11th revision Available via https://icd.who.int/en. Accessed 12 Dec 2020

Yang Q, Yang J, Zheng L et al (2021 Sep) (2021) Impact of home parenting environment on cognitive and psychomotor development in children under 5 years old: A meta-analysis. Front Pediatr. 28(9):658094. https://doi.org/10.3389/fped.2021.658094

Zachman L, Jorgensen C, Huisingh R et al (1984) TOPS—Test of problem solving. LinguiSystems, Moline, IL

Zadeh LM, Silbert NH, Sternasty K et al (2019) Extended high-frequency hearing enhances speech perception in noise. Proc Natl Acad Sci USA 116(47):23753–23759

Zafeiriou DI (2004) Primitive reflexes and postural reactions in the neurodevelopmental examination. Pediatr Neurol 31(1):1–8

Ziegler M, Danay E, Heene M et al (2012) Openness, fluid intelligence, and crystallized intelligence: toward an integrative model. J Res Personal 46(2):173–183

Zoccolotti P, Friedmann N (2010) From dyslexia to dyslexias, from dysgraphia to dysgraphias, from a cause to causes: a look at current research on developmental dyslexia and dysgraphia. Cortex 46(10):1211–1215

Zukowski A, Ratner NB (2024) Putting words together: Comprehension and production of morphology and syntax in the preschool years. Ch.5. In: Gleason JB, Ratner NB (eds) The development of language, 10th edn. Plural Publishing, Inc, San Diego, CA, pp 133–176

13 Special Kind of Literacy Development Disorders

Andrea Hasselbusch

13.1 Occupational Therapy Assessment of Written Communication and Handwriting in Children and Young People

Andrea Hasselbusch

13.1.1 Introduction

Occupational therapy (OT) as a profession focuses on enabling engagement in and performance of occupations within daily life (Townsend and Polatajko 2013). Within occupational therapy, the term 'occupations' refers to everything people do in the course of their daily life (Royal College of Occupational Therapists, RCOT 2015). Children's and young people's occupations include self-care activities such as dressing, eating a meal, using the toilet; work or being productive within school, college, university; and leisure, recreation and play such as socialising and playing with friends, participating in hobbies or sports (RCOT 2015; Townsend and Polatajko 2013). The role of occupational therapists with children and young people who experience difficulties in functional written communication or acquisition of handwriting skills is to enable performance of schoolwork activities and tasks, and by doing so facilitate their participation in everyday school life, as well as promote learning and independence.

A. Hasselbusch (✉)
Bournemouth University, Bournemouth, Dorset, UK
e-mail: ahasselbusch@bournemouth.ac.uk

13.1.2 An Occupational Therapy Perspective on Written Communication and Handwriting

Children and young people with developmental literacy disorders, developmental coordination disorder (DCD) or other childhood disabilities commonly experience difficulties with functional written communication throughout different lessons and in a range of typical school activities in a typical school day. Those difficulties impinge on their overall participation in school life and long-term academic success.

Handwriting is a complex and important functional task for school-age children and the primary way they express thoughts, ideas and knowledge (Pollock et al. 2018). Schoolwork entails many activities and tasks across different lessons and topic areas requiring written communication for a variety of purposes, such as producing written output, demonstrating learning, completing worksheets, copying from the board, recording and taking notes. Acquisition of functional handwriting skills is

A. am Zehnhoff-Dinnesen et al. (eds.), *Phoniatrics II*, European Manual of Medicine,
https://doi.org/10.1007/978-3-031-25175-7_13

an important part of primary school education. Children who acquire sound functional handwriting skills tend to perform at a higher level academically (Hoy et al. 2011; Pollock et al. 2018)). Handwriting problems are the most common referral reason for primary school-age children to require occupational therapy (Hoy et al. 2011). However, alternative forms of written communication, in particular use of technology, are increasingly available and more widely used within contemporary mainstream education. Occupational therapists advise on appropriate alternatives for children depending on their needs and abilities.

Growing evidence suggests that goal-directed occupational therapy focusing on functional improvements is effective (Hoy et al. 2011; Law and Darrah 2014), which in this case would be focusing on the development of functional written communication to promote participation in school life and academic learning. Collaborative goal setting, which actively engages the adult (school staff and parents) and young clients, is not a mere means to an end but a powerful therapeutic tool in itself (Poulsen et al. 2015). The occupational therapy assessment process requires the collection of data relevant to setting meaningful goals (Poulsen et al. 2015) as well as planning effective intervention consistent with the current evidence base (Cole 2023; Wallen et al. 2013). Occupational therapy intervention may focus on supporting the acquisition of handwriting abilities or use of alternative methods and strategies for written communication. Contemporary best practice in handwriting acquisition emphasises targeted and frequent practice (Hoy et al. 2011) using motor learning principles (Cole 2023; Zwicker and Harris 2009) or the Cognitive Orientation to Daily Occupational Performance (CO-OP) approach (Polatajko and Mandich 2004; Dawson et al. 2017). The effectiveness of these tailored interventions should be measured by the change they make to the child/young person's ability to engage in learning and perform functional schoolwork activities within daily school life.

13.1.3 Occupational Therapy Assessment

An occupational therapy assessment usually begins with identifying and prioritising occupations that a child 'wants to do, needs to do or is expected to do' but at present 'can't do, doesn't do or isn't satisfied with the way they do' (Law et al. 2014, p. 4). The Canadian Occupational Performance Measure (COPM) is commonly used by therapists with parents and possibly children and school staff to identify those priority areas (Law et al. 2014). Even though children may be referred because of handwriting problems, they frequently experience challenges in a range of everyday schoolwork and self-care, as well as leisure, recreation and play activities. Therefore, a wider assessment of a child's occupational needs and occupational performance problems may be necessary. In this assessment, the occupational therapist will identify and analyse multiple factors which may have an impact on a child's or young person's ability to carry out the prioritised occupations. Therapists are likely to use observation of the child or young person doing the actual activity prioritised (ideally in context), and if necessary additional standardised or non-standardised assessments, to identify contributing factors (see Fig. 13.1) (Frolek Clark et al. 2019). From the therapist's clinical reasoning, a general OT assessment or specialised handwriting assessment may be conducted on the basis of a child's needs, strength and wider contextual considerations.

13.1.4 Occupational Therapy Assessment of Written Communication and Handwriting

In terms of an assessment of difficulties in the area of written communication or handwriting, occupational therapists have access to a wide range of instruments for a more specialised assessment. Some of the traditional tools used by occupational therapist to assess handwriting are limited in their ability to assist the therapist in interpreting the results and determining the direc-

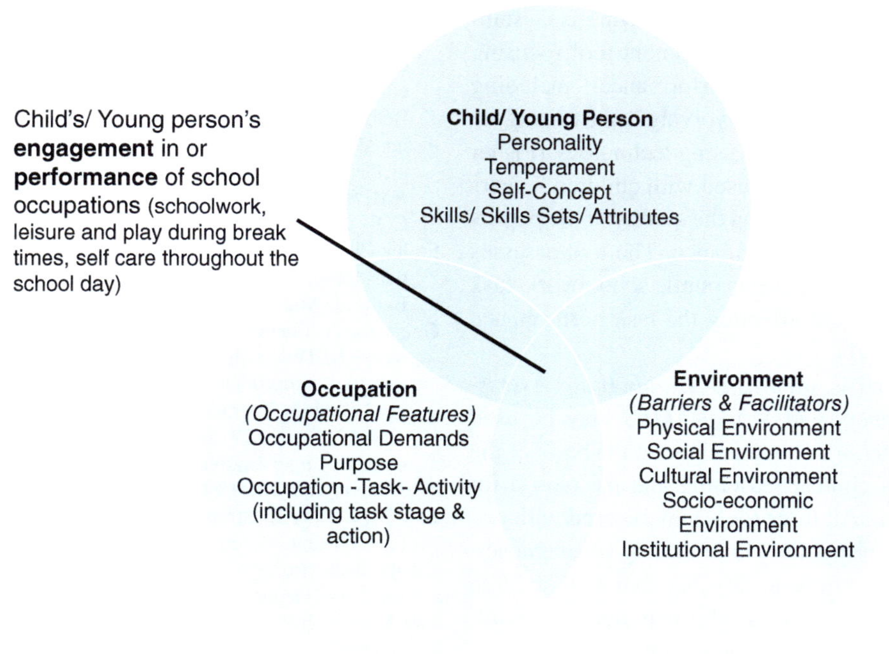

Fig. 13.1 A child's or young person's ability to perform a schoolwork occupation involving written communication (occupational performance) is the result of the interaction between personal, environmental and occupational factors (based on Law et al. 1996, Law et al. 2014; Townsend and Polatajko 2013)

tion of contemporary intervention. In particular, '*impairment or deficit-oriented approaches to assessment of underlying capacity*' of handwriting have been criticised (Wallen et al. 2013, p. 368). Contemporary OT assessment should focus on the actual process and output of handwriting (Wallen et al. 2013), if possible within the real-life school context (Frolek Clark et al. 2019).

Assessment tools such as the *Here's How I Write (HHIW)* (Goldstand et al. 2013), the *McMaster Handwriting Assessment Protocol* (3rd edn) (Pollock et al. 2018) and the *School Version of the Assessment of Motor and Process Skills* (School AMPS) (2nd edn) (Fisher et al. 2007) are consistent with contemporary best practice. The *HHIW*, *McMaster Handwriting Assessment Protocol* and *School AMPS* collect detailed information about different functional aspects of the writing process and the output produced. Additionally, all three tools offer opportunities actively to engage the child or young person, school staff and parents in the assessment process.

The ***HHIW*** is a criterion-referenced child's self-assessment and goal setting tool, actively engaging pupils from year 2 to year 5 in the assessment of their own handwriting and in setting goals for improvement (Goldstand et al. 2013). HHIW is a picture-card interview exploring the child's views alongside the teacher's perspective on various aspects of handwriting such as specific performance features of handwriting, the child's feelings about writing and physical factors contributing to writing. Engaging children in the goal setting process increases ownership and motivation, thus affecting intervention outcomes positively (Poulsen et al. 2015).

The ***McMaster Handwriting Assessment Protocol*** (3rd edn) is a structured framework for the assessment of handwriting of children from kindergarten to Grade 6 (Pollock et al. 2018). The assessment protocol and its individual components build on a comprehensive synthesis of evidence regarding factors contributing to handwriting difficulties. The assessment protocol is designed to facilitate the therapist's decision-making, assisting the identification of specific areas of difficulty and determine whether and where to intervene (Pollock et al. 2018).

The ***School AMPS*** (second edn) is a standardised observational assessment tool focusing on schoolwork task performance, including schoolwork activities involving handwriting or written communication using technology (Fisher et al. 2007). It may be used with children 3 years of age or older, assessing the quality of the pupil's schoolwork task performance. The tool assesses the interaction between pupil, schoolwork task and environment affecting the task performance (see Fig. 13.1).

The *HHIW*, *McMaster Handwriting Assessment Protocol* and *School AMPS* may be used individually or in conjunction, on the basis of the therapist's clinical reasoning and the reason for assessment. All three tools may be used with primary school pupils with a variety of diagnoses, special needs or disability, but also with children without any diagnosis who experience difficulties with written communication.

13.1.5 Conclusion

Handwriting and written communication is part of many important schoolwork activities and tasks that contribute to a child's school success. Children who have difficulties with functional written communication or handwriting are at risk of not achieving their academic potential. Research supports the effectiveness of occupational therapy interventions for writing issues. A specialised occupational therapy assessment process using tools consistent with the current evidence base should underlie the therapist's clinical decision making. Occupational therapy has an important role in assessing and improving written communication or handwriting abilities in children and young people.

References

Cole A (2023) Occupational Therapy Intervention to address handwriting deficit in elementary-aged school children: How to, how much, and how often? A scoping review. J Occup Ther Sch Early Interv 16(3):368–381. https://doi.org/10.1080/19411243.2022.205448

Dawson DR, McEwen SE, Polatajko HJ (2017) Cognitive orientation to daily occupational performance in occupational therapy: using the CO-OP approach the enable participation across the lifespan. AOTA Press, Bethesda MD

Fisher AG, Bryze K, Hume V et al (2007) School version of the assessment of motor and process skills (school AMPS), 2nd edn. Three Star Press Inc., Fort Collins CO

Frolek Clark G, Rioux JE, Chandler BE (2019) Best practices for occupational therapy in schools. AOTA Press, Bethesda MD

Goldstand S, Cermak S, Bissell J (2013) Here's how I write (HHIW): a child's self-assessment and goal setting tool—improving handwriting abilities in school-aged children. Therapro, Framingham MA

Hoy MMP, Egan MY, Feder KP (2011) A systematic review of interventions to improve handwriting. Can J Occup Ther 78(1):13–25

Law M, Cooper B, Strong S, et al (1996) The Person—Environment—Occupation Model: A transactive approach to occupational performance. Canadian Journal of Occupational Therapy, 63(1), 9–23.

Law M, Darrah J (2014) Emerging therapy approaches: an emphasis on function. J Child Neurol 29(8):1101–1107

Law M, Baptiste S, Carswell A et al (2014) Canadian occupational performance measure (COPM), 5th edn. Canadian Association of Occupational Therapists, Ottawa ON

Polatajko H, Mandich A (2004) Enabling occupation in children: the cognitive orientation to daily occupational performance (CO-OP) approach. Canadian Association of Occupational Therapists, Ottawa ON

Pollock N, Lockhart J, Boehm K et al (2018) Handwriting assessment protocol, 3rd edn. McMaster University/CanChild Centre for Childhood Disability Research, Hamilton, ON. Available via https://www.canchild.ca/en/shop/32-handwriting-assessment-protocol-3rd-edition. Accessed 9th Nov 2021

Poulsen AA, Ziviani J, Cuskelly M (2015) Goal setting and motivation in therapy: engaging children and parents. Jessica Kingsley Publishers, London

RCOT (Royal College of Occupational Therapists) (2015) Occupational therapy evidence fact sheet: occupational therapy with children and young people. Available via https://www.cot.co.uk/sites/default/files/commissioning_ot/public/OT-with-children-and-young-people-updated-April2015.pdf. Accessed 20 Aug 2015

Townsend E, Polatajko HJ (2013) Enabling occupation II: advancing an occupational therapy vision for health, Well-being and justice through occupation, 2nd edn. CAOT Publications ACE, Ottawa ON

Wallen M, Duff S, Goyen T et al (2013) Respecting the evidence: responsible assessment and effective intervention for children with handwriting difficulties. Aust Occup Ther J 60(5):366–369

Zwicker J, Harris S (2009) A reflection on motor learning theory in pediatric occupational therapy practice. Can J Occup Ther 76(1):29–37

14 Prevention of Literacy Development Disorders

Anja Fiori

14.1 Early Diagnosis of Specific Speech Deficits

Anja Fiori

14.1.1 Phonological Skills: Predictors of Reading and Writing Development

Broadly acknowledged in scientific discourse is the impact of specific phonological skills on later literacy development. Three components of phonological processing have proved to be robust predictors of later literacy: phonological awareness (Stackhouse 1997), auditory working memory (Brady 1991) and rapid automatised naming (Norton and Wolf 2012). A further predictive factor relevant for literacy acquisition, paired associate learning (PAL), is the ability to link unrelated stimuli via repeated learning.

14.1.2 Phonological Awareness

Phonological awareness is a meta-linguistic ability needed to ignore the meaning of a word and focus on its phonological form instead. For example, the estimation of word length ('which word is longer: worm or hosepipe?') requires phonological awareness.

Children successively learn to identify, analyse, synthesise and manipulate sublexical units of words, such as onset and rhyme, syllables and phonemes. For a systematic classification of aspects of phonological awareness regarding explicitness of operation and size of phonological unit, see Schnitzler (2008). The predictive value of phonological awareness and specific effects of preschool training in phonological awareness on later literacy have been shown in several longitudinal studies. Early deficits in phonological awareness predict later deficits in reading and writing acquisition (Bradley and Bryant 1983; Stackhouse 1997; Hulme et al. 2007). Preschool intervention programmes addressing phonological skills have been proved to have positive effects on later literacy in primary school (Bradley and Bryant 1983; Lundberg et al. 1988; Höse et al. 2016; Schneider et al. 1999; Goldstein et al. 2017).

Therefore, several screening tests focusing on phonological awareness to identify children at risk and on prevention programmes have been developed and evaluated. Examples of screenings and tests in English are the Comprehensive Test of Phonological Processing (Pennington and Bishop 2009), the Test of Phonological Awareness (Hendren et al. 2018) and the Woodcock Reading Mastery Test, third edition (Woodcock 2011).

A. Fiori (✉)
Münster Department of Health MDH, Münster University of Applied Science, Münster, Germany
e-mail: fiori@fh-muenster.de

A. am Zehnhoff-Dinnesen et al. (eds.), *Phoniatrics II*, European Manual of Medicine,
https://doi.org/10.1007/978-3-031-25175-7_14

14.1.3 Auditory Working Memory

Auditory working memory is crucial for keeping sequences of phonemes or words available for further processing. It is particularly required in sublexical processing, i.e. letter-by-letter reading and conversion of phonemes into graphemes. Children with deficits in working memory often show specific difficulty in acquiring the alphabetic strategy (Brady 1991). To prevent confounding influences of auditory working memory on tasks aiming at phonological awareness, items are often presented visually in addition to acoustic presentation (Knoop-van Campen et al. 2018). An example of a recent Test in English is The Comprehensive Assessment Battery for Children—Working Memory (CABC-WM) (Cabbage et al. 2017).

14.1.4 Rapid Automatised Naming

Rapid automatised naming (RAN) is the ability to identify rapidly a sequence of visually presented items (objects, colours, digits or letters), access phonological representations in the mental lexicon, plan articulatory motor actions and name the item in question in a highly effective and automatised manner. Though moderately intercorrelated with phonological awareness, it has been proved to have a differential effect on literacy acquisition. Children with RAN deficits show impaired automatised word recognition with an impact on reading fluency (Norton and Wolf 2012), and children with impaired phonological awareness tend to exhibit deficits in phoneme analysis and conversion into letters. According to the double deficit hypothesis (Wolf and Bowers 1999), children with difficulties in both domains develop most severe dyslexic symptoms.

Children showing deficits in these phonological processing domains can be considered to be at risk for developing difficulties in learning to read or write. They are given the chance of early specific intervention if identified early via preschool screenings. According to Bishop and Snowling (2004), subtypes of the 'phonological deficit' can be described: They differentiate between underspecified phonological representations, difficulty in segmentation, rapid decay of representations and difficulty in mapping phonology and orthography.

14.1.5 Paired Associate Learning

The last aspect mentioned is a further predictive factor relevant for literacy acquisition: paired associate learning (PAL), the ability to link unrelated stimuli via repeated learning. In a study by Hulme et al. (2007), correlations between visual–verbal PAL tasks and reading were stronger than those of reading with visual–visual or verbal–verbal tasks. Apart from phoneme-deletion, visual–verbal PAL was a unique predictor of single-word reading and irregular-word reading. The authors conclude that visual–verbal PAL is a specific task that can reveal differences in the ability to map orthographic to phonological material. This competence is considered to be important for developing word recognition skills. According to a comparative study by Jones et al. (2018), normally developing readers were superior to dyslexic readers in recalling novel phonological associates, and they also improved more with repetition. The authors assume that their superiority in reading acquisition may be explained by their better use of statistical contingencies to identify consistent stimulus features across multiple exposures (Jones et al. 2018).

14.2 Understanding the Importance of Early Diagnosis and Therapy of Language Impairment

Anja Fiori

14.2.1 Intervention as Early as Possible and as Long as Required!

> It is important to characterize children's reading and diagnose dyslexia early, because early intervention with targeted reading remediation can improve reading outcomes—Munzer et al. (2020)

Generally, the importance of early intervention is well accepted. In the evidence- and consensus-based guidelines of diagnostics and therapy of developmental dyslexia (DGKJP 2015), therapy from the first school grade—and even pre-school when deficits in phonological awareness are present—is recommended, as effects of specific intervention at this early stage of development are greater than those at later stages. Considering the psychosocial impact of the disorder, Schulte-Körne et al. (2007) argue 'there is an urgent need to intervene as early as possible in order to avoid the psychosocial consequences of this disorder'. In addition, a possible risk of missing critical periods in cortical development for language learning has to be taken into account (Schulte-Körne et al. 2007). For children at risk, van der Leij (2013) emphasises the importance of early, individualised intervention continuing from pre-school stages through grades 1–3 at school to prevent several 'threats' these children might meet in their individual development.

Screening tests aiming at identifying children at risk can be found in all languages. In the UK, early detection in school is monitored by the Department for Education at the national level (Colenbrander et al. 2018). Screening material is given out by the governmental Standards and Testing Agency: a recent version of the Early Years Foundation Profile (EYFP) was released in 2019 (Standards and Testing Agency 2019). A longitudinal study on the predictive value of screening tests in kindergarten in the USA was carried out by Catts et al. (2015). The authors describe the screening battery used for their study and point out that

> …measures of letter naming fluency, phonological awareness, rapid naming or non-word repetition accurately identified good and poor readers at the end of first grade.—Catts et al. (2015)

14.2.2 Speech and Language Development: Prerequisites of Learning to Read or Write

Owing to the general phonological foundation of written language in alphabetic orthographies, the focus on phonological processing in prevention and remediation seems self-evident. In addition, relationships between the development of general speech and language as a foundation of literacy acquisition are often assumed (Adlof and Hogan 2018). If language impairment is suspected in dyslexic children, diagnostics should include the assessment of receptive or expressive language disorders (DGKJP 2015).

Bishop and Snowling (2004) suggest that, apart from phonological language development, further ('non-phonological') aspects of language development should be taken into account as possible predictors of literacy: These are lexical development (comprehension as well as active vocabulary) and syntactic development. The authors consider subtypes of reading impairment relating to different types of language impairment and suggest a two-dimensional model of the relationship between dyslexia and specific language impairment (SLI). Lexical development can be seen as a prerequisite for written word recognition and understanding (Lundberg 2002; Hulme and Snowling 2014). There is also evidence for the influence of the extent and complexity of vocabulary on the accuracy of phonological representations, which have a positive impact on phonological awareness (Walley et al. 2004). Syntactic abilities seem to be crucial for the development of discourse skills and the ability to understand texts (Bishop and Snowling 2004). A study by Moll et al. (2016) further underlines the importance of considering both general language development and phonological skills in early identification and intervention of children at risk for developmental dyslexia.

14.2.3 Consequences for Diagnostics and Remediation

According to Bishop and Snowling (2004), syntax is not adequately covered by reading tests focusing on single-word reading. They suggest that tests of vocabulary development and grammatical sensitivity are useful for the assessment of non-phonological language skills. The authors warn professionals that neglecting verbal skills beyond phonology could raise the risk of leaving untreated the fundamental skills underlying decoding and reading comprehension.

In their review, Catts and Hogan (2003) point out the language basis of learning to read. Within their 'simple view of reading', they differentiate different types of dyslexia: difficulties in word decoding and difficulties in reading comprehension. They allocate a different underlying competence to each subtype. The authors suggest differential diagnosis and remediation that meet the individual strengths and weaknesses of the affected children.

References

Adlof SM, Hogan TP (2018) Understanding dyslexia in the context of developmental language disorders. Lang Speech Hear Serv Sch 49(4):762–773

Bishop DVM, Snowling MJ (2004) Developmental dyslexia and specific language impairment: same or different? Psychol Bull 130(6):858–886

Bradley L, Bryant PE (1983) Categorising sounds and learning to read—a causal connection. Nature 301(5899):419–421

Brady SA (1991) The role of working memory in reading disability. In: Brady SA, Shankweiler DP (eds) Phonological processes in literacy: a tribute to Isabelle Y. Erlbaum, Hillsdale, NJ, pp 129–151

Cabbage K, Brinkley S, Gray S et al (2017) Assessing working memory in children: the comprehensive assessment battery for children—working memory (CABC-WM). J Vis Exp 124:55121. https://doi.org/10.3791/55121

Catts HW, Hogan TP (2003) Language basis of reading disabilities and implications for early identification and remediation. Read Psychol 24(3–4):223–246

Catts HW, Nielsen DC, Bridges MS et al (2015) Early identification of reading disabilities within an RTI framework. J Learn Disabil 48(3):281–297

Colenbrander D, Ricketts J, Breadmore HL (2018) Early identification of dyslexia: understanding the issues. Lang Speech Hear Serv Sch 49(4):817–828

DGKJP (2015) Deutsche Gesellschaft für Kinder- und Jugendpsychiatrie, Psychosomatik und Psychotherapie e.V. Diagnostik und Behandlung von Kindern und Jugendlichen mit Lese- und/oder Rechtschreibstörung. Evidenz- und konsensbasierte Leitlinie (S3); AWMF-Registriernummer 028–044

Goldstein H, Olszewski A, Haring C et al (2017) Efficacy of a supplemental phonemic awareness curriculum to instruct preschoolers with delays in early literacy development. J Speech Lang Hear Res 60(1):89–103

Hendren RL, Haft SL, Black JM et al (2018) Recognizing psychiatric comorbidity with reading disorders. Front Psych 9:101. https://doi.org/10.3389/fpsyt.2018.00101

Höse A, Wyschkon A, Moraske S et al (2016) Prevention of dyslexia—short-term and intermediate effects of promoting phonological awareness and letter-sound correspondence with at-risk preschool children. Z Kinder Jugendpsychiatr Psychother 44(5):377–393

Hulme C, Snowling MJ (2014) The interface between spoken and written language: developmental disorders. Philos Trans R Soc B 369(1634):20120395

Hulme C, Goetz K, Gooch D et al (2007) Paired associate learning, phoneme awareness and learning to read. J Exp Child Psychol 96(2):150–166

Jones MW, Kuipers JR, Nugent S et al (2018) Episodic traces and statistical regularities: paired associate learning in typical and dyslexic readers. Cognition 177:214–225

Knoop-van Campen CAN, Segers E, Verhoeven L (2018) How phonological awareness mediates the relation between working memory and word reading efficiency in children with dyslexia. Dyslexia 24(2):156–169

Lundberg I (2002) The child's route into reading and what can go wrong. Dyslexia 8(1):1–13

Lundberg I, Frost J, Peterson OP (1988) Effects of an extensive program for stimulating phonological awareness in preschool children. Read Res Q 33:263–284

Moll K, Thompson PA, Mikulajova M et al (2016) Precursors of reading difficulties in Czech and Slovak children at risk of dyslexia. Dyslexia 22(2):120–136

Munzer T, Hussain K, Soares N (2020) Dyslexia: neurobiology, clinical features, evaluation and management. Transl Pediatr 9(Suppl 1):S36–S45

Norton ES, Wolf M (2012) Rapid automatized naming (RAN) and reading fluency: implications for understanding and treatment of reading disabilities. Annu Rev Psychol 63:427–452

Pennington BF, Bishop DVM (2009) Relations among speech, language, and reading disorders. Annu Rev Psychol 60:283–306

Schneider W, Ennemoser M, Roth E et al (1999) Kindergarten prevention of dyslexia: does training in phonological awareness work for everybody? J Learn Disabil 32(5):429–436

Schnitzler CD (2008) Phonologische Bewusstheit und Schriftspracherwerb (phonological awareness and written language acquisition). In: Springer L, Schrey-Dern D (eds) Forum Logopädie (forum speech therapy). Thieme, Stuttgart

Schulte-Körne G, Ludwig KK, el Sharkawy J et al (2007) Genetics and neuroscience in dyslexia: perspectives for education and remediation. Mind Brain Educ 1(4):162–172

Stackhouse J (1997) Phonological awareness: connecting speech and literacy problems. In: Hodson BW, Edwards ML (eds) Perspectives in applied phonology. Gaithersburg, MD, Aspen, CO, pp 157–196

Standards and Testing Agency (2019) Early years foundation profile. 2020 Handbook. Available via https://assets.publishing.service.gov.uk/government/uploads/system/uploads/attachment_data/file/858652/EYFSP_Handbook_2020v5.pdf. Accessed 29th Sept 2021 van der Leij A (2013) Dyslexia and early intervention: what did we learn from the Dutch Dyslexia Programme? Dyslexia 19(4):241–255

Walley AC, Metsala JL, Garlock VM (2004) Spoken vocabulary growth: its role in the development of phoneme awareness and early reading ability. Read Writ 16:5–20

Wolf M, Bowers P (1999) The double-deficit hypothesis for the developmental dyslexias. J Educ Psychol 91(3):415–438

Woodcock RW (2011) Woodcock reading mastery tests (3rd edn) (WRMT-III). Pearson, San Antonio, TX

15 Rehabilitation and Prognosis of Literacy Development Disorders

Tahany Abdul Karim Al-Sayed Ahmed,
Doris-Eva Bamiou, Nicole G. Campbell,
Mirela Duranovic, Anja Fiori, Manuel Föcker,
Reinhild Hofmann, Barbara Maciejewska,
David R. Moore, Rudolf Reiter, and Tony Sirimanna

Barbara Maciejewska and Manuel Föcker share equal first authorship

T. Abdul Karim Al-Sayed Ahmed (✉)
ENT & Audiology, COSMOMID CA Clinic,
Salmyia, Kuwait

D.-E. Bamiou
University College London, National Hospital for Neurology and Neurosurgery, London, UK
e-mail: d.bamiou@ucl.ac.uk

N. G. Campbell
University of Southampton, Southampton, UK
e-mail: N.G.Campbell@soton.ac.uk

M. Duranovic
Department of Speech and Language Pathology, University of Tuzla, Tuzla, Bosnia and Herzegovina

A. Fiori
Münster Department of Health MDH, Münster University of Applied Science, Münster, Germany
e-mail: fiori@fh-muenster.de

M. Föcker
University Hospital Münster, Department of Child and Adolescent Psychiatry, Münster, Germany
e-mail: manuel.foecker@ukmuenster.de

R. Hofmann
ICBF International Centre for the Study of Giftedness, University of Münster, Münster, Germany
e-mail: r.hofmann@uni-muenster.de

B. Maciejewska
Department and Clinic of Phoniatrics and Audiology, Poznan University of Medical Sciences,
Poznan, Poland
e-mail: barbaramaciejewska@ump.edu.pl

D. R. Moore
Cincinnati Children's Hospital Medical Center, Cincinnati, OH, USA
e-mail: david.moore2@cchmc.org

R. Reiter
Department of Otolaryngology, Section for Phoniatrics and Paedaudiology, University HNO Clinic, Ulm, Germany
e-mail: rudolf.reiter@uniklinik-ulm.de

T. Sirimanna
Audiological Medicine and Cochlear Implant Department, Great Ormond Street Hospital,
London, UK

A. am Zehnhoff-Dinnesen et al. (eds.), *Phoniatrics II*, European Manual of Medicine,
https://doi.org/10.1007/978-3-031-25175-7_15

15.1 Coordination of Rehabilitative Measures for Developmental Literacy Disorders

Barbara Maciejewska and Reinhild Hofmann

15.1.1 Management of Development Literacy Disorders

Within the proper management of developmental literacy disorders, the coordination of rehabilitative measures is an activity that follows the diagnostic process.

The composition of the multidisciplinary team may vary from country to country owing to national and regional policies, but the team needs specialists for the medical, psychological, pedagogic and therapeutic aspects of diagnosis and treatment of dyslexia. The coordinator of this team needs to fulfil the following *qualifications*, including having:

- A profound knowledge and regular update on the nature, causes, development and symptoms of developmental dyslexia, and on co-morbidities
- An understanding of the interaction of contributing risk and protective factors at the genetic, neural, cognitive and environmental levels on the overall functional outcome (Haft et al. 2016)
- State-of-the-art knowledge on valid screening and diagnostic instruments, and on evidence-based interventions (e.g. Galuschka et al. 2014, 2020; Huemer et al. 2019)
- A regular interdisciplinary exchange/communication with the involved professional areas (paediatric psychologist, child and adolescent psychiatrist, pedaudiologist/phoniatrician, ophthalmologist, speech language therapist/logopaedist, school teacher, occupational therapist, special education teacher)
- A detailed knowledge on the country-specific laws set up to compensate for the disadvantages of students with developmental dyslexia in school and vocational education
- Up-to-date knowledge on financing possibilities of the available treatment forms in the specific country/local area

Every individual with specific reading or writing problems is different. So is every country, culture and educational context (Smythe et al. 2005). These are the reasons that therapeutic procedures in dyslexia must be chosen individually; for different countries and for each child and its family background. Note that there are indications for starting the dyslexia treatment as early as class one, e.g. in the case of a severe phonological processing disorder that prevents sufficient progress in the school setting. Ideally, treatment takes place in single person or small group settings, and should directly address the dyslexic symptoms (e.g. Schulte-Körne and Galuschka 2015).

Not only is the diagnostic process a multidisciplinary one, but in most cases the therapeutic intervention is also. A challenge here is the gap in the research on evidence-based strategies for treating developmental disorders with accompanying comorbid conditions. The coordinating doctor has to decide whether to start with treating only one condition, or two or even more conditions simultaneously. Here, the severity of the symptoms, a realistic hypothesis on the individual roles of contributing factors, and last but not least, the resources of the child, the family and the environment will influence the decision.

In the case of an ocular dysfunction, which can—by definition—not be the cause of, but an additive factor in, developmental dyslexia, an appropriate treatment by the ophthalmologist should be the starting point of the intervention plan. The same approach should be taken for a discrete hearing disorder, which would be treated by the pedaudiologist/phoniatrician. Dyslexic children show changes in auditory potentials i.e. MMN, P300, P50, N1 and P2 waves. Therefore, the auditory processing disorder rehabilitation programme uses selective auditory attention tasks, which have significantly improved speech perception in noise and dichotic listening in dyslexic children (Maciejewska et al. 2013, Ghasemi et al. 2016, Panahi et al. 2023). The speech language therapist/special education teacher (country-specific) plays one of the more important roles in addressing the core dyslexic symptoms (see Sect. 12.5) and—if appropriate—an accompanying phonological processing disorder. A further important role is that of the paediatric psychologist/child and adolescent psychiatrist (or country-specific equivalent) if the child shows significant concomitant psychological/psychiatric symptoms (see Sects. 11.3, 12.1 and 15.5).

The focus of occupational therapy is on disorders of fine-motor skills, eye–hand coordination and concentration. Postural rehabilitation may also be useful. According to the current literature, dyslexic children have poor postural control and a poor motor coordination with respect to control age-matched children, which could be due to a cerebellar deficit in dyslexic children (Goulème et al. 2015). Including rehabilitation of cerebellar function in the therapy leads to increasing attention, as well as improving equilibrium, which are both impaired in individuals with learning disorders, especially in dyslexia (Delavarian et al. 2013). Note that, as in other multifactorial settings, more is not always better. A professional therapist of developmental literacy disorders always sees the bigger picture and may present some additional qualification beyond her or his core competence.

The coordinator's *tasks* in the rehabilitative process are to:

- Interpret the diagnostic findings
- Set up the intervention concept in consideration of the specific service options provided in the particular area/country and at the child's school
- Understand the needs and strengths of the individual child and its family (e.g. socio-economic situation, family language(s), parent–child interaction, family time beyond schooling and work) and incorporate these into the intervention concept
- Inform—and where appropriate involve—parents and child about the diagnosis and intervention concept
- Forward the diagnostic results and intervention concept to the treating professionals and ask for short regular reports, e.g. every 6 months

15.1.2 Counselling of Development Literacy Disorders

A well-performed initial counselling session can be the first step of the intervention: it may unburden parents and sometimes also the children with respect to seeing themselves (partly) responsible for the individual deficits in reading or writing. Therefore, the coordinator has to *counsel* parents and child on:

- The nature and causes of dyslexia: what it is and what it is not—here the most important information for the child, family and school is that children with dyslexia are as intelligent as children without dyslexia
- (If appropriate) additional conditions detected in the diagnostic process (e.g. attention-deficit disorder, anxiety disorder, dyscalculia) and their relation to the individual reading or writing problems
- The country-specific laws of compensation for the dyslexic disadvantage in school and vocational education
- A realistic expectation with regard to goals and time course of the treatment

A further important task of the coordinating doctor is to *monitor* the process of the ongoing treatment regularly. This monitoring comprises the re-application of diagnostic instruments, inter-relating the results with treatment reports and subjective reports of the child, parents and school. Proper therapy may minimise the educational, social, emotional and behavioural problems in children with dyslexia (De Jong et al. 2006; Facoetti et al. 2003; Walker and Norman 2010). If the expected progress is not reached or is even absent, the treatment plan should be updated according to the current findings. This could be the change of a single therapeutic approach or the whole intervention concept. If there is uncertainty about the underlying reasons for insufficient progress, a consultation or round-table meeting with other specialists of the multi-disciplinary team (and possibly the parents and child) may be indicated. In case the child reaches age-appropriate reading and writing skills, the treatment can be paused or terminated. However, very often therapy in developmental dyslexia is long-lasting and time-consuming, it is a process in time with constant observation (de Lima et al. 2017; Facoetti et al. 2003; Walker and Norman 2010). In cases of severe developmental dyslexia, reading or writing often remains a life-long challenge for the affected child and family, and may need repeated treatment intervals.

15.2 Neuropsychological Therapy Principles and Therapy Programmes for the Executive Functions Skill in Individuals with Dyslexia

Tahany Abdul Karim Al-Sayed Ahmed

15.2.1 Introduction

Neuropsychology is the study of the assessment, understanding and modification trajectories of brain–behaviour relationships, through the structure of neural networks and mental processes. Consequently, neuropsychology gives us the keys to be able to understand the importance of the executive functions and complex mental activities that we must use to achieve a goal in learning. It has been found that executive functions are a contributing factor to dyslexia (Akyurek and Bumin 2018). Executive function is an umbrella term for the complex cognitive processes that underlie flexible response inhibition, working memory and switching updating, switching and goal-directed learning (Goldstein and Naglieri 2015; Friedman and Miyake 2017). It also includes multiple cognitive domains such as accumulated knowledge, achievement, attention, working memory (WM), processing and processing speed, problem-solving and reasoning (Baddeley 2017; Decker and Roberts 2015). Furthermore, it involves planning, organising, decision-making, process evaluation, cognitive flexibility, the ability to concentrate on necessary stimuli and ignore irrelevant distractions, time management, emotion control, self-monitoring personality, thinking, learning, remembering and consciousness (Pani et al. 2013).

Different studies have shown a lack of executive functioning in children and adults with reading disabilities (RD) (Varvara et al. 2014). Booth et al. (2010) have emphasised that children with dyslexia have difficulties in various executive functions, which include sustaining associated information in the WM, reserving inappropriate information and retrieving material in long-term memory. Both verbal and visual-spatial components of WM have been found to be impaired in RD children (Menghini et al. 2011; Wang et al. 2017) and adults (Alloway and Alloway 2013; Morkena et al. 2017). It has been proposed by Kofler et al. (2019) that reading problems in children with AD(H)D are attributable, at least partly, to underdeveloped working memory, and that reading performance is linked to inattention (Plourde et al. 2018). To explain learning and reading difficulties, studies exploring working memory training have found transfer of training in adults (Jaeggi et al. 2014) and children (Karbach et al. 2015).

Furthermore, training effects are transferred to improved reading ability, reduced socio-emotional problems and increased capacity for self-regulation, as response inhibition is predictive of reading and socio-emotional problems associated with dyslexia (Doyle 2017; Wang and Yang 2014), and appear to be necessary for effective self-regulation and socio-emotional well-being (Bridgett et al. 2013; Snyder et al. 2015). Moreover, it has been found that response inhibition and updating appear to have compatible demands, and therefore have a facilitative interaction; inhibition can protect the contents of working memory from distractor interference and increase attentional focus. This enhances the ability to update information in working memory correctly (Friedman and Miyake 2017) and improves response inhibition, with possible training in dyslexia through the compensatory effects that are observed for children (Peng and Miller 2016); training also appears to result in direct improvements in the trained task in adults (Hartmann et al. 2016). Similarly, Horowitz-Kraus (2015) explored transfer of combined training (working memory, naming, speed, inhibition and flexibility) in children with ADHD and comorbid dyslexia–ADHD, and found differential effects in each subgroup. Training was transferred to improved reading ability, speed and spatial abilities in those with comorbid dyslexia–

ADHD, and improved working memory and speed, but not reading ability, in those with ADHD alone (Horowitz-Kraus 2015). An additional study by Peng et al. (2013) found that processing speed accounted for response inhibition and updating impairments in dyslexia, and a number of other researchers suggest that processing speed is a shared impairment in dyslexia and ADHD, accounting for the overlap (Peterson et al. 2016).

The knowledge base of neuropsychology bridges and integrates multiple disciplines that are very important for creating a therapy plan. Paediatric neuropsychologists are in a unique position to provide advanced assessment, treatment recommendations and advice to parents on the optimum accommodation for children with SLD conditions, on the basis of their knowledge of brain–behaviour relationships and learning difficulties with the cooperation of an educational team and school psychologist.

15.2.2 Neuropsychological Therapy Principles for Children/Adults with SLD

Before starting any neuropsychological therapy programme, we have to consider basic principles for treatment that should include:

Neuropsychological/Cognitive Assessments The results from these are fundamental in providing help to clinicians, psychologists and educators with a deeper description of the impairments of different cognitive and neuropsychological functions related to effective learning. Investigating profiles of people with specific learning disorders can help define interventions, even though debated (Fletcher and Miciak 2017). Correspondingly, they provide information on other cognitive functions more directly related to the learning of reading, such as phonological abilities, mainly during adolescence and adult life, where they seem to have a crucial role in learning difficulties (Alahmadi 2017; Smith-Spark et al. 2016).

The Effects of Intervention These can be from observing different neuropsychological and academic limitations (Holmes and Gathercole 2013; Karbach et al. 2015). Information gathered before will provide more insight into how children acquire, use and achieve mastery of academic abilities over developmental time. This will refine the professional's ability to determine the optimal timing and content of specific interventions for low performing children (D'Souza and Karmiloff-Smith 2017).

Theoretical Background of Programme Design This is important before applying neuropsychological therapy programmes. They should include cognitive developments and intellectual maturation of functional systems, their lateralisation and the axis of ontogenetic development that stem from inferior to superior structures, and from posterior to anterior structures (Rosselli et al. 2006).

Communicating to the Team This is similar to providing feedback to parents for a clinical evaluation. The communication should start with an all-purpose overview of parent and school district concerns and documented areas of discrepancy. The child's neuropsychological functioning should be revised with an emphasis on implications for the educational setting (Mason et al. 2012). In order to meet this goal, the report should provide an integration of the evaluation findings with specific eligibility criteria, as set out in each country's or state's special education rules and cultural diversity (Ortiz and Seymour 2017; Ortiz 2019).

Specific Functional Difficulties These should be known for each child in both the academic and behavioural spheres, with a clear understanding of the student's brain functioning, highlighting strengths and weaknesses (Miciak et al. 2018). It is important to document the child's neuropsychological strengths and weaknesses, and overall diagnostic impressions, which should guide the education team as they consider the child's educational needs, and explain which areas can be remediated and which areas require accommodation (Fuchs et al. 2017; Hanson et al. 2009). Research has suggested that adaptive training interventions are more effective than non-adaptive for improving working memory (Peng and Miller 2016; Schwaighofer et al. 2015).

Guiding the Development of Appropriate Recommendations This should relate to curricular modifications and support, remedial techniques, accommodation and compensatory strategies. Without an understanding of probable causes, it is difficult to select and tailor interventions that will address the student's unique learning needs (Ortiz and Artiles 2010).

Finding Rationale Solutions These are required for each requested accommodation, correlated with specific functional limitations and established through the evaluation process from test results and clinical observations (Miciak et al. 2018). An in depth explanation, supporting the necessity for every requested accommodation must be provided and correlated with specific functional limitations established through the evaluation process from test results and clinical observations (Burns et al. 2016).

Ineffective Interventions These include methods that are not obvious, often reinforced constructionist, discovering approaches (Seidenberg 2017). It is necessary to arrange activities in a hierarchical way, to give opportunities for task repetition, to adjust the plan once results are measured, and to use long-lasting treatments, as in cases of dyslexia (Duff et al. 2014).

Neuropsychological Therapies These are developed to support both phonological reading interventions and the teaching of specific word identification strategies, to compensate for working memory deficits, and have been demonstrated to lead to higher gains in reading performance and in the ability to maintain these gains after 1-year follow-up for children with severe RD (Morris et al. 2012).

Specific Processes of Self-Regulated Learning These are linked to reading comprehension, and include establishing objectives, activating information, following rules, using adequate cognitive and metacognitive strategies, monitoring one's own performance, time management, seeking help when necessary, self-efficacy, motivation, identifying factors that affect learning, and experiencing satisfaction with one's own efforts (Karbach et al. 2015).

Combination Training Approaches This training approach combines obvious instruction strategies and self-regulation. Strategy instruction involves six stages: (1) developing and activating the background knowledge; (2) discussing the strategy; (3) modelling the strategy; (4) memorising the strategy; (5) lending support to the strategy and (6) independent performance. Thus, the adults (parents, teachers and therapist) systematically transfer control and responsibility over the use of the strategy to the scholar (Mason et al. 2012; Fuchs et al. 2014). Recent findings suggest that metacognitive efficiency in one perceptual modality predicts meta-cognitive efficiency in others, and that they share electrophysiological markers (Faivre et al. 2018). Meta-cognitive efficiency is connected across vision and visual short-term memory, especially for features such as orientation (Samaha and Postle 2017).

Multisensory Integration This completely and explicitly registers linguistic information (phonological and other) in the learner's working memory by linking new learning to previously established skills. Its supremacy may derive from the mediating consequence of several sensory and motor experiences on attention and recall. Multisensory experiences with linguistic units may activate more circuitry than do uni-sensory experiences (or one experience) during language learning, by creating new neural networks through frequent activation (Fletcher et al. 2018).

Training Parents with their Children This should happen for at least one of the activities with their children in order to promote adherence to the intervention. Parents' awareness of executive functioning can help sustain the effects of the intervention in everyday life (Volckaert and Nöel 2015). Tamm et al. (2014) showed with a subgroup of 24 children that the intervention was achievable and widely accepted by the parents (with a high rate of assistance and adherence, low resistance and high satisfaction). In terms of efficacy, improvements were observed in executive functions (visual and auditory attention, working memory and cognitive flexibility) with their corresponding improvements in parents' ratings.

Optimising the Challenges Most successful interventions for improving executive functions, which avoid frustrating or boring the learner, involve a challenge that is neither too high nor too low, and that train these functions directly and support them indirectly as well. Indirect support includes reducing factors that seem to decrease executive functions, such as stress or sadness, and support factors that appear to enhance executive functions, such as joy and social support (Diamond and Ling 2016).

Training Executive Function (as Self-Regulation) It is difficult to make cogent reading intervention (Cirino et al. 2017) more effective. Moreover, training cognitive skills in isolation from academic content does not improve reading, maths or writing (Melby-Lervåg et al. 2016). Changes must be produced in areas that are important to the patient's daily life, that is, they must have ecological value (Rosenblum et al. 2014).

Importance of a Central Information Folder The therapy plan, practices, links of performance to intervention and follow up should be kept in a student folder to be used in family and school contexts for the exercise of strategies. Parents as well as teachers can keep track of the progress through the materials in the folder The objective of this module is to establish a system of reinforcement, to create conditions for reinforcing the target behaviour and adjusting intervention if needed (Decker et al. 2018; Mather and Jaffe 2016).

15.2.3 Therapy Programmes for the Executive Functions Skill in Individuals with Dyslexia

Implementing any therapeutic programme should be orientated directly towards ameliorating weaknesses in the Executive Functions (EF) of individuals with dyslexia, and be based on neuropsychological principles.

> There is no single 'ideal' developmental pathway for everyone; instead there are multiple pathways to healthy development, learning, academic success, and resilience.—Cantor et al. (2018), p. 9

This means that a therapy programme should be developed on an understanding of the dyslexic's individual powers and weaknesses (metacognitive awareness) and employ strategies that typically result in improved effort and perseverance, a positive self-concept and better results (Meltzer 2018). Furthermore, the therapy programme must help children achieve acceptable mental functions, academic activities and educational responsibilities (Tops et al. 2013). Likewise, we have to pay attention to adults with dyslexia; research suggests that they experience additional difficulties, including problems with memory and organisation (Smith-Spark et al. 2017).

Stimulating strategies towards EF to overcome reading difficulties may include

> reading strategies involving manipulation of information, response time, the capacity to inhibit distracting stimuli, as well as the alternation between different elements with different meanings—Medina et al. (2017), p. 450

That such an effective programme overcomes weakness areas is suggested by evidence that working memory and inhibitory control can be co-dependent and the significant relationship between components of working memory and reading decoding/reading fluency (Butterfuss and Kendeou 2018; Cirino et al. 2018; Peng et al. 2018). Training of executive functions should not be suspended for long because improvements in executive functions usually decrease with increasing time gaps between training sessions (Diamond and Ling 2016). However, we need a technique that develops the child's experience of rich text and creates occasions for acquiring world knowledge (Rappolt-Schlichtmann et al. 2018), as well as their motivation, self-efficacy, self-confidence, inter-individual characteristics and interest (Aro et al. 2018; Hwang 2019; Lou and Noels 2019; Pezoa et al. 2019).

In general, exertion executive functions helps to regulate behaviour in two ways. The first are executive functions for *mental purposes* and the second for *behaviour purposes* (Dawson and Guare 2018). See Tables 15.1 and 15.2.

Table 15.1 Executive functions skills for mental purposes. Description, strategies and suggested programmes (Abdul Karim©2021)

Executive functions for mental purposes				
Skills	Description	Language area	Strategies	Programmes and materials
Planning	Involves the ability to decide what is important, to create and make a road map to achieve a goal or complete a task. Allows the reader to direct attention and predict higher levels of reading comprehension in adults (Das and Misra 2015; Georgiou and Das 2018). Helps adults to take notes to plan and organise ideas before writing can act as an external memory, reducing the cognitive load during the writing task (Graham 2018), allows them to modify their attention between writing functions more enthusiastically	– Handwriting – Reading comprehension – Oral expression – Prosody – Intention	**Mind Map Strategy**: Is a visual graphical way to characterise ideas and concepts, arrange and simplify material, the better to analyse, comprehend, synthesise, recall and generate new ideas. Is a useful technique that supports learning, improves information-recording and expressing how different proofs and thoughts are related, and enhances creative problem-solving (Buzan and Buzan 2007) **Scheme**: To enhance understanding and construct meaning by thinking through the text with others. The scheme can be explained when encountering new information in the text, engaging with others, and gaining personal experience (Vacca et al. 2011) **Triple Note Tote Strategy**: Can be used to document a strategy for memorising information by using graphic organisers and three-column note-taking systems (Meltzer 2018) **Self-regulated Strategy Development**: Taking notes to plan and organise ideas before writing can act as an external memory, reducing the cognitive load during the writing task (Graham 2018) **Goal Setting and Planning**: Organising structural writing reduces WM load by providing steps to improve planning, organisation and setting goals, listing key points needed or writing paragraphs to include in their written work (Hebert et al. 2018a) **Text Structure Instruction**: An effective strategy for improving the expository reading and writing skills of individuals. The use of these skills through self-instruction involving defining the problem, focusing on attention and planning, engaging in writing, error correction, coping, and self-reinforcement (Roehling et al. 2017; Hebert et al. 2018b)	– Mind map: The British Dyslexia Association, www.bdadyslexia.org.uk – Planning: www.thepathway2success.com/games-to-improve-executive-functioning-skills – Graphic organisers, concept maps, flowcharts, timeline – **Livescribe**: An assistive technology that can help dysfluent writers keep up with note-taking. It is a smart pen that has a camera and a recording device. http://www.livescribe.com/en-us/

Organisation	The ability to design and maintain systems for upholding data (Logue and Gould 2014). It is the key to organising information, rearranging it to be easily understood and retained. Research supports the effectiveness of such intervention for good organisation and documentation for mental health promotion and well-being in adults with dyslexia (Armaou et al. 2020; Doyle and McDowall 2019)	– Vocabulary – Sentence drill and structure (parts of speech, capitalisation, punctuation) – Reading comprehension – Decoding unfamiliar words – Reading fluently – Reading accuracy – Writing skills	**Systematic and cumulative**: Organisations require organisation of language instruction and monitoring material in order, starting with the easiest concepts and most basic components and progress and must be systematically revised to reinforce memory (Birsh 2018) **Prioritising and Organising ideas**: Sequencing events or the different components of multistage projects after investigating sources **Direct Instructions**: Clear, explicit, methodical, systematic instruction with full descriptions (McArthur and Castles 2017) **Comprehensive Word Strategies**: Integration and synchronisation of the multiple sub-processes involved in reading, such as phonological, morphological and orthographic aspects of word reading, retrieval of knowledge and word meanings (lexicons) from long-term memory. Integrating prior knowledge with new information, pacing, reading self-questioning, story structure instruction, graphic, organisers, semantic and comprehension monitoring (Solis et al. 2012)	– A KWL grid (What I know, What I want to know) – A QUADS grid (Question, Answer, Detail, Source) – Calculator. – Speech-to-Text software – Text-to-Speech software – Electronic dictionary – Spelling checker – Grammar checker – Hamburger paragraph graphic organiser – Sequence chart graphic organiser – Note-taking
Time management	Includes the sense of time and approximating the duration of how long it takes to finish tasks. It is a problem related to understanding specialised literature, identifying the key ideas in a text, understanding instructions (e.g. in exams), taking notes, organising essays and reports, and expressing ideas in a written format (Webster 2016). Training time management decreases stress (Häfner et al. 2015)	– Writing – Reading – Listening – Comprehension – Processing speed – Reading accuracy – Reading fluently – Word retrieval – Spelling	**Flexible and changing**: By following a schedule with extended time allowing for more frequent breaks and changing the order of tasks or subtests **Skimming and Scanning**: These are very rapid reading methods, allowing rapid gathering of the most important information (Meltzer 2018) **Time Constrictions**: Students need to utilise 'brain breaks' where opportunities to move about and stretch are provided to assist in maintaining concentration and focus levels (Reid and Green 2014) **Self-awareness and Self-management**: A positive cognitive reframing of dyslexia, as a key success factor allows successful life experiences, proactivity at work and improves efficient functioning in everyday dyslexic adults (Gordon et al. 2018; Nukari et al. 2020)	– A family calendar – Visual checklists – An analogue clock – Be focused pro – Focus Timer app – Useful website with many ideas from students about how they organise and manage their time, record timetable in many ways to suit individual preferences; yearly planner, diary, calendar, paper template, outlook calendar, electronic diary, mobile phone, list etc. http://www.lexdis.org.uk/about/

(continued)

Table 15.1 (continued)

Executive functions for mental purposes				
Skills	Description	Language area	Strategies	Programmes and materials
Working memory	The ability to keep past information in the brain and recall as needed. It is explained by three mechanisms, which include maintenance of information in short-term storage, retrieving information from long-term memory, and attentional control (Shipstead et al. 2014; Yang et al. 2017). Holding and connecting ideas in the mind while reading, by constructing new neural networks through regular activation (Fletcher et al. 2018), and word decoding effects on reading comprehension (Jacobson et al. 2017)	– Auditory attention – Orthographic coding – Phonemic awareness – Phonological memory – Sound-symbol association – Syllabication – Spelling – Word decoding – Decoding unfamiliar words – Rapid naming – Word retrieval – Processing speed	**Retrieving and recalling Information**: Taking notes or outlining when completing independent reading, or studying by focusing on the big picture and the relevant supporting details (Meltzer et al. 2015) **Construction-Integration Model**: Integrating knowledge from the text with schemes in long-term memory (Kintsch 2019). **Multisensory Techniques**: Supports simultaneous brain learning (visual, auditory, kinaesthetic, tactile) in order to enhance memory and learning. The child looks at the word, says the word, pronounces the word slowly while tracing it, and then writes it from memory (Birsh 2018; Black 2016). **Literacy strategy**: An evidence-based literacy strategy can help students develop phonemic awareness by focusing on segmenting and blending the sounds in words. **Paragraph shrinking**: An evidence-based literacy strategy that a routine student can use to practise finding the main idea by summarising a text. Paragraph shrinking can be used with students of any reading level and with any text	– Orton-Gillingham based reading instruction interventions utilise multisensory, sequential, systematic phonics-based techniques to instruct reading in an explicit manner – Elkonin Sound Boxes – CogniFit Brain Training
Metacognition	Thinking about thinking. Includes self-monitoring and self-assessment to reflect or see how the problem can be solved from an individual's knowledge. Is linked with principles, attentiveness, knowledge, information, the sense of perception and the decision of learning, the theory of mind, metacognitive skills, high-order skills, comprehension monitoring, knowledge strategies, and self-regulation (Wang and Han 2017; Yang and Bai 2019). Metacognitive awareness promotes positive language learning (Zhang 2018). Effective learners use different strategies from ineffective learners (Zhang et al. 2019)	– Phonics and word identification – Phonological memory – Processing speed – Vocabulary – Decoding unfamiliar words – Spelling – Reading comprehension – Oral expression – Syntax – Prosody – Intention	**Metacognitive Strategies**: Help individuals understand their learning profiles—when to use which strategies (e.g. questioning, clarification, understanding, assessing connecting) and in what situations, as not all strategies work (Meltzer 2014; Cirino et al. 2017) **Modelling of sound-symbol memos**: Recording the sound of letters written on a transparency. **Self-concept and Critical Thinking**: Enhancing reading ability on the basis of previous knowledge, self-regulation and regulation of cognitive processing (Altıok et al. 2019; Helmstaedter et al. 2019; Wang and Han 2017) **Monitoring and Deploying Strategies**: For enhancing reading comprehension this depends upon the development of accurate and fluent word recognition, oral language development and background knowledge (Birsh 2018) **Reciprocal Reading and Spelling Skill Strategies**: For phonics, fluency, nonsense words, sight words, spelling to support upper level literacy (McArthur and Castles 2017) **Metacognitive Strategies and Critical Thinking**: When students' approximation of their comprehension shows that they have a belief in their ability to complete a task and monitor their comprehension (Zhang and Ardasheva 2019)	– Technology tools: https://www.region10.org/programs/dyslexia/techplan/ – Dragon voice recognition (http://www.nuance.com), aid students to transcribe their thoughts via speech-to text capabilities, bypassing difficulties in spelling and handwriting

Table 15.2 Executive functions skills for behaviour. Purposes, description strategies and suggested programmes (Abdul Karim©2021)

Executive functions for behavioural purposes				
Skills	Description	Language area	Strategies	Programmes
Sustained attention	Enhancing the ability to attend to a task in the presence of distraction, fatigue or boredom. Individuals with dyslexia deficits may have visual-spatial as well as verbal material in the temporary storage (Varvara et al. 2014; Lehongre et al. 2011)	– Auditory attention – Listening for comprehension. – Phonological processing – Phoneme/grapheme – Orthography – Reading comprehension	**Director—Visualising**: This strategy is concerned with building a good mental image for sentence practice and construction (parts of speech, capitalisation and punctuation) (McArthur and Castles 2017; Bucci 2019; Meltzer 2018) **Analytical Training**: By breaking down reading tasks (e.g. base word, prefix, root and suffix) this teaches how the whole word can be considered as its component parts (Birsh 2018) **Thinking Strategies**: This helps access to information that is implied but not directly stated, by the use of, e.g. Annotation, SQ3R, and KWL charts	– The Reading Rockets website is a good example of how speech-pathologists and teachers might develop this strategy with children: http://www.readingrockets.org/article/picture-using-mental-imagery-while-reading – Highlighting, mnemonics and colour code – SQ3R; KWL chart
Response inhibition	Pre-operative thinking capacity relates to the ability to resist automatic, common, dominant responses to stimuli, but support more specific context, task-appropriate responses and deciding behavioural attitudes (Meltzer 2010; Diamond 2014). Can control attention on information that is more important and ignore distracting or irrelevant information or unrelated data. Is a basic factor for a successful function (Cartwright 2015; Cartwright et al. 2019; Danielsson et al. 2010)	– Auditory attention – Listening for comprehension – Word recognition – Word decoding – Oral motor production – Rapid naming – Prosody	**Self-Monitoring**: Requires scholars/adults to develop personalised self-checking aides-memoire or cards to help them remember the core ideas in texts they read (Meltzer 2010). Checking work so that the end study reflects an understanding of the content **Reciprocal Reading Strategies**: By encouraging reading a few paragraphs of the assigned text selection, and training the summarising, questioning, predicting and clarifying strategies (Oczuks 2003) **Cueing and Directing**: Attention and immediate memory for reading words and connected text (McCloskey 2016) **Orthographic Coding**: Using memory for letters, letter clusters or whole words to recognise a learned word. Knowledge of irregular/exemption words (pint) or homophones (rose vs. rows) (Kilpatrick et al. 2015)	– Whispersync is an app for the kindle reader that allows the switching between reading and listening – Read and write software enables the user to read on-screen text aloud – Claro-read enables the user to read on-screen text – Predictive text software co-writer – Predictive text software sprint-plus – Mind-mapping Kidspiration
Task initiation	The ability to initiate a task and finish it at the right time. Dyslexic children may suffer from sluggish attentional shifting, i.e. engaging and disengaging attention (Laasonen et al. 2012)	Both spoken and written words: – Vowels – Consonants – Phonemes – Graphemes – Syllables – Reading comprehension	**Open-ended Tasks**: As in writing papers, projects or studying for tests **Building Blocks**: Encouraging the initiation and presentation of spoken and written words in vowels, consonants, phonemes, graphemes, syllables (McArthur and Castles 2017) **Self-Efficacy**: Individuals' beliefs in their ability to accomplish a task; is considered as self-efficacy (Zhang and Ardasheva 2019)	Programmes that help provide explicit phonemic and phonological skills – The *Reading Doctor* (2016), *Cracking* The ABC Code (Fawcett 2019) – *Spelfabet* (Clarke et al. 2016) – *Jolly Phonics* (Jolly Learning 1992–2018)

(continued)

Table 15.2 (continued)

Executive functions for behavioural purposes				
Skills	Description	Language area	Strategies	Programmes
Goal-directed	The capacity to follow and achieve goal setting and self-reinforcement and not to decrease main aim owing to other interests (Meltzer 2010, 2018; Zusho and Edwards 2011)	– Orthographic coding – Phonic/decoding – Phonological memory – Syllables analyse – Word meaning	**Goal setting**: Helps to set attainable goals, break goals down into smaller steps, and to identify ways of overcoming these difficulties **Practical Knowledge Strategy**: For alphabetic code in spelling direction and coordinate phonology, orthography, and morphology (Berninger 2015) **Direct Instruction Strategy**: Reduces orthographic deficits by encouraging use of more accurate words and repeated reading connected texts (Borre 2019). **Self-Efficacy and self-Confidence**: These can be developed through short training interventions and entail hope, resiliency, problem-solving, which are malleable for adults, a sense of personal control, goal setting and person–environment fit, their coping strategies (McLoughlin and Leather 2013; Costantini et al. 2019)	– MultiLit (Wheldall et al. 2015). An Australian programme for low progress readers consistent with international best practice in the area of literacy instruction
Flexibility	The ability to switch attention and adapt to altered conditions (Mental Health Daily 2017; Meltzer 2018). Requires rapid access to words and strategic search through lexical/ phonological and conceptual/ semantic memory (Baldo and Dronkers 2006)	– Speech sounds – Letter symbols – Phonological memory – Lexical/phonologic – Word meanings	**Shifting and Switching**: Between the different processes as in reading and writing (e.g. shifting between the main ideas and associated details and back, moving between delineating text to brief summary and back, or shifting between multiple-choice test questions to answering open-ended enquiries on tests (Meltzer 2010, 2018) **A multiple-Linguistic Methodology**: Practise and reviewing language contrivances—speech sounds, letter symbols and word meanings obviously identified and connected together (McArthur and Castles 2017) **Cueing Retrieval of Information**: Sustaining working memory resources from lexicons to reading words, connected text and constructing meaning from text (McCloskey 2016)	– School software: Word shark uses multisensory learning to help dyslexic students with spelling, reading, and writing. It uses more than 50 games to teach phonics, spelling rules, word sequencing, and word sounds

Emotional control (self-regulation)	The ability to direct emotions to achieve ultimate goals or to control, direct behaviour and self-regulate learning (Panadero 2017), behavioural self-regulation has been put forward as another important skill for reading acquisition (McClelland et al. 2014). Likewise, it has been found to predict word decoding considerably in middle childhood (Messer et al. 2016) and predict concurrent reading comprehension (Cirino et al. 2017)	Auditory attention and the six language systems: – Listening comprehension – Oral expression – Prosody – Intention – Reading comprehension – Written expression	**Bridging Strategies**: Cognitive specific executive function skill routines that can be practised by students to increase their ability for self-direction, direct perceptions, feelings, thoughts and self-talk strategies and discipline between external demands with internal desires to succeed goals (McCloskey et al. 2016) **Simultaneous and Involvement**: By enhancing four language systems: listening comprehension, oral expression, reading comprehension and written expression **Building Reliance and self-Esteem**: By training to focus on developing the students' adaptive coping skills. Instruction in seven main areas: defying self-defeating thoughts, knowledge, joining, coping strategies, identifying needs, seeking appropriate support, to build positive self-esteem by reflecting on their strengths and pride as a potential individualisation strategy (Borre et al. 2019; Boudah 2018; Karten 2015; Yang and Bai 2019) **Motivational and Self-Efficacy**: Encouraging learners to use strategies to create their own learning intentions, such as goals that are connected with further education, can help them to achieve goals and are predictors of the application of self-regulated motivation, the learner is more likely to complete tasks effectively by selecting and applying appropriate self-regulated motivation strategies (Paulino et al. 2016) **Practice Mindfulness**: Can help children and young adults feel calmer, improve focus, and manage emotions better. Translates as increases in student academic performances (Idler et al. 2017; Maynard et al. 2017)	– Beating Dyslexia (http://www.beatingdyslexia.com/) has additional strategies on developing self-help skills – Mindfulness Bundle—Distance Learning – Brain Futures 2019: enhances children's executive function skills with brain literacy via direct instruction, evidence-based computer-delivered cognitive skills training programmes, mindfulness programmes, and cognitive-physical activities

15.3 Logopaedics/SLP Therapy Principles: Principles of Pedagogic Training in Dyslexic and Dysgraphic Pupils; Principles of Computerised Rehabilitation

Anja Fiori

15.3.1 Introduction

Therapeutic intervention in developmental dyslexia needs a combination of technical, linguistically grounded principles with specific knowledge from the psychology of learning and educational science. In this spirit, Schulte-Körne et al. (2007) have indicated interdisciplinary cooperation as one of the main challenges in prevention and remediation. Therapy of developmental dyslexia is a time- and effort-consuming, complex long-term intervention. The following section is an attempt to give a structured overview of a holistic therapeutic approach to developmental dyslexia (in the sense of respect for the complexity of the issue). It moves from general educational and motivational considerations to therapeutic measures depending on the stage of acquisition, with linguistically based principles of intervention. The text does not focus on single published therapeutic programmes, as these are generally restricted to a specific language. It rather gives an overview of general cross-language principles of therapy. The last paragraph is about computer-based forms of exercise as an example of utilising motivating modern formats for intervention. The aim of this paragraph is to provide potential readers with quality criteria against which they can evaluate programmes relevant to their language. In order to provide readers with internationally usable information, and owing to the rapid development of ever newer offerings, examples of specific computer programmes are not given.

15.3.2 General Educational Considerations

Some general considerations are important with regard to the expectations of parents and children: one-dimensional or unambiguous causalities of developmental dyslexia are, from a scientific point of view, dubious and so are therapeutic methods that suggest quick and easy help and relief.
As Munzer et al. (2020) state:

> Because dyslexia is a chronic condition, management often requires a life-span approach.

Respectable forms of intervention are generally intensive, time-consuming and hard work for the dyslexic child. This should be made clear from the first contact on to assure the adherence and perseverance needed for successful intervention. The therapeutic intervention should be carried out interdisciplinarily until age-appropriate participation in everyday life is achieved. A recent evidence- and consent-based guideline developed by the German Association of Child and Youth Psychiatry in cooperation with several interdisciplinary professional associations (DGKJP 2015; Galuschka and Schulte-Körne 2016) gives a good overview of relevant international literature and practical recommendations for diagnosis and remediation. According to these authors, yearly follow-ups to check for therapeutic progress and re-assessing indication are recommended. Very informative is the clinical forum by Hogan (2018) offering evidence-based knowledge inter alia about the neurobiological basis of dyslexia and the current state of diagnostics and therapeutic approaches. This insight may be considered as official guidance by the American Speech-Language-Hearing Association (2018).

15.3.3 Motivation Is a Therapeutic Goal

Although early detection of specific difficulties in literacy acquisition is desirable (Schulte-Körne et al. 2007; Shaywitz et al. 2008; Snowling 2013), in clinical practice, dyslexic children often show a long individual history of discouraging and frustrating experience in the field of learning (not only in reading and writing) before referral to therapy.

> Most children suffering from dyslexia are diagnosed in the third grade. Depending on the schooling in the different countries, the children are between 7 and 9 years old—Schulte-Körne et al. (2007)

Secondary psychiatric comorbidities such as depression, reluctance to go to school, and anxiety are often described (Warnke et al. 2004; Munzer et al. 2020). In consequence, it seems self-evident that professionals working in the field of dyslexia therapy should show extreme sensitivity in dealing with such children. Therapists have to bear in mind that their clients have to be motivated to put great effort for a considerably long period into a field of personal frustration. Therefore, motivation itself is often an explicit therapeutic goal to be achieved before being able to work on specific linguistic topics. There are some general principles to be followed:

- Respect for the importance of the child's and parents´ consent to therapy, including necessary frequency and importance of homework.
- Transparency of general and specific therapeutic aims and methods for the treated child, and readjustment if in doubt about the child's consent.
- Avoidance of any discouraging or frustrating experience due to excessive demands; choosing exercise material that ensures working at the limit of no mistakes.
- Word and text material should be of interest and 'sensible' to the dyslexic child.
- Demands in school life should be considered and may be altered, upon agreement with teachers and pedagogic staff, in cases of interdisciplinary intervention. Munzer et al. (2020) mention the opportunity of individualised educational accommodation from secondary school on.

15.3.4 Psycholinguistic Considerations

From a psycholinguistic viewpoint, a symptom-orientated, individual therapeutic approach is recommended (Shaywitz et al. 2008; DGKJP 2015). Depending on the stage of reading and writing acquisition, and on the individual constellation of symptoms, different goals of intervention may be derived. In early stages, the main therapeutic aim is to establish the alphabetic principle via training of grapheme–phoneme correspondences and phonological analysis. Exercises should move from simple words to those of increasing phonological complexity and from high to low linguistic frequency. Depending on the results of further diagnostics, it may be crucial to train phonological abilities as a basis for further work with spelling exercises. It has to be noted though that prolonged isolated training of phonological awareness unconnected to written material is not recommended, as effects have proved to be non-specific for reading and writing (DGKJP 2015). The combination of phonological training with written material is highly recommended.

In children showing severe deficits in working memory, focusing only on a sublexical (letter-by-letter) strategy of literacy acquisition might be overtaxing. It may be advisable to include compensatory lexical (whole-word) strategies in the general sublexical approach. Again, these are not recommended as the only methods, but might be used in addition to phonologically orientated training. As shown in a recent systematic review on spelling interventions (Galuschka et al. 2020), phonics as well as orthographic and morphological instruction have been proven to have an impact on spelling performance. The following paragraphs explain general principles of how to combine these approaches in a sensible sequence.

15.3.5 First Principle: Alphabetic Skills First, Orthographic Rules Second

Before working on orthographic rules, the alphabetic principle should be well established, with only few mistakes changing the phonetic structure of a word (Ehri 2000). This means that, before addressing orthographic rules in remediation, phoneme and grapheme analysis, as well as grapheme–phoneme correspondences and phoneme–grapheme correspondences, should be well established via child-orientated exercises to ensure phonetically accurate writing and fluent reading as a first step. Only when the child has learned to spell out the speech-sounds and syllables that a spoken word consists of correctly, and to read out graphemes and syllables in their correct order and blend them to identify words, is the next step to introduce orthographic rules by explicit instructions in a child-orientated manner. Planning is based on the individual symptomatic profile derived from qualitative analysis of the incidence of the types of mistakes. An individual sequence of specific therapeutic goals in spelling can be derived. According to Ehri (2000), reading should never be taught independently from spelling, as both competences are intertwined in development.

15.3.6 Second Principle: Individualised Sequence of Orthographic Rules to Be Trained

As Galuschka et al. (2020) point out,

> understanding the principles of an orthography is beneficial for learners with dyslexia or spelling deficits.

The following principles may help to derive a useful sequential arrangement of orthographic topics. Linguistic frequency (which can be interpreted as an indicator of general relevance) and the individual's incidence of mistakes are the two general, sometimes competing, aspects that should be taken into account when deciding on the sequence of orthographic rules to be worked on. If orthographic rules are well-established in the therapeutic setting, the next step is generalisation to different contexts of increasing complexity.

15.3.7 Third Principle: Additional Helpful Strategies for Self-Monitoring and Comprehension

Establishing monitoring strategies (self-correction) in 'real life' is a further important therapeutic aim. Strategies enhancing text comprehension can be applied complementarily, if helpful for the individual child, but are not recommended as the sole method in reading disorders (Shaywitz et al. 2008; DGKJP 2015). However, according to a review by Stevens et al. (2019), targeted summarising and main idea identification have proven to be helpful reading comprehension strategies for poor readers. In children with reading difficulties, manipulation of text material (enlarged type size and line pitch and graphically augmented segmentation) can be used to give them additional support (DGKJP 2015).

15.3.8 Intervention for Children with Handwriting Difficulties

Dyslexic children often show handwriting difficulties in addition to their reading and spelling deficits (Montgomery 2007; Sumner et al. 2014; Hebert et al. 2018c; Gosse and Van Reybroeck 2020). The question of whether these difficulties arise from spelling or graphomotor deficits has no clear answer yet. According to Sumner et al. (2014), 'it is conceivable that spelling ability will influence rate of handwriting production' in children with dyslexia and beginning writers. They examined the influence of spelling ability and within-word pausing on handwriting production. They concluded that handwriting productivity relies on spelling capability and is not predicted by aspects of motor skill. Similar findings are described by Arfé et al. (2020) for children writing Italian. These authors compared the influence of script (cursive vs. manuscript) with that of orthographic complexity on writing tasks in dyslexic children compared with chronological and handwriting age-matched peers. They attribute the weaker writing performance of dyslexic children to the orthographic complexity of the writing tasks and not to the motor requirements. However, in a French study reported by Gosse and Van Reybroeck (2020), the authors conclude that graphomotor aspects of writing have a greater impact than orthographic complexity on dyslexic children's writing performance compared with (chronologically or writing) age-matched peers in writing tasks. Several authors give advice on treatment options for writing difficulties, each with a different focus: Montgomery (2007) argues that more attention should be paid to the spelling and writing process in the treatment of dyslexic children and gives a comprehensive overview of research in the field and specific therapeutic and teaching approaches. Andrews and Lombardino (2014) emphasise the importance of fluent and legible handwriting, and provide guidance in diagnostics and therapy for dyslexic children with handwriting difficulties. Hebert et al. (2018c) give advice on instructional strategies for handwriting, based on systematic searches and the examination of recent meta-analyses in the field. They report evidence of effective remedial and compensatory interventions.

15.3.9 Setting: Groups or Individuals?

In terms of therapeutic setting, no significant differences in outcome between individuals or small groups of up to five children have been found. Deciding in which setting the intervention is to be carried out should depend on possible co-morbidities or the individual symptomatic profile of the child (DGKJP 2015).

15.3.10 Using a Computer for Remediation

Computer-based reading or spelling programmes bring many advantages if used in addition to conventional face-to-face-therapy:

- Formats of exercises are usually motivating for the young clients.
- Exercises are highly structured in small steps of learning demand.
- Learning software allows immediate, impartial feedback.
- Given thorough supervision, it can be used for homework and thus ensure high frequency of exercises.
- It is usually possible to outline improvement of performance graphically.

Nevertheless, learning software cannot be substituted for conventional therapy or education. Studies on the efficiency of learning software in dyslexia therapy show that learning software can be an effective tool (Kast et al. 2011), but not superior to conventional therapy, although a positive effect on motivation and attention is noted (Zimdars and Zink 2006; Hartmann 2014).

As demand is high from parents, therapists and dyslexic children, new products of varying quality are constantly developed, and a critical review of the products available is recommended. Some general considerations and criteria used to judge the quality and benefit of typical formats are proposed:

- Computer programmes should be individually adaptable to a child's level of performance.
- The possibility of feeding the system with individual word material would be ideal.
- Specific difficulties in reading or writing should be addressed by specific material and exercises.
- To which stage of reading and writing development the software refers, and which specific goals can be obtained, should be documented.
- The choice of word material (if not individually adaptable) should be critically reviewed to avoid excessive demands through inadequate material.

Many therapeutic programmes offer learning software in addition to their conventional paper–pencil material, which is linguistically structured according to the programme's standards, and use the same word material. Therefore, making use of computer-based learning software can be recommended in addition to conventional therapy, provided that a critical view of the material, instruction and supervision is given by the supporting expert (Zimdars and Zink 2006).

15.3.11 Conclusion

The therapy of developmental dyslexia is interdisciplinary, symptom-orientated, individualised, linguistically structured, dependent on the developmental stage. It should be carried out by experts with special proficiency in literacy acquisition and enhancement who are experienced in dealing with children with circumscribed developmental disorders (DGKJP 2015).

15.4 Treatment of Auditory Processing Disorders

15.4.1 Rehabilitation and Prognosis for Children with Auditory Processing Disorder

David R. Moore, Nicole G. Campbell, Doris-Eva Bamiou and Tony Sirimanna

15.4.1.1 Introduction

Current intervention strategies can be divided into four main categories: (1) listening strategies, (2) modifying the listening environment, (3) auditory training and (4) compensatory strategies (BSA 2011, 2018; Chermak and Musiek 2013). The strategies listed under "Modifying the Listening Environment" are more evidence-based than the other strategies. Several "auditory training" approaches have been tested rigorously, with mixed results. "Compensatory strategies" are widely advocated but have not been well validated (BSA 2018). The lack of an agreed diagnostic procedure makes it more challenging to conduct traditional case-control studies in which those with the disorder are compared with carefully matched controls who lack the disorder. Also, there is no agreement on what the "gold standard" should be against which the sensitivity or specificity of a candidate intervention should be compared. Finally, the high co-occurrence of APD with other disorders can make the use of interventions for specific difficulties of limited general effectiveness. Nevertheless, there is no shortage of suggestions as to what may work (BSA 2011; Chermak and Musiek 2013), and there is increasing evidence that some approaches may improve listening in general.

New technologies, such as remote microphone devices (also referred to as assistive listening devices or wireless listening devices), personal sound amplification products ("PSAPs") and "apps", are promising (Smart et al. 2018) but require further investigation. Remote microphone devices are also proving to be beneficial to those with language and attention difficulties, as the technology allows better access to the primary signal, reducing background noise and reverberation (Schafer et al. 2014).

15.4.1.2 Listening Strategies

There is no doubt that fixating a speaking face improves speech perception (Everdell et al. 2007; Vo et al. 2012), but observation of normal-hearing listeners suggests that this is not something we all do routinely unless we are having difficulty hearing, in which case an individual will intuitively look directly at the speaker. For a person with a listening difficulty (APD), it is the simplest way to improve listening. For a child, it may be something they have never been taught to do (Truesdale 1990). Asking a speaker to direct speech towards a listener and to ensure their face is uncovered is also a good idea.

15.4.1.3 Modifying the Listening Environment

Increasing the signal (speech) level relative to that of the background noise (signal/noise ratio; S/N) will usually result in enhanced perception. This may be achieved in a low-tech way, for example, by sitting or standing closer to a speaker. Reducing the noise level of a listening environment may also be feasible and has been shown to be helpful, for example, in schools (Shield et al.

2015). In addition to reducing the level of a bothersome sound, reducing reverberation within an environment commonly used for communication is advised (Klatte et al. 2013). This may be achieved through passive acoustic methods such as carpets, curtains, doors, seals and rubber tips on furniture legs and the installation of noise-absorbent partitions or screens. Other aspects that can be considered are architectural design of buildings (e.g. double-glazed windows) and interventions to improve the S/N, including preferential seating (BSA 2018).

Wireless listening devices, also known as "FM systems", have been used for many years to improve the S/N. The principle of wireless listening devices is simple. A target sound source is amplified relative to prevailing noise. This can be achieved without creating an overloud signal by using a closed-loop system in which the listener wears headphones or other receiver (e.g. insert earphones), usually connected wirelessly to a microphone and transmitter, which may be worn by or placed close to the speaker. FM and "Bluetooth" (2.4 GHz) wireless listening devices are becoming simpler to use, more affordable and smaller. Recent evidence suggests that such systems can improve learning outcomes, auditory perception and the fidelity with which the auditory brainstem encodes speech signals (Hornickel et al. 2012; Smart et al. 2018). Although one of these studies targeted children with reading disorders (Hornickel et al. 2012), about half of those children were likely to have APD (Sharma et al. 2009). It may therefore be assumed that the improved outcomes observed would also be seen in children with APD.

15.4.1.4 Auditory Training

There is overwhelming evidence that auditory training results in "near" learning, hearing of stimuli that are the same as, or closely related to, those used during training (e.g. Ferguson et al. 2014). A systematic review (Loo et al. 2010) suggested that current software provides robust "on-task" learning of the exact skill trained, but little or no transfer of learning to untrained tasks or skills. However, a crucial issue in evaluating the rehabilitation benefits of training is whether the observed learning transfers to untrained tasks (Wright and Zhang 2009), especially those that cause difficulty in hearing and listening in everyday life. For example, does music training, or playing computer games involving simple acoustic stimuli (e.g. tones, phonemes), transfer to improved speech perception in noisy environments or reduced inattention of a child to the parent or teacher they need to communicate with? On this issue, the evidence is more equivocal (BSA 2018). There seems reasonable agreement that some short-term, computer-based sensorimotor training can transfer to untrained stimuli (Anguera et al. 2013), but there are also several examples of well-controlled studies where short-term training (i.e. less than about 3 months of daily or near-daily exercises) has been ineffective (Halliday et al. 2012; Murphy et al. 2015). Musical training has been found beneficial for learning important auditory skills and tuning underlying brain processes (Strait et al. 2013; Alain et al. 2014). However, the extent of benefit and transfer to real-world tasks and settings is controversial. In further research it is essential to control carefully for therapist-contact, and to use active control groups, and robust outcome measures to prevent false-positive results (Halliday 2014). It is important that intervention addresses core difficulties and results in improvement in daily functioning, rather than improvement in only a discrete skill that is trained and then remeasured.

15.4.1.5 Compensatory Strategies

Training in metacognitive and metalinguistic strategies can also be considered. These strategies include self-regulation and problem-solving, by identifying individual listening strengths and weaknesses and listening situations that are more challenging. Possible solutions include use of visual material, visual imagery or "chunking" to remember and recall verbal information or writing information down to stay focused and for remembering. Verbal rehearsal may be used to commit verbal information to memory. These strategies, though widely advocated, have not been scientifically tested (BSA 2018).

15.4.1.6 Long-Term Benefit

To the extent that good listening strategies and acoustic enhancement may be lifelong changes in behaviour, we can assume that the benefits of those interventions will persist. Persistence of benefit is likely to be enhanced by making tasks easier, more attractive or more accessible, but these requirements should be balanced against the need for close attention to and engagement with the speaker. Performance may even improve over time owing to long-term learning effects. Similarly, as with other forms of training, continuing engagement with relevant, demanding listening tasks, either during training or in the course of everyday life, may lead to benefits of the sort reported following prolonged musical or language training. There is evidence that various forms of perceptual learning are persistent (Molloy et al. 2012) and that skill acquisition or recovery, especially earlier in life, may be retained without further specific intervention. Finally, the activity for which there is the best evidence for the retention and enhancement of cognitive function, underpinning all aspects of hearing and listening, is aerobic exercise (Hillman 2014; Hillman et al. 2008), and higher physical activity is associated with reduced age-related hearing loss (Curhan et al. 2013). Research of the effect of exercise on children's listening skills could be fruitful. The APD MESHGuide, a new evidence-based resource, offers practical guidence (Campbell et al. 2019).

15.5 Comorbidities of Literacy and Attention-Deficit/Hyperactivity Disorders Leading to Close Cooperation with Child and Adolescent Psychiatrists

Barbara Maciejewska and Manuel Föcker

15.5.1 Dyslexia/Learning Disorders, Attention-Deficit/Hyperactivity Disorders and Comorbidity

Dyslexia (a specific learning disorder with impairment in reading, reading disorder (RD), a type of learning disability (LD)) and attention-deficit/hyperactivity disorder (ADHD) are both common developmental disorders diagnosed in childhood, with a high comorbidity rate (25–40%) (Willcutt et al. 2000; Willcutt and Pennington 2000a, b; DuPaul et al. 2013; Brimo et al. 2021). According to ICD-11 (WHO 2024), dyslexia is described as a developmental learning disorder with impairment in reading (6A03.0). It is assigned to the category developmental learning disorders along with developmental learning disorders with impairment in written expression (6A03.1), impairment in mathematics (6A03.2), other specified impairments of learning (6A03.3) and the unspecified form (6A03.Z).

Dyslexia is defined as a specific persistent failure to acquire reading skills in spite of a conventional learning process, normal intelligence and socio-cultural opportunities (for detailed diagnostic criteria, see Table 15.3) (Lyon et al. 2003; Schulte-Körne 2021). ADHD is characterised by excessive activity, short attention span and impulsivity. According to ICD-11 (WHO 2024), ADHD (6A05) is divided into three specified subtypes: predominantly inattentive presentation (6A05.0), predominantly hyperactive-impulsive presentation (6A05.1) and combined presentation (6A05.2). (For detailed diagnostic criteria, see Table 15.3, Sánchez-Morán et al. 2018; Drechsler et al. 2020.) Because the phenotypes of ADHD and dyslexia overlap, and the rate of comorbidity between these two disorders is high, ADHD is an often under- or mis-diagnosed disorder in children with LD such as dyslexia (Gnanavel et al. 2019).

Dyslexia may co-occur with other conditions, as shown in Table 15.4. Children with ADHD may have a comorbid developmental LD, neurodevelopmental disorders, physical diseases and health disorders (Patel et al. 2012; Hendren et al. 2018; Ijeoma and Chinelo 2019). Learning disorders including dyslexia show high levels of comorbidity with disruptive and emotional disorders such as ADHD, depression/depressed mood, anxiety and conduct disorder (CD) (Diakakis et al. 2008; Maughan and Carroll 2006; Nelson and Gregg 2012; Horbach et al. 2020). Much research has indicated a clear relationship and overlap between dyslexia and other developmental disorders: up to 85% of dyslexics suffer from dyspraxia, and 60% of dyslexics have symptoms of developmental coordination disorders (Puac 2005).

Table 15.3 Definitions and diagnostic criteria for developmental disorders and attention-deficit/hyperactivity disorders (Based on WHO (2024))

ICD-11 (2021)	Definition
Developmental learning disorder	Developmental learning disorder is characterised by significant and persistent difficulties in learning academic skills, which may include reading, writing or arithmetic. The individual's performance in the affected academic skill(s) is markedly below what would be expected for chronological age and general level of intellectual functioning, and results in significant impairment in the individual's academic or occupational functioning. Developmental learning disorder first manifests when academic skills are taught during the early school years. Developmental learning disorder is not due to a disorder of intellectual development, sensory impairment (vision or hearing), neurological or motor disorder, lack of availability of education, lack of proficiency in the language of academic instruction, or psychosocial adversity
Developmental learning disorder with impairment in reading	Developmental learning disorder with impairment in reading is characterised by significant and persistent difficulties in learning academic skills related to reading, such as word reading accuracy, reading fluency and reading comprehension. The individual's performance in reading is markedly below what would be expected for chronological age and level of intellectual functioning, and results in significant impairment in the individual's academic or occupational functioning. Developmental learning disorder with impairment in reading is not due to a disorder of intellectual development, sensory impairment (vision or hearing), neurological disorder, lack of availability of education, lack of proficiency in the language of academic instruction, or psychosocial adversity
ADHD	Attention-deficit hyperactivity disorder is characterised by a persistent pattern (at least 6 months) of inattention or hyperactivity-impulsivity or both that has a direct negative impact on academic, occupational or social functioning. There is evidence of significant inattention or hyperactivity-impulsivity symptoms before age 12, typically by early to mid-childhood, though some individuals may first come to clinical attention later. The degree of inattention and hyperactivity-impulsivity is outside the limits of normal variation expected for age and level of intellectual functioning. Inattention refers to significant difficulty in sustaining attention to tasks that do not provide a high level of stimulation or frequent rewards, distractibility and problems with organisation. Hyperactivity refers to excessive motor activity and difficulties in remaining still, most evident in structured situations that require behavioural self-control. Impulsivity is a tendency to act in response to immediate stimuli, without deliberation or consideration of the risks and consequences. The relative balance and the specific manifestations of inattentive and hyperactive-impulsive characteristics vary across individuals, and may change over the course of development. In order for a diagnosis to be made, manifestations of inattention or hyperactivity-impulsivity must be evident across multiple situations or settings (e.g. home, school, work, with friends or relatives), but are likely to vary according to the structure and demands of the setting. Symptoms are not better accounted for by another mental, behavioural or neurodevelopmental disorder, and are not due to the effect of a substance or medication

Approximately 80% of children suffer from ADHD, and 60% of children with reading disorders meet criteria for at last one additional psychiatric or somatic diagnosis (Germanò et al. 2010).

According to Patel et al. (2012),

'67% of ADHD children had at least one other mental health or neurodevelopmental disorder compared with 11% of children without ADHD'; of the 67% with ADHD, '33% have one comorbidity disorder, 16% have two, and 18% have three or more'.

ADHD (vs. no ADHD) is associated with following conditions: learning disorders (46% vs. 5%), conduct disorder (27% vs. 2%), anxiety (18% vs. 2%), depression (14% vs. 1%), speech problems (12% vs. 3%), autism spectrum disorder (6% vs. 0.6%), epilepsy/seizures (2.6% vs. 0.6%). The most frequent comorbidity of ADHD was oppositional defiant disorder (ODD) at 46.9%, followed by mood disorder (27.9%), conduct disorder (CD) and elimination disorder (EID) (18.5%), dyslexia (17.6%), anxiety (16.7%) and Tourette disorders (TD) (9.5%)

Table 15.4 Problems associated with RD and dyslexia as comorbid disorders (Based on Margari et al. (2013), Carotenuto et al. (2016), Moll et al. (2020), Peters et al. (2018), Patel et al. (2012), Hakim and Ghorbani (2015), Masi and Gignac (2015))

Psychiatric/psychological	Developmental	Physical	Social
Attention-deficit disorder (ADD)	Dyscalculia	Sleep-wake disorders	Loneliness
Attention-deficit hyperactivity disorder (ADHD)	Dysgraphia	Autoimmune diseases	Poor school integration
Anxiety	Dyspraxia	Allergies	Bullying
Mood disorder	Motor coordination disorder (Clumsiness)	Epilepsy	Low self esteem
Depression	Speech problems	Obesity and being overweight	
Impulse control disorders		Bulimia nervosa/binge eating disorder	
Conduct disorder (CD)			
Oppositional defiant disorder (ODD)			
Tics			
Substance abuse			
Autism spectrum disorders (ASD)			

(Patel et al. 2012). It is worth noting that ADHD symptoms persist from childhood into adulthood. However, there are differences between children and adolescents (Banaschewski et al. 2018).

As Moll et al. (2020) assumed, rates of comorbidity between RD and neurodevelopmental disorders range from 11% to 70% for RD and mathematics disorder, 20% to 50% for RD and behavioural disorders (ADHD and CD) and from 9% to 29% for RD and emotional problems. Although comorbidity rates vary widely between studies, they are higher than expected by chance, indicating that comorbidities between reading disorders and other neurodevelopmental disorders are the rule rather than an exception (Ijeoma and Chinelo 2019). Rates of comorbidity of ADHD and LD vary depending of the study (Sahoo et al. 2015).

Comorbidity depends on the diagnostic focus of the physician. If he or she performs diagnostics related to both ADHD and dyslexia, the rate of comorbidity is very high (McGrath and Stoodley 2019). Dyslexia and ADHD are two complex neurobehavioural disorders that co-occur more often than expected, so that RD has been linked to ADHD, especially the inattention symptoms (ADD) (Sánchez-Morán et al. 2018). Common consequences are poor school and social integration.

15.5.2 Theories of the Attention-Deficit/Hyperactivity Disorder: Reading Disability Comorbidity

ADHD and RD are complex childhood disorders that frequently co-occur, but the aetiology of this comorbidity remains unknown (Willcutt et al. 2010). Several theories have been put forward to explain the shared symptoms of these two neurobehavioural disorders. Both are considered complex disorders influenced by multiple genetic and environmental risk factors. There is strong evidence for shared genetic, neuropsychological and neural risk factors that contribute to the dyslexia-ADHD comorbidity (McGrath and Stoodley 2019).

15.5.2.1 Genetic Findings

ADHD and dyslexia are highly heritable, so they are thought to have a strong genetic component. Twin studies have reported a heritability from 40% to 60% for dyslexia (Fisher and DeFries 2002; Scerri and Schulte-Körne 2010) and 70% to 80% for ADHD (Faraone and Larsson 2019). Up to ten candidate genes may be associated with dyslexia (DYX1C1, KIAA0319, DCDC2, ROBO1, KIAA0319L: Couto et al. 2008) (CNTNAP2, MRPL19, C2ORF3, CEP63, NCAN: Grimm et al. 2020). Six candidate genes for ADHD were revealed in a meta-analysis across multiple studies: the serotonin transporter gene (5HTT), dopamine transporter gene (DAT1), D4 dopamine receptor gene (DRD4), D5 dopamine receptor gene (DRD5), serotonin 1B receptor gene (HTR1B) and a gene coding for a synaptic vesicle-regulating protein (SNAP25). Additionally, the dopamine transporter gene (SLC6A3) was found to be associated in several studies (for review, see Faraone and Larsson 2019).

A significant contribution of common genetic variants to dyslexia risk and novel genomic overlap with such psychiatric conditions such as ADHD, bipolar disorder, schizophrenia and cross-disorder susceptibility were found by Gialluisi et al. (2020). The use of gene network reconstruction and analysis methods is a powerful tool for investigating the molecular mechanisms of comorbidities. This method is used to predict genes that play a key role in the development of comorbidities, that is, it aims to assess genes for comorbid disorders: ADHD and dyslexia. There are approximately 20 genes with highest priority by average rank, implicated in the co-occurrence of dyslexia and ADHD. Out of highest-priority genes, e.g. OOPRM1, CHRNA4, SNCADRD2, DRD4, CNTNAP2 and GRIN2B are mentioned in the literature as being associated with the co-occurrence of ADHD and dyslexia. The most relevant genes were shown to be involved in biological processes related to signal transduction, positive regulation of transcription from RNA polymerase II promoters, chemical synaptic transmission, drug response, transmembrane ion transport, nervous system development, cell adhesion and neuronal migration (Hongyao et al. 2023). Ciulkinyte et al. (2024) confirmed the increased genetic relation concerning dyslexia and ADHD compared to other psychiatric traits and revealed novel pleiotropic variants affecting both traits.

15.5.2.2 Gene-Environmental Explanation

The gene-environmental interaction theory suggests that the environment or some event in the life of the foetus (elevated testosterone, nicotine, drugs, alcohol or infection) or child (low level of fatty acids, environmental toxicants, pollution, viruses, and sex chromosome composition) triggers a genetic predisposition to be expressed (Virolainen et al. 2023).

15.5.2.3 Neuropsychological Risk Factors

The partial genetic overlap in symptoms between RD and ADHD suggests that there may also be partial overlap between the disorders at the cognitive level (Gialluisi et al. 2019, 2020). A shared genetic risk factor may lead to a specific neuropsychological weakness that increases the susceptibility to both disorders (McGrath and Stoodley 2019). At the neuropsychological level, weaknesses in several cognitive domains are observed: phonological processing difficulties, deficits in processing speed and aspects of executive functioning, including working memory, inhibition and sustained attention, planning (Willcutt et al. 2010; Moura et al. 2017).

15.5.2.4 Neural Factors at the Neural Level of Analysis

At this level clear evidence for comorbidity is being sought and evaluated. Many brain areas are being investigated as neural correlates between dyslexia and ADHD. Some neural areas are suspected to be structural connections of comorbidity. For dyslexia, the most commonly implicated neural correlates involve a reading network such as the left occipito-temporal region, left temporo-parietal region and the left inferior frontal gyrus (Ramus et al. 2018). The prefrontal cortex and striatum are considered regions characteristically affected in ADHD (McCarthy et al. 2014; Hoogman et al. 2017). In the dyslexia and ADHD literature, the meta-analysis of Stoodley (2014) and Cunff et al. (2024) examined brain regions associated with both disorders in the cerebellum. Decreased grey matter in the right caudate as a region of statistically significant conjunction between ADHD and dyslexia was described by McGrath and Stoodley (2019) in a meta-analysis of voxel-based morphometry (VBM) studies. However, as there was no evidence of unequivocal neuroregional overlap, it is possible that overlap regions have received less attention because they are not part of these canonical regions. Other neuroimaging modalities may be sensitive to overlapping neural correlates.

From the discussion of the above mentioned pathophysiological aspects, the following mechanisms of comorbidity are suggested:

- Shared genetic or environmental risk—the two disorders share common risk factors, whether neurobiological, psychological, genetic or social.
- One disorder directly increases the risk for the other (behavioural problems may impede reading acquisition, or frustrations arising from learning difficulties may exacerbate the risk of behaviour problems).
- The comorbid condition is a separate entity, distinct from either 'pure' disorder.
- Epiphenomenal comorbidity—psychiatric problems as a secondary phenomenon accompanying LD and caused by it but not modifying the course of the main disorder.

15.5.3 Phenotypic Overlaps Between ADHD and Dyslexia

First, there are many other possibilities or explanations for hyperactive impulsive behaviour. A few of the conditions are learning disability (which leads to poor school performance), frustration and a behavioural pattern where the child stops paying attention or gives up. Attention lapses can be caused by obsessive thoughts, silent impulsive rituals or any kind of seizure. Children with ADHD may present staring episodes, which can be differentiated from partial complex seizures. Undiagnosed subclinical fits may lead to reading disorders or attention deficit or both. A middle ear infection, causing an intermittent hearing problem, interferes with a child's ability to respond to an orally presented request. Disruptive unresponsive behaviour can be due to anxiety, depression or bipolar disorders. Environmental factors or stresses, such as divorce in the family, can lead to restlessness or inattention (Ogundele 2018; Patel et al. 2012).

Secondly, the symptoms of ADHD may mimic another disease; for example many children with ADHD also have learning disorders. ADHD affects the ability to learn but is not a true learning disability. It is the impulsivity, hyperactivity and distractibility that interfere with the learning process The symptoms of ADHD and different conditions, for example literacy disorders, overlap, so there has been controversy over whether ADHD exists as primary disorder or only secondary to other psychiatric symptoms.

Thirdly, a high comorbidity rate is observed between ADHD and other disorders. Some children with ADHD display significantly a learning disability, obsessive compulsive disorder, compulsive disorder, anxiety disorder or depressive disorder, while others may show evidence of a co-occurring tic disorder; some show multiple comorbid disorders.

To sum up, the comorbidity may be explained by following hypothesis (Table 15.5):

- Common ethology—the two disorders share the same genetic background.
- Phenotype—dyslexics may mimic behaviour characterised for children suffering from ADHD (phenocopy), but without a neuroanatomical background specific for ADHD.
- Cross-assortment—dyslexia and ADHD run in families independently, and the comorbidity is only by chance.
- Cognitive subtype—there is no comorbidity, it is only cognitive subtype of ADHD.

A major step towards a better understanding of developmental disorders and their comorbidities was the shift from single-deficit models to multiple-deficit models (Pennington 2006). Single-deficit models are especially problematic for explaining the high comorbidity rates between disorders from different diagnostic groupings, such as the comorbidity between reading disorder and ADHD (heterotypic comorbidity); this is because the two disorders are characterised by clearly distinct core deficits (phonological deficits in the case of reading disorder and executive deficits in ADHD). First, there is increasing evidence that the aetiology of such disorders is multifactorial, and cannot be explained by single causes at the genetic, environmental, neurobiological or cognitive analytical levels. Secondly, single-deficit models do not explain the heterogeneity

Table 15.5 Model of comorbidity of ADHD and RD and levels of causation (Based on: Luo et al. (2019))

Level of pathology	Biological correlates		Observed consequences
Aetiology	Risk factors		Pathological functions of cells
	Genes	Environment	
Neurobiology	Central nervous system		Abnormal structures and activities of brain areas, incorrect level of neurotransmitters
Cognition	Attention deficit	Phonological deficit	Affected functions
Behaviour	Recognised diseases		Pathological symptoms
	AD(H)D	RD	

in symptomatology observed between individuals diagnosed with the same disorder. Finally, single-deficit models do not account for the high comorbidity rates observed between different neurodevelopmental disorders (Moll et al. 2020).

15.5.4 Psychological Problems and Psychiatric Disorders in Dyslexia: The Role of the Child and Adolescent Psychiatrist

Learning difficulties are described as an important risk factor for mental problems and psychological discomfort. A growing number of studies indicate that children with RD are at high risk of internalising and externalising problems. Dyslexia persists throughout life and is a complicating factor in adult life. Preliminary analysis has shown that negative emotional experiences related to dyslexia negatively affect self-esteem even in late adulthood (Carawan et al. 2016, Brunswick et al. 2022). Internalising symptoms are associated with depression, anxiety, low mood, socio-emotional withdrawal, whereas externalising problems are indicated by overactivity, aggression and anger (Mugnaini et al. 2009; Hendren et al. 2018; Boyes et al. 2016; Cederlof et al. 2017). Children and adolescents with dyslexia experience three times more behavioural disorders than healthy children and adolescents, and one-third of children with behavioural problems are affected by dyslexia (Huc-Chabrolle et al. 2010; Bäcker and Neuhäuser 2003; Horbach et al. 2020). They have more interpersonal problems, more conflicts with friends, more social anxiety, a depressed mood and weaker relationships. They often become victims of bullying, both direct (shoves, insults, derisions) and indirect (threats, gossip and group exclusion) (see Table 15.4) to a greater extent than those without LD (Mugnaini et al. 2009; Boyes et al. 2016), and are more likely to commit suicide (Mugnaini et al. 2009). If the Specific Learning Disorders (SLD) and Disorders Not Otherwise Specified (LD NOS) subgroups are considered separately regarding comorbidities, ADHD is present in 33%, anxiety disorder in 28.8%, developmental coordination disorder in 17.8%, language disorder in 11% and mood disorder in 9.4% of patients in the LSD subgroup (Margari et al. 2013). In the LD NOS subgroup, language disorder is present in 28.6%, developmental coordination disorder in 27.5%, ADHD in 25.4%, anxiety disorder in 16.4% and mood disorder in 2.1% of patients. Considering each comorbidity in the LSD subgroup, ADHD, anxiety and mood disorders comorbidity are more frequent with a statistically significant difference.

Two of the more common comorbid conditions in childhood are RD and ADHD (especially ADD) (Hendren et al. 2018; Margari et al. 2013; Sahoo et al. 2015; Sexton et al. 2012). ADHD per se is highly associated with psychiatric problems, emotional discomfort, behavioural problems (Spencer et al. 2007; Masi et al. 2020) (see Table 15.6).

The psychological and medical literature describes LD, as well as ADHD, as an important risk factor for current and future social-emotional or behavioural problems. As a result, children with RD who have comorbid ADHD, experience more depressive and anxious symptomatology

Table 15.6 ADHD and possible associated problems and disabilities (Based on Hendren et al. (2018), Margari et al. (2013), Sahoo et al. (2015), Sexton et al. (2012), Spencer et al. (2007), Masi et al. (2020))

Psychiatric	Medical	Developmental
Oppositional defiant disorder ODD	Obesity	Specific learning disorder/dyslexia
Conduct disorder CD	Sleep disorder	Developmental coordination disorder
Depression	Brain injury	Communication disorders
Disruptive mood dysregulation disorder (DMDD)	Epilepsy	
Addiction	Enuresis	
Addictive behaviour	Allergies	
Anxiety disorder		
Post-traumatic stress disorder		
Obsessive compulsive disorder (OCD)		
Tics		
Autistic spectrum disorder (ASD)		
Bulimia nervosa and binge eating disorder		
Borderline personality disorder		
Antisocial personality disorder		

than children without a comorbid condition (Mugnaini et al. 2009).

The presence of comorbid features complicates the clinical picture essential for working with children with ADHD, so that it can be challenging to identify and treat them. The prognostic and treatment effects of children with comorbid ADHD is worse than children with only ADHD (Masi and Gignac 2015). Close cooperation is needed between the phoniatrician and the child and adolescent psychiatrist to provide potential clinical benefits for children with LD and ADHD.

It is noteworthy that the incidence or occurrence of the specific comorbid disorders of ADHD change over a life span (Masi and Gignac 2015; Banaschewski et al. 2018). ODD, enuresis and language disorders are the most common comorbidities in early childhood. Middle-school age is characterised by anxiety and tics. Mood disorders, personality problems, substance-use disorders are usually observed at the beginning of adolescence. In children with developmental disorders ADHD is three times more common than in healthy ones. Moreover, comparison of Tables 15.3 and 15.5 shows that people with ADHD and RD share similar diseases and disabilities.

To ensure guideline-based treatment and diagnosis, children with ADHD or dyslexia should be presented to a child and adolescent psychiatrist. It is important to determine whether a child presents with comorbidity of dyslexia and ADHD, or presents with ADHD and has a secondary difficulty in reading because of inattention.

15.5.5 Treatment Comorbidity of LD and ADHD

The very frequent comorbidity of dyslexia and ADHD puts the child at high risk of psychopathology (Mugnaini and Fabiano 2006). There are some significant questions to be answered regarding comorbidity:

- Are reading interventions, which are known to be effective for children with pure disorders, as effective for those with comorbid disorders (Hendren et al. 2018; Sexton et al. 2012)?
- Should children with comorbid disorders receive one intervention for both disorders (complex therapy) or two different interventions?
- If two different therapies are chosen, should they be recommended in parallel or sequentially, and if the latter which should be the first?
- Are transfer effects possible?
- Does intervention with treatment for ADHD have a synergistic effect on reading outcomes (making the intervention more effective)?

A growing number of research articles indicate that a treatment programme for children with comorbid conditions should address the full range of problems (Galuschka and Schulte-Körne 2016). For example, when a child not also only shows the features of LD but also meets the diagnostic criteria for ADHD/ADD, treatment should focus on all the problems associated with each of these areas. Recent reports appear to confirm that when comorbid literacy and emotional/behavioural problems are detected, effective treatments in one domain will not necessarily result in improvements in the other; as a consequence, each disorder needs separate treatment (Maughan and Carroll 2006; Moll et al. 2020).Moll et al. (2020) examined several theories and came to the conclusion that:

> The treatment for attention and the intervention for reading had largely independent effects on attention and on aspects of reading fluency. On reading comprehension, the effects were however interestingly different in that the attention treatment had a more positive effective than reading intervention. On reading comprehension, the effects were however interestingly different in that the attention treatment had a more positive effective than reading intervention.

Children and adolescents with LD or dyslexia have higher rates of ADHD diagnoses, and both disabilities are frequently associated with psychological and emotional problems: anxiety disorders, social phobias, depression, low self-esteem (Hendren et al. 2018). Moreover, comorbid psychiatric diseases such as depression, disruptive, impulse-control, conduct and autism spectrum disorders, have been described in the literature as highly connected with both RD and ADHD. The increased psychiatric morbidity and functional impairment of children and adolescents with RD/ADHD highlight the importance of developing psychiatric care. The treatment of ADHD in children should be planned according to a multimodal comprehensive therapeutic concept, which includes psychosocial, psychotherapeutic and pharmacological interventions. The basis is a comprehensive psycho-education. Children below 6 years should primarily receive psychosocial/psycho-therapeutic interventions.

Pharmacological interventions should not be used below an age of 3 years. In mild cases psychosocial/psycho-therapeutic interventions should be the first choice. In severe cases pharmacotherapy should be offered. Pharmacotherapy and psychotherapy are often combined (Banaschewski et al. 2018). Various stimulants are used in the treatment of ADHD, which inhibit the re-uptake of dopamine and norepinephrine in the pre-synapse by blocking dopamine transporters. Comorbid disorders should be treated in line with the existing medical guidelines. The severity of the respective disease determines the priority of treatment. If pharmacotherapy or psychosocial/psycho-therapeutic interventions are effective in treating the core ADHD symptoms, it should be evaluated together with the patient or the parents if comorbid symptoms are ongoing (e.g. aggressive behaviour, anxiety, LD). These accompanying difficulties should be addressed in an individual treatment plan. Children with ADHD and the coexisting problems often benefit from behavioural therapy, social skill training, parent skill training and counselling, family therapy. The best results occur when a team approach is used, so treatment should be multi-disciplinary in nature, extensive and complex. Multidisciplinary medical cooperation is needed as well.

15.5.6 Conclusion

There is a high risk of comorbidity in learning-disabled children. Comorbidity is the rule not the exception (Kaplan et al. 2001; Ijeoma and Chinelo 2019). ADHD is also a highly comorbid disorder and it is the most frequent psychiatric disorder associated with dyslexia. It is worth noting that RD are mainly related to the inattentive type of ADHD rather than hyperactivity or impulsivity. Despite a strong association between RD and ADD, their co-occurrence is often under-recognised and under-treated. As a result:

- Comorbid mental and associated emotional problems may be inadequately integrated into intervention plans (Reale et al. 2017).
- Assessment and intervention for RD may be delayed in or absent from children with frequently co-occurring ADHD/ADD not fully responding to treatment (Serrallach et al. 2016).

The comorbidity of developmental dyslexia with both internalising and externalising disorders, as well as with other learning disabilities, underscores the need for complex medical, cognitive and behavioural approaches in the remediation programmes offered to dyslexic children. The phoniatrician can be an important member of the team that helps a child with RD and ADHD to maximise his or her potential and succeed in school and at home. However, a close cooperation with child and adolescent psychiatrists is needed. The final diagnosis of ADD/ADHD should always be confirmed by a child and adolescent psychiatrist who can rule out other medical problems and offer appropriate treatment and medical long-term care.

The very frequent comorbidity between dyslexia and ADHD leads to a high risk of psychopathology. As a result, effective treatment for children with LD and a comorbid ADHD/ADD needs specialist psychiatric care. Early diagnosis and intervention in children with LD/RD make a substantial improvement in self-confidence and social competence, which helps them in school and at further work.

Effective networking between mental health professionals, paediatricians, community-based health services and professionals from the education sector is essential in medical care of children with comorbid disorders.

15.6 Prognosis of Developmental Literacy Disorders

Mirela Duranović and Rudolf Reiter

15.6.1 Introduction

Dyslexia is a neurodevelopmental disorder with a probable genetic origin. The core difficulty in dyslexia is with word decoding, which in turn affects reading and spelling performance. Dyslexia is persistent *through* the lifespan (Snowling 2013) and does not resolve over time. Reading scores in children with dyslexia improve as they get older, but they are still below those of *normally achieving* readers (Shaywitz 2003). Although some young persons with dyslexia enter higher education, others leave school with minimum qualifications. Dyslexia in adults is manifested by slow reading, problems of spelling and difficulties with written expression. Working memory, attention and organisation can also be affected (Snowling 2013).

Dyslexia does not pose a temporary phenomenon at a certain childhood age but is a disturbance that influences the entire development and that persists into adulthood (Schulte-Körne 2004; Schleider 2009; Shaywitz et al. 1999; Vizzi et al. 2024). In some cases, deficits can be compensated for by a variety of strategies and a lot of practice, but in other cases, such compensatory strategies are *not sufficient* to remediate a *dyslexic's* difficulties. Dyslexia is not always detected and diagnosed; people with dyslexia need excessive hours of work in order to achieve what is easy for others, sometimes without realising why it is so hard for them (Lopez-Escribano et al. 2018).

There are mixed messages about dyslexia. While dyslexia has been associated with significant creative and artistic talents, some dyslexics may note that their academic opportunities are limited because of negative learning experiences (Bacon and Bennet 2012). Individuals with learning disabilities are three times more likely to drop out of school than the average student, 18.1% versus 6.5% (NCLD 2020). A higher unemployment rate (up to 26%) can be found which corresponds to 6–7 times higher than people without dyslexia (Esser and Wyschkon 2002; Schleider 2009). Adults with dyslexia encountered a wide range of challenges, such as mental exhaustian, discrimination, restricted access to support, and fatigue, which left them susceptible to job burnout (Wissell et al. 2022).

Hughes and Dawson (1995) observed that dyslexic adults often experience failure in school, which leads to *negative feelings* of low *self-esteem* and a belief that they are less worthy than others. This perception of low personal intelligence can affect various aspects of their lives, including social functioning and employment prospects. Even if dyslexics gain access to higher education, difficulties related to dyslexia can lead to problems with study skills such as learning from lectures, note taking, producing coursework and examination answers, and practicalities such as using the library or mastering keyboard skills (Mortimore and Crozier 2006).

15.6.2 Early Identification and Intervention of Dyslexia

Scientific research on dyslexia has made significant advances during the past 50 years, and there is a great deal of information on it: its nature, aetiology and assessment. It should be possible for educators now to recognise the signs, suggesting that a child is at risk of reading failure. Such early identification should allow interventions to be implemented before negative consequences of dyslexia can develop. To choose an effective programme or approach, professionals need to have an understanding of the principles of interventions and their suitability for different children (Snowling 2013). Identifying students with learning disabilities, such as dyslexia, at an early stage is essential for delivering timely support and helping them overcome challenges with reading (Daniel et al. 2024). There is strong evidence that intensive reading interventions are most effective in pre-school, kindergarten and first grade (Ozernov-Palchik and Gaab 2016; Ozernov-Palchik et al. 2016); therefore, early identification is crucial. Research has shown that children, who receive reading intervention early, in the first and second grades, make gains in foundational word reading skills relative to controls, almost twice those of children receiving intervention in the third grade (Lovett et al. 2017).

Unfortunately, teacher training institutions have largely been inadequate in preparing teachers to deliver research-based, effective reading instruction (Spear-Swerling et al. 2005). Information about dyslexia and its early identification is also lacking in most teacher training programmes. To teach students effectively, teachers need in-depth knowledge about the structure of language, including phonology, orthography, morphology, semantics and syntax. Similarly, to teach written expression effectively, teachers need a knowledge base about language structure, including sentence and discourse structure (IDA 2010). Pre-service teachers and teachers do not get enough information about basic language concepts and other components connected to reading instruction, which results in a lack of explicit knowledge of such concepts (Duranovic et al. 2014a; Washburn et al. 2010). In a study conducted by Duranovic et al. (2011), teachers expressed low self-esteem in supporting dyslexic children, which indicates a need for more training to be given to teachers about dyslexia.

Given that poor literacy has potential harmful consequences resulting in social inequality, it is crucial that the risk of reading failure is detected and improved as much and as early as possible. It is desirable for the risk of reading failure to be detected in pre-school, and possibly prevented before reading instruction (Protopapas 2019). The nature of the remedial educational intervention is crucial for efficient outcomes in children with dyslexia. The use of an intensive evidence-based reading intervention is important for development of the neural systems that underlie skilled reading. This intervention brings about significant and durable changes in brain organisation, so that brain activation patterns resemble those of typical readers (Shaywitz et al. 2004). The results of a study using fMRI to examine children who were struggling to read and learn, and who then received a year-long experimental reading programme, showed that not only were the right-sided auxiliary pathways much less prominent than before treatment, but that there was further development of the primary neural system on the left side of the brain. These activation patterns were comparable to these obtained from children who had always been good readers. This explains why children who receive effective early intervention develop into both accurate and fluent readers (Shaywitz 2003). Any sign of problems in learning to read, even very early, should be taken seriously. Early identification and early intervention can prevent most serious reading difficulties, or at least reduce the severity of them (Siegel 2006).

15.6.3 Dyslexic Adults in Higher Education

The number of students with dyslexia entering higher education has increased recently (Duranovic et al. 2014b), most likely owing to better assessment, guidance and remediation in primary and secondary education (Hadjikakou and Hartas 2008; Madriaga et al. 2010). In the United Kingdom in 2000, such students accounted for 1.2% of the student body; in 2016, they represented 5% of all students (Higher Education Statistical Agency HESA Free Online DATA Table, 2017). In the USA, students with disabilities represented nearly an estimated 11% of all postsecondary students in 2008, of whom less than 10% had specific learning disabilities (SpLDs) according to the National Postsecondary Student Aid Study (HESA 2017). Two longitudinal studies reviewed by the US Government Accountability Office estimated that students with SpLDs constituted 70% of the population of disabled students in higher education institutions (GAO 2009). Duranovic (2013) found that 4.4% of students were suspected of having dyslexia at different universities in Bosnia and Herzegovina.

Arguments about the progression of dyslexic students at university are mixed. Whereas some researchers have provided evidence that dyslexic students are more likely than non-dyslexics to withdraw from their studies during the first year and are less likely to complete their programmes of study (Richardson and Wydell 2003; Stampoltzis and Polychronopoulou 2008), others have shown that dyslexic students are just as likely to pass their first and second year exams and to progress through their studies as are non-dyslexic students (McKendree and Snowling 2011). Richardson and Wydell (2003) highlighted the importance of appropriate support, which can lead to completion rates of students with dyslexia matching those of students with no disabilities.

The chances of graduating with either a first class or an upper second-class degree for students with dyslexia are lower than those of non-dyslexic students, which again highlight the need for good, evidence-based support for students with dyslexia, to enable final degree results to be equivalent to those of non-dyslexic students (Brunswick 2012). Higher education lecturers must have adequate knowledge about dyslexia, in order to ensure the efficacy and quality of their pedagogic practices, as well as to allow them to engage fully with legislative and institutional policies aimed at securing fair and equal access to higher education for all students (Ryder and Norwich 2018). Universities ought to enhance support for their teaching staff by offering guidance and practical training, enabling their courses to be more inclusive and accessible to all students, including those with dyslexia (Cernickaja and Sokolova 2024).

15.6.4 Talents Among People with Dyslexia

The major focus of research on dyslexia has been orientated towards pathology. Researchers have been trying to find out what is ‘wrong’ with persons with dyslexia, exploring difficulties and trying to find resources of remediation (West 2005). However, there is also a view that persons with dyslexia are talented in visual-spatial areas (West 1997, 2005; Winner et al. 2001) and that dyslexia is not only associated with a deficit. An association between dyslexia and creative abilities has long been documented, suggesting that several eminent artists may have experienced difficulties associated with dyslexia (Chakravarty 2009). There are stories about famous people such as Winston Churchill, Albert Einstein, Thomas Edison and Leonardo de Vinci all having had great difficulties with linguistic skills, but who also had other talents and skills, enabling them to contribute a great deal to the world (Stowe 2000).

Geschwind and Galaburda (1987) found a high proportion of persons with dyslexia in professions such as engineering, art and architecture. Wolff and Lundberg (2002) noted more common symptoms and signs of dyslexia in students who studied at an art academy than in those at non-art universities; they found that 4% of art students were dyslexic as opposed to only 1.5% among non-art students. Studying and practising art had helped them to facilitate the development of a positive personal identity as an artist with dyslexia (Bacon and Bennet 2012). Therefore, dyslexia may often be present in careers that require high visual-spatial talents (Winner et al. 1991).

However, proof of the connection of visual-spatial talents with dyslexia is far from conclusive. A higher prevalence of dyslexia among those in spatial fields does not necessary mean that dyslexia is associated with visual-spatial strength (von Karolyi and Winner 2005). Research results have been inconsistent with respect to whether dyslexic visual-spatial abilities should be superior or inferior than those of non-dyslexics. Some results suggest relative strengths in visual-spatial areas, while others indicate spatial skills that are neither inferior nor superior to the rest of the population (Duranovic et al. 2015). Children with dyslexia exhibit notable strenghts and potential advantages in nonverbal creativity (Lam and Tong 2021), outperforming the control group in creativity and teamwork skills (Stampoltzis et al. 2023).

Linking dyslexia to talent gives a more optimistic direction than connecting dyslexia only with deficits. Talent discovery in people with dyslexia opens the door to more effective educational strategies and career choices in which they can be successful (von Karolyi et al. 2003). It is important to analyse visual thinking and creativity in persons with dyslexia better, to see their strengths and to detect how they can benefit from a new view of what we have long recognised mostly as a problem (West 2005).

References

Achenbach TM (1991) Integrative guide for the 1991 CBCL (4c18), YSR, and TRF profiles. University of Vermont, Department of Psychiatry, Burlington, VT

Achenbach TM (1998) Young adult self-report for the child behavior checklist. University of Vermont, Department of Psychiatry, Burlington, VT

Akyurek G, Bumin G (2018) Home literacy environment and occupational routines in children with dyslexia. Bozok Med J 8(3):16–23. [Turkish]

Alahmadi NA (2017) Cognitive control in children with learning disabilities: neuromarker for deficient executive function. Neuroreport 28:638–644

Alain C, Zendel BR, Hutka S et al (2014) Turning down the noise: the benefit of musical training on the aging auditory brain. Hear Res 308:162–173

Alloway TP, Alloway RG (2013) Working memory in the lifespan: a cross-sectional approach. J Cogn Psychol 25:84–93

Altıok S, Başer Z, Yükseltürk E (2019) Enhancing metacognitive awareness of undergraduates through using an e-educational video environment. Comput Educ 139(1):129–145

American Speech-Language-Hearing Association ASHA (2018) LSHSS clinical forum: what SLPs need to know about dyslexia. Guest post by Hogan T Available via https://academy.pubs.asha.org/2018/10/lshss-clinical-forum-what-slps-need-to-know-about-dyslexia/ Accessed 4 Oct 2021

Andrews JE, Lombardino LJ (2014) Strategies for teaching handwriting to children with writing disabilities. Perspect Lang Learn Educ 21:114–126

Anguera JA, Boccanfuso J, Rintoul JL et al (2013) Video game training enhances cognitive control in older adults. Nature 501(7465):97–101. https://doi.org/10.1038/nature12486

Arfé B, Corato F, Pizzocaro E et al (2020) The effects of script and orthographic complexity on the handwriting and spelling performance of children with dyslexia. J Learn Disabil 53(2):96–108

Armaou M, Konstantinidis S, Blake H (2020) The effectiveness of digital interventions for psychological Well-being in the workplace: a systematic review protocol. Int J Environ Res Public Health 17(1):255. https://doi.org/10.3390/ijerph17010255

Aro T, Viholainen H, Koponen T et al (2018) Can reading fluency and self-efficacy of reading fluency be enhanced with an intervention targeting the sources of self-efficacy? Learn Individ Differ 67(1):53–66

Bäcker A, Neuhäuser G (2003) Internalisierende und externalisierende Syndrome bei Lese- und Rechtschreibstörungen [Internalizing and externalizing syndrome in reading and writing disorders]. Prax Kinderpsychol Kinderpsychiatr 52(5):329–337

Bacon AM, Bennet S (2012) Dyslexia in higher education: the decision to study art. Eur J Spec Needs Educ 28(1):19–32

Baddeley A (2017) The concept of working memory: a view of its current state and probable future development. In: Baddeley A (ed) Exploring working memory: selected works of Alan Baddeley. Routledge/Taylor & Francis, Abingdon-on-Thames UK, pp 99–106

Baldo JV, Dronkers NF (2006) The role of inferior parietal and inferior frontal cortex in working memory. Neuropsychology 20(5):529–538

Banaschewski T, Hohmann S, Millenet S (2018) Attention-deficit/hyperactivity disorder (ADHD) in children, adolescents and adults. https://www.awmf.org/leitlinien/detail/ll/028-045.html

Berninger VW (2015) Interdisciplinary frameworks for schools: best professional practices for serving the needs of all students. American Psychological Association, Washington, DC

Birsh JR (2018) Connecting research and practice. In: Birsh JR (ed) Multisensory teaching of basic language skills, 4th edn. Paul H. Brookes Publishing, Baltimore, MD, pp 21–34

Black J (2016) Orthographic processing: a subcomponent or subtype of dyslexia? Address given at the Cullowhee Conference, Dallas, Texas, April 2016

Booth JN, Boyle JM, Kelly SW (2010) Do tasks make a difference? Accounting for heterogeneity of performance of children with reading difficulties on tasks of executive function: findings from a meta-analysis. Br J Dev Psychol 28:133–176

Borre AJ, Bernhard J, Bleiker C et al (2019) Preschool literacy intervention for low-income, ethnically diverse children: effects of the early authors program through kindergarten. J Educ Stud Placed Risk 24(2):132–153

Boudah DJ (2018) Evaluation of intensive reading strategies intervention for low performing adolescents with and without learning disabilities. Ins Learn Disabil 15(2):195–205

Boyes M, Leitao S, Claessen M et al (2016) Why are reading difficulties associated with mental health problems?: reading difficulties and child mental health. Dyslexia 22:263–266

Bridgett DJ, Oddi KB, Laake LM et al (2013) Integrating and differentiating aspects of self-regulation: effortful control, executive functioning, and links to negative affectivity. Emotion 13(1):47–63

Brimo K, Dinkler L, Gillberg C et al (2021) The co-occurrence of neurodevelopmental problems in dyslexia. Dyslexia 27(3):277–293

British Society of Audiology (2011) An overview of current management of auditory processing disorder. http://www.thebsa.org.uk/wp-content/uploads/2014/04/BSA_APD_Management_1Aug11_FINAL_amended17Oct11.pdf. Accessed 29 Dec 2015

British Society of Audiology APD SIG (2018) Practical Guidance: An overview of current management of auditory processing disorder. www.thebsa.org.uk/wp-content/uploads/2018/02/Position-Statement-and-Practice-Guidance-APD-2018-1.pdf. Accessed 12 Jul 2018

Brunswick N (2012) Dyslexia in UK higher education and employment: an introduction and overview. In: Brunswick N (ed) Supporting dyslexic adults in higher education and the workplace. Wiley-Blackwell, London

Brunswick N, Bargary S (2022) Self-concept, creativity and developmental dyslexia in university students: Effects of age of assessment. Dyslexia 28(3):293–308. https://doi.org/10.1002/dys.1722. Epub 2022 Jul 11. PMID: 35818173; PMCID: PMC9543102

Bucci MP (2019) Visual training could be useful for improving reading capabilities in dyslexia. Appl Neuropsychol Child 13:1–10

Burns MK, Petersen-Brown S, Haegele K et al (2016) Meta-analysis of academic interventions derived from neuropsychological data. Sch Psychol Q 31:28–42

Butterfuss R, Kendeou P (2018) The role of executive functions in reading comprehension. Educ Psychol Rev 30(3):801–826

Buzan T, Buzan B (2007) The mind map book. BBC Books, Edinburgh

Campbell NG, Grant P, Rosen S, Moore DR (2019) Auditory processing disorder in children, BATOD Foundation. Available at: http://www.meshguides.org/guides/node/1432

Cantor P, Osher D, Berg J et al (2018) Malleability, plasticity, and individuality: how children learn and develop in context. Appl Dev Sci 23(4):1–31

Carawan LW, Nalavany BA, Jenkins C (2016) Emotional experience with dyslexia and self-esteem: the protective role of perceived family suport in late adulthood. Aging Ment Health 20(3):284–294. https://doi.org/10.1080/13607863.2015.1008984. Epub 2015 Feb 9. PMID: 25660279

Carotenuto M, Esposito M, Cortese S et al (2016) Children with developmental dyslexia showed greater sleep disturbances than controls, including problems initiating and maintaining sleep. Acta Paediatr 105:1079–1082

Cartwright KB (2015) Executive function and reading comprehension: the critical role of cognitive flexibility. In: Parris SR, Headley K (eds) Comprehension instruction: research-based best practices, 3rd edn. Guilford Press, New York, NY, pp 56–71

Cartwright KB, Marshall TR, Huemer CM et al (2019) Executive function in the classroom: cognitive flexibility supports reading fluency for typical readers and teacher-identified low-achieving readers. Res Dev Disabil 88:42–52

Cederlof M, Maughan B, Larsson H et al (2017) Reading problems and major mental disorders - co-occurrences and familial overlaps in a Swedish nation-wide cohort. J Psychiatr Res 91:124–129

Černickaja K, Sokolova L (2024) Dyslexia in higher education – teacher's perspective: scoping review. Front Educ 9:1372699

Chakravarty A (2009) Artistic talent in dyslexia—a hypothesis. Med Hypotheses 73(4):569–571

Chermak GD, Musiek FE (2013) Handbook of central auditory processing disorder, comprehensive intervention, vol 2, 2nd edn. San Diego, CA, Plural

Cirino PT, Miciak J, Gerst E et al (2017) Executive function, self-regulated learning, and reading comprehension: a training study. J Learn Disabil 50:450–467

Cirino PT, Ahmed Y, Miciak J et al (2018) A framework for executive function in the late elementary years. Neuropsychology 32(2):176–189

Ciulkinyte A, Mountford HS, Fontanillas P et al (2024) Genetic neurodevelopmental clustering and dyslexia. Mol Psychiatry Advance Online Publication. https://doi.org/10.1038/s41380-024-02649-8

Clarke A, Weadman T, Galioto A et al (2016) Controversial dyslexia therapies [web log post]. Available via https://www.spelfabet.com.au/about-spelfabet/ Accessed 11 Oct 2021

Costantini A, Demerouti E, Ceschi A et al (2019) Evidence on the hierarchical, multidimensional nature of behavioural job crafting. Appl Psychol 70(1):311–341

Couto JM, Gomez L, Wigg K et al (2008) The KIAA0319-like (KIAA0319L) gene on chromosome 1p34 as a candidate for reading disabilities. J Neurogenet 22(4):295–313

Curhan SG, Eavey R, Wang M et al (2013) Body mass index, waist circumference, physical activity, and risk of hearing loss in women. Am J Med 126(12):1142.e1141–1142.e1148. https://doi.org/10.1016/j.amjmed.2013.04.026

Le Cunff AL, Dommett E, Giampietro V (2024) Neurophysiological measures and correlates of cognitive load in attention-deficit/hyperactivity disorder (ADHD), autism spectrum disorder (ASD) and dyslexia: A scoping review and research recommendations. Eur J Neurosci 59(2):256–282. https://doi.org/10.1111/ejn.16201. Epub 2023 Dec 18

D'Souza H, Karmiloff-Smith A (2017) Neurodevelopmental disorders. Wiley Interdiscip Rev Cogn Sci 8:1–10

Daniel J, Clucas L, Wang HH (2024) Identifying students with dyslexia: exploration of current assessment methods. Ann Dyslexia. https://doi.org/10.1007/s11881-024-00313-y. Epub ahead of print. PMID: 39198310

Danielsson H, Lucy H, Rönnberg J et al (2010) Executive functions in individuals with intellectual disability. Res Dev Disabil 31(6):1299–1304

Das JP, Misra SB (2015) Cognitive planning and executive functions: applications in management and education. Sage Publications, New Delhi

Dawson P, Guare R (2018) Executive skills in children and adolescents: a practical guide to assessment and intervention, 3rd edn. Guilford Publications, New York

De Jong CGW, Oosterlaan J, Sergeant JA (2006) The role of double dissociation studies in the search for candidate endophenotypes for the comorbidity of attention deficit/hyperactivity disorder and reading disability. Int J Disabil Dev Educ 53(2):177–193

de Lima RF, Azoni CAS, Ciasca SM (2017) Development of a neuropsychological rehabilitation program for executive functions in students with developmental dyslexia. Psychology 8(8):1110–1128

Decker SL, Roberts AM (2015) Specific cognitive predictors of early math problem solving. Psychol Sch 52:477–488

Decker SL, Strait JE, Roberts AM et al (2018) Cognitive mediators of reading comprehension in early development. Contemp Sch Psychol 22(3):249–257

Delavarian M, Afrooz G, Shahriar G (2013) The effect of visual and cerebellar exercises on dyslexia. J Neuropsychiatry Clin Neurosci 25:E31. https://doi.org/10.1176/appi.neuropsych.12020035

DGKJP (2015) Deutsche Gesellschaft für Kinder- und Jugendpsychiatrie, Psychosomatik und Psychotherapie e.V. Diagnostik und Behandlung von Kindern und Jugendlichen mit Lese- und/oder Rechtschreibstörung. Evidenz- und konsensbasierte Leitlinie (S3); AWMF-Registriernummer 028-044

Diakakis P, Gardelis J, Ventouri K et al (2008) Behavioral problems in children with learning difficulties according to their parents and teachers. Pediatrics 121:100–101

Diamond A (2014) Executive functions: insights into ways to help more children thrive. Zero to Three 35(2):9–17

Diamond A, Ling DS (2016) Conclusions about interventions, programs, and approaches for improving executive functions that appear justified and those that, despite much hype, do not. Dev Cogn Neurosci 18:34–48

Doyle C (2017) Executive function (EF) in dyslexia: examining an EF profile associated with dyslexia and comorbid dyslexia–ADHD and exploring the near and far transfer effects of EF training in dyslexia alone. PhD thesis, Dublin City University

Doyle N, McDowall A (2019) Context matters: a review to formulate a conceptual framework for coaching as a disability accommodation. PLoS One 14(8):e0199408

Drechsler R, Brem S, Brandeis D et al (2020) ADHD: current concepts and treatments in children and adolescents. Neuropediatrics 51(5):315–335

Duff FJ, Holme C, Grainger K et al (2014) Reading and language intervention for children at risk of dyslexia: a randomised controlled trial. J Child Psychol Psychiatry 55(11):1234–1243

DuPaul GJ, Gormley MJ, Laracy SD (2013) Comorbidity of LD and ADHD: implications of DSM-5 for assessment and treatment. J Learn Disabil 46(1):43–51

Duranovic M (2013) Supporting dyslexic adults in higher education in Bosnia and Herzegovina. In: Fawcett A, Saunders K (eds) The dyslexia handbook Bracknell. The British Dyslexia Association, Backnell, UK, pp 77–81

Duranovic M, Dedeic M, Huseinbasic M et al (2011) Teachers' attitudes about dyslexia: evidence from Bosnia and Herzegovina and Montenegro. Proceedings of Conference "learning disabilities at school: research and education", Locarno, Switzerland, Department Formation and Learning (DFA)

Duranovic M, Tinjak S, Kacka M (2014a) Teachers' knowledge of basic language concepts related to reading instruction. Bulgarian J Commun Disord 8(8):17–28

Duranovic M, Krco D, Tinjak S (2014b) A validation of the dyslexia adult screening test (DAST) for language with shallow orthography. Cash Sci Nat 23(5):2–24

Duranovic M, Dedeic M, Gavric M (2015) Dyslexia and visual-spatial talents. Curr Psychol 34(2):207–222

Ehri LC (2000) Learning to read and learning to spell: two sides of a coin. Top Lang Disord 20(3):19–36

Esser G, Wyschkon A (2002) Was wird aus Achtjährigen mit einer Lese- und Rechtschreibstörung? Ergebnisse im Alter von 25 Jahren (what happens to eight-year-olds with a reading and spelling disorder? Results at the age of 25). Z Klin Psychol Psychother 31(4):235–242

Everdell IT, Marsh HO, Yurick MD et al (2007) Gaze behaviour in audiovisual speech perception: asymmetrical distribution of face-directed fixations. Perception 36(10):1535–1545

Facoetti A, Lorusso ML, Paganoni P et al (2003) The role of visuospatial attention in developmental dyslexia: evidence from a rehabilitation study. Brain Res Cogn Brain Res 15(2):154–164

Faivre N, Filevich E, Solovey G et al (2018) Behavioral, modeling, and electrophysiological evidence for supramodality in human metacognition. J Neurosci 38:263–277

Faraone SV, Larsson H (2019) Genetics of attention deficit hyperactivity disorder. Mol Psychiatry 24(4):562–575

Fawcett L (2019) Cracking the ABC code. Available via http://crackingtheabccode.com/ Accessed on 9 Oct 2021

Ferguson MA, Henshaw H, Clark DP et al (2014) Benefits of phoneme discrimination training in a randomized controlled trial of 50- to 74-year-olds with mild hearing loss. Ear Hear 35(4):e110–e121. https://doi.org/10.1097/aud.0000000000000020

Fisher SE, DeFries JC (2002) Developmental dyslexia: genetic dissection of a complex cognitive trait. Nat Rev Neurosci 3(10):767–780

Fletcher JM, Miciak J (2017) Comprehensive cognitive assessments are not necessary for the identification and treatment of learning disabilities. Arch Clin Neuropsychol 32:2–7

Fletcher JM, Lyon GR, Fuchs LS et al (2018) Learning disabilities: from identification to intervention, 2nd edn. Guilford Press, New York, NY

Friedman NP, Miyake A (2017) Unity and diversity of executive functions: individual differences as a window on cognitive structure. Cortex 86:186–204

Fuchs D, Fuchs LS, Vaughn S (2014) What is intensive instruction and why is it important? Teach Except Child 46:13–18

Fuchs LS, Fuchs D, Malone AS (2017) The taxonomy of intervention intensity. Teach Except Child 50(1): 35–43

Galuschka K, Schulte-Körne G (2016) The diagnosis and treatment of reading and/or spelling disorders in children and adolescents. Dtsch Arztebl Int 113(16):279–286

Galuschka K, Ise E, Krick K et al (2014) Effectiveness of the treatment approaches for children and adolescents with reading disabilities: a meta-analysis of randomized controlled trials. PLoS One 9(2):e89900. https://doi.org/10.1371/journal.pone.0089900

Galuschka K, Görgen R, Kalmar J et al (2020) Effectiveness of spelling interventions for learners with dyslexia: a meta-analysis and systematic review. Educ Psychol 55(1):1–20

GAO (Government Accountability Office) (2009) Higher education and disability. Report to the Chairman, Committee on Education and Labor, House of Representatives. GAO-10-33, 2009. Available via http://www.gao.gov/new.items/d1033.pdf. Accessed November 2013

Ghasemi M, Hassanzadeh S, Shokoohi-Yekta M et al (2016) The effectiveness of central auditory processing rehabilitation program on speech reception in noise and dichotic listening in dyslexic students. Audit Vestib Res 25(3):183–193

Georgiou GK, Das JP (2018) Direct and indirect effects of executive function on reading comprehension in young adults. J Res Read 41(2):243–258

Germanò E, Gagliano A, Curatolo P (2010) Comorbidity of ADHD and dyslexia. Dev Neuropsychol 35(5):475–493

Geschwind N, Galaburda A (1987) Cerebral lateralisation. MIT Press, Cambridge

Gialluisi A, Andlauer TFM, Mirza-Schreiber N et al (2019) Genome-wide association scan identifies new variants associated with a cognitive predictor of dyslexia. Transl. Psychiatry 9(1):77. https://doi.org/10.1038/s41398-019-0402-0

Gialluisi A, Andlauer TFM, Mirza-Schreiber N et al (2020) Genome-wide association study reveals new insights into the heritability and genetic correlates of developmental dyslexia. Mol Psychiatry 26:3004. https://doi.org/10.1038/s41380-020-00898-x

Gnanavel S, Sharma P, Kaushal P et al (2019) Attention deficit hyperactivity disorder and comorbidity: a review of literature. World J Clin Cases 7(17):2420–2426

Goldstein S, Naglieri J (eds) (2015) Executive functioning handbook. Springer, New York, NY

Gordon HJ, Demerouti E, Le Blanc PM et al (2018) Individual job redesign: job crafting interventions in healthcare. J Vocat Behav 104:98–114

Gosse C, Van Reybroeck M (2020) Do children with dyslexia present a handwriting deficit? Impact of word orthographic and graphic complexity on handwriting and spelling performance. Res Dev Disabil 97:103553. https://doi.org/10.1016/j.ridd.2019.103553

Gouléme N, Gérard C-L, Bucci MP (2015) The effect of training on postural control in dyslexic children. PLoS One 10(7):e0130196

Graham S (2018) A writer(s) within community model of writing. In: Bazerman C, Berninger V, Brandt D et al (eds) The lifespan development of writing. National Council of English, Urbana, IL, pp 271–325

Grimm T, Garshasbi M, Puettmann L et al (2020) A novel locus and candidate gene for familial developmental dyslexia on chromosome 4q. Z Kinder Jugendpsychiatr Psychother 48(6):478–489

Hadjikakou K, Hartas D (2008) Higher education provision for students with disabilities in Cyprus. High Educ 55:103–119

Häfner A, Stock A, Oberst V (2015) Decreasing students' stress through time management training: an intervention study. Eur J Psychol Educ 30:81–94

Haft SL, Meyers CA, Hoeft F (2016) Socio-emotional and cognitive resilience in children with reading disabilities. Curr Opin Behav Sci 10:133–141

Hakim A, Ghorbani BA (2015) Prevalence of dyslexia among male students in primary schools and its relationship with obesity and being overweight in Ahvaz, Iran. Int J Community Based Nurs Midwifery 3:116–122

Halliday LF (2014) A tale of two studies on auditory training in children: a response to the claim that 'discrimination training of phonemic contrasts enhances phonological processing in mainstream school children' by Moore, Rosenberg and Coleman (2005). Dyslexia 20(2):101–118. https://doi.org/10.1002/dys.1470

Halliday LF, Taylor JL, Millward KE et al (2012) Lack of generalization of auditory learning in typically developing children. J Speech Lang Hear Res 55(1):168–181. https://doi.org/10.1044/1092-4388(2011/09-0213)

Hanson J, Sharman LA, Esparza-Brown J (2009) Pattern of strengths and weaknesses in specific learning disabilities: What's it all about? Technical Assistance Paper, Oregon School Psychologists Association

Hartmann E (2014) Möglichkeiten und Effektivität von computerbasierten Interventionen bei kindlichen Lese-Rechtschreibschwierigkeiten (LRS). Schweizerische Zeitschrift für Heilpädagogik 20:1

Hartmann L, Sallard E, Spierer L (2016) Enhancing frontal top-down inhibitory control with Go/NoGo training. Brain Struct Funct 221(7):3835–3842

Hebert M, Bohaty JJ, Nelson JR et al (2018a) Identifying and discriminating expository text structures: an experiment with 4th and 5th grade struggling readers. Read Write 31(9):2115–2145

Hebert M, Bohaty JJ, Nelson JR et al (2018b) Writing informational text using provided information and text structures: an intervention for upper elementary struggling writers. Read Write 31(9):2165–2190

Hebert M, Kearns DM, Hayes JB et al (2018c) Why children with dyslexia struggle with writing and how to help them. Lang Speech Hear Serv Sch 49(4):843–863

Helmstaedter C, Durch P, Hoppe C et al (2019) Is the computerized assessment of psychomotor speed more sensitive to cognitive effects of antiepileptic pharmacotherapy than tests with a focus on higher-order cognitive processing? Implications for the choice of sensitive test parameters. Eur Neuropsychopharmacol 29(11):1273–1281

Hendren RL, Haft SL, Black JM et al (2018) Recognizing psychiatric comorbidity with reading disorders. Front Psych 9:101. https://doi.org/10.3389/fpsyt.2018.00101

HESA (Higher Education Statistical Agency) (2017) 'Free online data table.' Available via https://www.hesa.ac.uk/data-and-analysis. Accessed 12 Aug 2017

Hillman CH (2014) I. An introduction to the relation of physical activity to cognitive and brain health, and scholastic achievement. Monogr Soc Res Child Dev 79(4):1–6. https://doi.org/10.1111/mono.12127

Hillman CH, Erickson KI, Kramer AF (2008) Be smart, exercise your heart: exercise effects on brain and cognition. Nat Rev Neurosci 9(1):58–65. https://doi.org/10.1038/nrn2298

Hogan TP (2018) What speech-language pathologists need to know about dyslexia. Lang Speech Hear Serv Sch 49(4):759–761

Holmes J, Gathercole SE (2013) Taking working memory training from the laboratory into schools. Educ Psychol 34:440–450

Hongyao HE, Chun JI, Xiaoyan G et al (2023) Associative gene networks reveal novel candidates important for ADHD and dyslexia comorbidity. BMC Med Genomics 16(1):208. https://doi.org/10.1186/s12920-023-01502-1. PMID: 37667328; PMCID: PMC10478365

Hoogman M, Bralten J, Hibar DP et al (2017) Subcortical brain volume differences in participants with attention deficit hyperactivity disorder in children and adults: a cross-sectional mega-analysis. Lancet Psychiatry 4(4):310–319

Horbach J, Mayer A, Scharke W et al. (2020) Comorbidities between Reading Disorders and other Developmental Disorders. Sci Stud Read 24(1):57–71. Published online: 15 Jul 2019; https://doi.org/10.1080/10888438.2019.1641504

Hornickel J, Zecker SG, Bradlow AR et al (2012) Assistive listening devices drive neuroplasticity in children with dyslexia. Proc Natl Acad Sci USA 109(41):16731–16736. https://doi.org/10.1073/pnas.1206628109

Horowitz-Kraus T (2015) Differential effect of cognitive training on executive functions and reading abilities in children with ADHD and in children with ADHD comorbid with reading difficulties. J Atten Disord 19(6):515–526

Huc-Chabrolle M, Barthez MA, Tripi G et al (2010) Psychocognitive and psychiatric disorders associated with developmental dyslexia: a clinical and scientific issue. Encéphale 36(2):172–179

Huemer SM, Pointner A, Schöfl M et al (2019) Evidenzbasierte LRS-Förderung. Bundesministerium für Bildung, Wissenschaft und Forschung Österreich, Wien doi: https://doi.org/10.13140/RG.2.2.19181.33767

Hughes W, Dawson R (1995) Memories of school: adult dyslexics recall their school days. Support Learn 10(4):181–184

Hwang H (2019) The role of science domain knowledge and reading motivation in predicting informational and narrative reading comprehension in L1 and L2: an international study. Learn Individ Differ 76(1):1–11

IDA (International Dyslexia Association) (2010) Professional standards and practices committee. Knowledge and practice standards for teachers of reading. International Dyslexia Association, Baltimore MD

Idler AM, Mercer SH, Starosta L et al (2017) Effects of a mindful breathing exercise during reading fluency intervention for students with attentional difficulties. Contemp Sch Psychol 21(4):323–334

Ijeoma AJ, Chinelo U (2019) Dyslexia, neurodevelopmental conditions and comobidity: a rule rather than an exception. Arch Neurol Neurosci 4(2):1–5

Jacobson LA, Koriakin T, Lipkin P et al (2017) Executive functions contribute uniquely to reading competence in minority youth. J Learn Disabil 50(4):422–433

Jaeggi SM, Buschkuehl M, Shah P et al (2014) The role of individual differences in cognitive training and transfer. Mem Cogn 42(3):464–480

Jolly Learning (2014) Jolly phonics. Available via https://www.jollylearning.co.uk/jolly-phonics/, Accessed 9 October 2021

Kaplan BJ, Dewey DM, Crawford SG et al (2001) The term comorbidity is of questionable value in reference to development disorder: data and theory. J Learn Disabil 34(6):555–565

Karbach J, Strobach T, Schubert T (2015) Adaptive working-memory training benefits reading, but not mathematics in middle childhood. Child Neuropsychol 21(3):285–301

Karten T (2015) In: Robb L (ed) Inclusion strategies that work! Scholastic Inc., Corwin, CA

Kast M, Baschera GM, Gross M et al (2011) Computer-based learning of spelling skills in children with and without dyslexia. Ann Dyslexia 61(2):177–200

Kilpatrick D, Kaufman A, Nadeen L (2015) Essentials of assessing, preventing, and overcoming reading difficulties. In: Kaufman A, Nadeen L (eds) . John Wiley & Sons, Inc., Hoboken, NJ

Kintsch W (2019) Revisiting the construction-integration model of text comprehension and its implications for instruction. In: Alvermann DE, Unrau NY, Ruddell RB (eds) Theoretical models and processes of literacy, 7th edn. Routledge, New York, NY, pp 178–203

Klatte M, Bergstrom K, Lachmann T (2013) Does noise affect learning? A short review on noise effects on cognitive performance in children. Front Psychol 4:578. https://doi.org/10.3389/fpsyg.2013.00578

Kofler M, Spiegel JA, Sot EF et al (2019) Do working memory deficits underlie reading problems in attention-deficit/hyperactivity disorder (ADHD)? J Abnorm Child Psychol 47:433–446

Laasonen M, Salomaa J, Cousineau D et al (2012) Project DyAdd: visual attention in adult dyslexia and ADHD. Brain Cogn 80(3):311–327

Lehongre K, Ramus F, Villiermet N et al (2011) Altered low-γ sampling in auditory cortex accounts for the three main facets of dyslexia. Neuron 72(6):1080–1090

Logue S, Gould T (2014) The neural and genetic basis of executive function: attention, cognitive flexibility, and response inhibition. Pharmacol Biochem Behav 123:45–54

Lam JHY, Tong SX (2021) Drawing a New Picture: Children with Developmental Dyslexia Exhibit Superior Nonverbal Creativity. Res Dev Disbil 116:104036

Loo JHY, Bamiou DE, Campbell N et al (2010) Computer-based auditory training (CBAT): benefits for children with language- and reading-related learning difficulties. Dev Med Child Neurol 52(8):708–717

Lopez-Escribano C, Sanchez JS, Carretero FL (2018) Prevalence of developmental dyslexia in Spanish university students. Brain Sci 8(5):82. https://doi.org/10.3390/brainsci8050082

Lou NM, Noels KA (2019) Promoting growth in foreign and second language education: a research agenda for mindsets in language learning and teaching. System 86(1):143–153

Lovett MW, Frijters JC, Wolf M et al (2017) Early intervention for children at risk for reading disabilities: the impact of grade at intervention and individual differences on intervention outcomes. J Educ Psychol 109(7):889914

Luo Y, Weibman D, Halperin JM et al (2019) A review of heterogeneity in attention deficit/hyperactivity disorder (ADHD). Front Hum Neurosci 13:42. https://doi.org/10.3389/fnhum.2019.00042

Lyon GR, Shaywitz SE, Shaywitz BA (2003) A Definition of Dyslexia. Ann Dyslexia 53:1–14

Maciejewska B, Wiskirska-Woznica B, Swidziński P, Michalak M (2013) Assessing Auditory Processing Disorders in Children with Developmental Dyslexia Using Auditory Cognitive Event-Related Potentials. Folia phoniatr logop 65:129–135. https://doi.org/10.1159/000354167

Madriaga M, Hanson K, Heaton C et al (2010) Confronting similar challenges? Disabled and non-disabled students' learning and assessment experiences. Stud High Educ 35(6):647–658

Margari L, Buttiglione M, Craig F et al (2013) Neuropsychopathological comorbidities in learning disorders. BMC Neurol 13:198. https://doi.org/10.1186/1471-2377-13-198

Masi L, Gignac M (2015) ADHD and comorbid disorders in childhood psychitaric problems, medical problems, leading disorders and developmantal coordination disorder. Clin Psychiatry 1:1–5

Masi G, Fantozzi P, Muratori P (2020) Emotional dysregulation and callous unemotional traits as possible predictors of short-term response to methylphenidate monotherapy in drug-naïve youth with ADHD. Compr Psychiatry 100. https://doi.org/10.1016/j.comppsych.2020.152178

Mason LH, Reid R, Hanagan JL (2012) Building comprehension in adolescents. Paul H Brooks, Baltimore, MD

Mather N, Jaffe LE (2016) Woodcock-Johnson IV: reports, recommendations, and strategies. John Wiley & Sons Inc., Hoboken NJ

Maughan B, Carroll JM (2006) Literacy and mental disorders. Curr Opin Psychiatry 19:350–354

Maynard BR, Solis M, Miller VL et al (2017) Mindfulness-based interventions for improving cognition, academic achievement, behavior, and socioemotional functioning of primary and secondary school students. Campbell Syst Rev 13(1):1–144

McArthur G, Castles A (2017) Helping children with reading difficulties: some things we have learned so far. NPJ Sci Learn 2:7. https://doi.org/10.1038/s41539-017-0008-3

McCarthy H, Skokauskas N, Frodl T (2014) Identifying a consistent pattern of neural function in attention deficit hyperactivity disorder: a meta-analysis. Psychol Med 44(4):869–880

McClelland MM, Cameron CE, Duncan R et al (2014) Predictors of early growth in academic achievement: the head-toes-knees-shoulders task. Front Psychol 5:599. https://doi.org/10.3389/fpsyg.2014.00599

McCloskey G (2016) Interventions for students with executive function difficulties directly related to reading problems" February, New Orleans, LA CDL. Cited in: Instruction and Intervention for Dyslexia and Other Reading ...www.pattan.net › 1. Intervention Development PowerPoint

McGrath LM, Stoodley CJ (2019) Are there shared neural correlates between dyslexia and ADHD? A meta-analysis of voxel-based morphometry studies. J Neurodev Disord 11(1):31. https://doi.org/10.1186/s11689-019-9287-8

McKendree J, Snowling MJ (2011) Examination results of medical students with dyslexia. Med Educ 45(2):176–182

McLoughlin D, Leather C (2013) The dyslexic adult: interventions and outcomes—an evidence-based approach, 2nd edn. John Wiley & Sons, Chichester

Medina GB, Minetto M, Guimarães SRK et al (2017) Funções executivasna dislexia do desenvolvimento: revendo evidências de pesquisas (Executive functions in development dyslexia: reviewing research evidence). Revista Brasileira de Educação Especial 23(3):439–454

Melby-Lervåg M, Redick T, Hulme C (2016) Working memory training does not improve performance on measures of intelligence or other measures of "far transfer" evidence from a meta-analytic review. Perspect Psychol Sci 11:512–534

Meltzer L (2010) Promoting executive function in the classroom. In: Harris KR, Graham S (eds) What works for special needs learners. Guilford Press, New York, NY

Meltzer LJ (2014) Teaching executive function processes: promoting metacognition, strategy use, and effort. In: Goldstein S, Naglieri J (eds) Executive functioning handbook. Springer, New York, NY, pp 445–474

Meltzer LJ (2018) Creating strategic classrooms and schools: embedding executive function strategies in the curriculum. In: Meltzer LJ (ed) Executive function in education: from theory to practice, 2nd edn. Guilford Press, New York, NY, pp 263–299

Meltzer LJ, Greschler M, Kurkul K et al (2015) Executive function and peer mentoring: fostering metacognitive awareness, effort, and academic success. In: Harris K, Meltzer L (eds) The power of peers in the classroom: enhancing learning and social skills. Guilford Press, New York, NY, pp 1–32

Menghini D, Finzi A, Carlesimo GA et al (2011) Working memory impairment in children with developmental dyslexia: is it just a phonological deficity? Dev Neuropsychol 36(2):199–213

Mental Health Daily (2017) What is cognitive flexibility. Available via https://mentalhealthdaily.com/2015/07/24/what-is-cognitive-flexibility/. Accessed 9 Oct 2021

Messer D, Henry LA, Nash G (2016) The relation between executive functioning, reaction time, naming speed, and single word reading in children with typical development and language impairments. Br J Educ Psychol 86(3):412–428

Miciak J, Taylor WP, Stuebing KK et al (2018) Simulation of LD identification accuracy using a pattern of processing strengths and weaknesses method with multiple measures. J Psychoeduc Assess 36:21–33

Moll K, Snowling MJ, Hulme C (2020) Introduction to the special issue "comorbidities between reading disorders and other developmental disorders". Sci Stud Read 24(1):1–6

Molloy K, Moore DR, Sohoglu E et al (2012) Less is more: latent learning is maximized by shorter training sessions in auditory perceptual learning. PLoS One 7(5):e36929. https://doi.org/10.1371/journal.pone.0036929

Montgomery D (2007) Spelling, handwriting and dyslexia: overcoming barriers to learning. Routledge, Milton Park, UK

Morkena F, Helland T, Hugdahl K et al (2017) Reading in dyslexia across literacy development: a longitudinal study of effective connectivity. Neuro Image 144:92–100

Morris R, Lovett M, Wolf M et al (2012) Multiple component remediation for developmental reading disabilities: IQ, socioeconomic status, and race as factors in remedial outcome. J Learn Disabil 45(2):99–127

Mortimore T, Crozier WR (2006) Dyslexia and difficulties with study skills in higher education. Stud High Educ 31(2):235–251

Moura O, Pereira M, Alfaiated C et al (2017) Neurocognitive functioning in children with developmental dyslexia and attention-deficit/hyperactivity disorder: multiple deficits and diagnostic accuracy. J Clin Exp Neuropsychol 39(3):296–312

Mugnaini D, Fabiano GA (2006) The evaluation of impairment in the attention deficit/hyperactivity disorder: the contribution of the impairment rating scale. Minerva Pediatr 58:159–166

Mugnaini D, Lassi S, La Malfa G et al (2009) Internalizing correlates of dyslexia. World J Pediatr 5(4):255–264

Munzer T, Hussain K, Soares N (2020) Dyslexia: neurobiology, clinical features, evaluation and management. Transl Pediatr 9(Suppl 1):S36–S45

Murphy CF, Moore DR, Schochat E (2015) Generalization of auditory sensory and cognitive learning in typically developing children. PLoS One 10(8):e0135422

NCLD (National Center for Learning Disabilities) (2020) Report. Available via https://www.ncld.org/news/newsroom/the-state-of-ld-understanding-the-1-in-5. Accessed 27 May 2020

Nelson JM, Gregg N (2012) Depression and anxiety among transitioning adolescents and college students with ADHD, dyslexia, or comorbid ADHD/dyslexia. J Atten Disord 16(3):244–254

Nukari JM, Poutiainen ET, Arkkila EP et al (2020) Both individual and group-based neuropsychological interventions of dyslexia improve processing speed in young adults: a randomized controlled study. J Learn Disabil 53(3):213–227

Oczuks L (2003) Reciprocal teaching at work: strategies for improving reading comprehension. (3rd edn) Foreword by John Hattie. International Reading Association, Newark, DE

Ogundele MO (2018) Behavioural and emotional disorders in childhood: a brief overview for paediatricians. World J Clin Pediatr 7(1):9–26

Ortiz SO (2019) On the measurement of cognitive abilities in English learners. Contemp Sch Psychol 23(1):68–86

Ortiz AA, Artiles AJ (2010) Meeting the needs of ELs with disabilities: a linguistically and culturally responsive model. In: Li G, Edwards P (eds) Best practices in ELL instruction. The Guilford Press, New York, NY

Ortiz SO, Seymour KL (2017) The culturally competent school psychologist. In: Thielking M, Terjesen MT (eds) Australian handbook of school psychology. Springer Books, New York, NY, pp 81–110

Ozernov-Palchik O, Gaab N (2016) Tackling the 'dyslexia paradox': reading brain and behavior for early markers of developmental dyslexia. Wiley Interdiscip Rev Cogn Sci 7(2):156–176

Ozernov-Palchik O, Yu X, Wang Y et al (2016) Lessons to be learned: how a comprehensive neurobiological framework of atypical reading development can inform educational practice. Curr Opin Behav Sci 10:45–58

Panadero E (2017) A review of self-regulated learning: six models and four directions for research. Front Psychol 8:422. https://doi.org/10.3389/fpsyg.2017.00422

Panahi R, Akbari M, Jarollahi F et al. (2023) Atypical function of auditory sensory gating in children with developmental dyslexia: Investigating its relationship with cognitive abilities. Dyslexia 29(4):426–440. https://doi.org/10.1002/dys.1754. Epub 2023 Oct 1. PMID: 37779260.

Pani P, Menghini D, Napolitano C et al (2013) Proactive and reactive control of movement are differently affected in attention deficit hyperactivity disorder children. Res Dev Disabil 34:3104–3111

Patel A, Patel M, Patel H (2012) ADHD and comorbid conditions. In: Norvilitis JM (ed) Current directions in ADHD and its treatment. IntechOpen, Rijeka Croatia, pp 25–46. Available via www.intechopen.com Accessed 13 Oct 2021

Paulino P, Sá I, Lopes da Silva A (2016) Self-regulation of motivation: contributing to students' learning in middle school. The European proceedings of social and behavioural sciences EpSBS. icCSBs J 8(4). https://doi.org/10.15405/epsbs.2016.05.1

Peng P, Miller AC (2016) Does attention training work? A selective meta-analysis to explore the effects of attention training and moderators. Learn Individ Differ 45:77–87

Peng P, Sha T, Li B (2013) The deficit profile of working memory, inhibition, and updating in Chinese children with reading difficulties. Learn Individ Differ 25:111–117

Peng P, Barnes M, Wang C et al (2018) A meta-analysis on the relation between reading and working memory. Psychol Bull 144(1):48–76

Pennington BF (2006) From single to multiple deficit models of developmental disorders. Cognition 101(2):385–413

Peters L, Bulthé J, Daniels N et al (2018) Dyscalculia and dyslexia: different behavioral, yet similar brain activity profiles during arithmetic. Neuroimage Clin 18:663–674

Peterson RL, Boada R, McGrath LM et al (2016) Cognitive prediction of reading, math, and attention: shared and unique influences. J Learn Disabil 50(4):408–421

Pezoa JP, Mendive S, Strasser K (2019) Reading interest and family literacy practices from prekindergarten to kindergarten: contributions from a cross-lagged analysis. Early Child Res Q 47(2):284–295

Plourde V, Boivin M, Brendgen M et al (2018) Cognitive mechanisms underlying the associations between inattention and reading abilities. Dev Neuropsychol 43:92–105

Protopapas A (2019) Evolving concepts of dyslexia and their implications for research and remediation. Front Psychol 10:2873. https://doi.org/10.3389/fpsyg.2019.02873

Puac R (2005) Comorbidity of dyslexia, dyspraxia, attention deficit disorder (ADD), attention deficit hyperactive disorder (ADHD), obsessive compulsive disorder (OCD) and Tourette's syndrome in children: a prospective epidemiological study. Clin Chiropractic 8:189–198

Ramus F, Altarelli I, Jednoróg K et al (2018) Neuroanatomy of developmental dyslexia: pitfalls and promise. Neurosci Biobehav Rev 84:434–452

Rappolt-Schlichtmann G, Boucher AR, Evans M (2018) From deficit remediation to capacity building: learning to enable rather than disable students with dyslexia. Lang Speech Hear Serv Sch 49(4):864–874

Reale L, Bartoli B, Cartabia M et al (2017) Comorbidity prevalence and treatment outcome in children and adolescents with ADHD. Eur Child Adolesc Psychiatry 26:1443–1457

Reid G, Green S (2014) 100+ ideas for supporting pupils with dyslexia. Bloomsbury, London

Richardson AJ (2006) Omega-3 fatty acids in ADHD and related neurodevelopmental disorders. Int Rev Psychiatry 18(2):155–172

Richardson JTE, Wydell TN (2003) The representation and attainment of students with dyslexia in higher education. J Read Writ 16(5):475–503

Roehling JV, Hebert M, Nelson JR et al (2017) Text structure strategies for improving expository reading comprehension. Read Teach 71(1):71–82

Rosenblum S, Frisch C, Deutsh-Castel T et al (2014) Daily functioning profile of children with attention deficit hyperactive disorder: a pilot study using an ecological assessment. Neuropsychol Rehabil 23:1–17

Rosselli M, Matute E, Ardila A (2006) Neuropsychological predictors of reading ability in Spanish Revista De Neurologia 42:202–210

Ryder D, Norwich B (2018) UK higher education lecturers' perspectives of dyslexia, dyslexic students and related disability provision. J Res Spec Educ Needs 19(3):161–172

Sahoo MK, Biswas H, Padhy SK (2015) Psychological co-morbidity in children with specific learning disorders. J Family Med Prim Care 4:21–25

Samaha J, Postle BR (2017) Correlated individual differences suggest a common mechanism underlying metacognition in visual perception and visual short-term memory. Proc Biol Sci 284(1867):20172035. https://doi.org/10.1098/rspb.2017.2035pmid:29167365

Sánchez-Morán M, Hernández JA, Duñabeitia JA et al (2018) Genetic association study of dyslexia and ADHD candidate genes in a Spanish cohort: implications of comorbid samples. PLoS One 13(10):e0206431

Scerri TS, Schulte-Körne G (2010) Genetics of developmental dyslexia. Eur Child Adolesc Psychiatry 19(3):179–197

Schafer EC, Florence S, Anderson C et al (2014) A critical review of remote-microphone technology for children with normal hearing and auditory differences. J Educ Audiol 20:1–11

Schleider K (2009) Lese- und Rechtschreibstörungen (Reading and spelling disorders). UTB Profile. Ernst Reinhardt Verlag, Munich, pp 79–83

Schulte-Körne G (2004) Lese-Rechtschreibstörung (reading and spelling disorder). In: Thome G (ed) Lese-Rechtschreibschwierigkeiten (LRS) und Legasthenie. Eine grundlegende Einführung (Reading and spelling difficulties (LRS) and dyslexia. A basic introduction). Beltz, Weinheim, pp 64–85

Schulte-Körne G (2021) Verpasste Chancen: die neuen diagnostischen Leitlinien zur Lese-, Rechtschreib- und Rechenstörung der ICD-11 [missed opportunities: the new ICD-11 diagnostic guidelines for reading, spelling and calculation disorders]. Z Kinder Jugendpsychiatr Psychother 5:1–5

Schulte-Körne G, Galuschka K (2015) Diagnostik und Behandlung von Lese- und/oder Rechtschreibstörung bei Kindern und Jugendlichen, S3-Leitlinie AWMF-Register-Nr. 028/044. Available via www.awmf.org/leitlinien/detail/ll/028-044.html. Accessed 5 Sept 2019

Schulte-Körne G, Ludwig KK, el Sharkawy J et al (2007) Genetics and neuroscience in dyslexia: perspectives for education and remediation. Mind Brain Educ 1(4):162–172

Schwaighofer M, Fischer F, Bühner M (2015) Does working memory training transfer? A meta-analysis including training conditions as moderators. Educ Psychol 50(2):138–166

Seidenberg M (2017) Language at the speed of sight: how we read, why so many can't, and what can be done about it. Basic Books, New York NY

Serrallach B, Groß C, Bernhofs V et al (2016) Neural biomarkers for dyslexia, ADHD, and ADD in the auditory cortex of children. Front Neurosci 10:324. https://doi.org/10.3389/fnins.2016.00324

Sexton CC, Gelhorn HL, Bell JA et al (2012) The co-occurrence of reading disorder and ADHD: epidemiology, treatment, psychosocial impact, and economic burden. Aust J Learn Disabil 45(6):538–564

Sharma M, Purdy SC, Kelly AS (2009) Comorbidity of auditory processing, language, and reading disorders. J Speech Lang Hear Res 52(3):706–722. https://doi.org/10.1044/1092-4388(2008/07-0226)

Shaywitz S (2003) Overcoming dyslexia. A new and complete science-based program for reading problems at any level. Alfred A. Knopf, New York, NY

Shaywitz SE, Fletcher JM, Holahan JM et al (1999) Persistence of dyslexia: the Connecticut longitudinal study at adolescence. Pediatrics 104(6):1351–1359

Shaywitz BA, Shaywitz SE, Blachman BA et al (2004) Development of left occipitotemporal systems for skilled reading in children after a phonologically-based intervention. Biol Psychiatry 55(9):926–933

Shaywitz SE, Morris R, Shaywitz BA (2008) The education of dyslexic children from childhood to young adulthood. Annu Rev Psychol 59:451–475

Shield B, Conetta R, Dockrell J et al (2015) A survey of acoustic conditions and noise levels in secondary school classrooms in England. J Acoust Soc Am 137(1):177–188. https://doi.org/10.1121/1.4904528

Shipstead Z, Lindsey DR, Marshall RL et al (2014) The mechanisms of working memory capacity: primary memory, secondary memory, and attention control. J Mem Lang 72:116–141

Siegel LS (2006) Perspectives on dyslexia. Paediatr Child Health 11(9):581–587

Smart JL, Purdy SC, Kelly AS (2018) Impact of personal frequency modulation systems on behavioral and cortical auditory evoked potential measures of auditory processing and classroom listening in school-aged children with auditory processing disorder. J Am Acad Audiol 29(7):568–586

Smith-Spark JH, Henry LA, Messer DJ et al (2016) Executive functions in adults with developmental dyslexia. Res Dev Disabil 53–54:323–341

Smith-Spark JH, Henry LA, Messer DJ et al (2017) Verbal and non-verbal fluency in adults with developmental dyslexia: phonological processing or executive control problems? Dyslexia 23(3):234–250

Smythe I, Everatt J, Salter R (2005) The international book of dyslexia: a guide to practice and resources. John Wiley & Sons Ltd, Hoboken NJ, pp 1–5

Snowling MJ (2013) Early identification and interventions for dyslexia: a contemporary view. J Res Spec Educ Needs 13(1):7–14

Snyder HR, Miyake A, Hankin BL (2015) Advancing understanding of executive function impairments and psychopathology: bridging the gap between clinical and cognitive approaches. Front Psychol 6:328. https://doi.org/10.3389/fpsyg.2015.00328

Solis M, Ciullo S, Vaughn S et al (2012) Reading comprehension interventions for middle school students with learning disabilities: a synthesis of 30 years of research. J Learn Disabil 45(4):327–340

Spear-Swerling L, Brucker PO, Alfano MP (2005) Teachers' literacy-related knowledge and self- perceptions in relation to preparation and experience. Ann Dyslexia 55(2):266–296

Spencer TJ, Biederman J, Mick E (2007) Attention-deficit/hyperactivity disorder: diagnosis, lifespan, comorbidities, and neurobiology. Ambul Pediatr 7:73–81

Stampoltzis A, Paradisi E, Theodosakis D (2023) Resilience, Mental Flourishing, Character Strengths and Job Satisfaction of Adults with Dyslexia Compared to a Control Group. EJPER 6(3):119–130

Stampoltzis A, Polychronopoulou S (2008) Dyslexia in Greek higher education: a study of incidence, policy and provision. J Res Spec Educ Needs 8(1):37–46

Stevens EA, Park S, Vaughn S (2019) A review of summarizing and main idea interventions for struggling readers in grades 3 through 12: 1978–2016. Remedial Spec Educ 40(3):131–149

Stoodley CJ (2014) Distinct regions of the cerebellum show gray matter decreases in autism, ADHD, and developmental dyslexia. Front Syst Neurosci 8:92. https://doi.org/10.3389/fnsys.2014.00092

Stowe CM (2000) How to reach and teach children and teens with dyslexia: a parent and teacher guide to helping students of all ages academically, socially and emotionally. Jossey-Bass, San Fransisco, CA

Strait DL, Parbery-Clark A, O'Connell S et al (2013) Biological impact of preschool music classes on processing speech in noise. Dev Cog Neurosci 6:51–56

Sumner E, Connelly V, Barnett AL (2014) The influence of spelling ability on handwriting production: children with and without dyslexia. J Exp Psychol Learn Mem Cogn 40(5):1441–1447

Tamm L, Nakonnezny PA, Hughes CW (2014) An open trial of a metacognitive executive function training for young children with ADHD. J Atten Disord 18(6):551–559

Tops W, Callens M, Van Cauwenberghe E et al (2013) Beyond spelling: the writing skills of students with dyslexia in higher education. Read Write 26:705–720

Truesdale SP (1990) Whole body listening: developing active auditory skills. Lang Speech Hear Serv Sch 21(3):183–184

Vacca RT, Vacca JL, Mraz ME (2011) Content-area reading: literacy and learning across the curriculum, 10th edn. Allyn and Bacon, Boston, MA

Varvara P, Varuzza C, Sorrentino ACP et al (2014) Executive functions in developmental dyslexia. Front Hum Neurosci 8:120. https://doi.org/10.3389/fnhum.2014.00120

Virolainen SJ, Von Handorf A, Viel KCMF et al. (2023) Gene–environment interactions and their impact on human health. Genes Immun 24, 1–11. https://doi.org/10.1038/s41435-022-00192-6

Vizzi F, Iaia M, Carlino MD et al (2024) The Enduring Challenge of Literacy Issues in Adulthood: Investigating Spelling Deficits among Dyslexic Italian University Students. Brain Sci 14(7):712

Vo ML, Smith TJ, Mital PK et al (2012) Do the eyes really have it? Dynamic allocation of attention when viewing moving faces. J Vis 12(13). https://doi.org/10.1167/12.13.3

Volckaert AM, Nöel MP (2015) Training executive function in pre-schoolers reduce externalizing behaviours. Trends Neurosci Educ 4:37–47

von Karolyi C, Winner E (2005) Investigations of visual-spatial abilities in dyslexia. In: Columbus F (ed) Focus on dyslexia research. Nova Science, Hauppauge, pp 1–25

von Karolyi C, Winner E, Gray W et al (2003) Dyslexia linked to talent: global visual-spatial ability. Brain Lang 85(3):427–431

Walker JE, Norman CA (2010) The neurophysiology of dyslexia: a selective review with implications for neurofeedback remediation and results of treatment in twelve consecutive patients. J Neurother 10(1):45–55

Wang Z, Han F (2017) Metacognitive knowledge and metacognitive control of writing strategy between high and low-performing Chinese EFL writers. Theory Pract Lang Stud 7(7):523–532

Wang L-C, Yang H-M (2014) Diverse inhibition and working memory of word recognition for dyslexic and typically developing children. Dyslexia 21(2):162–176

Wang L, Liu D, Chung KK et al (2017) Development of lexical tone awareness in Chinese children with and without dyslexia. Contemp Educ Psychol 49:203–214

Warnke A, Hemminger U, Plume E (2004) Lese-Rechtschreib-Störungen. Leitfaden Kinder- und Jugendpsychotherapie. Göttingen, Hogrefe

Washburn EK, Joshi RM, Binks-Centrell E (2010) Are preservice teachers prepared to teach struggling readers? Ann Dyslexia 61(1):21–43

Webster DM (2016) Listening to the voice of dyslexic students at a small, vocational higher education institution to promote successful inclusive practice in the 21st century. Int J Learn Teach 2(1):78–86

West TG (1997) In the mind's eye: visual thinkers, gifted people with dyslexia and other learning difficulties, computer images, and the ironies of creativity. Prometheus, Amherst, NY

West TG (2005) The gifts of dyslexia: talents among dyslexics and their families. Hong Kong J Paediatr 10:153–158

Wheldall K, Wheldall R, Rothwell I (2015) Reading tutor program. Multilit: a research initiative of Macquarie University. Available via http://www.multilit.com/programs. Accessed 9 Oct 2021

WHO (2024) ICD-11 for Mortality and Morbidity Statistics (Version: 01/2024) https://icd.who.int/browse11/l-m/en: Accessed 24th October 2024

Willcutt EG, Pennington BF (2000a) Psychiatric comorbidity in children and adolescents with reading disability. J Child Psychol Psychiatry 41:1039–1048

Willcutt EG, Pennington BF (2000b) Comorbidity of reading disability and attention deficit/ hyperactivity disorder: differences by gender and subtype. J Learn Disabil 33(2):179–191

Willcutt EG, Pennington BF, DeFries JC (2000) Twin study of the etiology of comorbidity between reading disability and attention-deficit/hyperactivity disorder. Am J Med Genet 96:293–301

Willcutt EG, Betjemann RS, McGrath LM et al (2010) Etiology and neuropsychology of comorbidity between RD and ADHD: the case for multiple-deficit models. Cortex 46(10):1345–1361

Winner E, Casey MB, DaSilva D et al (1991) Spatial abilities and reading deficits in visual art students. Empir Stud Arts 9(1):51–63

Winner E, von Karolyi C, Malinsky D et al (2001) Dyslexia and visual-spatial talents: compensation vs deficit model. Brain Lang 76(2):81–110

Wissell S, Karimi L, Serry T et al (2022) "You Don't Look Dyslexic": Using the Job Demands-Resource Model of Burnout to Explore Employment Experiences of Australian Adults with Dyslexia. Int J Environ Res Public Health 28;19(17):10719. https://doi.org/10.3390/ijerph191710719. PMID: 36078435; PMCID: PMC9518213

Wolff U, Lundberg I (2002) The prevalence of dyslexia among art students. Dyslexia 8(1):34–42

Wright BA, Zhang Y (2009) A review of the generalization of auditory learning. Philos Trans R Soc Lond B Biol Sci 364(1515):301–311. https://doi.org/10.1098/rstb.2008.026

Yang C, Bai L (2019) The use of metacognitive strategies by Chinese PhD students of social sciences in Australian universities. Int J Educ Res 97(1):43–52

Yang J, Peng J, Zhang D et al (2017) Specific effects of working memory training on the reading skills of Chinese children with developmental dyslexia. PlosOne 12(11):e0186114. https://doi.org/10.1371/journal.pone.0186114

Zhang L (2018) Metacognitive and cognitive strategy use in reading comprehension. A structural equation modelling approach. Springer, Cham

Zhang X, Ardasheva Y (2019) Sources of college EFL learners' self-efficacy in the English public speaking domain. English Specif Purp 53(1):47–59

Zhang LJ, Thomas N, Qin TL (2019) Language learning strategy research in system: looking back and looking forward. System 84(1):87–92

Zimdars K, Zink S (2006) Computergestützte Trainingsverfahren. In: von Suchodoletz W (ed) Therapie der Lese-Rechtschreib-Störung (LRS). Traditionelle und alternative Behandlungsmethoden im Überblick, 2nd edn. Kohlhammer, Stuttgart, pp 58–81

Zusho A, Edwards K (2011) Self-regulation of achievement goals in the college classroom. In: Bembenutty H (ed) Self-regulated learning: new directions for teaching and learning, no. 126. Jossey-Bass, San Francisco, CA, pp 21–31

Electronic Supplementary Material: Description of Video Examples and Audio Samples and Still Images of Videos for European Manual of Medicine Phoniatrics II

Katrin Neumann, Corinna Gietmann, and Antoinette am Zehnhoff-Dinnesen

Authors:

R. Shprintzen
Connecticut Children's (WDG), Farmington; and The Virtual Center for Velo-Cardio-Facial Syndrome (RJS), Manlius, NY, USA
e-mail: robert.shprintzen@vcfscenter.org

T. Fuhr
Fresenius University of Applied Sciences, Idstein, Germany
e-mail: tanja.fuhr@he-fresenius.de

S. Reinert
Interdisciplinary Centre for Cleft Palate and Craniofacial Malformations, Tuebingen University Hospital, Tuebingen, Germany
e-mail: siegmar.reinert@med.uni-tuebingen.de

M. Brunner
Department of Otorhinolaryngology, Head and Neck Surgery, Division of Phoniatrics and Pedaudiology, University of Heidelberg, Germany
e-mail: info@monikabrunner.eu

U. Sick
Ulrike Sick, Marianne Frostig School, Auf der Rosenhöhe 55, 63069 Offenbach am Main, Germany
e-mail: ulrike.sick@mfs-of.de

A. Wolff von Gudenberg
Institute of the Kassel Stuttering Therapy, Bad Emstal, Germany
e-mail: awvgudenberg@kasseler-stottertherapie.de

K. Neumann
Department of Phoniatrics and Pedaudiology, University Hospital Münster, University Münster, Germany
e-mail: Katrin.neumann@uni-muenster.de

1. **Case Study Video 1.1**: Three-dimensional assessment of velopharyngeal valving demonstrated by videofluoroscopy in multiple views

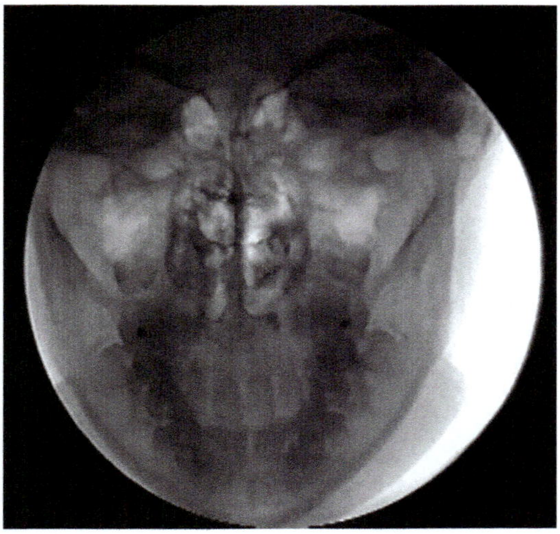

K. Neumann · C. Gietmann
A. am Zehnhoff-Dinnesen
Department of Phoniatrics and Pedaudiology, University Hospital Münster, University Münster, Münster, Germany

A. am Zehnhoff-Dinnesen et al. (eds.), *Phoniatrics II*, European Manual of Medicine,
https://doi.org/10.1007/978-3-031-25175-7

2. **Case Study Video 1.2**: Videofluoroscopy of velopharyngeal function in an English-speaking child in lateral view showing the primary place of closure at the adenoid pad

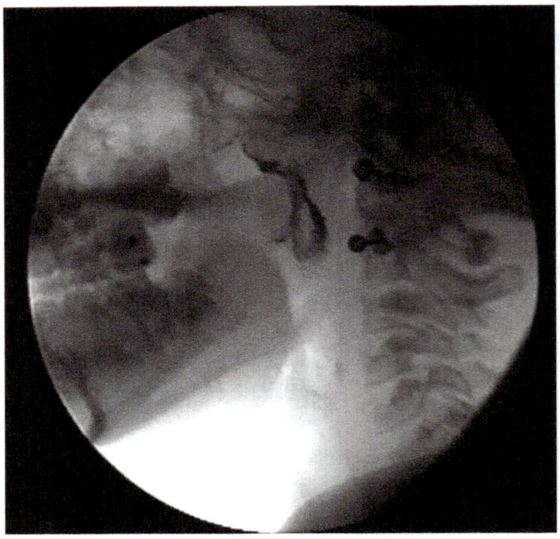

3. **Case Study Video 1.3**: English-speaking child with velopharyngeal closure insufficiency demonstrated by both nasopharyngoscopy and multi-view videofluoroscopy. The movement of the lateral pharyngeal walls cannot be determined from the endoscopic examination, but it can be seen excellently on frontal view videofluoroscopy (the second radiographic projection in the examination).

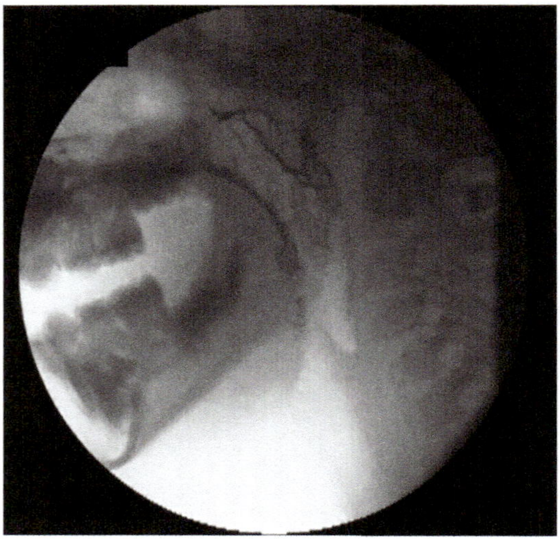

4. **Case Study Video 1.4**: Different patterns of velopharyngeal closure in three English-speaking adults with normal velopharyngeal function shown by nasopharyngoscopy

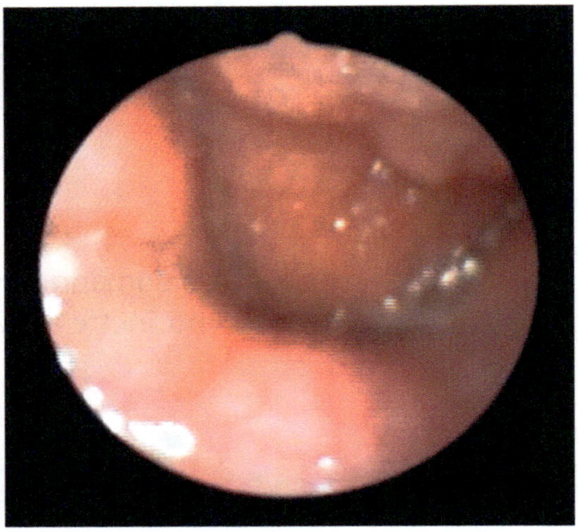

5. **Case Study Video 1.5**: Elevation of the velum by contraction of the levator veli palatini muscle in an adult with normal velopharyngeal function visualised by videofluoroscopy in lateral view. The posterio-superior movement of the velum to the posterior pharyngeal wall results in contact above the plane of the hard palate.

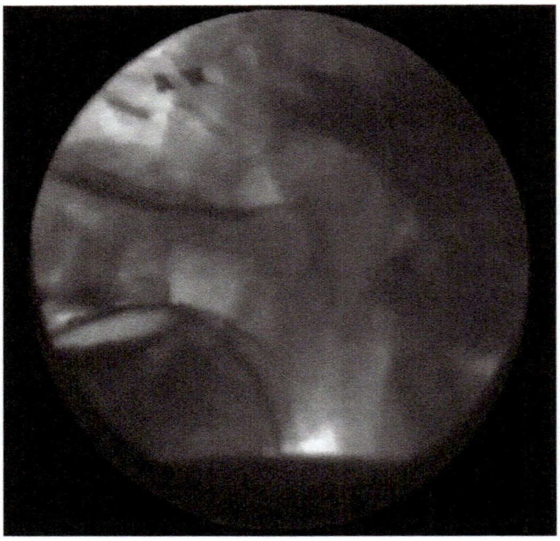

6. **Case Study Video 1.6**: Nasopharyngoscopy in an English-speaking man with normal velopharyngeal function shows how the belly of the levator veli palatini muscle dilates the opening of the Eustachian tube orifice

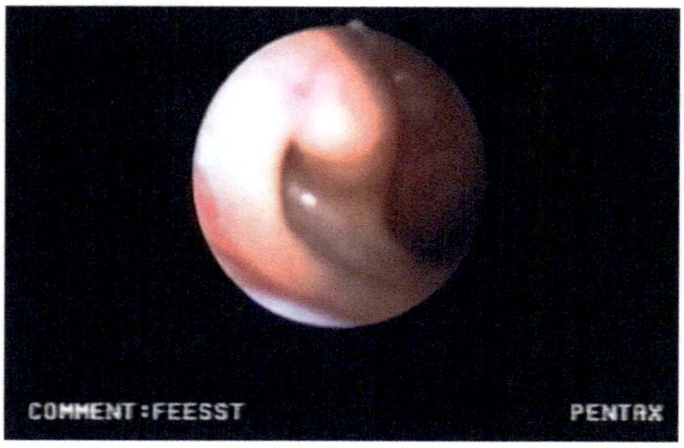

Source videos 1.1–1.6: R. Shprintzen

7. **Case Study Audio 3.1**: Lingual, labial and buccal dysglossia in a 41-year-old German-speaking man after treatment of a left mouth floor tumour; rigidity of the left buccinator, mylohyoideus and geniohyoideus muscles after 9-fold irradiation. Impairment of speech sounds, especially fricatives; left restricted protrusion of lips results in impaired quality of vowels /o/ and /u/, which are difficult to differentiate. Left-sided salivary flow is restricted.
Source audio: T. Fuhr
8. **Relation for Video 4.1 and 4.2 Source Kerstin Kerkhofs and Martine de Smit**:
Fat: 8. Relation for Videos 4.1 and 4.2:
Not fat: Part 1, Chapter 4, Section 4.2.4.
Video 4.1: Example of BOA responses.
Video 4.2: Recommended VRA procedure.
Fat: Source Videos 4.1 and 4.2: Kerstin Kerkhofs and Martine de Smit.
9. **Case Study Video 5.1**: Fibre-optic assessment of velopharyngeal function in an 8-year-old German-speaking girl with a left-sided cleft palate 1.5 years after velopharyngoplasty with a cranial-based pharyngeal flap made by the Sanvenero-Rosselli technique. This surgery is applied to reduce rhinophonia aperta and prevent nasal regurgitation. The video shows a fairly good velopharyngeal closure with only mild to moderate residual rhinophonia aperta and thus fairly good intelligibility (palatal dysglossia) and occasional retrograde regurgitation of mucus into the nasopharynx.
Source: S. Reinert

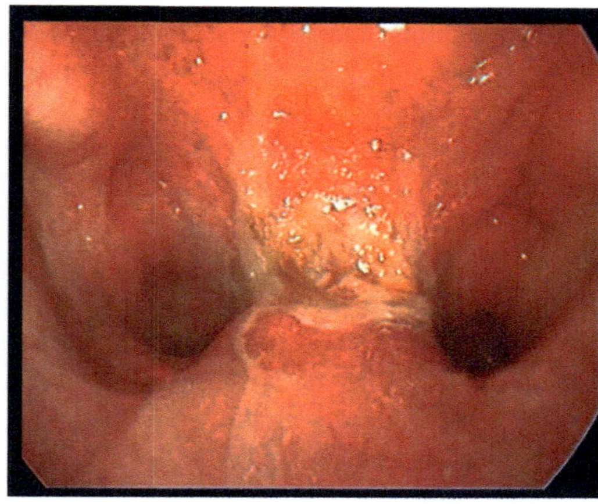

Case Study Videos 5.2a–c: Biofeedback therapy of inconsistent velopharyngeal closure during voiceless stop consonants in a ten-year-old German-speaking girl with childhood apraxia of speech (CAS) using flexible nasopharyngoscopy. The girl has difficulty in planning and programming movement sequences and regulating muscle tone. She often achieves good velopharyngeal closure on voiced stop sounds /b/d/g/, but no consistent closure on voiceless stop sounds /p/t/k/ (Video 5.2a). To compensate for her disability, she attempts to speak with an excessively loud voice and forced muscle tension, which is unhelpful in achieving full velopharyngeal closure (Video 5.2b). Conventional speech therapy for motor regulation has limited effectiveness.

Treatment method: Provided with the view of the velopharyngeal sphincter via flexible nasopharyngoscopy, the girl learns to use adequate muscle tension while pronouncing the voiceless stop sounds.

The treatment consists of four steps:

1. Introduction: learning the structures and function of the velopharyngeal closure while watching a video of a nasopharyngoscopy.

2. Experimentation: self-observation of articulation movements guided by therapeutic instructions to move from stop sounds with the best velopharyngeal closure (/b/d/g/) to those with the least closure (/p/t/k/) and slowly fuse them.
3. Coupling: merging visual and auditory perception with the help of guided relaxation.
4. Consolidation: transfer to spontaneous speech with the help of a diary.

The 20-min biofeedback sessions focus on training a target sound in isolation and during syllable production. After two sessions, the girl mastered motor speech planning and achieved complete velopharyngeal closure immediately and consistently during the pronunciation of voiceless stop sounds (Video 5.2c).

10. **Case Study Video 5.2a**: Pre-therapeutic inconsistent velopharyngeal closure for voiceless stop consonants

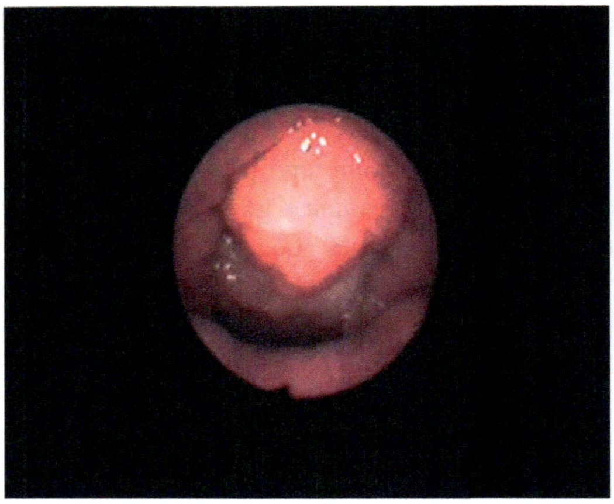

11. **Case Study Video 5.2b**: Pre-therapeutic compensation attempt of inconsistent velopharyngeal closure by overly loud voicing

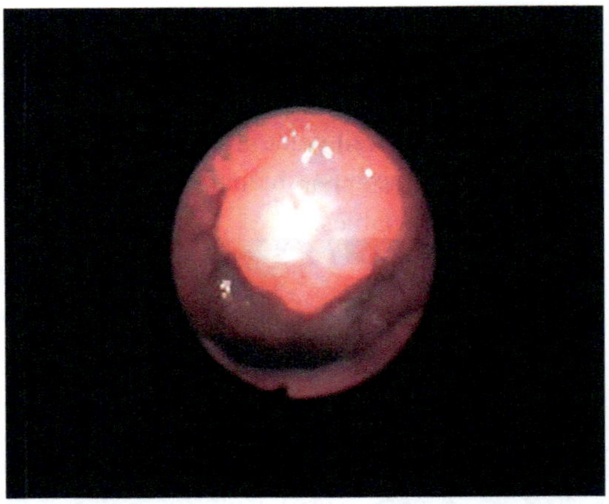

12. **Case Study Video 5.2c**: Sufficient velopharyngeal closure after biofeedback therapy by flexible nasopharyngoscopy

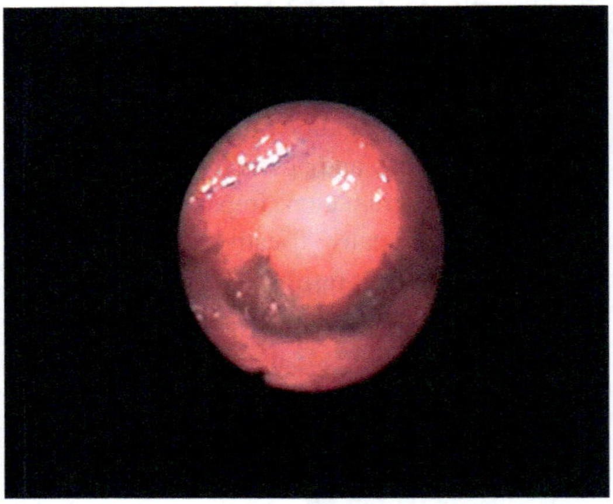

Source Videos 5.2a–c: M. Brunner

Case Study Videos 5.3.a–d: Velopharyngeal insufficiency in a 19-year-old German-speaking man with cleft lip and palate closed at one year of age. He had received speech therapy for about six years without learning to control the coordination of velopharyngeal closure sufficiently (Videos 5.3.a and b). Only nasopharyngoscopic feedback helped him (Videos 5.3.c and d).

13. **Case Study Video 5.3.a**: Pretherapeutic inconsistent velopharyngeal closure on sentences and syllables. Velopharyngeal closure examined nasopharyngoscopically is possible in principle but not coordinated with phonation.

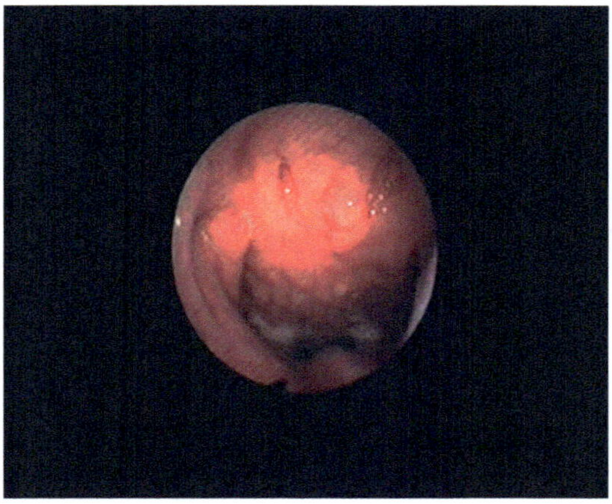

14. **Case Study Video 5.3.b**: Pretherapeutic inconsistent velopharyngeal closure for spontaneous speech. As demonstrated with nasopharyngoscopy, there is nearly no velopharyngeal closure and the sound is hypernasal.

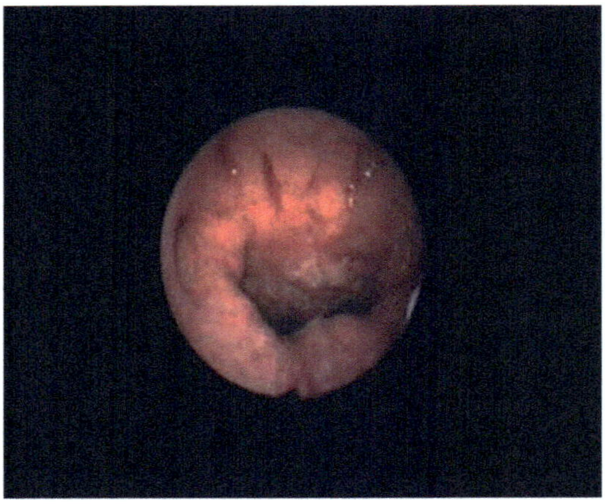

15. **Case Study Video 5.3.c**: Sufficient velopharyngeal closure for single sounds and syllables after biofeedback therapy by flexible nasopharyngoscopy. The patient has learned to coordinate the movement of the velopharynx with the sound production.

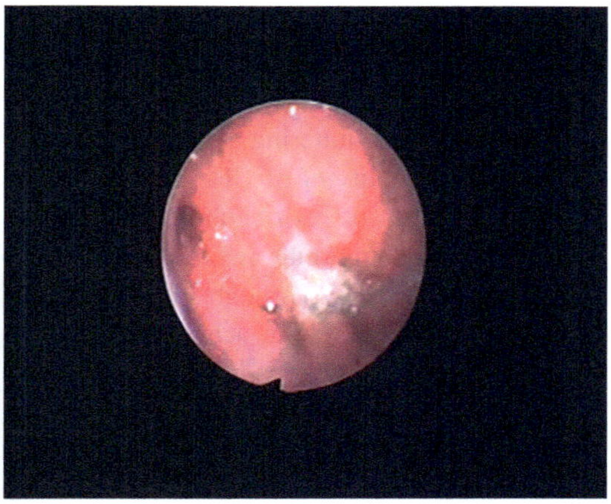

16. **Case Study Video 5.3.d**: Sufficient velopharyngeal closure for spontaneous speech after biofeedback therapy by flexible nasopharyngoscopy: The patient has learned to manage the velopharyngeal closure in spontaneous speech. The sound is no longer hypernasal.

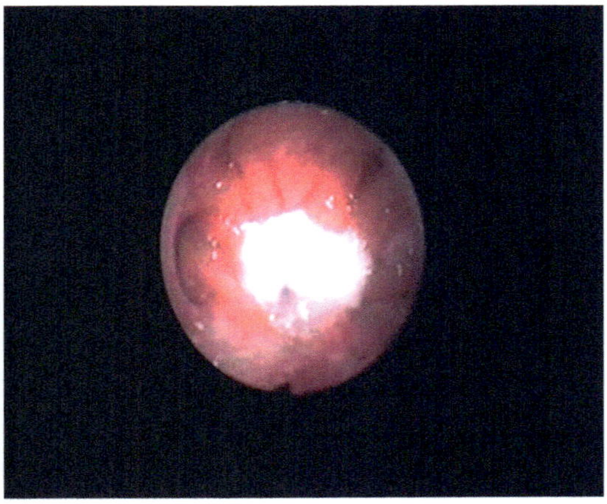

Source Videos 5.3a–d: M. Brunner

Case Study Videos 6.1 and 10.1a–c: A 24-year-old man with severe persistent developmental stuttering. He exhibits the core symptoms of stuttering such as repetitions, severe blocks and prolongations. Especially words with consonant clusters at the beginning of the word, such as /fr/ in "Freischuss" or /br/ in "Brauhaus", cause him difficulties.

In addition, he shows interjections, episodes of upward drifting of the voice pitch while speaking, physical concomitants and vegetative symptoms such as breathing irregularities, facial expressions, grimacing, turning of the head and movements of the hands and legs (Video 6.1). He suffers emotionally very much from his stuttering and is severely limited in his quality of life. He has spent more than 13 years of his childhood and adolescence undergoing stuttering treatments of different approaches. Through fluency shaping therapy, he was able to achieve fluency, but the new speech patterns he learned cost him constant attention and his way of speaking was perceived by him as alien and unnatural, so he did not use it in everyday life (Video 10.1a). Finally, a trial of deep brain stimulation—the first worldwide to be used specifically for stuttering—was successful (Videos 10.1b and 10.1c). With this approach, he improved his speech fluency by about 30% and got rid of most of the stuttering-accompanying behaviour. This enabled him to take up work as a lawyer in a law firm.

17. **Case Study Video 6.1**: Severe stuttering symptoms before a treatment trial with deep brain stimulation. Notice the long block in the word "Freischuss".

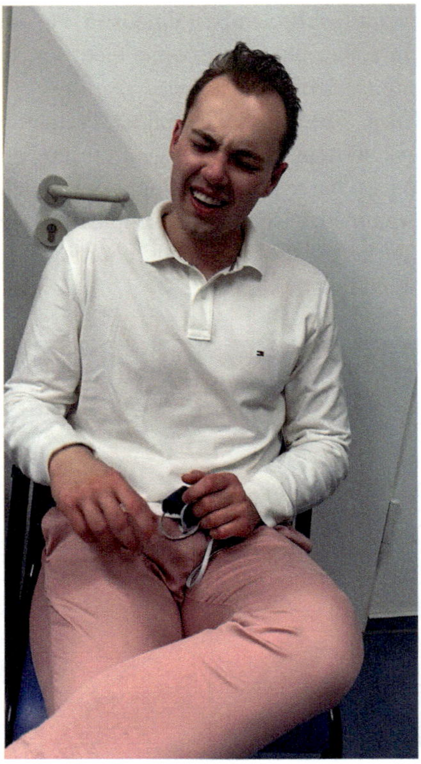

Source Videos 6.1 and 10.1a–c: K. Neumann

18. **Case Study 6.2**: Persistent developmental stuttering of a 4-year-old German-speaking boy which developed one year ago. Pro-

nounced physical concomitants such as turning the head away, interrupting eye contact when speaking and hypermobility must be interpreted as escape and avoidance behaviour to prevent or escape from stuttering.

Source: K. Neumann

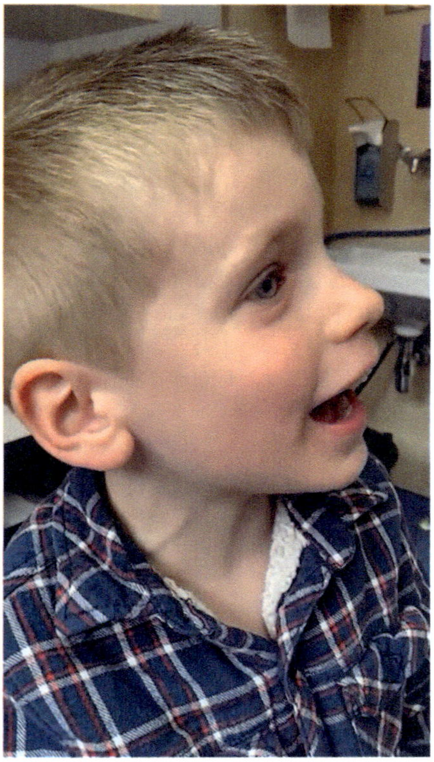

19. **Case Study 6.3**: Severe neurogenic stuttering of a German-speaking young men together with severe mixed spastic and ataxic dysarthria due to brain injury after a traffic accident

    Source: K. Neumann

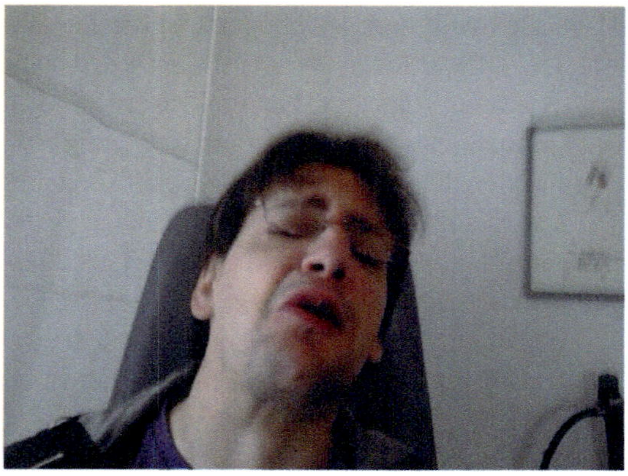

20. **Case Study 6.4**: Psychogenic stuttering of a German-speaking surgeon from Novosibirsk who had moved to Germany. He had to change jobs within Germany and was unhappy with his new work situation and under stress. Suddenly, he developed stutter-like symptoms and various neurological paralysis-like symptoms. Neurological causes were ruled out. He did not accept the diagnosis of a dissociative disorder and refused psychosomatic therapy, which would have been the therapy of choice here.

    Source: K. Neumann

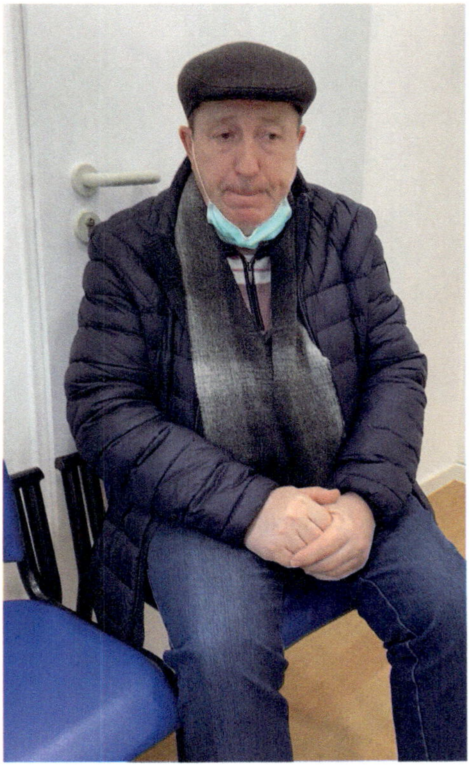

21. **Case Study 6.5**: Psychogenic stuttering and gait difficulties as symptoms of a dissociative neurological symptom disorder in a German-speaking girl. Both the stuttering and the gait difficulties had started suddenly 3 weeks earlier, together with headaches. A neurological cause could be ruled out. The stuttering shown in the video was characterised by loose syllable repetitions and had already improved at the time of the video recording. The girl underwent psychosomatic treatment, which is the therapy of choice here.

    Source: K. Neumann

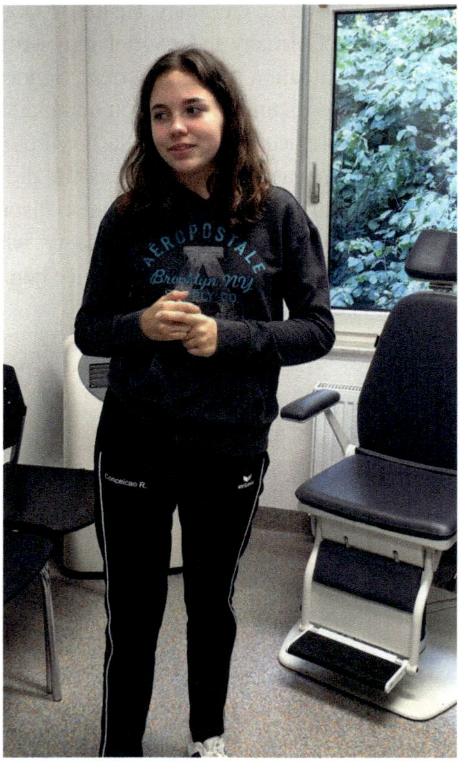

Case Study Audios 7.1a–c: German-speaking man who clutters: rapid and irregular speech tempo with irregularly occurring phonetic and phonological anomalies, contraction or omission of syllables, abnormal pauses, syllable stress and speech rhythm, as well as dysfluencies atypical of stuttering—symptoms that impair his intelligibility.

22. **Case Study Audio 7.1a:** Rapid and irregular speech tempo with irregularly occurring phonetic and phonological anomalies
23. **Case Study Audio 7.1b:** Man describes difficulty writing evenly
24. **Case Study Audio 7.1c:** Many dysfluencies atypical for stuttering

    Source audios 7.1a–c: U. Sick

25. **Relation for Video 8.1**: Part 2, Chapter 8, Section 8.4.4.

    Fat: Relation for Video 8.1:

    Not fat: Part 2, Chapter 8, Section 8.4.4.

    Video 8.1 Tips and tricks for laryngeal examination.

    Fat: Source Video 8.1: Tiina Pakka, Annika Laaksonen, Ahmed Geneid.

    Fat: Relation for Videos 8.2–8.10 and Case Study Video 8.4:

    Not fat: Part 2, Chapter 8, Section 8.4.6.

    Video 8.2 Stroboscopy of the lips: crescendo-decrescendo, French horn. Regular vibratory pattern of the lips.

    Video 8.3 Stroboscopy of the lips: musical scale, trumpet. Regular vibratory pattern of the lips.

    Case Study Video 8.4 Stroboscopy of the lips: flugelhorn player with stenosis of the spinal canal between C2 and C5.

    Video 8.4 Stroboscopy of the lips: single tones played with the trombone. The regular vibratory pattern of the lips is similar to the vocal fold vibration. The mucosa in the centre of the upper lip initiates the closure as a result of the Bernoulli effect.

    Video 8.5 Sonography of the lips: transversal b-mode scans of the upper lip. Orbicularis oris muscle visible as narrow black band.

    Video 8.6 Sonography of the lips: sagittal B-mode scans of the lips (upper lip left, lower lip right, cavum oris in between). Typical 'hockey stick' shape of the orbicularis oris muscle, visible as black band within the lip.

    Video 8.7 Kymography (high-speed line scanning) of the lips: broken chords, French horn (upper lip right, lower lip left).

    Video 8.8 Kymography (high-speed line scanning) of the lips: sound of tuba played at

Gflat0 (23 Hz). Because of this low frequency, the tone is hardly audible. The real-time video kymogram shows approximately one vibrational cycle per image. Solely the upper lip is visible from the right.

Video 8.9 Sonography of the tongue: mediosagittal scans (left) and simultaneous TM-mode scans (right) while playing the soprano recorder.

Video 8.10 Sonography of the tongue: mediosagittal scans (left) and simultaneous TM-mode scans (right) during trumpet playing.

Fat: Source Videos 8.2–8.10 and Case Study Video 8.4: Renate Haubrich and Wolfgang Angerstein.

26. **Case Study Audio 10.1a**: German-speaking man with severe stuttering characterised by many repetitions before stuttering therapy
27. **Case Study Audio 10.1b**: Same patient as in Audio 10.1a in the middle of a 3-week intensive therapy course of a fluency shaping therapy. He has achieved speech fluency using rhythmic speech with soft voice onsets, syllable binding and a specific breathing technique; however, speech naturalness has still to be trained.
28. **Case Study Audio 10.2a**: German-speaking man with severe stuttering characterised by long-lasting blocks before stuttering therapy
29. **Case Study Audio 10.2.b**: Same patient as in Audio 10.2a directly after a 3-week intensive therapy course of a fluency shaping therapy: he has achieved nearly complete speech fluency using rhythmic speech with soft voice onsets, syllable binding and a specific breathing technique. Moreover, his speech sound quite natural at the end of the therapy course.

Source audios 10.1a, b and 10.2a, b: A. Wolff von Gudenberg

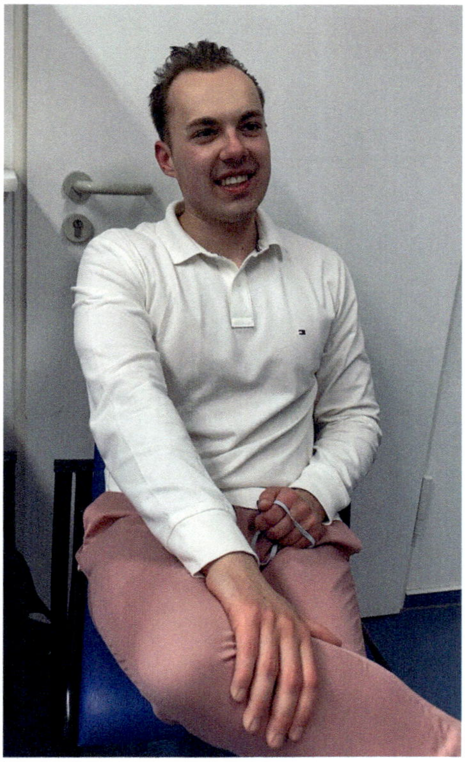

30. **Case Study Video 10.1a**: Significantly reduced stuttering symptoms through new speech patterns that the German-speaking patient from Video 6.1 had learned in a fluency shaping therapy course. However, he did not want to use the new speaking technique in everyday life because it costs him effort and seemed strange and unnatural to him. Notice the persistent tension in his face when speaking and the many co-movements of the hands with which he helps him overcome the impending speech disfluencies.

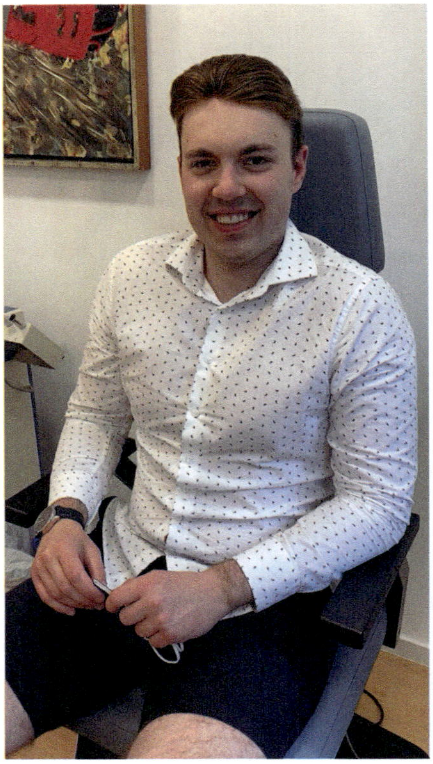

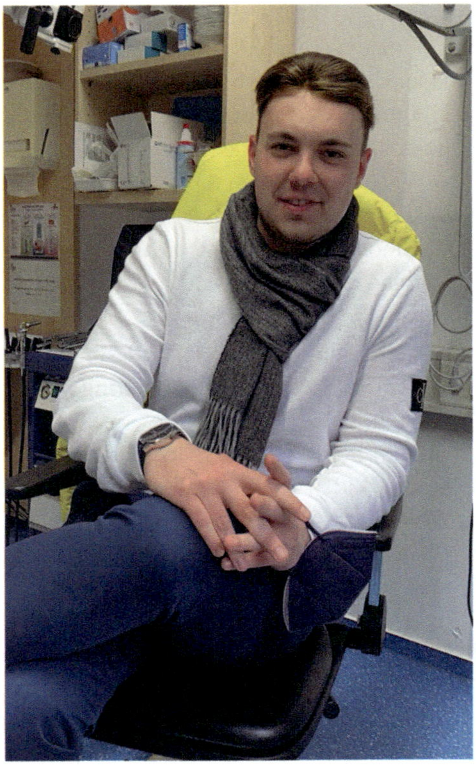

31. **Case Study 10.1b**: Significantly reduced stuttering symptoms a few weeks after the start of a treatment trial using deep brain stimulation (DBS) of the left ventral intermediate nucleus of thalamus (VIM) in the German-speaking patient from Video 6.1. The previously stuttered words such as "Freischuss" or "Brauhaus" can now be spoken fluently by the patient. The tension in his face and movements of his hands have reduced but are still present.
32. **Case Study 10.1c**: Significantly reduced stuttering symptoms some months after the start of a treatment trial using deep brain stimulation (DBS) of the left ventral intermediate nucleus of thalamus (VIM) in the German-speaking patient from Video 6.1. The previously stuttered words such as "Freischuss" or "Brauhaus" can now be spoken fluently by the patient. The tension in his face has clearly decreased compared to before treatment.

Source Videos 6.1 and 10.1a–c: K. Neumann

Index

A. am Zehnhoff-Dinnesen et al. (eds.), *Phoniatrics II*, European Manual of Medicine,
https://doi.org/10.1007/978-3-031-25175-7

B

C

GPSR Compliance

The European Union's (EU) General Product Safety Regulation (GPSR) is a set of rules that requires consumer products to be safe and our obligations to ensure this.

If you have any concerns about our products, you can contact us on ProductSafety@springernature.com

In case Publisher is established outside the EU, the EU authorized representative is:

Springer Nature Customer Service Center GmbH
Europaplatz 3
69115 Heidelberg, Germany

Batch number: 10621349

Printed by Printforce, the Netherlands